# Resilience Process and Its Personal and Social Bases

Chau Kiu Cheung

# Resilience Process and Its Personal and Social Bases

Springer

Chau Kiu Cheung
City University of Hong Kong
Hong Kong, China

ISBN 978-981-97-7390-9 ISBN 978-981-97-7391-6 (eBook)
https://doi.org/10.1007/978-981-97-7391-6



This Springer imprint is published by the registered company Springer Nature Singapore Pte Ltd.
The registered company address is: 152 Beach Road, #21-01/04 Gateway East, Singapore 189721, Singapore

# Contents

# Chapter 1
# Introduction

**Abstract** Chapter 1 introduces the conceptualization of resilience to elucidate the value of developing resilience. The conceptualization covers resilience as a process constituted by exposure, belief, action, and feeling regarding resilience, with the feeling marking the core state of resilience. Essentially, resilience means adjustment under adversity to indicate rebounding, recovering, or restoring to maintain normal living or functioning. As a primal concern of analytical functionalism, functioning necessitates the four functions of fulfillment, adaptation, integration, and latency. Four currencies are leveraged in functionalist mechanisms to achieve functions, power, utility, ideals, and norms. These mechanisms are integral to the analytical-functionalist framework for examining the development of resilience by various personal and societal conditions. These conditions include contextual, sociodemographic, peer, practice, social capital, and developmental. Their examination involved six datasets of 6948 cases surveyed in Chinese societies. Remarkably, the examination revealed the positive effects of societal caring, kindness, social capital, and ritualistic activity on resilience. Conversely, the examination found the inverse effects of societal exclusion, adversity, and peer adversity on resilience.

## Introduction

Resilience in the person is a valid concept understandable across cultures and backgrounds to indicate a person's recovery or bouncing back to normalcy after suffering from adversity (Hjemdal et al. 2015; Zheng et al. 2020). Such cross-cultural validity also holds in the developmental context of young people (Jowkar et al. 2010; Plouffe et al. 2020). In Western culture, resilience features accepting, active, altering, and independent in dealing with adversity (Xie and Wong 2021; Zheng et al. 2020). These features originate from Christianity and stoicism, emphasizing affirmative, managing, rational, responsible, and self-controlling (Jarrett 2013; Ramsey and Blieszner 1999). In Chinese culture, resilience similarly features accepting, adjusting, and harmonious dealing with adversity (Xie and Wong 2021). Particularly in the Chinese society of Hong Kong, resilience prevails through being optimistic and



C. K. Cheung, *Resilience Process and Its Personal and Social Bases*,
https://doi.org/10.1007/978-981-97-7391-6_1

persevering (Mak et al. 2019). Such features partly rest on the Buddhist emphasis on environmental connection and the Confucian emphasis on destiny (Mak et al. 2019; Xie and Wong 2021). In addition, resilience is also prominent in Islamic culture, which accentuates fasting as a developmental ritual (Annalakshmi and Abeer 2011). Nevertheless, despite the commonality of resilience across cultures, a complete understanding of resilience needs to accommodate some cultural differences, such as those between individualism or being independent and collectivism or being caring about and conforming to others, which underlies the importance of social relation (Xie and Wong 2021; Zheng et al. 2020). Evidence about resilience from East Asia, such as Hong Kong and its Chinese neighbors with collectivist tradition, which more broadly prevails in Asia, is thus indispensable to the complete understanding (Cohen et al. 2007; Mak et al. 2019; Zheng et al. 2020). The collectivist, Asian perspective, which is less researched, thus highlights social as well as personal bases for resilience (Chen et al. 2020, 2021).

Developing resilience or adjustment in the face of adversity is an increasing demand on the person, considering the growing adversity around the person (Goodman et al. 2017; Pangallo et al. 2015). The demand mushrooms with the individualization of risk and responsibility to disconnect adversity and resilience from social groups or bonds (Hall and Lamont 2013; Schwarz 2018). This individualization reflects the consolidation of narcissism or minimal self in contemporary society, which requires self-improvement or self-healing in the person (Braun 2019; De Vos 2010; Lasch 1984; Kilminster 2008). Individualization also indicates risk society, which popularizes risks and adversity in environmental, lifestyle, health, economic, political, institutional, interpersonal, and personal aspects (Babcicky and Seebauer 2017; Beck 1999; Lupton 2013). Notably, biotechnical risks are globally spreading and calamitous (Beck 2006; Strydom 2002). Facing such towering and pressing risks or adversity, the person experiences a mounting social expectation for maintaining resilience (Garrett 2016; Tierney 2015). The expectation rests on the notion of resilience as ordinary magic, which regards resilience as personally workable, executable, amenable, and developable (Masten 2014). This notion, nonetheless, is dissonant with the notion of risk society, which laments about social or environmental influence, determination, and manipulation over the person (Lupton 2013; Morton and Duck 2001). Social determination implies that social or societal conditions preempt, bridle, or override the personal development of resilience. The dissonance between personal growth and social determination thus poses critical questions about the grounds and viability of individual resilience.

The dissonance and critical questions are manifest in the resilience of such luminaries as Helen Keller (1880–1968) and Stephen William Hawking (1942–2018). Conceivably, the luminaries had their constitutional giftedness to flourish in their resilience and success despite adversity. The giftedness, moreover, only covers some of the life stories of the luminaries. Notably, the luminaries' beliefs, such as being irreligious and believing in human potential and autonomy in Hawking and socialism in Keller, underlay their endeavor to build resilience and success. Without endeavor and persistence, the luminaries might not be able to excel in the face of failure and criticism. That is, the luminaries were not perfect in their endowment and work.

Additional bases for resilience are social support, instruction, mentoring, and role modeling in the luminaries' surroundings (Einhorn 1998; Ferguson 2011; Hawking 2013; Herrmann 1998; Mialet 2012). They are social factors originating socially as empowering and norming and internalized by the luminaries as resources and norms. Given technical, financial, and familial aid, Hawking could concentrate his talents on scientific achievement (Ferguson 2011; Hawking 2013; Mialet 2012). Moreover, people glorifying resilience in society is a social factor that highlights, foregrounds, and probably inflates the luminaries' resilience and success. Society can be deterministic in selecting people to celebrate their resilience. Overall, the luminaries' resilience appears to be personally and socially grounded. Their extraordinary cases, critically questioned, require an empirical generalization to testify that individual resilience is ordinary and viable.

Critical questions concerning the development of resilience trigger the present work to address. Briefly, resilience refers to the state of adjustment or rebounding to normal conditions in the face of adversity (Pangallo et al. 2015). Resilience, here, is different from resiliency as a trait of ability or habit for adjustment in the face of adversity (Truebridge 2016). The issues about resilience development are those about its feasibility by personal, voluntaristic resources and its infeasibility or constraint due to social, deterministic factors (Schwarz 2018). Related issues are those about Western, ethnocentric, individualistic, and elitist ideals versus non-Western ideals (Cocking 2017; Schoon 2006; Schwarz 2018). In other words, the issues concern whether resilience development is shared across or is specific to contexts. Addressing the issues thus necessitates the investigation of personal and social influences in a non-Western but highly Westernized place, such as Hong Kong, a special administrative region of China. The investigation is essential because of the value of resilience, its development, and the confusion, ambiguity, and uncertainty in existing theory and research. Clarification of resilience and its contributors or predictors is thereby necessary. Briefly speaking, the clarification is valuable because of the value of resilience and its development. Specifically, resilience is valuable for health and well-being (Leigert and Reutter 2005). Resilience development is valuable for empowerment (Brodsky and Cattaneo 2013). Furthermore, resilience is relevant to counseling, education, and personal development (Richardson 2017). Overall, the focus on resilience registers a paradigm shift from pathology, deficit, and even well-being to their precursors or salutogenesis (Schoon 2006). That is, resilience is a basis or precondition for well-being. To promote well-being, advancing resilience is a necessary earlier step.

## Core and Constituents of Resilience

A necessary step to unraveling resilience applied to the person is untangling its core and constituents, representing the process of resilience. Accordingly, the core means the central, integral, and necessary definition of resilience to be most representative of resilience. The chosen core is a state or phenomenon demonstrating adjustment or rebounding to normalcy in adversity (Goodman et al. 2017; Pangallo et al. 2015). Adversity is a noxious condition involving challenge, trauma, risk, unsafety, loss, deprivation, stress, or crisis (Sandler 2001; Waller 2001). Thus, resilience happens when a patient feels comfortable, healthy, painless, or unworried. Hence, resilience is a state of adjustment under the condition of adversity. In brief, resilience is a total adjustment that is typically favorable. Such a core state is necessary to make resilience intelligible and manageable (Prince-Embury 2014a).

The state of resilience differs from alternatives to represent resilience as an ability or a trait of capability and resourcefulness generally (Chen et al. 2016; Cherry et al. 2018; Metzl and Morrell 2008; Truebridge 2018). This trait is a stable constellation of habit and style in many folds, including being accepting, adapting, competent, creative, enduring, faithful, flexible, hardy, hopeful, intelligent, mastering, open, optimistic, patient, resourceful, robust, spiritual, sustainable, strong, and tolerant (Celinski and Allen 2017; Connor et al. 2003; Cornum et al. 2011; Jayawardana et al. 2019; Jones and Jetten 2011; Metzl and Morrell 2008; Pangallo et al. 2015; Zautra 2014). Specifically, being intelligent includes making choices, taking others' perspectives, and being cohesive and empathic while remaining unique (Nemeth and Olivier 2017). The trait also involves being collaborative, courageous, honest, persistent, and self-regulating (Cornum et al. 2011). Furthermore, resilience as a trait encompasses the capacity for absorption in an activity, adaptation to the situation, learning from adversity, transforming oneself to circumvent adversity, and maintaining favorable anticipations (Jones and d'Errico 2019). In sustaining the trait, acquiring stable resources or energy from the organization, social relationships, and social status is habitual (Pangallo et al. 2015; Richardson 2002; Van Vliet 2008). They are necessary for coping, planning, staying coherent, efficacious, and mastering. As such, resilience is a trait that allows for resourceful acceptance, confrontation, and control of adversity (Celinski and Allen 2017; Jayawardana et al. 2019). All these alternatives, however, are better at representing resiliency rather than resilience (Truebridge 2018). They imply the potential of resilience rather than the fact or phenomenon of resilience. As such, resiliency or the traits of resilience are the constituents of resilience.

Resilience involves its constituents as well as its core state. A constituent is that necessary for, indispensable to, and therefore inalienable from resilience. The constituents include the behavior, belief, thought, or mindset, and motivation of resilience (Pangallo et al. 2015; Richardson 2017). The behavior or action suggests doing something to maintain or show resilience. It includes accepting, controlling, coping with, resisting, and understanding adversity (Connor et al. 2003; Mukherjee and Kumar 2017; Nemeth and Olivier 2017; Van Vliet 2008). These, in turn, embrace acting on, attaching to, connecting, expecting, engaging support for, keeping, learning, protecting, refocusing, restoring, and sustaining something. Eventually, resilient behavior transpires from being humorous, growing, and moderate. The behavior, simply put, is to lessen adversity or its adverse reaction and strengthen adjustment to it to achieve resilience. Meanwhile, the resilient mindset includes attribution and thought related to religion, spirituality, or ideology (Johnson et al. 2017). For instance, adherence to the religious tenets of being hopeful, self-controlling, and eternal constitutes resilience. As an additional constituent of resilience, motivation for resilience includes building character and staying honest, integral, kind, loyal, trustworthy, and moral (Richardson 2017). Eventually, the motivation is to secure connection, honor, respect, be intelligent, efficacious, and noble, and understand and plan to live. Motivation thus implies being planful or setting a goal for resilience. As such, resilience action, belief, and other factors represent resilience's constituents. Resilience belief, for instance, is evident in Hawking's relativistic thinking about contextual limits in the universe and everything (King 2003). This belief gives hope as opposed to fatalism. As such, reframing the context is conducive to resilience (King 2003; King et al. 2003). The core and constituents of resilience together represent the resilience process (Pangallo et al. 2015; Truebridge 2016). Specifically, the resilience process refers to the constitution of resilience by its constituents, comprising the development series from belief and action to feeling about resilience.

Regarding resilience as a state is preferable to regarding resilience as a trait. Relatedly, resilience as a state is more noteworthy than resiliency as a trait. Resilience is a state because it is transitory, situational, dynamic, changeable, and developable (Ni et al. 2016; Pangallo et al. 2015; Truebridge 2016; van Rensburg et al. 2019). One cannot be resilient all the time concerning everything. Resiliency as a trait represents an umbrella concept encompassing capability, resources, and habits for resilience (Pangallo et al. 2015; Truebridge 2016). Thus, resiliency means being adaptable, competent, flexible, hardy, mastering, optimistic, resourceful, spiritual, strong, and having many other resources, capabilities, and dispositions. This meaning suggests that resiliency involves persistently capable, powerful, omnipotent, and insuperable performance. The obvious problem with this coverage is that such resiliency is redundant to its associated concepts, such as adaptability and flexibility (Jayawardana et al. 2019). When the various concepts are unique and meaningful, the concept of resiliency is superfluous and confusing. Resiliency or resilience is a valuable concept only when it is distinguishable from other concepts. Resiliency can exist, but its distinctiveness or discriminant validity from other concepts is questionable. The availability of the many concepts downplays the conceptual significance of resiliency. Moreover, resiliency or the resilience trait is practically limited because it is mainly stable, unchangeable, and undevelopable (Boden et al. 2014). Identifying a trait without the possibility of development is frustrating to practice for advancing resilience and well-being (Truebridge 2016).

These concerns highlight resilience as a state for conceptualization, research, and practical focus. First, resilience as a state is distinguishable from the many concepts of capability, resources, dispositions, and other traits. It is also distinguishable from adjustment, adaptation, health, and well-being because it importantly necessitates the concept of adversity. That is, resilience means staying adjusted during adversity. Hence, resilience combines both adjustment and adversity. It is, therefore, different from adjustment or well-being alone. Specifically, resilience differs from positive emotions, such as attention and hope (Pangallo et al. 2015; Van Vliet 2008). This difference is because resilience entails the condition of adversity and is specific to maintaining adjustment under adversity. Essentially, resilience is a precursor to well-being and adjustment in general. Resilience, necessarily in the face of adversity, also counts as a form of adjustment or adaptation. Second, resilience can serve as an outcome or response that is predictable, malleable, or developable by other factors (Crane et al. 2019; Pangallo et al. 2015). Identifying resilience as a precursor to well-being is helpful. This identification, in turn, testifies to the value of predicting resilience. Understanding the prediction of or basis for resilience is, thereby, the mission of this work.

Two ways of examining resilience as a state are differentiable. They are the explicit and implicit or implied ways (Masten 2014). The explicit way means the usual way of defining resilience directly, typically subjectively, according to the personal understanding of resilience. That is, the way requires the person to report resilience or its details. By contrast, the implicit or implied way taps resilience indirectly as the concurrence of adjustment and adversity (Goodman et al. 2017). This tapping is to deny the direct measurement of resilience (Schoon 2006). That is, the way taps adjustment and adversity separately and infers resilience when adjustment and adversity happen simultaneously. A version of the implicit way takes the buffering of the deleterious impact of adversity as resilience (Johnson et al. 2017). Such buffering can arise from different buffers; thus, there are different resilience measures for different buffers. This version will only complicate the examination of resilience if it ascertains what resilience is precise. Hence, a viable implicit way to tap resilience is about the conjunction of adjustment and adversity measured separately rather than the buffering version.

Resilience and its development are valuable because of their benefits and other consequences. Supposedly, resilience is salutary as a basis for well-being. Hence, resilience has sustained health, life satisfaction, positive affect, and patience (Chen et al. 2016; Karoly and Ruehlman 2006; McKay et al. 2018). Resilience implies living a good life as it is conditional well-being under adversity. Moreover, resilience is vital as a precondition for the good life. Conversely, resilience has prevented anxiety, fear, depression, and the feeling of stress (Chen et al. 2016; Maltby et al. 2016; McKay et al. 2018). This prevention illustrates that resilience buffers the emotional harm of stress or adversity. Furthermore, resilience has buttressed coping and impeded involvement in crime, violence, and smoking (Fields and McNamara 2003; Hoffman 2003; Karoly and Ruehlman 2006;. Chen et al. 2016). These effects illustrate the indirect contribution of resilience to personal conduct and social harmony. Eventually, resilience has fostered the traits of controllability and sensitivity (Karoly and Ruehlman 2006). As such, resilience affords conditions, including time and stamina, for character development and consolidation. Meanwhile, resilience has diminished one's environmentalist activism and need for prescriptions (Karoly and Ruehlman 2006; Plutzer et al. 1998). The diminution of environmentalism means reducing discontent and rage and sustaining trust in government (Kanji and Nevitte 1997; Lubell 2003). As such, resilience fosters a socially cohesive and mutually supportive community.

Resilience is also intrinsically valuable due to its reflection on valuable factors. These factors include adaptation, capability, coping, functioning, heroism, maturation, morale, order, resourcefulness, and strengths (Allison et al. 2017; Charles and Carstensen 2009; Chen et al. 2016; Cherry et al. 2018; Huta 2017; Lawler et al. 2009; Pangallo et al. 2015; Peterson et al. 2008; Prilleltensky 2012; White 2014). Notably, resilience reflects law-abiding as it prevents involvement in crime (Hoffman 2006). By maintaining personal order, resilience is also conducive to social order (Lawler et al. 2009). For example, controlling temper is a desirable quality of resilience not to irritate others. Resilience also reflects connecting to, accepting, and integrating into society (Lau et al. 2008). That is, resilience is welcome among people as a socially desirable manner to secure friendship. This desire echoes the popularity of personal capability. Resilience is thus virtuous and represents a personal and socially valuable strength.

Resilience is also justifiable by the discourses of neoliberalism and strengths or positive psychology (Kristjansson 2013; Schwarz 2018). On the one hand, neoliberalism favors being rational, responsible, and living individually, independently, and autonomously concerning individualization, which secures freedom from traditional social constraints (Cocking 2017; Schwarz 2018). It thus champions individual resilience in tackling personal problems. Neoliberalism, in turn, is valuable as a reflection of and accommodation to commercialization and other ways of modernization, which effaces traditions with new development (Bellah et al. 1985; Smart 2003). As such, modernization and commercialization enable, endorse, and entail neoliberalism and individual resilience. In addition, strength discourse or positive psychology regards resilience as a strength or virtue to remain tranquil and equanimous (Kristjansson 2013). On the other hand, positive psychology, which stresses strengths, is justifiable by its compatibility with education, enlightenment, reflection, and proactive or agentic orientation (Christopher and Campbell 2008; Kristjansson 2013). In addition, strengths are meritorious in their connotations of being moral and even human (Petersen and Park 2009). Developing, fulfilling, and realizing one's strengths are moralistic. Strength discourse also posits the value of strengths or resilience because of its ubiquitous and distinctive nature (Petersen and Park 2009). That is, resilience is prevalent and feasible in characterizing the person and is valuable.

Paradoxically, the discourses and nature of resilience expose issues and controversies about resilience. The neoliberal, individualist, and strength discourses and other conceptions about resilience indicate that resilience is an elitist, exceptional, and ethnocentric phenomenon (Schoon 2006; Schwarz 2018). These discourses emphasize personal freedom, choice, decision-making, and application of available personal ability. This emphasis means resilience is not ordinary, prevalent, and universal, thus not prevailing in everyone. Resilience is a strength upheld, constructed, and reified to become possible and valuable in Western culture. The central counterargument is that resilience depends on social factors overruling its individualistic bases (Schwarz 2016). This counterargument emanates from ecological, poststructuralist, and socialist discourses (Schoon 2006; Schwarz 2018). Ecological discourse posits that resilience evolves from social or extra-personal factors as well as personal factors. Similarly, socialist discourse states that social or societal factors, including social construction, labeling, and institutionalization, affect resilience and its benefits and value. Social discourse furthermore disfavors these factors and their domination or oppression. Also similar is poststructuralist discourse, which regards resilience as a product of discourse or social construction. Hence, the discourse denies the reality and value of resilience. The discourse adds that resilience represents self-surveillance, which is undesirable. Essentially, the counterargument maintains that resilience results from deterministic rather than voluntaristic forces. Whether resilience is socially determined or personally developed is thus a critical concern. Specifically, when resilience is a deterministic result, it is not personally developable and does not reflect personal capability, resources, and other merits. In this case, deterministic factors suppress the effects of personal, voluntaristic factors. Personal development of resilience is thus futile, and resilience is not virtuous to represent the merit of personal striving. Conversely, when resilience results from a voluntaristic basis, it realizes humanity and its virtue, such that one makes one's world. This realization thus bolsters neoliberal, individualistic, and strength visions about enlightenment and modernization of the person.

The ecological discourse of resilience mainly envisions the socioecological (i.e., ecological in the human context) model, which essentially integrates personal or voluntaristic and extrapersonal or deterministic bases for resilience. This model emphasizes the acquisition or construction of meaningful resources cooperatively through social ecology transactions to sustain resilience, like adaptation and survival (Lerner et al. 2012; Ungar 2012; Xie and Wong 2021). In a broad sense, the resources comprise personal and social assets, opportunities, and meanings (Ungar 2012; Zautra et al. 2010). Personal resources crucially consist of personal strengths, whose self-regulation is most notable. Self-regulation is a cognitive or executive function regulation of one's action, body, deliberation, emotion, impulse, and temper (Gross 2015; Inzlicht and Schmeichel 2016; Koegl and Day 2019; Koole and Aldas 2016). The regulation maintains awareness, goals, and strategies to facilitate acceptance, orientation, and processing according to one's plan (Droutman et al. 2018; Koole and Aldas 2016). Other strengths include courage, curiosity, gratitude, grit, mindfulness, temperance, and wisdom (Banicki 2014; Goodman et al. 2017; Kristjansson 2013). When widely available and perceptible, these strengths make resilience ordinary magic (Masten 2014). In addition to personal resources are social resources such as social capital or networking and institutional provision or affordance (Lerner et al. 2012). Social capital refers to resources accessible through social relations (Ostrom 2009). Such resources accrue from others' accompanying, approving, befriending, exalting, helping, integrating, networking, sympathizing, understanding and/or being trustworthy to secure prestige (Halevy et al. 2019; Muskett 2012; Narayan and Cassidy 2001; Robison et al. 2002; Savelkoul et al. 2011; Tulin et al. 2018; Wakefield and Poland 2005; Wollebaek and Selle 2002; Wuthnow 2002). These resources are similarly available or accessible from institutions through empowerment, enforcement, institutionalization, and regulation (Lowndes and Roberts 2013; Scott 2008). All social and institutional resources may represent opportunities for the person who needs to negotiate with the social network and institution to acquire his or her resources (Ungar 2010, 2012). Personal and extrapersonal resources benefit the person only when they are meaningful in social ecology, encompassing the culture and institution. Furthermore, meaningful resources are particularly beneficial when they fit the person's needs and resources (Ungar 2012). For example, the resources need to be culturally understandable and approvable (Theron and Liebenberg 2015).

Such resources constitute a component of voluntaristic and deterministic bases in the analytical-functionalist framework.

## Voluntaristic and Deterministic Bases for Resilience

As an overview, personal demographic and other background characteristics, beliefs, practices, traits or dispositions, and the constituents of resilience are voluntaristic bases for resilience. In contrast, social or societal factors, such as social exclusion, social capital, social support, and societal values or norms, identify deterministic bases for resilience. Voluntaristic bases, thus, refer to those inherent in and usable by the person, whereas deterministic bases are those outside and uncontrollable by the person. Deterministic bases involve collective forces that can directly or indirectly influence the person through voluntaristic factors. Direct influence, without reliance on the person's voluntaristic bases, happens when others give or share something with the person. For example, allowances parents give their child become the child's income. A similar vicarious case occurs when a child shares homeownership status when living in a house owned by his or her parents.

The voluntaristic and deterministic bases constitute the analytical-functionalist framework, as enriched, consolidated, and leveraged extensively (Cheung 2018; Cheung and Yue 2020; Munch 1987; Parsons 1968; Turner 2013). This framework holds four requisite functions to sustain both voluntaristic and deterministic mechanisms. In the framework, a function is a componential action that is conducive to maintaining the whole system. Herein, society is a whole system buttressed by the interrelated functions of political, economic, communal, and cultural subsystems, which rest on their people's interrelated functions. This maintenance, accordingly, necessitates the four functions of goal attainment or fulfillment, adaptation, integration, and latency or pattern maintenance. Analytically, these functions are the products of two dimensions, internal–external or inside-environmental concerns and intrinsic-extrinsic or consummatory-instrumental concerns. These functions apply to different levels: personal, organizational, community, societal, national, and even global. At the personal level, concerns are internal and external to the person and consummatory, ultimate, or intrinsic, and instrumental to consummatory ones. For instance, the person has the personal resource of intelligence and the external resource of money and achieves the consummatory goal of resilience or sharpens the instrumental means of the action of resilience.

First, goal attainment or fulfillment function means applying internal or intrinsic resources to deal with the external environment. Resources, power, goals, or directions are bases for action. An example is the workings of the factory, which installs its goal, design, energy, and material to generate products. This function underlies the voluntaristic mechanism of power realization and the deterministic mechanism of empowering. For instance, money is powerful when spent to realize its power to attain its goal. Whereas the power realization mechanism means that personal resources, goals, or designs drive personal action, the empowering mechanism means that collective power drives personal action directly or indirectly through the power realization mechanism and other voluntaristic mechanisms. For example, personal power can be the goal or desire for resilience, whereas collective power can be training for resilience provided in society (Brodsky and Cattaneo 2013; Hassija and Cloitre 2014; Jayawardana et al. 2019; Lerner et al. 2012). The personal drives and educational support represent internal power and external empowerment, boosting the resilience of Helen Keller and Stephen Hawking.

Second, the function of adaptation means taking care of extrinsic concerns, such as those about monetary reward, in dealing with the external environment. That is, expected gain or incentive attracts action. An example is a chameleon adapting to the environment to optimize gains from hunting and protection. This function buttresses the voluntaristic mechanism of utility optimization and the deterministic mechanism of incentivizing. Whereas the utility optimization mechanism highlights extrinsic gains personally expected or received as causal factors, the incentivizing mechanism posits collective gains to induce collective action, including direct or indirect provisioning and sharing through voluntaristic mechanisms. When resilience is gainful, such as getting an award or praise, resilience is likely to happen (Masten et al. 2009). Awards offered and desired were nonetheless the external incentive and internal calculus, possibly attracting the resilience of Helen Keller and Stephen Hawking.

Third, the integration function means that intrinsic concerns are essential to deal with internal issues. Such intrinsic concerns are the personal tendencies of socializing, affiliation, social awareness, orientation, or interest, whereas internal issues concern maintaining social relationships to stabilize oneself. An example is a unanimous response to a fad. The function thus emphasizes social factors as causal factors. These factors constitute the voluntaristic mechanism of norm conformity and the deterministic mechanism of standardizing. Whereas the norm conformity mechanism accentuates that personally received or experienced social norms are influential, the standardizing mechanism maintains that collective or exotic social standards or norms influence the person directly, vicariously, or indirectly through various voluntaristic mechanisms. For instance, a peer norm for resilience induces individual resilience through contagion, modeling, and learning (Batone 2017; Cocking 2017). The norm can also be a standard for resilience, even unconsciously or unwittingly (Matusitz 2017). Mentoring or role modeling received by Helen Keller and Stephen Hawking could provide the external and internalized norm of resilience for cloning their resilience.

Fourth, the latency or pattern maintenance function emphasizes extrinsic or instrumental concerns for dealing with internal issues. Such concerns involve thinking, beliefs, ideals, or obsessions, whereas the issues deal with the self or internal integrity. An example is the faith and practices consistently maintained inside a church. The function props the voluntaristic mechanism of ideal or idealistic consistency and the deterministic mechanism of signifying. Thus, religious faith and practices maintain consistency due to common latent religious ideals. Whereas the ideal consistency or calibration mechanism cherishes personal beliefs, values, and attitudes as influential factors, the signifying mechanism foregrounds cultural factors as influential in affecting the person directly or indirectly through various voluntaristic mechanisms. Belief about resilience can translate into action for resilience and the state or feeling of resilience (Park 2017; Park and Slattery 2014). Such belief, when held and disseminated collectively to become a culture of resilience, can set a frame for screening and retaining individual resilience (Buzzanell 2010; Simon et al. 2005). Internally or personally, atheist and humanist and socialist beliefs thus underlay the respective career investment, success, and resilience of Stephen Hawking and Helen Keller. Additionally, societal favor for resilience might privilege and flaunt the resilience of Helen Keller and Stephen Hawking.

The analytical-functionalist framework can incorporate or explain all existing theories and research findings regarding resilience. In explaining resilience, the power realization mechanism covers attachment theory, broaden-and-build theory, capital or resource theory, self-regulation theory, and virtue theory. The utility optimization mechanism encompasses exchange, rational choice, and social-cognitive theories. Meanwhile, the norm conformity mechanism covers impact theory, social learning or social-cognitive theory, social constructionist theory, and discourse theory. In addition, the ideal consistency or calibration mechanism encompasses meaning-making theory, phenomenological theory, self-affirmation theory, self-reflection theory, and social identity theory.

The analytical-functionalist framework thereby explains resilience as an action or experience generated by the four voluntaristic mechanisms of power realization, utility optimization, norm conformity, and ideal consistency, and the four deterministic mechanisms of empowering, incentivizing, standardizing, and signifying. Voluntaristic mechanisms highlight personal influences, but deterministic mechanisms hinge on collective influences. Overall, the voluntaristic and deterministic mechanisms of the analytical-functional framework incorporate existing theories, such as the socioecological model and research findings of the formation of resilience.

Specifically, the voluntaristic mechanism of power realization posits that personal power, resources, strengths, goals, motivation, and/or design drive, activate, enable, or shape resilience. This mechanism highlights the driving force. For example, emotional intelligence, comprising being aware of the emotions of oneself and others, controlling or regulating emotions, expressing and managing emotions aptly, and even thinking and using emotions reasonably, has driven resilience (Armstrong et al. 2011). More specifically, humor and engaging with emotions are likely to uphold resilience. In addition, the power realization mechanism underlies the resilience process, notably from resilience action to resilience feeling. Herein, the state of resilience results from the realization of the power of resilience action. That is, one exerts one's power in action for resilience to produce the feeling of resilience. For instance, one needs to reframe the context to make it gainful to achieve resilience (King et al. 2003).

Alternatively, the voluntaristic mechanism of utility optimization specifies personal gains expected or experienced to attract resilience. This specification represents an attracting or gravitating force. For example, the experience of trauma may attract resilience to optimize the gain from relieving the trauma (Cherry et al. 2018). This positive influence is opposite to the negative influence based on the power realization mechanism, which holds trauma as disabling. As such, the challenge of adversity can activate resilience to quell any adverse effect.

The voluntaristic mechanism of norm conformity emphasizes the personal experience of the norm of the corresponding group or collective practice and the personal practice of learning and conformity as influences on resilience. This emphasis represents the assimilating or contagious force. For instance, the experience of resilience in the family has been conducive to resilience (Jones and d'Errico 2019). That is, the family sets a norm for individual resilience in the family member.

The voluntaristic mechanism of ideal consistency emphasizes the causal roles of beliefs, values, attitudes, and behavior or habit for inducing resilience. This emphasis represents the rationalizing force. Belief about resilience has been conducive to resilience (Truebridge 2016). Coping has also been predictive of resilience (Corbin and Hall 2019). Furthermore, the value of affiliation or connectedness has contributed to resilience, possibly because of consistency between the value and resilience (Chua et al. 2019). Such belief, practice, and value are compatible and share common ground with resilience in being socially desirable. Notably, the ideal consistency or calibration mechanism is responsible for contributing resilience belief to resilience action and feeling in the resilience process. Resilience action and feeling result from maintaining ideational consistency with resilience belief (Lee et al. 2010; Truebridge 2016). Similarly, beliefs in growth and a just world have predisposed the feeling of resilience in the youth (Wu et al. 2011; Zeng et al. 2016). Hawking's relativistic belief exemplifies resilience (King 2003).

The deterministic mechanism of empowering emphasizes the causal origin of resilience in collective or surrounding power or resources. Herein, family wealth, assets, and the number of income sources have sustained individual resilience (Jones and d'Errico 2019). The provision of resources by others maintains subsistence and energy for resilience.

The deterministic mechanism of incentivizing influences individual resilience through collective incentive or gain. For instance, a youth's resilience has been stronger when his or her parents have been more caring, involved, warm, and active in monitoring the youth (Kim-Cohen et al. 2004; Masten et al. 2009; Ungar et al. 2005). Conversely, a youth's resilience has been low when his or her parents have been neglectful (Fang Hong et al. 2019). That is, reward from the parent or other attracts the youth's resilience or its action and feeling specifically.

The deterministic mechanism of incentivizing influences individual resilience through collective incentive or gain. For instance, a youth's resilience has been stronger when his or her parents have been more caring, involved, warm, and active in monitoring the youth (Kim-Cohen et al. 2004; Masten et al. 2009; Ungar et al. 2005). Conversely, a youth's resilience has been low when his or her parents have been neglectful (Fang Hong et al. 2019). A reward from the parent or other attracts the youth's resilience or its action and feeling specifically.

The deterministic mechanism of standardizing operates when collective or even exotic norms or practices influence individual resilience. Hence, family resilience has influenced individual resilience even without personal awareness about family resilience (Jones and d'Errico 2019; Masten et al. 2009). Accordingly, family resilience can help sustain individual resilience directly or vicariously, or indirectly through various voluntaristic mechanisms, including norm conformity and others. The direct or vicarious way means that one adopts family resilience for oneself. Herein, resilience is something, such as an ideal or label, provided by the family and adopted by the person.

The deterministic mechanism of signifying or framing accentuates the influences of culture or collective beliefs, values, attitudes, habits, and other characteristics on individual resilience. Parents' faith, talent, and skill in drawing meaning in life and regulating themselves have contributed to the youth's resilience (Masten et al. 2009). Similarly, teachers' self-efficacy has buttressed students' resilience (Sosa and Gomez 2012). The proactive atmosphere or culture parents or teachers create shapes the youth's resilience. These contributions show consistency between individual resilience and contextual characteristics.

## Issues to Address

The development of individual resilience is a general issue to address. First, development means that across the lifespan, not just confined to childhood or youth, as resilience is ordinary and changing everywhere in the lifespan (Masten 2014; Weine et al. 2012). Second, the development registers a process comprising a sequence of belief, action, and feeling about resilience in the person. The process realizes the production of resilience with its resources regarding ability, strengths, and traits (Pangallo et al. 2015). Third, the development hinges on contextual, ecological, or social inputs, considering the socioecological model within the analytical-functionalist framework. The development is meaningful only in a social context, notably concerning the interaction or fit between personal and extrapersonal factors. The social context can range from peers to society. Peers have something in common and are an important reference group for comparison and connection (King 2003). For instance, peers are those attending the same service unit, implying they have the same need and/or background. Peers constitute an interpersonal context in social ecology (Zautra et al. 2010).

Particularly, whether individual resilience is developable by personal or social factors is a critical issue to address. The general issue prevails because of the need for more empirical evidence about the development of resilience. Notably, the evidence needs to be complete to exhibit the effects of various sociodemographic characteristics, traits, experiences, practices, attitudes, and feelings on resilience. This incompleteness in knowledge especially happens to the ordinary person who is not a patient, service user, older person, or person with a disability. That is, resilience is vital for everyone with or without disability or service needs. For a thorough understanding of resilience, research needs to cover a full range of people. More specifically, existing empirical evidence cannot help address the issue of the effects of personal and social factors on individual resilience. This issue arises from the doubt and challenge that resilience stems from personal ability, effort, and other characteristics (Cocking 2017; Schoon 2006; Schwarz 2018). The challenge criticizes the individualist and elitist bias, which regards the person as able and responsible for achieving resilience. This bias blames the victim for being incompetent, irresponsible, and lazy to be resilient. The challenge, instead, cherishes a deterministic view that social or personally uncontrollable factors determine resilience and override the effects of personal factors. That is, social or non-personal factors predominate and nullify personal effects. As such, the challenge or criticism faults and downplays resilience as infeasible personally. The criticism maintains that when resilience is infeasible, it cannot be a goal for promotion and advocacy to raise personal development. Hence, if resilience is not personally developable, it will lose its value. Such criticism evolves from poststructuralist or social constructionist views that social factors such as surveillance are deterministic (Schwarz 2018). The view furthermore criticizes resilience as self-surveillance, which is undesirable. On the contrary, neoliberal and positive psychology or strength discourses champion individual resilience (Kristjansson 2013; Schwarz 2018). These perspectives insist that individual resilience is feasible and desirable because of the availability and desirability of personal strengths and freedom. Such antagonistic discourses foreground the issue concerning the personal development of individual resilience. Clarifying the effects of personal and social factors on resilience is thus necessary to address the issue.

Personal factors comprise sociodemographic characteristics, traits, practices, attitudes, and feelings. Among demographic characteristics, age is an essential, visible, and thus important one. Age is likely to hinder resilience, considering the power realization mechanism. Accordingly, age denotes the decline of power, strength, energy, and thus the ability to achieve resilience. This decline implies that young age enables resilience. This possible effect supports the relevance of the positive factor to resilience. However, the possible adverse effect of age reveals a problem in resilience development, such that resilience dwindles with age. This possible negative effect thus casts doubt on individual resilience development and, hence, the infeasibility of resilience. By contrast, according to the power realization mechanism, age can generate a positive effect on resilience, such that age accumulates experience and knowledge, thus consolidating power. This possible positive effect endorses individual resilience development and, hence, the feasibility of resilience. Whether negative or positive, the effect of age needs to rest on empirical evidence.

Apart from demographic factors, personal factors include personality traits, experiences, practices, attitudes, and feelings. Traits include extraversion and functional disability, whereas attitudes include benevolent world belief, experience includes Westernization, and practices include being kind, compensatory, self-aware, using experience in coping, socializing, and religious. In addition, extraversion is a personality trait that drives assertiveness, boldness, liveliness, enthusiasm, ambition, and joy (Witt and Revelle 2009). Extraversion has thus shaped satisfaction, self-esteem, self-efficacy, hedonic balance, and other aspects of well-being (Frederick et al. 2016; Judge et al. 2002; Quilty et al. 2006; Schimmack et al. 2002). Hence, extraversion likely sets the resilience plan, considering the power realization mechanism. This mechanism also explains the contributions of functional ability, self-awareness, and religious and other practices to resilience. According to the power realization mechanism, the contributions happen because of power and production by the ability and practices. Self-awareness means agency or the ability to self-understand (Morin 2011). Practices also include coping in hard or confrontative ways, such as problem-solving, and soft or compromising ways, such as humor, which influence resilience (Cherry et al. 2018; McKay et al. 2018). Meanwhile, the ideal consistency mechanism also explains the contributions of benevolent world belief, self-awareness, experience-based coping, religious practice, and Westernization to resilience. Herein, resilience happens because of its consistency with proactive beliefs and practices. Notably, Westernization favors individualism and independence, consistent with agency emphasized in individual resilience (Fu and Chiu 2007).

The significance of personal factors would also be transparent in the resilience process, involving the contribution of belief about resilience to learning, action, and feeling about resilience as a phenomenon successively. That is, belief about resilience sustains learning and action about resilience, and the learning and action engender feeling of resilience. The contributions of belief about resilience or its learning, such as the value and efficacy of resilience, realize the ideal consistency mechanism. Accordingly, the belief and learning are consistent with resilience. Such belief has been predictive of resilience (Truebridge 2016). Learning resilience represents self-empowerment, which has been predictive of resilience (Stewart and Yuen 2011). More generally, socioemotional learning about being aware of oneself and others, being skillful in relating to others, and being responsible for making decisions has been conducive to resilience (Merrell 2009). Moreover, belief is generally the basis for action (Cooke and Sheeran 2004; Jenkins and Dragojevic 2011). The contribution of resilience action to resilience applies the power realization mechanism, such that the action harnesses the power to produce resilience. Resilience action such as coping has been predictive of resilience (Corbin and Hall 2019; Graber et al. 2016).

Social factors comprise experiences with other people and contextual conditions. Whereas the experiences influence individual resilience through the voluntaristic mechanisms of norm conformity, power realization, and utility optimization, other people's or contextual factors determine individual resilience through various deterministic mechanisms. Generally, social experiences like group ones have been conducive to individual resilience (Corbin and Hall 2019). Experiences of social support and mentoring have also championed individual resilience (Cherry et al. 2018; Notter et al. 2008). These contributions work through the power realization mechanism, such that the experiences are about power or resources accruing by others. Mentoring can enhance individual resilience through training or skill learning. Mentoring can also motivate individual resilience by showing the gain from resilience concerning the utility optimization mechanism. Experiences of family and community resilience or their norms have encouraged individual resilience (Masten et al. 2009; Ungar et al. 2005). This encouragement reflects the norm conformity mechanism. Family wealth, income source variety, assets, and adaptability have propped individual resilience even without personal experience of the family factors (Jones and d'Errico 2019). The contributions of these factors emanate from the empowering mechanism, such that the factors represent power or resources for family members to use and share to enhance each member's resilience. Moreover, collectivism in society has raised individual resilience (Wu et al. 2011). The raising also represents the deterministic mechanism of empowering, as collectivism embraces mutual support and thus empowering (Triandis 1995). In addition, teacher self-efficacy has been conducive to the student's resilience (Sosa and Gomez 2012). This contribution embodies the deterministic mechanism of signifying, such that teacher self-efficacy cues students' resilience, strengthening each student's resilience through sharing. Herein, self-efficacy is consistent with and conducive to resilience personally (Masten et al. 2009; Ungar et al. 2005). Hence, self-efficiency and resilience should also be consistent collectively.

Social factors also include experiences of caring, peace, violence, pragmatism, social capital, social exclusion in society, and other people's kindness, sociability, aid, demand, and social inclusion. Experiences of caring, peace, social capital, kindness, sociability, and aid are likely to undergird individual resilience through the power realization mechanism. Accordingly, these experiences make the person feel supported and robust, which enables the person's resilience. These factors' contributions echo the social support received (Cherry et al. 2018; Ungar et al. 2005). More specifically, experiences or reception of other caring and prosocial behavior have buttressed individual resilience (Masten et al. 2009; von Soest et al. 2010). Social capital has fostered individual resilience (Li et al. 2018). Notably, the experience of family cohesion has been conducive to individual resilience (Aitcheson et al. 2017; White et al. 2008). Conversely, experiences of violence and social exclusion in society are likely to impede individual resilience through the power realization mechanism. At this juncture, the experiences reduce personal resources and power for resilience. Furthermore, the experience of others' demand for one's resilience is likely to boost one's resilience through the power realization mechanism. Herein, others' demand represents an external force to strengthen personal power to maintain resilience. The contribution is consistent with that of social challenge on resilience (Godwin et al. 2015). However, others' demand for one's resilience is also likely to undercut one's resilience through the utility optimization mechanism, as compliance with the demand makes one less autonomous, intrinsically motivated, and thus self-determined. The negative effect echoes the youth's lower resilience when his or her parent is more overly protective (von Soest et al. 2010). Individual resilience is likely to be lower when society counts as more pragmatic, given the power realization mechanism. People are calculative and self-oriented in a pragmatic society and thus withhold mutual support. Hence, a pragmatic society does not generate collective support for one's resilience. The negative effect of a pragmatic society thus echoes that of others' neglect of individual resilience (Hong et al. 2018). Conversely, sharing culture experienced in society is conducive to individual resilience (Theron et al. 2011). These societal experiences represent empowering (or disempowering) in the deterministic mechanism to enable individual resilience.

The aggregates (i.e., averages) of social factors in peers in the service unit represent peer factors. Such aggregation thus identifies action, learning, belief, and demand about resilience, kindness, sociability, adversity, disability, and others in peers. The peers characterize a socioecological factor to exert main and interaction effects on the person's resilience process. Herein, the interaction effects are due to the interaction or fit between personal and peer factors. One possibility is that the fit indicates that the peer factor amplifies the effect of the personal factor predicated. For instance, the peer acceptance of one's action for resilience, such as trying something new, heightens the effectiveness of the action. According to the analytical-functionalist framework, the heightening of the effectiveness represents the deterministic mechanism of empowering through peer acceptance on the voluntaristic mechanism of power realization through resilience action. Moreover, the experience of fit may induce the feeling of resilience through the voluntaristic mechanism of ideal consistency. A notable fit is that with culture to bring honor for buttressing resilience (Panter-Brick 2015). This bringing is consonant with the contribution of the experience of balance between various ideals to resilience (Cantor et al. 2002). In addition, the fit represents complementarity between peer acceptance and individual resilience action. Complementarity means the multiplication of contributions of two factors (Bao et al. 2017; Wang and Busemeyer 2015). This multiplication again represents the enhancement of the power realization mechanism.

Given the paucity and incompleteness of current research findings, the impacts of personal and social factors on individual resilience require further investigations. This requirement is because those suggested personal and social factors have slipped from rigorous examination. Remarkably, most personal demographic factors and resilience process factors have been personal factors neglected in existing investigations. Moreover, the suppression of the influences of personal factors by social factors has yet to be a focus of the existing investigation. Elucidating the impacts of personal factors and their suppression by social factors is necessary to address the issue of the infeasibility and futility of the development of resilience. When personal factors influence individual resilience, resilience is feasible in the presence of social factors, and personal factors are effective rather than futile. Meanwhile, gauging the influences of social factors is necessary to establish social factors as dominant conditions for resilience.

A developmental approach to resilience is also a concern, particularly for secondary school pupils. Such an approach means a formal, organized, and planned strategy for coaching, counseling, or educating to develop resilience or its ability and belief through disciplining (Hue 2011; Thompson 2006). Disciplining notably functions as an inoculation to accept suffering and thus prepare for resilience (Jarrett 2013). The development includes practices in sports, adventuring, volunteering, and religious, carnival, musical, ritualistic, and nation-related activities. These practices aim to enhance physical and spiritual strengths through empowering, framing, and normalizing to learn or strengthen capabilities and internalized or normative beliefs (First et al. 2018; Masten 2014; Thompson 2006). Specifically, sport exemplifies physical and spiritual strengthening (Eccles and Barber 1999). The sport features physical strengthening with fitness and skill in disciplined or organized activity to comply with specific rules to induce achievement and enjoyment (Hendry et al. 1993; Larson et al. 2006; Prins et al. 2014; Stafford 2000). In practice, the sport is functional through challenge, discipline, fairness, and investment of effort (Larson et al.

2006; Shields and Bredemeier 2008; Spreitzer 1994). The functions of sport transpire in building character, efficacy, self-esteem, and social relationships (Eccles and Barber 1999; Eitle and Eitle 2002; Kavussanu and Roberts 2001; Marsh 1993). Eventually, the sport has developed conformity, health, self-control, self-esteem, higher education studies, and teamwork (Baron 2007; Eccles and Barber 1999; Marsh 1993; Snyder and Spreitzer 1992; Takano and Sogon 2008). In addition, religion and its ritualistic practices exemplify spiritual strengthening. Religious practice means a collective activity to impose social control by providing spiritual resources of faith, grace, and hope (Regnerus 2003; Sagy et al. 1999). Such practice, possibly involving music, rituals, and volunteering, seeks to cultivate cultural and social capital, skills in coping, leadership, and community to facilitate social networking (Mayrl and Uecker 2011; Regnerus 2003). Eventually, religious practice has nurtured such strengths as conscientiousness, self-control, social capital, social, teamwork, and other competencies or skills (Crystal and DeBell 2002; Larson et al. 2006; Kneezel and Emmons 2005; Ward et al. 2015). Religious practice has thus sustained resilience (Crawford et al. 2005). Notably, religious or ritualistic practices such as fasting are a discipline that builds resilience (Annalakshmi and Abeer 2011). Like religion, other institutions such as schools and states can organize collective and ritualistic activities to discipline and thus foster resilience (Hue 2011; Sant and Hanley 2018).

## Databases for Clarifying Resilience

Six databases for clarifying resilience are those on the public regarding poverty, violence, service users, elders, youths, and people with visual impairment in Hong Kong, China. In other words, they were data from the poverty study in 2011 ($N = 1526$), violence study in 2014 ($N = 1099$), service study in 2014 ($N = 2340$), elder study in 2011 ($N = 340$), youth study in 2008 ($N = 3564$), and visual impairment study in 2016 ($N = 704$). These databases contain data from 6948 Chinese people, including those with or without a need for help. They also included young, mid-age, and older people with disabilities. That is, mid-age service users were those using rehabilitation services, and older users of elderly services have various levels of functional disability. The data cover the personal and social factors mentioned, including personal background and resilience factors. Most of the databases contain more than 700 cases, which are enough to ensure a weak effect ($r = 0.1$) at least with 95% confidence and 75.6% statistical power. At most, the most extensive database had 3564 cases, enough to ensure a weak effect ($r = 0.1$) at least with 95% confidence and 100% statistical power. Alternatively, they can test a feeble effect ($r = 0.047$) with 95% confidence and 80% statistical power. Thus, the databases are substantive enough for statistical analysis to generate combinable findings and understand resilience thoroughly. In addition, 85.7% of the service users had economic, familial, and/or health adversity in the previous year for applying their resilience.

Hong Kong is a metropolis suitable for consolidating and advancing knowledge about resilience. This suitability is because of the general compatibility of Hong

Kong with Western and other places where knowledge evolves and improves. The compatibility stands on the globalization and cosmopolitan orientation of Hong Kong, as opposed to being provincial and ethnocentric (Forestier and Crossley 2015; McNeill 2014). Notably, Hong Kong cherishes the interchange of knowledge with other places (Forestier and Crossley 2015). More specifically, Hong Kong is economically compatible with Western and other places through global economic linkages (Fung 2014). Furthermore, Hong Kong shares merit with other places, such as economic competitiveness and free markets, and drawbacks, such as economic inequality and crises (Delang and Lung 2010; Li 2012; Smart and Smart 2008). Politically, Hong Kong shares neoliberalism with the West and other places to emphasize the free market, managerialism, democracy, and judicial procedures (Cheung 2011; Hui and Au 2016; Oksanen 2011). Hong Kong establishes strong bureaucracies, legal systems, and legislative and consultative structures in its political or administrative arenas to maintain economic freedom. Culturally, Hong Kong shares desire with the West and other places for capitalism, consumerism, cosmopolitanism, English use, freedom, globalization, individualism, justice, the rule of law, openness, pluralism, pragmatism, and Americanization (Brooks 2011; DeGolyer 2001; Ho 2013; Irazabal and Chakravarty 2007; Ma 2011b; Overholt 2004; Richardson 2018; Sin and Chu 2000). The colonial heritage of Hong Kong also maintains its compatibility with the West (Ku 2012). Hong Kong culture harbors adoration for the West (Chan and Cheng 2012). Admittedly, Hong Kong is culturally different from the West and other places in its anti-patriotic, amoral, and antitraditional flavors (Lee et al. 2014; Richardson 2018; Sing 2004; Zheng and Keat 2007). However, Hong Kong culture favors resilience (Li 2012). All the international compatibility and uniqueness of Hong Kong thereby warrant its distinctive contribution to supplementing and advancing knowledge about resilience internationally.

Hong Kong is a bustling metropolis that provides a fertile ground for investigating resilience. Such investigation has illuminated the resilience process, including its belief, action, and feeling (Chan and Chan 2011; Cheung and Kam 2012; Cheung and Yue 2013; Lee et al. 2010; Lou and Ng 2012). Belief about resilience rests on Chinese culture, notably embracing Buddhism, Confucianism, and Daoism (Chan and Chan 2011; Lou and Ng 2012; Xie and Wong 2021). Buddhist belief emphasizes connection with the environment, endurance, and transcendence beyond the person, Confucian belief emphasizes destiny, and Daoist belief emphasizes inaction. They all treasure acceptance of adversity, adjustment, character building, and harmony with nature and people, as exemplified in familism or valuation of the extended family. Nevertheless, such features of accepting, adjusting, enduring, and transcending have their counterparts in other places (Greene et al. 2012; Jones and Jetten 2011; Pangallo et al. 2015; Walsh 2002; Yorgason et al. 2007). Consistent with belief about resilience belief, action and feeling about resilience in Hong Kong have featured accepting, accommodating, accompanying, adjusting, affiliating, managing oneself, outperforming, persisting, relaxing, relying on oneself, selecting life goals, solving problems, and being interdependent and open (Chan and Chan 2011; Cheung and Kam 2012; Lou and Ng 2012). These are compatible with similar features of action and feeling about resilience in other places (Celinski and Allen 2017; Cornum et al. 2011; Hrostowski and Rehner 2012; Langer 2004; Schwager and Rothermund 2014; Taylor et al. 2005; Van Vliet 2008). Additionally, resilience has displayed the following features in Hong Kong. First, resilience has been predictable by prior resilience (Lee et al. 2010). Second, belief about resilience has underlain resilience or resiliency (Cheung and Kam 2012; Qu et al. 2021). Third, belief about resilience has been particularly conducive to feeling of resilience in the face of adversity (Lee et al. 2010). Fourth, social isolation has impeded resilience (Cheung and Kam 2012). Conversely, the migrant's connectedness with Hong Kong locals has been conducive to the migrant's resilience (Cheung and Yue 2013). They are consistent with the socioecological model and voluntaristic and deterministic mechanisms of the analytical-functionalist framework of resilience. Moreover, Hong Kong's resilience has dampened depression (Cheung and Yue 2013). Resiliency has also impeded depression and sustained personal growth in the migrant to Hong Kong (Qu et al. 2021; Yu et al. 2014).

To unfold the empirical study covering young, mid-age, and older people located in schools, social service units, or their homes in Hong Kong, essential tasks proceed with investigations of background bases for resilience processes, societal impacts on resilience, resilience processes, and their social influences, practical bases for resilience, and social capital bases for resilience. Notably, resilience processes comprise demand received for resilience, belief about resilience, learning about resilience, action for resilience, and resilience resultantly. The tasks thus serve to scrutinize the impacts of personal and social factors on resilience. The impacts or effects refer to statistical terms estimated by regression analysis, which control for background and response characteristics (Karpinski 1990). In the analysis, predictors are those reported to precede (e.g., past year) outcomes (e.g., recent month). With such a specification of the temporal order, the correlational design provides a way for estimating the effects of earlier predictors on later outcomes (Jaeger 2008; Luo et al. 2010; Van der Stede 2014). Although the data stemmed from Hong Kong Chinese people, a counterfactual adjustment applies to derive findings for the Westernized people (Morgan and Winship 2007). Specifically, the adjustment weights data on a person with the person's report of Westernization experienced to overplay data from Westernized people. The analysis can, therefore, illustrate differentials in findings due to Westernization or cultural differences.

## Subsequent Chapters

Chapter 2 recites the resilience process connecting exposure, belief, action, and feeling regarding resilience. Resilience exposure conveys the integration function of social norms or demand. Resilience belief embodies the latency function of defining ideals. Resilience action, comprising learning and handling, represents the adaptation function to tackle adversity to acquire utility. Resilience feeling constitutes the fulfillment function to set goals and power. These resilience factors were distinguishable from adjustment, aid received, and sincerity experienced. The factors maintained positive correlations among themselves and with adjustment, aid received, and sincerity experienced, and inverse correlations with adversity experienced. More specifically, resilience feeling depended on resilience action, which depended on resilience belief.

Chapter 3 displays a fundamental attempt to address feasibility and reasonableness in developing resilience based on the person's background characteristics. Background characteristics include personal, sociodemographic, and socioeconomic characteristics such as age, gender, education, birthplace, and residency. Concerning the analytical-functionalist framework, background characteristics are influential through their functions for the voluntaristic mechanisms of power realization, utility optimization, norm conformity, and ideal consistency. Resilience processes comprise feeling, action, belief, learning, and demand received about resilience. Analysis of poverty survey data on the public revealed that age was the only significant background characteristic eroding resilience. Meanwhile, analysis of violence survey data on the public showed that marriage was the only significant background characteristic buttressing resilience. In this connection, the effect of age was positive but not significant. Analysis of survey data on social service users revealed that age, earnings, and living with parents significantly upheld resilience. Meanwhile, family size significantly diminished resilience. Moreover, age, education, and living with offspring significantly positively affected action for resilience. Living with the spouse, parents, and private housing significantly positively affected learning resilience. Similarly, age, female gender, education, living with siblings, and living with parents positively impacted belief about resilience. By contrast, age significantly negatively affected the demand received for resilience. Nevertheless, analysis of survey data on elders showed that no background characteristic had a significant effect on resilience. In addition, analysis of survey data on people with visual impairment indicated that family income per capita, social welfare, and having a birthplace in Hong Kong significantly positively affected resilience. By contrast, visual impairment severity, visual impairment duration, education, being an employee, being self-employed, being unemployed, and living in rental public housing significantly negatively affected resilience. Hence, the person's age, education, marriage, earnings, living with parents, family income, and even reception of social welfare tend to prop resilience. As these characteristics represent human, financial, and social resources, their contributions to resilience embody the power realization mechanism. The contributions testify to the feasibility and reasonableness because the characteristics are more inherent and accessible to the person. That is, no external force appears to inhibit or displace the contributions. Hence, resilience evolves from the voluntaristic use of personal background characteristics, which, for instance, provides power or resources to sustain the process of resilience. That is, static power is necessary for the dynamics of action.

Chapter 4 critically attempts to gauge societal impacts on individual resilience and thus the involuntary basis, infeasibility, and unreasonableness of resilience. Societal impacts examined were those of caring, social exclusion, peace, violence, and pragmatism perceived in society and social inclusion experienced. Notably, pragmatism is relevant to resilience because it furnishes the orientation toward solving problems or tackling adversities. These impacts reflect the deterministic mechanisms of the analytical-functionalist framework. Analysis of poverty survey data on the public showed that caring in society had a significant and strong positive effect on resilience, and social exclusion in society exerted a significant and strong negative effect on resilience. Moreover, social inclusion experienced did not manifest a significant effect on resilience. That is, the effects of caring and social exclusion in society preempted the effect of social inclusion experienced. Meanwhile, analysis of violence survey data on the public revealed that pragmatism in society, but not peace and violence in society, exerted a significant inverse effect on resilience. Overall, the significant societal impacts reflect the deterministic force on resilience. This force demonstrates the social influences on resilience.

Chapter 5 further attempts to gauge the social, deterministic, and personal, voluntaristic development of resilience processes. Such processes comprise the voluntaristic formation of resilience, including its action, learning, belief, and resilience demand received successively. Moreover, the related behavior, belief, and character include self-awareness, compensation, benevolent world belief, and kindness. Other social factors reflect deterministic development, including aid received and the sociability and kindness of other people. These factors notably included those aggregated for peers in the service unit. According to the vision of the resilience process, resilience evolves from factors progressively emerging at different points. Analysis of survey data on social service users showed that kindness, the sociability and kindness of other people, and aid received, apart from background characteristics, were the earliest contributors to resilience and its resilience, learning, and belief. Furthermore, beliefs about resilience and a benevolent world were earlier significant contributors to resilience, resilience action, and resilience learning. In addition, resilience action, learning resilience, self-awareness, and compensation later contributed to resilience. However, the demand for resilience manifested adverse effects on resilience, resilience action, resilience learning, and resilience belief. Thus, the process of resilience from learning and belief about resilience to action and feeling about resilience successively was demonstrable. This process reflects the voluntaristic mechanism of ideal consistency in the analytical-functionalist framework. Similarly, the contributions of other behaviors, beliefs, and dispositions illustrate the same voluntaristic mechanism. By contrast, the impacts of social factors on individual resilience represent the deterministic mechanisms, which focus on the suprapersonal or group determinants of the analytical-functionalist framework. For instance, a significant peer influence was the positive effect of peers' disabilities on resilience. This effect indicates that individual resilience was higher than in poorer peers' conditions. Such contrast reflects the deterministic mechanism of incentivizing to show one's distinctiveness from others. Hence, the deterministic basis for developing the resilience process is evident. Nevertheless, the deterministic basis is unlikely to override the voluntaristic process. Resilience and its process are feasible and reasonable because of their voluntaristic basis.

Chapter 6 examines the voluntaristic basis for resilience, emphasizing personal and peer practices, including experience-based coping, socializing, engaging with pets, religious practice, hardening, and softening. Hardening means forceful, confronting, proactive practice, whereas softening means acting tenderly, compromising, and withdrawing. The aggregates (averages) of personal practices in the service unit identify peer or contextual practices. Besides these personal and peer practice factors, advice received, and Westernization represents social deterministic factors. Survey data analysis on elders showed that experience-based coping, hardening, and softening significantly sustained resilience. Meanwhile, functional disability significantly impeded resilience. These impacts represent the voluntaristic mechanism of power realization, goal attainment, or transforming resources, capabilities, and/or efforts in production. The impacts also reflect the voluntaristic mechanism of ideal consistency, such that the practices are consonant with resilience. By contrast, advice received and Westernization did not consistently deliver significant effects on resilience. This nonsignificance does not bolster the deterministic mechanism. Hence, the voluntaristic mechanism outperforms the deterministic mechanism in developing resilience. Nevertheless, socializing, religious practice, and pet engagement did not indicate significant effects on resilience. These practices are thus inconsistent with and/or incapable of generating resilience concerning the voluntaristic mechanisms of ideal consistency and power realization. In addition, some interactions between personal and peer practice manifested significant effects on resilience. For instance, resilience was higher when peer advice was higher despite higher personal adversity. This effect indicates the effectiveness of peer advice sharing among peers. Additionally, this reflects the deterministic mechanism of empowering, particularly in the case of powerlessness due to adversity. Furthermore, Westernization did not affect the effects of the personal and social factors on resilience, thus showing that the effects are stable across Westernized and non-Westernized people. The findings are thus likely not specific to Hong Kong Chinese people.

Chapter 7 attempts to elaborate on the social, deterministic influence on resilience. Accordingly, the social factors concerned are social capital and empowerment. Social capital arises from two sources, associations (e.g., parental associations) and friends, which comprises structural (i.e., relational), functional (e.g., aid), and substantive or resource (e.g., wealth) forms in the sources. In addition, extraversion is a personal factor in registering the voluntaristic mechanism of power realization. Analysis of survey data on people with visual disabilities revealed that associational social capital, friend structural social capital, friend functional social capital, and friend social capital integrated significantly sustained resilience. This sustenance demonstrates the deterministic mechanism of empowering. However, empowerment did not significantly elevate resilience, thus tempering support for the deterministic mechanism of empowering. By contrast, friend substantive social capital significantly negatively affected resilience. This effect reveals the deterministic mechanism of incentivizing, such that friends' resources devalue and discourage the personal development of resilience. In addition, extraversion displayed a significant positive effect on resilience. This effect reflects the voluntaristic mechanism of power realization. Overall, social or deterministic factors, as well as the personal factor of extraversion, influence resilience. Deterministic factors do not displace personal factors, and these factors maintain their unique contributions.

Chapter 8 additionally focuses on a survey of 3564 junior secondary school pupils in the Chinese cities of Hong Kong, Macau, and Guangzhou to clarify the impacts of developmental conditions on resilience. Such conditions include individual sports, collective sports, sports coaching, adventuring, volunteering, religious activity, carnival activity, musical activity, and ritualistic and nation-related activity. They contribute to resilience through the voluntaristic mechanism of power realization, following empowerment through individual or collective activity. Such power includes physical, spiritual, and social ones buttressed by religion and the nation, reflecting coaching and nurturing generally. They provide disciplining, training, and support to confront difficulties to develop resilience. As such, the developmental effect of such practices starts with social or collective empowerment, notably involving rituals. Nevertheless, the effectiveness of such practices hinges on their fostering of voluntarism or self-determination to raise personal power to realize the voluntaristic mechanism. The fostering, in turn, benefits from the assimilation of social norms according to the voluntaristic mechanism of norm conformity. As such, ritualistic activity can respectively inculcate the religious and national norms of resilience. Furthermore, nation-related activity is more normative and empowering for resilience in Guangzhou than in Macau and Hong Kong.

Chapter 9 reveals that resilience and its processes have personal and social bases that are simultaneously explicable by the analytical-functionalist framework. The personal bases are evident in the resilience process, with resilience belief successively generating resilience learning, resilience action, and resilience feeling. Moreover, the personal bases are demonstrable in the contributions of the practical bases of hardening and softening to resilience. Other personal factors affect resilience, including marriage, earnings, extraversion, kindness, and functional disability. Meanwhile, the social bases are evident in the influences of caring, peace, violence, pragmatism, and social exclusion experienced in society. Moreover, kindness, sociability, social inclusion, and social capital experienced interpersonally testify to the significance of social bases. The simultaneous influences of personal and social factors thus dispel the suspicion that social factors exert predominant influences on resilience and its processes. Hence, resilience is personally developable, notably through the personal practices of hardening and softening. Nevertheless, social factors such as social capital, caring, and social exclusion in society also exerted enormous influences on resilience. For the pupil, ritualistic and other social activities develop resilience. Voluntaristic and deterministic mechanisms for the functions of goal attainment, integration, and latency are, therefore, particularly influential on resilience.

# Chapter 2
# Resilience Process

**Abstract** This Chapter recites the resilience process connecting exposure, belief, action, and feeling regarding resilience. Resilience exposure conveys the integration function of social norms or demand. Resilience belief embodies the latency function to define ideals. Resilience action, comprising learning and handling, represents the adaptation function to tackle adversity to acquire utility. Resilience feeling constitutes the fulfillment function to set goals and power. These resilience factors were distinguishable from adjustment, aid received, and sincerity experienced. The factors maintained positive correlations among themselves and with adjustment, aid received, and sincerity experienced, and inverse correlations with adversity experienced. More specifically, resilience feeling depended on resilience action, which in turn depended on resilience belief.

The personal resilience process as a broad definition of resilience comprises the feeling, action, belief, and exposure regarding resilience. Notably, resilience feeling, felt, or self-perceived is resilience in its proper form as a state (Lock et al. 2020; Pangallo et al. 2015). Meanwhile, resilience action indicates the behavioral constituent; resilience belief indicates the cognitive constituent; and resilience exposure, such as to others' demand for resilience, indicates the social-normative constituent of resilience. Overall, the process conception of resilience reflects the developmental and dynamic properties of resilience (Bowers et al. 2017). Accordingly, resilience is changeable, modifiable, and responsive to intrapersonal and extrapersonal or environmental influences. These influences register fulfillment or goal attainment by resilience action, adaptation, and latency or pattern maintenance by resilience belief, and integration by exposure to others' demand, corresponding to the requisite functions of analytical functionalism. Accordingly, resilience action employs power or resources to produce resilience as a way of fulfillment, goal attainment, or power realization. Resilience belief sustains resilience with belief, expectation, or experience embracing the instrumental and/or substantive or intrinsic value of resilience through adaptation or utility optimization, and/or latency or ideal calibration. Meanwhile, resilience exposure to others' demand for resilience indicates the social-normative basis for resilience through integration or norm conformity. In other

 
C. K. Cheung, *Resilience Process and Its Personal and Social Bases*,
https://doi.org/10.1007/978-981-97-7391-6_2

words, resilience action drives resilience, resilience exposure assimilates resilience, and resilience belief attracts or rationalizes resilience in the resilience process.

Resilience, defined as a feeling of bouncing back from a temporary setback to normality, such as feeling calm under pressure, is the proper outcome of the resilience process (Lock et al. 2020; Pangallo et al. 2015). This state reflects that resilience is emergent and dynamic (Bowers et al. 2017). Hence, resilience is not a trait (Rutter 2012; Truebridge 2016). Whereas resilience is a state, resiliency is a trait, characteristic, or quality (Prince-Embury et al. 2017; Richardson 2002). Resilience is a real outcome felt or experienced. This outcome results from the behavior or action, belief, and at least exposure to the resilience process (Ungar 2012). As a real feeling, experience, or outcome, resilience is not an ability, asset, capability, capacity, capital, resource, or strength that is hypothetical or potential. The feeling means the coupling of adjustment and adversity or risk (Cole et al. 2022; Luthar et al. 2000). Hence, resilience can either be direct without the coupling or inferred feeling with or based on the coupling (Metzl and Morrell 2008; Schoon 2006). As a feeling state, resilience is unique and thus nonredundant to resiliency, commonly known as adaptability, adaptivity, flexibility, grit, hardiness, optimism, or perseverance (Godwin et al. 2015; Rojas and Tyler 2018; Woodier 2011).

## Resilience and Its Constituents

The resilience process holds resilience or its feeling as the outcome of resilience action, belief, and exposure to others' demand for resilience. More specifically, resilience exposure is a constituent of resilience belief, action, and feeling, resilience belief is a constituent of resilience action and feeling, and resilience action is a constituent of resilience feeling.

### *Resilience Feeling*

Resilience or its feeling covers fulfillment, goal attainment, or power realization, adaptation or utility optimization, integration or norm conformity, and latency or ideal consistency to demonstrate analytical functionalism. Altogether, feeling fulfilling or powerful, adaptive, socially integrative, and intrinsically consistent or congruent sustains the functioning of resilience.

Resilience feelings of fulfillment concern goals, power, strength, and their attainment or realization. Fulfillment or goal attainment most crucially flows in bouncing back, goal direction, recovery, and restoration (Celinski and Allen 2017; Zautra et al. 2010). Alternatively, fulfillment happens as adjustment under adversity or risk (Hariharan and Rana 2017; Nemeth and Olivier 2017). Adjustment means fulfilling needs and performance in compatible ways to uphold self-esteem and vitality (Deci et al. 2006; Ramadier 2017). Power realization transpires in character building, commitment, continuity, control, endurance, expression, functioning, maintenance, meaning-making, persistence, production, safety maintenance, self-regulation, and sustainability (Brodsky and Cattaneo 2013; Castro and Murray 2010; Celinski and Allen 2017; Jayawardana et al. 2019; Kent and Davis 2010). Meanwhile, feelings of power characterize activeness, agency, competence, mastery, maturity, potentiality resource acquisition or mobilization, resourcefulness, robustness, spontaneity, stability, strength, tenacity, uniqueness, and vitality (Corbin and Hall 2019; Jones and d'Errico 2019; Jones and Jetten 2011; Nemeth and Olivier 2017; Pangallo et al. 2015; Richardson 2017; Schwager and Rothermund 2014; Ungar 2010; Xie and Wong 2021; Zautra 2014). Goals are prominent in choice and purposefulness (Connor et al. 2003; Friedman and Robbins 2012). Particularly in the youth, fulfillment feelings additionally highlight achievement, autonomy, certainty, credit, equanimity, excellence, goal orientation, hope, influence, meaningfulness, normality, overcoming, planfulness, problem resolution, relaxation, resolve, self-efficacy, and self-reliance (Artuch-Garde et al. 2017; Brooks and Brooks 2014; Callegari et al. 2016; Eccles and Gootman 2002; Kim 2015; Li et al. 2018; Olsson et al. 2003; Prince-Embury 2014a; Ramasubramanian 2017; von Soest et al. 2010; Wong and Chui 2017; Wang et al. 2015; Wright and Masten 2015). In the elder, fulfillment feelings additionally include affirmation, busyness, engagement, independence, living, mobility, proactiveness, resistance, routinization, and self-management (Greene et al. 2012; Langer 2004; Lou and Ng 2012; Nakashima and Canda 2005; Nelson-Becker 2006; Ramsey and Blieszner 1999; Sawyer and Allman 2010; Tanner 2007; Wiles et al. 2012). For the patient or service user, fulfillment feelings additionally embrace determination, self-sufficiency, stress management, and structure (Godwin et al. 2015; Dageid and Gronlie 2015; Hines et al. 2005). In the working person, fulfillment additionally resides in the power of mindfulness and stamina (McCray et al. 2016). These feelings concern the goal, power, or their use or meeting.

Resilience feelings of adaptation or utility optimization include absorption, acceptance, adjustment, altering, flexibility, growth, learning, negotiation, openness, patience, reframing, reorientation, tolerance, transformation, and understanding (Celinski and Allen 2017; Connor et al. 2003; Jones and d'Errico 2019; Kent and Davis 2010; Maltby et al. 2019; Nemeth and Olivier 2017; Pangallo et al. 2015; Richardson 2017; Schwager and Rothermund 2014; Ungar 2010; Xie and Wong 2021). Adaptation feelings in the youth transpire in cultural fit, information seeking, and open-mindedness (Kim et al. 2018; Prince-Embury 2013b; Ungar et al. 2007). In the elder, adaptation feelings additionally highlight accommodation, improvisation, modification, and self-redefinition (Gergen and Gergen 2010; Lou and Ng 2012; Moen et al. 2010; Nelson-Becker 2006). To the patient or service user, resilience additionally indicates adaptation or optimization with problem-solving and turning (Echezarraga et al. 2018; Godwin et al. 2015). For the minority person, adaptation additionally transpires in legality (Payne 2011). These feelings reflect change in response to the environment.

Resilience feelings of integration or norm conformity transpire in social attachment, benevolence, cohesion, collaboration, communication, community, connection, correspondence, empathy, engaging support, harmony, loyalty, perspective taking, reintegration, relatedness, responsiveness, sociality, and teamwork (Connor et al. 2003; Cornum et al. 2011; Friedman and Robbins 2012; Nemeth and Olivier 2017; Pangallo et al. 2015; Richardson 2017; Solomon and Roloff 2018; Xie and Wong 2021; Walsh 2002; Zautra 2014; Zautra et al. 2010). Particularly in the youth, integration feelings additionally encompass social adherence, appreciation, care, commonality, conformity, discipline, fidelity, justice, love, mentoring, prosociality, responsibility, role-taking, sharing, social orientation, trust, and trustworthiness (Brooks and Brooks 2014; Gardner et al. 2008; Kim et al. 2018; Li et al. 2018; Markstrom et al. 2000; Ni et al. 2016; Prince-Embury 2014a; Ungar 2015; von Soest et al. 2010; Wang et al. 2015). In the elder, integration feelings additionally include affiliation, band formation, companionship, confluence, friendliness, gratitude, interdependence, and mutuality (Gergen and Gergen 2010; Greene et al. 2012; Lou and Ng 2012; Manning 2014; Ramsey and Blieszner 1999). For the patient or service user, integration feelings additionally concern social inclusiveness (Liebenberg and Moore 2018). In the minority person, integration additionally features in belongingness, bonding, closeness, collectivism, and reciprocity (Holleran and Waller 2003; Johns et al. 2014; Payne 2011). These feelings emphasize social concern, assimilation, or conformity.

Resilience feelings of latency or rationalization happen in authenticity, honesty, genuineness, integrity, and self-actualization (Friedman and Robbins 2012; Richardson 2017). Moreover, resilience manifests consistency with bouncing back, coherence, continuation, endurance, expressiveness, keeping, maintenance, perseverance, recovery, robustness, sustainability, and tenacity as opposed to disruption (Brodsky and Cattaneo 2013; Castro and Murray 2010; Celinski and Allen 2017; Greeff and van der Merwe 2004; Jayawardana et al. 2019; Jones and d'Errico 2019; Jones and Jetten 2011; Kent and Davis 2010; Mak et al. 2019; Nemeth and Olivier 2017; Richardson 2002; Yu and Zhang 2007; Zautra et al. 2010). Particularly in the youth, latency feelings additionally include coherence, commitment, self-acceptance, self-awareness, self-expression, and self-righting (Brooks and Brooks 2014; Davis and Paster 2000; Joseph 1994; Johnson et al. 2015; Li et al. 2018; Svetina 2014). In the elder, resilience additionally exhibits consistency in continuity, self-affirmation, and staying (Tanner 2007). These feelings highlight ideal, belief, or value consistency.

## *Resilience Action*

Resilience action or behavior works for fulfillment, adaptation, integration, and latency to champion resilience functioning expected in analytical functionalism. Such action encompasses accepting, adapting, appraising, attributing, controlling, coping, and enduring (Corbin and Hall 2019; Jones and Jetten 2011; Johnson et al. 2017; Kent and Davis 2010; Lock et al. 2020; Maltby et al. 2019; Nemeth and Olivier 2017; Van Vliet 2008). Resilience action thus functions as buffering to avoid or lessen delay or disruption to facilitate recovery (Boden et al. 2014; Bowers et al. 2017; Johnson et al.

2017). Such action also includes interactions with adversity, the environment, and others (Pangallo et al. 2015). To the youth, resilience action particularly characterizes adjusting, flourishing, and learning (Cole et al. 2022; Jowkar et al. 2010; Fredrickson and Losada 2005). In the patient or service user, resilience action mainly counts as a defense (mechanism) and transformation to maintain homeostasis (Davydov et al. 2010; Norris et al. 2008; Tebes et al. 2004). Simply put, resilience means steeling (Rutter 2012).

Resilience action for fulfillment operates as character building, challenging, committing, goal striving, monitoring, hoping, joking, keeping, meaning-making, negotiating, persevering, persisting, planning, problem-solving, producing, purpose sustaining, resisting, resource mobilizing, restoring, and self-regulating (Castro and Murray 2010; Connor et al. 2003; Cornum et al. 2011; Corbin and Hall 2019; Kent and Davis 2010; Mak et al. 2019; Nemeth and Olivier 2017; Pangallo et al. 2015; Richardson 2017; Schwager and Rothermund 2014; Ungar 2010; Van Vliet 2008; Xie and Wong 2021). In the youth, resilience action for fulfillment additionally displays aspiring, confronting, future orientation, goal orientation, relaxing, self-acceptance, and self-relying (Brooks and Brooks 2014; Kim 2015; Ramasubramanian 2017; Shibue and Kasai 2014; Sun and Stewart 2007; von Soest et al. 2010). For the elder, resilience action for fulfillment additionally emphasizes acquiring, busying, creating (poems, songs, or stories), moving, purpose maintaining, self-affirming, striving, and tricking (Greene et al. 2012; Manning 2014; Sawyer and Allman 2010; Tanner 2007). To the patient, resilience action for fulfillment additionally includes eating and patience (Godwin et al. 2015; Woodier 2011; Williams et al. 2011). These actions demonstrate acquiring, developing, or realizing goals or power for attainment or sustenance.

Resilience action for adaptation unfolds as acceptance, adjusting, altering, attending, flexibility, learning, openness, reflection, refocusing, reframing, reorienting, self-righting, transforming, tolerating, training, and understanding (Brodsky and Cattaneo 2013; Connor et al. 2003; Kent and Davis 2010; Nemeth and Olivier 2017; Pangallo et al. 2015; Richardson 2017; Schwager and Rothermund 2014; Van Vliet 2008; Xie and Wong 2021). In the youth, resilience action for adaptation additionally exhibits appreciating, information seeking, novelty seeking, and self-improving (Ma et al. 2022; Prince-Embury 2013b; Shibue and Kasai 2014; von Soest et al. 2010). For the elder, resilience action for adaptation consists in self-redefining (Nelson-Becker 2006). To the patient or service user, resilience action for adaptation additionally features normalizing (Henry 2001; Simon et al. 2005). These actions seek to achieve adaptation.

Resilience action for integration emerges as altruism, attaching, cohesion, collaborating, communicating, compassion, connecting, empathizing, engaging support, harmonizing, humanizing, perspective taking, reintegrating, servicing, and teamworking (Cornum et al. 2011; Jones and d'Errico 2019; Kent and Davis 2010; Nemeth and Olivier 2017; Richardson 2002; Solomon and Roloff 2018; Walsh 2002; Xie and Wong 2021; Zautra 2014). In the youth, resilience action for integration additionally happens in adhering, conforming, forgiving, role-taking, social orientation, and trusting (Kim et al. 2018; Prince-Embury 2014a; Ungar 2015; von Soest et al. 2010).

For the elder, resilience action for integration additionally displays accompanying, affiliating, banding, caring, and helping (Greene et al. 2012; Pentz 2005; Lou and Ng 2012). These actions sustain and benefit from social integration.

Resilience action for latency emphasizes self-actualizing (Friedman and Robbins 2012). In the youth, resilience action for latency highlights authenticity and self-expression (Callegari et al. 2016; Davis and Paster 2000). For the elder, resilience action for latency underlies reminiscing (Pentz 2005). These actions highlight rationalizing based on one's perspective.

As a prominent form of resilience, coping embraces fulfillment, adaptation, integration, and latency for functioning based on analytical functionalism. Essentially, coping represents protracted effort or planning to respond to adversity, risk, or stress (Kleinke 2007). Thus, coping registers a challenge to natural and social environments (Nelson-Becker 2005). Nevertheless, coping is in flux and ineffective (Kleinke 2007; Towsley et al. 2007). Coping effectiveness can depend on the breach experienced, responsibility, urgency, and the reconciliation of acceptance and remorse (Pollio et al. 1997). This dependence reflects the power realization mechanism of the voluntaristic framework of analytical functionalism, such that reconciliation, responsibility, and urgency indicate the power to counter resistance from the breach and attain the goal of coping. Similarly, coping effectiveness has risen with the controllability of stressors (Hampel and Petermann 2005). Such effectiveness also reflects the power realization mechanism in realizing power to attain the goal of controlling stressors. Thus, effective coping ensues when power controls or overcomes the breach or stressors.

Coping for fulfillment operates in activeness, approaching, confronting, engaging purposively, focusing positively, planning, reciprocating, repairing, problem-solving, threat minimizing, thinking wishfully, and venting (Kleinke 2007; Major and Townsend 2010; Pollio et al. 1997; Rodebaugh and Heimberg 2008; Wills 1997). In the youth, coping for fulfillment additionally manifests focusing positively, negotiation, and opposition (Frydenberg 2008; Zimmer-Gembeck and Skinner 2015). In the minority person, coping for fulfillment additionally figures in self-relying (Lee and Chan 2009). These actions exercise power to attain goals.

Coping for adaptation unfolds in acceptance, avoiding, detracting, disengaging, distancing, doping, redefining, escaping, exercising, flexibility, moving, reappraising positively, reinterpreting, self-repression or self-suppression, and working (Kleinke 2007; Major and Townsend 2010; Rodebaugh and Heimberg 2008; Tam and Ip 2017; Wills 1997). In the youth, coping to achieve adaptation additionally upholds indifference and recreational activity (Frydenberg 2008; Vandoninck and d'Haenens 2015). To the elder, coping to achieve adaptation additionally breeds compensation (Clare 2002). These actions uphold changes, including forgoing goals, in response to adversity, constraint, or threat. The actions, nonetheless, may need to be more adaptive and effective.

Coping for integration transpires in collaborating, comparing with others downwardly, community making, dependency, forgiving, and recourse (Loriol 2016; Pargament 1997; Pollio et al. 1997; Wills 1997). In the youth, coping to achieve integration additionally embraces socializing (Frydenberg 2008). These actions integrate socially to cope with or share adversity.

Coping for latency happens by acting according to religion, meditating, and rationalizing (Kleinke 2007; Pollio et al. 1997; Wyer and Abbarracin 2014). In the youth, coping to achieve latency additionally raises demonizing, ruminating, and sanctifying (Mahoney et al. 2005; Zimmer-Gembeck and Skinner 2015). To the elder, coping to achieve latency additionally highlights praying and scripture reading (Nelson-Becker 2005). For the patient or service user, coping to achieve latency additionally emphasizes resisting discursively (Nelson-Becker 2005). In the minority person, coping to achieve latency additionally unfolds by acting according to conscience and making sense of adversity (Lee and Chan 2009; Pan et al. 2008). These actions leverage personally held beliefs and reasoning.

Resilience action also proceeds as learning about resilience, comprising its power, utility, ideals, and norms for fulfillment, adaptation, latency, and integration functions, respectively. Power including or stemming from competence, efficiency, goals and motivation for goal attainment, and self-efficacy for resilience derives from learning about attribution, communication or dialogue, comparison, consideration, criticalness, emotional intelligence, empathy, evaluation, examination or testing including trial and error, excusing or rationalization, investment, justification, labeling, learnability, problem-solving, protection, prudence, reasoning, self-regulation, and support received (Bouton et al. 2001; Clark and Janevic 2013; Gadsden 2008; Huesmann 2018; Krahe 2001; Maltseva 2016; Mesirow 2003; Mussweiler et al. 2006; O'Brien 2014; Power and Dalgleish 2008; Schunk and Usher 2019; Thomas 1997; Zurbriggen 2013). Utility or expectancy from resilience hinges on in learning about conditions for success, controllability, predictability, reward or reinforcement (Aiken 2002; Bardo et al. 2003; Bouton et al. 2001; Leander and Chartrand 2017; Mruk 2019; Schunk and Usher 2019; Thomas 1997). Ideals or values for resilience emanate from learning about adaptation, agency, agreement, coherence, complementarity, decency, empiricism, euphemism, morality, open-mindedness, pragmatism, responsibility, and understanding (Bandura 2012; Bussey 2020; Gadsden 2008; Mesirow 2003; Pohling et al. 2010; Schunk and Usher 2019; Zurbriggen 2013). Norms for resilience based on communication, imitating, interaction, and observing congeal from learning about social consensus and others' efficacy (Achterkamp et al. 2016; Clark and Janevic 2013; Gadsden 2008; Krahe 2001; Schunk and Usher 2019).

## *Resilience Belief*

Belief in resilience incorporates ideals favoring and justifying the fulfillment, adaptation, integration, and latency of resilient functioning, as predicated on analytical functionalism. Such belief functions as an asset or resource for the functioning (Berger 2015; Truebridge 2016). Remarkably, resilience belief means heroism (Allison et al. 2017). Such belief also provides legal and moral bases, causes, morale, and meanings for resilience and its mechanisms (Goodman et al. 2017; Hoffman 2003; Peterson et al. 2008; Schwager and Rothermund 2014; Zautra et al. 2010). More broadly, resilience belief reflects personality (Metzl and Morrell 2008). To the youth, resilience belief furthermore warrants the dignity, honor, or respectfulness of resilience (Panter-Brick 2015). Specifically, resilience belief connects resilience to self-esteem (Di Fabio et al. 2015). For the patient or service user, resilience belief maintains the desirability of resilience (Zhao and Fu 2022).

Resilience belief unfolds as four functional bases for resilience and its action on goals or power, utility or instrumental value, social norms, and mindsets or intrinsic value. Notably, goals and power are established factors to express or realize intrinsic value, follow social norms during the resilience process, and achieve utility afterward. These bases warrant fulfillment or power realization, adaptation or utility optimization, integration or norm conformity, and latency or ideal consistency.

Resilience belief traces resilience to goals or needs covering adaptation, competition, growth, recovery, and survival, particularly healthily (Celinski and Allen 2017; Evans and Sewell 2013; Leigert and Reutter 2005; Nemeth and Olivier 2017; Richardson 2017; Zautra et al. 2010). Growth for resilience, particularly for the youth, applies to achievement, altruism, attachment, autonomy, belongingness, courage, generosity, independence, and mastery (Brandtro and Larson 2004). To the youth, goals set for resilience additionally concern achievement, goal orientation, normality, outperforming, and performance (Sattler and Font 2018; Supkoff et al. 2012; von Soest et al. 2010; Wang et al. 2015; Wong 2008). In the elder, goals for resilience additionally specify accommodation, friendship, generativity or nurturing or providing for younger generations, independence, and self-management (Greene et al. 2012; Lou and Ng 2012; Nelson-Becker 2006). Living or surviving is a particularly vital goal for the elder (Greene et al. 2012; Tanner 2007). Meanwhile, loss, particularly neuronally, is a crucial risk to the elder (Boerner et al. 2005; Lavretsky and Irwin 2007). Resilience belief furthermore justifies goals and needs with the conditions of crisis, disability, disconnection, discrimination, exploitation, hardship, inequality, injustice, insecurity, manipulation, monopoly, pandemics, risk, stigmatization, and victimization (Dunn 2013; Hall and Lamont 2013; Paul et al. 2022; Lamont et al. 2013; Tierney 2015). Such conditions particularly prevail in minority status (Mak et al. 2019). Additionally, resilience belief regards resilience as need-matching (Sandler 2001). Overall, resilience belief about goals highlights their driving for resilience to secure goal attainment.

Resilience belief rests resilience on power, resources, or means to attain goals emphasizing attractiveness, capability, competence, courage, creativity, empowerment, faith, health, intelligence, learning, mastery, mindfulness, resourcefulness, self-confidence, self-efficacy, self-esteem, self-potency, skill, social status, spirituality, strength, support received socially, wisdom, and capital in a human, financial, physical, or social form (Brodsky and Cattaneo 2013; Castro and Murray 2010; Cohn and Fredrickson 2009; Connor et al. 2003; Fields and McNamara 2003; Johnson et al. 2017; Jones and d'Errico 2019; Kent and Davis 2010; Leigert and Reutter 2005; Metzl and Morrell 2008; Pangallo et al. 2015; Richardson 2017; Schwager and Rothermund 2014; Truebridge 2016; Van Vliet 2008; White 2014; Xie and Wong 2021). Competence notably includes its social arm (Hjemdal et al. 2015). Such power furthermore includes that for discussion, negotiation, and persuasion (Ungar

2010). Intelligence for resilience covers automaticity, choice, cohesion, empathy, perspective-taking, and working (Nemeth and Olivier 2017; Zautra 2014). Resources or their accessibility for resilience include adaptability, agency, education, exercising, functioning, hardiness, health, hope, mastery, optimism, responsivity, security, and self-efficacy (Nemeth and Olivier 2017; Pangallo et al. 2015; Zautra et al. 2010). Additionally, resourcefulness for resilience transpires in acceptance, awareness, confronting, controlling, deliberation, integration, and intentionality (Celinski and Allen 2017; Jayawardana et al. 2019). Strength in character for resilience includes courage, honesty, leadership, optimism, persistence, self-regulation, and teamwork (Cornum et al. 2011). In the youth, strength additionally emanates from cheerfulness, honesty, kindness, perseverance, and responsibility (Li et al. 2018). Human capital for resilience includes expressiveness, insight, optimism, productivity, self-confidence, warmth, and capacity for self-regulation (Castro and Murray 2010). Virtue underlying resilience includes courage, commitment, forgiveness, integrity, open-mindedness, perseverance, transcendence, trustworthiness, and wisdom (Kim et al. 2018). Wisdom for resilience strategizes acceptance, adjustment, character-building, and meaning-making (Nemeth and Olivier 2017). Such belief furthermore emphasizes agency, counseling, education, and teaching received, resource acquisition, support engaging, and their viability (Connor et al. 2003; Richardson 2017; Sandler 2001). In the youth, resilience power, resources, or strengths additionally include curiosity, humor, recourse, self-praising, and virtue (Davis and Paster 2000; Kim et al. 2018; Prince-Embury 2014a; von Soest et al. 2010). Particularly in the youth, social resources additionally arise from appreciation, cohesion, encouragement, help, and material received (Olsson et al. 2003; von Soest et al. 2010). For the elder, wisdom for resilience additionally concerns altering, managing, modifying, or redefining identities, relationships, situations, tension, or strain (Moen et al. 2010). To the patient or service user, resilience belief for power or strength additionally emphasizes defense mechanisms, gentleness, gratitude, honesty, justice, love, patience, peacefulness, services received, self-reliance, serenity, social capital, stability in emotion, and truthfulness (Bottrell 2009; Davydov et al. 2010; Dominguez et al. 2015; Frimpong-Manso 2018; Godwin et al. 2013; Mota and Matos 2015, Rajan-Rankin 2014; Sanders et al. 2015; Woodier 2011). For the minority person, resilience belief for resilience resources additionally relishes community, especially co-ethnic community (Johns et al. 2014). Eventually, resilience belief about power reveals power as the basis for resilience through power realization or use.

Resilience belief envisions the contribution of resilience to utility, highlighting advancement, consumption, productivity, reward, satisfaction, self interest, and well-being (Evans and Sewell 2013; Hall and Lamont 2013; Schwarz 2018; Tierney 2015; Van Haaften et al. 2004). Such belief justifies utility with commodification or market value, efficiency, and meritocracy (Hall and Lamont 2013; Schwarz 2018; Son Hag 2013). In the youth, resilience utility additionally emphasizes flourishing (Fredrickson and Losada 2005). To the elder, utility derived from resilience additionally concerns dementia prevention, dying positively, hospice care, and their strength based on knowledge, relatedness, spirituality, and talent (Harris 2008; Nakashima and Canda 2005; Nelson-Becker 2006). Such strengths comprise meaning-making, openness, and philosophizing for preparing for dying (Nakashima and Canda 2005). Accordingly, resilience belief about utility justifies resilience through utility optimization.

Resilience belief bases resilience on social norms foregrounding acceptance, adjustment, connection, flexibility, following destiny, harmony with nature and others, hope, inactivity, self-competence, and transcendence (Nemeth and Olivier 2017; Xie and Wong 2021). In the youth, such social norms particularly concern achievement, coping, creativity, flexibility, identity, quality, and self-esteem (Wang et al. 2015). These social norms rest on belief in social awareness, cohesion, collectivity, community, connection, ecology, interdependence, and organization (Brodsky and Cattaneo 2013; Friedman and Robbins 2012; Lamont et al. 2013; Nemeth and Olivier 2017; Richardson 2017; Schoon 2006; Van Vliet 2008). To the youth, resilience belief favoring social norms particularly emphasizes social adherence, conformity, discipline, normalization, orientation, and trust (Ni et al. 2016; Plouffe et al. 2020; Ungar 2015; von Soest et al. 2010; Wright and Masten 2015). In the patient or service user, resilience belief about social norms additionally concerns contextual cohesion, connectedness, flexibility, inclusion, love, problem resolution, resource identification, and supportiveness (Dageid and Gronlie 2015; Liebenberg and Moore 2018; Simon et al. 2005). For the minority person, resilience belief about resilience norms additionally emphasizes social closeness and consideration (Holleran and Waller 2003). Overall, resilience belief about social norms recognizes social conditions for resilience through assimilation or conformity.

Resilience belief rationalizes resilience with mindsets, ideals, or values prioritizing autonomy or self-determination, character building, choice, entrepreneurship, individuality, liberalism or freedom, positivity, proactivity, salutogenesis, self-responsibility, stoicism, transcendence, and voluntarism (Dunn 2013; Evans and Sewell 2013; Hall and Lamont 2013; Kristjansson 2013; Schoon 2006; Tierney 2015; Xie and Wong 2021). Positivity, optimism, or positive thinking rests on cognitive assets, reasoning, and stoicism, favoring the preventability of problems (Garrett 2016; Kristjansson 2013). Similarly, solutogenesis cherishes positivity and its causal roles as opposed to pathology and deficit (Schoon 2006). Stoicism treasures assenting, desensitization, detachment, equanimity, and tranquility as opposed to choosing, sensitivity, and emotionality, notably characterized by anger, compassion, and sadness (Kristjansson 2013). In the youth, ideals in the resilience process additionally specify authenticity, dignity, honor, respectability, self-esteem, and stability (Callegari et al. 2016; Panter-Brick 2015; Wang et al. 2015; Zolkoski and Bullock 2012). For the elder, resilience ideals additionally include accountability, assimilation, coherence, directedness, externalizing problems, harmony, hope, integrity, learning, livability, morality, movement, openness, purposiveness, reconciliation, reconstruction, revising, rewriting, successful aging, transcendence, and vitality (Harris 2008; Randall and McKim 2008). Successful aging hails compensation, coping, health, proactivity, and optimization (Harris 2008). Moreover, the elder particularly embraces religiosity or spirituality as a basis for resilience (Nelson-Becker 2006; Pentz 2005). Religiosity or spirituality for resilience emphasizes affirmation, contact with god, divine support, faith, gifting, gratitude, growth, hope, interdependence, learning, love, nurturing, and sharing (Manning 2014; Pentz 2005; Ramsey and Blieszner 1999), faith notably sustains community, connectedness, peacefulness, power to work, and reflection (Ramsey and Blieszner 1999). To the patient or service user, resilience belief for rationalization additionally embraces magical thinking, critical reflection, and self-construction (Norris et al. 2008; Ungar 2004; Woollett et al. 2016). In the minority person, resilience belief for rationalization additionally highlights acceptance, collectivism, forgiveness, reciprocity, self-sacrifice, sharing, and freedom from desire and obsession (Johns et al. 2014). Hence, resilience belief indicates ideals for achieving resilience through ideal consistency or rationalization.

More systematically, resilience belief adduces Buddhism, Daoism, humanism, individualism, scholarism (i.e., Confucianism), and spirituality (Friedman and Robbins 2012; Kent and Davis 2010; Xie and Wong 2021). In the youth, resilience belief additionally emphasizes Islamism (Annalakshmi and Abeer 2011). To the elder, resilience belief additionally hails religiosity (Nelson-Becker 2006; Pentz 2005). For the working person, resilience belief additionally boosts stoicism (Jarrett 2013). In the minority person, resilience belief additionally resides in collectivism (Jia Li et al. 2018). Notably, spirituality encompasses Buddhism, Christianity, Daoism, existentialism, Hinduism, Islamism, Jainism, Judaism, paranormal belief, religiosity, Shintoism, Sikhism, and Zoroastrianism (Harris et al. 2018; MacDonald and Friedman 2002; Patch 2012; Richards 2012). Spirituality can happen in awareness, belief, experience, faith, involvement, motivation, opinion, and practice, including a search concerning meaning or spirit (Dalby 2006; Gorsuch and Miller 1999; Hall and Edwards 2002; Harris et al. 2018; Kalkstein and Tower 2009; Pargament and Mahoney 2009; Schwartz 2012). Meanwhile, religiosity incorporates belief in axioms or gospels, experience, faith, grouping, identity, institutionalization, orientation, status, value, and practice, including sacrificing and searching for sacredness (Harris et al. 2018; Leung et al. 2002; Peifer 2010; Wuthnow 2011; Saucier and Skrzypinska 2006; Tenorio and Lo 2011). These beliefs or ideologies sustain resilience by specifying goals and power, utility, norms, and ideals through the functionalist mechanisms of power realization, utility optimization, norm conformity, and ideal consistency.

Spirituality highlights such goals for resilience as the afterlife, incarnation, and sacredness (Harris et al. 2018; Schwartz 2012; Shek 2010). In the elder, spirituality adds the goals of love and truth-seeking (Wang et al. 2008).

Spirituality reveals such power or strength for resilience as forgiveness, health, hope, and optimism (Sanderson and Linehan 1999; Shek 2010; Yahne and Miller 1999). Additionally, such spiritual power arises from such aspects of spirituality as collaboration, connectedness, contemplation, faith, meaning-making, mindfulness, meditation, prayer, self-reflection, service, and worship (Gorsuch and Miller 1999; Harris et al. 2018; Shek 2010; Vess et al. 2009). In the youth, spirituality additionally highlights the power of self-discovery and wisdom (Hart 2005; Verona 2006). Spirituality adds recourse to the patient or service user to acquire resources (Parviniannasab et al. 2022).

Spirituality registers such utility for resilience as meaningfulness, purposefulness, and worthiness (Harris et al. 2018; Shek 2010). In the youth, spirituality added the utility of belongingness and connectedness (Wagener and Malony 2006).

Spirituality maintains such ideals for resilience as acceptance, compassion, ethicalness, forbearance, grandiosity, growth, integrity, love, morality, serenity, stability, and surrendering. transcendence as opposed to disappointment (Cole and Pargament 1999; Connors et al. 1999; Gorsuch and Miller 1999; Hall and Edwards 2002; MacDonald and Friedman 2002; Sanderson and Linehan 1999; Shek 2010). Spiritual ideals also inhere in such practices as challenging, overcoming, and struggling (Harris et al. 2018; Kelly 2012; Schmidt and Little 2007). In the youth, spirituality adds the ideals or practices of facing, equanimity, openness, questioning, and self-responsibility (Gehrke 2008; Hay et al. 2006; Heiden Rootes et al. 2010). For the elder, spirituality adds the ideals of efficiency, endurance, independence, journeying, peacefulness, productivity, relaxation, resistance, selectivity, self-definition, solitude, and tranquility as opposed to fear and self-centeredness (Dalby 2006; Johnson 2009; Wang et al. 2008). To the patient or service user, spirituality adds the ideals of fatalism and self-management (Unantenne et al. 2013).

Religiosity dictates such goals for resilience as sacredness (Ager and Ager 2011). In the youth, religiosity additionally highlights the goal of redemption (van Dyke and Elias 2007).

Religiosity gathers such power, strength, or its sources for resilience as affiliation, attachment to religion, divine relatedness, forgiveness, prayer, and service (Marks 2004; Myers 2014; Shorey et al. 2018; Tenorio and Lo 2011; Wuthnow 2004). In the youth, religiosity additionally emphasizes divine or supernatural power (Lerner et al. 2006). To the patient or service user, religiosity additionally accentuates the power of closeness to god and community (Dobson and Wong 2008).

Religiosity identifies such utility for resilience as belongingness, community, maturity, meaningfulness, and subsistence as opposed to pathology (Ager and Ager 2011; Dy-Liacco et al. 2009; Harris et al. 2018; Paterson 2018; Tenorio and Lo 2011; Wuthnow 2004). In the minority person, religiosity added the utility of health (Zhan et al. 2013).

Religiosity defines or treasures such ideals or obsessions for resilience as acceptance, activism, adherence, agency, assertiveness, autonomy, caring, compassion, coping, ethicalness, grandiosity, love, obedience, reflexivity, self-actualization, and voluntarism (Ager and Ager 2011; Maliepaard and Phalet 2012; O'Brien 2015; Rip et al. 2012; Rowatt et al. 2009; Saroglou and Anciaux 2004; Simpson et al. 2008; Tenorio and Lo 2011). In the case of a patient or service user, religiosity additionally cherishes the ideals of controlling and finding meaning (Dobson and Wong 2008).

Buddhism dictates such goals as nirvana, purity, perfection, and truthfulness for resilience (Woo 2008). For resilience, Buddhism identifies such power or strength as comprehension or enlightenment, insight, vigor, and wisdom as opposed to desiring, multiplicity, and resistance (Hocksmann 2004; Patch 2012; Richards 2012). Comprehension or enlightenment clarifies aging, blessing, craving, emptiness, existence cyclically, happiness, impermanence, liberation, passion, sense, serenity, suffering, and wholeness (Gowans 2003; Hocksmann 2004; Patch 2012;

Woo 2008). Buddhism posits such power sources as concentration, contemplation, meditation, mindfulness, prayer, reflection, and reasoning (Gowans 2003; Hocksmann 2004; Lin et al. 2021; Weiberg-Salzmann 2014; Woo 2008). Meanwhile, Buddhism prioritizes the ideals of abandoning, appreciation, comforting, compassion or self-compassion, deliverance, discipline, emptiness, endlessness, generosity, harmony, moderation, patience, peacefulness, purifying the mind, respect, sacrificing, selflessness, simplicity, service, sharing, tolerance, transcendence, and unity for resilience as opposed to clinging, craving, delusion, greed, hatred, selfishness, and violence (Chaiwutikornwanich 2015; Fang 2006; Gowans 2003; Ho and Li 2022; Hocksmann 2004; Orjuela 2020; Richards 2012; Woo 2008).

Christianity highlights such goals as redemption and salvation for resilience (Browning and Cooper 2004). For the goals, Christianity emphasizes following, obeying, and submitting to god, and prayer to get power or vitality through revelation for resilience (Browning and Cooper 2004; Chaiwutikornwanich 2015; Collier 2001; Richards 2012). Christianity inculcates such ideals for resilience as agape or love, chivalry, compassion, contentment, courage, faith, gratitude, hope, hospitality, humility, peacefulness, perseverance, poverty, reconciliation, responsibility, sacrificing, and struggling as opposed to idleness, oppression, and violence (Browning and Cooper 2004; Chaiwutikornwanich 2015; Collier 2001; Paterson 2018; Pedersen 2018; Reynolds 2015).

Collectivism identifies such goals as social order and solidarity for resilience. For goal attainment, collectivism traces the source of power in recourse (Oyserman et al. 2002). Collectivism identifies such utility as belongingness and connectedness from resilience (Oyserman et al. 2002; Triandis 1995). Meanwhile, collectivism prioritizes such ideals for resilience as caring, conformity, cooperation, dutifulness, harmony, self-reduction, self-transcendence, and sharing as opposed to self-enhancement (Firat 2021; Oyserman et al. 2002; Singelis and Triandis 1995; Triandis 1995).

Daoism preaches such ideals for resilience as adjustment and readjustment, childishness, complacency, effortlessness, far-sightedness, femininity, forgetting, following, harmony, humility, inactivity, meekness, middling, playing, plainness, quietude, relaxation, respect, restraint, selflessness, self-control, self-effacement, self-generation, self-realization, simplicity, softness like water, spontaneity, suppleness, tolerance, transcendence, and weakness as opposed to aggression, arrogance, competition, credit claiming, desiring, intellectualism, and self-righteousness (Brooks 2020; Coleman 2002; Moeller 2006; Richards 2012; Wawrytko 2005; Zheng 2008). Meanwhile, Daoism treasures such a goal as freedom for resilience (Zheng 2008). Daoism gathers power for resilience through contemplation, matching complementarily, meditation, and reflection (Coleman 2002; Tan 2008).

Existentialism highlights such goals as existence or living for resilience (Cox 2012). For goal attainment, existentialism emphasizes such power or its sources as friendship, humor, willpower, and wittiness (Cox 2012; Solomon 2003). Existentialism prizes such utility as meaningfulness as opposed to nihilism from resilience (Solomon 2003). Existentialism boosts such ideals for resilience as activeness, affirmation, artistry, atheism, assertiveness, authenticity, choice, engagement, enthusiasm, heroism, love, mastery, morality, nobility, obligation, reasoning, security, solidarity, and vibrance as opposed to blaming, conformity, cowardice, dependency, desiring, despair, humility, mediocrity, romance, and slave mentality (Cox 2012; Solomon 2003). Specifically, existentialism identifies virtues for resilience in contribution, courage, courtesy, directedness, expression, fullness, generosity, honesty, insight, integrity, justice, playfulness, politeness, responsibility, risking, solitude, sympathy, temperance, and toughness (Solomon 2003).

Hinduism prized such ideals for resilience as deserving, devotion, oneness or unity, responsibility, and self-detachment, as opposed to dependence on chance (Cast and Stets 2016; Richards 2012; Smith 1991). Besides, Hinduism articulates such virtues as autonomy, calmness, chastity, community, creativity, discipline, harmony, humbleness, loving, obedience, patience, peacefulness, scholarship, self-efficacy, self-sacrificing, shame, studying, temperance, tolerance, and truthfulness (Banavathy and Choudry 2014; Thomas 1997). Meanwhile, Hinduism highlights getting power from enlightenment, worship, and yoga (Richards 2012; Smith 1991).

Humanism weighs such utility from utility as dignity, enlightenment, freedom, honor, knowledge, order, relatedness, self-actualization, self-realization, and vitality, as opposed to alienation, ignorance, and pleasure (Browning and Cooper 2004; Fuchs 2020; Selznick 2008; Visher 1997; Waterman 2013). For the utility, humanism emphasizes such ideals for resilience as achievement, acceptance, affirmation, agency, aiding, arguing, attachment, authenticity, autonomy, choice, coherence, collectivity, concreteness, cooperation, construction, creativity, critical thinking, empathy, friendship, logical thinking, loving, morality, objectivity, rationality, reasoning, reflection, respect, responsibility, self-control, self-denial, self-improvement, sharing, toleration, working, and worldliness as opposed to conflict, desiring, indulgence, manipulation, neutrality, passion, prayer, and worship (Doane 2017; Fuchs 2020; Selznick 2008; Visher 1997).

Individualism emphasizes such utility for resilience as achievement, consumption, contribution, finance, freedom, identity, leisure, privilege, privacy, success, superiority, uniqueness, and worth as opposed to community and embeddedness (Bunge 1996; Davis and Robinson 1999; Krys et al. 2019; Norris and Inglehart 2009; Sullivan et al. 2015). For the utility, individualism extols such ideals, beliefs, and practices as agency, autonomy, character, choice, competition, demonstration, education, hedonism, independence, Protestantism, reasoning, reflexivity, responsibility, restlessness, science, self-actualization, self-centrality, self-construction, self-development, self-interest, self-knowledge, self-restraint, sentimentality, utilitarianism, voluntarism, and working as opposed to prejudice and superstition (Braun 2011; Coffe and Geys 2007; Davis and Robinson 1999; Oishi et al. 2007; O'Brien 2015; Oyserman et al. 2002; Speed et al. 2018; Sullivan et al. 2015; Sun and Wang 2010). Hedonism boosts such utility for resilience as carefreeness, comfort, enjoyment, freedom, fun, joyfulness, pleasure, satisfaction, self-enhancement, and self-preservation (Huta 2017; Son and Wilson 2012). Moreover, hedonism prioritizes ideals for resilience, such as presentism and self-love (Huta 2017; Kerstein 2002). Protestantism prides such ideals for resilience as acceptance, asceticism, computation rationally, future orientation, guilt, production, repression, sacrificing, suppression, and trust as opposed to desire and fear (Fjellvang 2011; Gill 2004; Kim and

Cohen 2017; Seabach 2017). To gain power, Protestantism highlights a connection with god (Gill 2004). Utilitarianism highlights such utility from resilience as benefit, enjoyment, gratification, merit, perfection, satisfaction, security, and stability as opposed to exploitation (Shaw 1999). For the utility, utilitarianism treasures such ideals for resilience as arguing, benevolence, cooperation, fairness, forward-looking, hedonism, impartiality, instrumentality, liberty, long-termism, objectivity, rationality, realism, and truthfulness as opposed to dedication and deservingness (Hample 2018; Shaw 1999; Yeager 2001).

Islamism cherishes such ideals for resilience as brotherhood, communality, community, conformity, discipline, fairness, fatalism, honesty, machismo, martyrdom, procreation, self-realization, striving, struggle, submission to god, thrift, and working as opposed to alcoholism, arrogance, doping, gambling, greed, self-esteem, suicide, and violence (Braun 2011; Esposito 2002; Richards 2012; Scruton 2014). Specifically, Islamism accentuates such virtues for resilience as courage, courtesy, forgiveness, gentleness, kindness, humility, moderation, modesty, and repentance (Thomas 1997). Meanwhile, Islamism traces the source of power in connection with the divine (Esposito 2002).

Jainism honors such ideals for resilience as asceticism, enlightenment, and meditation (Richards 2012). More specifically, Jainism proclaims virtues for resilience in agreeableness, altruism, calmness, candidness, chastity, fidelity, forgiveness, generosity, honesty, humility, kindheartedness, moderation, temperance, truthfulness, and veracity (Thomas 1997).

Judaism hails such virtues for resilience as courtesy, humanitarianism, respect, and self-directedness as opposed to gossiping, littering, lying, murdering, punishing, and randomness (Thomas 1997). Humanitarianism accentuates utility, dignity, and freedom (Ager and Ager 2011; Vestergaard 2013). For such utility, humanitarianism favors such ideals as caring, consent, entitlement, faith, impartiality, individualism, reasoning, responsibility, and self-determination as opposed to discipline (Ager and Ager 2011; Bendixsen 2018; Brigg 2018; Burchardt 2013; Hoekstra 2021; Mitchell 2017; Mitoma and Bystrom 2013). Meanwhile, Judaism detests force, sex, speech, and wealth as vices (Thomas 1997). Judaism regards prayer and worship as sources to gain power (Richards 2012).

Shintoism prizes the utility of enjoyment and preaches the ideals of cleanliness, nature appreciation and closeness, and purification (McDowell and Brown 2009; Richards 2012). Sikhism honors discipline, faith, humility, love, martyrdom, and mercy (McDowell and Brown 2009; Richards 2012). However, Sikhism opposes mind-altering, sacrifice, and seclusion (McDowell and Brown 2009). Zoroastrianism treasures meditation and prayer (Richards 2012). Additionally, Zoroastrianism emphasizes struggling as a goal (McDowell and Brown 2009).

Stoicism valorizes such utility as dignity, honor, and knowledge (Holowchak 2008; Mitsis 2003). For the utility, stoicism advocates such ideals for resilience as accepting, attaching, calmness, choice, conservation, controlling, cosmopolitanism, delaying, education, enduring, equanimity, exercising, harmony, indifference, invincibility, justice, kindness, logical thinking, magnanimity, naturalism, obligation, perfectionism, preparation, poverty, purity, rationality, resolve, planning, reasoning, sacrificing, self-control, self-direction, self-love, self-preservation, simplicity (Holowchak 2008; Martin 2016; Mitsis 2003). Cosmopolitanism favors reflection (Holowchak 2008). Naturalism extols such utility as freedom (Hocksmann 2004). For such utility, naturalism cherishes such virtues as impartiality, naturalness, peacefulness, quietness, and resting as opposed to competition, coercion, desire, and intervention (Cooper 1999; Hocksmann 2004). Perfectionism pursues such virtues for resilience as autonomy, capacity, collaboration, complexity, curiosity, development, elevation, effectiveness, eudaimonia, flourishing, meaningfulness, morality, positivity, productivity, purposiveness, relational ease, satisfaction, self-esteem, and self-knowledge (Sirgy 2012). Eudaimonia encompasses such virtues as acceptance, accomplishment, actualizing, aliveness, appreciation, authenticity, autonomy, balance, belongingness, commitment, competence, concern, congruence, contemplation, contribution, controlling, coping, courage, creativity, development, efficacy, engagement, excellence, expressiveness, fairness, functioning, generativity, generosity, grit, growth, hardiness, identity, insight, integration, integrity, intimacy, justice, knowledge, love, meaningfulness, maturity, moderation, mastery, mindfulness, morality, organizing, perseverance, planning, prosociality, purposiveness, reasoning, reflectiveness, relatedness, resonance, respect, responsibility, rightness, salvation, self-discovery, self-realization, self-regulation, understanding, volition, vitality, welcoming, and wisdom (Huta 2017; Meadows 2014; Phillips 2006; Sirgy 2012; Waterman 2008). Positivity upholds such virtues as acceptance, authenticity, autonomy, confidence, contentment, contribution, ecstasy, faith, gratification, growth, hope, integration, mastery, meaningfulness, morality, optimism, pleasure, pride, purposiveness, relaxation, satisfaction, serenity, and trust (Burnett 2012; Sirgy 2012). Contrariwise, however, stoicism scorns such ideals as chance, convenience, desire, emotion, easiness, expression, future orientation, leisure, and pleasure (Holowchak 2008).

## *Resilience Exposure*

Resilience exposure concerns other people's advice on or demand for resilience (Brodsky and Cattaneo 2013; Celinski and Allen 2017). Such exposure primarily functions as socially taken power to drive resilience belief, action, and feeling. This function thus rests on integrating power realization and norm conformity for fulfillment and integration in analytical functionalism.

Resilience exposure manifests its function of power realization in cognition, insight, and understanding regarding resilience (Castro and Murray 2010; Celinski and Allen 2017; Nemeth and Olivier 2017; Richardson 2017). In the youth, resilience exposure unfolds as consciousness, curiosity, knowledge, and mastery regarding resilience (Boulton and Macaulay 2022; Brooks and Brooks 2014; Hays-Grudo et al. 2021; Plouffe et al. 2020; Prince-Embury 2014a). For the patient or service user, resilience exposure additionally happens in faith as opposed to ambiguity and doubt (Dziengel 2015; Woodier 2011). In the working person, resilience exposure additionally resides in mindfulness (McCray et al. 2016).

Resilience exposure as norm conformity transpires in attention, learning, negotiating, perspective taking, and receiving education, empowerment, power, resources, support, training, and warning regarding resilience (Brodsky and Cattaneo 2013; Jones and d'Errico 2019; Kent and Davis 2010; Nemeth and Olivier 2017; Ungar 2010; Van Vliet 2008; Walsh 2002; Zautra 2014). In the youth, resilience exposure to social norms additionally hinges on communication with, conformity to, connection with, empathy with, fitting to, disciplining from, influence from, listening to, mentoring from, parenting from, participation with, protection from, psychoeducation as a way of counseling from, recourse to, role-taking from, seeking information from, sharing with, and social interaction including visiting from others regarding resilience (Davis and Paster 2000; Gardner et al. 2008; Joseph 1994; Li et al. 2018; Masten et al. 2009; Ni et al. 2016; Prince-Embury 2013b, 2014a; Sun and Stewart 2007; Thompson 2006; Ungar et al. 2007; von Soest et al. 2010; Wang et al. 2015; Zolkoski and Bullock 2012). To the elder, resilience exposure to social norms additionally involves accommodating with, affiliation with, benefitting from, confluence with, companionship with, contact with, interdependence with, modeling after, and openness to others (Gergen and Gergen 2010; Lou and Ng 2012; Nakashima and Canda 2005; Ramsey and Blieszner 1999). In the patient or service user, resilience exposure to social norms additionally implicates social cohesion, collaboration, and inclusion (Dageid and Gronlie 2015; Godwin et al. 2015; Liebenberg and Moore 2018). To the minority person, resilience exposure to social norms additionally springs from collective or social advocacy, assimilation, bonding, closeness, collectivism, and trust (Cheng et al. 2021; Holleran and Waller 2003; Johns et al. 2014; Payne 2011).

Advice, coaching, counseling, and mentoring are thus the primary and systematic communication sources of social norms for resilience and general healthy development (Fawcett 2012). Such developmental communication demands resilience, including its goals, needs, motivation, and related power for fulfillment, goal attainment or realization, utility for adaptation or optimization, norms for conformity or integration, and beliefs, ideologies, mindsets, or lifestyles for latency or maintaining consistency to thrive based on analytical functionalism.

Developmental communication highlights the goals or needs of resilience, including acceptance, bearing, calming, commitment, fortitude, grit, normalization or normalizing, neutralization, recovery, repair or reparation, tolerance or toleration (Boorman et al. 2012; Brazier 1995; Bussolari and Goodell 2009; Caputo et al. 2018; Evans 1996; Hayes 2014; Proyer et al. 2013; Lintz et al. 2019; Littman-Ovadia et al. 2014; Semple and Hott 2012; Sperry 2012; Sympson and Elder 2000; Vallejos et al. 2016). More generally, such communication emphasizes goals, aspirations, and dreams (Law 2007; Lloyd and Dallos 2008).

Developmental communication consolidates fulfillment or goal attainment (Fall et al. 2004). Fulfillment covers achievement, breakthrough, performance, progressing, resolution, self-fulfillment, and success (Bachkirova 2018; Bussolari and Goodell 2009; Caputo et al. 2018; Cheavens 2000; Hayes 2014; Proyer et al.

2013; van Deurzen 2012; Western 2017). Conversely, such communication laments deflection and incompletion (Allan and Whybrow 2007; Ellis and Smith 2012).

Developmental communication affirms power for goals (Paul 2012). Power encompasses adaptability, agency, agility, artistry, capability, competence, consciousness, creativity, insight, intelligence, knowledge, learnability, mastery, memory, potentiality, repertoire, resolute, resourcefulness, skill, self-efficacy, strengths, volition, willpower, and wisdom (Bachkirova 2018; Blum et al. 2006; Braun 2020; Caputo et al. 2018; Donohoe and Ricketts 2012a; Drake 2018; Geldard and Geldard 2012a; Joseph and Bryant-Jefferies 2007; Kast 2006; Kelly 1997; Koerner 2012; Midtgaard et al. 2007; Miguel and Pino-Juste 2021; Pett 2000; Rowan 1998; Semple and Hott 2012; Savickas 2015; Schwartz 2012; Spence and Grant 2014; Sympson and Elder 2000; Turner and Conkel 2010; Williams et al. 2012). Such communication furthermore indicates that power stems personally from breathing, broadening, camping, catharsis, centeredness, curiosity, discharge, enlightenment, exercising, meditation, mindfulness, motivation, ownership, recreation, relaxation, release, self-discovery, self-nurturing, vacation, yoga, and zest (Baim 2012; Boorman et al. 2012; Brown 2011; Fall et al. 2004; Heenan 2012; Kwong et al. 2019; Mytton 2012; Potash et al. 2019; Samuels 1985; Totton 2012; Western 2017). This communication also avers that power derives externally or socially from alliances, bonding, connection, education, encouragement received, exploration, learning, meandering, mobilizing, networking, prayer, relationships, support received, training, treatment, upskilling, and watching (Bennett and Campone 2017; Brazier 1995; Carlson et al. 2006; Gergen and Gergen 2006; Jones-Smith 2014; McLeod 2012; Oades et al. 2014; Proyer et al. 2013; Schwartz 2012; Turner and Conkel 2010; VanFleet et al. 2010). Conversely, such communication denies one's dependence, incapability, difficulty, limitation, subjugation, and uncertainty (Farber 2010; Fink 1995; Ghitterbuck et al. 2017; Goldstein 2001; Spinelli 2018; Toporek and Cohen 2017).

Developmental communication advocates power realization or actualization (Western 2017). Such communication furthermore indicates that power realization personally engages abstraction, action, activation, affirmation, application, autonomy, chanting, choice, construction, coping, dancing, deconstruction, decision making, desensitization, devotion, difference making, exception building, expression, fantasy, improvisation, interpretation, meaning making, opportunity use, preparation, prevention, problem-solving, production, protection, pursuit, rehearsal, risking, scheduling, sense making, simplification, strength use, striving, struggle, symbolization, unfoldment, and work (Braun 2020; Blum et al. 2006; Bullough 2012; Donohoe and Ricketts 2012a; Egan 2012; Fawcett 2012; Francis and Zarecky 2017; Grawe 2004; Jones-Smith 2014; Koerner 2012; Midtgaard et al. 2007; Proyer et al. 2013; Timulak 2015). Particularly, power realization centers on the self through self-compassion, self-congratulation, self-control, self-description, self-determination, self-direction, self-help, self-monitoring, self-love, self-overcoming, self-reliance, and self-soothing (Brown 2011; Bennett and Campone 2017; Carlson et al. 2006; Dryden 2003; Jamison and Schuttler 2017; Law 2007; Pett 2000; Vallejos et al. 2016). That communication also finds power realization socially in advocacy, appraisal, arguing, battling, articulation, assertiveness, challenging, clarification, condemnation, confrontation or facing, controlling, defense, discussion, domination, leadership, monitoring, negotiation, regulation, reauthoring, restorying or retelling, storytelling, surveillance (Bimrose 2012; Caputo et al. 2018; Fall et al. 2004; Fink 1995; Goldstein 1995; Hayes 2014; Heenan 2012; Kwong et al. 2019; Leitner and Epting 2015; Miguel and Pino-Juste 2021; Mytton 2012; O'Connell 2012; Passmore and Whybrow 2007; Sitzer and Stockwell 2015; Strong 2002; Turner and Conkel 2010; Waines 2012; Williams et al. 2012; Zimmerman and Dickerson 1996). Conversely, such communication questions aversion, avoidance, compromise, denial, defusing, disjunction, distancing, elimination, ending, foreclosure, ignoring, reciprocity, repression, splitting, and withdrawal (Carlson et al. 2006; Goldstein 2001; Silvester 2000).

Developmental communication encourages adaptation (Bussolari and Goodell 2009). On the one hand, adaptation works personally in adjustment, alternative taking, change, compensation, displacement, diversion, flexibility, integration, letting go, modifying, multiplicity, newness, redirection, redefining, reframing, reforming, reorientation, restructuring, reversal, self-transformation, shifting, transformation, and transition (Bachkirova 2018; Basseches 2003; Brazier 1995; Donohoe and Ricketts 2012a; Craig 2007; Fall et al. 2004; Grawe 2004; Harris and Laidlaw 2012; Savickas 2015; Stuart and Robertson 2003; Timulak 2015; Williams et al. 2012). On the other hand, adaptation operates socially in accommodation, attunement, balance, co-construction, equilibrium, fitting, moderation, openness, open-mindedness, resocialization, synthesis, and unity (Baim 2012; Bullough 2012; Brodsky and Stanley 2013; Boorman et al. 2012; Braun 2020; Caputo et al. 2018; Grant and Cavanagh 2018; Greenberg 2004; Hayes 2014; Bimrose 2012; Kang and Gottfredson 2015; Schwartz 2012; Smith and Hawkins 2018; Totton 2012). Conversely, such communication disapproves of anger, arousal, and resistance (Braun 2020; Williams et al. 2012).

Developmental communication specifies utility, expectancy, or worth (Dybicz 2011; Swales and Dunkley 2012; Watts et al. 2004). Utility emanates personally from cheerfulness, comfort, confidence, contentment, enjoyment, equanimity, hope, identity, laughing, leisure, living, meaningfulness, nutrition, order, perfection, play, pleasure, positivity, purposiveness, savoring, satisfaction, selfhood, self-actualization, self-esteem, self-sufficiency, serenity, and survival (Basseches 2003; Brown 2011; Craig 2007; Fawcett 2012; Jones-Smith 2014; Kwong et al. 2019; Miguel and Pino-Juste 2021; Parker 2011; Pryor and Bright 2007; Spence and Grant 2014; van Deurzen 2012; Walker 2012). Moreover, utility derives socially from belongingness, blessing, connectedness, emancipation, freedom, growth, happiness, health, independence, interestedness, intimacy, liberation, love, recognition, rights, safety, security, sex, superiority, uniqueness, and warmth (Boniwell and Kauffman 2018; Browning and Cooper 2004; Dybicz 2011; Heenan 2012; Koerner 2012; Lieneman et al. 2017; Mruk 2019; Phipps and Vorster 2011; Shapiro 2016; Shoukry 2017; Sperry 2012). Conversely, such communication detests alienation or estrangement, anxiety, boredom, compulsion, constriction, death, depression, disruption, distress, disturbance, doubt, emptiness, fear, futility, grief, guilt, hate, harm, illness, isolation, loneliness, nihilism, objectification, oppression, pain, pathology, poverty, rejection, sadness, self-blame, self-criticism, self-fragmentation, self-punishment, shame, stagnation, stigma, symptoms, tension, and trauma (Carlson et al. 2006; Gergen and Gergen 2006; Goldstein 2001; Goodman et al. 2016; Proyer et al. 2013; Koerner 2012; Lieneman et al. 2017; Miguel and Pino-Juste 2021; Proyer et al. 2013; Schneider 2000; Semple and Hott 2012; Shapiro 2016; Stuart and Robertson 2003; Tew 2002; Timulak 2015; Toporek and Cohen 2017; Watson and Bohart 2015).

Developmental communication favors utility optimization, working personally, including analogy, analysis, anticipation, conceptualization, concretization, consideration, contemplation, cost–benefit analysis, costing, designing, differentiation, discernment, evaluation, examination, externalization, goal setting, holism, imagination, investigation, justifying, mentalization, processing, reappraisal, reattribution, reflection, reflexivity, restructuring, self-talk, thinking, validation, and visualization (Baim 2012; Brodsky and Stanley 2013; Duignan 2007; Jinks 2012; Koerner 2012; Mytton 2012; Samuels 2006; Spence and Grant 2014; Timulak 2015; Williams et al. 2012). Additionally, utility optimization proceeds socially through exposure, attentiveness, comparison, dialogue, discovery, experimenting, exploration, niche finding and relocation, observing, projection, questioning, relearning, responsiveness, sensitivity or sensitization, surfing, and testing (Boorman et al. 2012; Donohoe and Ricketts 2012a; Fall et al. 2004; Greenberg 2004; Kang and Gottfredson 2015; Kwong et al. 2019; Ladany and O'Shaughnessy 2014; Sitzer and Stockwell 2015; Savickas 2015; Stelter 2017; Turner and Conkel 2010; Williams 2012). Conversely, such communication refutes absolutism, arbitrariness, catastrophizing, confusion, dichotomization, distortion, double standard application, emotionality, impulsivity, labeling, overgeneralization, partiality, perfectionism, personalization or self-centeredness, polarization, preoccupation, ruminating, stereotyping (Brodsky and Stanley 2013; Fall et al. 2004; Bimrose 2012; MacPherson et al. 2013; Mytton 2012; Shapiro 2016).

Developmental communication appreciates norm conformity, including social agreement, assimilation, cohesion, confluence, following, imitation, modeling, piety, respect, role-taking, and submission (Allan and Whybrow 2007; Bachkirova 2018; Barlow and Burlingame 2006; Bratter 2003; Braun 2020; Caputo et al. 2018; Ellis and Smith 2012; Fall et al. 2004; Kwong et al. 2019; Ladany and O'Shaughnessy 2014; Lieneman et al. 2017; Savickas 2015; Swales and Dunkley 2012; Turner and Conkel 2010; Yang 2017). Such communication furthermore indicated that norm conformity stems from social admiration, affiliation, attachment, collaboration, communication, community, contact, contracting, conversation, cooperation, embeddedness, empathy, harmony, grouping, interaction, interest, involvement, similarity, socializing, and trust (Bachkirova 2018; Bratter 2003; Braun 2020; Brown 2011; Caputo et al. 2018; Carlson et al. 2006; Egan 2012; Fall et al. 2004; Goldstein 1995; Inskipp 2012; Kwong et al. 2019; Ladany and O'Shaughnessy 2014; McLeod 2012; Savickas 2015; Stuart and Robertson 2003; Swales and Dunkley 2012; Turner and Conkel 2010). Conversely, such communication discourages social blaming, conflict, competition, criticism, defense, demanding, dispute, dominance, hostility, scapegoating, and separaton (Bachkirova 2018; Bratter 2003; Braun 2020; Caputo et al. 2018; Fall et al. 2004; Goldstein 2001; Kwong et al. 2019; Ladany and O'Shaughnessy 2014; Passmore and Whybrow 2007; Savickas 2015; Stuart and Robertson 2003; Swales and Dunkley 2012; Turner and Conkel 2010).

Developmental communication preaches such ideals or virtues (Caputo et al. 2018; Goldstein 1995; Passmore and Whybrow 2007; Sperry 2012; Yang 2017). Ideals or virtues stand personally in conduct, contrition, easygoing, emptying, faith, femininity, freshness, inactivity, integrity, newness, optimism, playfulness, prudence, purifying, quietness, rationality, science, self-cultivation, simplicity, spirituality, spontaneity, teleology, temperance, and water mentality (Bachkirova 2018; Baim 2012; Brazier 1995; Browning and Cooper 2004; Craig 2007; Dybicz 2011; Fawcett 2012; Grant and Cavanagh 2018; Hayes 2014; Kelly 1997; Koerner 2012; Pryor and Bright 2007; Sperry 2012; Strong 2002; J. Yang 2017). Additionally, ideals ring socially in as accountability, altruism, caring, charity, circulating, citizenship, compassion, compliments, contribution, equality or equalizing, ethicality, fairness, forgiveness, generosity, gentleness, gratitude, hierarchy, humility, humor, informing, justice, kindness, loving, mothering, nature, noninterference, participation, praise, reciprocity, responsibility, revolution, service, self-disclosure, sharing, solidarity, sympathy, transcendence, truthfulness, trustworthiness, and understanding (Barak 2016; Bimrose 2012; Boorman et al. 2012; Brodsky and Stanley 2013; Caputo et al. 2018; Carlson et al. 2006; Cheavens and Guter 2018; Dryden 2003; Ellis and Smith 2012; Fall et al. 2004; Guilfoyle 2005; Geldard and Geldard 2012b; Heenan 2012; Kwong et al. 2019; Parker 2011; Shapiro 2016; Sieler 2018; Stelter 2017; Western 2017). Particularly, such communication advocates such ideal systems or ideologies as atheism, familism, fatalism, gradualism, hedonism, holism, individualism, materialism, objectivism, pragmatism, presentism or nowness, relativism, realism, supernaturalism, theism, traditionalism, universalism (Bachkirova 2018; Barak 2016; Baim 2012; Bimrose 2012; Boorman et al. 2012; Brodsky and Stanley 2013; Caputo et al. 2018; Carlson et al. 2006; Cheavens and Guter 2018; Craig 2007; Dybicz 2011; Ellis and Smith 2012; Fall et al. 2004; Fawcett 2012; Guilfoyle 2005; Hayes 2014; Heenan 2012; Kelly 1997, Kwong et al. 2019; Koerner 2012; O'Connell 2012; Pryor and Bright 2007; Shapiro 2016; Stelter 2017; Yang 2017). However, some other communication questions aggression, ambivalence, awfulizing, damnation, demand, desire, depreciation, delusion, destruction, egalitarianism, egoism or egotism, evilness, foreclosure, greed, idealization, indulgence, narcissism, nonsense, perfectionism, rationalism, sexuality, social comparison, utopianism (Allan and Whybrow 2007; Brazier 1995; Browning and Cooper 2004; Craig 2007; Goldstein 2001; Dryden 2003; Fall et al. 2004; Parker 2011; Sperry 2012; Stuart and Robertson 2003; Yang 2017).

Developmental communication upholds ideal consistency or rationalization (Shapiro 2016). Consistency furthermore engages authenticity, congruence, coherence or self-cohesion, concordance, genuineness, sticking (Fall et al. 2004; Francis and Zarecky 2017; Goldstein 1995; Heenan 2012; Koerner 2012; Jinks 2012; Leitner and Epting 2015; Shapiro 2016). Conversely, such communication disdains intrapsychic gaps or discrepancies (Brown 2011).

## *Dynamics of the Resilience Process*

The dynamics of the resilience process chiefly function in the development of resilience through its exposure, belief, action, and feeling sequentially. Specifically, exposure to social demand for resilience activates resilience belief, action, and feeling, resilience belief underlies resilience action and feeling, and resilience action generates resilience feeling. In other words, resilience feeling builds on resilience exposure, belief, and action. According to the voluntaristic lens of analytical functionalism, resilience action sets goals and power for resilience for fulfillment through power realization, resilience belief determines utility and ideals for adaptation through utility optimization, and resilience exposure to social demand constitutes social norms for integration through norm conformity.

## *Resilience Constituted by Its Action*

Resilience or its feeling is a product of resilience action, which installs or consolidates goals and power for resilience, based on the power realization mechanism to achieve fulfillment or goal attainment from the functionalist perspective. Typical resilience action embraces coping, restoring, and returning (Corbin and Hall 2019; Crane et al. 2019; Kent and Davis 2010; Nemeth and Olivier 2017; Pangallo et al. 2015; Park and Slattery 2014; Schwager and Rothermund 2014). They represent the goal and power for resilience to secure conditions or resources for achieving resilience or its feeling. In more detail, resilience action operates personally or socially.

In theory, such action happens personally in broadening and building mental commitment, converting resources, coping, defense, distracting, meaning-making, processing, reappraising, relaxation, restoring resources, restructuring cognitively, risking such as challenging risks, self-affirmation, self-reflection, self-regulation, and transportation to a virtual world (Bowen et al. 2013; Crane et al. 2019; Gallo et al. 2004; Hassija and Cloitre 2014; Matusitz 2017; Mikulincer and Shaver 2014; Park and Slattery 2014; Paul et al. 2022; Schwager and Rothermund 2014; Schoon 2006; Shaver and Mikulincer 2012; Sherman and Cohen 2006). Broadening and building apply to intellectual interest and problem-solving skills (Graham and Donaldson 1999; Taylor and Pancer 2007). Coping effectively includes joking, problem-solving, and religious activities (Cherry et al. 2018). Meaning-making includes applying a culturally derived conclusion, offering a lesson, and realizing the consequence of not following a social rule (Sanderson et al. 2016). Restructuring features finding a new faith, going along with fate, and making light of the situation (Martin et al. 2007). Self-reflection features thinking about oneself and daydreaming about oneself (Lindwall 2004). Self-regulation comprises attention, changing, developing, modifying, modulating, processing, and selecting (Boden et al. 2014; Schwager and Rothermund

2014). Attention embraces distracting, focusing, opening, and processing, encompassing positive thinking and reasoning, including wishful thinking and problem-focusing (Schwager and Rothermund 2014). Transportation to a cyber world engages expressing, gaming, identity building, immersion, and playing (Fuchs 2008; Ho and Ng 2022; Sun et al. 2008). Besides, learning and life styling have been effective personal resilience action (Buikstra et al. 2010).

Furthermore, resilience action can operate socially in accommodating, attention, communication, fitting, helping, negotiating, networking, regulation, and storytelling and restorying (Buzzanell 2010; Cocking 2017; Hassija and Cloitre 2014; Park 2017; Park and Slattery 2014; Schwager and Rothermund 2014; Ungar 2012; Van Vliet 2008). Additionally, effective resilience social action has been cultural or ceremonial activity and distancing from non-supporting sources (Corbin and Hall 2019).

In the youth, additional resilience action working personally includes exercising or sporting, initiative taking, meditating, planning, self-enhancing, self-protecting, self-talking, striving, time management and use constructively, and ventilating (Eisenberg et al. 2004; Griciute 2015; Kaplan 2012; Lipsitt and Demick 2012; Prince-Embury 2013c; Thompson 2006; Ungar et al. 2005). Striving aims at accommodation, generativity, growth, independence, intimacy, and positivity (Seaton and Beaumont 2015). Generativity includes advising, contributing to society, and teaching (Marks et al. 2004). Conversely, resilience personal action precludes avoiding, doping, and externalizing (Graber et al. 2016; Markstrom et al. 2000; Ungar et al. 2005). Externalizing includes disturbing, fidgeting, and hurting (Puig et al. 1999).

In the youth, additional resilience action operating socially includes attaching, recourse, and role-taking (Graber et al. 2016; Masten 2014; Ungar et al. 2005). Conversely, resilience social action precludes aggression, being absent, and gossiping (Prince-Embury 2013c; Shure and Aberson 2012; Ye et al. 2021).

In the elder, additional resilience action functioning personally includes compensation, coping heroically, optimization, and selection (Dubovska et al. 2017; Roberto 2009). Compensation involves the self, environment, social support, and technology. Optimization proceeds with initiating, practicing, reframing, and regulating. Selection applies to activity, functioning, health, and relationships. Conversely, personal resilience action precludes smoking (Sawyer and Allman 2010). Meanwhile, additional resilience action operating socially includes family management, grandparenting, social contact, and volunteering (Bailey et al. 2013; Taylor et al. 2005; Visaria et al. 2023). Grandparenting comprises modeling, nurturing, and storytelling (Taylor et al. 2005).

In the patient or service users, additional resilience action includes capitalizing or building on strengths, controlling, resource managing, self-cultivating, self-empowering, and training (Davydov et al. 2010; Jamison et al. 2017; Lawton Smith 2017; Wong et al. 2018). Moreover, resilience action emphasizes coping that is active, appraising, confronting, courageous, redefining, reformulating, and using social support (Parviniannasab et al. 2022; Stewart and Yuen 2011; Yin et al. 2022; Zhao and Fu 2022).

In the working person, additional resilience action includes acting proactively, caring, cooperating, preparing, reconciling, and responding (Biggart et al. 2017;

Portnoy et al. 2018; Schilbach et al. 2021; Vandsburger et al. 2012; Wilson and Ferch 2005). Reconciling applies to conflict, differences, and dilemmas.

Resilience action can generate power for resilience to activate the power realization mechanism. Such generation hinges on internal or personal and external social resource building, notably through such resilience action as cultural or literary practice, protesting, and volunteering (Hofstetter et al. 1999; Isham et al. 2006; Liang and Lee 2022).

Personally, resilience action can draw power from establishing arguments, control, courage, dominance, goals, guilt, humility, magnanimity, modesty, responsibility, and temperance (Dillard 2004; Keltener et al. 2008; ten Brinke and Keltner 2020). Goal establishment engages affect management, conversation management, identity building, impression management, obligation, orientation, and recourse (Dillard 2004). Impression management involves honesty, open-mindedness, and following rules (Paulhus 1991).

Socially, resilience action can accrue power through social alignment, association, cooperation, engagement, mobilization, reputation, solidarity, and status (Keltener et al. 2008); Matthewman 2011; Munro 2009; ten Brinke and Keltner 2020). Additionally, resilience action can muster external power through connecting with god spiritually, information gathering, and technology use (Engelstad 2009; Gass and Seiter 2004; Munro 2009). Conversely, resilience strengthens social power by precluding gossip (Keltener et al. 2008).

## *Resilience Constituted by Its Belief*

Resilience or its feeling is also a product of resilience belief, which defines utility, ideals, power, and norms regarding resilience. Resilience belief about utility indicates utility for optimizing through resilience. Alternatively, resilience belief about ideals or habits specifies ideals rationalizing resilience to maintain ideal consistency. Resilience belief regarding power or its motivational sources in dispositions, goals, or needs highlights power or capability for realizing resilience. Additionally, resilience belief regarding norms or their demand or pressure foregrounds norms for assimilating or conforming to resilience.

Belief about utility notably involves attribution and expectancy about resilience, that is, about the causes and impacts of resilience. Such defining capitalizes on utility optimization and ideal consistency mechanisms in the voluntaristic lens of the functionalist perspective. These mechanisms work internally or personally and externally or socially to boost resilience. Accordingly, the utility of resilience attracts resilience or its feeling, whereas ideals rationalize resilience or its feeling through compatibility or similarity. Rationalizing based on ideal consistency rests on the idealistic property of resilience, such as adaptation, heroism, legality, meaningfulness, strength, and well-being (Allison et al. 2017; Bowers et al. 2017; Hoffman 2003; Rutter 2012; Van Haaften et al. 2004; Zautra et al. 2010). Additionally, power realization for resilience operates in belief in such resilience bases as assets, capability, capacity, resources, and strength (Berger 2015; Truebridge 2016; White 2014; Zheng et al. 2020). Resources include social support received (Truebridge 2016). Furthermore, power derives from belief in, consciousness about, or self-awareness about dispositions or traits predisposing to or structuring resilience (Sawyers et al. 2020).

Resilience belief about the personal utility of resilience emphasizes courage demonstration, distress management, efficacy demonstration, health, livability, religious responsiveness, resource demonstration, and self-confidence demonstration (Cherry et al. 2023; Shaver and Mikulincer 2012). Moreover, resilience belief about the social utility of resilience foregrounds adaptation (Leigert and Reutter 2005; Bowers et al. 2017; Ungar 2012).

Resilience belief about ideals personally emphasizes agency, development, growth, mastery, normalcy, positivity, reactivity, relaxation, restructuring cognitively, resolution, self-regulation, and virtuousness (Cocking 2017; Dwivedi 2017; Gallo et al. 2004; Gilligan 2009; Buzzanell 2010; Prince-Embury et al. 2017; Simon et al. 2005; Van Vliet 2008). Mastery comprises adaptability, self-efficacy, and optimism (Prince-Embury et al. 2017). Virtuousness embraces appreciation, flourishing, gratitude, hope, humor, spirituality, and wisdom (Dwivedi 2017). Spirituality encompasses contemplation, meditation, and prayer (Dwivedi 2017). Conversely, resilience belief discounts reactivity or sensitivity (Prince-Embury et al. 2017). In the youth, resilience belief adds such personal ideals as self-acceptance, self-discipline, and self-understanding (Kaplan 2012; Shibue and Kasai 2014). For the elder, resilience belief additionally emphasizes such personal ideals as coherence, engagement, enjoyment, functioning, independence, pleasure, religiosity, self-esteem, stability, and younghood (Dubovska et al. 2017; Fry and Debats 2010). Religiosity encompasses discipleship, fellowship, missions, and worship (Fry and Debats 2010; Roberto 2009). To the patient or service user, resilience belief additionally highlights such personal ideals as challenging, coping, pride, responsibility, satisfaction, and success (Lawton Smith 2017; Simon et al. 2005; Woollett et al. 2016).

Resilience belief about social ideals hails social agreement, communality, relatedness or interconnectedness, solidarity, trustworthiness, and validation (Cocking 2017; Prince-Embury et al. 2017; Simon et al. 2005). Relatedness encompasses tolerance, trust, social comfort, and support received (Prince-Embury et al. 2017). In the youth, resilience belief adds such social ideas as social or cultural practicing, justice in the world, progress, and responsiveness to the world (Manglos-Weber and Avelis 2019; Shibue and Kasai 2014; Wu et al. 2011). For the elder, resilience belief additionally favors such ideals as luck and relatedness with significant others (Dubovska et al. 2017; Fry and Debats 2010). To the patient or service user, resilience belief additionally embraces such social ideals or obsessions as fatalism, fitness to environment, and trust (Dageid and Gronlie 2015; Jaffee et al. 2007; Woollett et al. 2016).

Resilience belief about power, capability, competence, or its dispositional sources for resilience covers access, adaptability, assets, attractiveness, capital, controllability, courage, drives, faithfulness, flexibility, hardiness, influence, openness, optimism, patience, perseverance, resources, resourcefulness, robustness, self-efficacy, self-esteem, skills, social status, spirituality, strengths, tenacity, and yearning (Connor et al. 2003; Corbin and Hall 2019; Hjemdal et al. 2015; Jayawardana et al. 2019; Jones and d'Errico 2019; Kent and Davis 2010; Mak et al. 2019; Nemeth and Olivier 2017; Pangallo et al. 2015; Richardson 2017; Van Vliet 2008; Yu and Zhang 2007). Access applies to education, healthcare, housing, and potential realization (Nemeth and Olivier 2017). Capital comprises financial, human, and social capital, which includes political capital (i.e., politically relevant social capital) (Castro and Murray 2010; Jones and d'Errico 2019). Human capital encompasses confidence, expressiveness, goal directionality, insight, optimism, productivity, responsibility, self-regulation capacity, and warmth (Castro and Murray 2010). Courage stands on senses of battling, dignity, endurance, leadership, heroism, persistence, pride, protecting, resistance, saving, stoicism, and voluntarism (Cheng and Huang 2017; Gruber 2011; McGurk and Castro 2010; Osswald et al. 2010; Roller and Zimbardo 2017; Wein 2007), Drives are characterological or intellectual (Richardson 2017). Characterological drives comprise honesty, honor, integrity, kindness, loyalty, morality, self-efficacy, self-esteem, and trustworthiness, whereas intellectual drives operate in planning and understanding (Richardson 2017). Other drives include creativity, energy, faithfulness, genuineness, humor, openness, playfulness, and spontaneity (Richardson 2017). They underlie connecting, eating, living, moving, risking, and surviving (Richardson 2017). Hardiness or toughness comprises challenging commitment, confidence, and control (Perry et al. 2013). Resources stem from adaptability, agency, education, exercising, family coherence, hardiness, optimism, relatedness, self-efficacy, and volunteerism (Hjemdal et al. 2015; Kent and Davis 2010; Pangallo et al. 2015; Zautra et al. 2010). Resourcefulness transpires in comprehensibility, controllability, courage, and intentionality (Celinski and Allen 2017). Strengths embrace collaboration, courage, honesty, leadership, optimism, persistence, and self-regulation (Cornum et al. 2011).

Beliefs sustaining resilience have appeared to embrace such power or its dispositional sources as agreeableness, conscientiousness, emotional intelligence, emotional stability, extraversion, openness, purposiveness, and self-esteem (Armstrong et al. 2011; Buikstra et al. 2010; Yu and Zhang 2007). Agreeableness musters power for resilience through communality, intimacy, solidarity, and unity (Graziano and Tobin 2009). Conscientiousness exhibits power in cautiousness, control, decisiveness, orderliness or organization, planning, and reliability or dependability (Bogg 2008; Roberts et al. 2009). Emotional intelligence comprises awareness of self and others, expression, self-control, managing of self and others, and reasoning about emotion (Armstrong et al. 2011). Such intelligence demonstrates power in attention, clarifying, empathy, recognizing, regulating, and repairing emotions (Ghorbani et al. 2002; Zeidner et al. 2009). Extraversion manifests power in achieving activeness, ambitiousness, boldness, assertiveness, enthusiasm, expressiveness, and liveliness (Foschi and Lauriola 2014; Witt and Revelle 2009). Openness registers power in excitement and flexibility (Curtin et al. 2010).

Resilience belief also features spiritual, religious, and ideological beliefs such as communitarianism, fatalism, individualism, and stoicism. They mark the viability of resilience.

Spiritual belief specifies the utility of resilience as communion with god, existence, growth, health, and meaningfulness (Gorsuch and Miller 1999; Harris et al. 2018; Kelly 2012; Schmidt and Little 2007; Shek 2010) In the youth, spiritual belief additionally indicates the utility of resilience for purposiveness (Shek and Zhu 2018).

Spiritual belief champions such ideals congenial to resilience as asceticism, calmness, compassion and self-compassion, faith, forbearance, forgiveness, hope, openness, optimism, overcoming, serenity, and transcendence (Connors et al. 1999; Gorsuch and Miller 1999; Kelly 2012; Patch 2012; Richards 2012; Sanderson and Linehan 1999; Schmidt and Little 2007; Shek 2010; Yahne and Miller 1999). Asceticism involves fasting, self-control, and self-cultivation. Conversely, spiritual belief holds ideals to denounce self-criticism (Choi 2012). In the youth, spiritual belief additionally endorses the ideal of equanimity (Gehrke 2008). To the elder, spiritual belief additionally installs such ideals as commitment, endurance, peacefulness, relaxation, resistance, self-redefinition, and tranquility (Johnson 2009; Nelson-Becker et al. 2006; Wang et al. 2008). For the patient or service user, spiritual belief additionally establishes such ideals or obsessions as fatalism and harmony (Chan et al. 2000; Unantenne et al. 2013). Fatalism treasures acceptance and self-management (Unantenne et al. 2013).

Religious belief posits the utility of resilience as character development, dignity, and meaningfulness (Harris et al. 2018; Horell 2014; Medvedovski and Allison 2017). To the patient or service user, religious belief regards the utility of resilience as adjustment (Ano and Vasconelles 2005).

Religious belief maintains ideals compatible with resilience, such as agency, autonomy, discipline, forgiveness, maturity, and stability (Dy-Liacco et al. 2009; Muluk et al. 2013; Myers 2014; O'Brien 2015; Turner 2009). To the youth, religious belief additionally emphasizes such ideals as faith and positivity (Exline et al. 2012; Kozlowski et al. 2014).

Communitarian belief foregrounds the utility of resilience for cleanliness (i.e., acceptable to people) and the commonweal (Frazer 1999). Meanwhile, such belief embraces ideals compatible with resilience, such as dutifulness, obligation or responsibility, and self-discipline (Delanty 2009; Frazer 1999; Moore 2010).

Individualist belief regards the utility of resilience as achievement or success, character development, meaningfulness, self-construction, self-development, self-worth, and uniqueness (Fevre 2006; Norris and Inglehart 2009; Oyserman et al. 2002; Speed et al. 2018; Sun and Wang 2010). Meanwhile, individualist belief emphasizes ideals compatible with resilience, such as responsibility and working (Braun 2011; Davis and Robinson 1999).

Stoicism honors the utility of resilience for dignity, harmony, satisfaction or contentment, and self-preservation (Holowchak 2008; Mitsis 2003). Meanwhile, stoicism champions such ideals congenial to resilience as acceptance, controlling and self-control, endurance, equanimity or calmness, fearlessness, hardship, indifference, invincibility, magnanimity, obligation or dutifulness, resolve, self-direction, self-sufficiency, self-love, silence, and steadfastness (Holowchak 2008; Martin 2016).

### Resilience Action Constituted by Resilience Belief

Resilience belief primarily identifies the utility of resilience action and ideals consistent with the action to constitute resilience action. The constitution by utility belief capitalizes on utility optimization to achieve adaptation from the analytical functionalist perspective. Meanwhile, the constitution by ideal belief hinges on idea consistency to sustain latency from the perspective. The constitution of resilience action by resilience belief operates like the constitution of resilience feeling. Additionally, coping as resilience action constituted by resilience belief is noteworthy.

Coping has built on belief about coping or resilience utility, such as curing, effectiveness, and incrementality or improvability (McClaran et al. 2022; Sutherland and Rehman 2018). In the youth, belief about coping utility has concerned malleability (Kneeland and Dovidio 2019). Conversely, coping has subsided with belief about barriers (Byars-Winston and Fouad 2008). To the patient or service user, coping has sprung from belief about medication and problem controllability (De Smedt et al. 2012).

Coping has hinged on belief about power enhanced by religious faith or social support or motivated by the need to tackle stress or trauma (Pargament et al. 2011). In the youth, coping has risen from belief about challenge, competence, urgency, victimization, and family adaptability to generate power for coping (Dai et al. 2015; Kochenderfer-Ladd 2004; Ma et al. 2022; Prelow et al. 2006). For the elder, coping has ensued from belief about death, religious faith, and spirituality to generate power for coping (Cobb 2001; Lowis et al. 2007). To the patient or service user, coping has depended on belief about divine control, relatedness, patient status, and problem chronicity and severity to breed the need or power for coping (De Smedt et al. 2012; Johnson et al. 2013; Umezawa et al. 2012). In the minority person, coping has evolved from belief about prejudice to install the need or power for coping (Frey and Roysircar 2006).

### Resilience Constituted by Its Exposure

Exposure to others' resilience or demand for it constitutes the social norm to assimilate resilience through norm conformity in the voluntaristic theory of analytical functionalism. Such conformity meets the requisite function of social integration. The assimilation or integration hinges on social influence, such as communication and modeling, regarding resilience or normalcy (Buzzanell 2010; Shaver and Mikulincer 2012). In the youth, others' adaptation, skills, and success additionally influence resilience (Thompson 2006; Ungar 2018; Wessells 2018). The influence heightens with social accommodating, agreement, anchoring, attachment, attention, civility, commonality, connectedness or relatedness, identification, information processing, interaction, fitting, followership, networking, sharing, solidarity, trust, and validation (Afifi et al. 2016; Batone 2017; Buzzanell 2010; Cocking 2017; Jayawardana et al.

2019; Matusitz 2017; Park 2017; Schwager and Rothermund 2014; Ungar 2012). To the youth, social conformity, demand, impact, and learning about resilience are additionally crucial (Masten 2014; Thompson 2006; Ungar 2018; Wessells 2018). In the minority person, social proximity is additionally relevant (Juang et al. 2018). This heightening demonstrates power realization in voluntaristic theory to gather power to activate social influence.

Resilience has risen from exposure to others' innovation (Buikstra et al. 2010). Herein, innovation reflects acceptance, adaptation, coping, flexibility, health, and persistence germane to resilience (Charyton et al. 2009; Gu et al. 2016; Kreitler and Casakin 2009; Montgomery et al. 2004; Whitton 2018). In the youth, exposure to others' resilience and related abidance, competence, flexibility, organization, norm, and stability have induced resilience (Boulton and Macaulay 2022; Masten et al. 2009; Ungar et al. 2005). Others' demand for adaptation can raise the youth's resilience (Ungar 2018; Wessells 2018).

## Original Findings

Original findings on the resilience process evolved from analyzing 2211 Chinese persons in Hong Kong. These persons participated in the study through the support of some social service units for youth, mid-age people, and older adults. Hence, the persons were service users. These persons had an average of 46.8 years in age, 7.6 years in education, and 3.1 persons in the family (see Table 2.1). Among them, 69.5% were female, 35.0% were youth aged below 25 years, 28.1% were mid-age aged from 25 to 59 years, 36.9% were older aged 60 years or above, 29.0% lived with spouses, 31.5% lived with children, 26.3% lived with siblings, 39.0% lived with friends, 39.5% completed the survey by self-administration, and 31.9% completed the survey by interviewing. The average response credibility rated by interviewers was 84.7 on a 0–100 scale (Table 2.1)

The survey measured adjustment in the recent week ($M = 69.1$ on a 0–100 scale, see Table 2.1; Costa-Requena 2009), resilience (feeling) in the recent week ($M =$ 51.0, Shek et al. 2007), resilience action in the past month (M = 62.7, Shek et al. 2007) with multiple items, resilience belief ($M = 67.2$, Shek et al. 2007), resilience demand received or exposure to resilience in the past six months ($M = 48.0$, Shek et al. 2007), sincerity experience in the past six months ($M = 62.2$, Noronha 2002), aid received in the past six months ($M = 61.3$, Hendrick and Hendrick 1989), adversity in the past year ($M = 23.9$, Pan et al. 2008), and functional disability in the past year ($M = 12.7$, Bass et al. 1999). These items, including negatively keyed ones, loaded substantially on their respective factors to sustain factorial validity, comprising convergent and discriminant, in confirmatory factor analysis (see Table 2.3). The validity was warrantable with the good fit of the analysis ($L^2$ (695) = 5695, $SRMR =$ 0.042, $RMSEA = 0.061$, $CFI = 0.914$), given the 40 items input to the analysis. Hence, resilience, adjustment, sincerity, aid, adversity, and disability were distinguishable.

**Table 2.1** Means and standard deviations (service dataset) ($N = 2211$)

| Variable | Scoring | *M* | *SD* |
|---|---|---|---|
| Adjustment, recent week | 0–100 | 69.1 | 14.6 |
| Resilience, recent week | 0–100 | 51.0 | 19.1 |
| Resilience action, past month | 0–100 | 62.7 | 15.3 |
| Resilience belief, past 3 months | 0–100 | 67.2 | 16.4 |
| Resilience demand reception, past 6 months | 0–100 | 48.0 | 21.0 |
| Sincerity experience, past 6 month | 0–100 | 62.2 | 19.7 |
| Aid reception, past 6 months | 0–100 | 61.3 | 20.5 |
| Adversity, past year | 0–100 | 23.9 | 18.6 |
| Functional disability, past year | 0–100 | 12.7 | 20.1 |
| Age | Years | 46.8 | 25.0 |
| Youth | 0, 100 | 35.0 | 47.7 |
| Mid-age | 0, 100 | 28.1 | 45.0 |
| Older | 0, 100 | 36.9 | 48.3 |
| Education | Years | 7.6 | 4.8 |
| Female | 0, 100 | 69.5 | 46.1 |
| Earnings (US$1 = HK$7.8) | ln(HK$) | 1.9 | 3.6 |
| Family size | Persons | 3.1 | 2.3 |
| Family income per capita | ln(HK$) | 8.1 | 1.8 |
| Housing: public (rental) | 0, 100 | 49.7 | 50.0 |
| SOS (purchased public housing) | 0, 100 | 15.5 | 36.2 |
| Private flat | 0, 100 | 31.5 | 46.5 |
| Aged home | 0, 100 | 0.2 | 4.3 |
| Hostel | 0, 100 | 1.3 | 11.5 |
| Divided apartment | 0, 100 | 1.5 | 12.1 |
| Coresident: spouse | 0, 100 | 29.0 | 45.4 |
| Child | 0, 100 | 31.5 | 46.5 |
| Sibling | 0, 100 | 26.3 | 44.0 |
| Parent | 0, 100 | 39.0 | 48.8 |
| Friend | 0, 100 | 10.4 | 30.6 |
| Survey administration: fellow | 0, 100 | 0.3 | 5.6 |
| Service worker | 0, 100 | 0.8 | 9.0 |
| Self | 0, 100 | 39.5 | 48.9 |
| Interviewer | 0, 100 | 31.9 | 46.6 |
| Credibility | 0, 100 | 84.7 | 15.7 |
| Reply date | Date | 2014.0 | 0.3 |

**Table 2.2** Means by age (service dataset)

| Variable | Young | Mid | Old | All |
|---|---|---|---|---|
| Adjustment, recent week | 67.0 | 65.4 | 74.1 | 69.2 |
| Resilience, recent week | 51.0 | 50.0 | 52.0 | 51.1 |
| Resilience action, past month | 58.0 | 58.7 | 70.3 | 62.8 |
| Resilience belief, past 3 months | 61.9 | 62.7 | 76.2 | 67.4 |
| Resilience demand reception, past 6 months | 53.3 | 49.0 | 42.0 | 47.9 |
| Sincerity experience, past 6 month | 59.1 | 58.7 | 68.5 | 62.4 |
| Aid reception, past 6 months | 59.6 | 55.8 | 67.6 | 61.5 |
| Adversity, past year | 22.2 | 30.0 | 20.5 | 23.8 |
| Functional disability, past year | 5.9 | 15.7 | 17.3 | 12.9 |
| Age | 19.0 | 44.3 | 75.0 | 46.8 |
| Youth | 100.0 | 0.0 | 0.0 | 35.0 |
| Mid-age | 0.0 | 100.0 | 0.0 | 28.1 |
| Older | 0.0 | 0.0 | 100.0 | 36.9 |
| Education | 11.0 | 8.6 | 4.3 | 7.6 |
| Female | 52.3 | 68.8 | 85.5 | 69.2 |
| Earnings (logged, US$1 = HK$7.8) | 3.0 | 2.6 | 0.2 | 1.9 |
| Family size | 3.8 | 3.4 | 2.3 | 3.1 |
| Family income per capita | 8.5 | 8.0 | 7.8 | 8.1 |
| Housing: public (rental) | 48.6 | 56.3 | 45.4 | 49.6 |
| SOS (purchased public housing) | 16.6 | 15.6 | 13.9 | 15.3 |
| Private flat | 31.9 | 21.1 | 40.1 | 31.9 |
| Aged home | 0.1 | 0.5 | 0.0 | 0.2 |
| Hostel | 1.4 | 2.7 | 0.0 | 1.2 |
| Divided apartment | 1.3 | 3.1 | 0.6 | 1.5 |
| Coresident: spouse | 2.2 | 48.9 | 38.9 | 28.9 |
| Child | 1.6 | 53.8 | 41.7 | 31.1 |
| Sibling | 62.6 | 13.4 | 1.8 | 26.3 |
| Parent | 93.7 | 21.6 | 0.6 | 39.1 |
| Friend | 3.8 | 11.6 | 16.5 | 10.6 |
| Survey administration: fellow | 0.8 | 0.2 | 0.0 | 0.3 |
| Service worker | 1.2 | 1.0 | 0.1 | 0.8 |
| Self | 54.6 | 55.6 | 12.5 | 39.4 |
| Interviewer | 1.1 | 3.0 | 85.7 | 32.9 |
| Credibility | 92.3 | 86.8 | 83.9 | 84.8 |
| Reply date | 2013.8 | 2014.0 | 2014.0 | 2014.0 |

**Table 2.3** Standardized factor loadings from the 7-factor model

| Variable | Trait |
|---|---|
| Adjustment, recent week ($\alpha = 0.821$) | 0.670 |
| Being happy | 0.679 |
| Turning good | 0.491 |
| (Not) Losing control | 0.298 |
| (Not) Losing hope for life | 0.424 |
| (Not) Worrying | 0.506 |
| (Not) Having some loss | 0.446 |
| (Not) Giving up some ideas | 0.457 |
| Resilience, recent week ($\alpha = 0.788$) | 0.777 |
| Being able to face even difficult circumstances | 0.598 |
| Feeling calm under pressure | 0.449 |
| Liking yourself when making a mistake | 0.344 |
| Recovering soon even if frustrated | 0.792 |
| Being able to remain calm when facing tremendous pressure | 0.776 |
| Being able to remain calm even in a terrible environment | 0.629 |
| Resilience action, past month ($\alpha = 0.894$) | 0.811 |
| Releasing yourself | 0.706 |
| Daring to try | 0.363 |
| Thinking of something funny | 0.675 |
| Dong the best | 0.571 |
| Trying to do a good job | 0.616 |
| Putting things down | 0.649 |
| Accepting adversity | 0.522 |
| Forgiving others | 0.591 |
| (Not) Caring small matters | 0.412 |
| (Not) Being persistent | 0.325 |
| Resilience belief, past 3 months ($\alpha = 0.918$) | 0.801 |
| Having ups and downs in life | 0.584 |
| Being fine to have a clear conscience | 0.673 |
| Friends' being good to you | 0.776 |
| Living, learning, and working | 0.741 |
| Needing to break through the frame of questions | 0.384 |
| Things getting better | 0.442 |
| Suffering necessarily existing in the world | 0.387 |
| Wanting someone to remind you | 0.387 |
| Resilience demand reception, past 6 months ($\alpha = 0.807$) | 0.779 |
| Others wanting you to hold on | 0.549 |

(continued)

**Table 2.3** (continued)

| Variable | Trait |
|---|---|
| Others wanting you to accept adversity | 0.727 |
| Others wanting you to do your best | 0.794 |
| Aid reception, past 6 months ($\alpha = 0.796$) | 0.923 |
| Someone giving you good advice | 0.600 |
| Someone having a good time with you together | 0.705 |
| Someone loving you | 0.796 |
| Someone understanding difficulties that you face | 0.618 |
| Sincerity experience, past 6 month ($\alpha = 0.622$) | 0.563 |
| Speakers being for your own good | 0.618 |
| Speakers speaking from the heart | 0.741 |

$L^2$ (695) = 5695, $SRMR = 0.042$, $RMSEA = 0.061$, $CFI = 0.914$

The resilience process was demonstrable by significant positive correlations among resilience (feeling), resilience action, resilience belief, and resilience exposure or demand received (partial $r$ = 0.055–0.525, see Table 2.4, controlling the method artifact of acquiescence). Nevertheless, the correlations between resilience exposure or demand and resilience feeling, action, and belief were slight (partial $r$ = 0.055–0.084). Meanwhile, the resilience process significantly positively correlated with adjustment, aid received, and sincerity experienced and significantly negatively correlated with adversity.

An alternative, inferred measure of resilience was the product of adjustment and adversity, that is, adjustment despite adversity (Hariharan and Rana 2017; Son Hag 2013). Such resilience was significantly positively correlated with resilience feeling, action, belief, and exposure (partial $r$ = 0.123–0.477, see Table 2.5, controlling for acquiescence and adversity). Moreover, inferred resilience significantly positively correlated with adjustment, aid received, and sincerity experienced (partial $r$ = 0.292–0.399).

The resilience process was evident in regression analysis controlling for all background and earlier factors Accordingly resilience feeling in the recent week was significantly positively predictable by resilience action in the past month ($\beta = 0.469$, see Table 2.6). Furthermore, resilience action in the past month was significantly positively predictable by resilience belief in the past three months ($\beta = 0.347$). However, resilience exposure to others' demand in the past six months did not significantly predict resilience feeling, action, or belief. Resilience belief in the past three months, contrary to expectation, displayed a significant negative effect on resilience feeling in the recent week ($\beta = -0.092$), given the control for resilience action and others.

The resilience process thus consists of connections between resilience exposure, belief, action, and feeling to sustain resilience functioning. According to the voluntaristic theory of analytical functionalism, such functioning rests on resilience action for transmitting power for power realization, resilience belief to identify utility and

**Table 2.4** Partial correlations

| Correlate | (1) | (2) | (3) | (4) | (5) | (6) | (7) |
|---|---|---|---|---|---|---|---|
| Adjustment (1) | 1.000 | | | | | | |
| Resilience (2) | 0.399** | 1.000 | | | | | |
| Resilience action (3) | 0.578** | 0.453** | 1.000 | | | | |
| Resilience belief (4) | 0.402** | 0.198** | 0.525** | 1.000 | | | |
| Resilience demand received (5) | 0.126** | 0.055* | 0.084** | 0.060** | 1.000 | | |
| Aid received (6) | 0.485** | 0.247** | 0.494** | 0.415** | 0.280** | 1.000 | |
| Sincerity experienced (7) | 0.370** | 0.203** | 0.407** | 0.411** | 0.257** | 0.612** | 1.000 |
| Adversity | – 0.298** | – 0.216** | – 0.275** | – 0.236** | – 0.048* | – 0.325** | – 0.243** |

*Note* Controlling for acquiescence
*$p < 0.05$, **$p < 0.01$

**Table 2.5** Partial correlations additionally controlling for adversity

| Correlate | (1) | (2) | (3) | (4) | (5) | (6) | (7) |
|---|---|---|---|---|---|---|---|
| Adjustment (1) | 1.000 | | | | | | |
| Resilience (2) | 0.359** | 1.000 | | | | | |
| Resilience action (3) | 0.541** | 0.419** | 1.000 | | | | |
| Resilience belief (4) | 0.358** | 0.155** | 0.493** | 1.000 | | | |
| Resilience demand received (5) | 0.117** | 0.046* | 0.074** | 0.051* | 1.000 | | |
| Aid received (6) | 0.429** | 0.191** | 0.445** | 0.369** | 0.280** | 1.000 | |
| Sincerity experienced (7) | 0.321** | 0.159** | 0.364** | 0.375** | 0.254** | 0.581** | 1.000 |
| Resilience as adjustment × adversity | 0.916** | 0.309** | 0.477** | 0.305** | 0.123** | 0.399** | 0.292** |

*Note* Controlling for adversity and acquiescence
*$p < 0.05$, **$p < 0.01$

ideals for utility optimization and ideal consistency, and resilience exposure to social norms for norm conformity. Resilience or its feeling represents the core of resilience, and covers adaptation, adjustment, bouncing back, buffering, functioning, growth, maturity, recovery, restoration, and sustainability under adversity (Bowers et al. 2017; Celinski and Allen 2017; Corbin and Hall 2019; Maltby et al. 2019; Nemeth and Olivier 2017; Xie and Wong 2021; Zautra et al. 2010). Presently, resilience feeling

**Table 2.6** Standardized effects about the resilience process

| Predictor | Resilience | Resilience action | Resilience belief |
|---|---|---|---|
| Resilience action | 0.469*** | | |
| Resilience belief | − 0.092* | 0.347*** | |
| Resilience demand received | 0.012 | − 0.048 | − 0.043 |

*Note* Controlling for background and earlier factors
*$p < 0.05$, ***$p < 0.001$

involved calmness, recovering, and self-liking under adversity. Resilience action operates as accepting, acquiring resources, adapting, adjusting, altering, appraising, attaching, choosing, collaborating, coping, controlling, enduring, engaging, facing, learning, maintaining, mobilizing resources, moderating, planning, perspective-taking, preventing, protecting, realizing potential, reflecting, refocusing, reframing, reorienting, striving, sustaining, training, understanding regarding resilience, self-actualizing, and self-regulating (Brodsky and Cattaneo 2013; Celinski and Allen 2017; Cocking 2017; Connor et al. 2003; Corbin and Hall 2019; Cornum et al. 2011; Friedman and Robbins 2012; Hjemdal et al. 2015; Jones and Jetten 2011; Kent and Davis 2010; Mak et al. 2019; Maltby et al. 2019; Mukherjee and Kumar 2017; Nemeth and Olivier 2017; Pangallo et al. 2015; Schwager and Rothermund 2014; Solomon and Roloff 2018; Ungar 2010; Van Vliet 2008; Xie and Wong 2021; Zautra 2014). Presently, resilience action included relaxing, trying, thinking of something funny, doing the best, putting things down, accepting adversity, and forgiving. Such action generates and transmits resilience power, assets, capacity, capital, competence, drives, insight, motivation, resources, skill, or strength covering adaptability, agency, creativity, directedness, empathy, flexibility, hardiness, humor, intelligence, intentionality, learnability, mastery, openness, optimism, patience, perseverance, productivity, reliability, resourcefulness, robustness, self-compassion, self-efficacy, self-regulation, spirituality, tenacity, tolerance, and transformability (Castro and Murray 2010; Celinski and Allen 2017; Connor et al. 2003; Jayawardana et al. 2019; Jones and d'Errico 2019; Kent and Davis 2010; Mak et al. 2019; Metzl and Morrell 2008; Nemeth and Olivier 2017; Pangallo et al. 2015; Richardson 2017; Van Vliet 2008; Yu and Zhang 2007; Zautra 2014; Zautra et al. 2010). Presently, such power arose from social support. Resilience belief highlights such utility of resilience as achievement, attractiveness, fearlessness, health, meaningfulness, transcendence, and well-being generally (Kent and Davis 2010; Leigert and Reutter 2005; Nemeth and Olivier 2017; Van Haaften et al. 2004; Van Vliet 2008; Xie and Wong 2021). Conversely, utility also means that resilience is feasible, not costly or formidable (Vanderplaat 2016). Presently, such utility arose from belief about the acceptability of adversity and others and the changeability or improvability of events. Furthermore, resilience belief aligns resilience with such ideals as adaptation, agency, autonomy, choice, competitiveness, confidence, courage, empowerment, entrepreneurship, freedom, individuality, proactiveness, rationality, responsibility, self-reliance, and virtuousness (Brodsky and Cattaneo 2013; Dunn 2013; Evans and Sewell 2013; Friedman and Robbins 2012; Garrett 2016; Hall and Lamont 2013; Leigert and Reutter 2005; Richardson 2017; Son Hag 2013; Schwarz 2018; Tierney 2015). Presently, such ideals include breaking through, conscience, seeking advice, and the trio of learning, living, and working. Resilience exposure to others' demand reflects collective, communal, cultural, ecological, or social appropriateness, cohesiveness, collaboration, construction, integration, interaction, and legitimacy regarding resilience (Berger 2015; Bowers et al. 2017; Celinski and Allen 2017; Cocking 2017; Hoffman 2003; Nemeth and Olivier 2017; Pangallo et al. 2015; Schwarz 2018). Overall, the resilience process functions with resilience feeling, action, belief, and exposure to mingle power realization, utility optimization, idea consistency, and norm conformity.

Resilience was correlated with adjustment, reflecting that resilience is conditional adjustment under adversity. Alternatively, adjustment under adversity infers resilience (Cole et al. 2022; Hariharan and Rana 2017; Son Hag 2013). Adjustment means congruence and fitness with the environment, characterized by compatibility, self-esteem, and vitality as opposed to depression and distress (Deci et al. 2006; Ramadier 2017). From the functionalist perspective, adjustment centers on fulfilling needs and performance (Ramadier 2017).

On the one hand, adjustment has built on resilience (Khodabakhsh and Ooi 2022). From the voluntaristic theory of analytical functionalism, such building relies on power realization, utility optimization, ideal consistency, and norm conformity generated by resilience. Power generated by resilience for realizing adjustment derives from approaching, coping, homeostasis, resolution or problem solving, security, self-regulation, and stability (Baylis 2005; Gall et al. 2005; DeNeve and Cooper 1998; Matthews 1997; Meyer and Frost 2013; Mikulincer and Shaver 2014; Sheldon and Kasser 2001; Sirgy 2012; Sovereign and Walker 2021; Zhan et al. 2022). In the youth, resilience power additionally stems from commitment, defense, vitality, and skills specifically for problem-solving and resilience as opposed to disruption and withdrawal (Gfellner and Cordoba 2017; Guroglu et al. 2007; Kern et al. 2015; Lee and Lee 2020; Meeus et al. 2005; Migerode et al. 2012; Moneta et al. 2001). As such, adjustment is realizable with power. Utility for optimizing adjustment emanates from such resilience qualities as confidence, optimism, religiosity, and spirituality as opposed to pessimism (Bailey et al. 2007; Diener et al. 2009; Kimhi et al. 2021; Reeskens and Vandecasteele 2017). In the youth, resilience bases for adjustment utility additionally include free will, malleability, and struggling (Eryilmaz 2013; Li et al. 2017; Smith et al. 2018). For the patient or service, utility that has attracted adjustment has stemmed from resilience expectancy for work (Vansteenkiste et al. 2005). To the working person, such resilience utility as work benefit and the balance between effort and reward can sustain adjustment (Huffman et al. 2015; Huynh et al. 2012). Accordingly, adjustment is gainful and worthy. Ideals championed by resilience for maintaining consistency with adjustment evolve from courage, flexibility, forgiveness, grit, hardiness, militancy, persistence, recovery, and self-determination as opposed to vegetativeness (Chirkov et al. 2003; DeNeve and Cooper 1998; Diener and Lucas 1999; Diener et al. 2009; Goodman et al. 2017; Kuiper and Borowicz-Sibenik 2005; Schulz 1995; Sovereign and Walker 2021; Watkins 2016).

In the youth, resilience ideals conducive to adjustment additional include authenticity, leadership, open-mindedness, responsibility, and zest (Fan et al. 2021; Shimai et al. 2006). For the elder, an additional resilience ideal for adjustment has been continuity (Atchley 1999b). To the working person, such a resilience ideal as conservation can be conducive to adjustment (Preston 2018). Accordingly, adjustment is ideal, as congenial to other ideals. Social norms propagated by resilience for conforming to sustain adjustment congeal from others' optimism (Aspinwall and Taylor 1992).

On the other hand, adjustment has buttressed resilience or its process including action, belief, and exposure related to coping (Buikstra et al. 2010; Johnson et al. 2013; Yu and Zhang 2007). According to the voluntaristic theory of analytical functionalism, such buttressing hinges on adjustment power realized for driving resilience, adjustment utility optimized for attracting resilience, adjustment ideals aligned for rationalizing resilience, and adjustment norms conformed for assimilating resilience. Such adjustment power stems from controlling, humor, meditation, prayer, relaxation, restructuring cognitively, self-regulation including emotion regulation (Boden et al. 2014; Cherry et al. 2018; Dwivedi 2017; Gallo et al. 2004; Sherman and Cohen 2006; Van Vliet 2008). Adjustment power conducive to resilience also emanated from such dispositions or goals as agreeableness, openness, and stability (Lock et al. 2020; Yu and Zhang 2007). Emotion regulation comprises cognitive change, attention development, modifying situations, modulating responses, and selecting situations (Boden et al. 2014). In the youth, power derived from adjustment additionally rests on adaptiveness or adaptation skill, defense, easy temperament, emotional intelligence, industriousness, managing emotions, persevering, problem-solving ability or skill, reappraisal positively, reflection, reflexivity, responsiveness, safety, security, self-protecting, self-organization, spirituality, and ventilating or expressing emotions (Annalakshmi and Abeer 2011; Artuch-Garde et al. 2017; Kaplan 2012; Lipsitt and Demick 2012; Luthar et al. 2000; Manglos-Weber and Avelis 2019; Masten 2014; Masten et al. 2009; Migerode et al. 2012; Prince-Bmbury 2013c, 2014a; Shibue and Kasai 2014; Svetina 2014; Ungar et al. 2005; van Aken 1994). To the elder, power involved in adjustment for facilitating resilience additionally derives from compensation, enjoyment ability, health, optimization, plasticity, reminiscing, resistance, restorying, and selection (Dubovska et al. 2017; Hardy and Gill 2004; Hertzog and Jopp 2010; Langer 2004; Roberto 2009). In the patient or service user, adjustment power boosting resilience additionally includes coping ability, determination, introspection, self-cultivation, and self-empowerment (Stewart and Yuen 2011; Woollett et al. 2016; Zhao and Fu 2022). For the work person, adjustment power activating resilience additionally arises from proactiveness and the need to manage shock (Powley 2009; Vandsburger et al. 2012). Accordingly, power involved in adjustment facilitates resilience. Utility derived from adjustment to optimize resilience derives from hope or optimism and religiosity such as divine blessing and solvability (Buikstra et al. 2010; Crane et al. 2019; Dwivedi 2017; Truebridge 2016). In the youth, adjustment utility sustaining resilience has additionally sprung from belief in a just world, positivity expected, and trust (Masten et al. 2009; Wu et al. 2011; Svetina 2014). To the elder, utility based on adjustment for elevating resilience additionally emanates from luck belief (Dubovska et al. 2017).

Accordingly, utility generated by adjustment induces resilience. Ideals engendered by adjustment for rationalizing resilience uphold accommodation, balance, congruence, fitness, flexibility, flourishing, normalcy, positivity, self-affirmation (Buzzanell 2010; Dwivedi 2017; Hassija and Cloitre 2014; Cantor et al. 2002; Park 2017; Schwager and Rothermund 2014; Sherman and Cohen 2006; Ungar 2012). In the youth, ideals based on adjustment to induce resilience additionally favor courage, integrity, sufficiency, and transcendence (Kim et al. 2018; Ungar et al. 2005). To the elder, ideals based on adjustment to lift resilience additionally highlight acceptance, adequacy, coherence, continuity, engagement, enjoyment, independence, life, reconciliation, responsibility, self-reliance, tolerance, and working (Cheung and Kam 2012; Dubovska et al. 2017; Fry and Debats 2010; Roberto 2009; Visaria et al. 2023). In the patient or service users, adjustment ideals rationalizing resilience additional include fatalism or belief in fate, goal orientation, and pragmatism (Woollett et al. 2016). Accordingly, ideals based on adjustment rationalize resilience. Norms identified by adjustment for assimilating resilience evolve from others' flexibility, hardiness, potential for growth, and resource identification or resourcefulness (Batone 2017; Simon et al. 2005). In the youth, social norms based on adjustment to induce resilience additionally rest on others' abidance, coherence, flexibility, organization, perseverance, resilience, success, and stability (Aitcheson et al. 2017; Boulton and Macaulay 2022; Masten et al. 2009; Ungar et al. 2005). To the elder, social norms derived from adjustment for sustaining resilience additionally include others' strengths (Visaria et al. 2023). For the working person, the adjustment norm encouraging resilience has additionally arisen from others' reflections (McCray et al. 2016). As such, adjustment as a social norm assimilates resilience.

In sum, the resilience process internally builds on the voluntaristic mechanisms of power realization, utility optimization, ideal consistency, and norm conformity. According to the voluntaristic theory of analytical functionalism, power drives, utility attracts, ideals rationalize, and norms assimilate resilience for fulfillment, adaptation, latency, and integration, respectively. Power for resilience can include assets, capacity, capital, resources, and skill (Berger 2015; Brodsky and Cattaneo 2013; Hassija and Cloitre 2014; Jayawardana et al. 2019; Lerner et al. 2012; Ungar 2012; Xie and Wong 2021). These various forms of power can stem from agency, attachment, cognitive functioning, commitment, companionship, empowerment, humor, mindfulness, readiness, realization, opportunity, positivity, safety, security, self-awareness, self-efficacy, spirituality, support received, and wisdom (Bowen et al. 2013; Brodsky and Cattaneo 2013; Dwivedi 2017; Gilligan 2009; Hassija and Cloitre 2014; Kent and Davis 2010; Metzl and Morrell 2008; Matusitz 2017; Mikulincer and Shaver 2014; Park and Slattery 2014; Tugade and Fredrickson 2004). Power can also consolidate due to the goals or needs of challenge, congruence, development, excellence, fitness, flourishing, meaningfulness, narrating or storytelling (Crane et al. 2019; Dwivedi 2017; Hassija and Cloitre 2014; Schoon 2006; Ungar 2012). Utility from resilience can arise from hope or optimism (Dwivedi 2017). Ideals for resilience can embrace absorption, accommodation, flexibility, coping, meaning-making, negotiation, restructuring, self-affirmation, self-reflection, self-regulation, including emotion regulation, and solution focus (Crane et al. 2019; Gallo et al.

2004; Hassija and Cloitre 2014; Kent and Davis 2010; Park 2017; Park and Slattery 2014; Paul et al. 2022; Sherman and Cohen 2006; Ungar 2012). Norms for resilience can spring from others' alternative logic, challenge, flexibility, gratitude, growth, hardiness, normalcy, positivity, and resourcefulness (Buzzanell 2010; Dwivedi 2017; Simon et al. 2005). Normative influence can hinge on commonality, communication, discourse, interaction, participation, relatedness or connectedness, sharing, and social construction (Afifi et al. 2016; Batone 2017; Buzzanell 2010; Cocking 2017; Matusitz 2017; Simon et al. 2005; Ungar 2012).

# Chapter 3
# Personal Background Bases for the Resilience Process

**Abstract** This Chapter displays a fundamental attempt to address feasibility and reasonableness in developing resilience based on the person's background characteristics. Background characteristics include personal, sociodemographic, and socioeconomic characteristics such as a person's age, gender, education, birthplace, and residency. Concerning the analytical-functionalist framework, background characteristics are influential through their functions for the voluntaristic mechanisms of power realization, utility optimization, norm conformity, and ideal consistency. Resilience processes comprise feeling, action, belief, learning, and demand received about resilience. Analysis of poverty survey data on the public revealed that age was the only significant background characteristic eroding resilience. Meanwhile, analysis of violence survey data on the public showed that marriage was the only significant background characteristic buttressing resilience. In this connection, the effect of age was positive but not significant. Analysis of survey data on social service users revealed that age, earnings, and living with parents significantly upheld resilience. Meanwhile, family size significantly diminished resilience. Moreover, age, education, and living with offspring significantly positively affected action for resilience. Living with the spouse, parents, and private housing significantly positively affected learning resilience. Similarly, age, female gender, education, living with siblings, and living with parents positively impacted belief about resilience. By contrast, age significantly negatively affected the demand received for resilience. Nevertheless, analysis of survey data on elders showed that no background characteristic had a significant effect on resilience. In addition, analysis of survey data on people with visual impairment indicated that family income per capita, social welfare, and having a birthplace in Hong Kong significantly positively affected resilience. By contrast, visual impairment severity, visual impairment duration, education, being an employee, being self employed, being unemployed, and living in rental public housing significantly negatively affected resilience. Hence, the person's age, education, marriage, earnings, living with parents, family income, and even reception of social welfare tend to prop resilience. As these characteristics represent human, financial, and social resources, their contributions to resilience embody the power realization mechanism. The contributions testify to the feasibility and reasonableness because the characteristics are more inherent and accessible to the person. That is,

 
C. K. Cheung, *Resilience Process and Its Personal and Social Bases*,
https://doi.org/10.1007/978-981-97-7391-6_3

no external force appears to inhibit or displace the contributions. Hence, resilience evolves from the voluntaristic use of personal background characteristics, which, for instance, provides power or resources to sustain the process of resilience. That is, static power is necessary for the dynamics of action.

Personal backgrounds are likely the basis for the resilience process. Herein, personal characteristics include the person's age, gender, birthplace, education, residency, marital status, living arrangement, family size, housing, employment, income, welfare reception, religious faith, and impairment. The resilience process includes resilience or feeling, resilience action (including learning), resilience belief, and resilience exposure to others' demand for resilience. This process builds on personal characteristics according to the voluntaristic mechanisms of power realization, utility optimization, norm conformity, and ideal consistency in analytical functionalism. Power realization employs power provided by personal characteristics to drive the resilience process. Power encompasses capacity, capability, competence, and energy and evolves from knowledge, skills, resources, goals, needs, motivation, and action. Utility optimization gravitates to the resilience process based on resilience utility expected from personal characteristics. Utility means experiences, beliefs, or perceptions regarding benefit, feasibility, gain, reward, and success as opposed to cost, difficulty, and loss. Conversely, disutility discouraging resilience involves frustration, loss, and punishment from resilience or related action. Ideal consistency rationalizes the resilience process by ideals consonant with resilience stemming from personal characteristics. Ideals include evaluations, satisfaction, values, and beliefs about something good, proactive, or self-enhancing. Conversely, scruples or lacking ideals for achievement, adaptation, flexibility, independence, or security resist resilience. Likewise, ideals for destruction or suicide contradict and impede resilience. Norm conformity assimilates the resilience process through social norms sustained by personal characteristics. Norms refer to those widespread, prevalent, or shared in the group, social network, community, society, and social environment in general, covering goals and ideals.

To drive resilience, power has evolved from (dispositions in) agreeableness, conscientiousness, emotional intelligence and stability, extraversion, friendship, goal-setting, groupness, learning, mentorship, openness, purposiveness, religiosity or belief in divine support, self-esteem, sensation seeking, supportive services, and social support (Armstrong et al. 2011; Buikstra et al. 2010; Cherry et al. 2023; Corbin and Hall 2019; Lock et al. 2020; Lou et al. 2018; Notter et al. 2008; Wong and Chui 2017; Yu and Zhang 2007). Conversely, power has drained by neuroticism, and trauma (Cherry et al. 2023; Yu and Zhang 2007). The sinews of power rest on such conditions as association, attachment to God, coercion, dominance, education, employment, engagement, enrollment, family, income, kinship, membership, religious faith, reputation, solidifying, status, and violence (Cialdini 2016; Emerson 1986; Engelstad 2009; Hofstetter et al. 1999; Isham et al. 2006; Keltener et al. 2008; Matthewman 2011; Ross and Mirowsky 2009; ten Brinke and Keltner 2020;

Thye et al. 2006). Power also evolves from desires, goals, needs, or motivation for argumentation, change, control, dominance, explicitness, face, fame, gain, giving, identity, incentive, management, obligation, relating, resources, rights, self-interest, and sharing (Cialdini 2016; Dillard 2004; ten Brinke and Keltner 2020). Additionally, power derives from dispositions or qualities such as attractiveness or beauty, conservatism, courage, fluency, happiness, knowledge, responsibility, selectivity, and self-control (Keltener et al. 2008; Engelstad 2009; Gass and Seiter 2004; Hofstetter et al. 1999; Jimenez-Anca 2013; Matthewman 2011; ten Brinke and Keltner 2020). Power also develops through action or effort, such as attention, cooperation, performance, protesting, resolving, technology use, and volunteering (Cialdini 2016; Isham et al. 2006; Liang and Lee 2022; Matthewman 2011; Ten Brinke and Keltner 2020; Thye et al. 2006). In rationalizing or maintaining consistency with resilience, ideals have transpired in (beliefs in) balance, coping, and the values of affiliation or connectedness (Buikstra et al. 2010; Cantor et al. 2002; Chua et al. 2019). In attracting resilience, utility from resilience has arisen from beliefs in growth and the just world and optimism (Buikstra et al. 2010; Wu et al. 2011; Zeng et al. 2016). For assimilating resilience, social norms have hailed abidance, flexibility, innovation, resilience, resourcefulness, stability, and success (Boulton and Macaulay 2022; Buikstra et al. 2010; Masten et al. 2009; Ungar et al. 2005). Such power, utility, ideals, and norms derive from personal background characteristics.

## Existing Knowledge

Existing knowledge based on research findings and theorizing explains the impacts of personal background characteristics on resilience. These characteristics include the person's age, gender, birthplace, education, residency, marital status, living arrangement, family size, housing, employment, income, welfare reception, religious faith, and impairment. Meanwhile, resilience manifests a process constituted by resilience exposure, belief, action, and feeling.

### *Age*

Resilience has increased with age (Cherry et al. 2023). This increase also happened in the youth and patient or service user (Aldwin et al. 2009; Cole et al. 2022). Bases for the increase are likely to involve power, utility, norms, and ideals regarding resilience growing with aging.

Power increasing with age for realizing to drive resilience includes companionship, controlling or mastery, cultural and human capital and its investment, intelligence, learning, marriage, optimization, reasoning, relational closeness, selection or concentration, self-determination, self-regulation including emotion regulation and its ability, social contribution, and strength integration (Charles and Carstensen 2009;

Consedine 2011; Fulle-Iglesias et al. 2009; Holstein and Gubrium 2000; Kuntla et al. 2013; Morgan and Robinson 2013; Pena 2020; Penningroth and Scott 2012; Ramsey and Gentzler 2015; Von Krogh and Wallin 2011). Marriage signifies power from spousal beneficial support (Solomon 2006). Relational closeness accesses or earns power based on help, identity, and social support (Georgas et al. 1997; Levitt et al. 1994; Sharabany 1994). Self-determination reflects power or resources (Stavrova and Ehlebracht 2018). Self-regulation registers robust functioning (Inzlicht and Schmeichel 2016). According to functionalist theory, social contribution sustains society and thus draws power from societal support (Holstein and Gubrium 2000). Moreover, such power increases with the decline in fear through aging (Morgan and Robinson 2013). Power also rises from the goal or motivation for resilience due to functional decline and increased stress with age (Charles and Carstensen 2009; Howe 2010). Additionally, such power has stemmed from affordability, community attachment, knowledge, leisure, organizational membership, religiosity, and religious activity, spirituality, and trust (Fung et al. 2008; Goerres 2007; Hallerod 2006; Howe 2010; MacDonald 2000; Marcum 2013; Molana and Adams 2019; Price et al. 2006; Sneed et al. 2006). Community attachment is part of social capital used to access resources and support (Saegert and Winkel 2004). Organizational membership is a basis for flourishing and generating belongingness, closeness, identity, and self-esteem, and diminishing anxiety (Baumeister and Leary 1995; Goodman et al. 2017; Hampton 2007; Malloy 2018). Religiosity implies access to the divine and the religious community's power or support (Kay et al. 2008; Peifer 2010). Spirituality similarly implies power (Shek 2010). Trust is a component of social capital that allows access to resources and support (Sundquist and Yang 2007). Need for resilience has grown with age (Hallerod 2006). Moreover, this goal has grown with anxiety, distress, illness, stagnation, and attention to negativity (Ruffman et al. 2016; Siu-man Ng et al. 2006; Schaie 2013). Conversely, this goal has grown with declining functioning and health (Goerres 2007; Ruffman et al. 2016). In the youth, the sources of power for resilience additionally include increased academic achievement, autonomy, compromise, conflict resolution, creativity, identity achievement, intimacy, maturity, meaningfulness, self-esteem, and sociability, and reduced loneliness and susceptibility with aging (Ahmed et al. 2020; Froiland et al. 2015; Krauss et al. 2014; Monahan et al. 2013; Owens et al. 2005; Pratt and Matsuba 2018; Rostan 1997; Schneider 1993; Shen 2009; Steger et al. 2008; Wires et al. 1994). In the youth, autonomy implies getting others' support. To become powerful (Schenke et al. 2015). Compromise and conflict resolution represent goals to generate or reflect such power as creativity, rationality, and security (Dorjee 2013; Simmons 2020). In the youth, creativity is mental ability or power (Tacher and Readdick 2006). Intimacy in the youth draws social support to become assertive (Roth and Assor 2012). Maturity embraces such power as efficacy in the youth (Cordeiro et al. 2015). Meaningfulness is motivational to consolidate power in the youth (Sanderson et al. 2016). Self-esteem reflects such power as competence in the youth (Wilkinson 2010). Moreover, self-esteem constitutes the resiliency trait and, thus the resilience process or state (Di Fabio et al. 2015). To the youth, sociability is a basis for receiving social support to enhance such power as competence (Collins and van Dulmen 2006; Nilsen et al. 2013). Susceptibility reflects powerlessness (Biagas and Bianchi 2016).

Utility or expectancy from resilience has stemmed from the youth's increased confidence and hope and reduced frustration with aging (Drummond et al. 2011; Garst et al. 2021; Gummerum and Keller 2008; Han and Grogan-Kaylor 2012).

Resilience is an ideal growing with age (Charles and Carstensen 2009). Other ideals growing with age for rationalizing resilience include accommodation, adaptation, balancing, compensation, continuity, and present orientation (Consedine 2011; Marcum 2013; Morgan and Robinson 2013; Ramsey and Gentzler 2015; Von Dras and Blumenthal 2000). Additionally, other ideals for resilience increasing with age have included appraisal or emotion, problem-focused coping, self-reliance, stability, and the values of conservation, transcendence, trust, and work (Caplan and Schooler 2007; Charles and Carstensen 2009; Chen and Davey 2009; Consedine 2011; Datler et al. 2013; Daniel et al. 2022; Ferssizidis et al. 2010; Howe 2010; Kiecolt 2003; Roberts and DelVecchio 2000; Sneed et al. 2006; Steger et al. 2009; Tomas et al. 2013), Conversely, those against resilience declining with age have included anger, depression, negative affect, and strain (Caplan and Schooler 2007; Charles and Carstensen 2008; Consedine 2011; Stanley et al. 2014). Negative affect has included regret, sadness, and intrusiveness felt (Consedine 2011; Wrosch et al. 2005). In the youth, ideals for resilience growing with age additionally include the value of competence (Coie et al. 1990).

Resilience norms have evolved with aging through increased family cohesion or solidarity and functioning (Smith and Hamon 2012). Conversely, family strain or stress has declined with the youth's age (Hay 2003).

## *Gender*

Resilience has appeared to be lower in the girl than the boy (Armfield et al. 2021; Freitas et al. 2017). Similarly, resilience has fared lower in the female working person than the male one (Portnoy et al. 2018). According to the voluntaristic theory of analytical functionalism, the gender difference stems from differences in power, utility, norms, and ideals to sustain the resilience functions of fulfillment, adaptation, integration, and latency.

Power lower in the woman than in the man for realizing to drive resilience rests on health, mastery, leisure, motivation for power, self efficacy, self-esteem, and social achievement, dominance, independence, influence, resources, and status (Carli 2004; Gattino et al. 2015; Davey et al. 2009; Goldberg 1993; Guo et al. 2008; Lu and Kao 2002; Renfrow and Howard 2013; Rundman and Glick 2008; Straughn and Andriot 2011; Thapa et al. 2021; Tomas et al. 2013; Valiente 2018). Social achievement is a power source through social integration, leadership, and others (Chung 2000; Praszkier 2018; Ullrich et al. 2007). Moreover, the woman's lower power is attributable to her higher anxiety, depression, dependence on medicine, distress, gullibility, illness, role overload, stagnation, subordination or oppression, and victimization received than the man (Betz et al. 2013; de Coster 2005; Fischer and Evers 2013; Fyall and Gazley 2015; Ng et al. 2006; Schaie 2013; Teunisse et al. 2020; Thapa et al. 2021). Victimization induces difficulty to deprive power (Michalski 2005). Weaker power for resilience in the girl than in the boy has additionally stemmed from her higher anomia, control by others, discomfort, hurt by others, impulsivity, neuroticism, rejection by others, sadness, stress felt (Adnanes 2007; Ahadi et al. 1993; Cornell et al. 2014; Costello and Hope 2016; Esteban 2006; Lessard et al. 2011; Pedersen et al. 2017; Thunberg and Kallstrom 2018). Conversely, power for resilience lower in the girl than in the boy has additionally stemmed from concentration, courage, defensiveness, and entrepreneurship (Mundia 2011; Muris et al. 2010; Nash et al. 2004; Schmitt-Redermund and Vondracek 2002).

Utility or expectancy lower in the woman than in the man stems from the benefit or reward received and instrumentality and relational satisfaction (Carli and Bukatko 2000; Diekman and Schneider 2010; Mau 2005a; Franklin 2012; Wong et al. 2011). Relational satisfaction strengthens power through social integration (Imamoglu 2003). Conversely, disutility such as risk perceived has been higher in the woman than in the man (Lemyre et al. 2006). Utility for resilience has been lower in the girl than in the boy (Gabay-Egozi et al. 2010).

Ideals for resilience such as agency, assertiveness, heroism, independence, responsibility, and self-enhancement are lower in the woman than in the man (Daniel et al. 2022; Diekman and Schneider 2010; Feingold 1994; Fyall and Gazley 2015; Guo et al. 2008; Jakobsen 2010; Weimann and Brosius 1994). Self-enhancement safeguards personal resources and well-being (Sarpila 2014). Conversely, ideals or obsessions disfavoring resilience such as passivity and traditionalism are higher in the woman than in the man (Batalha and Reynolds 2013; Caprara and Vecchione 2017; Eagly et al. 2004). These ideals have been distressful (Brynin et al. 2009). Ideals for resilience lower in the girl than in the boy additionally include humor and self-reliance (Myers et al. 1997; Zupancic et al. 2014). Humor has buttressed resilience (Ungar et al. 2005). Conversely, ideals impeding resilience higher in the girl than in the boy have additionally included aspiration and suicidal ideation (Davis and Shlafer 2016; Vrangalova and Savin-Williams 2011). In the youth, aspiration breeds floundering, thus impairing resilience (Rojewski and Kim 2003). Suicidal ideation is harmful and risky, hence hindering resilience (Lacourse et al. 2001).

Resilience norms disfavoring resilience higher in the girl than in the boy include dependence and emotionality (Sumter et al. 2013; Zupancic et al. 2014). In the youth, emotionality defies self-regulation as required for resilience (Zhang and Cross 2011).

## *Migrant Status*

The immigrant or migrant patient or service user has exhibited lower resilience than the native counterpart (Theron et al. 2011). This difference is attributable to the migrant's lower power, utility, norms, and ideals for resilience, based on voluntaristic theory in analytical functionalism.

The migrant has been lower than the native in power driving resilience stemming from community attachment, employment, health, marital status, neighborhood support received, social capital, and social trust (Anton and Lawrence 2014; Brown et al. 2014; Fanning et al. 2011; Islam et al. 2006; Kurz et al. 2005; Lilly et al. 2011; Ravanera et al. 2003). Community attachment upholds such power as knowledge, mastery, resourcefulness, and self-efficacy (Notter et al. 2008; Ohmer 2007). Social trust implies power based on cooperation and social capital received to sustain health and survival (Barefoot et al. 1998; Brown et al. 2014; Six 2014). Conversely, the migrant has been lower than the native in power due to higher dysfunction or functional limitation, poverty, social exclusion, and unemployment experienced (Bask 2005; Herd et al. 2008; Kurz et al. 2005; Posthumus et al. 2013). Among youth, the immigrant has been lower than the native in power due to higher discrimination experienced and lower coping, coping efficacy, and self-esteem (Lipshits-Braziler and Tatar 2012; Steinhausen et al. 2009; Tam and Lam 2005; Ullman and Tatar 2001).

The migrant has been higher than the native in the ideal or obsession favoring suicide to impend resilience (Hassan 1995). Suicide contradicts living, including resilience (Cheng et al. 2017; Sahin et al. 1994). Conversely, the migrant has secured a lower ideal in life satisfaction to bolster resilience (Ambrey and Fleming 2014). Among youth, the immigrant has been lower than the native in ideals for resilience, including adjustment, independence, positivity, and self-control (Chirkov et al. 2005; Liu and Liu 2016). Conversely, the immigrant youth has been higher than the immigrant native in ideals contradicting resilience, including avoidance and worry (Steinhausen et al. 2009; Tam and Lam 2005).

The immigrant has been lower than the native in social norms experienced for resilience favoring acceptance, coping efficacy, obligation, and social support (Lipshits-Braziler and Tatar 2012; Phinney et al. 2000; Steinhausen et al. 2009). Obligation sustains power for resilience through assertiveness and enthusiasm (Lavigne et al. 2013). Conversely, the immigrant youth has been higher than the native youth in encountering the social norm of rejection to impede resilience (Steinhausen et al. 2009). The youth's experience of rejection has fomented depression, disorders, and loneliness, as opposed to comfort, effort, and self-esteem (Sommer et al. 2001; Tani and Schneider 1997; Witkow 2005).

## *Residency*

The youth's residency has raised resilience (Armfield et al. 2021). Such raising is attributable to power, utility, norms, and ideals regarding resilience engendered by residency, considering the voluntaristic theory of analytical functionalism.

Residency has secured such power sources to drive resilience as community attachment and involvement, health, religious attendance, self-esteem social capital including that stemming from associations and friendship, social support received, and social trust (Anton and Lawrence 2014; Apinunmahakul and Devlin 2008; Jorgensen et al. 2010; Marschall and Stolle 2004; Palmer et al. 2011; Patulny and Morris 2012; Prouteau and Wolff 2008). Moreover, residency has sustained power by fostering intimacy and preventing unemployment in the youth (Aberg and Hedstrom 2011; Chang et al. 2008). Intimacy has fostered such power and power sources for resilience as competence and social trust in the youth (Henderson et al. 2009).

Residency has boosted such utility attracting resilience as satisfaction with healthcare, housing, and the neighborhood (Greenwald et al. 2004; Oliver 2003; Spelman 2004). Among youth, residency has boosted utility for resilience concerning development and meaningfulness (Cheung and Ngai 2004).

Residency has consolidated social norms experienced to sustain resilience, such as morale (Wulfhorst and Kranich 1999). Morale is a power basis for resilience resting on confidence, devotion, enthusiasm, leadership, optimism, purposiveness, and trust (Peterson et al. 2008).

## *Education*

Resilience has increased with education in the elder and patient or service user (Sawyer and Allman 2010; Visaria et al. 2023; Yin et al. 2022). This increase benefits from power, utility, norms, and ideals regarding resilience raised by education, predicated on the voluntaristic theory of analytical functionalism.

Education is power known as ability, expertise, human capital, knowledge, learning, resources, self-esteem, and skill (Fiske et al. 1990; Kung 2003; Nordin 2011; Papastephanon 2015; Straughn and Andriot 2011; Verba et al. 1995). Power based on education for resilience involves challenging, controlling, creativity, cultural capital, earnings, enlightenment, functioning, health, home equipment, income, insurance coverage, intelligence, interest, marriage, mastery, memory, organizational membership, security, self-discovery, self-efficacy, social status, social support received, social trust, and youthfulness (Apinunmahakul and Devlin 2008; Bullock 2021; Cerin and Leslie 2008; Corcoran et al. 2011; Hraba et al. 2001; Holbrook et al. 2003; Horowitz 2018; Knab et al. 2008; Kuppens et al. 2018; Lam et al. 1999; Miyata et al. 2008; Papastephanon 2015; Pratt et al. 1996; Schnittker and Behrman 2012; Shin 2012; Stavrova and Ehlebracht 2018; Stevens et al. 2001; Yair 2003; Yienprugsawan et al. 2010; van Praag and Frijters 1999; Whyte and Gao 2009). Interest, as goal-setting to generate power or motivation, has bred coping, creativity, knowledge, and self-efficacy (Charyton et al. 2009; Dai et al. 2015; Forster et al. 2017; Garriott et al. 2017b; Wen and Cui 2014). Such breeding hinges on persistence and self-regulation (Cohen and Gelbrich 1999). Moreover, education has boosted power for resilience by preventing distress, discrimination experienced, poverty, social exclusion experienced, somatization, threat experienced, victimization experienced, and vulnerability (Al-krenawi et al. 2011; Backman and Nilsson 2011; Kessler et al. 1999; Kaukinen 2004; Langenderfer and Shimp 2001; Raijman et al. 2003; Snyder et al.

2020; Wang et al. 2013). In the youth, education additionally lifts power for resilience through cognitive apprenticeship, creativity, and innovativeness (Flogie et al. 2018; Furnham-Diggory 1992; Giambra 2018). Cognitive apprenticeship embraces articulation or verbalization, competition, cooperation, exploration, learning, modeling, motivation, and reflection concerning problem-solving strategy (Furnham-Diggory 1992). Innovativeness applies to decision-making, interpretability, transparency, and technicality (Flogie et al. 2018). Conversely, education has additionally sustained power for resilience by lessening fear, and loneliness in the youth (Thompson and Norris 1992; Valdivia et al. 2005).

Education has lifted utility, benefit, and expectancy from resilience by realizing justice, opportunity, life quality or standards, and satisfaction with safety and security in society (Barker and Tinnick 2006; Emler and Frazer 1999; Helwig 2004; Mau 2005a). Conversely, education has sustained utility from benefits by reducing constraint and punishment (Furman and Buhrmester 1992; Stavrova and Ehlebracht 2018).

Education has developed ideals for resilience such as acceptance, autonomy, choice, deliberation, dutifulness, health maintenance, independence, meritocratism, openness, persistence, reasoning, and working (Armon and Dawson 2003; Fjellvang 2011; Evans et al. 2010; Jacobs et al. 2009; James and Amato 2013; James and Luo 1999; Lin et al. 2008; Lo and Jim 2012; Mirowsky and Ross 2001; Rossi 2001; Stone and Buttice 2010; Weimann and Brosius 1994; Whyte and Gao 2009; Xiao 2000). Furthermore, education has sustained power for resilience for diminishing the ideals or obsessions for alienation, hazards, paranoia, and psychoticism (Al-krenawi et al. 2011; Cerin and Leslie 2008; Coffe and Geys 2007), In the youth, education has additionally raised such ideals for resilience as adjustment, fitness, learning, need fulfillment, self-determination (Giambra 2018; Liu and Chen 2010; Seitz et al. 2022).

Education has sustained social norms for resilience by finding fewer problems and risks in society (Sjoberg 2003; Staples et al. 1999; Treno and Holder 1997).

## *Marriage*

Marriage is likely to secure resilience through power, utility, norms, and ideals from the voluntaristic theory of analytical functionalism. Accordingly, marriage is beneficial and counts as a solution to problems (Lichter et al. 2002; Solomon 2006). Conversely, divorce and widowhood are likely to weaken resilience.

Marriage is a power source for resilience in providing intimacy and support to fulfill needs (Carbery and Buhrmester 1998). The source has hinged on the contribution of marriage to closeness, community attachment and involvement, financial adequacy, health, living standards, mental health, religiousness or religious activity, self esteem, social capital, social integration, social support received, social trust, and socioeconomic status (Apinunmahakul and Devlin 2008; Chang 2009; Hou et al. 2015; Immerzeel and van Tubergen 2013; Lelli 2008; Lindstrom and Rosvall 2012; Lizardo 2006; Mata and Pendakur 2014; McCabe 2014; Molana and Adams 2019;

Prezza et al. 2001). Social capital is accessible from friends, kin, neighbors, and other affiliations or bonding sources (Apinunmahakul and Devlin 2008; Cornwall 2009; Volker et al. 2007). Socioeconomic status features homeownership as opposed to poverty and welfare dependence (London 2003; Manturuk et al. 2010; Vartanian 1999). Conversely, marriage has sustained power for resilience by preventing depression, disability or limitations, discrimination and social exclusion experienced, fear, loneliness, and victimization experienced (Carr and Friedman 2005; Koromeckyj-Cox et al. 2007; Li and Chung 2008; Moore and Shepherd 2006; Ross and Mirowsky 2009; Wright et al. 2015; Yienprugsawan et al. 2010). Furthermore, divorce or spousal decease has weakened power for resilience by raising stagnation (Ng et al. 2006).

Marriage has achieved utility in relational or interactional quality and life satisfaction to attract resilience (McMullin and Cairney 2004). Life satisfaction has enhanced well-being, including health, hope, and self-efficacy as opposed to loneliness, to raise resilience (Celso et al. 2003; Corcoran et al. 2011; Oishi et al. 2000; Rocke and Lachman 2008; Neto and Barros 2003).

Marriage has evolved ideals for resilience, such as the value of working (James and Luo 1999; Obucina 2013). Conversely, divorce has led to ideals against resilience, such as reliance on others (Cox and Paley 1997). Likewise, divorce has attenuated ideals for resilience, such as dependability (Allemand et al. 2015). Spousal decease has also eroded life satisfaction as an ideal for resilience (Tiliouine et al. 2006).

## *Living Alone*

Living alone weakens such currencies as power, utility, ideals, and norms for upholding resilience. These currencies are requisite to run the voluntaristic mechanisms of power realization, utility optimization, ideal calibration, and norm conformity to achieve the functioning expected in analytical functionalism.

Power to drive resilience drained by living alone has rested on health, sleep quality, and social capital (Gu et al. 2010; Murayama et al. 2019; Sundquist and Yang 2007). Social capital has fostered well-being, including flourishing, happiness, health, life satisfaction, pride, and the sense of community to safeguard resilience (Chua et al. 2021; Yetim and Yetim 2014). Conversely, living alone has bred alcoholism, depression, distress, psychopathology, and suicide to dampen power to drive resilience (Cook and Moore 2001; Lofors and Sundquist 2007; Oshio and Kan 2019; Schneider et al. 2014). Alcoholism has fomented illness, injury, and pathology, thus disempowering (Brotchie et al. 2004; Haapanen-Niemi et al. 1999). Attempted suicide has induced anxiety to obstruct resilience (Cheng et al. 2017).

Utility to attract resilience blocked by loving alone has resided in benefits received and life satisfaction (Lou and Chi 2008; Richards 2016). Conversely, living alone has incurred loss to dampen utility and thus its attraction to resilience (Krause-Parello and Gulick 2013).

Ideals to rationalize resilience discouraged by living alone have emphasized responsibility and volunteering (Shtudiner et al. 2017). Responsibility has advanced wisdom to facilitate resilience (Spengler et al. 2018). Volunteerism has raised well-being, including health, life satisfaction, mastery, morale, positive affect, and self-esteem as opposed to depression, loneliness, and mortality (Borgonovi 2008; Gillath et al. 2005; Li and Ferraro 2006; Midlarsky and Kahana 1994; Oman et al. 1999; Thoits and Hewitt 2001; Zotti et al. 2016).

The norm to assimilate resilience that has dismissed living alone has concerned earnings (Hughes 2003). This norm has assimilated personal earnings (Flap and Volker 2008). Earnings have buttressed mastery and satisfaction and eroded depression and strain to safeguard resilience (Conger et al. 2000; O'Neill and Evans 1999; Schyns 2000).

## *Family Size*

Family size is likely to impede resilience due to difficulties in power, utility, deals, and norms for resilience. According to the voluntaristic theory of analytical functionalism, power, utility, ideals, and norms are requisite for realizing, optimizing, maintaining consistency, and conformity to drive, attract, assimilate, and rationalize resilience.

Family size has restricted power or its sources for resilience including health, neighborhood amenities and social relationships, and trust in professionals (Ahern and Hendryx 2003; Bonaiuto et al. 1999; Roy and Chaudhuri 2008). Conversely, family size has led to welfare dependence to diminish power for resilience (Mitrut and Wolff 2011). In the elder, family size has heightened functional disability and service need to indicate power inadequacy for resilience (Calsyn et al. 1998; Giraldez-Garcia et al. 2013). To the elder, family size has sustained health, wealth, and social support reception, and reduced hospitalization to furnish power for resilience (Bernheim et al. 2001; Giraldez-Garcia et al. 2013; Roy and Chaudhuri 2008; Zimmer and Kwong 2003).

Family size has eroded ideals for resilience, including fulfillment of need, satisfaction with finance and life, and willingness to pay (Guardiola and Garcia-Munoz 2011; Hui 1999; Knies 2012; Mitrut and Wolff 2011). Conversely, family size has fomented ideals against resilience, including violence (Farrington 2007).

## *Homeownership*

Homeownership or living in purchased housing is likely to champion resilience through power, utility, norms, and ideals. Such housing contrasts with rental private or public housing, hostels, and aged homes. Housing is influential because of its endurability, necessity for living or ontological security, and sizable stake (Henretta 1987; La Grange and Pretorius 2000).

Homeownership has secured power or its sources for resilience in community attachment and involvement, financial adequacy, friendship, health, marriage, social capital, and social trust (Anton and Lawrence 2014; Gibson-Davis 2009; McCabe 2014; Manturuk et al. 2010; Mirowsky and Ross 1999; Putnam 2007; Roy and Chaudhuri 2008; Tsai 2006; Wilson and Hammer 2001). Social capital notably included neighbors' support (Shaw 2005). Meanwhile, social capital rises with social interaction facilitated by homeownership (Degenne et al. 2004; Manturuk et al. 2010). Conversely, homeownership has maintained power by preventing depression, divorce, and victimization (Congdon 2010; Michalski 2005; Thornton et al. 2007; Woldoff and Ovadia 2009). To the elder, homeownership has raised aspiration, social support received, and volunteering to secure power for resilience (Chou et al. 2003; Principi et al. 2016; Shaw 2005). Conversely, homeownership has reduced the elder's dysfunction, illness, poverty, and welfare dependency to preserve power for resilience (Elder and Powers 2006; Forward et al. 2023; Haveman et al. 2003; Roy and Chaudhuri 2008). To the patient or service user, homeownership has enabled savings and family income to muster power for resilience (Ssewamala et al. 2006). For the working person, homeownership has boosted cooperation and prevented poverty to secure power for resilience (Haveman et al. 2007; Tillmar and Lindkvist 2007). To the minority person, homeownership has boosted aspiration, employment, and social integration to provide power for resilience (Baker et al. 2000; Rumbaut 1997; Sassler 2006). For the patient or service user, homeownership constitutes power stemming from aspiration and self-efficacy as opposed to poverty to facilitate resilience (Barnes and Janet 2003).

To the patient and service user, homeownership signifies individualism as an ideal to maintain resiliency (Barnes and Janet 2003). Individualism has reflected pride to prop resilience (Suhay 2015).

Homeownership has raised achievement experience, family quality, and neighborhood quality and helpfulness to sustain utility expected from resilience in the patient or service user and satisfaction with housing and the neighborhood (Granzin and Haggard 2000; Harris 2001; Zhan and Sherraden 2003). To the user, homeownership also embodies hope and upward social mobility to consolidate utility from resilience (Barnes and Janet 2003).

## *Social Class*

Reflecting social class, work hours have elevated resilience in the youth (Hartley 2013). Such class means the ownership of financial capital, expertise, and authority for production (Todorova 2013; Wright 1997). Its position descends from the employer down to the self-employed, middle-class, working-class, surplus class or nonworking, and underclass or unemployed, welfare-dependent, or incarcerated person (Buckingham 1999). Social class embodies a central social relation, notably based on production (Flemming 2013). It can boost resilience through power, utility, norms, and ideals, as central to buttress functions required in analytical functionalism.

Social class (high vs. low) has generated power or its sources for resilience, including health, patience, and positive affect or emotion (Chen et al. 2016; Karoly and Ruehlman 2006; McKay et al. 2018). Conversely, social class has maintained power for resilience by relieving anxiety, depression, fear, stress, symptoms, and need for medicine (Karoly and Ruehlman 2006; Lock et al. 2020; Mak et al. 2019; Sawyers et al. 2020; Zheng et al. 2020). In the youth, social class has strengthened power or its sources for resilience, additionally including social capital and social support received (Tolonen 2008; Wong 2017). For the working person, social class has sustained power by additionally raising commitment, education, effort, housing quality, human capital, income, and training (Anderson and Miller 2003; Camp 1990; Hult and Svallfors 2002; Kohn et al. 1997; Lin and Wu 2009; Owens 1992; Tam and Chiu 2010). Conversely, social class has maintained power by additionally reducing alienation, conflict, distress, and risk (Green and Thorogood 1998; Gronlund and Oun 2012; Mirowsky and Ross 1989; Thompson et al. 1999). In the youth, familial social class has facilitated power for resilience, including knowledge and mastery (Cetin et al. 2010; Reichert and Print 2017).

Social class raises utility from resilience in controllability and life satisfaction (Karoly and Ruehlman 2006; McKay et al. 2018). In the youth, such utility has happened in achievement and success (belief or experience) (Bjarnason 2000; Tolonen 2008). In the working person, such utility has additionally evolved from benefits received and meritocratic expectations that are rewarding (Jackson 2007; Walder 1995).

Social class erodes ideals against resilience, including coping and reliance on professionals (Karoly and Ruehlman 2006). Coping has included ignorance, persistence, and self-talk (Karoly and Ruehlman 2006). To the working person, social class has advanced ideals for resilience additionally, including controlling, flexibility, self-direction, and the value of autonomy (Kohn et al. 1990, 1997; Kohn et al. 2004; Mirowsky and Ross 1990). To the youth, familial social class has established ideals for resilience through impulse control and self-esteem (Cetin et al. 2010).

In the working person, social class buttresses social norms for resilience, including flexibility (Gersitel and Clauson 2014).

## *Personal Income*

Personal income has sustained resilience in the elder, patient or service user, working person, and minority person (Nee and Sanders 2001; Portnoy et al. 2018; Sawyer and Allman 2010; Yin et al. 2022). Such sustenance reflects the contributions of power, utility, norms, and ideals for resilience, following the voluntaristic theory of analytical functionalism.

Personal income has escalated power (Rijken and Groenewegen 2008). Moreover, personal income has secured power bases for resilience, including aspiration, community involvement, cultural capital, family income, financial adequacy, health, insurance coverage knowledge, religiousness or belief in divine support, security, self-efficacy, skill, sleep, social capital, social integration, social support received, social well-being, and quality in the family, housing, and neighborhood (Beaudoin and Thorson 2006; Carpiano 2008; Corcoran et al. 2011; Frei et al. 2009; Glaeser and Gottlieb 2006; Gross and Brammli-Greenberg 2004; Hallerod 2006; Hraba et al. 2001; Kerrissey and Schofer 2013; Lelli 2008; Logan et al. 1999; Patulny and Morris 2012; Price et al. 2006; Skerkat and Ellison 1999; Son and Wilson 2012; Van Zandt and Rohe 2006; Vartanian 1999). Furthermore, such power or bases have derived from reducing alienation, anxiety, death risk, depression, deprivation experienced, discrimination experienced, distress, dysfunction or limitations, fear, homelessness, loneliness, stagnation, social exclusion experienced, threat experienced, and victimization experienced by personal income (Buck 2001; Clarke et al. 2011; Hou et al. 2015; Kessler et al. 1999; Kaukinen 2004; Lantz et al. 2005; Lelli 2008; Li and Chung 2008; Ng et al. 2006; Rijken and Groenewegen 2008; Schneider 2007; Weakliem and Borch 2006).

Personal income has furnished ideals for resilience, including acceptance, adaptation, controlling, deliberation, dutifulness, institutional and social trust, self-esteem, tolerance, and satisfaction with the country, finance, government, health, housing, individualism, job, income, leisure, life, marriage, neighborhood, and need fulfillment (Granzin and Haggard 2000; Guardiola and Garcia-Munoz 2011; Herreros 2009; Jacobs et al. 2009; Kadushin and Jones 1992; Khattab and Fenton 2009; Kluegel and Smith 1986; Lo and Jim 2012; Prenda and Lachman 2001; Schyns 2001; Sengupta and Sibley 2019; Sun and Wang 2012; Tiliouine et al. 2006; Tsou and Liu 2001; Yeh et al. 2013; van Praag and Ferrer-I-Carbonell 2004; Van Praag et al. 2010; Weimann and Brosius 1994; Zimmerman and Reyna 2013). For the youth, personal income has bolstered power for resilience by preventing illness and pressure (Conger et al. 1997; Gibson 2001).

Personal income has secured utility from resilience based on justice perception (Liebig and Mau 2007). In the youth, personal income has raised achievement to sustain resilience utility (Berends et al. 1999).

Personal income has diminished the perception of social norms impeding resilience, including conflict and risk (Anciaes et al. 2017; Lewin-Epstein et al. 2003).

## *Family Income*

Family income or wealth has facilitated resilience (Jones and d'Errico 2019). Similarly, family socioeconomic status has buttressed the youth's resilience (von Soest et al. 2010). According to the voluntaristic and deterministic theories of analytical functionalism, family income boosts resilience through power, utility, ideals, and social norms.

Family income has elevated power or its sources for resilience in financial adequacy, health, living standards, mastery, mental health, neighborhood quality, self-efficacy, and self-esteem (Cerin and Leslie 2008; Oshio and Kobayashi 2010;

Powdthavee 2009; Thoits and Hewitt 2001; Woldoff and Ovadia 2009; Whyte and Gao 2009). Conversely, family income sustained power for resilience by impeding strain (Becchetta 2010). In the youth, family income has strengthened power additionally by raising aspiration, cognitive ability, commitment, competence, education, family interaction quality, family resources, health maintenance, intelligence, knowledge, leadership, learning, parental attachment and closeness, school attachment, skill, sociability, social integration, and trust (Bradstreet and Parent 2018; Campbell and Eggerling-Boeck 2006; Catalano et al. 2003; Cheadle and Goosby 2010; Elliott et al. 2006; Henderson et al. 2007; Jaeger 2012; McCormick et al. 2016; Moore and Aweiss 2003; Morris et al. 2017; Park et al. 2017; Tepper 2001; Vander Ven et al. 2001; Wen et al. 2020; Yeung et al. 2002). Conversely, family income has sustained power by additionally diminishing anomie or normlessness or aimlessness and financial strain, problems, stress or pressure, unemployment, and welfare dependence in the youth (Adnanes 2007; Gutman et al. 2005; Votruba-Drzal 2006; Yeung et al. 2002; Yuji 2007).

Family income has secured utility to attract resilience and satisfaction with finance, friendship, housing, jobs, leisure, life, marriage, and neighborhood (Ambrey and Fleming 2014; Harris 2001; Kwok et al. 2015; Louis and Zhao 2002; van Praag et al. 2003). In the youth, family income has raised utility from resilience through achievement and gain in the youth (Dunifon and Kowaleski-Jones 2003; Gutman et al. 2005; Muller 1998; Wen et al. 2020). Moreover, In the youth, family income has secured control, entrepreneurship, self-regulation, and the value of studying as ideals for resilience (Brody et al. 1995; Dehejia et al. 2009; Heyns 1996; Wen et al. 2020).

Family income has bolstered norms for resilience, emphasizing aspiration and mental health in the youth (Johnston et al. 2013; Wen et al. 2020).

## *Welfare Reception*

Welfare reception is likely to sustain resilience through service access (Jones and d'Errico 2019). Such access or reception provides power, utility, ideals, and norms to execute the voluntaristic mechanisms of analytical functionalism. Specifically, public welfare or services cover childcare, employment, food, healthcare, and housing (Benitez-Silva et al. 2010; Currie and Grozer 2001; Latimer 1999; Monroe and Tiller 2001).

Welfare reception has facilitated power or its sources for resilience through education, health, insurance coverage, and social support received (Bjornberg and Latta 2007; Campbell 2003; Knab et al. 2008). Conversely, welfare reception has sustained power by preventing poverty (Iceland and Kim 2001). For the youth, welfare reception has raised power for resilience through neighbor interaction (Duncan et al. 2001).

Welfare reception has attained utility in satisfaction to attract resilience (Mitrut and Wolff 2011). Alternatively, welfare reception has championed ideals for resilience through acceptance (Funk 2000). In the youth, welfare reception has fostered ideals for resilience through fate control (Duncan et al. 2001).

## Disability or Impairment

Disability or impairment, such as functional disability and visual impairment, is likely to impede resilience. Such impedance stems from the erosion of power, utility, ideals, and norms in the voluntaristic mechanism of analytical functionalism.

Impairment has diminished power or its sources for resilience in employment, health, self-efficacy, social capital, and social trust (Gastil 2000; Cornwall 2009; Ross and Mirowsky 1995; Zanin et al. 2013). Conversely, impairment has deprived power by raising distress (Phongsavan et al. 2006).

Impairment has reduced utility from resilience by weakening belief in resilience efficacy (Gastil 2000). In the youth, impairment has impeded utility from resilience additionally by reducing achievement experienced and raising punishment received (Lemaire and Mallik 2002).

Impairment has dispelled such ideals for resilience as the values of cheerfulness and responsibility (Konarska 2005).

## Adversity

Adversity has impeded resilience (Cherry et al. 2023). This impedance has also specifically happened in the youth (Lee et al. 2010; Wilks and Spivey 2010). According to the voluntaristic mechanisms of analytical functionalism, the impendence arises from the reduction of power, utility, ideals, and norms for resilience by adversity. Notably, adversity includes challenge, disorders, failure, hassles, health problems, hostility, indignation, pandemics, ressentiment, stigma, trauma, and uncontrollability experienced or received (Berger 2015; Demertzis 2020; Garfin et al. 2015; Khoo et al. 2021; Kleiman and Riskind 2014; Su et al. 2021; Walen and Lachman 2016; Zheng et al. 2020).

Adversity has declined power or its sources for resilience, including health, meaningfulness, positive affect, social integration, social support received, and social trust (Alesina and La Ferrara 2002; Dunkel-Schetter and Bennett 1990; Garcia and Herrero 2004; Mathis et al. 2016; Mroczek 2004). Conversely, adversity has removed power for resilience by fomenting depression, disability, distress, health complaints, and memory loss (Lantz et al. 2005; Lupien et al. 2009; Raposa et al. 2016; Shrira 2012; Snyder et al. 2020; Wallenius 2006). In the youth, adversity has impeded power for resilience by additionally instigating anxiety, illness, and worry (Cohen et al. 2013; Misra and Castillo 2004; Taylor and Snyder 2022). Conversely, adversity has weakened power for resilience by additionally undermining coping and financial well-being in the youth (Heiman and Kariv 2004; Norvilitis et al. 2003).

Adversity has eroded an ideal for resilience, including forgiveness (Toussaint et al. 2016; Parkes et al. 2002). Conversely, adversity has bred ideals or obsessions against resilience, including alcoholism, deviance, doping, maltreatment, suicide, and violence (Atkinson et al. 2005; Backman and Nilsson 2011; Dutton et al. 2016; Grzywacz and Almeida 2008; Hatch 2007; Song et al. 2017). In the youth, adversity has impeded ideals for resilience additionally including adjustment, controlling, coping resources, responsibility, and working (Kaye-Tzadok and Davidson-Arad 2017; Printz et al. 1999; Strauser et al. 2006; Wintre and Yaffe 2000; Vollhardt and Staub 2011). Conversely, adversity has fomented ideals or obsessions against resilience additionally including anger, dependence, indecision, internalizing, psychopathology, recourse, and rumination in the youth (Broidy 2001; Collins and Feeney 2000; Dorahy et al. 2003; Hillman 2008; E. Kim et al. 2003; Nakashima et al. 2013; Taylor and Snyder 2022).

Adversity has dampened utility for resilience in life quality and life and neighbor satisfaction (Baumeister et al. 2013; Zotti et al. 2016). In the youth, adversity has diminished utility from resilience by raising frustration (Tam and Taki 2007). Conversely, adversity has eroded utility from resilience by impeding achievement experienced and hope in the youth (Kaye-Tzadok and Davidson-Arad 2017; Kennedy and Tuckman 2013).

Adversity has highlighted social norms about conflict and risk to contradict resilience (Dutton et al. 2016; Macias 2015). In the youth, adversity has accentuated the social norm about problems to impede resilience (Flook and Fuligni 2008).

## Original Findings

Original findings supported 19 of the 44 hypothesized effects of personal backgrounds on the resilience process (see Table 3.1). On the one hand, support happened to the positive effects of native status, residency, marriage, living with parents, earnings, personal income, family income per capita, and welfare reception. On the other hand, support materialized in the inverse effects of female gender, family size, public housing, rental private housing, lower class positions, and visual impairment and its duration. The original findings evolved from the analysis of six datasets covering the resilience process, including resilience (feeling) and adjustment, resilience action including handling and learning, resilience belief, and resilience exposure or advice or demand received.

### *Resilience*

In analyzing data from the poverty study, only age exhibited a significant negative effect on resilience (feeling) ($\beta = -0.370$, see Table 3.2). This effect contradicted

**Table 3.1** Personal background effects on resilience

| Characteristic | Expected | Currently found | | | |
|---|---|---|---|---|---|
| | | Feeling | Action | Belief | Exposure |
| Age | + | ? | + | + | – |
| Female | – | – | 0 | + | 0 |
| Born in Hong Kong | + | + | 0 | 0 | 0 |
| Born in Mainland China | – | 0 | 0 | 0 | 0 |
| Residency | + | + | 0 | 0 | 0 |
| Education | + | – | + | + | 0 |
| Married | + | + | 0 | 0 | 0 |
| Divorced | – | 0 | 0 | 0 | 0 |
| Widowed | – | 0 | 0 | 0 | 0 |
| Living with the spouse | + | 0 | 0 | 0 | 0 |
| Living with offspring | + | 0 | + | 0 | 0 |
| Living with siblings | + | 0 | 0 | + | 0 |
| Living with parents | + | + | + | + | 0 |
| Living with other relatives | + | 0 | 0 | 0 | 0 |
| Living alone | – | 0 | 0 | 0 | 0 |
| Family size | – | – | 0 | 0 | 0 |
| Owned public housing | – | 0 | 0 | 0 | 0 |
| Rental public housing | – | – | 0 | 0 | 0 |
| Owned private housing | – | – | 0 | 0 | 0 |
| Private housing | – | 0 | 0 | + | 0 |
| Private flat | – | 0 | 0 | 0 | 0 |
| Rental private housing | – | – | 0 | 0 | 0 |
| Rental private room | – | 0 | 0 | 0 | 0 |
| Divided rental private flat | – | – | 0 | 0 | 0 |
| Hostel | – | 0 | 0 | 0 | 0 |
| Aged home | – | 0 | 0 | 0 | 0 |
| Employer | – | 0 | 0 | 0 | 0 |
| Self-employed | – | – | 0 | 0 | 0 |
| Employee | – | – | 0 | 0 | 0 |
| Both employer and employee | + | 0 | 0 | 0 | 0 |
| Managerial role | – | 0 | 0 | 0 | 0 |
| Unemployed | – | – | 0 | 0 | 0 |
| Earnings | + | + | 0 | 0 | 0 |
| Personal income | + | + | 0 | 0 | 0 |
| Family income | + | 0 | 0 | 0 | 0 |
| Family income per capita | + | + | 0 | 0 | 0 |

(continued)

**Table 3.1** (continued)

| Characteristic | Expected | Currently found | | | |
|---|---|---|---|---|---|
| | | Feeling | Action | Belief | Exposure |
| Poor family | – | 0 | 0 | 0 | 0 |
| Receiving social welfare | + | + | 0 | 0 | 0 |
| Receiving social welfare formerly | + | 0 | 0 | 0 | 0 |
| Irreligious | + | 0 | 0 | 0 | 0 |
| Functional disability / Visual impairment | – | – | – | 0 | 0 |
| Visual impairment duration | – | – | 0 | 0 | 0 |
| Adversity | – | – | – | – | – |

*Note* +: positive effect; –: negative effect; ?: mixed effects; 0: no effect

the hypothesized positive effect of age. Meanwhile, the other 18 effects of personal backgrounds did not indicate significant effects.

**Table 3.2** Standardized effects on resilience (poverty dataset)

| Predictor | Resilience |
|---|---|
| Income | 0.053 |
| Living in owned private housing | – 0.189 |
| Irreligious | 0.019 |
| Residency | 0.293 |
| Born in Hong Kong | – 0.168 |
| Born in Mainland China | – 0.095 |
| Education | – 0.058 |
| Employer versus nonworking | – 0.112 |
| Employee versus nonworking | – 0.097 |
| Both employer and employee versus nonworking | 0.060 |
| Self-employed versus nonworking | 0.180 |
| Unemployed versus nonworking | 0.010 |
| Family size | 0.123 |
| Poor | – 0.007 |
| Married | 0.066 |
| Divorced | – 0.011 |
| Widowed | 0.065 |
| Age | – 0.370* |
| Female | – 0.273 |
| $R^2$ | 0.658 |

$^{*}p < 0.05$

**Table 3.3** Standardized effects on resilience (violence dataset)

| Predictor | Resilience |
|---|---|
| Female | – 0.043 |
| Age | 0.162 |
| Locally born | 0.009 |
| Residency | – 0.069 |
| Education | 0.075 |
| Managerial role | – 0.116 |
| Married | 0.151* |
| $R^2$ | 0.100 |

$^*p < 0.05$, $^{**}p < 0.01$, $^{***}p < 0.001$

Analysis of data from the violence study revealed that marriage was the only personal background generating a significant positive effect on resilience (feeling) ($\beta = 0.151$, see Table 3.3). This effect matched the hypothesized positive effect. Meanwhile, the other six effects of personal backgrounds did not give significant effects.

Analysis of data from the resilience study revealed the significant positive effects of age ($\beta = 0.164$, see Table 3.4), living with parents ($\beta = 0.093$), and earnings ($\beta = 0.054$) on resilience (feeling). By contrast, family size ($\beta = -0.069$), female gender ($\beta = -0.087$), functional disability ($\beta = -0.053$), and adversity ($\beta = -0.211$) exhibited significant negative effects on resilience. Notably, the analysis controlled for response characteristics including acquiescence ($\beta = -0.209$), interviewing ($\beta = -0.083$), and others.

Some personal backgrounds manifested significant effects on resilience only in the youth, mid-age adult, or elder. Unique to the youth were the positive effects of living with parents and earnings ($\beta = 0.075$ and 0.095, see Table 3.4). Hence, youth enhanced the contributions of earnings and living with parents on resilience. Specific to the mid-ager were the effects of age, family size, and private housing ($\beta = 0.132$, – 0.093, and 0.078). As such, mid-age strengthened the effects of age, family size, and private housing on resilience. Distinctive to the elder was the negative effect of functional disability ($\beta = -0.082$). Thus, old age strengthened the deleterious effect of functional disability on resilience.

Analysis of data from the elder resilience study unfolded the significant negative effects of adversity and functional disability on resilience (feeling) ($\beta = -0.182$ and – 0.217, see Table 3.5). These two effects remained significant in the analysis of data weighted by the elder's Westernization ($\beta = -0.125$ and – 0.138). Additionally, this weighted analysis revealed that living with the spouse emerged to have a significant positive effect on resilience ($\beta = 0.134$). Hence, the contribution of the spouse was likely to happen in the West when Westernization strengthened the contribution. Meanwhile, other personal backgrounds did not display a significant effect on resilience in the elder.

**Table 3.4** Standardized effects on resilience (service dataset)

| Predictor | Youth | Mid-age | Elder | All |
|---|---|---|---|---|
| Living with the spouse | 0.061 | 0.005 | – 0.060 | 0.005 |
| Living with offspring | – 0.013 | – 0.057 | 0.009 | – 0.006 |
| Living with siblings | – 0.010 | 0.022 | – 0.004 | – 0.004 |
| Living with parents | 0.075* | 0.064 | – 0.022 | 0.093* |
| Living with other relatives | 0.021 | – 0.015 | – 0.030 | – 0.027 |
| Education | 0.030 | 0.065 | 0.048 | 0.048 |
| Family size | – 0.051 | – 0.093* | 0.026 | – 0.069** |
| Owned public housing | 0.024 | – 0.028 | – 0.018 | – 0.016 |
| Private housing | – 0.007 | 0.078* | – 0.003 | – 0.006 |
| Hostel | – 0.002 | – 0.030 | 0.057 | – 0.013 |
| Divided private flat | – 0.057 | – 0.010 | – 0.010 | – 0.021 |
| Age | 0.017 | 0.132** | 0.005 | 0.164** |
| Female | – 0.127*** | – 0.041 | – 0.082* | – 0.087*** |
| Earnings | 0.095* | 0.027 | – 0.007 | 0.054* |
| Family income per capita | – 0.026 | 0.012 | 0.013 | 0.009 |
| Survey assisted by fellows | – 0.047 | 0.031 | – | – 0.008 |
| Survey assisted by service workers | – 0.016 | – 0.021 | – 0.016 | – 0.019 |
| Interviewed | – 0.019 | – 0.014 | 0.006 | – 0.083* |
| Survey date | – 0.001 | – 0.102 | 0.229 | – 0.027 |
| Wave 2 | 0.084* | 0.073 | – 0.212 | 0.040 |
| Repeated response | 0.029 | 0.022 | 0.040 | 0.032 |
| Acquiescence | – 0.285*** | 0.347*** | 0.047 | – 0.209*** |
| $R^2$ | 0.146 | 0.260 | 0.079 | 0.124 |
| Functional disability | 0.022 | – 0.039 | – 0.082* | – 0.053* |
| Adversity | – 0.133*** | – 0.234*** | – 0.213*** | – 0.211*** |
| $R^2$ | 0.153 | 0.309 | 0.131 | 0.169 |

*Note* Reference categories were living alone, living in rental public housing, and self-administered response
$^{*}p < 0.05$, $^{**}p < 0.01$, $^{***}p < 0.001$

Analysis of data from the visual impairment study unfolded 11 significant personal background effects on resilience (feeling). Among these backgrounds, native or locally born status ($\beta = 0.264$, see Table 3.6), welfare reception ($\beta = 0.109$), and family income per capita ($\beta = 0.126$) displayed positive effects. By contrast, rental public housing ($\beta = -0.133$), rental private housing ($\beta = -0.081$), education ($\beta$

**Table 3.5** Standardized effects on resilience (elder dataset)

| Predictor | Unweighted | Weighted by Westernization |
|---|---|---|
| Living with the spouse | 0.044 | 0.134* |
| Living with the offspring | 0.038 | – 0.009 |
| Education | 0.068 | 0.020 |
| Personal income | 0.048 | 0.031 |
| Family income | – 0.083 | – 0.073 |
| Rented public housing | – 0.061 | 0.038 |
| Owned public housing | 0.027 | 0.069 |
| Private flat | 0.088 | 0.107 |
| Aged home | – 0.097 | 0.038 |
| Hostel | – 0.027 | – 0.039 |
| Age | – 0.015 | 0.094 |
| Female | – 0.044 | – 0.029 |
| Response assisted by fellows | 0.037 | 0.021 |
| Response assisted by staff | 0.005 | – 0.015 |
| Response month | 0.029 | 0.011 |
| Acquiescence | 0.035 | 0.024 |
| $R^2$ | 0.049 | 0.038 |
| Adversity | – 0.182** | – 0.125* |
| Functional disability | – 0.217*** | – 0.138* |
| $R^2$ | 0.120 | 0.065 |

*Note* Reference categories were living alone, atypical housing, and response by oneself
$*p < 0.05$, $**p < 0.01$, $***p < 0.001$

= – 0.169), employee status ($\beta$ = – 0.086), self-employed status ($\beta$ = – 0.114), unemployed status ($\beta$ = – 0.091), visual impairment ($\beta$ = – 0.124), and its duration ($\beta$ = – 0.094) sent negative effects on resilience. The analysis controlled for the response characteristics of acquiescence ($\beta$ = 0.471).

Analysis of data from the youth play study revealed five significant personal background effects on resilience (feeling). Among these backgrounds, female gender ($\beta$ = 0.033, see Table 3.7), maternal education ($\beta$ = 0.062), and family income ($\beta$ = 0.123) manifested positive effects. By contrast, age ($\beta$ = – 0.046) and family size ($\beta$ = – 0.054) exhibited negative effects on resilience. The analysis controlled for the response characteristics of acquiescence and social desirability ($\beta$ = – 0.086).

Analysis of data from the resilience study revealed three significant personal background effects generally on inferred resilience as a product of adjustment and adversity. Among them, private housing ($\beta$ = – 0.062, see Table 3.8) and functional disability ($\beta$ = – 0.055) exhibited negative effects. By contrast, adversity ($\beta$ = 0.816) demonstrated a positive effect on inferred resilience, to which adversity was a

**Table 3.6** Standardized effects on resilience (visual impairment dataset)

| Predictor | Resilience |
|---|---|
| Visual impairment | – 0.124*** |
| Rental public housing | – 0.133* |
| Owned public housing | – 0.030 |
| Rental private housing | – 0.081* |
| Owned private housing | – 0.003 |
| Irreligious | 0.007 |
| Residency | 0.010 |
| Born in Hong Kong | 0.264* |
| Norn in Mainland China | 0.168 |
| Education | – 0.169*** |
| Employer versus nonworking | – 0.015 |
| Employee versus nonworking | – 0.086* |
| Self-employed versus nonworking | – 0.114** |
| Unemployed versus nonworking | – 0.091** |
| Family size | – 0.071 |
| Receiving social welfare | 0.109** |
| Receiving social welfare formerly | – 0.044 |
| Married | 0.006 |
| Divorced/separated | 0.023 |
| Widowed | – 0.057 |
| Age | 0.065 |
| Visual impairment duration | – 0.094** |
| Female | – 0.040 |
| Family income per capita | 0.126** |
| Acquiescence | 0.471*** |
| $R^2$ | 0.308 |

*$p < 0.05$, **$p < 0.01$, ***$p < 0.001$

defining constituent. The analysis controlled for response characteristics, including acquiescence and interviewing ($\beta = -$ 0.198 and – 0.158).

Some background effects happened significantly only in the mid-ager. Unique to the mid-ager were the negative effects of living in owned public housing ($\beta =$ – 0.126, see Table 3.8) and living in private housing ($\beta =$ 0.098) on inferred resilience. Hence, mid-age strengthened the negative effects of living in owned public housing and living in private housing on inferred resilience.

Analysis of data from the elder resilience study revealed six significant personal background effects on inferred resilience as a product of adjustment and adversity. Among the backgrounds, family income ($\beta = 0.129$, see Table 3.9), adversity ($\beta =$ 0.807), and functional disability ($\beta = 0.091$) displayed positive effects. By contrast,

**Table 3.7** Standardized effects on resilience, past month ($N = 3564$) (youth dataset)

| Predictor | All |
|---|---|
| Age | – 0.046** |
| Female | 0.033* |
| Irreligious | 0.006 |
| Family size | – 0.054** |
| Living with parents | 0.021 |
| Paternal education | – 0.019 |
| Maternal education | 0.062** |
| City residency | 0.006 |
| Living with young sisters | 0.035 |
| Family income | 0.123*** |
| Social desirability | – 0.086*** |
| Acquiescence | – 0.010 |
| $R^2$ | 0.039 |

*$p < 0.05$, **$p < 0.01$, ***$p < 0.001$

living with the spouse ($\beta = -0.132$) and female gender ($\beta = -0.187$) indicated negative effects on inferred resilience. The analysis controlled for such response characteristics as acquiescence ($\beta = 0.309$).

The significant background characteristics held in the analysis were weighted by the elder's Westernization. Hence, the effects were not specific to the West or Westernization.

## *Adjustment*

Analysis of data from the resilience study revealed eight significant personal background effects generally on adjustment. Among the backgrounds, living with parents ($\beta = 0.112$, see Table 3.10), education ($\beta = 0.087$), and age ($\beta = 0.117$) manifested positive effects. By contrast, living with relatives other than the spouse, offspring, siblings, or parents ($\beta = -0.047$), family size ($\beta = -0.060$), living in a divided private flat ($\beta = -0.039$), functional disability ($\beta = -0.088$), and adversity ($\beta = -0.214$) delivered negative effects on adjustment. The analysis controlled for such response characteristics as acquiescence ($\beta = -0.248$).

Some significant personal background effects were unique to the youth, mid-ager, or elder. For the youth, such an effect sprang from living in a divided private flat ($\beta = -0.116$). Hence, youth enhanced this negative effect. Distinctive to the mid-ager, was the effect of education ($\beta = 0.146$). Hence, mid-age lifted the contribution of education. Specific to the elder were the effects of living in a hostel ($\beta = 0.094$), female gender ($\beta = -0.120$), and earnings ($\beta = -0.098$).

**Table 3.8** Standardized effects on inferred resilience (service dataset)

| Predictor | Youth | Mid-age | Elder | All |
|---|---|---|---|---|
| Living with the spouse | – 0.060 | – 0.059 | 0.024 | – 0.044 |
| Living with offspring | 0.035 | – 0.023 | 0.054 | – 0.008 |
| Living with siblings | – 0.012 | – 0.026 | 0.041 | – 0.011 |
| Living with parents | 0.012 | 0.002 | 0.017 | – 0.008 |
| Living with other relatives | – 0.029 | 0.049 | 0.057 | 0.029 |
| Education | – 0.061 | 0.012 | – 0.008 | 0.002 |
| Family size | – 0.035 | 0.011 | – 0.074 | – 0.014 |
| Owned public housing | 0.051 | – 0.126** | – 0.017 | – 0.038 |
| Private housing | – 0.046 | – 0.098* | – 0.017 | – 0.062** |
| Hostel | 0.021 | – 0.061 | 0.046 | – 0.009 |
| Divided private flat | – 0.046 | 0.052 | 0.031 | 0.016 |
| Age | 0.029 | 0.047 | 0.012 | 0.088 |
| Female | 0.018 | – 0.025 | – 0.069 | – 0.027 |
| Earnings | 0.042 | – 0.012 | – 0.059 | 0.004 |
| Family income per capita | 0.031 | 0.047 | – 0.018 | 0.021 |
| Survey assisted by fellows | – 0.022 | – 0.015 | – | – 0.027 |
| Survey assisted by service workers | 0.026 | – 0.024 | 0.010 | 0.000 |
| Interviewed | – 0.025 | – 0.094* | – 0.097* | – 0.158*** |
| Survey date | – 0.041 | 0.082 | – 0.031 | – 0.001 |
| Wave 2 | 0.022 | – 0.118 | 0.025 | – 0.001 |
| Repeated response | 0.023 | 0.009 | 0.008 | 0.012 |
| Acquiescence | – 0.122** | – 0.155** | – 0.292*** | – 0.198*** |
| $R^2$ | 0.069 | 0.091 | 0.140 | 0.073 |
| Functional disability | – 0.022 | – 0.086** | – 0.050* | – 0.055*** |
| Adversity | 0.853*** | 0.793*** | 0.744*** | 0.816*** |
| $R^2$ | 0.769 | 0.629 | 0.604 | 0.663 |

*Note* Reference categories were living alone, living in rental public housing, and self-administered response

*$p < 0.05$, **$p < 0.01$, ***$p < 0.001$

## *Depression*

Analysis of data from the elder resilience study unfolded three significant personal background effects on depression. Among the backgrounds, living with the spouse ($\beta = -0.248$, see Table 3.11) indicated a negative effect. By contrast, adversity ($\beta =$

**Table 3.9** Standardized effects on inferred resilience (elder dataset)

| Predictor | Unweighted | Weighted by Westernization |
|---|---|---|
| Living with the spouse | – 0.132* | – 0.207*** |
| Living with the offspring | 0.078 | 0.101 |
| Education | – 0.043 | – 0.005 |
| Personal income | – 0.100 | – 0.003 |
| Family income | 0.129* | 0.123* |
| Rented public housing | – 0.024 | – 0.061 |
| Owned public housing | 0.163 | 0.270 |
| Private flat | 0.103 | 0.206 |
| Aged home | 0.152 | 0.263 |
| Hostel | – 0.038 | – 0.012 |
| Age | – 0.026 | – 0.066 |
| Female | – 0.187** | – 0.205** |
| Response assisted by fellows | 0.003 | 0.108* |
| Response assisted by staff | – 0.092 | – 0.117* |
| Response month | 0.170** | 0.211*** |
| Acquiescence | 0.309*** | 0.224*** |
| $R^2$ | 0.194 | 0.221 |
| Adversity | 0.807*** | 0.809*** |
| Functional disability | 0.091** | 0.099** |
| $R^2$ | 0.713 | 0.706 |

*Note* Reference categories were living alone, atypical housing, and response by oneself
*$p < 0.05$, **$p < 0.01$, ***$p < 0.001$

0.126) and functional disability ($\beta = 0.126$) presented positive effects on depression. The analysis controlled for the response characteristic of acquiescence.

Analysis with data weighted by the elder's Westernization showed four significant personal background effects. Among them, living with the spouse ($\beta = -0.273$, see Table 3.11) and personal income ($\beta = -0.162$) held negative effects. By contrast, family income and adversity manifested a positive effect on depression ($\beta = 0.131$ and 0.222).

## *Resilience Action*

Resilience action comprised resilience handling and resilience. Notably, resilience handling referred to externalizing to act on something whereas learning referred to internalizing to absorb something. Such action was comparable to self-awareness which did not concern resilience specifically.

**Table 3.10** Standardized effects on adjustment (service dataset)

| Predictor | Youth | Mid-age | Elder | All |
|---|---|---|---|---|
| Living with the spouse | − 0.024 | 0.028 | − 0.016 | 0.004 |
| Living with offspring | − 0.050 | − 0.078 | 0.087 | 0.002 |
| Living with siblings | − 0.022 | − 0.001 | 0.000 | − 0.016 |
| Living with parents | 0.055 | 0.084 | 0.062 | 0.112** |
| Living with other relatives | − 0.016 | − 0.047 | − 0.012 | − 0.047* |
| Education | 0.027 | 0.146*** | 0.037 | 0.087** |
| Family size | − 0.046 | − 0.075 | 0.020 | − 0.060** |
| Owned public housing | 0.027 | − 0.014 | − 0.007 | 0.006 |
| Private housing | − 0.020 | 0.040 | 0.036 | 0.021 |
| Hostel | 0.002 | 0.001 | 0.094** | 0.017 |
| Divided private flat | − 0.116** | − 0.040 | 0.023 | − 0.039* |
| Age | − 0.069 | 0.089 | − 0.001 | 0.117* |
| Female | − 0.014 | 0.036 | − 0.120** | − 0.024 |
| Earnings | 0.060 | 0.013 | − 0.098** | 0.008 |
| Family income per capita | 0.041 | 0.031 | 0.058 | 0.039 |
| Survey assisted by fellows | − 0.047 | − 0.011 | – | − 0.020 |
| Survey assisted by service workers | 0.037 | 0.019 | − 0.029 | 0.016 |
| Interviewed | − 0.035 | − 0.014 | 0.063 | 0.023 |
| Survey date | 0.010 | − 0.064 | 0.009 | − 0.060 |
| Wave 2 | 0.010 | 0.059 | 0.041 | 0.077 |
| Repeated response | 0.023 | − 0.012 | − 0.023 | − 0.010 |
| Acquiescence | − 0.245*** | − 0.368*** | − 0.061 | − 0.248*** |
| $R^2$ | 0.153 | 0.273 | 0.104 | 0.199 |
| Functional disability | − 0.044 | − 0.079* | − 0.100** | − 0.088*** |
| Adversity | − 0.116** | − 0.226*** | − 0.298*** | − 0.214*** |
| $R^2$ | 0.159 | 0.324 | 0.201 | 0.250 |

*Note* Reference categories were living alone, living in rental public housing, and self-administered response
$^*p < 0.05$, $^{**}p < 0.01$, $^{***}p < 0.001$

Analysis of data from the resilience study revealed four significant personal background effects on resilience handling generally. On the one hand, living with offspring ($\beta = 0.055$, see Table 3.12) and age ($\beta = 0.116$) displayed positive effects. On the

**Table 3.11** Standardized effects on depression (elder dataset)

| Predictor | Unweighted | Weighted by Westernization |
|---|---|---|
| Living with the spouse | – 0.248*** | – 0.273*** |
| Living with the offspring | – 0.075 | – 0.065 |
| Education | – 0.101 | – 0.029 |
| Personal income | – 0.041 | – 0.162** |
| Family income | 0.051 | 0.131* |
| Rented public housing | 0.021 | – 0.086 |
| Owned public housing | 0.007 | – 0.034 |
| Private flat | – 0.034 | – 0.102 |
| Aged home | 0.024 | – 0.129 |
| Hostel | – 0.021 | – 0.048 |
| Age | – 0.009 | – 0.002 |
| Female | – 0.080 | – 0.044 |
| Response assisted by fellows | – 0.009 | 0.017 |
| Response assisted by staff | – 0.008 | 0.006 |
| Response month | 0.037 | 0.103 |
| Acquiescence | – 0.035 | – 0.087 |
| $R^2$ | 0.080 | 0.108 |
| Adversity | 0.126* | 0.222*** |
| Functional disability | 0.159** | 0.110 |
| $R^2$ | 0.117 | 0.153 |

*Note* Reference categories were living alone, atypical housing, and response by oneself
*$p < 0.05$, **$p < 0.01$, ***$p < 0.001$

other hand, adversity ($\beta = -\ 0.185$) and functional disability ($\beta = -\ 0.050$) exhibited positive effects on resilience handling. The analysis controlled for such response characteristics as acquiescence ($\beta = -\ 0.259$).

Some personal background effects were specific to the youth, mid-ager, and elder. Specific to the youth was the negative effect of family size ($\beta = -\ 0.073$). Hence, youth enhanced the detrimental effect of family size on resilience handling. Unique to the mid-ager was the positive effect of age ($\beta = 0.093$). Hence, mid-age raised the age contribution. Distinctive to the elder were the effects of living with offspring ($\beta = 0.105$) and functional disability ($\beta = -\ 0.071$). Thus, old age strengthened the effects of offspring and functional disability.

Analysis of data from the resilience study showed four significant personal background effects on resilience learning generally. On the one hand, living with offspring ($\beta = 0.059$, see Table 3.13) and parents ($\beta = 0.080$), and education ($\beta = 0.083$) exhibited positive effects. On the other hand, adversity ($\beta = -\ 0.162$) induced a negative effect on resilience learning. The analysis controlled for such response characteristics as acquiescence ($\beta = -\ 0.063$).

**Table 3.12** Standardized effects on resilience handling (service dataset)

| Predictor | Youth | Mid-age | Elder | All |
|---|---|---|---|---|
| Living with the spouse | 0.067 | 0.041 | 0.001 | – 0.002 |
| Living with offspring | – 0.056 | 0.021 | 0.105* | 0.055* |
| Living with siblings | 0.042 | 0.056 | 0.026 | 0.034 |
| Living with parents | 0.046 | 0.053 | 0.004 | 0.069 |
| Living with other relatives | – 0.010 | 0.007 | 0.011 | – 0.031 |
| Education | 0.023 | 0.105** | 0.101** | 0.094*** |
| Family size | – 0.073* | – 0.006 | – 0.008 | – 0.024 |
| Owned public housing | – 0.001 | – 0.014 | 0.063 | 0.010 |
| Private housing | 0.007 | 0.071 | 0.021 | 0.026 |
| Hostel | 0.010 | – 0.013 | 0.019 | 0.009 |
| Divided private flat | – 0.051 | – 0.007 | 0.056 | – 0.002 |
| Age | 0.044 | 0.093* | 0.022 | 0.116* |
| Female | – 0.044 | 0.011 | 0.014 | – 0.016 |
| Earnings | 0.067 | 0.045 | – 0.028 | 0.036 |
| Family income per capita | 0.010 | – 0.011 | – 0.020 | – 0.007 |
| Survey assisted by fellows | – 0.031 | – 0.017 | – | – 0.013 |
| Survey assisted by service workers | 0.002 | – 0.059 | – 0.006 | – 0.016 |
| Interviewed | 0.013 | 0.020 | 0.106** | 0.064 |
| Survey date | – 0.033 | – 0.063 | 0.166 | – 0.033 |
| Wave 2 | 0.039 | – 0.005 | – 0.048 | 0.053 |
| Repeated response | 0.002 | 0.005 | – 0.051 | – 0.006 |
| Acquiescence | – 0.281*** | – 0.383*** | – 0.054 | – 0.259*** |
| $R^2$ | 0.164 | 0.269 | 0.137 | 0.268 |
| Functional disability | – 0.012 | – 0.048 | – 0.071* | – 0.050* |
| Adversity | – 0.100*** | – 0.233*** | – 0.233*** | – 0.185*** |
| $R^2$ | 0.174 | 0.321 | 0.194 | 0.302 |

*Note* Reference categories were living alone, living in rental public housing, and self-administered response

*$p < 0.05$, **$p < 0.01$, ***$p < 0.001$

Some personal backgrounds indicated their effects on resilience learning specific to the youth and mid-ager. Specific to the youth was the positive effects of living with the spouse ($\beta = 0.095$, see Table 3.13) and parents ($\beta = 0.098$). As such, youth strengthened the contribution of living with the spouse and parents to resilience learning. Unique to the mid-ager was the positive effect of female gender ($\beta =$

**Table 3.13** Standardized effects on resilience learning (service dataset)

| Predictor | Youth | Mid-age | Elder | All |
|---|---|---|---|---|
| Living with the spouse | 0.095* | 0.020 | 0.000 | 0.040 |
| Living with offspring | – 0.012 | 0.029 | 0.067 | 0.059* |
| Living with siblings | 0.005 | 0.017 | 0.033 | 0.006 |
| Living with parents | 0.098* | 0.029 | 0.047 | 0.080* |
| Living with other relatives | 0.016 | 0.018 | – 0.011 | – 0.008 |
| Education | 0.011 | 0.084* | 0.102** | 0.083** |
| Family size | – 0.050 | 0.037 | 0.004 | – 0.001 |
| Owned public housing | 0.031 | 0.006 | – 0.030 | – 0.001 |
| Private housing | 0.048 | 0.053 | – 0.035 | 0.029 |
| Hostel | – 0.050 | – 0.015 | 0.011 | – 0.013 |
| Divided private flat | – 0.032 | 0.007 | – 0.004 | 0.003 |
| Age | 0.069 | 0.043 | – 0.063 | 0.049 |
| Female | – 0.047 | 0.087* | 0.017 | 0.025 |
| Earnings | 0.036 | 0.041 | – 0.063 | 0.018 |
| Family income per capita | – 0.042 | – 0.012 | – 0.027 | – 0.023 |
| Survey assisted by fellows | – 0.076* | – 0.018 | – | – 0.036 |
| Survey assisted by service workers | – 0.093** | – 0.066 | 0.055 | – 0.043* |
| Interviewed | – 0.027 | – 0.010 | 0.044 | 0.008 |
| Survey date | – 0.062 | – 0.036 | 0.078 | – 0.041 |
| Wave 2 | 0.058 | 0.006 | – 0.085 | 0.022 |
| Repeated response | – 0.029 | 0.052 | 0.058 | 0.036 |
| Acquiescence | – 0.181*** | – 0.246*** | 0.196*** | – 0.063** |
| $R^2$ | 0.082 | 0.138 | 0.159 | 0.071 |
| Functional disability | 0.017 | 0.016 | – 0.066 | – 0.027 |
| Adversity | – 0.090** | – 0.208*** | – 0.143*** | – 0.162*** |
| $R^2$ | 0.090 | 0.175 | 0.185 | 0.097 |

*Note.* Reference categories were living alone, living in rental public housing, and self-administered response
*$p < 0.05$, **$p < 0.01$, ***$p < 0.001$

0.087). Hence, mid-age sustained the contribution of female gender to resilience learning.

Analysis of data from the resilience study showed five significant personal background effects generally on self-awareness as a concomitant of resilience learning. On the one hand, living with the spouse ($\beta = 0.072$, see Table 3.14) and parents

($\beta = 0.080$), education ($\beta = 0.155$), and private housing ($\beta = 0.055$) unfolded positive effects. On the other hand, adversity ($\beta = -0.161$) fomented a negative effect on self-awareness. The analysis controlled for such response characteristics as acquiescence ($\beta = -0.206$), interviewing ($\beta = 0.080$), and the study wave ($\beta = 0.076$).

**Table 3.14** Standardized effects on self-awareness (service dataset)

| Predictor | Youth | Mid-age | Elder | All |
|---|---|---|---|---|
| Living with the spouse | 0.087* | 0.040 | 0.101* | 0.072** |
| Living with offspring | – 0.059 | – 0.047 | 0.125** | 0.023 |
| Living with siblings | 0.018 | 0.016 | 0.063 | 0.023 |
| Living with parents | 0.093* | 0.039 | – 0.005 | 0.080* |
| Living with other relatives | 0.055 | – 0.063 | 0.013 | – 0.018 |
| Education | 0.017 | 0.190*** | 0.146*** | 0.155*** |
| Family size | – 0.055 | – 0.009 | – 0.071 | – 0.034 |
| Owned public housing | 0.015 | – 0.013 | 0.040 | 0.016 |
| Private housing | 0.029 | 0.103* | 0.022 | 0.055* |
| Hostel | 0.023 | – 0.016 | 0.060 | 0.019 |
| Divided private flat | – 0.090* | 0.010 | 0.040 | – 0.010 |
| Age | 0.030 | 0.049 | – 0.101* | – 0.001 |
| Female | 0.000 | 0.070 | 0.060 | 0.035 |
| Earnings | 0.014 | 0.005 | 0.001 | 0.008 |
| Family income per capita | – 0.028 | – 0.036 | 0.008 | – 0.020 |
| Survey assisted by fellows | – 0.047 | 0.002 | – | – 0.017 |
| Survey assisted by service workers | – 0.016 | – 0.044 | 0.009 | – 0.021 |
| Interviewed | 0.037 | 0.022 | 0.073 | 0.080* |
| Survey date | 0.000 | – 0.047 | 0.058 | – 0.070 |
| Wave 2 | 0.024 | 0.008 | – 0.012 | 0.076* |
| Repeated response | 0.009 | – 0.013 | – 0.007 | 0.007 |
| Acquiescence | – 0.193*** | – 0.293*** | – 0.072* | – 0.206*** |
| $R^2$ | 0.090 | 0.237 | 0.157 | 0.142 |
| Functional disability | – 0.021 | – 0.018 | – 0.027 | – 0.031 |
| Adversity | 0.057 | – 0.253*** | – 0.123*** | – 0.161*** |
| $R^2$ | 0.094 | 0.293 | 0.172 | 0.167 |

*Note* Reference categories were living alone, living in rental public housing, and self-administered response

*$p < 0.05$, **$p < 0.01$, ***$p < 0.001$

Some personal backgrounds indicated their effects on self-awareness specific to the youth, mid-ager, and elder. Specific to the youth were the positive effects of living with parents ($\beta = 0.093$, see Table 3.14) and the negative effect of living in a divided private flat ($\beta = -0.090$). As such, youth strengthened the contribution of living with parents and the divided private flat. Unique to the mid-ager was the positive effect of private housing ($\beta = 0.103$). Hence, mid-age sustained the contribution of private housing to self-awareness. Distinctive to the elder was the negative effect of age on self-awareness ($\beta = -0.101$). Accordingly, old age turned the age effect negative, reflecting the aging decline.

## *Resilience Belief*

Analysis of data from the resilience study revealed seven significant personal background effects generally on resilience belief. On the one hand, positive effects arose from age ($\beta = 0.123$, see Table 3.15), education ($\beta = 0.113$), living and parents ($\beta = 0.080$) and siblings ($\beta = 0.052$), private housing ($\beta = 0.078$), and female gender ($\beta = 0.069$). On the other hand, adversity ($\beta = -0.153$) displayed a negative effect on resilience belief. The analysis controlled for such response characteristics as acquiescence ($\beta = -0.178$) and interviewing ($\beta = 0.150$).

Some personal backgrounds indicated their effects on resilience belief specific to the youth, mid-ager, and elder. Specific to the youth were the positive effects of living with siblings ($\beta = 0.082$, see Table 3.15). As such, youth highlighted the contribution of living with siblings. Unique to the mid-ager were the positive effect of private housing ($\beta = 0.088$) and female gender ($\beta = 0.131$). Hence, mid-age facilitated the contribution of private housing and female gender to resilience belief. Distinctive to the elder was the positive effect of owned public housing on resilience belief ($\beta = 0.085$). Accordingly, old age enhanced the contribution of owned public housing.

Analysis of data from the resilience study revealed five significant personal background effects generally on benevolent world belief as an associate of resilience belief. On the one hand, positive effects arose from age ($\beta = 0.171$, see Table 3.16), living and parents ($\beta = 0.101$), and female gender ($\beta = 0.065$). On the other hand, adversity ($\beta = -0.146$) and functional disability ($\beta = -0.067$) exhibited negative effects on benevolent world belief. The analysis controlled for such response characteristics as acquiescence ($\beta = -0.265$).

Some personal backgrounds indicated their effects on benevolent world belief specific to the elder. These effects were positive from age ($\beta = 0.137$, see Table 3.16), living in owned public housing ($\beta = 0.067$), living in a hostel ($\beta = 0.081$), and family income per capita ($\beta = 0.064$). As such, old age consolidated the contributions of age, living conditions, and family income.

**Table 3.15** Standardized effects on resilience belief (service dataset)

| Predictor | Youth | Mid-age | Elder | All |
|---|---|---|---|---|
| Living with the spouse | 0.011 | 0.042 | – 0.020 | 0.019 |
| Living with offspring | 0.022 | 0.015 | – 0.013 | 0.024 |
| Living with siblings | 0.082* | 0.057 | 0.021 | 0.052* |
| Living with parents | 0.048 | 0.065 | 0.040 | 0.080* |
| Living with other relatives | 0.024 | – 0.045 | 0.042 | – 0.015 |
| Education | 0.070 | 0.164*** | 0.079* | 0.113*** |
| Family size | – 0.073 | – 0.001 | 0.056 | 0.001 |
| Owned public housing | – 0.005 | – 0.003 | 0.085* | 0.028 |
| Private housing | 0.067 | 0.088* | 0.071 | 0.078** |
| Hostel | – 0.076* | 0.015 | 0.068* | – 0.007 |
| Divided private flat | – 0.053 | 0.051 | 0.006 | 0.013 |
| Age | – 0.005 | 0.058 | 0.063 | 0.123* |
| Female | 0.055 | 0.131** | – 0.017 | 0.069** |
| Earnings | 0.038 | – 0.071 | – 0.033 | – 0.010 |
| Family income per capita | 0.036 | – 0.001 | 0.000 | 0.010 |
| Survey assisted by fellows | 0.009 | – 0.029 | – | – 0.001 |
| Survey assisted by service workers | – 0.003 | – 0.046 | 0.006 | – 0.023 |
| Interviewed | 0.024 | 0.032 | 0.127** | 0.150** |
| Survey date | 0.012 | – 0.074 | 0.180 | 0.038 |
| Wave 2 | – 0.044 | – 0.084 | – 0.082 | – 0.037 |
| Repeated response | 0.008 | 0.042 | 0.028 | 0.024 |
| Acquiescence | – 0.121*** | – 0.270*** | – 0.109*** | – 0.178*** |
| $R^2$ | 0.092 | 0.246 | 0.192 | 0.285 |
| Functional disability | – 0.032 | 0.006 | – 0.007 | – 0.031 |
| Adversity | – 0.098** | – 0.187*** | – 0.212*** | – 0.153*** |
| $R^2$ | 0.103 | 0.275 | 0.230 | 0.308 |

*Note* Reference categories were living alone, living in rental public housing, and self-administered response

*$p < 0.05$, **$p < 0.01$, ***$p < 0.001$

## *Resilience Exposure*

Analysis of data from the resilience study revealed two significant personal background effects generally on exposure to resilience demand. Accordingly, age ($\beta =$

**Table 3.16** Standardized effects on benevolent world belief (service dataset)

| Predictor | Youth | Mid-age | Elder | All |
|---|---|---|---|---|
| Living with the spouse | – 0.016 | 0.028 | – 0.048 | – 0.010 |
| Living with offspring | – 0.018 | 0.000 | – 0.065 | 0.005 |
| Living with siblings | 0.017 | 0.009 | – 0.021 | – 0.008 |
| Living with parents | 0.066 | 0.026 | 0.005 | 0.101** |
| Living with other relatives | 0.000 | – 0.015 | – 0.006 | – 0.032 |
| Education | 0.052 | 0.059 | 0.009 | 0.045 |
| Family size | – 0.077* | 0.011 | 0.092* | – 0.003 |
| Owned public housing | – 0.054 | – 0.033 | 0.067* | – 0.018 |
| Private housing | 0.030 | 0.061 | 0.006 | 0.038 |
| Hostel | – 0.008 | – 0.014 | 0.081* | 0.000 |
| Divided private flat | – 0.096** | 0.025 | – 0.002 | – 0.004 |
| Age | 0.022 | 0.036 | 0.137*** | 0.171*** |
| Female | 0.095** | 0.092* | – 0.036 | 0.065** |
| Earnings | 0.044 | – 0.066 | – 0.028 | – 0.001 |
| Family income per capita | 0.050 | – 0.008 | 0.064* | 0.033 |
| Survey assisted by fellows | 0.008 | – 0.001 | – | 0.005 |
| Survey assisted by service workers | – 0.025 | – 0.004 | – 0.009 | – 0.013 |
| Interviewed | 0.000 | 0.021 | 0.042 | 0.084 |
| Survey date | 0.068 | – 0.038 | 0.068 | – 0.006 |
| Wave 2 | – 0.022 | – 0.055 | – 0.022 | 0.010 |
| Repeated response | 0.035 | 0.000 | 0.011 | 0.013 |
| Acquiescence | – 0.159*** | – 0.363*** | – 0.252*** | – 0.265*** |
| $R^2$ | 0.104 | 0.262 | 0.311 | 0.301 |
| Functional disability | – 0.038 | – 0.074 | – 0.030 | – 0.067** |
| Adversity | – 0.100** | – 0.185*** | – 0.185*** | – 0.146*** |
| $R^2$ | 0.115 | 0.299 | 0.508 | 0.328 |

*Note* Reference categories were living alone, living in rental public housing, and self-administered response

*$p < 0.05$, **$p < 0.01$, ***$p < 0.001$

– 0.101, see Table 3.17) and adversity ($\beta = 0.061$) showed negative effects. The analysis controlled for such response characteristics as acquiescence ($\beta = 0.081$).

Some personal backgrounds indicated their effects on exposure to resilience demand specific to the youth, mid-ager, and elder. Specific to the youth was the negative effects of living in a hostel ($\beta = – 0.090$, see Table 3.17). As such, youth

**Table 3.17** Standardized effects on resilience demand (service dataset)

| Predictor | Youth | Mid-age | Elder | All |
|---|---|---|---|---|
| Living with the spouse | – 0.068 | 0.034 | – 0.035 | 0.005 |
| Living with offspring | – 0.047 | 0.026 | – 0.020 | – 0.007 |
| Living with siblings | 0.023 | 0.005 | 0.007 | 0.013 |
| Living with parents | – 0.036 | 0.012 | 0.018 | 0.002 |
| Living with other relatives | 0.034 | 0.056 | – 0.080 | – 0.020 |
| Education | – 0.019 | 0.011 | – 0.035 | – 0.001 |
| Family size | 0.011 | 0.001 | – 0.008 | 0.017 |
| Owned public housing | – 0.065 | 0.016 | 0.000 | – 0.026 |
| Private housing | 0.041 | – 0.021 | – 0.083* | – 0.034 |
| Hostel | – 0.090* | 0.103* | 0.034 | 0.029 |
| Divided private flat | 0.025 | 0.012 | 0.029 | 0.025 |
| Age | 0.060 | – 0.083 | – 0.041 | – 0.101* |
| Female | 0.003 | – 0.011 | – 0.060 | 0.000 |
| Earnings | – 0.007 | 0.084* | – 0.058 | 0.031 |
| Family income per capita | 0.057 | – 0.008 | 0.056 | 0.039 |
| Survey assisted by fellows | 0.000 | 0.006 | – | 0.005 |
| Survey assisted by service workers | 0.000 | – 0.029 | – 0.026 | – 0.010 |
| Interviewed | – 0.022 | 0.001 | 0.044 | 0.036 |
| Survey date | – 0.053 | – 0.071 | – 0.175 | – 0.045 |
| Wave 2 | 0.014 | 0.016 | 0.134 | 0.010 |
| Repeated response | – 0.004 | 0.099* | 0.015 | 0.027 |
| Acquiescence | 0.049 | – 0.025 | 0.166*** | 0.081** |
| $R^2$ | 0.041 | 0.118 | 0.110 | 0.114 |
| Functional disability | 0.010 | 0.064 | – 0.041 | 0.006 |
| Adversity | – 0.056 | – 0.043 | – 0.042 | – 0.061** |
| $R^2$ | 0.044 | 0.122 | 0.113 | 0.117 |

*Note* Reference categories were living alone, living in rental public housing, and self-administered response
*$p < 0.05$, **$p < 0.01$, ***$p < 0.001$

turned the hostel effect negative. By contrast, living in a hostel ($\beta = 0.103$) and earnings ($\beta = 0.084$) displayed positive effects on exposure to resilience demand in the mid-ager. Hence, mid-age turned the hostel and earnings effects positive on exposure to resilience demand. Distinctive to the elder was the negative effect of private housing on exposure to resilience demand ($\beta = -0.083$). Apparently, old age foregrounded the isolation effect of private housing.

## *Age Effects*

Age displayed inconsistent effects on the resilience process, including feeling, action, belief, and exposure. The effects were positive and negative on resilience feeling, positive on resilience action and belief, and negative on exposure to resilience demand. Thus, the negative effect of age is noteworthy for diminishing power, utility, ideals, and norms for resilience from the voluntaristic perspective of analytical functionalism. Such an inverse effect would offset the positive effect of age based on increasing power, utility, ideals, and norms for resilience. Notably, the negative effect primarily applied to resilience feeling and exposure.

Power for resilience declining with age arises from assimilation, accommodation, communication, controlling future orientation, information searching, knowledge acquisition, physical function, and self-esteem (Charles and Carstensen 2008; Frazier et al. 2007; Morgan and Robinson 2013). The decline has also arisen from increasing illness and negative affect with age (Alea et al. 2004; Schaie 2013). Conversely, power for resilience declining with age has involved achievement need, cognitive ability, emotional intelligence, exploring, functioning, future goal setting, income, marriage, meaning search, memory, motivation, openness, optimizing, rationality, responsibility, sleeping, social integration, sporting, and tolerance (Freund 2006; Howe 2010; Penningroth and Scott 2012; Ferssizidis et al. 2010; Gerstorf et al. 2006; Goerres 2007; Karuza et al. 1990; Ruffman et al. 2016; Isaacowitz et al. 2003; Inglehart 2003; Larrick et al. 1993; Marcum 2013; Plagnol and Easterlin 2008; Ruffman et al. 2016; Steger et al. 2009; Stevens et al. 2001; Yee 2006). Sleep is a basis for health (Dregan and Armstrong 2009). Sporting has contributed to health, income, and social capital and has reduced depression (Growiec and Growiec 2010; Kunovich and Hudson 1999; Lee 2020; Luschen et al. 1996; Meeus 2019). In the youth, power for resilience has eroded with age in increasing alcoholism, anxiety, depression, distress, doping, emotionality, loneliness, regret, and victimization experienced (McCormack and Feeney 2015; Meeus 2019; Niditch and Varela 2011; van de Rakt et al. 2012; Vitaro et al. 2005; Wright et al. 2009; Zysberg 2012). Alcoholism and doping are debilitating to the youth's resilience (Wong 2008). Likewise, distress has weakened power for resilience in the youth (Tett and Wang 2005). The youth has also shown declining aspiration, attachment, bonding, and closeness to parents, care received, family relationship quality, health, social capital from parents, social support received, and task orientation with age to sustain power for resilience (Bankston and Zhou 2002b; Boyd and Yin 1996; Campbell and Eggerling-Boeck 2006; Gil and Molina 2007; Fasang et al. 2014; Schoeni and Ross 2005; Shek 2002; Stokes and Regnerus 2008; Tapia 2011; Yee et al. 1990). Such attachment, caring, social capital, and social support have been power bases for the youth's resilience (Shibue and Kasai 2014; Ungar et al. 2005). In the elder, aging means decline and deficiency (Alain et al. 2019). With increasing age, the elder's power for resilience erodes, involving cognitive ability, employment, and mastery (Alain et al. 2019; Friedman et al. 2001; Menec and Chipperfield 1997). Conversely, the elder's aging has raised fear, neuroticism, and disability and its functional form to impede power for resilience (Atchley 1999; Houts and Kassals 1997; Small et al. 2003; Sugisawa et al. 1994). In the elder, aggressiveness has increased with aging as a goal or orientation countering resilience (Cohen-Mansfield and Werner 1998). For the patient or service user, aging has eroded power for resilience based on housing quality (Biswas-Diener and Diener 2001).

Utility from resilience diminishing with age has resided in belief in social responsiveness, confidence in social institutions, and satisfaction with health and safety (Emery et al. 2015; Goerres 2007; Howe 2010). The youth has displayed eroding resilience utility derived from achievement experience and institutional trust with age (Niemi and Klingler 2012; Pong and Chen 2010). Conversely, the youth has shown decreasing resilience utility due to increasing arrest and failure experienced with age (Gil and Molina 2007; Tapia 2011). In the elder, aging has raised uncontrollability as disutility to impede resilience (Brandstadter and Baltes-Gotz 1990).

Ideals for resilience subsiding with age has included the values of independence, openness, and working (Chen and Davey 2009; Daniel et al. 2022; Davey et al. 2009; Fjellvang 2011; Howe 2010; James and Luo 1999). The youth has shown declining satisfaction with life and others, self-esteem, and values in achievement and independence with age to impede ideals for resilience (Fahmy 2006; Marsh et al. 2007; Watkins et al. 2000; Zupancic et al. 2014). Conversely, the youth has increased suicidal ideation with age as an ideal against resilience (Campbell and Eggerling-Boeck 2006).

Norms for resilience, covering family cohesion and functioning or resilience, have declined with age in the youth (Baer 2002; He et al. 2022; Shek 2002). That is, reduced family resilience would assimilate reduced personal resilience with increasing age in the youth.

Moreover, aging attenuates power, utility, ideals, and norms for exposure to resilience demand. Aging has retarded power for exposure in raising inhibition and stagnation and reducing attentional, communication, community, diversity, exploratory, search, social integration, and socializing goals or practices (Goerres 2007; Howe 2010; Isaacowitz et al. 2003; Marcum 2013; Ng et al. 2006; Stalker 2008; Steger et al. 2009; Van den Broeck et al. 2015). Conversely, aging champions the ideal or obsessions for conservatism and value in conservation, disengagement, and emotional and social distancing to reduce exposure (Charles and Carstensen 2009; Cornelis et al. 2009; Daniel et al. 2022; Marcum 2013). Hence, aging particularly impeded exposure to resilience demand.

By contrast, aging enables resilience action and belief particularly by mobilizing power, utility, ideals, and norms for them. The enabling of action has stemmed from the enhancement of controlling, coping, discriminating by aging, ecologically relevant action, environmental negotiation and protection, housework, influencing others, media use, organization activity, religious activity, self-construction or subjectivation, self-regulation, sharing, and volunteering (Angermeyer et al. 2014; Boulianne et al. 2022; Caplan and Schooler 2007; Charles and Carstensen 2009; Cheung and Chiu 2021; Datler et al. 2013; Doumas and Krampe 2015; Elvestad and Blekesaune 2008; Hamermesh 2019; Howe 2010; Inglehart 2003; Isaacowitz et al. 2003; Nussio 2019; Sarpila 2014; Schaie 2013; Tam 2014). Meanwhile, aging has increased beliefs regarding duty, conservatism, materialism, meritocracy, moralism, neoliberalism, and religiosity to boost resilience belief (Clark 2004a; Cornelis et al. 2009; Evans et al. 2010; Goerres 2007; Kurata 2015; Norris and Inglehart 2009). Herein, resilience has arisen from beliefs regarding religion (Cherry et al. 2023). Conservatism embraces attachment, balancing, conformity, discipline, flexibility, responsibility, saving, security, self-direction, and toleration as opposed to change and decay to induce resilience belief (Heilman and Kusev 2020; Kekes 1998; Scruton 2014; Sidanius and Pratto 1999; Yoos 2007). Materialism emphasizes the defense of one's interest to maintain resilience belief (Davis and Dooley 1999). Meritocracy support prizes agency, choice, control, deservingness, earning, freedom, mastery, responsibility, smartness, and striving to enhance resilience belief (Sandel 2020). Moralism accentuates divinity, dutifulness, rule abidance, and virtuousness to insist on one's resilience belief (Garner 1994). Neoliberalism dictates flexibility, freedom, meritocracy, self-interest, self-responsibility, and striving to consolidate resilience belief (Campbell 2019; Smart 2003; Zucker and Bay-Cheng 2021). Religiosity maintains certainty, dignity, divinity, faith, identity, ethicalness, sacredness, stability, and strictness to consolidate resilience belief (Donnelly 2013; Harris et al. 2018; Malka and Soto 2011; Peifer 2010; Petrovic et al. 2020; Requena and Stanek 2014; Tenorio and Lo 2011).

## *Gender Effects*

The resilience process was generally lower in the woman than in the man. The exception appeared in resilience belief, which was higher in the woman than in the man. According to the voluntarist theory of analytical functionalism, power, utility, ideals, and norms supporting resilience belief is higher in the woman than in the man. Power drives, utility attracts, ideals rationalize, and norms assimilate resilience belief. Resilience belief upholds ability, capacity, capability, or strength, coping, endurance, functioning, growth, heroism, meaningfulness, morale, opportunity, resourcefulness, social networking, social support received, and steeling for resilience (Allison et al. 2017; Huta 2017; Bowers et al. 2017; Pangallo et al. 2015; Prilleltensky 2012; Rutter 2012; Truebridge 2016; Walsh 2002; Zautra et al. 2010; Zheng et al. 2020). Conversely, resilience belief discourages disruption (Boden et al. 2014). Resilience belief builds on religious and spiritual beliefs (Cherry et al. 2023; Dwivedi 2017; Kent and Davis 2010; Taylor and Distelberg 2016).

Power higher in the woman than in the man for resilience belief transpires in language and verbal abilities (Motschenbacher 2010; Straughn and Andriot 2011). Language and verbal abilities include comprehensibility and fluency to defend and formulate resilience belief (Magi et al. 2018). Moreover, such power stems from agreeableness, attachment, commitment, endurance, expressiveness, longevity, purposefulness, and relatedness higher in the woman than in the man to sustain resilience belief (Caprara and Vecchione 2017; Diekman and Schneider 2010; Franklin 2012; Hepper et al. 2020; Hopcroft 2016; Ferssizidis et al. 2010). Attachment and relatedness have drawn power to enhance commitment (Patwardhan et al. 2019; Sharma 2003). Purposefulness has raised such power as aspiration (Morgan and Robinson 2013). Relatedness is a basis for stability (Fingerman et al. 2011).

Utility higher in the woman than in the man realized for resilience belief rests on satisfaction with democracy, government, life, and relationships, and security experienced (Hraba et al. 2001; Norris 2011; Prins et al. 1993; Tiliouine et al. 2006; van der Toorn et al. 2010). Security experienced has sustained confrontation and spirituality (Hall and Edwards 2002; Lavy et al. 2010). Conversely, utility from resilience belief has been higher in the woman than in the man when risk perceived and stress experienced has been lower in the woman than in the man (de Coster 2005; Trumbo et al. 2008). Risk perceived has impaired self-determination (Shippee 2012).

Ideals higher in the woman than in the man for resilience belief evolve from agreement, approval, religiosity, support for meritocracy and security, and values for conservation, security, and transcendence (Caprara and Vecchione 2017; Daniel et al. 2022; Evans et al. 2010; Immerzeel and van Tubergen 2013; Rentziou et al. 2011; Maule and Goidel 2003; Mondak and Hurwitz 2012). Conversely, such ideals have been higher in the woman than in the man when aggression, cynicism, and protesting have fared lower in the woman than in the man (Kirk and Papachristos 2011; Lee and Chan 2016; Lippa 2005). Aggression reflects panic (Petrou and Kandylis 2016). Such ideals have also been higher in the woman than in the man when alienation was lower in the woman than in the man (Weakliem and Borch 2006).

Norms exposed for resilience belief have been higher in the woman than in the man when the violence norms perceived have been lower in the former (Scharrer 2008). Such norms stem from higher norm conformity and obedience in the woman than in woman (Barber 2004; Fer 2012).

## *Education Effects*

Education displayed positive effects on resilience action and belief as expected, but a negative effect on resilience feeling. The latter effect reflects reduced power, utility, ideals, and norms for resilience feeling, following the voluntaristic theory of analytical functionalism. Power drives resilience feeling for the fulfillment function. Utility attracts resilience feeling for the adaptation function. Ideals rationalize resilience feeling for the latency function. Norms assimilate resilience feeling for the integration function. Resilience feeling highlights acceptance, adaptation, adjustment, bouncing back, coherence, commitment, continuation, control, development, endurance, faith, growth, functioning, homeostasis, hope, humor, improvement, maintenance, mastery, meaningfulness, morale, optimism, patience, recovery, resistance, return, robustness, stability, sustainability, tenacity, and tolerance despite adversity (Boden et al. 2014;

Bowers et al. 2017; Brodsky and Cattaneo 2013; Celinski and Allen 2017; Connor et al. 2003; Crafter et al. 2019; Greeff and van der Merwe 2004; Huta 2017; Jayawardana et al. 2019; Kent and Davis 2010; Nemeth and Olivier 2017; Pangallo et al. 2015; Peterson et al. 2008; Rutter 2012; Schwager and Rothermund 2014; Taylor and Distelberg 2016; Xie and Wong 2021; Yu and Zhang 2007; Zautra et al. 2010). Conversely, resilience feeling precludes fear and curtails disruption, loss, risk, and threat (Hariharan and Rana 2017; Kent and Davis 2010; Nemeth and Olivier 2017; Sherman and Cohen 2006). Power driving resilience feeling has stemmed from agreeableness, conscientiousness, coping, emotional intelligence and stability, learning, and mentoring and supportive services received (Armstrong et al. 2011; Buikstra et al. 2010; Corbin and Hall 2019; Lock et al. 2020; Notter et al. 2008; Yu and Zhang 2007). Utility attracting resilience feeling has rested on balance experienced and optimism (Buikstra et al. 2010; Cantor et al. 2002). Ideals rationalizing resilience feeling have covere4 purposiveness, religiosity, and self-esteem (Buikstra et al. 2010; Cherry et al. 2023; Yu and Zhang 2007). Norms assimilating resilience feelings have concerned adaptation and safety (Jones and d'Errico 2019).

Power for resilience feeling reduced by education has stemmed from personal care, recourse, self-esteem, and social trust (Gershuny 2000; Rochelle 2015; Su and Feng 2013). Conversely, education has raised depression, stagnation, and susceptibility to weaken power for resilience feeling (Ng et al. 2006; Opp 1989). Education has also fomented power by protesting to contradict the feeling of resilience (Grasso 2014). Protesting has invoked anger and worry to counter resilience feeling (Boehnke and Wong 2011; Landmann and Rohmann 2020). Conversely, protesting has eroded hope, thus impairing resilience feeling (Paez et al. 2015).

Utility from resilience feeling dampened by education has been individualist attribution, belief in collective efficacy, perception about equal opportunity, justice, social impact, and state efficiency, satisfaction with achievement and living standards, and trust in government and police (Bullock 2021; Chan 2014; Jasso 2015; Kwak et al. 2010; Larsen 2006; Perkins and Long 2002; Sikora 2005; Silbereisen et al. 2010). Conversely, education has raised aspiration, discrimination perceived, and victimization experienced to lessen utility from resilience feeling (Kluegal and Bobo 2001; Norris 2011; Pratt et al. 2010)

Ideals for resilience feeling attenuated by education have been approval, Buddhism, religiosity, support for security, and values for diligence and survival (Bullock 2021; Chen and Davey 2009; Datler et al. 2013; Immerzeel and van Tubergen 2013; Mondak and Hurwitz 2012; Tang 2009; Tang 2001; Tomas et al. 2013; Yienprugsawan et al. 2010).

Norms for resilience impeded by education have covered civility (Ferriss 2002). Conversely, education has raised the perceived norm for violence to weaken resilience feeling (Scharrer 2008).

Hence, education has fueled such feelings as depression, dissatisfaction with achievement, democracy, economic status, living standards, and nationhood, self-doubt about the family, and stagnation to weaken resilience feeling (Chen and Davey 2009; Ng et al. 2006; Norris 2011; Tiliouine et al. 2006; Yienprugsawan et al. 2010). In the youth, education has raised such feelings as anomia, identity confusion, life dissatisfaction, self-doubt about the body, and self-diffidence to dampen resilience feeling (Holden et al. 2002; Menard 1995; Liu and Chen 2010; Zhang et al. 2014). Education has also impeded development and health statuses, thus eroding resilience status (Benson et al. 2011; Kwan 2010). Similarly, in the elder, education has induced such feelings as depression, life disaffection, and loneliness to diminish resilience feeling (Bookwala 2014; van Hiel and Vansteenkiste 2009; Yang and Victor 2008). Education has also dampened the elder's health and raised the elder's mental illness, thus impeding resilience status (Helmchen et al. 1999; Sereny 2011). In the patient or service user, education has elevated distress and job dissatisfaction to impede resilience feeling (Hammer 2007; Kershaw et al. 2004). To the working person, education has impeded such feelings as happiness and satisfaction with the job and organization, thus attenuating resilience feeling (Hustinx and Handy 2009; Rego et al. 2009; Stater and Stater 2019). For the minority person, education has dampened such feelings as adjustment and life satisfaction, thus constraining resilience feeling (Harker 2001; Sellers and Neighbors 2008). Conversely, the minority person's education has fomented such feelings as depression and worry about economic conditions, thus eroding resilience feeling (Lai 2011; Wu et al. 2003). Such feelings reinforce each other through the voluntaristic mechanism of ideal consistency or rationalization to achieve the latency function.

Contrariwise, education has fostered such actions as applying skills, choosing, distancing, exercising, expressing, maintaining health, persisting, preventing, protecting, sporting, and studying to propel resilience action (Bekkers et al. 2008; Foster et al. 2001; Horowitz 2018; Leung et al. 2005; Lin et al. 2008; Mirowsky and Ross 2001; Morenoff et al. 2008; Pallas 2002; Scherger 2009; Stone and Buttice 2010; Tsai 2006). Hence, education has sustained activeness for resilience action (Yang et al. 2012). To the elder, education has generally buttressed activities to sustain resilience action (Lawton et al. 2002). More specifically, the elder's education has activated such actions as approaching, caring and self-caring, exercising, expressing, gathering information, maintaining health, planning, and studying for resilience action (Benjamins et al. 2004; Kincade et al. 1998; Krause 2010; Prenda and Lachman 2001; Reitzes and Mutran 2004; Satariano et al. 2002; Sorensen et al. 2014; Tang and Morrow-Howell 2008; Timmer and Aartsen 2003). In the youth, education has fostered such actions as elaborative processing, exercising, learning, and planning for life to facilitate resilience action (Hellevik and Settersten 2013; Jakoubek and Swenson 1993; Park et al. 2018; Tepper 2001). Conversely, the youth's education has inhibited such actions as delinquency, externalizing problems, and risking, thus safeguarding resilience action (Chui and Cheng 2017; Goldman and Peleg 2010; Reid et al. 1999). For the patient or service user, education has raised such actions as desistance from crime, exercising, vaccination, and working to foster resilience action (Coups et al. 2009; Jennings 2004; Kohlhammer et al. 2007; Lee 2009). Conversely, education in the patient or service e user has impeded such actions as abusing substances, dropping out from services, risking, and suicide, thus safeguarding resilience action (Kim and Zurlo 2007; Romanowicz et al. 2013; Rabin 2011; Ryb et al. 2006). For the working person, education has activated such actions as controlling, maintaining health, performance, planning, and self-directing to facilitate resilience action (Curl and Ingram 2013; Grzywacz and Marks 2001; Kohn et al. 1983; Roch and Sai 2015; Shane 2013). Conversely, the working person's education has prevented such actions as abusing substances, exiting work, slacking, and striking, thus buttressing resilience action (Akkerman 2013; DiPrete et al. 2001; Headey et al. 2001; Seeman and Seeman 1992). To the minority person, education has diminished such action as crime to sustain resilience action (Kaplan et al. 2002). Reinforcements among resilience and other actions build on the voluntaristic mechanism of ideal consistency or rationalization to secure the latency function.

Education has fostered such beliefs in capitalism, deliberation, democracy, duty, equity, freedom, maturity, and self-interest to consolidate resilience belief (Gibson 2013; Hraba et al. 2001; Jacobs et al. 2009; Reeskens and van Oorschot 2013; Van Oorschot 2000; Velladics et al. 2006; Weimann and Brosius 1994; Welzel 2013). Capitalism favors beliefs in earning, individualism, rationalization, and self-interest to propel resilience belief (Bernstein 2012). Individualism hails beliefs in achievement and success, character development, choice, competition, freedom, independence, reasoning, responsibility, restlessness, self-construction, self-development, self-interest, self-worth, and working to underlie resilience belief (Braun 2011; Davis and Robinson 1999; Fevre 2006; Norris and Inglehart 2009; Oyserman et al. 2002; Speed et al. 2018; Sullivan et al. 2015; Sun and Wang 2010). Democracy necessitates beliefs in agency, assertiveness, autonomy, argumentation, choice, competition, confrontation, criticalness, deliberation, independence, inquiry, negotiation, rationality, reasoning, responsibility, self-cultivation, self-determination, self-development, struggle, tolerance, and working to achieve resilience belief (Blokker 2018; Caciagli 2003; Caprara and Vecchione 2017; Christians et el. 2009; Fishkin 2018; Festenstein 2010; King 2008; Levi 2003; Kim 2018; Minogue 2010; O'Neill 2000; Peng et al. 2017; Ringen 2007; Steiner 2012; Talisse 2009; Warren 2011). Belief in equity emphasizes exchange, negotiation, and trading to guide resilience belief (Skitka et al. 2915). Meanwhile, belief in freedom or liberalism cherishes agency, authenticity, autonomy, choice, competition, creativity, criticalness, empowerment, innovation, inquiry, negotiation, openness, rationality, self-realization, and tolerance to sustain resilience belief (Gustavsson 2012; Delanty 2009; Flanagan and Lee 2003; Morriss 2009; Ramsay 1997; Scruton 2014; Yoos 2007). Maturity encompasses autonomy, conscientiousness, discipline, hope, openness, persistence, stability, and vigor facilitating resilience belief (Hendry and Kloep 2012; van Scheppingen et al. 2016). Education also secures such beliefs as expressivism, humanism, individualism, liberalism, and meritocratism to buttress resilience belief (Evans et al. 2010; Sotirovic 2000; Welzel 2013; Yuchtman-Yaar 2002). Humanism champions beliefs in agency, argumentation, autonomy, authenticity, choice, conflict resolution, creativity, criticalness, freedom, independence, intelligence, isolation, knowledge, rationality, reasoning, self-control, self-improvement, self-realization, survival, toleration, vitality, voicing, and working to foster resilience belief (Browning and Cooper 2004; Doane 2017; Fuchs 2020; Selznick 2008; Visher 1997; Waterman 2013). Education furthermore upholds values for autonomy, independence, reasoning, and working to rationalize resilience belief (Armon and Dawson 2003; Fjellvang 2011;

James and Luo 1999; Xiao 2000). Hence, resilience and other beliefs reinforce each other according to the voluntaristic mechanism of ideal consistency or rationalization to secure the latency function.

# Chapter 4
# Societal Impacts on Resilience

**Abstract** This Chapter critically attempts to gauge societal impacts on individual resilience and thus the involuntary basis, infeasibility, and unreasonableness of resilience. Societal impacts examined were those of caring, social exclusion, peace, violence, and pragmatism perceived in society and social inclusion experienced. Notably, pragmatism is relevant to resilience because it furnishes the orientation toward solving problems or tackling adversities. These impacts reflect the deterministic mechanisms of the analytical-functionalist framework. Analysis of poverty survey data on the public showed that caring in society had a significant and strong positive effect on resilience, and social exclusion in society exerted a significant and strong negative effect on resilience. Moreover, social inclusion experienced did not manifest a significant effect on resilience. That is, the effects of caring and social exclusion in society preempted the effect of social inclusion experienced. Meanwhile, analysis of violence survey data on the public revealed that pragmatism in society, but not peace and violence in society, exerted a significant inverse effect on resilience. Overall, the significant societal impacts reflect the deterministic force on resilience. This force demonstrates the social influences on resilience.

Societal impacts evolve from societal conditions, including caring, social inclusion, social exclusion, peace, violence, pragmatism, and Westernization. The impacts also stem from different societies, including Guangzhou, Hong Kong, and Macau in China. Society refers to an enduring human institution achieving the functions of goal attainment or fulfillment, adaptation, integration, and latency or pattern maintenance, predicated on analytical functionalism. The fulfillment function relies on authority, constitution, government, justice, and law (Campbell 1981; Krossa 2013; MacKay 2017; Scaff 2014). The function of adaptation unfolds in exchange or trading, healthcare, industry, science, and technology (Campbell 1981; MacKay 2017; Schroeder 2013). The function of integration features in autonomy, charity, civil society, media, and mores (Ardalan 2016, Campbell 1981; Krossa 2013; Neuhouser 2000; Scaff 2014; Schroeder 2013). Civil society functions to consolidate association, charity, civility, compassion, cooperation, discipline, equality, esteem, freedom, harmony, justice, mutuality, networking, partnership, respect, responsibility, rights, social



C. K. Cheung, *Resilience Process and Its Personal and Social Bases*,
https://doi.org/10.1007/978-981-97-7391-6_4

capital, social movements, solidarity, tolerance, and volunteerism (DeLue and Dale 2009; Novak 2001; O'Mahony 2013; Powell 2007; Teets 2014). The function of latency engages civilization, education, and religion (Campbell 1981; Krossa 2013; Morody and Giza-Poleszczuk 2018).

Societal care, inclusion, peace, pragmatism, and Westernization are likely to foster personal resilience, whereas societal exclusion and violence are likely to disturb personal resilience. Such fostering and disturbing hinge on the direct and indirect deterministic mechanisms of analytical functionalism. Direct mechanisms comprise sharing privately and vicariously, whereas indirect mechanisms engage mediation by voluntaristic mechanisms. The engagement is fourfold. For the fulfillment function, the indirect deterministic mechanism of empowering activates the voluntaristic mechanism of power realization. Power, capability, capital, resources, or strength for resilience has stemmed from future orientation, grouping, learning, mentoring received, purposiveness, services received, relational aspiration, religiosity, self-esteem, sensation seeking, and social support received (Buikstra et al. 2010; Cherry et al. 2023; Corbin and Hall 2019; Lou et al. 2018; McKay et al. 2018; Notter et al. 2008; Yu and Zhang 2007). Conversely, power for resilience has diminished due to trauma experienced (Cherry et al. 2023). For the adaptation function, the indirect deterministic mechanism of incentivizing entrains the voluntaristic mechanism of utility optimization. Utility attracting resilience has included optimism (Buikstra et al. 2010). For the integration function, the indirect deterministic mechanism of normalizing or standardizing triggers the voluntaristic mechanism of norm conformity. Norms for resilience have upheld balancing and innovation (Cantor et al. 2002; Sawyers et al. 2020). For the latency function, the indirect deterministic mechanism of framing or signifying ignites the voluntaristic mechanism of ideal consistency. Ideals for resilience have included agreeableness, balancing, coping, distancing from adversity, emotional stability, humor, openness, and problem-solving (Corbin and Hall 2019; Lock et al. 2020; McKay et al. 2018; Notter et al. 2008; Yu and Zhang 2007).

## Existing Knowledge

Existing knowledge drawn from research findings and theorizing explains the impacts of societal conditions on personal resilience. These conditions include caring, social inclusion, social exclusion, peace, violence, pragmatism, and Westernization. Moreover, the three Chinese societies of Guangzhou, Hong Kong, and Macau make a difference in personal resilience.

## *Societal Care*

Societal care is likely to raise personal resilience through direct and indirect deterministic and voluntaristic mechanisms. Direct deterministic mechanisms engage care sharing privately and vicariously. Herein, care features altruism, compassion, empathy, protection, and service (Kent and Davis 2010; Mukherjee and Kumar 2017). Care shared privately or personally has fostered resilience (Buikstra et al. 2010; Cherry et al. 2023). Alternatively, care shared vicariously or in others without personal access has also raised resilience (Jones and d'Errico 2019). Additionally, indirect deterministic mechanisms provide power for empowering, incentives for incentivizing, norms for normalizing or standardizing, and ideals for framing or signifying. Furthermore, voluntaristic mechanisms reflected in awareness about societal care collaborate with indirect deterministic mechanisms to champion resilience. Voluntaristic mechanisms hinge on power, utility, norms, and ideals underlying the awareness to engender resilience.

Power, capital, or resources generated by societal care for empowering personal resilience rests on attachment and security, friendship or friendliness, helpfulness, meanings, purposes, self-efficacy, self-esteem or mattering, social control or regulation, social integration, social support reception, and togetherness (Feeney and Collins 2018; Filip et al. 2006; Ganster and Victor 1988; Godoy et al. 2007; Hofferth et al. 1999; Holliman et al. 2021; Makarios and Sams 2013; Thoits 2011). Attachment and security can foster discovery and independence to empower resilience, especially when under distress or when there is a need in the person (Feeney and Collins 2018). Togetherness can facilitate coping to strengthen resilience (Feeney and Collins 2018). Societal care can work as a regulation to empower resilience, particularly collectively, through social interaction, conversation, and gossip (Feeney and Collins 2018; Lakey and Orehek 2011). Moreover, societal care has strengthened community attachment and identification, competence, functioning, health, medical service use, purposefulness, recourse, relational quality, self-efficacy, self-esteem, social capital, and social trust as power bases for empowering personal resilience (Bishop et al. 2002; Bloom et al. 1991; Gorman et al. 2010; Kasen et al. 2006; Kim et al. 2012; Klein and Milardo 2000; Kouzis and Eaton 1998; Logan and Cobb 2013; Navarra et al. 2018; Palmer et al. 2011; Schwarzer and Knoll 2007; Young and Willmont 1957). Conversely, societal care has diminished symptoms, thus empowering personal resilience (Glendinning et al. 2003).

Incentives created by societal care for incentivizing personal resilience are fairness or fair exchange, hope, optimism, and life and relational satisfaction for resilience (Harber et al. 2005; Turner 2013). Accordingly, societal care is a return to meet personal dependence to incentivize resilience (Turner 2013).

Ideals highlighted by societal care for framing personal resilience include acceptance, care or flexibility, prevention problem-solving, responsiveness, sensitivity, tolerance for or openness to adversity or suffering (Biglan 2018, Biglan and Prinz 2017; Binder et al. 2012; Collins et al. 2011; Davis-Lipman et al. 2007; Feeney and Collins 2018; Harber et al. 2005; Lakey and Orehek 2011; Patulny and Morris

2012; Stewart 1989). Accordingly, responsiveness and satisfaction represent ideals to frame resilience (Feeney and Collins 2018; Lakey and Orehek 2011). Moreover, societal care has generated such ideals as autonomous motivation, control, coping, forgiveness, health maintenance, persistence, planning, pleasure, self-determination to frame personal resilience (Holliman et al. 2021; Hui et al. 2013; Lincoln et al. 2003; Peterson and Seligman 2004; Pierce and Quiroz 2018; Prenda and Lachman 2001; Schwarzer and Knoll 2007; Thrasher et al. 2004; Walen and Lachman 2016; Williams et al. 2006; Xi and Hwang 2011). Coping raised by societal coping has included problem-solving and religious approaches (Goodwin et al. 2001; Pargament et al. 2011). Health maintenance elevated by societal care included exercising (Cerin and Leslie 2008). Conversely, societal care has alleviated anger, anxiety, avoidance, depression, distress, substance abuse, suicide, and unemployment, thus lessening framing ideals against resilience (Besser and Priel 2008; Brown and Zoorob 2022; Dutton et al. 2016; Kafetsio and Sideridis 2006; Krug and Prechsl 2020; Lee and Robbins 1998; Lowe et al. 2009; Ozbay 2008).

Norms shared by societal care for normalizing personal resilience have registered societal civility, social integration, success, and wellness (Garcia and Herrero 2004; Greeff and van der Merwe 2004; Paez et al. 2007; Pavlova and Silbereisen 2015). Such normalizing work through social comparison and interaction (Coulson 2019; Ganster and Victor 1988; Helgeson 2003). Conversely, societal care prevented anomie or normlessness and such norms as societal alienation, disconfirmation, illness, problems, and stress normalizing against resilience (Grundy and Sloggett 2003; Kendler et al. 2006; Levitt et al. 1994; Myer et al. 2008; Ross and Mirowsky 1989; Stewart 1989).

Power reflected in awareness of societal care to drive resilience rests on affordance and attachment (Bloom et al. 1991; Collins et al. 2011; Coulson 2019). Affordance to learn about societal care covers adaptation, connection, exploration, narration, and self-presentation to secure power (Coulson 2019). Attachment facilitates safety and security and supports reception to attain power (Collins et al. 2011). Furthermore, societal care awareness has reflected such power bases as bonding, education, employment, health and mental health, income, marriage, organizational affiliation, pleasure, safety, social capital, social class, and social networking including friendship and organizational connection to enable resilience (Binder et al. 2012; Lennartsson 2010; Marti et al. 2017; Mata and Pendakur 2014; Mitchell and Moos 1984; Patulny and Morris 2012; Pena-Lopez and Sanchez-Santos 2016; Wetterbeng 2007). Conversely, societal care awareness has reflected freedom from isolation and psychiatric disorders disabling resilience (Magliano et al. 2006; Viry et al. 2009).

Utility reflected in societal care awareness to attract resilience has resided in distributive and procedural justice perceived (Davis-Lipman et al. 2007). Justice perceived has buttressed accommodation, health, life satisfaction, and self-esteem (Bjornskov et al. 2013; Dalbert 2001; Lipkus and Bissonette 1998; Lucas et al. 2013; Pena-Lopez and Sanchez-Santos 2016). Conversely, justice perceived has reduced anger, depression, and ruminating (Benson and Ritter 1990; Dalbert 1998; Rothmund et al. 2014).

Societal care awareness has diminished fatalism as an ideal inhibiting resilience (Goodwin et al. 2001). Fatalism has sprung from low education and income, thus lacking power to sustain resilience (Bynner and Parsons 2002; Speed et al. 2018).

## *Societal Inclusion*

Societal inclusion is likely to lift personal resilience through direct and indirect deterministic and voluntaristic mechanisms. Direct deterministic mechanisms spread inclusion privately and publicly so that societal members can experience inclusion personally and vicariously. Herein, inclusion characterizes resilience featuring acceptance (Pangallo et al. 2015). Inclusion experienced personally has elevated resilience (Corbin and Hall 2019). Moreover, indirect deterministic mechanisms provide power for empowering, incentives for incentivizing, norms for normalizing or standardizing, and ideals for framing or signifying. Additionally, voluntaristic mechanisms reflected in awareness about societal inclusion collaborate with indirect deterministic mechanisms to prop resilience. Voluntaristic mechanisms apply power, utility, norms, and ideals reflected in the awareness to sustain resilience. These mechanisms additionally operate when societal inclusion raises social inclusion experienced personally.

Based on the deterministic mechanism, power inherent in societal inclusion to empower personal resilience emanates from cooperation (Graeff and Svendsen 2013). Furthermore, societal inclusion can set the developmental goal to empower or motivate personal resilience (Poku and Whitman 2011). Societal inclusion can also foster economic and environmental or natural (capital) development, production, and public resources to facilitate personal resilience (Foster et al. 2001; Fukuyama 1999; Milner 2002; Pretty and Ward 2001). Such development hinges on synergy and transaction cost reduction through societal inclusion (Foster et al. 2001; Pretty and Ward 2001; Varda 2011). Furthermore, societal inclusion secures power bases to empower resilience by embracing associational affiliation and activism, bonding and bridging social capital including social trust, caring and compassion, communitarianism, community building and services, education, empowerment, housing, institutionalization, mutual aid, networking, proximity, social integration, solidarity, therapy, volunteering, and welfare (Bailey 2005; Dwyer and Guiso et al. 2004; Hardill 2011; Hileman et al. 2018; Lie et al. 2009; Norris 2002; Pawson 2002; Paz-Fuchs 2008; Percival 2009; Raffo and Gunter 2008; Ridley-Duff 2007; Varda 2011; Wearing 2011; Williams and Windebanh 2000; Wong 2007; Zhong 2009). Moreover, societal inclusion has sustained neighborhood quality and health and trust in government and medicine to empower personal resilience (Ahern and Hendryx 2003; Han et al. 2017; Fujisawa et al. 2009; Olson et al. 2016). Societal inclusion has also built on societal education, empowerment, homeownership, government quality, and stability as power bases to empower resilience (Coffe and Geys 2006; Cummings 2000; Petro 2001; Puntscher et al. 2016).

Based on the deterministic mechanism, incentives embraced by societal inclusion to incentivize personal resilience encompass and stand on justice (Raffo and

Gunter 2008; Munch 2012; Semenova et al. 2020), justice has buttressed such resilience rewards or utility as belongingness, health, life satisfaction, and self-esteem (Bjornskov et al. 2013; Dalbert 2001; Lucas et al. 2013; van Prooijen et al. 2008). Conversely, justice has lessened such disutility as anger and depression (Benson and Ritter 1990; Rothmund et al. 2014). Societal inclusion has also benefitted from the societal incentive for social capital construction to incentivize resilience (Petro 2001).

Based on the deterministic mechanism, ideals buttressed by societal inclusion to frame personal resilience include acceptance and openness (Bailey 2005; Semenova et al. 2020). Conversely, societal inclusion prevents crime as an obsession that hinders resilience (Coffe and Geys 2006; Zhong 2009). Crime opposes such resilience ideals as order, protection, responsibility, safety, self-control, stability, and tolerance (de Castro-Rodrigues and Sacau 2015; Wright and DeLisi 2016). Moreover, societal inclusion has raised satisfaction with life and the neighborhood and success experience to frame resilience (Cramm et al. 2012; Furstenberg and Hughes 1995; Sampson 1991). Success incorporates such resilience ideals as order, stability, and survival (Chung 2000; Craig et al. 2020; Furstenberg and Hughes 1995). Conversely, societal inclusion has prevented personal violence as an ideal frame against resilience (Wright et al. 2015). Contrary to resilience, violence means destruction, disruption, incompliance, painfulness, and tension (Farrington 2007; Murer and Schwarze 2022; Nassauer 2019; Pulkkinen 2018).

Based on the deterministic mechanism, norms upheld in societal inclusion to normalize personal resilience arise from societal or community resilience, continuity, competitiveness, coordination, responsibility, and working (Alexiadou 2002; Glendinning 2008; Jones et al. 2011; Long and Bramham 2006; Ungar 2011). Such normalizing hinges on reducing anomie or normlessness to sustain resilience (Munch 2012). Additionally, societal inclusion stands on energy, fame, health, and tolerance norms to normalize personal resilience (Fox 1996; Norris 2002; Zhong 2009).

Based on the voluntaristic mechanism, power or resources raised by social inclusion to drive resilience stem from aautonomy, belongingness, health, marriage, social status, and social support received (Dinerstein 2010; Wilson 2000; Wilson and Musick 1997; Rippl et al. 2010; Skerkat and Ellison 1999; Steinkamp and Kelly 1987). Conversely, power raised by social inclusion reduces poverty and thus its impedance to resilience (Dinerstein 2010). Social inclusion also embraces social attachment and closeness, collaboration, connection, friendship, networking, production or working, and trust to breed power to drive resilience (Chan et al. 2014; Isham et al. 2006; Lineres 2004; Myers 1999; Stolz 2011; Tindall and Wellman 2001). Additionally, social inclusion has diminished depression, thus sustaining power to drive resilience (Mullins and Dugan 1991). Moreover, social inclusion builds on employment, knowledge, resources, and social capital as power to prop resilience (Stolz 2011; Gundert and Hohendanner 2015; Naveed and Wang 2021; Tsai 2006). Social inclusion has also built on education, employment, friendship, health and mental health, income, marriage, organizational membership, pleasure, resources, security, social support received, and wealth as power bases to drive resilience (Chan et al. 2014; Frei et al. 2009; Gundert and Hohendanner 2015; Lizardo 2006; Molm

2008; Myers 1999). Conversely, social inclusion has reflected low anger, depression, deprivation, disability, discrimination, stress experienced to retain power to drive resilience (Chan et al. 2014; Garcia and Herrero 2004; Gundert and Hohendanner 2015; Molm 2008).

Based on the voluntaristic mechanism, utility generated by social inclusion to attract resilience covers reciprocity (Wong et al. 2011). Conversely, social inclusion lessens punishment as disutility, which impedes resilience (Hammer et al. 2009). Moreover, social inclusion depends on rewards received as utility to attract resilience (Tyler et al. 1997). Conversely, social inclusion has hinged on low risk to sustain utility to attract resilience (Hammer et al. 2009).

Based on the voluntaristic mechanism, ideals fostered by social inclusion to ratio nalize resilience emphasize voluntariness (Gerometta et al. 2005). Voluntariness cherishes control, engagement, self-regulation, and vitality to align with resilience (Cosme and Berkman 2018; Emirbayer and Mische 1998; Pfundmair and Mahr 2022; Sieber et al. 2019). Moreover, social inclusion has depended on harmony as an ideal to rationalize resilience (Chan et al. 2014). Harmony embraces adjustment, attunement, balance, coherence, control, mindfulness, order, peace, safety, stability, and well-being to induce resilience (Arat and Kerelian 2019; Kjell et al. 2016).

Based on the voluntaristic mechanism, norms created by social inclusion to assimilate resilience concern prosperity or development (Semenova et al. 2020). Prosperity generally registers happiness, satisfaction, and well-being, as opposed to crisis constitutes norms to induce resilience (Peet and Hatwick 2009; Wolff and Resnick 2012). Conversely, social inclusion has rested on lacking the stress norm, thus sustaining resilience (Garcia and Herrero 2004).

## *Societal Exclusion*

Societal exclusion is likely to impede personal resilience. Such exclusion has resulted from inadequate resilience (Maltby et al. 2019). The impedance can engage direct and indirect deterministic and voluntaristic mechanisms in analytical functionalism. Direct deterministic mechanisms share exclusion privately and publicly to affect resilience personally and vicariously. Herein, the exclusion contradicts resilience characterized by acceptance (Pangallo et al. 2015). Indirect deterministic mechanisms provide power to empower, incentives to incentivize, norms to normalize, and ideals to frame personal resilience through voluntaristic mechanisms. Voluntaristic mechanisms hinge on power to drive, utility to attract, norms to assimilate, and ideals to rationalize resilience.

Power, capability, or resources reduced by societal exclusion operate through abandoning, deprivation, discrimination, disorganization, segregation, and stigmatization (Bask 2005; Gallie 2004; Kane 2019; Peruzzi 2014; Reardon and Bischoff 2011; Wacquant 2008). Consequently, societal exclusion induces anxiety, difficulty, distress, fear, isolation, painfulness, poverty, unemployment, violence experienced, and welfare dependence to weaken power for empowering resilience (Backman and

Nilsson 2011; Bask 2005; Buck 2001; Botti and D'Ippoliti 2014; Delanty 2008; Gallie 2004; MacDonald and Leary 2005; Maltby et al. 2019; Stanley et al. 2011; Takahashi et al. 2015). Conversely, societal exclusion disrupts attachment, belongingness, creativity, education, employment, health, housing, knowledge, meaning redefining, production, safety, security, services received, social capital, social proximity, social status, trust, and well-being as power bases for resilience (Backman and Nilsson 2011; Botti and D'Ippoliti 2014; Kane 2019; Lin et al. 2013; Maxwell et al. 2013; Peruzzi 2014; Phillips 2006; Reicher et al. 2010). Moreover, societal exclusion has raised negative mood to weaken power to empower resilience (Williams et al. 2000). Conversely, societal exclusion has impaired deliberation or reasoning to diminish power to empower resilience (Guillen et al. 2011). Additionally, societal exclusion arises from competition, conflict, deviance, and exploitation to deprive or drain power to empower resilience (Leary and Cottrell 2013). Conversely, societal exclusion reflects low education, resources, and solidarity to weaken power to empower resilience (Backman and Nilsson 2011; Gallie 2004; Long and Bramham 2006). Furthermore, societal exclusion has stemmed from inadequate conscientiousness, emotional well-being, employment, fluency, health and mental health, income, knowledge, marriage, safety, savings, and social status to reduce power for empowering resilience (Backman and Nilsson 2011; Buck 2001; Lin et al. 2013; Maltby et al. 2019; Pachankis et al. 2020; Peruzzi 2014; Ross and Mirowsky 2009; Secker et al. 2009; Wojcieszak and Mutz 2009). Conscientiousness facilitates cautiousness, control, dependability, and planning (Roberts et al. 2009). Moreover, conscientiousness has enhanced attachment, autonomy, life satisfaction, mastery, purposefulness, and self-acceptance (Fraley et al. 2011; Hounkpatin et al. 2015). Conversely, societal exclusion has resulted from alcoholism, deprivation, economic hardship, poverty, psychopathology, and other problems weakening power for empowering resilience (Backman and Nilsson 2011; Dhal et al. 2008; Peruzzi 2014; Ross and Mirowsky 2009). Alcoholism has fomented illness, injury, and pathology, thus disempowering (Brotchie et al. 2004; Haapanen-Niemi et al. 1999).

Incentives reduced by societal exclusion for incentivizing resilience lie in justice experienced (McGhee 2003). Justice experience has attracted belongingness, cooperation, life satisfaction, and self-esteem (Bjornskov et al. 2013; Dalbert 2001; van Prooijen et al. 2008). Conversely, justice experience has discouraged anger, depression, and protesting (Benson and Ritter 1990; Rothmund et al. 2014; Wenzel 2000). Protesting has provoked anger and discontent to erode resilience (Landmann and Rohmann 2020).

Ideals or obsessions upheld by societal exclusion to impede resilience concern blaming, dependency, poverty, risking, singleness, and worklessness (Cleaver 2005; Peruzzi 2014; Phillips 2006). Blaming reflects infirmity and victimization to divert resilience (Braman and Lambert 2001; Salazar et al. 2003). Singleness signifies deficiency, deviance, and self-blame to erode resilience (Reynolds et al. 2007; Sharp and Ganong 2011). Conversely, societal exclusion erodes such ideals as reflection and tolerance for framing resilience (Wojcieszak and Mutz 2009). Moreover, societal exclusion has eroded life satisfaction to weaken framing for resilience (Lin et al. 2013). Societal exclusion has also stemmed from crime, deviance, hostility, and restlessness, which disrupt ideals for framing resilience (Backman and Nilsson 2011; McPherson et al. 2006). Hostility has incurred anger, anxiety, and sadness to impede resilience (Vandervoort 2006). Conversely, societal exclusion has arisen from inadequate risk avoidance, thus dispelling ideals for framing resilience (Peruzzi 2014).

A norm reflected by societal exclusion for normalizing against resilience has emphasized disorder (Ross and Mirowsky 2009). The disorder norm normalizes deprivation, incivility, poverty, and stress (Brown et al. 2004; Congdon 2010; Vartanian 1999; Williams et al. 1999). This norm has sustained depression, economic hardship, normlessness, poverty, and victimization (Like 2011; Pei and Kim 2017; Ross and Mirowsky 2009; Whelan and Maitre 2013). Conversely, the norm has eroded earnings, happiness, pleasantness, safety, social capital, working, and general well-being (Congdon 2010; Hackman et al. 2019; Kanan and Pruitt 2002; van Praag and Frijters 1999; Vartanian 1999).

## *Societal Peace*

Societal peace is likely to sustain personal resilience through direct and indirect deterministic and voluntaristic mechanisms in analytical functionalism. Direct deterministic mechanisms share peace privately and publicly to induce resilience personally and vicariously. Herein, peace is a property of resilience featuring adaptation, order, safety, and stability (Boden et al. 2014; Bowers et al. 2017; Jones and d'Errico 2019; Lawler et al. 2009). Indirect deterministic mechanisms employ societal peace to provide power to empower, incentives to incentivize, norms to normalize, and ideals to frame personal resilience through voluntaristic mechanisms. Voluntaristic mechanisms capitalize on peace to generate power to drive, utility to attract, norms to assimilate, and ideals to rationalize resilience.

Power reflected in societal peace to empower resilience resides in cognitive or reasoning ability and trust (Stein 2013). Cognitive ability preempts bias in conservativism, consistency maintenance or dissonance avoidance, dispositional blaming, and self-defense and self-serving (Stein 2013). Trust indicates resources (Six 2014). It has sustained health and survival (Barefoot et al. 1998). Conversely, societal peace manifests the lack of external brutalization and threat to disempower resilience (Mgbeoji 2006; Stein 2013).

Incentives underlying societal peace to incentivize resilience cover equity and justice (Finkel and Rule 1986). Conversely, societal peace builds on removing frustration and thus its disincentive to resilience (Bartos and Wehr 2002). Justice experienced is activating and motivating, notably for cooperation, to uphold resilience (Campbell 2010; Dalbert 2001; van Prooijen et al. 2008). Moreover, justice experienced has sustained belongingness, health, life satisfaction, and self-esteem and eroded anger and depression, thus conducive to resilience (Bjornskov et al. 2013; Dalbert 2001; Lucas et al. 2013; Rothmund et al. 2014; van Prooijen et al. 2008).

Ideals held in societal peace to frame resilience embrace balance, confidence, easing, humanizing, harmony, maturity, mercy, and respect (Broome 2013; Davis 2006; Loukakis and Portos 2020). Conversely, societal peace erases conflict, crime, crises, hatred, protesting, rebellion, and violence, thus countering their framing against resilience (Anderson et al. 2019; Bebber 1995; Broome 2013; Dahlum and Wig 2019; de Soysa 2011; Somma and Medel 2019; Turner 2013; Yagci 2017). Societal peace has also strengthened happiness as an ideal for framing resilience (Ouweneel and Veenhoven 2016). Alternatively, societal peace builds on such ideals as continuity, individuality, prudence, and tolerance to frame resilience (Davis 2006). The ideal for individuality espouses human or self-development, autonomy, reasoning, responsibility, self-enhancement, and success to safeguard resilience (Church 2010; Davis and Robinson 1999; Fevre 2006; Krys et al. 2019; Norris and Inglehart 2009; Sun and Wang 2010). Moreover, societal peace reflects alternative thinking, openness, satisfaction, settlement, and success to furnish ideals for framing resilience (Bueno de Mesuita et al. 2002; Geller and Singer 1998; Sobek 2009; Stein 2013). Conversely, societal peace has stood by dispelling polarization or opposition, thus removing its framing against resilience (Geller and Singer 1998). Peace also prevails through appreciation, contemplation, enlightenment, meditation, minimizing differences, nonviolence, rationality, and redefinition, which are ideals to frame resilience (Barge and Andreas 2013; Dorjee 2013; Simmons 2020). Rationality has prevented aggression, anxiety, avoidance, depression, and disorders to safeguard resilience (DiGiuseppe et al. 2017).

Norms built by societal peace highlight balance, compatibility, development, openness, responsibility, social integration, and stability to normalize resilience (Bartos and Wehr 2002; Clarke and Shyu 1991; Hechter and Okamoto 2001; Shandra et al. 2003). Social integration prevented depression and suicide (Duberstein et al. 2004; Mullins and Dugan 1991). Such integration has also fostered cooperation (Lepkowski and Couper 2002). Conversely, societal peace reflects the insignificance of norms for alienation, atrocity, conflict, crisis, deprivation, disturbance, grievance, hostility, and strain to normalize against resilience (Bartos and Wehr 2002; Fuller 2000; Kellner 1989; Meyerson 1991; Van Dyke and Soule 2002).

## *Societal Violence*

Societal peace is likely to hinder personal resilience through direct and indirect deterministic and voluntaristic mechanisms in the analytical-functionalist framework. Direct deterministic mechanisms share violence privately and publicly to preempt resilience personally and vicariously. Herein, violence is antithetical to resilience, dispelling chaos and disruption, and upholding legality and order (Boden et al. 2014; Hoffman 2003; Lawler et al. 2009). Indirect deterministic mechanisms maintain societal violence to disempower, disincentivize, normalize against, and frame against personal resilience through voluntaristic mechanisms. Voluntaristic mechanisms hold violence shared in society to generate power, utility, norms, and ideals against resilience or constrain power, utility, norms, and ideals for resilience.

Based on the deterministic mechanism of empowering, societal violence incurs death and victimization to disempower personal resilience (Browning et al. 2004; Males 2010). Conversely, societal violence has eroded societal quality and resources to empower personal resilience (Sampson and Raudenbush 2004). Societal violence also reflects societal crowding, disadvantage, poverty, and strain as the loss of power, thus disempowering resilience (Browning et al. 2004; Hipp et al. 2009; Warner and Fowler 2003). Conversely, societal violence has risen from inadequate societal control, income, and stability, thus disempowering resilience (Browning et al. 2004; Hipp et al. 2009; Warner and Fowler 2003).

Based on the deterministic mechanism of framing, societal violence fosters violence as an obsession for framing against resilience (Douglas 2006). The ideal for violence has bred depression and stress in the youth (Muradwij and Allwood 2022).

Based on the deterministic mechanism of normalizing, societal violence has established norms for competition, confusion, deregulation, and protesting to normalize against resilience (Rogers and Pridemore 2018; Smidt 2020). Moreover, societal violence reflects anomie, challenge, competition, and inequality as norms to normalize something against resilience (Browning et al. 2004; Cuesta 2013; Hipp et al. 2009; Warner and Fowler 2003). Societal violence has also reflected norms for crime and deviance to normalize against resilience (Browning et al. 2004; Kwon and Baack 2005).

Based on the voluntaristic mechanism of power realization, violence breeds pain, social isolation, tension, and victimization, thus eroding power for resilience (Eatough et al. 2008; Krahe 2013; Murer and Schwarze 2022; Nassauer 2019). Violence also involves alienation, dysphoria, fear, suspicion, and trauma to weaken power for resilience (Heyman et al. 2013; Krahe 2013; Ruggiero 2020). Alienation involves meaninglessness, normlessness, and powerlessness (TenHouten 2017). It has engendered depression, detachment, and diminished social support received (Bishop et al. 2002; Loscocco and Spitze 1990). Trauma has raised depression, disability, distress, memory loss, substance abuse, and suicide (Dutton et al. 2016; Grzywacz and Almeida 2008; Lantz et al. 2005; Lowe et al. 2009; Lupien et al. 2009; Snyder et al. 2020). Conversely, trauma has eroded health, life quality, life, neighbor, and police satisfaction, and social integration, support received, and trust (Alesina and La Ferrara 2002; Garcia and Herrero 2004; Mathis et al. 2016; Parkes et al. 2002; Shrira 2012; Sun and Wang 2012; Zotti et al. 2016). Victimization experienced has induced anxiety, depression, distress, fear, helplessness, neuroticism, powerlessness, and symptoms to weaken power for resilience (Krahe 2013; Krulichova 2019; Lincoln et al. 2003; Lineres 2004; Ross and Mirowsky 2009; Wager 2012). Conversely, victimization experienced has impaired safety experienced and self-respect or self-worth to erode resilience (Fernandes 2018; Krahe 2013). Furthermore, violence has incurred depression, illness, injury, poverty, and unemployment to attenuate power for resilience (Krahe 2013; Wright et al. 2015). Violence also reflects alcoholism, deficiency, deprivation, disability, difficulty experienced, doping, irrationality, powerlessness, social detachment, discrimination, distrust, exclusion or rejection, marginalization or subordination, oppression, repulsion, segregation, desocialization, threat, unemployment to drain power for resilience (Espelage et al. 2007; Gelles 2007; Hattery and Smith 2012; Heitmeyer and Anhut 2008; Heyman et al. 2013; Hoffman and Edwards 2004; Johnson and Ferraro 2000; Krahe 2013; Kruesi 2007; MacDonald et al. 2005; Milner and Myers 2007; Mishna 2012; Pauwels and De Waele 2014; Ruggiero 2020; Stott et al. 2017; White et al. 2015). Irrationality encompasses awfulizing, dichotomous thinking, magnification or minimization, filtering for negatives, musterbation or expectation for gain, overgeneralization, and personalization or specializing oneself (Milner and Myers 2007). Conversely, violence arises from inadequate coping, interpersonal, and problem-solving skills, income, resources, security, self-control, solutions, social connection, inclusion, integration, and support received, and social class, prestige, or status to acquire power for resilience (Agnew 2007; Bornstein 2006; Diamond and Blair 2018; Gelles 2007; Heitmeyer and Anhut 2008; Kirkpatrick et al. 2002; Krahe 2001; Milner and Myers 2007; Palacios 2013; Pauwels and De Waele 2014). Furthermore, violence has grown from depression, disadvantage, distress, emotionality, neuroticism, psychoticism, strain, tension, troublesomeness, and vulnerability to constrain resilience (Farrington 2018; Gelles 2007; Gotzsche-Astrup 2020; Krahe 2013; Pauwels and De Waele 2014; Pulkkinen et al. 2009; Reilly et al. 2004; Savage 2014; Wright et al. 2015). Conversely, violence has followed low attachment, education, income, intelligence, mastery, self-control, and social class and inclusion, thus unable to drive resilience (Broom et al. 2013; Farrington 2018; Felson and Outlaw 2007; Gelles 2007; Pulkkinen et al. 2009; Kirkpatrick et al. 2002; Stogner et al. 2014).

Based on the voluntaristic mechanism of utility optimization, violence involves perceptions of injustice as disutility against resilience (Eatough et al. 2008). Moreover, violence reflects complaint, demand, discipline, nattering, punishment, and refusal received, and demonizing, disruption, failure, frustration or thwarting, humiliation or disgrace, and maltreatment or mistreatment experienced as disutility discouraging resilience (Berkowitz 2012; Eddy et al. 2018; Farrington 2007; Gelles 2007; Hoffman and Edwards 2004; Leander and Chartrand 2017; Mishna 2012; Ray 2014; Schinkel 2010; Ward 2002). Punishment received has bred alienation, distress, externalizing behavior, failure, relationship problems, and violence to contradict resilience (Antunes et al. 2014; Xing et al. 2011; Woodward and Fergusson 1999; Zalewski et al. 2017). Conversely, violence reflects inadequate favoritism, life quality, and recognition received to sustain utility for resilience (Heitmeyer and Anhut 2008; Hoffman and Edwards 2004).

Based on the voluntaristic mechanism of ideal consistency, violence fosters anger, antisociality, crying, grievance, harming, and violation as obsessions to discourage resilience (Eatough et al. 2008; Emjaian et al. 2018; Pinker 2011; Spitzberg 2013). Conversely, violence erodes compliance as an ideal for rationalizing resilience (Pulkkinen 2018). Moreover, violence rests on obsessions with fanaticism and panic to interfere with resilience (Petrou and Kandylis 2016; Ruggiero 2020). Violence also embraces obsessions with crime, destruction, hate, hostility, rage, revenge or retaliation, sadism, satanism, suicide, and unpleasure to contradict the ideal of resilience

(Aleksandrowicz 2009; Caplan 2006; Juni 2009; Krahe 2013; Pinker 2011; Ratelle and Souleimanov 2017; Ruggiero 2020). Alternatively, violence reflects obsessions or rationalizations with absolutism, anger, blaming, brutalization, conflict, crying, death, dehumanization, destruction, imbalance, impulsivity, inferiority, loss, mismatch, narcissism, polarization, resentment, shyness, stigma, stress, superiority, terror, and uncertainty to obstruct resilience (Cano and Vivian 2003; Collins 2012a; Eatough et al. 2008; Farrington 2007; Gelles 2007; Gotzsche-Astrup 2020; Grasner 2013; Heitmeyer and Anhut 2008; Krahe 2013; Johnson and Ferraro 2000; Messner et al. 2008; Palacios 2013; Ray 2014; Rogers et al. 2007; Ruggiero 2020; Schinkel 2004; Ward 2002). Narcissism accentuates exhibitionism, grandiosity, mastery, self-defense, self-omnipotence, self-preservation, self-sufficiency, and norm disidentification (Baumeister et al. 1996; Palacios 2013). In practice, narcissism underlies aggression, depression, misbehavior, and violence, thus impeding resilience (Lasch 1984; Tracy et al. 2009). Conversely, violence arises from inadequate conventionality or normativity, pleasure, morality, responsibility, satisfaction, and self-esteem, thus disrupting ideals for resilience (Hattery and Smith 2012; Heitmeyer and Anhut 2008; Milner and Myers 2007; Palacios 2013). Morality opposes psychopathology, which impedes resilience (Narvaez 2014). Furthermore, violence has sprung from criminality, disappointment, dissatisfaction, extremism, hyperactivity, risking, substance abuse, and violation, which contradict resilience (Farrington 2018; Krahe 2013; Pauwels and De Waele 2014; Pulkkinen et al. 2009; Santoro and Broidy 2014; Stogner et al. 2014; Vignansky and Timor 2017). Violence has also arisen from low compliance, contentment, happiness, meaningfulness, openness, religiosity, self-regulation, and stability, thus incongruous with resilience (Gotzsche-Astrup 2020; Huesmann 2018; Pulkkinen et al. 2009; Santoro and Broidy 2014; Vignansky and Timor 2017).

Based on the voluntaristic mechanism of norm conformity, violence reflects disapproving norms for social integration to impair resilience (Messner et al. 2008). Conversely, violence stems from exposure to and learning norms for antisociality, crime, or deviance, opposition, polarization, terrorism, and violence to resent resilience (Abrahms 2008; Ahmad and Monaghan 2019; Bjarnegard et al. 2019; Heitmeyer and Anhut 2008; Hoffman and Edwards 2004; Jensen 2007; Markowitz 2001; Ward 2002). Violence has also emerged from perceived norms favoring antagonism, conflict, delinquency, discrimination, and rowdiness and disfavoring arrest, order, and religiosity, thus discouraging resilience (Berger 2005; Collins et al. 2007; Emery et al. 2015; Krahe 2001; Krahe 2013; Pauwels and De Waele 2014). Normative influence increases with the expectation and perceived appropriateness of the norms (Ward 2002).

## *Societal Pragmatism*

Societal pragmatism is likely to champion personal resilience through direct and indirect deterministic and voluntaristic mechanisms in analytical functionalism. Pragmatism cultivates experimental and scientific problem-solving practices to realize the good and truth (Frega 2012; Knight and Johnson 2011; Ray 2004). Direct deterministic mechanisms share pragmatism privately and publicly to create resilience personally and vicariously. Pragmatism notably characterizes resilience (Dunn 2013). Moreover, pragmatism is a property of resilience upholding adaptation, adjustment, coping, functioning, and managing (Bowers et al. 2017; Crafter et al. 2019; Huta 2017; Prilleltensky 2012). Indirect deterministic mechanisms employ societal pragmatism to provide power to empower, incentives to incentivize, norms to normalize, and ideals to frame personal resilience through voluntaristic mechanisms. Voluntaristic mechanisms engage pragmatism to draw power to drive, utility to attract, norms to assimilate, and ideals to rationalize resilience.

Power derived from societal pragmatism rests on capitalism, creativity, education, and industrialization to empower resilience (Ray 2004; Stuhr 2003). Capitalism embraces creativity, experimentation, freedom, human capital, individualism, openness, rationality, self-regulation, wealth, and working to facilitate resilience (Furnham 1990; Hudson 2019; Novak 1993; Schram 2015; Wright 2019). Moreover, pragmatism champions effort and intelligence to generate power to empower resilience (Emirbayer and Mische 1998; Silver 2011. Eventually, societal pragmatism has generated power to empower resilience (ten Brinke and Keltner 2020).

Incentives generated from societal pragmatism uphold hope and meliorism or belief in amelioration to incentivize resilience (Stuhr 2003). Meanwhile, societal pragmatism posits that adversity is fallible and temporary, thus incentivizing resilience (Knight and Johnson 2011; Mahoney 2004).

Ideals promulgated from societal pragmatism embrace adaptation, choice, development and growth, diligence, diversity, expediency, experimentation, flexibility, freedom, inquiry, plurality, realism, reasoning, reconstruction, reflection or reflexivity, resolution or problem-solving, tolerance, transformation, and youthfulness to frame resilience (Matsueda and Grigoryeva 2014; Gross 2009; ten Brinke and Keltner 2020; Webb 2007). Choice has buttressed competence, effort and performance, life and neighborhood satisfaction, motivation, and self-determination to safeguard resilience (Day 2013; Gagne and Deci 2005; Helliwell et al. 2010; Patall et al. 2008). Realism favors security to furnish resilience (Bell 2010). Resolution engages creativity, deliberation, generativity, imagination, meditation, rationality, and security to facilitate resilience (Barge and Andreas 2013; Dorjee 2013; Simmons 2020). Creativity has sustained meaningfulness to frame resilience (Turner 2013). Reflexivity involves information processing ability and knowledge, planning, resolution, and self-actualization to uphold resilience (D'Cruz et al. 2007). Youthfulness emphasizes activeness, agency, autonomy, or self-determination, choice, creativity, development or growth, education, exploration, flexibility, fluidity, monitoring, positivity, reflexivity, self-control, vitality, and working to champion resilience (Coffey and Farrugia 2014; Cote 2014; Heinz 2009; Tanner and Arnett 2009). Self-control has eroded anxiety, crime, depression, risking, victimization experienced, violence, and vulnerability, thus favoring resilience (Koegl and Day 2019; Langenderfer and Shimp

2001; Marchetti et al. 2018; Zavala and Guadalupe-Diaz 2019). Conversely, self-control has boosted self-esteem to frame resilience (Armstrong et al. 2011). Furthermore, societal pragmatism sustains ideals for affordance, attuning, defense, purposefulness, rationality, self-determination, and tenacity to frame resilience (Emirbayer and Mische 1998; Mangion 2011; Matsueda and Grigoryeva 2014; Silver 2011). Conversely, societal pragmatism dissolves such ideals or obsessions as absolutism, dogmatism, and moodiness to frame resilience (Bromley 2004; Frega 2012; Knight and Johnson 2011; Mahoney 2004; Ray 2004; Silver 2011; Stuhr 2003; Webb 2007). Absolutism and dogmatism involve aggression, anger, anxiety and fear, closure, conflict, despair, fragility, intolerance, and self-indulgence to impede resilience (Ellis 2022; Johnson 2009). Moodiness has bred anxiety, depression, hostility, loneliness, and worry to hinder resilience (Hounkpatin et al. 2015; Maltby et al. 2016; Melton 2016; Neto and Barros 2003; Rossi 2004a). Conversely, moodiness has impeded autonomy, growth, health, purposefulness, relational quality, satisfaction with appearance, friendship, life, and weight, self-acceptance, self-compassion, and self-determination, thus blocking resilience (Austin et al. 2005; Finggerman et al. 2008; Frederick et al. 2016; Hounkpatin et al. 2015; Richards 2016). Additionally, societal pragmatism dispels ideals or obsessions such as formality, idealism, predetermination, and skepticism to frame resilience (Knight and Johnson 2011; Mahoney 2004; Webb 2007).

Norms fostered by societal pragmatism promote societal acceptance, deliberation, inquiry, justification, and understanding for normalizing resilience (Bromley 2004; Knight and Johnson 2011; Ray 2004). Notably, norms for management and planning have contributed to the youth's resilience (Ungar et al. 2005).

## *Westernization*

Westernization is likely to cultivate personal resilience through direct and indirect deterministic and voluntaristic mechanisms in analytical functionalism. Direct deterministic mechanisms share Westernization privately and publicly to create resilience personally and vicariously. Herein, Westernization constitutes resilience characterized by adaptation, choice, freedom, and individuality (Evans and Sewell 2013; Garrett 2016; Dunn 2013; Schwarz 2018). Indirect deterministic mechanisms employ Westernization to raise power to empower, incentives to incentivize, norms to normalize, and ideals to frame personal resilience through voluntaristic mechanisms. Voluntaristic mechanisms hold Westernization to breed power to drive, utility to attract, norms to assimilate, and ideals to rationalize resilience.

Power generated by Westernization rests on industrialization and technology to empower resilience (Ma 2019; Sternberg et al. 2011). Westernization has also reflected competence to empower resilience (Guan et al. 2010). Technology has sustained employment, environmental quality, income, and other resources to empower resilience (Florida 2005; Goetz et al. 2011; Welzel 2013).

Incentives from Westernization emphasize liberalization and meritocracy to incentivize resilience (Epstein 1997; Shortall and Warner 2010). Liberalization has fostered flexibility, prosperity, and life satisfaction to facilitate resilience (Abbott et al. 2011; Thelen 2012; Van 2017). Meritocracy champions agency, education, freedom, mastery, performance, responsibility, smartness, and working, effort, or striving to enhance resilience (Evans et al. 2010; Klein 2015; Sandel 2020).

Ideals fostered by Westernization favor controlling and mastery, creativity, safety, and tolerance to frame resilience (Hill 2000; Ma 2019; Narvaez 2014; Taplin et al. 2013). Westernization has also rested on the ideal for self-enhancement to frame resilience (Guan et al. 2010).

Norms fostered by Westernization emphasize choice, freedom, individuality, intelligence or knowledge, and relaxation to normalize resilience (Park et al. 2015; Sternberg et al. 2011; Zee 2022). Notably, normalization or standardization is a Westernization norm (Narvaez 2014).

## *Hong Kong, Guangzhou, and Macau*

Among the three Chinese societies, Hong Kong is likely to sustain resilience more than Guangzhou and Macau based on societal features to exercise direct and indirect deterministic and voluntaristic mechanisms in analytical functionalism. Hong Kong is renowned as a global, international, world metropolis returning to China in 1997 characterized by globalization, information communication and technology, dependence on Mainland China, and social risk (Chan 2006; Fung and Fong 2019; Holliday et al. 2004; Law 2014; Liu 2019; McNeill 2014; Wong et al. 2010). Macau is a microcity that returned to China in 1999 and is characterized by liberalization and integration with Mainland China (Chun 2019; Kwong and Wong 2017; Lam and Greenlees 2017). Guangzhou is a provincial capital in South China and is renowned as the forerunner for China (Chiu 2012). Direct deterministic mechanisms distribute societal features privately and publicly to create resilience personally and vicariously. Exactly, Hong Kong popularizes resilience (Li 2012). Indirect deterministic mechanisms apply societal features to raise power to empower, incentives to incentivize, norms to normalize, and ideals to frame personal resilience through voluntaristic mechanisms. Voluntaristic mechanisms employ societal features to breed power to drive, utility to attract, norms to assimilate, and ideals to rationalize resilience.

Power derived from Hong Kong rests on societal affluence, caring and social support, education, technology, and urbanization for empowering resilience (Chan and Cheng 2012; Delang and Lung 2010; Estes 2002; Lee and Chan 2023; Li 2012; Ma 2009; Nip 2010; Oksanen 2011; Overholt 2004). Education in society has buttressed health, intelligence, employment, income, social capital or trust, and volunteering to empower resilience (Herian et al. 2014; Lipford and Yandle 2009; Portes and Vickstrom 2011; Robert and Bukodi 2005; Schaie 2013; Uslaner and Brown 2005). Conversely, education in society has diminished illness, obesity, poverty, protesting, and violence, disempowering resilience (Dahlum and Wig 2019;

Goetz et al. 2011; Herian et al. 2014; Poveda 2011). Urbanization has enhanced medical care and the norm for control to sustain resilience (Khoshneviss and Benford 2018; Mapelli 1993).

Incentives fostered in Hong Kong highlight societal equality, inclusiveness, justice, legalism, liberty, life quality, opportunity, safety, security, and upward mobility for incentivizing resilience (Brooks 2011; Kleinman et al. 1999; Lai 2023; Lo 2018b; Ma 2011b; Sin and Chu 2000). Societal equality has sustained health, homeownership, life satisfaction, self-direction, social capital, and trust to raise resilience (Bond and Lun 2014; Kim and Kawachi 2007; Martin 2000; Meulemann 2010; Nilson 1981; Oishi et al. 2011; Portes and Vickstrom 2011). Moreover, societal equality has dampened anxiety, death, disability, and poverty, thus buttressing resilience (Kawachi et al. 1997; Kim and Kawachi 2007; Schwartz and Melech 2000). Societal justice has boosted prosperity to secure resilience (Rindermann 2008). Societal legalism, or the rule of law, has dampened radicalism and violence, thus buttressing resilience (Muthuswamy 2022; Sabia and Bass 2017). Radicalism has bred distrust, protesting, and violence to erode resilience (Levi and Strker 2000; Pauwels and De Waele 2014). Societal life quality has sustained health to empower resilience (Hadden et al. 2003). Conversely, Hong Kong dismisses paternalism as a disincentive against or obstacle to resilience (Ma 2011b). Paternalism is challenging, insulting, interfering, and overriding to disincentivize resilience (Arneson 2005; Hanna 2018; Kullgen 1995).

Ideals upheld in Hong Kong emphasize choice, creativity, entrepreneurialism, freedom, flexibility, growth, individualism, pluralism, repair, responsibility, stability, success, and sustainability to frame resilience (Chen and Pun 2007; Ku 2009; Lee et al. 2014; Lo 2012; Ma 2011b; Oksanen 2011; Yuen 2015), choice has fostered competence, effort and performance, income, life and neighborhood satisfaction, motivation, self-determination, and general well-being to induce resilience (Abbott and Sapsford 2006; Day 2013; Gagne and Deci 2005; Growiec and Growiec 2010; Helliwell et al. 2010; Patall et al. 2008). Entrepreneurialism embraces toughness and raises income to facilitate resilience (Ahmetoglu et al. 2011; Zietsma et al. 2019). Pluralism embraces or induces adjustment, agency, autonomy, compromise and tradeoff, deliberation, diversity, experimentation, individualism, innovation, liberty, openness, peace, receptiveness, respect, self-discipline, and tolerance to consolidate resilience (Connolly 2005; Galston 2005; Herman 2021; Moffitt 2018). Notably, Hong Kong hails rationalization to substantiate the framing mechanism (Forestier and Crossley 2015). Societal sustainability has propped life quality, security, and satisfaction and diminished homelessness, illness, and poverty to enable resilience (Bonini 2008; Thin 2002).

Norms shared in Hong Kong favor societal autonomy, independence, self-determination, self-direction, capitalism, entrepreneurship, freedom, individualism, innovation, openness, optimism, pragmatism, self-discipline, self-enhancement, self-help, and success, and Westernization to normalize resilience (Brooks 2011; DeGolyer 2001; Guan et al. 2010; Kwong and Wong 2017; Lai et al. 2014; Li 2012; Luk-Fong 2007; Ma 2009, 2011b; Ng and Wong 1999; Richardson 2018; Veg 2017; Yu 2020). Capitalism emphasizes diligence and success to secure resilience

(Ng and Wong 1999). Individualism favors effort, entrepreneurship, liberty, and self-enhancement to initiate resilience (Guan et al. 2010). Self-enhancement covers achievement, pleasure, and power to boost resilience (Guan et al. 2009). Westernization advances law, opportunity, optimism, rights, and voluntariness to enhance resilience (DeGolyer 2001). Conversely, Hong Kong maintains the norm against fatalism, thus safeguarding resilience (Lau and Kuan 1988).

Power inadequate for empowering resilience in Macau stems from societal class disparity, dependence on Mainland China, and fragmentation (Greenwood and Dwyer 2017; Hao 2015; Wu and Vong 2017). Dependence has weakened coping and health, thus eroding resilience (Bekker et al. 2011; Roy and Chaudhuri 2008). Conversely, Macau is inadequate in societal belongingness, counseling, economic capability and endogenous growth, education, professionalization, staffing, trust, and welfare and its generosity and universal provision, thus inadequate to empower resilience (Chen 2012; Greenwood and Dwyer 2017; Ho and Lam 2015; van Schalkwyk and Sit 2013; Yu 2020).

Incentives inadequate for incentivizing resilience or disincentives against resilience in Macau stem from gaming or gambling in rewarding (Lam and Greenlees 2017). Gambling can be pathological and reflect depression, bias or illusion in control, and low income, thus impending resilience (Chang 2005; Oei et al. 2008). Moreover, gambling means uncertainty, which incurs dissatisfaction and tension and inhibits resilience (Miyazaki et al. 1999; Theiss 2018).

Ideals inadequate for framing resilience in Macau dismiss planning and pluralism (Choi 2016; Lai 2017; Greenwood and Dwyer 2017). Planning has reflected achievement, education, health, and optimism to afford resilience (Hellevik and Settersten 2013; Poynton et al. 2015). Conversely, planning has weakened with disability, sickness, and unemployment, thus impeding resilience (Hellevik and Settersten 2013).

Norms inadequate for normalizing resilience in Macau favor hedonism and protest (Greenwood and Dwyer 2017; Ho 2015; Suntikul and Jachna 2016). Hedonism is associated with anomia and normlessness to inhibit resilience (Adnanes 2007). Moreover, hedonism has bred depression, shoplifting, substance abuse, and suicide and lowered self-esteem, thus impeding resilience (Bjarnason 2009). Conversely, norms inadequate for normalizing resilience in Macau discount self-worth (van Schalkwyk and Sit 2013).

Power is inadequate due to poverty to empower resilience in Mainland China (Gao et al. 2009). Conversely, Mainland China provides inadequate societal human capital and welfare to empower resilience (He and Wu 2009; Lu and Feng 2008).

Incentives inadequate to incentivize resilience in Mainland China stem from societal inequity, punishment, and stigmatization (Biddulph and Xie 2008; Wong and Chiu 1997). Stigmatization experienced stems from poverty to impede resilience (Chan et al. 2022). Conversely, Mainland China dispels liberalism, thus disincentivizing resilience (Gilley and Holbig 2009). Societal liberalism has increased equality and employment to secure resilience (Hicks and Kenworthy 2003).

Ideals inadequate to frame resilience in Mainland China dismiss happiness, individualism, innovation, self-help, and tolerance (Cao et al. 2016; Davey 2012; Lo

2021; Kachiga 2021; Zhang with Stening 2010). Innovation has reflected satisfaction and self-efficacy to prop resilience (Wang et al. 2013). Conversely, Mainland China fosters hostility as an ideal or necessity, thus weakening resilience (Chow 2016). Hostility has activated anger, anxiety, irrationality, and sadness to hinder resilience (Vandervoort 2006).

Norms inadequate to normalize resilience in Mainland China highlight societal dependence and self-defeating (Chen and Martin 2007; Peterson et al. 2006). Conversely, Mainland China holds norms dismissing creativity, heteronomy, individualism, self-enhancing, self-esteem, Westernization, and willpower, thus blocking resilience (Chen and Martin 2007; Rudowicz and Yue 2002; Sun and Bitter 2012). Willpower embraces acceptance, aspiration, continuation, deliberation, individualism, and self-control or self-regulation to propel resilience (Baumeister et al. 2007; Droutman et al. 2018; Heyman et al. 2013; Hoyle and Davison 2016; Ray 2017). Conversely, willpower dismisses impulsivity and risking to sustain resilience (Koegl and Day 2019). Impulsivity has bred stress and reduced purposiveness, thus impairing resilience (Hample 2018; Pompili et al. 2007). Risking has weakened health and raised crime and violence, thus blocking resilience (Farrington 2018; Pulkkinen et al. 2009; Wickrama et al. 1995). Furthermore, willpower has secured self-esteem to facilitate resilience (Armstrong et al. 2011). Conversely, willpower has dampened anxiety, crime, depression, victimization experienced, violence, and vulnerability, thus sustaining resilience (Marchetti et al. 2018; Cheung et al. 2014).

## Original Findings

Original findings supported five of the nine expected effects of societal conditions on resilience (see Table 4.1). On the one hand, support concerned the effects of societal caring, exclusion, Westernization, and Hong Kong versus Guangzhou and Macau. On the other hand, findings contradicted and refuted the hypothesis about the contribution of societal pragmatism to resilience. Additionally, hypotheses concerning societal inclusion, peace, and violence did not obtain support.

In the analysis of data from the poverty study, factorial or structural validity was evident in the factors of resilience, income, societal care perceived (Taylor and Curtis 2018), societal exclusion perceived (Geeraert and Demoulin 2013), and societal inclusion experienced (Boone and Leadbeater 2006; Secker et al. 2009). Accordingly, the indicators of the factors identified or loaded on their respective factors exclusively and substantively (see Table 4.2). The factors and their indicators were thus discriminable from each other and the method factor of acquiescent rating. Such convergent and discriminant validity constituted factorial or structural validity. Such validity transpired in the goodness of fit of confirmatory factor analysis.

In the analysis of data from the violence study, factorial or structural validity held for the factors of resilience, societal peace perceived (Miller 1983; Moos and Lemke 1996), societal violence perceived (Muradwij and Allwood 2022; Schmid 2012),

**Table 4.1** Societal effects on resilience

| Societal condition | Expected | Currently found |
|---|---|---|
| Caring | + | + |
| Inclusion | + | 0 |
| Exclusion | − | − |
| Peace | + | 0 |
| Violence | − | 0 |
| Pragmatism | + | − |
| Westernization | + | + |
| Guangzhou versus Hong Kong | − | − |
| Macau versus Hong Kong | − | − |

*Note* +: positive effect; −: negative effect; ?: mixed effects; 0: no effect

**Table 4.2** Standardized factor loadings (poverty dataset)

| Factor/Indicator | Trait | Method |
|---|---|---|
| *Societal care or caring in society, past 3 months ($\alpha = 0.603$)* | | |
| (No) Indifference of Hong Kong people to decrepit or wounded people | 0.429 | − 0.434 |
| Care of Hong Kong people to poor people | 0.799 | − 0.061 |
| Care of Hong Kong people experiencing privation | 0.431 | 0.323 |
| Hong Kong people just taking care of themselves | 0.432 | − 0.126 |
| Care of Hong Kong people to new arrivals | 0.436 | − 0.069 |
| *Societal exclusion in society, past 3 months ($\alpha = 0.547$)* | | |
| Income (in)equality in Hong Kong | 0.304 | − 0.147 |
| Hong Kong people's (in)ability to buy private housing | 0.578 | − 0.148 |
| (No) Disparity between the rich and the poor in Hong Kong | 0.695 | 0.085 |
| (No) Opportunity for Hong Kong people to get rich | 0.315 | − 0.108 |
| Poverty in Hong Kong | 0.645 | 0.259 |
| *Societal inclusion experienced, past 3 months ($\alpha = 0.559$)* | | |
| Chance to make friends with Hong Kong people | 0.375 | − 0.068 |
| Chance to rise at work and society | 0.356 | 0.174 |
| (No) Barriers to your personal development in society | 0.422 | − 0.497 |
| *Resilience, recent month ($\alpha = 0.612$)* | | |
| Facing difficulties actively | 0.794 | 0.247 |
| (Not) Feeling anxious at the time of pressure | 0.847 | − 0.207 |
| Keeping calm in the face of pressure | 0.598 | 0.289 |
| *Income* | | |
| Personal income | 0.945 | |
| Family income per capita | 1.052 | |

$L^2$ (918) = 4144, *SRMR* = 0.039, *RMSEA* = 0.017, *CFI* = 0.946

and societal pragmatism perceived (Cartwright et al. 2009; Lee 2010). Accordingly, the indicators of the factors converged into their respective factors, which were discriminable from each other and the method factor of acquiescent rating (see Table 4.3). Such convergence and discriminant validity underpinned factorial or structural validity. The validity stood on the goodness of fit of confirmatory factor analysis.

The regression analysis of resilience in the recent month from the poverty study revealed a significant positive effect of societal care perceived in the past three months ($\beta = 0.524$, see Table 4.4) and a significant negative effect of societal exclusion perceived in the past three months ($\beta = -0.584$). Meanwhile, the effect of societal inclusion in the past three months on resilience in the recent month was nonsignificant. Notably, the analysis controlled for personal characteristics.

The regression analysis of resilience in the recent month from the violence study exhibited a significant negative effect of societal pragmatism perceived in the past two months ($\beta = -0.269$, see Table 4.5). This effect contradicted the hypothesis about the contribution of societal pragmatism to resilience. Meanwhile, societal peace and violence in the past two months did not display significant effects on resilience in the recent month.

**Table 4.3** Standardized factor loadings (violence dataset)

| Factor/Indicator | Trait | Method |
|---|---|---|
| *Resilience, recent month ($\alpha = 0.622$)* | | |
| Being able to face adverse circumstances | 0.458 | 0.443 |
| Facing difficulties actively | 0.549 | 0.339 |
| Keeping calm in the face of pressure | 0.500 | 0.437 |
| *Societal peace awareness, past 2 months ($\alpha = 0.751$)* | | |
| Discussing peacefully | 0.735 | 0.218 |
| Discussing rationally | 0.669 | 0.270 |
| Being negotiable | 0.631 | 0.264 |
| *Societal violence awareness, past 2 months ($\alpha = 0.850$)* | | |
| Assaulting government facilities | 0.468 | 0.579 |
| Enclosing and blocking public facilities | 0.402 | 0.530 |
| Opposing police | 0.578 | 0.531 |
| Disrupting councils | 0.604 | 0.560 |
| Assaulting officials | 0.532 | 0.549 |
| *Pragmatism awareness, past 2 months ($\alpha = 0.548$)* | | |
| Paying attention to feasibility | 0.588 | 0.227 |
| Paying attention to adjustment to changing conditions | 0.538 | 0.292 |
| Suiting the remedy to the case | 0.505 | 0.269 |
| Stressing practicality | 0.460 | 0.303 |

$L^2$ (324) = 427, $SRMR = 0.027$, $RMSEA = 0.017$, $CFI = 0.958$

**Table 4.4** Standardized effects on resilience (poverty dataset)

| Predictor | Resilience |
|---|---|
| Caring in society | 0.524* |
| Social exclusion in society | – 0.584* |
| Social inclusion experienced | – 0.020 |
| $R^2$ | 0.658 |

*Note* Regression analysis controlled for background characteristics
*$p < 0.05$

**Table 4.5** Standardized effects on resilience (violence dataset)

| Predictor | Resilience |
|---|---|
| Peace awareness | 0.003 |
| Violence awareness | – 0.106 |
| Pragmatism awareness | – 0.269* |
| $R^2$ | 0.100 |

*Note* Regression analysis controlled for background characteristics
*$p < 0.05$

The regression analysis of resilience in the recent month from the elder resilience study showed a significant contribution of Westernization in the past four months, but only after weighting by Westernization ($\beta = 0.124$, see Table 4.6). This effect showed Westernization sustained resilience in a highly Westernized or Western context, as weighted by Westernization. Notably, the weighting simulated a Western context having Westernized elders mostly. That is, the effect was not strong enough to be significant in the Hong Kong context, when not weighted by Westernization to represent the Western context.

The regression analysis of inferred resilience in the recent month, which meant the lack of depression under adversity, from the elder resilience study did not find a significant effect from Westernization in the past four months. Weighting by Westernization to simulate the Western context did not make the effect significant (Table 4.7).

**Table 4.6** Standardized effects on resilience (elder dataset)

| Predictor | Unweighted | Weighted by Westernization |
|---|---|---|
| Westernization | 0.111 | 0.124* |
| $R^2$ | 0.176 | 0.112 |

*Note* Regression analysis controlled for background characteristics
*$p < 0.05$

**Table 4.7** Standardized effects on inferred resilience (elder dataset)

| Predictor | Unweighted | Weighted by Westernization |
|---|---|---|
| Westernization | 0.018 | 0.032 |

*Note* Regression analysis controlled for background characteristics

**Table 4.8** Standardized effects on depression (elder dataset)

| Predictor | Unweighted | Weighted by Westernization |
|---|---|---|
| Westernization | – 0.142 | – 0.055 |
| $R^2$ | 0.151 | 0.178 |

*Note* Regression analysis controlled for background characteristics

**Table 4.9** Standardized effects on resilience ($N =$ 3564) (youth dataset)

| Predictor | All |
|---|---|
| Guangzhou vs. Hong Kong | – 0.053** |
| Macau versus Hong Kong | – 0.056** |
| $R^2$ | 0.039 |

*Note* Regression analysis controlled for background characteristics
$^{**}p < 0.01$

The regression analysis of depression in the recent month from the elder resilience study manifested a significant inverse effect of Westernization in the past four months, but only before weighting by Westernization ($\beta = -0.142$, see Table 4.8). This effect showed Westernization eroded resilience in the Hong Kong context not weighted by Westernization.

The regression analysis of resilience from the play study indicated that resilience in the recent month was significantly lower in Guangzhou and Macau than Hong Kong ($\beta = -0.053$ and $-0.056$, see Table 4.9). These effects supported the hypothesis about the higher resilience in Hong Kong than in the two other Chinese societies.

## *Societal Pragmatism Effect*

The inverse effect of societal pragmatism reflects analytical-functionalist mechanisms opposite to the expected ones. These mechanisms encompass deterministic and voluntaristic ones emphasizing power, incentives or utility, ideals, and norms to achieve the functions of fulfillment, adaptation, latency, and integration. Hence, alternative power, incentives, ideals, and norms disempower, disincentivize, frame against, and normalize against resilience, respectively. The mechanisms unfolded in societal pragmatism, as indicated by paying attention to feasibility and adjustment to changing conditions, suiting the remedy to the case, and stressing practicality (see Table 4.3).

Ideals or beliefs upheld in societal pragmatism for change, criticalness or problematizing, debating, disagreement, or agonism, fallibility, contingency, uncertainty, or indeterminacy, incompliance, suspicion, and temporality frame against resilience (Bromley 2004; Farrelly 2007; Frega 2012; Hoover 2016; Mahoney 2004; Ralph 2018; Ziegler 1994). Societal change poses anxiety, challenge, clash, conflict, crises, discontinuity, disloyalty, marginalization, pathologization, and terror to weaken resilience (Adams 2007; Harper and Leicht 2011; Schmidt 2010; Turner 2003). Moreover, societal change has diminished social trust and welfare, thus disempowering resilience (Harper and Leicht 2011). Societal change has also bred migration to undermine resilience (Greenfield 2009). Additionally, change means stress featuring adversity, disorders, failure, and hassles to suppress resilience (Garfin et al. 2015; Kleiman and Riskind 2014; Shrira 2012; Walen and Lachman 2016). Debating manifests problematizing, strife, and struggle to upset resilience (Chilton 2004; Strydom 2002). Criticalness or disagreement has eroded well-being, thus impairing resilience (Cheung and Leung 2011). Fallibility or uncertainty has raised diffidence, dissatisfaction, and tension to jeopardize resilience (Theiss 2018). Disloyalty breeds conflict, passivity, and withdrawal to impede resilience (Guerrero 2015). Furthermore, disloyalty has eroded motivation and self-acceptance, thus compromising resilience (Agronick and Duncan 1998; Ferssizidis et al. 2010). Conversely, disloyalty has impeded achievement, emotional intelligence, and socioeconomic status, including income, thus preempting resilience (Agronick and Duncan 1998; Hagan et al. 1996; Seaton and Beaumont 2008). Noncompliance rejects acceptance and permissiveness, thus disrupting resilience (Marien and Hooghe 2011; Vermunt and Steensma 2016). Conversely, noncompliance manifests ignorance to block resilience (Zitek and Jordan 2019). Noncompliance has also invoked protesting, stress, and violence to weaken resilience (Molz et al. 2013; Morselli and Passini 2018; Pulkkinen et al. 2009). Conversely, incompliance has impaired adaptation and pleasantness, thus hindering resilience (Littlejohn et al. 2017; Turner 2006). Temporality, opposite to continuity, persistence, and stability, has reflected hardship and inadequate education, thus impeding resilience (Mirowsky and Ross 2001). Moreover, temporality rejects growth, thus antithetical to resilience (Chishima and Wilson 2021; Mrazek et al. 2018).

Conversely, pragmatism dispels naturalism and spirituality as ideals, thus framing against resilience (Gregg 2003; Stuhr 2003). Naturalism upholds freedom, joy, peace, reversal, silence, and softness to cultivate resilience (Hocksmann 2004; Moeller 2004). Conversely, naturalism rejects violence, thus buttressing resilience (Hocksmann 2004). Spirituality emphasizes calmness, compassion and self-compassion, meaningfulness, purposefulness, serenity, and tolerance to champion resilience (Connors et al. 1999; Harris et al. 2018; Kalkstein and Tower 2009; Kelly 2012; MacDonald and Friedman 2002; Richards 2012). Moreover, spirituality has sustained coping, forgiveness, joy, and general well-being to foster resilience (Mullet et al. 2005; Saroglou and Anciaux 2004; Seidlitz et al. 2002). Conversely, spirituality has dwindled guilt feeling, hostility, and sadness to maintain resilience (Seidlitz et al. 2002). As such, pragmatism discounts resilience by dispelling naturalism and spirituality.

## *Societal Inclusion Effect*

Societal inclusion did not display the expected contribution to resilience. Herein, social inclusion covered friendship, working, and personal development in society (Boone and Leadbeater 2006; Secker et al. 2009). Hence, social inclusion means involvement in society, including its arena, business, ecology, economy, market, polity, and socialization (Semenova et al. 2020; Ungar 2011). The lack of contribution reflects the inverse impact of societal inclusion in offsetting the contribution to resilience. This impact rides on deterministic and voluntaristic mechanisms of analytical functionalism to complete the functions of fulfillment, adaptation, latency, and integration. These mechanisms run with power, incentives or utility, norms, and ideals to disempower, disincentivize, frame against, and normalize against resilience.

Power sparked by societal inclusion to disempower resilience arises from societal competition (Alexiadou 2002; Inglehart and Welzel 2005). Societal competition has stemmed from societal protesting, thus hindering resilience (Brancati 2016). Competition has also eroded enjoyment, thus blocking resilience (Frederick-Recascino and Schuster-Smith 2003). Conversely, societal inclusion enables deprivation, stress, and victimization as societal power to disempower resilience (Hansen-Nord et al. 2014; Myer et al. 2008; Smith and Newman 2001). Deprivation has dampened social trust and general well-being, thus impeding resilience (Clark et al. 2008; Layte et al. 2000; Stephens et al. 2014). Conversely, deprivation has bred fatalism, illness, isolation, pressure experienced, strain, and suicide, thus hindering resilience (Ahnquist et al. 2012; Stephens et al. 2014; Swanson et al. 1992; Walker et al. 2010). Societal inclusion has also raised poverty to disempower resilience (Mayer 2003). Likewise, societal inclusion has reflected inadequate societal income to empower resilience (Coffe and Geys 2006).

Ideals fostered by societal inclusion to frame against resilience embrace activism and consumerism (Norris 2002; Semenova et al. 2020). Activism can breed criminality and failure to frame against resilience (Louis et al. 2020; Watts 2020). Similarly, activism incorporates antagonism, antisociality, conflict, defiance, disruption, fear, hostility, and violence to resist resilience (Renger et al. 2020; Castells 2012; Hammond 2015; Jost et al. 2012; Passini and Morselli 2011; Swart et al. 2020; Tan and Snow 2015; Wieloch 2002). Furthermore, activism has eroded hope, thus attenuating resilience (Paez et al. 2015). Conversely, activism has manifested impulsivity to distract resilience (Vestergren et al. 2017). Consumerism or consumptionism engages hedonism and irrationality to hinder resilience (Himes 2007). Moreover, consumerism has emerged from inadequate relaxation, thus contradictory to resilience (Wansink and van Itterum 2012). Meanwhile, social inclusion has eroded ideals for liberalism, thus framing against resilience (Brody and Lovrich 2002).

Norms incubated from societal inclusion to normalize against resilience highlight opposition (Smith and Newman 2001). Opposition opposes acceptance, thus impeding resilience (Takahashi and Gaber 1998). Furthermore, opposition features disruption, militancy, and violence to resist resilience (Ewick and Silbey 2003; Saxton and Benson 2006).

## *Societal Peace Effect*

Societal peace did not exhibit the expected contribution to resilience. Herein, societal peace happens in discussion and negotiation. The lack of contribution reflects the inverse impact of societal peace to offset the contribution to resilience. This impact draws on deterministic and voluntaristic mechanisms of analytical functionalism to complete the functions of fulfillment, adaptation, latency, and integration. These mechanisms engage power, incentives or utility, norms, and ideals to disempower, disincentivize, frame against, and normalize against resilience.

Societal peace emerges when societal development, prosperity, and resources, including education, revenue, and technology, are inadequate to invoke competition and conflict, thus also inadequate to empower resilience (Bueno de Mesuita et al. 2002; Dahlum and Wig 2019; Heaphy 2007; Hechter and Okamoto 2001; Sobek 2009; Stein 2013; Tao 2015; Yagci 2017). That is, societal development, including technology, has facilitated societal strife to disrupt societal peace. Societal development has advanced health to empower resilience (Hadden et al. 2003). Similarly, societal prosperity has raised education, health, life satisfaction, knowledge, relationship quality, self-efficacy, social trust, and value for independence to facilitate resilience (Baldacci et al. 2003; Bonini 2008; Fjellvang 2011; Fridberg and Kangas 2008; Miller 2015; Norris 2011; Traunmuller 2011). Conversely, societal prosperity has reduced personal illness and societal anomie, risk, and threat, thus sustaining resilience (Fridberg and Kangas 2008; Schneider 2007; Schwartz and Melech 2000; Teymoori et al. 2016). Societal education has boosted health, intelligence, social capital, and trust to empower resilience (Herian et al. 2014; Portes and Vickstrom 2011; Schaie 2013; Uslaner and Brown 2005). Conversely, societal education has diminished violence, thus maintaining resilience (Poveda 2011). Societal technology has fostered employment and income to empower resilience (Florida 2005; Goetz et al. 2011). Moreover, societal peace reflects inadequate societal trust and willpower to gather disruptive power and empower resilience (Beetham 1985; Inglehart 1997). Willpower has sustained self-esteem and dampened anxiety, depression, crime, risking, violence, victimization experienced, and vulnerability to uphold resilience (Armstrong et al. 2011; Cheung et al. 2014; Koegl and Day 2019; Langenderfer and Shimp 2001; Marchetti et al. 2018; Welch et al. 2008; Zavala and Guadalupe-Diaz 2019). Hence, societal peace can offset its power to empower resilience.

Societal peace dispels ideals for defense, religiosity, and self-regarding, thus framing against resilience (Brubaker 2015; Lichbach 1988; Stein 2013; Wuthnow 2004). Defense has stemmed from education, employment, fearlessness, self-efficacy, and knowledge to maintain resilience (Asencio et al. 2014; Bish and Michie 2010). Religiosity sustains flourishing, health, harmony perceived, mastery, meaningfulness, positive affect, relationship quality, satisfaction with finance and life, security perceived, self-esteem, social capital and trust, and general and socioemotional well-being to boost resilience (Chang 2009; Clemence 2001; Demerath 2002; Dy-Liacco et al. 2009; Dyck 2012; Flouri and Buchanan 2002; Helliwell and

Putnam 2005; Levin and Chatters 1998; Moschis and Ong 2011; Ng and Fisher 2016; Schieman 2001; Urbatsch 2014; Van Praag et al. 2010; Wuthnow 2004). Flourishing comprises altruism, purposiveness, and self-actualization (Dy-Liacco et al. 2009). Conversely, religiosity has lessened depression, fear, and loneliness, thus safeguarding resilience (Ellison et al. 2001; Hui et al. 2007; Lauder et al. 2006). Self-regarding has sustained equanimity, happiness, optimism, and positive affect to champion resilience (Barnard and Curry 2011). Conversely, self-regarding has dismissed anger, anxiety, catastrophizing, depression, negative affect, and rumination, thus maintaining resilience (Barnard and Curry 2011). Hence, societal peace can weaken ideals to offset framing resilience.

Societal peace or its maintenance has contradicted, reduced, or reduced societal norms for freedom and openness, thus normalizing against resilience (Hechter and Okamoto 2001; Moller and Skaaning 2014). Societal freedom champions autonomy, individuality, satisfaction, and self-realization to enable resilience (Bavetta et al. 2014). Moreover, societal freedom has raised economic well-being, life satisfaction, trust, and societal prosperity to facilitate resilience (Abbott et al. 2011; Mookerjee and Beron 2004; Rindermann 2008; Wong et al. 2016). Freedom perceived has sustained health, life satisfaction, self-esteem, and general well-being to enhance resilience (Gehring 2013; Glendinning et al. 2003; Haller and Hadler 2006). Conversely, freedom perceived has lessened depression and symptoms to safeguard resilience (Glendinning et al. 2003). Hence, societal peace can downplay norms to offset normalizing resilience.

## *Societal Violence Effect*

Societal violence did not manifest the expected harm to resilience. Herein, societal violence tapped assaulting government facilities, enclosing and blocking public facilities, opposing police, disrupting councils, and assaulting officials (see Table 4.3). The lack of harm reflects the contribution of societal violence to offset the harm to resilience. This contribution rides on deterministic and voluntaristic mechanisms of analytical functionalism to complete the functions of fulfillment, adaptation, latency, and integration. These mechanisms involve power, incentives or utility, norms, and ideals to disempower, disincentivize, frame against, and normalize against resilience.

Power generated by societal violence to empower resilience has rested on exercising and extraversion (Morenoff et al. 2008; van Hemert et al. 2002). Exercising has sustained well-being, thus empowering resilience (Sargent-Cox et al. 2015). Extraversion has shaped autonomy and self-determination, coping, emotional intelligence, growth, humor, mastery, positive affect, purposefulness, relatedness, satisfaction with appearance, life, and weight, security experienced, self-acceptance, self-efficacy, social support received, spirituality, and uplift experience to facilitate resilience (Anusic et al. 2014; Becker et al. 1997; Bishop 2015; Celso et al. 2003; Frederick et al. 2016; Hounkpatin et al. 2015; Ingledew et al. 2004; Judge et al. 2002; MacDonald and Friedman 2002; Matthews et al. 2012; Maybery et al. 2006;

Quilty et al. 2006; Richards 2016; Vernon et al. 2008). Conversely, extraversion has prevented anxiety, danger perceived, depression, and hostility, thus buttressing resilience (Becker et al. 1997; Hounkpatin et al. 2015; Sibley and Duckitt 2009). More generally, violence builds on power, capacity, or resources to empower resilience (Hattery and Smith 2012; Kivimaki 2012). Specifically, violence rides on power stemming from activeness, employment, financial well-being, mastery, self-esteem, social capital, socioeconomic status, and striving to empower resilience (Baumeister et al. 1996; Bartusevicius 2021; Fox et al. 2002; Gelles 2007; Kirkpatrick et al. 2002; Ozbay 2008; Pulkkinen et al. 2009; Song et al. 2017). Financial well-being has sustained life satisfaction and self-confidence to safeguard resilience (Lee and Lee 2019; Sahi 2017). Socioeconomic status has sustained coping, health, interaction quality, life satisfaction, self-esteem, and general well-being (Al-krenawi et al. 2011; Caplan and Schooler 2007; Molana and Adams 2019; Staudinger et al. 1999). Conversely, violence emerges from low burnout and dependence as power to empower resilience (Collins 2012a; Hattery and Smith 2012). Burnout means strain comprising cynicism, depersonalization, detachment, exhaustion, failure, fatigue, inauthenticity, and inefficacy (Cicognani et al. 2009; Fyhn et al. 2016; Maslach et al. 2001; Tumkaya 2007). Essentially, burnout has reflected inadequate resilience (Griffin and Sun 2018; Maltby et al. 2019). Moreover, burnout stems from loss, stress, threat experienced, and workload received to block resilience (Maslach et al. 2001; Pervez and Halbesleben 2017; Vaccaro et al. 2021). Conversely, burnout reflects inadequate aspiration, hope, resources, social support received, and willpower, thus hindering resilience (Barunstein-Bercovitz 2013; Halbesleben 2006; Schwartz et al. 2007). Furthermore, burnout has arisen from inadequate autonomy, competence, coping, equity experienced, hardiness, emotional intelligence, religiosity, reward received, security experienced, stability, trust, and well-being including enjoyment, health, positive affect, self-efficacy, and self-esteem, thus weakening resilience (Acker and Lawrence 2009; Chan 2006; Cicognani et al. 2009; de Henestrosa et al. 2023; Erickson and Ritter 2001; Fyhn et al. 2016; Kulik 2007; Lau et al. 2005; Maltby et al. 2019; McCarthy et al. 2022; Miner-Rubino and Reed 2010; Van welsch et al. 2001; Willis et al. 2008; Wright and Hobfoll 2004; Yan and Tang 2002). Conversely, burnout has originated from alienation, ambiguity, challenge, coercion, conflict, constraint, demand, imbalance, pressure, and stress experienced to impede resilience (Dawson et al. 2016; de Henestrosa et al. 2023; Griffin and Sun 2018; McCarthy and Frieze 1999; Moen et al. 2013; Powell 1994; Willis et al. 2008). Meanwhile, dependence has worsened health to disempower resilience (Roy and Chaudhuri 2008). Dependence also originates from inadequate development or maturity, thus jeopardizing resilience (Bornstein 2009).

Incentives reflected by societal violence to incentivize resilience stem from meritocracy (Schinkel 2004). Meritocracy motivates less capable people's violence and more capable people's resilience. Furthermore, meritocracy incentivizes agency, control, earning, education, freedom, mastery, performance, smartness, and working, effort, or striving to strengthen resilience (Evans et al. 2010; Sandel 2020).

Ideals fostered by societal violence to frame resilience have favored or reflected stability and tolerance (Douglas 2006; Hipp et al. 2009; Messner et al. 2008). Stability and tolerance constitute resilience (Boden et al. 2014; Connor et al. 2003; Lock et al. 2020; Prince-Embury et al. 2017). Societal violence also fosters or reflects individualism as an ideal to frame resilience (Cuesta 2013; Ray 2017; Stott et al. 2017). Moreover, violence builds on meaningfulness and success ideology as ideals to frame resilience (Ray 2014; Vignansky and Timor 2017). Meaningfulness has buttressed aspiration, engagement, happiness, health, life satisfaction, and positive affect to sustain resilience (Morgan and Robinson 2013; Steger et al. 2009). Conversely, meaningfulness has reduced depression and negative affect, thus lifting resilience (Steger et al. 2009). Success ideology embraces mastery to strengthen resilience (Chang et al. 1997).

Norms upheld by societal violence to normalize resilience popularizing defense and honor (Bufacchi 2007; Hipp et al. 2009; Triandis and Suh 2002). Defense has enabled humor and self-enhancement to safeguard resilience (Erickson and Feldstein 2007). Honor stands on choice, education, freedom, religiosity, security, and self-determination to boost resilience (Chong 2014; Preda 2013; Welsch 2002; Woods 2014). Honor dismisses discrimination, enslavement, persecution, and torture experienced, thus upholding resilience (Chong 2014). Moreover, honor has raised income to facilitate resilience (Welsch 2002).

## *Societal Westernization Effect*

Westernization in the context or societal Westernization amplified the contribution of personal Westernization to resilience but weakened the inverse effect of personal Westernization on depression (see Tables 4.6 and 4.7). The contribution of personal Westernization to resilience works with the voluntaristic mechanism of idealistic consistency, with Westernization rationalizing resilience. Such rationalizing stems from the emphases of Westernization on controlling, creativity, individualism, mastery, and tolerance (Ma 2019; Narvaez 2014; Taplin et al. 2013). Conversely, the inverse effect of personal Westernization on depression shows that Westernization rationalizes against depression. However, the feature of individualism in Westernization contributes to depression (Constantino et al. 2006; Karuza et al. 1990). Herein, societal individualism breeds competition, disintegration, helplessness, loneliness, isolation, and separation to incur depression (Bauman 2001; Beck and Beck-Gernsheim 2002; Burgess 2018; Riad and Norris 1992; Ritschel and Sheppard 2018). Hence, Westernization has its individualism exerting a positive effect on depression to offset the inverse effect of other Westernization features. Westernization thus exhibits a weak inverse effect on depression.

The amplification moderation effect of societal Westernization on the positive effect of personal Westernization on resilience reflects the contribution of the fit between societal and personal Westernization to power to strengthen the empowering or driving effect of personal Westernization. Herein, fit or alignment between the person and environment generates power according to functionalist and ecological perspectives (Georgiades et al. 2013; Ketelaars et al. 2017; Mahoney et al. 2009). Fit strengthens power for empowering through cooperation, coordination, and synergy (Brewer 1996; Riley et al. 2011).

The attenuation of the inverse effect of personal Westernization on depression by societal Westernization or the Westernized context is due to the conflict between personal and societal Westernization on depression. On the one hand, personal Westernization diminishes depression through controlling, creativity, individualism, tolerance, and working (Narvaez 2014; Taplin et al. 2013). Individualism has fostered self-enhancement (Church 2010). Self-enhancement has dampened depression (Bang et al. 2020). Depression has also declined with controlling (Xi and Hwang 2011). On the other hand, societal Westernization increases depression because of competition, disintegration, helplessness, loneliness, isolation, and separation (Bauman 2001; Beck and Beck-Gernsheim 2002; Burgess 2018; Riad and Norris 1992; Ritschel and Sheppard 2018). Conflict has weakened power or been disempowering (Schaie 2013). The conflict thus engenders a countervailing, resistant effect (Cooper et al. 2021; Herman-Kinney 2003). Such an effect is disempowering, based on the deterministic mechanism of analytical functionalism.

# Chapter 5
# Peer Influences on the Resilience Process

**Abstract** This Chapter exhibits a further attempt to gauge the social, deterministic, and personal, voluntaristic development of resilience processes. Such processes comprise the voluntaristic formation of resilience, including its action, learning, belief, and resilience demand received successively. Moreover, the related behavior, belief, and character include self-awareness, compensation, benevolent world belief, and kindness. Reflective of deterministic development are other social factors, including aid received and the sociability and kindness of other people. These factors notably included those aggregated for peers in the service unit. According to the vision of the resilience process, resilience evolves from factors progressively emerging at different points. Analysis of survey data on social service users showed that kindness, the sociability and kindness of other people, and aid received, apart from background characteristics, were the earliest contributors to resilience and its resilience, learning, and belief. Furthermore, beliefs about resilience and a benevolent world were earlier significant contributors to resilience, resilience action, and resilience learning. In addition, resilience action, learning resilience, self-awareness, and compensation later contributed to resilience. However, the demand for resilience manifested adverse effects on resilience, resilience action, resilience learning, and resilience belief. Thus, the process of resilience from learning and belief about resilience to action and feeling about resilience successively was demonstrable. This process reflects the voluntaristic mechanism of ideal consistency in the analytical functionalist framework. Similarly, the contributions of other behaviors, beliefs, and dispositions illustrate the same voluntaristic mechanism. By contrast, the impacts of social factors on individual resilience represent the deterministic mechanisms, which focus on the suprapersonal or group determinants of the analytical-functionalist framework. For instance, a significant peer influence was the positive effect of peers' disabilities on resilience. This effect indicates that individual resilience was higher than poorer peers' condition. Such contrast reflects the deterministic mechanism of incentivizing to show one's distinctiveness from others. Hence, the deterministic basis for developing the resilience process is evident. Nevertheless, the deterministic basis is unlikely to override the voluntaristic process. Resilience and its process are feasible and reasonable because of their voluntaristic basis.

 
C. K. Cheung, *Resilience Process and Its Personal and Social Bases*,
https://doi.org/10.1007/978-981-97-7391-6_5

Peer influences spring from interaction or reception directly and exposure or affiliation indirectly. Herein, peers refer to those in the same service units or involved in interaction or communication. Direct interaction with or reception from peers includes aid, advice, kindness, and sociability experienced during interaction. Exposure or affiliation for indirect influence is peer norms concerning such interaction, adversity, functional disability, and resilience, which comprises feeling, action, belief, and exposure. All the influences can proceed with the deterministic and voluntaristic mechanisms of analytical functionalism. These mechanisms engage power or resources, incentives or utility, ideals or beliefs, and norms to achieve the requisite functions of fulfillment, adaptation, latency, and integration. For the integral functioning of resilience, power has stemmed from agreeableness, conscientiousness, emotional intelligence, extraversion, learning, mentoring received, openness, purposiveness, self-esteem, and social support received (Armstrong et al. 2011; Buikstra et al. 2010; Cherry et al. 2023; Notter et al. 2008; Yu and Zhang 2007). Conversely, power for resilience has weakened with neuroticism (Yu and Zhang 2007). Utility from resilience has arisen from optimism (Buikstra et al. 2010). Ideals for resilience emphasize coping, humor, religiosity, resolution, stability, and survival or sustainability (Cherry et al. 2023; Corbin and Hall 2019; Lock et al. 2020; Lou et al. 2018; McKay et al. 2018). Norms for resilience have popularized adaptation, balance, innovation, and trauma (Buikstra et al. 2010; Cantor et al. 2002; Cherry et al. 2023; Jones and d'Errico 2019).

## Existing Knowledge

Peer influence works through providing power for empowerment and power realization, incentive or utility for incentivizing and utility optimization, ideals for framing or signifying and ideal calibration, and norms for normalizing and norm conformity, with direct and indirect mechanisms to complete functions in analytical functionalism. Power in peer influence fuels or resides in peer coercion, cognitive development, disagreement or challenge, educating, elaboration, guidance, induction, knowledge conservation and construction, offering, supporting, and tutelage (Aiken 2002; Brandenberger 2005; Collier 1997; Donaldson et al. 1994; Gibbs 2014; Gibbs et al. 2007; Hagan and McCarthy 1997; Simons et al. 1991; Windle 1992). Utility in peer influence benefits from peers' acceptance, appraisal, approval, comparability, cohesion, quality, reinforcement, resource provision, and satisfaction, as opposed to aggression, hostility, and tension (Ennett et al. 2008; Hoffmann and Dufur 2018; Kloep 1999; SunWolf 2008; Vega et al. 1993). Ideals in peer influence engage peers' defining to invoke one's interpretation, justification, self-construction, self-monitoring, self-organizing, and self-validating (Bennett and Segerberg 2012; Brandenberger 2005; Kabiri et al. 2020; Wei and Liu 2022; Wong and Lau 1993). Norms in peer influence hinge on association, attachment, collaboration or co-production, commitment, comparison, confluence, connection, discussion, equilibration or maintaining equal cognitive development, imitating, ingratiation, interaction, involvement, learning, networking, obligation, reciprocity, responsiveness, and role-taking regarding peers (Bennett and Segerberg 2012; Brandenberger 2005; Costello and Hope 2016; Fukushima et al. 2009; Gibbs 2014; Kabiri et al. 2020; Kutnick and Kington 2005; Kornienko et al. 2018; Thomas 1997; Zeidner and Matthews 2011), Meanwhile, peers influence with power, utility, ideals, and norms through peers' communication, curation, expectation, humiliation, integration, maintenance, preservation, questioning, rejection, sharing, sorting, and transmission (Bennett et al. 2014; Gibbs 2014; Hoffmann and Dufur 2018; Juvonen 1991; Wagenaar and Perry 1994). As such, peer influence is a priority (Costello and Hope 2016). Peers have also directly raised the youth's resilience (Cole et al. 2022; Masten et al. 2009).

Peer power to empower resilience stems from peer enhancement of cognitive capability, collaboration, knowledge, mental health, perspective-taking, reasoning, and responsibility (Aiken 2002; Collier 1997; Gibbs 2014; Kutnick and Kington 2005). Collaboration fosters happiness and reflects reasoning and virtue to activate resilience (Van Lange et al. 2014). Furthermore, collaboration has enhanced attachment to empower resilience (Tak 2017). Knowledge has underlain power, prevention, protection, satisfaction, self-efficacy, spirituality, tolerance, economic resources, and social resources and trust to facilitate resilience (Chang and Hsu 2016; Cheng and Ng 2006; Ertz et al. 2021; Mutz and Mondak 2006; Norris 2011; Nunkoo 2015; Pattie et al. 2004; Bish and Michie 2010; Rothwell et al. 2016). Conversely, knowledge has reduced the perception of risk and vulnerability, thus safeguarding resilience (Langenderfer and Shimp 2001; Shi et al. 2003). Perspective-taking has installed social trust to empower resilience (Fett et al. 2014). Reasoning has dampened aggressiveness, anxiety, dependence, depression, disorders, and self-defeating, thus upholding resilience (DiGiuseppe et al. 2017; Karuza et al. 1990). Responsibility has advanced wisdom to facilitate resilience (Spengler et al. 2018). Moreover, peers have fostered competence, creativity, critical thinking, development, intelligence, social attachment, and social support received as power to empower resilience (Ahmed et al. 2010; Berkowitz et al. 2006; Gu et al. 2014, Misra 1997, Stebleton et al. 2014; van Rijsewijk et al. 2016; Wen et al. 2020). Development or maturity has buttressed success to induce resilience (Spengler et al. 2018). Conversely, peers have dampened anxiety, depression, and distress, thus empowering resilience (Banks and Weems 2014; McGinley and Evans 2020; Oberle et al. 2019).

Peer incentives to incentivize resilience arise from peers' acceptance, approval and one's achievement, gain, popularity, quality evaluation, satisfaction, and success (Andrews 2020; Costello and Hope 2016; Galian et al. 2018; Owusu-Agyeman and Amoakoheme 2021; Vega et al. 1993). Such satisfaction has covered various life domains (Oberle et al. 2019). Obtaining acceptance or popularity has fostered positive affect and self-esteem to elevate resilience (Reich et al. 2018). Achievement or success has buttressed acceptance or tolerance, development, education, health, income, life quality, satisfaction, self-efficacy or competence, self-esteem, and social support received to induce resilience (Cook et al. 2002; Donnellan et al. 2005; Gibbs et al. 2015; Mackinnon 2012; Morgan and Streb 2001; Murray 2009; Pabilonic 2001;

Tompson and Dass 2000; Xiao et al. 2009). Conversely, achievement or success has dampened alienation, crime or delinquency, depression, distress, doping, and internalizing behavior, thus safeguarding resilience (Defoe et al. 2013; Fredricks and Eccles 2005; Lord et al. 2011; Menard and Mose 1984; Masten et al. 2005). Meanwhile, peers lessen conflict and isolation, thus incentivizing resilience (Kilian et al. 2013). Conflict has fomented distress, suicide, and violence to weaken resilience (Dutton et al. 2016; Farrington 2018; Li and Leung 2012). Conversely, conflict has eroded emotional intelligence, satisfaction, and social trust to inhibit resilience (Kunovich and Hodson 1999; Mikula et al. 2012; Schaie 2013). Isolation has bred a negative mood and impeded life satisfaction and reasoning to dampen resilience (Guillen et al. 2011; Lin et al. 2013; Williams et al. 2000).

Peer ideals to frame resilience involve raising individuation and social integration (Berndt and Keefe 1996; Caldas and Pounder 1990; Kloep 1999; McNeal 1997; Reis and Buhl 2008; SunWolf 2008). Individuation has fostered self-enhancement to boost resilience (Church 2010). Social integration has lessened depression and suicide, thus safeguarding resilience (Duberstein et al. 2004; Mullins and Dugan 1991). Conversely, peers reduce problem behavior and tension as ideals or obsessions, thus framing resilience (SunWolf 2008). Moreover, peers have induced adjustment, effort, future orientation, recourse, self-esteem, self-interest, task orientation, and tolerance for frustration as ideals to frame resilience (Franklin 1995; Israelashvili 1999; Petress 1995; Ridenour et al. 2006; Song et al. 2009; Stake 2006; Stoddard and Pierce 2018). Future orientation has fostered control and social trust to facilitate resilience (Prenda and Lachman 2001; Uslaner 2002). Recourse has alleviated distress, thus safeguarding resilience (Tracey et al. 1986). Conversely, peers have dampened crime, delinquency, externalizing behavior, indecision, and internalizing behavior as ideals or obsessions, thus framing resilience (Ridenour et al. 2006; Guay et al. 2006; Tanner-Smith et al. 2013). Furthermore, peer association has reflected self-esteem as an ideal to frame resilience (Kokkinos and Hatzinikolaou 2011).

Peer norms to normalize resilience have emphasized sociability, tolerance, and toughness (Ridenour et al. 2006; Schwendinger and Schwendinger 1985; Waterman et al. 2022). Sociability embodies cooperation, enjoyment, friendship, relational well-being, and trust to foster resilience (Donati and Archer 2015; Foschi and Lauriola 2014).

More specifically, peers can influence resilience through advice, aid, kindness, sociability, adversity, functional disability, and resilience. Such influence is prevalent due to peer interaction, including affiliation, collaboration, connection, grouping, and pressure (Hendry and Kloep 2012; Hospers and Jansen 2005; Moshman 2003; Rudkin et al. 1994; Sussman and Ames 2001; Wright 2016). Moreover, peers create their norms to exert influence (Livingstone et al. 2007; Waterman et al. 2022).

## *Peer Sociability*

Sociability manifests extraversion, relationship seeking, surgency, social interaction, and understanding of others in social interaction (Foschi and Lauriola 2014; Keightley et al. 2006). Peers' sociability is likely to sustain resilience through the voluntaristic mechanisms of power realization, utility optimization, ideal consistency, and norm conformity. Moreover, peer sociability influences using the deterministic mechanisms directly and indirectly through empowering, incentivizing, framing, and normalizing. As such, peer sociability lifts personal sociability, notably through deterministic mechanisms, including normalizing (Hoglund and Leadbeater 2004). Personal sociability, in turn, sustains resilience (Eisenberg et al. 2002). Accordingly, the influence capitalizes on the voluntaristic mechanisms of analytical functionalism. These mechanisms engage power, incentives or utility, ideals, and norms to boost resilience.

Power generated from sociability to drive resilience hinges on cooperation, enjoyment, empathy, friendship, relationship building, responsibility, self-control, social support received, social trust, and understanding of others (Barrera et al. 2018; Donati and Archer 2015; Flynn et al. 2019; Foschi and Lauriola 2014; Keightley et al. 2006; Zhou 2008), cooperation has facilitated social integration to secure power to drive resilience (Tak 2017). Responsibility has engendered wisdom to drive resilience (Spengler et al. 2018). Self-control has buttressed self-esteem and dampened anxiety, depression, criminal behavior, risking, victimization experience, violence, and vulnerability to facilitate resilience (Armstrong et al. 2011; Cheung et al. 2014; Koegl and Day 2019; Langenderfer and Shimp 2001; Marchetti et al. 2018; Welch et al. 2008; Zavala and Guadalupe-Diaz 2019). Moreover, sociability embraces communication, conflict management, cooperative skill (Tak 2017), friendship-making ability, and relational closeness to draw power or resources to drive resilience (Barry and Wigfield 2002; Giordano et al. 2006; Junttila et al. 2006; Larson et al. 2007). Relationship closeness has facilitated humor and social support received to lift resilience (Martin et al. 2003). Sociability has furthermore maintained belongingness, creativity, education, friendship quality, relationship satisfaction, and security to gather power to drive resilience (Anderson-Butcher et al. 2008; Collins and van Dulmen 2006; Ghayas and Malik 2013; Hintsanen et al. 2011; Larson et al. 2007). Belongingness has strengthened rewards to induce resilience (Nelson-Coffey et al. 2023). Conversely, sociability has prevented distress, poverty, and strain, thus maintaining power to drive resilience (De Bruyn and Boom 2005; Donati and Archer 2015; Larson et al. 2007). Besides, sociability stands on collaboration and its skill, conflict resolution skill, divergent thinking, knowledge, and mindfulness to furnish power to drive resilience (Kim et al. 2017; Ting-Toomey 2004). Mindfulness has boosted emotion regulation, positive affect, life satisfaction, and reduced depression to uphold resilience (Andrade et al. 2019; Droutman et al. 2018; Linares et al. 2016). Sociability has also sprung from conscientiousness, cognitive and executive functioning, emotional intelligence, maturity demand, popularity, rationality, self-regulation, and social integration to facilitate resilience (Allen et al. 2005; Bernard et al. 2017;

Brackett et al. 2006; de Bruyn et al. 2003; Davis et al. 2009; Keightley et al. 2006; Kim et al. 2017; Raitakari et al. 2016). Conscientiousness has propped autonomy, life satisfaction, mastery, purposefulness, relatedness, and self-acceptance, and diminished avoidance and anxiety to secure resilience (Fraley et al. 2011; Hounkpatin et al. 2015). Emotional intelligence has buttressed agreeableness, coping, defense, enthusiasm, friendship, intelligence, openness, optimism, self-control, success, and well-being to facilitate resilience (Goldenberg et al. 2006; Matthews et al. 2012; Mayer et al. 2004, 2008). Coping elevated by emotional intelligence has included cognitive restraint, problem-focused, and rational coping (Goldenberg et al. 2006; Kluemper 2008). Well-being raised by emotional intelligence has included adaptation, happiness, health, positive mood, life satisfaction, relatedness, relationship quality, and self-esteem as opposed to depression, distress, and symptoms (Ciarrochi et al. 2000; Goldenberg et al. 2006; Kluemper 2008; Matthews et al. 2012; Mayer et al. 2008; Schutte et al. 2002). Conversely, emotional intelligence has dampened abuse, deviance, disorders, neuroticism, problems experienced, social disconnection, and stress, thus maintaining resilience (Brackett and Mayer 2003; Kluemper 2008; Matthews et al. 2012; Mayer et al. 2008). Meanwhile, sociability has arisen from the lack of strain, symptoms, and victimization experienced to keep power for driving resilience (De Bruyn and Boom 2005; Leung and McBride-Chang 2013; Tan and Camras 2011). Victimization experienced has eroded well-being and enhanced risk, thus impeding resilience (Graham et al. 2010; McNeeley and Yuan 2017).

Utility sustained by sociability for attracting resilience involves achievement and reward (Hintsanen et al. 2011; Newby et al. 2000). Reward has sustained health maintenance, recourse, satisfaction, trust, and general well-being to induce resilience (Grimes 2006; Helgeson et al. 2006; Kasparian et al. 2009; Vogel et al. 2006; Wong and Lam 2016). Conversely, reward has diminished anger, anxiety, and depression, thus propping resilience (Helgeson et al. 2006; Wells et al. 1999).

Ideals maintained by sociability to rationalize resilience embrace positivity, self-help, and self-esteem (Gorbett and Kruczek 2008; Flynn et al. 2019). Positivity has buttressed benefits experienced, coping, curability, and survival to enable resilience (Clarke et al. 2000; Nes and Segerstrom 2006). Coping includes approach coping, covering acceptance, activeness, expression, growth, planning, reinterpretation, restructuring, recourse, task orientation, and venting (Nes and Segerstrom 2006). Self-help has elevated confidence, enthusiasm, functioning, positive affect, power, satisfaction, self-esteem, and skill to uplift resilience (Anderson-Butcher et al. 2004; Cameron 2002; Hatzidimitriadou 2002; Kelly et al. 2019; Kondo and Wada 2009; Schiff and Bargal 2000). Conversely, self-help has alleviated disorders, impairment, and substance abuse, thus restoring resilience (Devine et al. 1997; Kelly et al. 2019; Peterson et al. 2001). Sociability has sustained adjustment, control, ego development, meaningfulness, problem-solving, self-management, and general well-being as ideals to rationalize resilience (Booker and Dunsmore 2017; Finne and Svartdal 2017; Hintsanen et al. 2011; Larson et al. 2007; Lenz et al. 2010; Webster-Stratton and Lindsay 1999). Ego development embraces coping using flexibility, openness, problem-solving, responsiveness, and sensitivity to lift resilience (Walker and Hennig 1999). Conversely, sociability has lessened violence, thus safeguarding resilience

(Collins and van Dulmen 2006). Besides, sociability has built on agreeableness, cheerfulness, emotional stability, humor, openness, and satisfaction or need meeting to install ideals to rationalize resilience (Keightley et al. 2006; Stein et al. 2013; Yip and Martin 2006). Emotional stability has buttressed control, forgiveness, intelligence, spirituality, success, uplift experience, and well-being to raise resilience (Hounknatin et al. 2014; Lincoln et al. 2003; Maltby et al. 2016; Maybery et al. 2006; Mullet et al. 2005; Schaie 2013; Steca et al. 2017). Well-being has included autonomy, health, positive affect, purposiveness, relatedness, relationship quality, satisfaction with appearance, friendship, life, and weight, self-acceptance, self-compassion, and self-determination (Anusic et al. 2014; Austin et al. 2005; Finggerman et al. 2008; Frederick et al. 2016; Hounkpatin et al. 2015; Ingledew et al. 2004; Pfattheicher et al. 2017; Richards 2016). Conversely, well-being rejects anxiety, depression, hostility, loneliness, and worry (Anusic et al. 2014; Maltby et al. 2016; Neto and Barros 2003; Rossi 2004a). Meanwhile, sociability has arisen from the lack of avoidance, behavioral problems, delinquency, and negative reactivity, thus maintaining ideals to rationalize resilience (Barnett et al. 2010; Bartusch and Matsueda 1996; Hounkpatin et al. 2015; Hoglund and Leadbeater 2004; Tan and Camras 2011).

Norms sustaining sociability for assimilating resilience have emphasized self-determination (Serna et al. 2000). Self-determination has maintained commitment, effectiveness, performance, and well-being to boost resilience (Delhey 2010; Gagne and Deci 2005; Hui et al. 2013; Weinstein and Ryan 2010). Well-being has encompassed life satisfaction, mastery, relatedness, and relational quality, as opposed to anxiety and depression (Delhey 2010; Hui et al. 2013; Schieman and Plickert 2008; Schwartz and Melech 2000; Sheldon and Bettencourt 2002; Sieber et al. 2019; Weinstein and Ryan 2010). Conversely, sociability has emanated from the lack of conflict as a norm, thus maintaining resilience (Florsheim 1997). Conflict has dampened emotional intelligence, harmony perception, satisfaction, and trust to impede resilience (Kunovich and Hodson 1999; Mikula et al. 2012; Schaie 2013; Wong and Shik 2011). Conversely, conflict has fomented distress and violence, thus hindering resilience (Farrington 2018; Lau et al. 2017).

Extraversion as a basis for sociability furnishes power, utility, ideals, and norms to raise resilience through the voluntaristic mechanisms of analytical functionalism. Herein, extraversion embraces activity, assertiveness, ambition, emotionality, closeness, and potency (Foschi and Lauriola 2014; Witt and Revelle 2009). Notably, extraversion includes sociability, indicated by being confident, dramatic, energetic, entertaining, enthusiastic, romantic, warm, and the center of attention (Cassano et al. 2009). Moreover, extraversion has championed resilience directly (Campbell-Sills et al. 2006; Plouffe et al. 2020).

Power generated by extraversion to drive resilience emanates from activity and social activity, ambition, assertiveness, boldness, enthusiasm, positive affect and emotion, social closeness, and potency (Foschi and Lauriola 2014; Witt and Revelle 2009). Assertiveness has sustained life satisfaction and self-esteem to foster resilience (Diener and Fujita 1995; Menard and Offman 2009). Boldness champions breaking through, endurance, living now, persistence, openness, pride, resistance, self-acceptance, self-esteem, and stoicism to prop resilience (Cheng and

Huang 2017; Putman 2010; Roller and Zimbardo 2017; Wein 2007; Woodard 2010). Stoicism honors accepting, calmness or equanimity, conservation, controlling, dignity, enduring, invincibility, magnanimity, rehabilitation, resolve, self-control, self-direction, self-love, self-preservation, self-sufficiency, and simplicity to boost resilience (Holowchak 2008; Martin 2016; Mitsis 2003). Social closeness has invited social support to buttress resilience (Gant et al. 1999). Extraversion has also boosted autonomy and self-determination, aspiration, intelligence and emotional intelligence, mastery, relatedness or relationship quality, security, self-efficacy, social capital, social support received, spirituality, and uplift experience to secure power to drive resilience (Becker et al. 1997; Bishop 2015; Cassidy and Lynn 1991; Cheng et al. 2019; Hounkpatin et al. 2015; Ingledew et al. 2004; MacDonald and Friedman 2002; Maybery et al. 2006; Rasmussen et al. 2018; Siegling et al. 2012; Webster et al. 2014). Uplift experience has raised life satisfaction and positive affect to safeguard resilience (Maybery et al. 2006). Conversely, extraversion has dampened anxiety, depression, distress, loneliness, social exclusion experienced, and stress thus maintaining power to buttress resilience (Antonukis and Dietz 2011; Becker et al. 1997; Kim 2017; Maltby et al. 2019; Weinberg et al. 2021).

Utility facilitated by extraversion to attract resilience involves achievement, hope, and success (Colbert et al. 2012; Mascaro and Rosen 2005; Witt and Revelle 2009). Hope has buttressed health, life satisfaction, self-esteem, and general well-being as opposed to depression and suicide to induce resilience (Bronk et al. 2009; Frazier et al. 2007; Henry et al. 1993; Hull and Mendolia 1991; Myers 2008; Schindler et al. 2015). Conversely, extraversion has reduced the danger perceived, thus sustaining utility to encourage resilience (Sibley and Duckitt 2009).

Ideals maintained by extraversion for rationalizing resilience have evolved from well-being (Witt and Revelle 2009). Extraversion has also boosted control, coping, courage, dominance, flourishing, growth, happiness, humor, purposefulness, satisfaction, self-acceptance, self-esteem, and transcendence to build ideals for rationalizing resilience (Cassidy and Lynn 1991; Celso et al. 2003; Hounkpatin et al. 2015; Li et al. 2017; Lincoln et al. 2003; Quilty et al. 2006; Schnell and Becker 2006; Vernon et al. 2008; Waterman et al. 2010; Witt and Revelle 2009). Control has uplifted health maintenance, optimism, power, prevention, social trust, and well-being to elevate resilience (Cheng and Ng 2006; Etezadi and Pushkar 2013; Keltener et al. 2008; Moore and Aweiss 2003; Smith and Stasson 2000; Steinhardt 2012). Well-being has included health and life satisfaction, as opposed to anger and depression (Cundiff et al. 2015; Orlowski and Wicker 2015; Rose 2000; Xi and Hwang 2011). Dominance has escalated self-advancement to achieve resilience (Sinn and Hayes 2018). Satisfaction has covered appearance, life, marriage, and weight (Frederick et al. 2016; Li et al. 2017; Solomon and Jackson 2014). Transcendence has maintained life satisfaction and meaningfulness and impeded anxiety, depression, and stress to enhance resilience (Fishbein et al. 2020). Conversely, extraversion has lessoned avoidance, delinquency, deviance, eating disorders, hostility, preoccupation, and resentment as obsessions to impede resilience (Becker et al. 1997; Eggert et al. 2007; Fraley et al. 2011; Hounkpatin et al. 2015; Morizot and Le Blanc 2007; Mullet et al. 2005; Wright and DeLisi 2016).

Norms reflected by extraversion to enhance resilience have embraced religiosity (van Hemert et al. 2002). The religious social norm has incubated personal religiosity (Pollack and Pickel 2007; Skerkat and Ellison 1999; Stavrova and Siegers 2014). Religiosity has buttressed coping, friendship, forgiveness, harmony perceived, health maintenance, institutional and social trust, optimism, social capital, and well-being to raise resilience (Chang 2009; Clemence 2001; Furnham 1997; Hakhverdian and Mayne 2012; Myers 2008; Saroglou and Anciaux 2004; Wuthnow 2004; Zanin 2017). Well-being has included adjustment, flourishing, health, mastery relationship quality, satisfaction, self-esteem, and socioemotional well-being as opposed to depression, fear, and loneliness (Dy-Liacco et al. 2009; Ellison et al. 2001; Flouri and Buchanan 2002; Helliwell and Putnam 2005; Hui et al. 2007; Lauder et al. 2006; Moschis and Ong 2011; Schieman 2001; Skerkat and Ellison 1999; Wuthnow 2004). Satisfaction has covered democracy, police, finance, and life (Kwak et al. 2010; Lim and Putnam 2010; Marx 2014; Van Praag et al. 2010). Conversely, religiosity has prevented crime, deviance, doping, illness, poverty, protesting, and suicide, thus safeguarding resilience (Andrews et al. 2015; Duberstein et al. 2004; Hatch 2007; Muennig et al. 2013; Skerkat and Ellison 1999; Urbatsch 2014).

## *Peer Kindness*

Peer kindness associates with peers' altruism, caring, charity, collaboration, contribution, cooperation, donating, educating, empathy, generosity, helping, heroism, mutuality or reciprocity, politeness, regard, sharing, solidarity, supporting, and volunteering (Allidina et al. 2019; Bierhoff 2002; Nelson-Coffey et al. 2023; Coyne et al. 2018; Jirsaraie et al. 2019; Kafashun et al. 2017; Luria et al. 2019; Maltseva 2016; Mastain 2007; Matts et al. 2009; Miles 2015; Premo et al. 2018; Stagnaro et al. 2017; Walkowitz 2021; Wong and Yang 2022; Worley and Samp 2019; Yip and Martin 2006; Zhao et al. 2017). Helping includes advising, caregiving, consoling or reassuring, emergency intervention, neighboring, and providing (Bjornberg and Ekbrand 2008; Feeney and Collins 2001; Mata and Pendakur 2014). Conversely, peer kindness rejects aggression, competition, complaining, individualism, loneliness, punishment, selfishness, and sinning (Barber 2004; Coyne et al. 2018; Stagnaro et al. 2017; Van Lange et al. 2012; Worley and Samp 2019). Peer kindness has also raised responsibility to generate power to empower resilience (Shahzalal and Adnan 2022). Responsibility has elevated wisdom to drive resilience (Spengler et al. 2018). Kindness stands on religion and ethics such as Confucianism (Chen et al. 2022; Drezner 2013). Essentially, kindness embodies benefitting, developing, self-motivation, social fitting and orientation, and voluntariness (Clark et al. 2015; Dik et al. 2012; Froh et al. 2010; Mesurado et al. 2018; Zeng et al. 2020). Remarkably, peer kindness has raised resilience (Cherry et al. 2018; Cole et al. 2022; Masten et al. 2009). Such raising hinges on power, incentives, ideals, and norms through the deterministic and voluntaristic mechanisms of empowering and power realization, incentivizing and utility optimization, framing and ideal calibration, and normalizing and norm conformity. These mechanisms constitute personal and social functioning predicated on analytical functionalism.

Power stemming from peer kindness for empowering resilience has emanated from competence, creativity, critical thinking, development, education, self-efficacy, and social attachment (Ahmed et al. 2010; Berkowitz et al. 2006; Crysdale et al. 1999; Estell and Perdue 2013; Gu et al. 2014; Kristensen et al. 2023; Liu and Ngai 2019; Misra 1997). Conversely, peer kindness has eroded anxiety, depression, and distress as powerlessness, thus empowering resilience (Ahmed et al. 2010; Banks and Weems 2014). Furthermore, peer kindness raises power based on attachment, resources or energy, security, and togetherness to empower resilience (Feeney and Collins 2018). Besides, peer kindness has boosted power based on control, health and its maintenance, healthcare use, motivation, recourse, social capital, social integration, and social trust to empower resilience (Garcia and Herrero 2004; Gorman et al. 2010; Lincoln et al. 2003; Kouzis and Eaton 1998; Navarra et al. 2018; Palmer et al. 2011; Steinhardt 2012; Thrasher et al. 2004; Williams et al. 2006). Conversely, peer kindness has reduced illness, marital problems, and stress to maintain power, thus empowering resilience (Grundy and Sloggett 2003; Kendler et al. 2006; Myer et al. 2008). Illness has eroded functionality, health and mental health, knowledge, optimism, security, vitality, and general well-being, thus disempowering resilience (Benitez-Silva et al. 2010; Carrieri 2012; Korkeila et al. 2004; Price et al. 2006; van Dijk et al. 2008). Peer kindness has also reflected bonding, employment, mental health, organizational membership, safety, social class, and social and organizational networking as power to empower resilience (Lennartsson 2010; Marti et al. 2017; Mata and Pendakur 2014; Patulny and Morris 2012; Pena-Lopez and Sanchez-Santos 2016; Wetterbeng 2007). Organizational membership has raised outcome expectancy and reduced stress, thus boosting resilience (Nelson-Coffey et al. 2023). In the youth, peer kindness has additionally sustained relatedness as power to empower resilience (Levesque-Bristol et al. 2011; Phipps 2003). Conversely, the youth's peer kindness has additionally prevented psychopathology, thus retaining power to empower resilience (Tsai and Rosenheck 2012). Moreover, the youth's peer kindness has reflected the lack of social neglect and rejection, thus securing power to empower resilience (Wentzel 2003).

Incentives or utility provided by peer kindness for incentivizing resilience have involved achievement and success (Greeff and van der Merwe 2004; Larose et al. 1998; Wentzel and Caldwell 1997). Achievement or success embodies acceptance, capability, income, leadership, mental health, prestige, satisfaction, social integration, social status, stability, subordinating, victory, and wealth to shape resilience (Chung 2000; Ullrich et al. 2007; Furstenberg and Hughes 1995; Oettingen and Chromick 2018; Praszkier 2018; Schutte 2015; Spengler et al. 2018; Swartz 2013). Conversely, achievement or success precludes criminal activity or offense, distress, and violence, thus upholding resilience (Craig et al. 2020; Furstenberg and Hughes 1995). Peer kindness has also reflected justice perception as an incentive to incentivize resilience (Davis-Lipman et al. 2007). Justice perception reduces aggression and frustration, thus safeguarding resilience (Vermunt and Steensma 2016). Conversely, justice perception elevates acceptance, controllability, cooperation, meaningfulness, predictability, security, and trust to champion resilience (Dalbert 2001; Hafer and Sutton 2016; Vermunt and Steensma 2016). Moreover, justice perception has escalated accommodation, belongingness, health, life satisfaction, self-esteem, and social trust to boost resilience, (Bjornskov et al. 2013; Dalbert 2001; Hu 2013; Lipkus and Bissonette 1998; Lucas et al. 2013; van Prooijen et al. 2008). Conversely, justice perception has eroded depression and protesting, thus maintaining resilience (Benson and Ritter 1990; Wenzel 2000).

Ideals created by peer kindness for framing resilience have highlighted adjustment, self-esteem, and self-interest (Lan and Wang 2019; Petress 1995; Stake 2006). Self-interest fosters identity construction as an ideal to frame resilience (Toma 2017). Conversely, peer kindness has inhibited alcoholism, deviance, delinquency, doping, indecision, and violence as obsessions, thus framing resilience (Criss et al. 2017; Duncan et al. 2006; Guay et al. 2006; Menesini et al. 2003; Walters 2019). Alcoholism has caused aggression, illness, injury, and pathology to impede resilience (Brotchie et al. 2004; Haapanen-Niemi et al. 1999). Furthermore, peer kindness fosters ideals for or beliefs in independence, satisfaction, and general well-being to frame resilience (Feeney and Collins 2018; Lakey and Orehek 2011). Additionally, peer kindness has installed ideals for or beliefs in coping, emotional well-being, functioning, persistence, planning, pleasure, relational quality, self-determination, social well-being, and general well-being to frame resilience (Bishop et al. 2002; Bloom et al. 1991; Holliman et al. 2021; Logan and Cobb 2013; Peterson and Seligman 2004; Prenda and Lachman 2001; Vilhjalmsson and Thorlindsson 1998; Walen and Lachman 2016; Williams and Galliher 2006; Xi and Hwang 2011). Coping has included problem-solving and religious coping (Goodwin et al. 2001; Pargament et al. 2011). Functioning involves problem-solving, satisfaction, and success to facilitate resilience (Feldman 2018; Hahn et al. 2010; Swann 2012). Conversely, peer kindness has diminished anger, substance abuse, avoidance, suicide, and symptoms as obsessions, thus framing resilience (Brown and Zoorob 2022; Dutton et al. 2016; Glendinning et al. 2003; Kafetsio and Sideridis 2006; Ozbay 2008). Peer kindness has furthermore reflected life satisfaction as an ideal to frame resilience (Pena-Lopez and Sanchez-Santos 2016). Conversely, peer kindness has reflected resistance to obsessions for fatalism and schizophrenia, thus framing resilience (Goodwin et al. 2001; Magliano et al. 2006). In the youth, peer kindness has additionally fostered achievement, autonomy, conduct, enjoyment, exploration, future orientation, happiness, and self-orientation as ideals to frame resilience (Ahmed et al. 2010; Dietrich and Kracke 2009; Hitlin 2006; Iyer et al. 2009; Johnson et al. 2016; Levesque-Bristol et al. 2011; Phipps 2003). Exploration has buttressed self efficacy to facilitate resilience in the youth (Cabras and Mondo 2018; Harre 2007). Future orientation involves hope, interest or motivation, openness, optimism, persistence, and purposiveness to enhance resilience in the youth (Cabras and Mondo 2018; Ginevra et al. 2018; Oshri et al. 2018; Stoddard and Pierce 2018). Besides, future orientation has raised achievement, adaptability, control, health maintenance, learning effort, self-esteem, safety favor, and general well-being to boost resilience in the youth (Bradstreet and Parent 2018; Cabras and Mondo 2018; Jackman and MacPhee 2017; Mahajna 2017b; Steger et al. 2008; Stoddard and Pierce 2018). Conversely, future orientation has reduced doping expectancy and normativity, externalizing behavior, indecision, procrastination, and risking in the youth, thus safeguarding resilience (Chen and Vazsonyi 2013; Ginevra et al. 2016; Stoddard and Pierce 2018). Meanwhile, the youth's peer kindness has additionally reduced conflict, disorders, loneliness, and misconduct as obsessions, thus framing resilience (Bernardon et al. 2011; Hopson et al. 2014; Nieuwenhuis et al. 2017; Skomoravsky et al. 2006). Conflict has eroded life satisfaction, purposiveness, and general well-being in the youth to inhibit resilience (Hill et al. 2019). Conversely, conflict has bred anxiety, depression, somatization, and stress in the youth to impede resilience (Boudreaux and Ozer 2013; Hill et al. 2019).

Norms evolving from peer kindness to upgrade resilience have emphasized wellness and civic duty or engagement (Paez et al. 2007; Pavlova and Silbereisen 2015). Civic dutifulness has sustained health, mental health, and general well-being and eroded stress to advance resilience (Hample 2018; Tsai et al. 2018). Likewise, civic engagement fosters capacity, empowerment, and social capital to facilitate resilience (Speer and Hughey 1995; Stoll 2001; Smith 1997). Furthermore, civic engagement has incubated conflict resolution, education, happiness, health, income, individualism, life satisfaction, security normativity, social attachment, capital, integration, and trust, tolerance, and general well-being to advance resilience (Coffe and Geys 2007; Goren 2005; Growiec and Growiec 2010; Kroll 2011; Li and Walder 2001; Myers 1999; Pena-Lopez and Sanchez-Santos 2016; Posel and Casale 2011; Tak 2017; Tang 2011; Wallace and Pichler 2009; Welzel 2013; van Ingen and Bekkers 2015; Vincens et al. 2018). Conversely, civic engagement has reduced alcoholism, depression, and suicide, thus safeguarding resilience (Helliwell 2006; Ozbay 2008; Yu and Chiu 2016). Meanwhile, the youth's peer kindness has eroded the norm for delinquency, thus sustaining resilience (Ayers et al. 1999). Delinquency has jeopardized achievement, coping, education, mastery, life satisfaction, relational quality, self-efficacy, self-esteem, social attachment, and social capital in the youth to impede resilience (Carroll et al. 2009; Chung and Elias 1996; Compas et al. 1988; Fasang et al. 2014; Gault-Sherman 2012; Shek 2005). Conversely, delinquency has triggered disadvantage, distress, strain, suicide, and victimization experience to impair resilience in the youth (Cheung and Cheung 2006; Cutler et al. 2001; Hay 2003; Shek 2005).

Essentially, peer kindness is a norm to normalize personal kindness (de Groot and Steg 2009; Steg and de Groot 2010). Thus, the norm has underlain personal kindness (Greitemeyer et al. 2006; Wade-Benzoni and Tost 2009). Personal kindness, in turn, raises resilience with nuanced power, utility, ideals, and norms through the deterministic and voluntaristic mechanisms of analytical functionalism.

Power generated by kindness to drive resilience arises from competence, religiosity, and well-being (Dovidio et al. 2006; Hawley 2014; Mastain 2007). Furthermore, kindness has raised power through connectedness, empathy, and self-efficacy (Marsh and Dik 2021; Nai et al. 2018; Nelson-Coffey et al. 2023; Yao and Enright 2019). Connectedness has mitigated stress and negative emotion, thus upholding resilience (Nelson-Coffey et al. 2023). Empathy has facilitated communication quality and alleviated discontent and resentment to activate resilience (Redmond 2018). Conversely, kindness has diminished impulsivity, loneliness, and negative emotion as hurdles to resilience (Hample 2018; Nelson-Coffey et al. 2023). Impulsivity has fomented stress, thus weakening resilience (Hample 2018). In the youth, kindness has additionally sustained autonomy, ego strength, friendship quality, meaningfulness, relatedness, safety, soft or socioemotional skill, social attachment, and well-being to generate power to drive resilience (Bergin 2014; Dallago et al. 2009; Markiewicz et al. 2001; Martela and Ryan 2016; Na and Paternoster 2019). Ego strength covers coping to establish resilience in the youth (Walker and Hennig 1999). Friendship quality covers helpfulness, satisfaction, and security to maintain resilience in the youth (Leung and McBride-Chang 2013). Socioemotional skill has championed achievement, creativity, education, relational satisfaction, self-esteem, and social support received to boost resilience in the youth (Collins and van Dulmen 2006; de Bruyn et al. 2003; Ghayas and Malik. 2013; Larson et al. 2007; Nilsen et al. 2013). Conversely, socioemotional skill has diminished distress, insecurity, strain, and violence, thus restoring resilience in the youth (Collins and van Dulmen 2006; De Bruyn and Boom 2005; Larson et al. 2007; Pettit et al. 2006). Meanwhile, the youth's kindness has additionally prevented distress and loneliness, thus maintaining the power to drive resilience (Chen et al. 2022; Stotsky et al. 2019). Additionally, kindness reflects belongingness, education, emotion regulation, homeownership, income, intelligence, perception ability, social class, and wealth to furnish power to drive resilience (Degenne et al. 2004; Dovidio et al. 2006; Grant and Gino 2010; Greitemeyer et al. 2006; Hersberger-Langloh et al. 2022; Laguna et al. 2020; Thielmann and Hilbig 2019; Van de Vyver and Abrams 2018). Emotion regulation covers acceptance and impulsive control to advance resilience (Droutman et al. 2018). Such regulation has boosted self-esteem and weakened anxiety, depression, criminal behavior, risking, victimization experience, violence, and vulnerability to facilitate resilience (Armstrong et al. 2011; Cheung et al. 2014; Koegl and Day 2019; Langenderfer and Shimp 2001; Marchetti et al. 2018; Welch et al. 2008; Zavala and Guadalupe-Diaz 2019). Conversely, kindness hinges on the lack of impulsivity to maintain power to drive resilience (Thielmann et al. 2020).

Utility raised by kindness to attract resilience has emanated from achievement and success, benefit, hope, life satisfaction, and reward experienced (Bergin 2014; Layous et al. 2012; Marsh and Dik 2021; Mestre et al. 2019; Wentzel and Caldwell 1997). Achievement involves acceptance experienced, capability, homeownership, income, mental health, satisfaction, self-fulfillment, social integration, and wealth to foster resilience (Chung 2000; Craig et al. 2020; Furstenberg and Hughes 1995; Oettingen and Chromick 2018; Scabini and Cigoli 1997; Swartz 2013; Ullrich et al. 2007). Conversely, achievement precludes abuse, distress, criminal behavior, fighting, and offending, thus championing resilience (Craig et al. 2020; Furstenberg and Hughes 1995). Meanwhile, utility arises from the low cost experienced for attracting resilience (Bierhoff 2002).

Ideals nurtured by kindness to rationalize resilience have highlighted meaningfulness, protection, self-determination, and work value (Curry et al. 2018; Dinic and Bodroza 2021; Marsh and Dik 2021; Weinstein and Ryan 2010). In the youth, kindness has additionally fostered liking by others, popularity, self-clarity, and self-satisfaction as ideals to rationalize resilience (Bond and Kwan 2000; Crocetti et al.

2016; Umino and Dammeyer 2016). Conversely, youth's kindness has additionally dispelled delinquency, stigma, truancy, and violence as obsessions, thus safeguarding resilience (Eccles and Barber 1999; Hurd et al. 2011; Mesch 2009; Schulte 2002). Furthermore, kindness arises from agency, agreeableness, conservation value, coping, forgiveness, openness and its value, relief, and transcendence as ideals to rationalize resilience (Bayram 2016; Bierhoff 2002; Grant and Gino 2010; Heilman and Kusev 2020; Thielmann et al. 2020). Agency has maintained mastery, relational quality, satisfaction, and vitality to facilitate resilience (Delhey 2010; Hui et al. 2013; Ross and Drentea 1998; Sieber et al. 2019). Conversely, kindness arises from rejecting avoidance, dependence, narcissism, greed, and risking as obsessions, thus rationalizing resilience (Collins and Feeney 2004; Heilman and Kusev 2020; Thielmann et al. 2020). Dependence has eroded health, thus impeding resilience (Roy and Chaudhuri 2008). Narcissism has activated aggression, depression, misbehavior, and relational dissatisfaction, thus eroding resilience (Tracy et al. 2009). Risking has impaired health and activated criminal behavior and violence, thus weakening resilience (Farrington 2018; Pulkkinen et al. 2009; Wickrama et al. 1995).

Norms underlying kindness for normalizing resilience have hailed individualism (Hersberger-Langloh et al. 2022). Individualism embraces achievement, character, education, independence, reasoning, responsibility, and self-construction to sustain resilience (Davis and Robinson 1999; Fevre 2006; Oyserman et al. 2002). Hence, individualism has raised self-enhancement to advance resilience (Church 2010). Conversely, kindness has weakened peer or societal delinquency and uncertainty avoidance as norms, thus sustaining resilience (Layous et al. 2012; Na and Paternoster 2019).

## *Peer Advice*

Peer advice tackles adulthood, aging, anger, anxiety, panic, or phobia, bereavement, the body, cancer, career, chaos, courage, emotion, goals, meaning search, needs, obsession, oppression, recovery, sexuality, trauma, values, victimization, and well-being (Bachkirova 2018; Blum et al. 2006; Brown 2019; Bussolari and Goodell 2009; Donohoe and Ricketts 2012a; Fava and Ruini 2014; Goodman et al. 2016; Harper et al. 2003; Harris and Laidlaw 2012; Ladany and O'Shaughnessy 2014; Sieroda 2012; Syme 2012; Timulak 2015; Totton 2012; Oades et al. 2014; Ricketts and Donohoe 2012; Schneider 2000; Stelter 2017; Walker 2012; Williams et al. 2012). Such advice can raise resilience by generating power, incentives or utility, ideals, and norms to capitalize on the deterministic and voluntaristic mechanisms of analytical functionalism. Power empowering or driving resilience stands on social capital, social support received, spirituality, and strengths (Bottrell 2009; Dominguez et al. 2015; Mullin and Arce 2008). Moreover, resilience involves power based on competence, confidence, health, learning, and social attachment (Davydov et al. 2010; Orthner et al. 2004; Sitzer and Stockwell 2015; Ungar 2004; Williams et al. 2011). Resilience has benefited from power derived from coping ability, education, hardiness, income, learning, mastery, mentoring received, mindfulness, relatedness, religious faith, resources and their management, responsibility, self-efficacy, self-empowerment, self-esteem, social networks (Coholic 2011; Osterling et al. 2006; Jamison et al. 2017; Merrell 2009; Stewart and Yuen 2011; Theron et al. 2011; Woollett et al. 2016; Yin et al. 2022; Zhao and Fu 2022). Conversely, resilience has declined with power loss from anxiety, challenges experienced, and doping (Jaffee et al. 2007; Walker and Longmire-Avital 2013; Zhao and Fu 2022). Incentives incentivizing or attracting resilience build on finding benefits and optimism (Aldwin et al. 2009; Veronese and Barola 2018). Resilience has also arisen from utility stemming from hope (Stewart and Yuen 2011). Ideals framing or rationalizing resilience hail adaptation, controlling, defense, downward social comparison, and homeostasis (Davydov et al. 2010; Mullin and Arce 2008; Norris et al. 2008; Zhao and Fu 2022). Moreover, resilience involves ideals for coping, growth, happiness, meaning-making, recovery, satisfaction, self-care, self-construction, sustainability, and tolerance (Aldwin et al. 2009; Davydov et al. 2010; Helgeson et al. 2009; Henry 2001; Park 2009; L. Smith 2017; Ungar 2004; Veronese and Barola 2018). Resilience has also sprung from ideals for acceptance, challenge, forgiveness, humor, self-cultivation, self-reliance, temperance, and transcendence (Sitzer and Stockwell 2015; Stewart and Yuen 2011; Woollett et al. 2016; Zhao and Fu 2022). Norms normalizing or assimilating resilience emphasize flexibility, hardiness, normalization, resolution, and sharing (J. Simon et al. 2005; Theron et al. 2011). Conversely, resilience has stood on the social norm against crime (Jaffee et al. 2007). Notably, advice received has buttressed resilience (Greeff and van der Merwe 2004; Osterling et al. 2006; Regev and Ehrenberg 2012; Veronese and Barola 2018).

Power generated by advice received to raise resilience stems from adulthood, andragogy, or maturity and self-determination, attachment or bonding, consciousness, ego and self-development, interpersonal functioning, learning, mindfulness, rationality, responsibility, resolution, problem-solving, or solutions, self-esteem, skill, spirituality, and strength building (Bachkirova 2018; Bennett and Campone 2017; Brown 2011; Dryden 2012; Geldard and Geldard 2012a; Goldstein 1995, 2001; Mytton 2012; Nezu et al. 2013; Robinson and Dyson 2012; Ryan and Deci 2017; Schwartz 2012; Semple and Hott 2012; Shoukry 2017; Tudor and Sills 2012; Waines 2012; Williams et al. 2018). Such advice covers autonomy, creativity, reflection and self-reflection, relaxation, responsiveness, and self-monitoring (Fall et al. 2004; Potash et al. 2019; Sitzer and Stockwell 2015). Conversely, advice manages anger, anxiety, panic, phobia, and oppression experienced, thus retaining power to drive resilience (Brown 2019; Donohoe and Ricketts 2012a; Williams et al. 2012). For the youth, advice additionally establishes power based on identity (Raskin 1989). Advice has raised power to drive resilience by activating recourse (Vogel et al. 2006). To the patient or service user, advice has enhanced power based on health and emotional health and functioning, help received, intimacy, positive affect, and social skill to drive resilience (Boulton et al. 2001; Goertz-Dorten et al. 2017; Kwong et al. 2019; Lucas 2012; Jamison and Schuttler 2017;). Eventually, advice has boosted the power to secure the patient's or service user's resilience (Sitzer and Stockwell 2015). Social skill has covered emotion, knowledge, and nonverbal behavior (Koning et al. 2013).

Conversely, advice to the patient or service user has retained power to drive resilience by removing anxiety or phobia and society anxiety, depression, disorders, disturbance, and impulsivity (Erford et al. 2011; Goertz-Dorten et al. 2017; Herbert et al. 2005; Murphy et al. 2017). To the youth, advice received has raised employability, safety experience, self-efficacy and emotion regulation such as reappraisal to enhance power to drive resilience (Donald et al. 2019; Guntzviller et al. 2017; Lapan et al. 2001; Strepparava et al. 2016). Conversely, advice to youth has diminished symptoms, thus retaining power to drive resilience (Strepparava et al. 2016). To the elder, advice has also dampened depression to maintain power to drive resilience (Horowitz et al. 2005).

Power advised for adulthood or maturity rests on autonomy and self-determination, choice, competence, control, creativity, fitting, fulfillment, harmonizing, individuality, immediacy in action, intimacy, meaningfulness, mindfulness, negotiation, reflection, relatedness, responsibility, self-fulfillment, self-transformation, spontaneity, tolerance, trust, volition, and understanding (Bachkirova 2018; Fawcett 2012; Perlman 2000; Ryan and Deci 2017; Tudor and Sills 2012). Conversely, such advice rejects conflict, dependency, hostility, illusion, and playing (Bachkirova 2018; Gray 2017). Such advice unfolds acceptance, adulthood, authenticity, challenge, complementarity, contracting, feedback, interest, reasoning, regard, support, and transparency (Napper and Newton 2018; Ryan and Deci 2017). Conversely, such advice eschews childhood or immaturity, parenthood, and resistance (Napper and Newton 2018). Parenthood includes demanding and structuring (Napper and Newton 2018).

Power advised for attachment evolves from affect regulation, attunement, autonomy, clarification, collaboration, connection, control, curiosity, empathy, insight, intimacy, love experience, problem-solving, safety, secure bases, self-esteem, supporting (Goldstein 2001; Brown 2011; Schwartz 2012). Conversely, such advice removes acting out, aggression, aloneness, anger, blaming, boredom, conflict, defense, differentiation, distortion, disturbance, guilt, indulgence, narcissism, perfectionism, scapegoating, self-punishment, separation, and stimulation (Goldstein 2001; Brown 2011). Defense includes dissociation from self, idealization, projection, and splitting, contradiction, or inconsistency (Goldstein 2001). Such advice relies on confrontation, containment, empathy, exploring, hope, insight, integrity, intuition, neutrality, questioning, and reparation (Fall et al. 2004; Goldstein 2001; Brown 2011; Lipschitz-Elhawi 2009; McWilliams 2011). Hope covers activeness, control, positivity, and realism (Lipschitz-Elhawi 2009). Integrity embodies compromise, friendship, love, trust, warmth, and wholeness (Gross 2001). Interpretation concerns defense and resistance (Brown 2011; Yakeley 2012). Conversely, such advice avoids directiveness, regression, shaming, and shortness (Carlson et al. 2006; Izzard 2000; McWilliams 2011). Such advice has enhanced self-understanding and social recognition and reduced anxiety and interpersonal problems (Connolly and Crits-Christoph 1999).

Power advised for strengthening consciousness hinges on balancing, catharsis, choice, coherence, control, creativity, curiosity, differentiation, ego strength, empathy received, exploration, freedom, generativity, individuation, imagination, insight, mentalization, realization or reality awareness, self-regulation, reflection, resolution, self-acceptance, self-application, self-awareness, self-discovery, self-understanding, tolerating (Braun 2020; Brown 2011; Caputo et al. 2018; Geller 2014; Goldstein 2001; Kast 2006; Lee 2018; Samuels 2006; Williams 2012; Yakeley 2012). Conversely, such advice discourages competition, compromise, congestion, defense, depression, fixation, nihilism, and resistance (Braun 2020; Caputo et al. 2018; Fall et al. 2004; Fawcett 2012; Goldstein 2001; Semple and Hott 2012). Defense includes projection, regression, and repression concerning impulses (Goldstein 2001; Roberts and Brunning 2007). Such advice works with acceptance, anonymity, boundary setting, clarification, confrontation, detachment, insight, interpretation, self-reflection, and understanding (Brown 2011; Fawcett 2012; Goldstein 2001; McWilliams 2011; Segal 2012). Essentially, such advice aims to strengthen resilience (McWilliams 2011).

Power for ego or self-development advised evolves from adaptability, agency, admiration, autonomy, connectedness in mind, empathy, enjoyment, reflection, coping, defense, fitting, hope, insight, learning, meaning, mobilizing purpose, resources, narration, presentness, reflectiveness, resolution or problem-solving, responsibility, safety and security, self-acceptance, self-actualization, self-cohesion, self-esteem, synthesis or integration, testing, thinking, and understanding (Bachkirova 2022; Goldstein 1995, 2001). Conversely, such advice discourages aloneness, conflict, destructiveness, idealization, impulsivity, narcissism, omnipotence, perfection, self-deficit, and self-fragmentation (Goldstein 2001). Such advice exhibits acceptance, affirmation, attunement, consistency, empathy, explanation and interpretation, genuineness, humanness, immersion, repairing, responsiveness, soothing, understanding, and validation (Fall et al. 2004; Goldstein 2001). Conversely, such advice eschews confrontation and inquiry (Goldstein 2001).

Power based on interpersonal functioning arising from advice received springs from interpersonal attachment, involvement, need meeting, neutralization, quality, security, sharing, skill, support, trust, and validation (Evans 1996; Stuart and Robertson 2003). Conversely, such advice discourages interpersonal ambivalence, avoidance, crises or stress, and rejection (Stuart and Robertson 2003). Such advice proceeds with directive questioning, empathic and reflective listening, spontaneous discussion, and security or a secure base (Stuart and Robertson 2003).

Power regarding learning involves application, examination, autonomy and self-direction, collaboration, consequences, experiencing, exploration, mirroring, ownership, reappraising, relearning, and transformation (Bennett and Campone 2017, Williams et al. 2012). Experiencing encompasses conceptualization, experimentation, observation, reflection, resolution, self-management, and sense-making (Bennett and Campone 2017). Self-direction, resting on individualism, comprises autonomy, self-actualization, self-determination, and self-transformation (Bennett and Campone 2017). Transformation necessitates clarification, exploration, meaning-making, reflection, reframing, restructuring, and self-direction (Bennett and Campone 2017).

Power accruing from meaning search advised hinges on acceptance or coming to terms with the complexity of life, creating an ideal model, inner voice, self-reflection, self-responsibility, superconsciousness, synthesis, integration, or unifying, and will (Sieroda 2012; Silvester 2000; Waines 2012). Conversely, such advice minimizes denial, disconnection, identification, and splitting or contradiction (Sieroda 2012; Silvester 2000). Such advice works with altruistic love and empathic support (Sieroda 2012; Silvester 2000).

Power for mindfulness advised builds on analysis, breathing, acceptance, describing, eating, intuiting and reasoning, meditation, music listening, observing, one-mindedness, repertoire realizing, walking, and writing (Brodsky and Stanley 2013; McCay et al. 2015; Semple and Hott 2012; Swales and Dunkley 2012; Vega et al. 2014). Conversely, such advice rejects judging (Semple and Hott 2012).

Power advised to raise rationality covers and stems from alternative thinking, anticipating, attention, challenging, differentiating, experimenting and testing, goal setting, modifying, monitoring, realistic thinking, and restructuring beliefs, comprehension, interpretation, perception, prioritizing, questioning, self-awareness, self-talk (Donohoe and Ricketts 2012a; Fall et al. 2004; Jinks 2012; Mytton 2012; Williams et al. 2012, 2018; Waines 2012). Conversely, such advice maintains power for resilience by removing automaticity, disruption or interference encountered, and logical errors (Fawcett 2012; Mytton 2012; Parker 2002). Logical errors or distortions include awfulizing or catastrophizing, demanding or peppering, dichotomizing, filtering, magnification, maximization or minimization, overgeneralization, perfectionism, phoneyism, and personalization (Fall et al. 2004; Fawcett 2012; Mytton 2012; Williams et al. 2018). Such advice has maintained adjustment, coping, emotion regulation, and social support received to buttress resilience (Derella et al. 2020; Yang et al. 2018). Conversely, such advice has reduced anxiety, anger, depression, distress, eating disorders, misconduct, opposition, and stress (DeBar et al. 2013; Derella et al. 2020; Habigzang et al. 2013; O'Callaghan et al. 2013; Yang et al. 2018). Such advice hinges on disputation and experimentation (Donohoe and Richetts 2012b).

Power for resolution or problem-solving advised rests on adaptation, acting, cooperation, coping, deferment, expertise, learning, planfulness, self-direction, self-efficacy, self-regulation, self-talk, simplification, slowing, thinking, variety (Lloyd and Dallos 2008; Nezu et al. 2013; O'Connell and Palmer 2007). Adaptation comprises acceptance, optimism, and self-efficacy (Nezu et al. 2013). Self-talk covers arguing, challenging, and questioning as opposed to catastrophizing, judging, and overgeneralizing (Nezu et al. 2013). Slowing achieved by counting, breathing, exercising, imagining, praying, smiling, talking, and yawning (Nezu et al. 2013). Conversely, such advice precludes arbitrariness, avoidance, emotion, magnification and minimization, and overgeneralization (Nezu et al. 2013). Such advice applies acceptance, alliance building, brainstorming, competence seeking, complimenting, exception building, exploring, externalization or displaying information, feedback, flexibility, future visualizing, goal-setting, gradualism, hope, optimism, and positivity, listening, pragmatism, problem-free talk, questioning, reframing, the repertoire, respect, and success focus (Grant and Cavanagh 2018; Lloyd and Dallos 2008; Michael et al. 2000; Nezu et al. 2013; O'Connell 2012). Conversely, such advice discards presentness and problems (Grant and Cavanagh 2018; O'Connell 2012).

Power regarding skill strengthened by advice comprises desensitizing toward adversity, arousal reduction, attention, catharsis, expressing, imitation, joking or humor, relating, releasing or self-freeing, relaxing, and yoga (Bachkirova 2022; Fawcett 2012; Jinks 2012; Mytton 2012; Radley et al. 2014; Vallejos et al. 2016; VanFleet et al. 2010; Williams et al. 2012). Yoga involves breathing, calming, meditation, relaxing, posture, and vocalization, including chanting and dancing (Vallejos et al. 2016). For such strengthening, advice highlights exposure, rehearsal, modeling, monitoring, and scheduling (Fall et al. 2004; Jamison and Schuttler 2017). Such advice embodies acceptance, empathy, friendliness, rapport, recognition, respect, safety, and structuring (VanFleet et al. 2010). Conversely, such advice avoids asking, helping, hurrying, judging, and limiting (VanFleet et al. 2010).

Power from spirituality advised stands on balance, contemplation, devotion, fantasy, forgiveness, identity, newness and serendipity, questioning, meandering, meditation, prayer, reflection, relatedness, service, yoga, and wisdom (Fall et al. 2004; Sperry 2012; Western 2017). Such advice applies mirroring (Western 2017).

Power for building on strength advised accrues from accountability, affirmation, agency, assertiveness, awareness, balance, blessings, competence, collaboration and partnership, curiosity, forgiveness, goal-setting, gratitude, harmony, health, hope and optimism, humor, identity, leadership, letting go and in, meaningfulness, progressing, recovery, reframing, relatedness, relaxation, satisficing, savoring, self-concordance, self-determination, self-efficcy, self-esteem, solutions, spirituality, strength use, virtues, and zest (Boniwell and Kauffman 2018; Jones-Smith 2014; Littman-Ovadia et al. 2014; Mruk 2019; Proyer et al. 2013; Rashid 2014; Toporek and Cohen 2017). Goal-setting covers finance, health, leisure, life skills, living arrangements, occupation, recovery, relationships, and resources (Jones-Smith 2014). Health stands on living skill, nutrition, physical activity, and security (Jones-Smith 2014). Recovery manifests hope, planfulness and purposiveness, resourcefulness, respect, responsibility, self-direction, spirtuality, support reception, and work (Jones-Smith 2014). Conversely, recovery discards stigma (Jones-Smith 2014). Vittues additionally include chaity, faith, fortitude, justice, prudence, and temperance (Sperry 2012). Additionally, strengths transpire in analysis, character, creativity, education, finance, self-management, social support received, and wisdom (Jones-Smith 2014). Conversely, such advice dispels alienation and estrangement, anger, deficit, harm, pathology, and vices, including narcissism and self-indulgence (Jones-Smith 2014; Proyer et al. 2013; Sperry 2012; Toporek and Cohen 2017). Such advice realizes authenticity, genuineness, compliment, encouragement, relatedness, regard, respect, and support (Boniwell and Kauffman 2018; Jones-Smith 2014). Practically, such advice has raised curiosity, gratitude, hope, humor, positive mood, satisfaction, and zest (Proyer et al. 2013).

Utility induced by advice received to attract resilience draws on chance, hope, positivity in uncertainty, and workability (Boorman et al. 2012; Cheavens and Guter 2018; Pryor and Bright 2007). To the youth, advice has enhanced achievement and effectiveness experienced to secure utility and attract resilience (Fox and Butler 2009; Lapan et al. 2001).

Utility based on hope induced by advice emphasizes agency, clarification, competency, directiveness, interpretation, meditation, pathways, relaxation, self-talk, strengths, and success (Cheavens and Guter 2018; Lopez et al. 2000; Michael et al. 2000; Sympson and Elder 2000). Clarification concerns goals, subgoals, and their approach, commitment, and power gained from social networking (Cheavens and Guter 2018).

Ideals extolled by advice received to rationalize resilience prize acceptance and commitment, affirmation, confrontation, Confucianism, consistency, constructivism, or life designing, development, dialecticism, existentialism, feminism, forgiveness, holism, humanism, idealism, individuality or individualism, liberation, naturalism, positivity, postmodernism, poststructuralism, pragmatism, realism, social interest, stoicism, and zen (Bachkirova 2022; Bailly 2012; Boniwell and Kauffman 2018; Bratter 2003; Brazier 1995; Brodsky and Stanley 2013; Bryant-Davis 2007; Carlson et al. 2006; Craig 2007; Ellis and Smith 2012; Grawe 2004; Greenberg and Meneses 2019; Grimley 2007; Hayes 2014; Heenan 2012; Jarrett 2013; Leitner and Epting 2015; Lintz et al. 2019; McLeod 2012; Millar and Warner 2012; Nezu et al. 2013; Pett 2000; Savickas 2015; Shoukry 2017; Spinelli 2018; Strong 2002; Wubbolding et al. 2004; Yang 2017). For the youth, advice additionally nurtures ideals regarding Confucianism or scholarism (Luk-Fong 2006). To the patient or service user, advice has strengthened ideals for information processing, normalizing, and well-being or life quality to rationalize resilience (Goertz-Dorten et al. 2017; Lintz et al. 2019; Regev and Ehrenberg 2012). Conversely, advice to the patient or service user has lessened obsessions for aggression, doping, and oppositional behavior or defiance, thus upholding resilience (Erford et al. 2014; Goertz-Dorten et al. 2017; Lintz et al. 2019). To the youth, advice has buttressed ideals for rationalizing resilience by raising relationship quality, satisfaction, and general well-being (Lapan et al. 2001; Streparava et al. 2016).

Ideals for acceptance and commitment advised treasure choice, defusing problems, flexibility, knowledge, learning, meditation, mindfulness, and pragmatism (Boorman et al. 2012; Hayes 2014; Semple and Hott 2012). Conversely, such advice discourages avoidance, self-centeredness, and stickiness (Boorman et al. 2012; Hayes 2014).

Ideals for confrontation advised emphasize accepting responsibility, articulation, evaluation, mobilizing resources, and realizing the direction (Bratter 2003).

Ideals for Confucianism or scholarism advised extol acceptance, consanguinity, cooperation, equanimity, familism, filial piety, holism, hierarchy, openness, order, role fulfilling, self-cultivation, submission, and tradition (Yang 2017). Conversely, such advice minimizes desire, egalitarianism, and rationality as ideals (Yang 2017).

Ideals for consistency advised accentuate clarification, complementarity, monitoring feedback, and need fulfillment (Grawe 2004). Conversely, such advice dispels conflict and dissonance (Grawe 2004).

Ideals for constructivism advised treasure action, alternatives, change intentionally, completeness, coherence, mindfulness, narrative, possibility, reflexivity, self-characterizing, self-monitoring, tradeoff, and inquiry about living for explanation, prediction, and control (Fransella and Winter 2012; Kang and Gottfredson

2015; Leitner and Epting 2015; McIlveen 2015; Simon and Whitfield 2000; Stelter 2017). Such advice valorizes disequilibrium, distance communication, and listening (Duignan 2007; Fransella and Winter 2012).

Ideals for development advised value beauty, approach, autonomy, choice, competence, decidedness, exploration, goal setting, individuality, insight, modernism, negotiating, planning or planfulness, role-taking, self-efficacy, self-implementation, transition, working (Bachkirova 2022; Ladany and O'Shaughnessy 2014; Savickas 2015). Modernism advised treasures absolutism, deduction, evidence, objectivity, positivism, and science (Bachkirova 2022).

Ideals for dialecticism advised highlights analysis, accepting, accommodation, balance, collaboration, dialogue, distracting, easygoing, evaluation, equilibrium, flexibility, gentleness, mindfulness, multiplicity, negotiation, problem-solving, self-monitoring, synthesis or integration, tolerance for ambiguity, truthfulness, wholeness (Basseches 2003; Koerner 2012; McCay et al. 2015). Conversely, such advice dispels absolutism, apology, dichotomization, dilemmas, negative thinking, polarization, ruminating, and simplification (Brodsky and Stanley 2013; MacPherson et al. 2013). Such advice has instilled self-esteem and prevented depression (McCay et al. 2015).

Ideals for existentialism advised favor acceptance, acknowledgment, authenticity, autonomy, self-determination, and freedom, awareness, battling, bearing like a camel, breaking through, certainty experienced, choice, confrontation or facing, control, courage, creativity, difference-making, discovery, exploration and searching, functioning, generosity, growth, humor, identity, individualism or individuation, intimacy, investigation, loneliness, meaning, openness or tolerance, order experienced, predictability experienced, presentness, project engagement, purposiveness, responsibility and accountability, safety or security experienced, self-actualization, self-overcoming, self-reflection, self-sufficiency, self-understanding, sharing, superiority, uniqueness, and wisdom (Bachkirova 2022; Milton 2000; Shapiro 2016; van Deurzen 2012; Waines 2012). Acknowledgment covers acceptance, belonging, domination, and love as opposed to condemnation, hate, isolation, and rejection (van Deurzen 2012). Authenticity covers acceptance, courage, and relatedness (Fall et al. 2004). Autonomy covers confidence, identity, integrity, and perfection as opposed to disintegration, confusion, doubt, and imperfection (van Deurzen 2012). Awareness covers anxiety, consistency, death or mortality, defense, freedom, isolation, limits, meaning, predictability, presentness, security, and tension concerning fear, freedom, guilt, security, and stagnation (Shapiro 2016). Freedom rejects compulsion, constriction, and duties (Watson and Bohart 2015). Safety concerns death, health, illness, life, pleasure, pain, and poverty (van Deurzen 2012). Wisdom covers meaning, serenity, and purpose as opposed to evil, futility, and guilt (van Deurzen 2012). Conversely, such advice removes avoidance, confusion, emptiness, foreclosure, preoccupation, rejection, and weaknesses (Shapiro 2016). Moreover, such advice proceeds with attribution, collaboration, confrontation, empathy, flexibility, liberating, mirroring, privacy, questioning, respect, toughness, and understanding (Shapiro 2016; Spinelli 2018; Watson and Bohart 2015).

Ideals for feminism advised involve gender equality and justice, female activism and participation, agency, anger, assertiveness, awareness and knowledge, choice, collaboration, community service, competence, consent, empowerment, external attribution, grouping, growth, independence, and self-reliance, liberalization or liberation, normalizing, politics and power (Bimrose 2012; Brown 2019; Heenan 2012; Sympson and Elder 2000; Williams et al. 2012). Conversely, such advice rejects female domination, oppression, and stereotyping experienced (Bimrose 2012; Heenan 2012).

Ideals for forgiveness advised embrace acceptance, assertiveness, authenticity, compassion and self-compassion, dialogue, disregarding thoughts, distancing or clearing a space, emotion regulation, empathy, expressing emotions, generosity, goodwill, loving, responsiveness, safety and security experienced, and self-exploration (Greenberg 2004; Greenberg and Meneses 2019; Timulak 2015). Such advice disapproves anger or rage, hostility, punishment, resentment, self-criticism, and shame (Greenberg and Meneses 2019).

Ideals for holism advised foreground awareness, creativity, curiosity, discernment or discrimination, experimenting, responsibility, and self-aggression (Allan and Whybrow 2007; Bluckert 2018; Stelter 2017). Awareness avoids deflection, egotism, and self-aggression (Allan and Whybrow 2007; Bluckert 2018). Conversely, such advice rejects assimilation, incompleteness, and self-harm (Ellis and Smith 2012). Such advice runs with actuality, authenticity, dialogue, experiments, exploration, immediacy, presentness, responsibility, self-balance and self-regulation, self-support and self-trust, and wholeness (Ellis and Smith 2012; Fall et al. 2004; Rowan 2001). Actuality covers acceptance, awareness, insight, and presentness (Fall et al. 2004). Dialogue covers confirmation, inclusion, presence, and trust (Ellis and Smith 2012). Experiments concern the body, language, and work (Ellis and Smith 2012).

Ideals for humanism advised emphasizes agency, assertiveness, authenticity, awareness, catharsis, consciousness, coping, creativity, development, empathy, exploration and self-exploration, improvisation, individualism, insight, meaning, motivation, ownership, playfulness, presentness, purposiveness, reflection, relatedness, resistance, role-taking, self-acceptance, self-actualization, self-determination, self-integration, self-respect, spontaneity, striving, subjectivity, and understanding (Aspy et al. 2000; Bachkirova 2022; Baim 2012; Farber 2010; Friedman and MacDonald 2006; Joseph Bryant-Jefferies 2007; Lintz et al. 2019; Miguel and Pino-Juste 2021; Shapiro 2016; Tudor 2012; Williams et al. 2012). Development covers growth, breakthrough, catharsis, competence, enlightenment, ecstasy, and self-direction (Farber 2010; Rowan 1998; Watts et al. 2004). Growth concerns ego enhancement, liberation, and self-actualization (Farber 2010). Individualism covers authenticity, freedom, self-awareness, self-determining, and uniqueness (Rowan 1998). Motivation evolves from the ideal pursuit and experiences in affirmation, collaboration, discussion, empathy, rapport, and support as opposed to criticism (Brown 2011; Passmore and Whybrow 2007). Reflection covers freedom, intentionality, meaningfulness, purposefulness, relatedness, responsibility, and self-consciousness (Kelly 1997). Self-determination covers responsibility, self-actualization, self-development, self-direction, self-education, self-evaluation, and self-knowledge (Levitt et al. 2005; Rowan 1998). Subjectivity covers creativity, meaningfulness, potentialities, purposefulness, self-acceptance, self-determination, self-worth, transcendence, and uniqueness (Kelly 1997; Watts et al. 2004). Conversely, such advice dispels conformism, conflict, incongruence between self and reality, discomfort, reliance, and stereotyping (Barak 2016; Miguel and Pino-Juste 2021; Shapiro 2016; Tudor 2012). Such advice proceeds with affection, authenticity, awareness, caring, clarification, collaboration or allying, congruence between awareness and experience, connectedness or relationship building, creativity, innovation, or novelty, democracy, emotional intelligence, evocation, explanation and interpretation, flexibility, focusing, genuineness, helpfulness, hope, imaging, inquiry, liberation, listening, openness, praise, realism, reflection, regard, responsiveness, spontaneity, understanding, variety, and wholeness (Aspy et al. 2000; Bryant-Jefferies 2007; Brown 2011; Doucete 2004; Farber 2010; Joseph 2018; Rowan 1998; Stiles 2012; Wampold 2007; Watts et al. 2004; Tudor 2012). Democracy involves collaboration, co-creation, consensus, and equity (Rowan 1998). Inquiry concerns self-reflection and whole-person assessment (Farber 2010). Novelty concern choice, empathy, feedback, genuineness, growth, justice, resonance, responsiveness, self-disclosure, space, and warmth (Aspy et al. 2000; Farber 2010; Rowan 1998). Reflection covers awareness, monitoring, observation, and self-assessment (Farber 2010)). Wholeness covers the body, feeling, intellect, soul, and spirit (Rowan 1998). Conversely, such advice avoids authoritarianism, conformity, diagnosis, directiveness or directionality, theory, and transference (Aspy et al. 2000; Bryant-Jefferies 2007; Eliason et al. 2010; Rowan 1998).

Ideals for individualism or individuality advised prioritize acceptance, adaptation, assimilation, belongingness, capability, collaboration or cooperation, compensation, connecting, consciousness, contribution, courage, creativity, dominating, growth, hope, humanness, idealism, individuation, subjectifying, insight, knowledge producing, meaningfulness, optimism, positivity, prevention, purposefulness, reciprocity, recognition received, resource recognition, responsibility, science, superiority, understanding, and wholeness (Carlson et al. 2006; Fall et al. 2004; Fink 1995; Gullatz 2010; Parker 2011). Remarkably, such advice idealizes resilience (Carlson et al. 2006). Conversely, such advice discourages alienation and domination experienced, complaining, foreclosure, nonsense, obedience, projection by others, separation and subjugation experienced, servitude, withdrawal, and influence by others' desire (Carlson et al. 2006; Fink 1995; Parker 2011). Such advice proceeds with alliance building, confrontation, democracy, directiveness, diversity appreciation, education, encouragement, egalitarianism, flexibility, humor, interpretation, interrogating, interrupting, metaphorizing, peppering, redemption, reflection, reorientation, and respect (Carlson et al. 2006; Fink 1995; Parker 2011). Conversely, such advice abandons anxiety and resistance (Parker 2011).

Ideals for liberation or liberalism advised prize feminism, justice, liberty, and need fulfillment (Brown 2019, Bryant-Davis 2007). Conversely, such advice detests oppression (Bryant-Davis 2007).

Ideals for life designing advised foreground adaptability, hope, identity, learning, mattering, preparedness, and volition (Savickas 2015).

Ideals for naturalism advised cover attunement, compassion, emptying, equanimity, kindness, loving, moderation, natural resource use, nowness, purifying, softness, spontaneity, sympathy, and transcendence (Brown 2019; Craig 2007; Lee 2003). Conversely, such advice minimizes egoism or egocentrism, fighting, and inference (Lee 2003).

Ideals for postmodernism advised emphasize discourse, diversity, meaning-making, and self-determination (Brown 2019). Conversely, such advice dispels dogmatism (Brown 2019; Strong 2002). Conversely, such advice discourages authority and discipline (Bachkirova 2022). Such advice manifests trustworthiness (Strong 2002).

Ideals for poststructuralism advised underscore aspiration, dream, hope, authenticity, desire, mindfulness, resolution, self-recreation, strengths, and uniqueness through narration, restorying, or retelling, including reauthoring (Bailly 2012; Gergen and Gergen 2006; Law 2007; McLeod 2012; Richert 2002; Zimmerman and Dickerson 1996). Mindfulness involves acceptance, meditation, and repertoire building (Vega et al. 2014). Strengths include caring, collaboration, expectancy, and hope (Dybicz 2011). Narration prizes its actionability, agility, articulation, believability, broadening and thickening, externalizing causes and problems, self-disclosure, and self-reflection (Drake 2018; Gergen and Gergen 2006; Guilfoyle 2005; McLeod 2012; Phipps and Vorster 2011; Vega et al. 2014). Conversely, narration precludes guilt, rationality, and self-blame (Guilfoyle 2005; Gergen and Gergen 2006). Such advice realizes collaboration, decentering, familiarity, listening, reciprocity, social inclusion, trust, and witness (Drake 2018; Gergen and Gergen 2006; McLeod 2012; Phipps and Vorster 2011; Theobald 2016).

Ideals for pragmatism advised foreground acuity, choice, flexibility, goal-setting, outcomes, positivity, questioning, resolution or problem-solving, and transformation (Bridoux and Weaver 2000; Cooper and Seal 2012; Grimley 2007, 2018). Questioning concerns how, what, when, and where to avoid distortion and generalization (Grimley 2018). Such advice proceeds with acceptance, metaphor, rapport, reframing, and support (Bridoux and Weaver 2000; Grimley 2018).

Ideals for realism advised accentuate altruism, assertiveness, choice, clarifying, comfort, confrontation, control, humor, planning, positive thinking, presentness, relatedness, responsibility, safety, and self-evaluation (Fall et al. 2004; Howatt 2001; Wubbolding et al. 2004). Planning needs to be attainable, immediate, measurable, and simple for improvement (Wubbolding et al. 2004). Conversely, such advice discourages excusing and giving up (Fall et al. 2004). Such advice manifests acceptance, congruence between awareness and experience, empathy, regard, and trust (Howatt 2001).

Ideals for social interest advised favor flexibility, learning, responsibility, and strengths (Millar and Warner 2012). Such advice presents democracy and equality, empathy, interest, warmth, interdependence, mistake uncovering, modeling, and strength identifying (Millar and Warner 2012).

Ideals for stoicism advised treasure controlling, generalizing, interpreting, peace or tranquility, precision, rationality, self-acceptance, self-actualization, self-control, self-direction, self-help, and teaching (Browning and Cooper 2004; Dryden 2003;

Fall et al. 2004; Jarrett 2013). Rationality includes acceptance, self-acceptance, creativity, flexibility, interest, responsibility, scientificity, and tolerance (Browning and Cooper 2004; Dryden 2012). Conversely, irrationality includes awfulizing, depreciation, dogmatism, rigidity, self-criticism, short-termism, and utopianism (Browning and Cooper 2004; Dryden 2012). Conversely, such advice discounts passion, religiosity, and social comparison (Browning and Cooper 2004). Religiosity discounted includes dependence and sacrifice (Browning and Cooper 2004). Such advice demonstrates acceptance or tolerance, alternative thinking, argumentation, cost–benefit analysis, dialogue, directiveness, education, empathy, experimentation, flooding or total exposure, goal-setting, humor, imagery, immediacy, listening mistakes, pragmatism, questioning, and rationality (Dryden 2003, 2012; Fall et al. 2004). Conversely, such advice eschews awfulizing, damnation, demand, depreciation, shaming, and warmth (Fall et al. 2004).

Ideals for zen advised hail awakening and enlightening, breaking through, compassion and kindness, congruence, consciousness, cosmopolitanism, empathy, emptiness and self-surrender, forgiving, freshness, generosity, grit, harmony, honesty, liberation, loss, love and giving, meditation and quietness, open-mindedness and mind expansion, nature fitting, presentness, radiance, respect, self-examination, self-responsibility, simplicity, spirituality, transcendence, unity, will and goodwill, and wisdom (Brazier 1995). Cosmopolitanism upholds globalism and multiculturalism as opposed to nativism (Sorge 2008; Watts and Feldman 2001). Meditation emphasizes concentration, groupness, mindfulness, and walking (Brazier 1995). Conversely, such advice rejects compulsion, demand, delusion, greed, harm, hate, humanism, ignoring, self-actualization, self-supporting, sexuality, and shallowness (Brazier 1995). Humanism rejected includes conflicting and self-seeking (Brazier 1995).

Norms shared by advice received to assimilate resilience endorse autonomy, change, clarity and directness, connectedness, existentialism, fairness, holism, humanism, interpersonal functioning, leadership, rationality, and skill development (Barlow and Burlingame 2006; Fall et al. 2004; Paul 2012; Shechtman et al. 2002). To strengthen assimilation, advice emphasizes cohesiveness, conformity, empathy, feedback giving and receiving, interpersonal relevance, normativity, and social acceptability (Paul 2012). Such norms have engendered intimacy featuring attachment, frankness, giving, helping, loyalty, sensitivity, spontaneity, and trust to uplift resilience (Shechtman et al. 2002).

## *Peer Adversity*

Peer adversity is likely to impede resilience by diminishing power, utility, ideals, and norms favorable to resilience predicated on the analytical functionalist framework. This framework proposes power to empower or drive resilience for the fulfillment function, utility or incentives to incentivize or attract resilience for the adaptation function, ideals to frame or rationalize resilience for the latency function, and norms to normalize or assimilate resilience for the integration function. More specifically, peer adversity sustains the fulfillment function by raising agency (Soller et al. 2017). Alternatively, peer adversity bolsters the integration function with conformity, contagion, and controlling socially (Deptula and Cohen 2004; Prinstein and Wang 2005). Contagion comprises selection and training, including modeling and reinforcement (Prinstein and Wang 2005).

Peer adversity generally, including distress, emotionality, and withdrawal, has dampened life satisfaction and security experienced to impede resilience (Dost-Gozkan 2019; Mikulincer and Selinger 2001). Conversely, peer adversity has bred victimization experience to disrupt resilience (Schreck et al. 2007). Peer adversity thus has shrunk power and ideals for resilience. Additionally, peer deviance, as a case of peer adversity, has also eroded power, utility, ideals, and norms for resilience.

Power driving resilience reduced by peer deviance has involved conformity, prosocial behavior, and self-efficacy (Ma et al. 2007; Nivette et al. 2021; Soller et al. 2017). Conformity has furnished achievement and its pressure, mastery-goal setting, social closeness and support received, and tolerance to benefit resilience (Feldman 2003; Jiang et al. 2015; Magnuson et al. 2006). Conversely, conformity has mitigated conflict, distress, doping, externalizing behavior, and violence thus lifting resilience (Cohen and Fromme 2002; Jiang et al. 2015; Magnuson et al. 2006). Prosocial behavior has upheld the feelings of autonomy, competence, meaningfulness, satisfaction, self-clarity, and social well-being conducive to resilience (Crocetti et al. 2016; Layous et al. 2012; Martela and Ryan 2016; Umino and Dammeyer 2016). Social well-being comprises social adjustment and integration (Froh et al. 2010; Schludermann et al. 2000). In practice, prosocial behavior has enabled to optimize resilience (Bond and Kwan 2000). Prosocial behavior has also sustained the experiences of achievement, liking, and popularity, and safety (Bond and Kwan 2000; Wentzel and Caldwell 1997). Furthermore, prosical behavior has secured the disposition of religiosity to buttress resilience (Barry et al. 2012). Conversely, prosocial behavior has lessened delinquency, distress, ego depletion, loneliness, and violence, thus bolstering resilience (Ma et al. 2011; Martela and Ryan 2016; Mesch 2009; Stotsky et al. 2019). Self-efficacy has raised the quality of life, satisfaction, self-esteem, and general well-being to safeguard resilience (Forgeard and Benson 2019; Luszczynska and Gutierrez-Dona 2005). Satisfaction has covered coping, life, school, and study (Burger and Samuel 2017; Kanno and Koeske 2010; Kryshko et al. 2023). Conversely, self-efficacy has mitigated the feelings of anger, anxiety, depression, distress, and negative affect, thus bolstering resilience (Forgeard and Benson 2019; Fosco and Feinberg 2015; Luszczynska and Gutierrez-Dona 2005). In practice, self-efficacy has secured recourse, resource management, self-regulation, and self-regulated learning to achieve resilience (Brackney and Karabenick 1995; Garland and Zigler 1994; Kryshko et al. 2023; Schunk and Zimmerman 1996; Shell and Husman 2008). Self-efficacy has conduced to the experiences of achievement and learning to foster resilience (Kennedy and Tuckman 2013; Wang et al. 2017). Conversely, self-efficacy has lessened the experience of stress, thus securing resilience (Kennedy and Tuckman 2013). Self-efficacy has also consolidated the dispositions of creativity, entrepreneurship, optimism, and skill to enable resilience (Forgeard and Benson

2019; Rawlings 2012; Milioni et al. 2015; Schmitt-Redermund and Vondracek 2002). Hence, self-efficacy has maintained resilience (Milioni et al. 2015). Conversely, peer deviance has fomented aggression and violence, delinquency and theft, externalizing behavior, recidivism, risk, social rejection experienced, victimization experienced, and substance abuse, including alcoholism and doping to realize power against resilience or weaken power for driving resilience (Bhochhibhoya et al. 2021; Carlo et al. 2014; Deptula and Cohen 2004; German et al. 2009; Grant et al. 2019; Jackman and MacPhee 2017; Low and Shortt 2017; Paige et al. 2022; Walters 2020; Wilhoit and Goodnight 2023). Externalizing or problem behavior has included antisocial behavior and gang involvement (Aizer 2009; Lansford et al. 2003; Zimmermann and Bingenheimer 2002). Risk has generated feelings of anxiety, depression, and distress to erode resilience (Gerard and Buehler 2004; Muris and van den Berg 2003; Prelow et al. 2006). In practice, risk has raised delinquency and doping to impede resilience (Wright et al. 2016). Risk has also fomented the experiences of social rejection and victimization to erode resilience (Sanderson et al. 2016; Viola et al. 2016). Furthermore, risk has boosted the disposition of suicidality to impair resilience (Light et al. 2003). Conversely, risk has attenuated achievement experienced, hope, relational quality meaning-making, self-esteem, and social support received, thus forbidding resilience (Krishnakumar and Black 2003; Sanderson et al. 2016; Schoon 2006). Moreover, peer deviance has arisen from abusive experience, alienation experience, anger, harshness and punishment experienced, impulsivity and sensation seeking, isolation experienced, social deficit and withdrawal, and stigmatization experienced to disrupt power for resilience (Benda 2002; Gao et al. 2015; Johnson et al. 2004; Menard and Mose 1984; Morris et al. 2015; Yoon et al. 2020; Wilhoit and Goodnight 2023). Alienation experienced has fomented feelings of depression, guilt, internalizing, loneliness, negative emotion, resentment, and stupidity to disturb resilience (Sommer et al. 2001; Tani and Schneider 1997; Witkow 2005). In practice, alienation experienced has provoked aggression and conduct disorders as opposed to cooperation and effort, thus undermining resilience (Tani and Schneidner 1997; Witkow 2005). Alienation experienced has also generated experiences of frustration, rejection, and threat to belongingness, meaning, and self-esteem, thus impairing resilience (Sommer et al. 2001). Conversely, alienation experienced has attenuated self-esteem, thus disrupting resilience (Sommer et al. 2001). Punishment received has incurred alienation felt, distress, externalizing behavior, relational problems, and violence to erode resilience (Antunes et al. 2014; Woodward and Fergusson 1999; Xing et al. 2011; Zalewski et al. 2017; Zhang and Messner 1994). Conversely, punishment received has diminished achievement, thus disrupting resilience (Lee 2011). Impulsivity has fomented the experiences of persecution and stress to weaken resilience (Hample 2018). Isolation or social deficit has impeded self-esteem, thus disrupting resilience (Young and Bagley 1982). Withdrawal has fomented conflict to impair resilience (Debus et al. 2019). Meanwhile, peer deviance has ensued from inadequate power drawn from agreeableness, conscientiousness, relational quality, religiosity, self-control and self-regulation, social attachment, bonding, and support received, and socioeconomic status, thus dampening resilience (Ayers et al. 1999; Benda 2002; Brezina and Piquero 2007; Costello and Vowell 1999; Kendler et al. 2015; Lee et al.

2017; Paige et al. 2022; Price et al. 2019). Agreeableness has raised attachment and its security to enable resilience (Carver 1997). Conversely, agreeableness has prevented risking, thus safeguarding resilience (Howard and Alipour 2014). Conscientiousness has activated achievement, attachment and its security, controlling, prevention, and prudence to achieve resilience (Beutler and Gudmunson 2012; Carver 1997; Crede et al. 2010; Trapman et al. 2007).

Utility attracting resilience undermined by peer deviance has rested on effectiveness experienced (Peterson and Esbensen 2004). Moreover, peer deviance has stood on belief in reward from antisocial behavior to disincentivize resilience (Ayers et al. 1999). Antisocial belief has generated violence to disrupt resilience (Kornienko et al. 2018).

Ideals rationalizing resilience dismissed by peer deviance favor safety (Jackman and MacPhee 2017). Safety has maintained achievement, life quality, mental health, and sufficiency experienced to foster resilience (Crume et al. 2019). Conversely, safety has prevented aggression, anxiety, depression, internalizing, opposition, risking, and victimization experienced, thus safeguarding resilience (Barbarin and Richter 2001; Crume et al. 2019; Jackman and MacPhee 2017). Meanwhile, peer deviance has induced antisocial belief to rationalize against resilience (Carson 2013). Furthermore, peer deviance has evolved from inadequate ideals for humanitarianism, prosocial identification, and social preference, thus weakening resilience (Garnier and Stein 2002; Na and Paternoster 2019; Prinstein and Wang 2005). Humanitarianism hails and rests on protection, religiosity, and self-determination to sustain resilience (Ager and Ager 2011; Brigg 2018; Chouliaraki 2013). Meanwhile, peer deviance has ensued from obsessions for delinquency favor and violence belief to impede resilience (Morris et al. 2015; Walters 2016).

Norms assimilating resilience shielded by peer deviance have resided in social and parental control, education, monitoring, responsiveness, and supervision (Benda 2002; Elliott and Wilson 1996; Warr 2005; Weaver and Prelow 2005). These norms have reduced arrest experience, delinquency, failure expected, misconduct, problems, and substance abuse, thus upholding resilience (Cheung 2014; Kerr and Stattin 2000; Parker and Benson 2004; Soenens and Beyers 2012). Conversely, these norms have secured relational quality to boost resilience (Kerr and Stattin 2000). Meanwhile, peer deviance has evolved from norms for disorder and risking, thus impeding resilience (Low and Shortt 2017; Vander Ven et al. 2001). These norms have diminished earnings, safety, social capital, attachment, and trust, and well-being, thus eroding resilience (Brown et al. 2004; Congdon 2010; Kanan and Pruitt 2002; Ross and Mirowsky 2009; van Praag and Frijters 1999; Vartanian 1999). Well-being has included happiness and positive emotion (Hackman et al. 2019). Conversely, the norms have bred depression, economic hardship, normlessness, poverty, and victimization experienced to hurt resilience (Like 2011; Pei and Kim 2017; Ross and Mirowsky 2009; Vartanian 1999; Whelan and Maitre 2013). Moreover, social disorder encompasses deprivation, incivility, instability, poverty, and stress to weaken resilience (Brown et al. 2004; Brossard 2019; Congdon 2010; Vartanian 1999; Williams et al. 1999).

### *Peer Resilience*

Peer resilience is likely to raise personal resilience through empowering or driving, incentivizing or attracting, framing or rationalizing, and normalizing or assimilating, predicated on the analytical functionalist framework. This framework highlights power, incentives or utility, ideals, and norms for achieving the functions of fulfillment, adaptation, latency, and integration necessary to maintain the structural whole. Power engendered by peer resilience to drive personal resilience has rested on competence, security experienced, and self-efficacy (Bissell-Havran and Loken 2009; Dash and Anderson 2015; Markiewicz et al. 2001). Conversely, peer resilience has weakened antisocial behavior, thus retaining power for or weakening power against resilience (Criss et al. 2017). The ideal sustained by peer resilience values studying to rationalize resilience (Bissell-Havran and Loken 2009). Study valuation has facilitated achievement, career aspiration, education, and study engagement conducive to resilience (Anderman 2003; Liu and Yu 2016; Martin 2009). Conversely, study valuation has prevented delinquency, thus maintaining resilience (Hoffmann and Dufur 2008).

## Original Findings

Among the 16 hypothesized peer effects, 11 obtained support from the original findings based on the statistical analysis of the Chinese datasets (see Table 5.1). Peer effects that were not statistically significant originated from advice received, peer resilience demand received, peer relational kindness, peer resilience handling, and peer self-awareness.

Peer and personal factors involved in the peer effects each combined a set of rating items. Notably, some peer factors were the averages of the corresponding personal factors in the service unit. For instance, peer functional disability was the average functional disability of persons in the service unit. Besides, relational kindness, speaker sociability, and aid and advice received also originated from peers.

| |
|---|
| *Adversity, past year* ($\alpha = 0.723$) |
| Grief of the death of family |
| Pain from accident |
| Pain of economic loss |
| Pain of failure of school or work |
| Pain of broken marriage of family |
| Pain of illness |
| *Functional disability, past year* ($\alpha = 0.942$; Bass et al. 1999) |
| Walking up and down stairs |
| Bathing |

(continued)

(continued)

| |
|---|
| Taking transportation |
| Shopping |
| Walking half an hour |
| *Kindness, past 6 months ($\alpha = 0.925$;* Isaacowitz et al. 2003*)* |
| Using a good attitude toward your family |
| (Not) Using a bad attitude toward your family |
| Using a good attitude toward service staff |
| (Not) Using a bad attitude toward service staff |
| Using a good attitude toward friends |
| (Not) Using a bad attitude toward friends |
| *Relational kindness, past 6 months ($\alpha = 0.918$;* Isaacowitz et al. 2003*)* |
| Family using a good attitude toward you |
| Family (not) using a bad attitude toward you |
| Service staff using a good attitude toward you |
| Service staff (not) using a bad attitude toward you |
| Friends using a good attitude toward you |
| Friends (not) using a bad attitude toward you |
| *Speaker sociability, past 6 months ($\alpha = 0.912$;* de Bruyn et al. 2003*)* |
| Being with a group of people |
| Acting in concert with a group |
| Being close to you |
| Meeting you every day |
| Sharing your interests |
| Sharing similar experiences with you |
| Being good for you |
| Speaking out of the heart |
| Being easygoing |
| Being talkative |
| Standing in your position |
| Supporting your approach |
| Talking being pertinent |
| Saying the truth |
| *Aid reception, past 6 months ($\alpha = 0.796$;* Cheung and Chan 2010*)* |
| Someone helping you with your daily chores |
| Someone giving you good advice |
| Someone having a good time with you together |
| Someone loving you |
| Someone understanding difficulties that you face |

(continued)

(continued)

| |
|---|
| *Advice received, past 6 months ($\alpha = 0.716$;* Cheung and Chan 2010*)* |
| Experts teaching you how to overcome adversity |
| Friends teaching you how to overcome adversity |
| Other elders teaching you how to overcome adversity |
| Religious people teaching you how to overcome adversity |
| Family members teaching you how to overcome adversity |
| Social workers teaching you how to overcome adversity |
| People in the media teaching you how to overcome adversity |
| *Resilience exposure: demand reception, past 6 months ($\alpha = 0.807$)* |
| Others wanting you to hold on |
| Others wanting you to accept adversity |
| Others wanting you to do your best |
| *Resilience handling, past month ($\alpha = 0.894$)* |
| Releasing yourself |
| Daring to try |
| Thinking of something funny |
| Dong the best |
| Trying to do a good job |
| Putting things down |
| Accepting adversity |
| Forgiving others |
| (Not) Caring small matters |
| (Not) Being persistent |
| *Resilience learning, past month ($\alpha = 0.709$)* |
| Try hard to learn how to deal with adversity |
| Having fun in learning to deal with adversity |
| *Self-awareness, past month ($\alpha = 0.874$;* Kramer and Frazer 1990*)* |
| Appreciating your good side |
| Making good use of spare time |
| Being aware of your strengths |
| *Resilience belief, past 3 months ($\alpha = 0.918$)* |
| Having ups and downs in life |
| Being fine to have a clear conscience |
| Friends' being good to you |
| Living, learning, and working |
| Needing to break through the frame of questions |
| Things getting better |
| Suffering necessarily existing in the world |

(continued)

(continued)

| |
|---|
| Wanting someone to remind you |
| (Not) Being miserable |
| *Benevolent world belief, past 3 months (α = 0.917*; Janoff-Bulman 1992*)* |
| The world being beautiful |
| People being kind |
| People being helpful |
| *Resilience, recent week (α = 0.698)* |
| Being able to face even in difficult circumstances |
| Feeling calm under pressure |
| Liking yourself when making a mistake |
| Recovering soon even if frustrated |
| Being able to remain calm when facing tremendous pressure |
| Being able to remain calm even in a terrible environment |
| (Not) Having difficulty to face adversity |
| (Not) Being anxious in a stressful environment |
| *Adjustment, recent week (α = 0.821;* Costa-Requena 2009*)* |
| Being happy |
| Turning good |
| (Not) Losing control |
| (Not) Losing hope for life |
| (Not) Worrying |
| (Not) Having some loss |
| (Not) Giving up some ideas |
| *Resilience, recent month (α = 0.728)* |
| Keeping calm when faced with stress |
| Rolling with the punches |
| Actively facing difficulties |
| Being able to face adversity |
| (Not) Feeling anxious when stressed |
| (Not) Having difficulty to recover from setbacks |
| (Not) Worrying under pressure |
| (Not) Having difficulty to deal with problems |
| *Depression, recent month (α = 0.834*; Crawford and Henry 2003*)* |
| (Not) Living happily |
| Fearing |
| Feeling sad |
| Feeling lonely |
| Being depressed |

(continued)

| (continued) |
| --- |
| (Not) Being in the same good mood as others |
| (Not) Being happy |
| (Not) Having confidence in the future |

## Resilience Feeling

Regression analysis of resilience from the resilience study dataset revealed the significant positive effect of peer functional disability, speaker sociability, relational kindness, aid received, peer aid received, peer benevolent world belief, and peer resilience learning on resilience (see Table 5.2). Among the effects, that of peer benevolent world belief was the strongest ($\beta = 0.223$). Other weak positive effects were from speaker sociability and peer aid received ($\beta > 0.10$). Meanwhile, peer adversity, peer speaker sociability, and peer resilience belief delivered significant inverse effects on resilience. Among them, the inverse effect of peer speaker sociability was the strongest, at a moderate level ($\beta = -0.290$). The inverse effects of peer speaker sociability and peer resilience belief contradicted the corresponding hypotheses.

Regression analysis of resilience from the elder resilience dataset indicated that advice received did not have a significant effect on resilience (see Table 5.3). This null effect failed to support the corresponding hypothesis.

Regression analysis of inferred resilience or adjustment under adversity from the resilience study dataset showed the significant positive effects of speaker sociability, aid received, peer kindness, peer benevolent world belief, and peer resilience learning (see Table 5.4). Among the effects, that of speaker sociability was the strongest ($\beta = 0.214$). Other weak positive effects emanated from aid received, peer kindness, and peer benevolent world belief ($\beta > 0.10$). Conversely, only peer adversity displayed a significant but slight inverse effect on inferred resilience ($\beta = -0.070$).

Regression analysis of inferred resilience or non-depression under adversity from the elder resilience dataset indicated that advice received did not have a significant effect on resilience (see Table 5.5). This null effect failed to support the corresponding hypothesis.

## Adjustment and Depression

Regression analysis of adjustment from the resilience study dataset showed the significant positive effects of peer functional disability, peer kindness, peer benevolent world belief, and peer resilience learning (see Table 5.6). Among the effects, that of peer kindness was the strongest ($\beta = 0.202$). Another weak positive effect arose from peer benevolent world belief ($\beta > 0.10$). Conversely, peer adversity and peer resilience

**Table 5.1** Peer effects on resilience

| Peer condition | Expected | Currently found | | | |
|---|---|---|---|---|---|
| | | Feeling | Action | Belief | Exposure |
| Speaker sociability | + | + | + | + | |
| Relational kindness | + | + | + | + | |
| Aid received | + | + | + | + | |
| Advice received | + | 0 | | | |
| Peer functional disability | − | + | + | 0 | + |
| Peer Adversity | − | − | − | − | − |
| Peer resilience demand received | + | 0 | 0 | 0 | |
| Peer speaker sociability | + | − | − | + | |
| Peer relational kindness | + | 0 | − | − | |
| Peer aid received | + | + | 0 | − | |
| Peer kindness | + | 0 | + | + | |
| Peer resilience belief | + | − | + | | |
| Peer benevolent world belief | + | + | + | | |
| Peer resilience learning | + | + | | | |
| Peer resilience handling | + | 0 | | | |
| Peer self-awareness | + | 0 | | | |

*Note* +: positive effect; −: negative effect; ?: mixed effects; 0: no effect

belief displayed a significant but slight inverse effect on inferred resilience ($\beta = -0.096$ and $-0.150$). The latter effect contradicted the corresponding hypothesis.

Regression analysis of depression adversity from the elder resilience dataset did not find a significant effect of advice receive (see Table 5.7). This null effect failed to support the corresponding hypothesis.

## *Resilience Action*

Regression analysis of resilience handling from the resilience study dataset showed the significant positive effects of peer functional disability, speaker sociability, relational kindness, aid received, and peer benevolent world belief (see Table 5.8). Among the effects, that of speaker sociability was the strongest, at a moderate level ($\beta = 0.266$). Meanwhile, aid received and peer benevolent world belief gave weak positive effects ($\beta > 0.10$). Conversely, peer adversity, peer relational kindness, and peer resilience belief displayed significant inverse effect on resilience handling. The latter two effects contradicted the corresponding hypotheses.

Regression analysis of resilience learning from the resilience study dataset revealed the significant positive effects of peer functional disability, peer kindness,

**Table 5.2** Standardized effects on resilience (service dataset)

| Predictor | All |
|---|---|
| Peer functional disability | 0.089** |
| Peer adversity | – 0.148*** |
| $R^2$ | 0.136 |
| Speaker sociability | 0.200*** |
| Relational kindness | 0.085* |
| Aid received | 0.092** |
| Peer resilience demand received | 0.029 |
| Peer speaker sociability | – 0.290*** |
| Peer relational kindness | – 0.029 |
| Peer aid received | 0.124** |
| Peer kindness | 0.086 |
| $R^2$ | 0.228 |
| Peer resilience belief | – 0.178* |
| Peer benevolent world belief | 0.223** |
| $R^2$ | 0.259 |
| Peer resilience handling | – 0.039 |
| Peer self-awareness | 0.069 |
| Peer resilience learning | 0.056* |
| $R^2$ | 0.425 |

*Note* Regression analysis controlled for background characteristics
$*p < 0.05$, $**p < 0.01$, $***p < 0.001$

**Table 5.3** Standardized effects on resilience (elder dataset)

| Predictor | Unweighted | Weighted by Westernization |
|---|---|---|
| Advice received | 0.056 | 0.030 |
| $R^2$ | 0.176 | 0.112 |

*Note* Regression analysis controlled for background characteristics

and peer benevolent world belief (see Table 5.9). Among the effects, that of peer kindness was the strongest, at a moderate level ($\beta = 0.281$). Meanwhile, peer benevolent world belief gave a weak positive effect ($\beta > 0.10$). Conversely, peer adversity and peer speaker sociability exhibited significant inverse effects on resilienxe learning ($\beta = -0.064$ and $-0.221$). The latter contradicted the corresponding hypothesis.

Regression analysis of self-awareness from the resilience study dataset revealed the significant positive effects of peer functional disability, speaker sociability, relational kindness, aid received, peer kindness, and peer benevolent world belief (see Table 5.10). Among the effects, that of peer benevolent world belief was the strongest, albeit at a weak level ($\beta = 0.216$). Besides, speaker sociability, relational kindness, aid received, and peer kindness displayed weak positive effects on self-awareness

**Table 5.4** Standardized effects on inferred resilience (service dataset)

| Predictor | All |
|---|---|
| Peer functional disability | 0.023 |
| Peer adversity | – 0.070*** |
| $R^2$ | 0.661 |
| Speaker sociability | 0.214*** |
| Relational kindness | – 0.052 |
| Aid received | 0.125*** |
| Peer resilience demand received | 0.006 |
| Peer speaker sociability | – 0.054 |
| Peer relational kindness | – 0.099 |
| Peer aid received | 0.038 |
| Peer kindness | 0.121* |
| $R^2$ | 0.722 |
| Peer resilience belief | – 0.090 |
| Peer benevolent world belief | 0.105** |
| $R^2$ | 0.740 |
| Peer resilience handling | – 0.013 |
| Peer self-awareness | 0.044 |
| Peer resilience learning | 0.036* |
| $R^2$ | 0.776 |

*Note* Regression analysis controlled for background characteristics
*$p < 0.05$, **$p < 0.01$, ***$p < 0.001$

**Table 5.5** Standardized effects on inferred resilience (elder dataset)

| Predictor | Unweighted | Weighted by westernization |
|---|---|---|
| Advice received | – 0.059 | – 0.071 |
| $R^2$ | 0.717 | 0.710 |

*Note* Regression analysis controlled for background characteristics

($\beta > 0.10$). Conversely, peer adversity, peer relational kindness, and peer resilience belief revealed significant inverse effects on self-awareness. Notably, the inverse effect of peer resilience belief was at a moderate level ($\beta = -0.278$). The effects of peer relational kindness and peer resilience belief contradicted the corresponding hypotheses.

**Table 5.6** Standardized effects on adjustment (service dataset)

| Predictor | All |
|---|---|
| Peer functional disability | 0.053* |
| Peer Adversity | – 0.096*** |
| $R^2$ | 0.220 |
| Peer resilience demand received | 0.016 |
| Peer speaker sociability | – 0.106 |
| Peer relational kindness | – 0.135 |
| Peer aid received | 0.049 |
| Peer kindness | 0.202*** |
| $R^2$ | 0.388 |
| Peer resilience belief | – 0.150* |
| Peer benevolent world belief | 0.174** |
| $R^2$ | 0.437 |
| Peer resilience handling | 0.036 |
| Peer self-awareness | 0.025 |
| Peer resilience learning | 0.065* |
| $R^2$ | 0.537 |

*Note* Regression analysis controlled for background characteristics
*$p < 0.05$, **$p < 0.01$, ***$p < 0.001$

**Table 5.7** Standardized effects on depression (elder dataset)

| Predictor | Unweighted | Weighted by Westernization |
|---|---|---|
| Advice received | 0.024 | 0.051 |
| $R^2$ | 0.151 | 0.178 |

*Note* Regression analysis controlled for background characteristics

## *Resilience Belief*

Regression analysis of resilience belief from the resilience study dataset unfolded the significant positive effects of speaker sociability, relational kindness, aid received, peer speaker sociability, and peer kindness (see Table 5.11). Among the effects, that of speaker sociability was the strongest, approaching a moderate level ($\beta = 0.246$). Besides, relational kindness, peer speaker sociability, and peer kindness displayed weak positive effects on self-awareness ($\beta > 0.10$). Conversely, peer adversity and peer aid received displayed significant inverse effects on resilience belief. The latter contradicted the corresponding hypothesis.

**Table 5.8** Standardized effects on resilience handling (service dataset)

| Predictor | All |
|---|---|
| Peer functional disability | 0.099*** |
| Peer adversity | – 0.142*** |
| $R^2$ | 0.274 |
| Speaker sociability | 0.266*** |
| Relational kindness | 0.058* |
| Aid received | 0.121*** |
| Peer resilience demand received | 0.025 |
| Peer speaker sociability | 0.026 |
| Peer relational kindness | – 0.177* |
| Peer aid received | 0.004 |
| Peer kindness | 0.123 |
| $R^2$ | 0.454 |
| Peer resilience belief | – 0.180** |
| Peer benevolent world belief | 0.116* |
| $R^2$ | 0.515 |

*Note* Regression analysis controlled for background characteristics
*$p < 0.05$, **$p < 0.01$, ***$p < 0.001$

**Table 5.9** Standardized effects on resilience learning (service dataset)

| Predictor | All |
|---|---|
| Peer functional disability | 0.068* |
| Peer adversity | – 0.064* |
| $R^2$ | 0.058 |
| Speaker sociability | 0.155 |
| Relational kindness | 0.144 |
| Aid received | 0.055 |
| Peer resilience demand received | 0.140 |
| Peer speaker sociability | – 0.221** |
| Peer relational kindness | – 0.182 |
| Peer aid received | 0.030 |
| Peer kindness | 0.281** |
| $R^2$ | 0.160 |
| Peer resilience belief | – 0.095 |
| Peer benevolent world belief | 0.157* |
| $R^2$ | 0.189 |

*Note* Regression analysis controlled for background characteristics
*$p < 0.05$, **$p < 0.01$

**Table 5.10** Standardized effects on self-awareness (service dataset)

| Predictor | All |
|---|---|
| Peer functional disability | 0.042 |
| Peer adversity | – 0.099*** |
| $R^2$ | 0.201 |
| Speaker sociability | 0.206*** |
| Relational kindness | 0.123*** |
| Aid received | 0.106*** |
| Peer resilience demand received | – 0.050 |
| Peer speaker sociability | – 0.027 |
| Peer relational kindness | – 0.236** |
| Peer aid received | 0.079 |
| Peer kindness | 0.212** |
| $R^2$ | 0.341 |
| Peer resilience belief | – 0.278*** |
| Peer benevolent world belief | 0.216*** |
| $R^2$ | 0.365 |

*Note* Regression analysis controlled for background characteristics
$*p < 0.05$, $**p < 0.01$, $***p < 0.001$

**Table 5.11** Standardized effects on resilience belief (service dataset)

| Predictor | All |
|---|---|
| Peer functional disability | 0.030 |
| Peer adversity | – 0.079** |
| $R^2$ | 0.278 |
| Speaker sociability | 0.246*** |
| Relational kindness | 0.130*** |
| Aid received | 0.066** |
| Peer resilience demand received | 0.045 |
| Peer speaker sociability | 0.138* |
| Peer relational kindness | – 0.107 |
| Peer aid received | – 0.076* |
| Peer kindness | 0.136* |
| $R^2$ | 0.467 |

*Note* Regression analysis controlled for background characteristics
$*p < 0.05$, $**p < 0.01$, $***p < 0.001$

**Table 5.12** Standardized effects on resilience demand (service dataset)

| Predictor | All |
|---|---|
| Peer functional disability | 0.129*** |
| Peer adversity | – 0.065* |
| $R^2$ | 0.080 |

*Note* Regression analysis controlled for background characteristics
*$p < 0.05$, ***$p < 0.001$

## *Resilience Exposure*

Regression analysis of exposure to resilience demand from the resilience study dataset unfolded the significant positive effect of peer functional disability (see Table 5.12). This effect contradicted the corresponding hypothesis. Meanwhile, peer adversity exhibited a signficaint negative effect on resilience.

## *Effects not Supporting the Hypotheses*

Effects not supporting the hypotheses were those of advice received on resilience feeling, peer functional disability, peer resilience demand received, peer speaker sociability on resilience feeling and action, peer relational kindness, peer aid received on resilience action and belief, peer kindness on resilience feeling, peer resilience belief on resilience feeling, peer resilience handling on resilience feeling, and peer self-awareness on resilence feeling. Among them, the effects of peer functional disability, peer speaker sociability, peer relational kindness, peer aid received, and peer resilience belief contradicted the hypotheses.

### Peer Functional Disability

Peer functional disability displayed significant positive effects on resilience feeling, action, and exposure. According to analytical functionalism, the effects build on power, utility, ideals, and norms conveyed by peer functional disability to sustain resilience functioning.

Power raised by peer functional disability to drive resilience has been caring, networking for caring, and social support or supportiveness (Cornwall 2009; Logan and Spitze 1994; Smith et al. 2006). Caring engages devotion, meaningfulness, protection, reparation, responsibility, and social solidarity for resilience (Featherstone and Morris 2012; Fine 2007). Moreover, caring reflects attachment, safety, and security to buttress resilience (Collins et al. 2011). Meanwhile, networking sustains identity and self-esteem to incubate resilience (Malloy 2018). Conversely, networking reduces anxiety, thus safeguarding resilience (Baumeister and Leary 1995). Networking has also drawn benefits and alleviated stress, hence sustaining resilience (Nelson-Coffey et al. 2023). Likewise, networking has rested on happiness, life satisfaction, mindfulness, popularity, self-acceptance, self-esteem, and success experience to enhance resilience (Flett 2018; Gountas et al. 2012; Stadtfeld and Pentland 2015; Utz and Breuer 2017). Conversely, networking has diminished due to anxiety, depression, and stress, thus enabling resilience (Flett 2018). Supportiveness has fostered connectedness, hope, life satisfaction, meaningfulness, protection, religiosity, self-efficacy, and work value to facilitate resilience (Dinic and Bodroza 2021; Marsh and Dik 2021; Nelson-Coffey et al. 2023; Shahzalal and Adnan 2022; Yao and Enright 2019). Conversely, supportiveness has removed impulsivity, loneliness, and other negative emotions, thus enabling resilience (Hample 2018; Nelson-Coffey et al. 2023).

Ideas disseminated by peer functional disability to rationalize resilience have emphasized caring, cheerfulness, and responsibility (Gastil 2000; Knoarska 2005). Responsibility boosts sustainability, hence resilience (Shamir 2008). Moreover, responsibility has developed wisdom (Spengler et al. 2018). Responsibility has also rested on affordability and income, assets, savings, and wealth, education and literacy, individualism, religiosity, self-control, social class, and toleration to afford resilience (Chan 2012; Gelissen 2002; He 2019; Jakobsen 2010; Killian and Ganong 2002; Rudolph and Popp 2009; Shtudiner et al. 2017).

## Peer Sociability

Peer sociability diminished resilience feeling and action while enhancing resilience belief. According to analytical functionalism, such diminishment involves power, utility, ideals, and norms and their deterministic and voluntaristic mechanisms of empowering and power realization, incentivizing and utility optimization, framing and ideal calibration, and normalizing and norm conformity. As such, peer sociability diminished resilience by eroding its power, utility, ideal, and norm bases. Such erosion hinges on peer crime, delinquency, deviance, externalizing behavior, and violence created by peer sociability (Bartusch and Matsueda 1996; Collins and van Dulmen 2006; Larson et al. 2007). Such creation stems from the intimidation and self-promotion components of sociability for impression and self-management (Finne and Svartdal 2017; Gulliford et al. 2019). Peer deviance has undermined power, utility, ideals, and norms conducive to resilience (Carson 2013; Peterson and Esbensen 2004; Soller et al. 2017; Vander Ven et al. 2001). Likewise, peer sociability has reflected peer defiance and maladjustment (Stein et al. 2013; Tracey and Rohlfing 2010). Peer defiance and maladjustment can induce personal defiance and maladjustment (Nivette et al. 2021; Reitz et al. 2006; Sacker et al. 2002, Zimmermann and Bingenheimer 2002). This inducement reflects normalizing and assimilation. Peer sociability has also provoked and transmitted stressful and demanding experiences (Bellingtier et al. 2022; Hintsanen et al. 2011). Such transmission again realizes normalizing and assimilation.

Defiance and stress can impede resilience by reducing power, utility, ideals, and norms for resilience. The reduction runs according to the voluntaristic mechanisms of analytical functionalism.

Power driving resilience reduced by defiance has rested on adaptation, attentiveness, mastery-goal setting, maturity, pleasantness, and social closeness and support received (De Bruyn et al. 2003; Jiang et al. 2015; Littlejohn et al. 2017; Nelson et al. 2004). Attentiveness has hinged on education, income, and positive affect to facilitate resilience (Carreras 2018; Kitayama 1997). Mastery-goal setting has rested on growth belief to sustain resilience (Muenks et al. 2021). Conversely, defiance has diminished power for resilience by activating anxiety, arousal, conflict, crime, deviance, distress, doping, externalizing behavior, protesting, stress experienced, and violence (Cohen and Fromme 2002; de Courville Nicol 2011; Hatcher et al. 2018; Jiang et al. 2015; Magnuson et al. 2006; Molz et al. 2013; Pulkkinen et al. 2009; Raab 2019). Defiance also reflects antagonism, blaming, deficiency in cognition, depression, deprivation experienced, grievance, stigmatization experience, threat experience, and withdrawal to hinder power for resilience (Foy et al. 2014; Glasberg and Contributors 2018; Jenkins and Dragojevic 2011; Saxton and Benson 2006). Antagonism has fomented anger, anxiety, irrationality, and sadness to disrupt resilience (Vandervoort 2006). Blaming has reflected conflict perception and distress as opposed to compromise to impede resilience (Bagci and Celebi 2017; Recchia and Howe 2010; Wayment et al. 2010). Stigmatization experience concerns poverty and social problems that inhibit resilience (Chan et al. 2022). Threat experienced has fomented anxiety, avoidance, conflict, depression, fear, and hate to disrupt resilience (Edwards and Arnon 2021; MacLeod 2017; Moore and Shepherd 2006; O'Neill and Evans 1999; Rick et al. 2006; Ruiter et al. 2003). Conversely, the threat experienced has weakened meaningfulness, social capital, and inclusion experienced, tolerance, and general well-being, thus undermining resilience (Petersen et al. 2011; Raijman et al. 2008; Rothschild and Keefer 2022; Savelkoul et al. 2015; Schmid and Muldoon 2015). Withdrawal has fomented conflict to impair resilience (Debus et al. 2019). Meanwhile, defiance shrinks by power and social status to impair resilience (Foy et al. 2014). Moreover, defiance has diminished due to education, quality of life, religiosity, and social class, which weaken resilience (Hagan et al. 2016; Lubbers et al. 2006). Conversely, defiance has reflected disadvantaged status to weaken power to sustain resilience (Foy et al. 2014).

Utility attracting resilience attenuated by defiance has resided in achievement and effectiveness experienced (Magnuson et al. 2006; Uslaner 2008). Moreover, defiance shrinks by agreement experienced, and success experienced as utility, thus weakening resilience (Foy et al. 2014). Conversely, defiance reflects attack experience, discrepancy expected, deficit experienced, failure experienced, hegemony experienced, and violation experienced as disutility to distract resilience (Dilts 2017; Foy et al. 2014; Jenkins and Dragojevic 2011; Littlejohn et al. 2017; Thye and Kalkhoff 2014; Wendt 2001). Attack experience has bred antisocial behavior, depression, dysfunction, problems, stress, victimization experienced, and violence to impair resilience (Barber et al. 2016; Berger 2005; Ehrensuft et al. 2003; Krahe 2013). Conversely, attack experience has lessened quality of life, satisfaction, security, and tolerance, thus shaking resilience (Barber et al. 2016; Barkan and Cohn 2005; Sampson and Raudenbush 2004). Discrepancy experienced has dampened adjustment, thus disrupting resilience (Denson and Bowman 2015). Hegemony perceived has invoked distress, injury, and violence to erode resilience (Felson and Outlaw 2007; Overall et al. 2020).

Ideals rationalizing resilience diminished by defiance emphasize defense and tolerance (Feldman 2003; Schwartz et al. 2014). Defense reduces risk to sustain resilience (Erickson and Feldstein 2007). Moreover, defense hinges on resolution or problem-solving to uphold resilience (Dinic and Bodroza 2021). Defense also builds on confidence, education, efficacy belief, employment, knowledge, self-efficacy, and trust to maintain resilience (Bish and Michie 2010; Warner et al. 2022). Meanwhile, tolerance has sustained health, life satisfaction, and social trust to enhance resilience (Appleton and Song 2008; Stafford et al. 2005; Uslaner 2002).

Norms assimilating resilience dampened by defiance popularize development and growth (Sabet and Khaksar 2022). Development has facilitated success experienced to attract resilience (Spengler et al. 2018). Additionally, development stems from attachment and its safety and security, goal-setting, optimization, resourcefulness, social affiliation, and strengths as opposed to loss to uphold resilence (Hendry and Kloep 2012; Skinner et al. 2019). Strengths include courage, honesty, hope, optimism, mastery, perseverance, and skill (Hendry and Kloep 2012). Development has also stood on employment, memory integration, and self-tolerance to generate resilience (Bauer et al. 2005; Bleidorn et al. 2013; Ho and Li 2022). Moreover, defiance stems from norms for competition and protest to disrupt resilience (Watts and Feldman 2001; Ziv 2018).

Power driving resilience dampened by stress experienced rests on attention and control (Gatersleben and Griffin 2017). Moreover, stress experienced has attenuated brain functioning, intelligence, knowledge, memory, social integration, support received, and trust, and well-being as power bases for resilience (Alesina and La Ferrara 2002; Baumeister et al. 2013; Dunkel-Schetter and Bennett 1990; Garcia and Herrero 2004; Leiser et al. 2010; Lupien et al. 2009; Macias 2015). Intelligence has enhanced social capital and diminished criminality and depression, thus facilitating resilience (Cornwall 2009; Feinstein and Bynner 2006). Knowledge has secured health value, power, satisfaction, savings, self-efficacy, social resources, and spirituality to lift resilience (Ertz et al. 2021; Norris 2011; Chang and Hsu 2016; Nunkoo 2015; Rothwell et al. 2016; Sturgis et al. 2005). Social integration has prevented depression and suicide to buttress resilience (Duberstein et al. 2004; Mullins and Dugan 1991). Well-being has included eudaimonia, health, hedonia, meaningfulness, quality of life, and satisfaction with life and neighbors (Mathis et al. 2016; Parkes et al. 2002; Shrira 2012; Su et al. 2021; Zotti et al. 2016). Stress also shrinks by such power bases as activeness, coping ability, resources, self-determination, skill, social class, and understanding, thus disempowering resilience (Auerbach et al. 2011; Bellingtier et al. 2022; Carr and Umberson 2013; Ritchie 2012, van Deurzen 2021). Furthermore, stress has diminished by such power bases as agreeableness, assertiveness, coping, conformity, education, emotional intelligence, exercising, extraversion, income, neighborliness or bonding experienced, religiosity, self-esteem, social capital or networking, thus hindering resilience (Aytac et al. 2015; Beaudoin 2009; Boyes et al. 2017; Chen et al. 2015; Constantino et al. 2006; Extremera et al. 2007; Frank et al. 2014; Garfin et al. 2015; Gitto et al. 2020; Hair et al. 2007; Bellingtier et al. 2022; Molz et al. 2013; Weinberg et al. 2021; Zheng et al. 2020). Assertiveness has maintained life satisfaction and self-esteem and prevented risking to foster resilience (Diener and Fujita 1995; Menard and Offman 2009; Morokoff et al. 2009). Conformity can enhance adaptation and pleasantness and diminish anxiety to enhance resilience (de Courville Nicol 2011; Littlejohn et al. 2017). Emotional intelligence has sustained well-being, including adaptation, happiness, health, life satisfaction, positive mood, optimism, relational quality and relatedness, and self-esteem, as opposed to depression and distress to boost resilience (Goldenberg et al. 2006; Matthews et al. 2012; Mayer et al. 2008). Additionally, emotional intelligence has facilitated agreeableness, coping, defense, friendship, intelligence, openness, self-control, and success to lift resilience (Goldenberg et al. 2006; Matthews et al. 2012; Mayer et al. 2004, 2008; Van Rooy and Viswesvaran 2004). Conversely, emotional intelligence has impeded deviance, social disconnection, and substance abuse, thus retaining resilience (Matthews et al. 2012; Mayer et al. 2008). Exercising has raised well-being, including function and health (Sargent-Cox et al. 2015). Extraversion has fostered well-being, including autonomy, growth, hedonic balance, mastery, mattering, positive affect, purposefulness, relatedness, satisfaction with appearance, life, marriage, and weight, self-acceptance, self-determination, self-efficacy, and self-esteem, to facilitate resilience (Flett 2018; Frederick et al. 2016; Hounkpatin et al. 2015; Li et al. 2017; Ingledew et al. 2004; Quilty et al. 2006; Rasmussen et al. 2018; Schimmack et al. 2002; Solomon and Jackson 2014; Tiwari et al. 2021). Conversely, extraversion has dampened anxiety, distress, and hostility, thus safeguarding resilience (Becker et al. 1997; Hounkpatin et al. 2015; Weinberg et al. 2021). Meanwhile, stress incurs anxiety, conflict, crises, depression, deviance, distress, dysfunction, errors, frustration, irritability, sacrifice, substance abuse, suicide, and violence to drain power for resilience (Backman and Nilsson 2011; Berger 2015; Cano and Vivian 2003; Dutton et al. 2016; Gatersleben and Griffin 2017; Grzywacz and Almeida 2008; Hatch 2007; Lantz et al. 2005; Lupien et al. 2009; Segrin and Flora 2019; Sherkat and Ellison 2007). Frustration has incurred avoiding and withholding to impair resilience (Vanhee et al. 2018). Stress also stems from disadvantaged status, helplessness, hopelessness, negativity, and overload to impede resilience (Carr and Umberson 2013; Kleiman and Riskind 2014). Furthermore, stress has evolved from constraint, demand experienced, dependency and its experience, emotionality or neuroticism, hostility, illness, loss, risk, sociability, and strain to disturb power bases for resilience (Aytac et al. 2015; Bellingtier et al. 2022; Cepulic et al. 2022; Fenwick and Tausig 1994; Holman et al. 2011; Jonsson et al. 2003; Kachadourian et al. 2013; Mandel et al. 2018; Molz et al. 2013; Snyder et al. 2020; Weinberg et al. 2021). Demand experienced has eroded well-being, including job and life satisfaction as opposed to anxiety, burnout, and distress to attenuate resilience (Clark et al. 2013; De Moortel et al. 2015; Dust et al. 2020; Moen et al. 2013; Xie 1996). Dependency has raised illness and suicide and eroded health and mastery, thus shaking resilience (Bornstein 2012; Lu and Kao 2002; Roy and Chaudhuri 2008). Emotionality or neuroticism has worsened well-being, including autonomy, growth, health, positive affect, purposefulness, relatedness, satisfaction, self-acceptance, self-compassion, and self-determination, to resist resilience (Anusic et al. 2014; Hounkpatin et al. 2015; Ingledew et al. 2004; Pfattheicher et al. 2017; Richards 2016; Webster et al. 2014). Conversely, emotionality or neuroticism has sustained anxiety, depression, hostility, loneliness, and worry to impair resilience (Hounkpatin et al. 2015; Melton 2016, Maltby et al. 2016; Neto and Barros 2003; Rossi 2004a). Loss has incurred anger and depression and diminished income and marital satisfaction to dampen resilience (Boyce et al. 2013; Mehlsen et al. 2003; Wells et al. 1999).

Utility attracting resilience weakened by stress experience has derived from optimism (Extremera et al. 2007). Optimism has boosted benefits received, such as coping, curability, and survival, as opposed to barriers experienced to uphold resilience (Clarke et al. 2000; Nes and Segerstrom 2006). Conversely, stress incurs discrepancy or mismatch feeling as disutility to impede resilience (Berger 2015). Mismatch feeling has impeded cohesive and compliant behavior and knowledge, thus disrupting resilience (Guan et al. 2021; Richey 2009; Yoon et al. 2013). Stress has also evolved from pessimism to discourage resilience (Extremera et al. 2007).

Ideals rationalizing resilience dismissed by stress experienced emphasize forgiveness (Toussaint et al. 2016). Stress also dampens tolerance as an ideal, thus weakening resilience (Gatersleben and Griffin 2017). Tolerance has championed well-being, including health, life satisfaction, and social trust, to facilitate resilience (Appleton and Song 2008; Stafford et al. 2005; Uslaner 2002). Conversely, stress has shrunk by ideals for agreeing, tolerance, and working, thus weakening resilience (Bardeen et al. 2016; Jonsson et al. 2003). Agreeing has fostered growth, life satisfaction, mastery, purposefulness, relatedness, and acceptance as opposed to hostility to furnish resilience (Hounkpatin et al. 2015). Moreover, stress stems from blaming to retard resilience (van Deurzen 2021). Blaming has stemmed from conflict perceived and distress as opposed to compromise to retard resilience (Bagci and Celebi 2017; Recchia and Howe 2010; Wayment et al. 2010). Stress has also raised violence as an ideal to impede resilience (Song et al. 2017). Idealizing violence has evolved from anger and contempt as opposed to self-efficacy to resist resilience (Tausch et al. 2011).

Norms assimilating resilience prohibited by stress experience. Conversely, stress has foregrounded norms for risk and strain to resist resilience (Macias 2015; Walen and Lachman 2016). The norm for risk perceived has eroded adjustment, happiness, life satisfaction, positive affect, self-determination and sustained anxiety and fear, depression, negative affect, and sadness, thus undermining resilience (Prelow et al. 2004; Schoon 2006; Schwartz and Melech 2000; Shippee 2012; Vuori 2015). Additionally, the norm has impaired knowledge, social trust, and socioeconomic status to obstruct resilience (Herek et al. 2005; Lindstrom and Rosvall 2015). Conversely, the norm has raised protests and threats experienced to impede resilience (McLaren 2003; Scafuto and La Barbera 2016).

However, peer sociability enhanced resilience belief while reducing resilience feeling and action. Here, belief differs from feeling and action in that the latter two specifically concern oneself, whereas the former concerns all people. That is, resilience feeling and action mean that resilience happens to oneself, but resilience belief does not mean so. This difference allows peer sociability to have divergent impacts on resilience feeling, action, and belief. The contribution of sociability to resilience belief has transpired in the contribution of extraversion to just world belief (Bollmann et al. 2015; Nudelman 2013). Herein, sociability is a component of extraversion (Witt and Revelle 2009). Alternatively, sociability manifests extraversion (Foschi and Lauriola 2014). Meanwhile, just world belief foregrounds resilience (Dalbert 2001; Hafer and Sutton 2016).

### Peer Kindness and Aid Received

Peers' experience of relational kindness displayed inverse effects on resilience action and belief, contradicting the hypothesis. Similarly, peers' aid received showed an inverse effect on resilience belief. These effects reflected those of peer advantage or privilege to create personal disadvantage relatively, following the adaptation function of analytical functionalism. Accordingly, peer advantage raises the standard of achievement, thus incurring personal disadvantage or relative deprivation (Schmitt et al. 2010). That is, personal advantage becomes more difficult and costlier to reach the higher advantage standard. Hence, societal, economic growth, employment and its growth, income, and wage have incurred relative deprivation or disadvantage (Brady 2005; Clain 2007; Fan et al. 2004; Gundersen and Ziliak 2004; Knack 2002). This deprivation hinges on the deterministic mechanism of incentivizing or disincentivizing such that peer advantage raises the difficulty to achieve, thus, the disincentive for achievement. Notably, peer advantage is a disincentive or disutility rather than power, an ideal, or a norm to create a disadvantage. Such a disadvantage would attenuate power, utility, ideas, and norms to dampen resilience by applying the voluntaristic mechanisms of analytical functionalism.

Power driving resilience diminished by disadvantage arises from investment (Donnellan et al. 2013). Disadvantage has also eroded insurance coverage, social connection, and trust, thus weakening power driving resilience (Holl et al. 2005; Stephens et al. 2014). Insurance has conveyed education, health, and income to buttress resilience (Anderson and Eamon 2004; Gross and Brammli-Greenberg 2004). Investment has strengthened social capital to facilitate resilience (Hlasny and Lee 2020). Furthermore, disadvantage has shrunk by health, intelligence, and religiosity, thus dampening power to drive resilience (Dekkers 2008; Fischer et al. 1996; Urbatsch 2014). Conversely, disadvantage hastens impulsivity, pressure experienced, and stress experienced to undermine resilience (Donnellan et al. 2013; Simpson et al. 2011). Impulsivity has created stress to retard resilience (Hample 2018). Disadvantage has also incurred illness, isolation and social exclusion experienced, imprisonment experience, pressure experienced, strain, and suicide to weaken power, thus impeding resilience (Dhal et al. 2008; Fischer et al. 1996; Stephens et al. 2014; Swanson et al. 1992; Walker et al. 2010). Isolation or social exclusion experienced has installed negative mood and diminished life satisfaction, thus impairing resilience (Lin et al. 2013; Williams et al. 2000). Moreover, disadvantage springs from crises experienced, disability, hardship, illness, insecurity, and loneliness, thus alleviating power for resilience (Dekkers 2008; Dewilde 2003; Leu et al. 2016; Muffels and Fouarge 2004; Whelan et al. 2004). Crises experienced have weakened well-being, including health and life satisfaction, to hurt resilience (Baumeister et al. 2013; Mathis et al. 2016; Zotti et al. 2016). Disability has incurred distress and dampened health, life satisfaction, and self-efficacy, thus eroding resilience (Distante 2013; Gastil 2000; Michalos et al. 2000; Phongsavan et al. 2006).

Utility attracting resilience reduced by disadvantage emerges from reinforcement or reward (Mithaug 2000). Reinforcement has raised well-being, including satisfaction, to boost resilience (Helgeson et al. 2006; Wong and Lam 2016). Conversely, reinforcement has lessened anger, anxiety, and depression, thus sustaining resilience (Helgeson et al. 2006; Wells et al. 1999).

Ideals rationalizing resilience dismissed by disadvantage concern studying (James and Luo 1999). The ideal for studying has boosted achievement to engage resilience (Liu and Yu 2016). This ideal has also embodied identity achievement and satisfaction to foster resilience (Perez et al. 2014; Wilder et al. 2000). Conversely, disadvantage has bred fatalism as ideas against resilience (Layte et al. 2000). Fatalism has declined by education, income, and meaningfulness, thus sustaining resilience (Bynner and Parsons 2002; Speed et al. 2018; Steger et al. 2008). Conversely, fatalism has reflected idleness or withdrawal to impede resilience (Bynner and Parsons 2002). Moreover, disadvantage stems from atypicality or deviance as an ideal to block resilience (Curley 2005). Atypicality has eroded health and raised social exclusion experience, thus hurting resilience (Backman and Nilsson 2011).

Norms assimilating resilience blocked by disadvantage highlight education, health, income, quality of life, security, wage, welfare, and youth (Brady 2005; Clain 2007; Knack 2002; Moller et al. 2003; Sanders 1990; Vartanian 1999). Youth has buttressed health to facilitate resilience (Gluck et al. 2005). Conversely, disadvantage has reflected norms for inequality, risk, and unemployment to weaken resilience (Gundersen and Ziliak 2004; Knack 2002; Lipford and Yandle 2009; Vartanian and McNamara 2004). The norm for inequality stems from adversity and impairs resilience (Whyte and Gao 2009). Similarly, the norm for unemployment has bred disability, emotional problems, and illness to cripple resilience (Benitez-Silva et al. 2010).

## Peer Resilience Belief

Peers' resilience belief exhibited an inverse effect of resilience feeling, thus contradicting the hypothesis. Such belief would be a disincentive to raise the standard and thus make it difficult for resilience. This belief, hence, applies the deterministic mechanism of incentivizing or disincentivizing to shape resilience. The disincentivizing creates standards and demands to breed relative deprivation or disadvantage to deprive resilience. Such demands deprive power, utility, ideals, and norms upholding resilience. Alternatively, a disincentive emerges from depreciation due to inflation, such that one's resilience tarnishes when resilience is common. As such, deprivation works through the voluntaristic mechanisms of power realization, utility optimization, ideal calibration, and norm conformity.

Power driving resilience deprived by demand experienced has rested on creativity, mastery orientation, self-control, social support received, well-being, and work commitment (de Henestrosa et al. 2023; De Moortel et al. 2015; Moen et al. 2013; Nalis et al. 2022; Schieman 2006; Simons et al. 2021). Creativity has sustained happiness, meaningfulness, positive mood, satisfaction, and general well-being (Henderson 2004; Tavares 2016; Schneck 2014). Well-being as a power source has included health and job and life satisfaction as opposed to anxiety, burnout, and distress (Clark et al. 2013; Dust et al. 2020; Moen et al. 2013; Xie 1996). Mastery orientation has declined due to exhaustion, thus sustaining resilience (Vander Elst et al. 2014). Social support received has facilitated creativity to secure resilience (Chen et al. 2022). Work commitment has boosted self-efficacy and self-esteem to facilitate resilience (Bakker et al. 2008). Moreover, demand experienced declined due to autonomy and self-efficacy as power sources, thus eroding resilience (Schieman 2013; Smoktunowicz et al. 2017). Autonomy has raised well-being, including energy, health, mastery, meaningfulness, positive affect, pride, satisfaction, self-efficacy, and self-esteem, to boost resilience (Au and Cheung 2004; De Moortel et al. 2015; Erickson 2008; Garcia et al. 2017; Gahlawat et al. 2019; Hodson 1996; Martela and Riekki 2018; Schieman 2002; Schieman and Narisada 2014; Yoon 2001). Conversely, autonomy has prevented burnout, thus safeguarding resilience (Peeters and Rutte 2005). Self-efficacy has facilitated acceptance, creativity, and satisfaction to uplift resilience (De Moulin 1993). Demand experienced has also diminished by ability and competence, comfort, control, coping, health, positive affect, quality of life, recourse, satisfaction, self-efficacy, self-esteem, self-help, social support received, teamwork, training, trust, and work engagement as power bases, thus hurting resilience (Acker and Lawrence 2009; Conti et al. 2006; Gallie et al. 1998; Furnham 1997; Hair et al. 2007; Kane-Frieder et al. 2013; Liu et al. 2010; Mak and Mueller 2000; Moen et al. 2016; Nahum-Shani et al. 2014; Paoline and Lambert 2012; Swanson and Power 2001). Teamwork has enhanced capability use to maintain resilience (Steijn 2001). Conversely, demand experienced has generated conflict, hindrance experienced, minority or marginalization status, overload experienced, and stress to erode power for resilience (Duxbury and Halinski 2018; Haslam et al. 2004; Kraimer et al. 2022; Rantanen et al. 2021; Schieman and Young 2010; Smoktunowicz et al. 2017). Imbalance experienced has fomented anxiety, depression, and life dissatisfaction to hinder resilience (Grzywacz and Bass 2003; Landolfi et al. 2021). Demand experienced has also reflected control experienced, deficiency experienced, interference experienced, noise experienced, shame, and strain as power loss to weaken resilience (Conti et al. 2006; Duxbury et al. 2021; Furnham 1997; Gallie et al. 1998; Hair et al. 2007; Raper et al. 2019). Interference experienced has harmed adjustment, health and mental health, satisfaction, and self-efficacy, thus undermining resilience (Hechanova et al. 2003; Gao and Jin 2015; Yucel and Fan 2019). Conversely, interference experienced has fomented anxiety, burnout, depression, distress, and strain to hinder resilience (Grandley and Cropanzano 1999; Griffin and Sun 2018; Grzywacz and Bass 2003).

Utility attracting resilience deprived by demand experienced has covered success experience (Maume 2006). Moreover, demand experienced deprives fitness experienced and gain experience as utility to attract resilience (Edwards et al. 1998; Preston 2018). Fitness experienced has sustained health, life satisfaction, morale, and power to raise resilience (Li 2006; Pereyra-Rojas et al. 2017; Xie 1996). Conversely, fitness experienced has eroded anxiety, depression, strain, and stress, thus safeguarding resilience (Sutherland and Fogarty 1995; Xie 1996). Demand experienced has also shrunk by autonomy and discretion experienced, development experienced, and justice experienced, thus posing disunity to hinder resilience (Dbaibo et al. 2010; Furnham 1997; Gallie et al. 1998; Schieman 2013). Justice experienced has lifted positive mood, life satisfaction, and self-esteem to sustain resilience (Dalbert 2001). Conversely, justice experienced has reduced depression and self-doubt, thus protecting resilience (Dalbert 2001). Meanwhile, demand experienced springs from inconsistency experienced, deviation experienced, imbalance experienced, and loss experienced as disutility to hinder resilience (Cummings and Cooper 1998; Duxbury et al. 2021; Nahum-Shani et al. 2014; Tsutsumi and Kawakami 2004). Imbalance experienced has fomented anxiety and depression and eroded life satisfaction, thus shaking resilience (Grzywacz and Bass 2003; Landolfi et al. 2021). Loss experience has raised anger, depression, and suicide, and preempted life satisfaction and positive affect, thus impeding resilience (Boyce et al. 2013); Henry et al. 1993; Steverink and Lindenberg 2006; Wells et al. 1999). Additionally, demand experienced has reflected blame and challenge received, incongruence experienced, and risk experience as disutility discouraging resilience (Conti et al. 2006; Dbaibo et al. 2010; Gallie et al. 1998; Schieman 2013). Incongruence experienced has dampened adjustment, thus impairing resilience (Denson and Bowman 2015).

Ideals rationalizing resilience deprived by demand experienced concern social identification (Haslam et al. 2004). Social identification has fostered cooperation and relational quality to advance resilience (Haesevoets et al. 2015; Jorgensen and Nelson 2018). Conversely, social identification has prevented substance abuse, thus safeguarding resilience (Jorgensen and Nelson 2018). Moreover, demand experienced has diminished by professionalism as an ideal, thus jeopardizing resilience (Paoline and Lambert 2012). Professionalism has reflected autonomy and benefits received to sustain resilience (Giffords 2009).

Norms assimilating resilience deprived by demand experienced highlight friendliness (Gallie et al. 1998). These norms have sustained happiness and satisfaction and eroded distress, thus maintaining resilience (Cannuscio et al. 2004; Helliwell et al. 2009; Piercy 2000). Conversely, demand experienced has reflected norms for tension and undermining to disrupt resilience (Westman 1999). The tension norm has fomented complaints, distress, and powerlessness, and reduced self-esteem, thus attenuating resilience (Furnham 1997; Gerber et al. 2010).

By contrast, peer resilience belief demonstrated a positive effect on resilience action. This effect might reflect the contribution of peer resilience belief to personal resilience belief through the deterministic mechanism of normalizing. Resilience belief has sustained resilience action (McClaran et al. 2022; Sutherland and Rehman 2018). This sustenance can provide power, utility, ideas, and norms to capitalize on the voluntaristic mechanisms of power realization, utility optimization, ideal calibration, and norm conformity.

Power driving resilience action raised by resilience belief evolves from cooperation, meaningfulness, respect experienced, security, self-esteem, and trust (Dalbert 2001; Hafer and Sutton 2016; Vermunt and Steensma 2016). Cooperation has enhanced social attachment to raise power to drive resilience action (Tak 2017). Respect received has rested on education and health to generate power to drive resilience action (Malat 2001). Resilience belief has also fostered belongingness and social support received as power bases to activate resilience action (Davis-Lipman et al. 2007; van Prooijen et al. 2008). Belongingness has reduced negative emotions and stress to sustain resilience action (Nelson-Coffey et al. 2023). Moreover, resilience belief reflects existential motivation and freedom experienced as power bases to drive resilience action (Schmidtz 2006; van der Toorn et al. 2010). Freedom has enabled well-being, including health, life satisfaction, and self-esteem, as opposed to depression and symptoms to facilitate resilience action (Abbott et al. 2011; Glendinning et al. 2003; Haller and Hadler 2006). Furthermore, resilience belief has stemmed from agreeableness, conscientiousness, extraversion, honesty-humility, income, and social class and status to maintain power to drive resilience action (Bollmann et al. 2015; Liebig and Mau 2007; Nudelman 2013; Viewiebe and Wegener 2000; Whyte and Gao 2009). Conversely, resilience belief prevented aggression and frustration, thus safeguarding power for resilience action (Vermunt and Steensma 2016). Frustration has incurred avoidance to impede resilience action (Vanhee et al. 2018). Resilience belief has also diminished anger and depression, thus maintaining power bases for resilience action (Benson and Ritter 1990; Rothmund et al. 2014). Furthermore, resilience belief has shrunk by adversity experienced, coercion received, fear, and minority status, thus retaining power to drive resilience action (Shank 2012; Singer et al. 2019; Taylor et al. 2015; Whyte and Gao 2009).

Utility attracting resilience action furnished by resilience belief involves controllability, fairness, and predictability (Dalbert 2001; Hafer and Sutton 2016). Predictability reduces anger and blaming, thus upholding resilience action (Evans 2013). Resilience belief also reflects benefits received to generate utility to attract resilience action (Liebig and Mau 2007). Similarly, resilience belief has stemmed from appreciation received, life quality, and opportunity experienced to sustain utility to attract resilience action (Mikula et al. 2009; van Prookjen et al. 2004). Conversely, resilience belief has dropped because of inequality experienced, marginalization experienced, and neuroticism, thus upholding utility to attract resilience action (Eriksson et al. 2015; Nudelman 2013; Wright 2001). Inequality experienced has provoked crime and strain to hinder resilience action (Kyriacou 2020).

Ideals rationalizing resilience action forged by resilience belief concern acceptance and agency (Dalbert 2001; Vermunt and Steensma 2016). Agency has boosted autonomy, mastery, performance, and vitality and diminished anxiety and depression to sustain resilience action (Gagne and Deci 2005; Ross and Drentea 1998; Schwartz and Melech 2000; Sheldon and Bettencourt 2002; Sieber et al. 2019; Weinstein and Ryan 2010). Moreover, resilience belief has secured accommodation, fairness value, individualism, internal attribution, and life satisfaction as ideals to induce resilience action (Bjornskov et al. 2013; Burgoyne et al. 1999; Lipkus and Bissonette 1998; Monroe et al. 2021; Olson and Hafer 2001). Individualism has raised self-enhancement to secure resilience action (Church 2010). Resilience belief has also evolved from individualism and satisfaction to secure ideals rationalizing resilience action (Liebig and Mau 2007; Viewiebe and Wegener 2000). Conversely, resilience belief has impeded blaming and protesting as ideals, thus buttressing resilience action (Lodewijkx et al. 2008; Maes 1998). Protesting has bred anger, impulsivity, and worry to defuse resilience action (Boehnke and Wong 2011; Landmann and Rohmann 2020; Vestergren et al. 2017).

Norms assimilating resilience action exposed by resilience belief highlight fairness and justice (Gibson 2008; Ng and Allen 2005). These norms have championed cooperation and prevented protesting, thus sustaining resilience action (van Prooijen et al. 2008; Wenzel 2000). Resilience belief has also reflected the norm for effectiveness to assimilate resilience action (Taylor et al. 2015). This norm dampens anger, blaming, and retribution, thus enabling resilience action (Evans 2013). Conversely, resilience belief has diminished the norm for risk (Tyler et al. 1997). Resilience belief has also shrunk by the norm for exploitation, thus encouraging resilience action (Ng and Allen 2005). This norm has bred anger, fear, and sadness to impede resilience action (Landmann and Rohmann 2020).

## Peer Advice and Demand

Peer advice and demand did not raise resilience, thus refuting the hypotheses. The refutation may result from the balance of positive and negative effects of peer advice and demand to neutralize any effect. That is, the inverse effects of advice and demand received would offset the positive effect of advice and demand received on resilience. Such inverse effects would reflect reducing power, incentives or utility, ideals, and norms for resilience, according to their respective deterministic and voluntaristic mechanisms of analytical functionalism. This reduction suggests that advice and demand received are futile, inappropriate, ineffective, questionable, and temporary (Erford et al. 2011; Holstein and Gubrium 2000; Lipschitz-Elhawi 2009; Marquis et al. 2011).

Power for resilience reduced by advice or demand received has rested on controlling, friendship, and kindness (Aryee and Kang 1999; Proyer et al. 2013; Woods et al. 2013). Controlling has facilitated health maintenance, optimism, prevention, social trust, and well-being to generate power for resilience (Cheng and Ng 2006; Etezadi and Pushkar 2013; Moore and Aweiss 2003; Smith and Stasson 2000; Steinhardt 2012). Friendship has fostered gratitude to boost resilience (Rotkirch 2014). Well-being has included health and life satisfaction (Heidemeier and Staudinger 2012; Rose 2000). Conversely, controlling has reduced anger, depression, and stress, thus safeguarding resilience (Cundiff et al. 2015; Khoo et al. 2021; Xi and Hwang 2011). Conversely, advice or demand received has invoked delinquency, depression, gambling, indecisiveness, service need, and stress, thus countering power to drive resilience (Davis et al. 1998; Eaton et al. 2001; Farrington and Welsh 2007; Fenwick and Tausig 1994; Griffiths 1999; Perdrix et al. 2012). Gambling has raised negative feelings and suicide to erode resilience (Ladouceur et al. 1999; Peacock et al. 1999). Indecisiveness has bred anxiety and difficulty to impend resilience (Kelly and Lee 2002; Vertsberger and Gati 2016). Service need has reflected depression to erode resilience (Golberstein et al. 2008). Alternatively, advice or demand received has arisen from avoidance, anxiety, bullying experienced, conflict, depression, disorders, illness, minority status, stigmatization experienced, substance abuse, suicide attempt, and victimization experienced thus weakening power to drive resilience (Cummings 2014; Gowdy et al. 2020; Meng and Chen 2014; Myers and Harper 2004; Turner et al. 2007). Avoidance has impaired coping and well-being, including mindfulness and satisfaction, to hinder resilience (Barber et al. 2010; Basabe et al. 2002; Linares et al. 2016; Seaton and Beaumont 2008). Conversely, avoidance has fomented anger, anxiety, depression, and loneliness (Cheng and Cheung 2005; Kafetsio and Sideridis 2006; Linares et al. 2016). Stigmatization experienced has stemmed from phobia to weaken resilience (Yao et al. 2021). Advice or demand received also arises from uncertainty to block resilience (Oglensky 2008). Uncertainty has arisen from dissatisfaction to forestall resilience (Noack et al. 2001).

Utility for resilience diminished by advice or demand received has involved achievement (Soodak and Podell 1994). Achievement has fostered health, life quality, satisfaction, self-efficacy, and self-esteem as opposed to alienation, depression, and distress to uphold resilience (Donnellan et al. 2005; Fredricks and Eccles 2005; Menard and Mose 1984; Murray 2009; Piko et al. 2006; Tompson and Dass 2000; Xiao et al. 2009). Conversely, advice or demand has arisen from gaps experienced as disutility to discourage resilience (Kutsyuruba 2012). Gaps experienced have incurred anxiety, depression, and strain and diminished health, morale, and satisfaction, thus impending resilience (Sutherland and Fogarty 1995; Li 2006; Pereyra-Rojas et al. 2017; Xie 1996).

Ideals for resilience dismissed by advice or demand received applaud satisfaction and work commitment (Clark et al. 2013; Crawford et al. 2010; Dust et al. 2020). Work commitment has raised self-efficacy and self-esteem to enable resilience (Bakker et al. 2008).

Norms countering resilience raised by advice or demand received have emphasized competition, conflict, or struggle (Gowdy et al. 2020). Such norms have eroded happiness, thus hindering resilience (Ouweneel and Veenhoven 2016). Moreover, such norms have evolved from fraud and protesting as opposed to prosperity, thus impairing resilience (Brancati 2016).

# Chapter 6
# Practical Bases for Resilience

**Abstract** This chapter examines the voluntaristic basis for resilience, emphasizing personal and peer practices, including experience-based coping, socializing, engaging with pets, religious practice, hardening, and softening. Hardening means forceful, confronting, proactive practice, whereas softening means acting tenderly, compromising, and withdrawing. The aggregates (averages) of personal practices in the service unit identify peer or contextual practices. Besides these personal and peer practice factors, advice received and Westernization represent social deterministic factors. Analysis of survey data on elders exhibited that experience-based coping, hardening, and softening significantly sustained resilience. Meanwhile, functional disability significantly impeded resilience. These impacts represent the voluntaristic mechanism of power realization, goal attainment, or transforming resources, capabilities, and/or efforts in production. The impacts also reflect the voluntaristic mechanism of ideal consistency, such that the practices are consonant with resilience. By contrast, advice received, and Westernization could have consistently delivered significant effects on resilience. This nonsignificance does not bolster the deterministic mechanism. Hence, the voluntaristic mechanism outperforms the deterministic mechanism in developing resilience. Nevertheless, socializing, religious practice, and pet engagement did not indicate significant effects on resilience. These practices are thus inconsistent with and/or incapable of generating resilience concerning the voluntaristic mechanisms of ideal consistency and power realization. In addition, some interactions between personal and peer practice manifested significant effects on resilience. For instance, resilience was higher when peer advice was higher despite higher personal adversity. This differential indicates the effectiveness due to sharing peer advice among peers. Additionally, this reflects the deterministic mechanism of empowering, particularly in the case of powerlessness due to adversity. Furthermore, Westernization did not affect the effects of the personal and social factors on resilience, thus showing that the effects are stable across Westernized and non-Westernized people. The findings are thus likely not specific to Hong Kong Chinese people.

 
C. K. Cheung, *Resilience Process and Its Personal and Social Bases*,
https://doi.org/10.1007/978-981-97-7391-6_6

Practical bases for resilience include kindness, experience-based coping, socializing, pet engagement, religious practice, hardening, and softening. Kindness means holding a good attitude toward others. Socializing means deepening relationships with other people. Hardening means confronting and striving, thus applying hard tactics for living. Softening means calming and easygoing, thus using soft tactics for living. Religious practice means relying on the supernatural. Pet engagement means relating to pets. Experience-based coping means using experience to cope. Westernization means adopting Western culture. These practices are likely to champion resilience by raising power, utility, ideals, and norms to leverage the voluntaristic mechanisms of power realization, utility optimization, ideal calibration, and norm conformity to achieve the four requisite functions of fulfillment, adaptation, latency, and integration upheld in analytical functionalism. From this functionalist perspective, kindness represents a practice for the fulfillment function to realize power or the corresponding disposition or goal, hardening and softening represent practices for the adaptation function to optimize utility, Westernization, pet engagement, religiosity, and socializing represent practices for integration to conform to norms, and experience-based coping represents a practice for the latent function to calibrate ideals. Notably, Westernization embodies integration with Western culture, pet engagement embodies integration with animal nature, religiosity embodies integration with the supernatural, and socializing embodies integration with people. Meanwhile, hardening and softening adapt to opportunity and risk to optimize gain.

## Existing Knowledge

The practices of kindness, hardening, softening, Westernization, socializing, religiosity, pet engagement, and experience-based coping are likely to champion resilience by acquiring power, utility, ideals, and norms to leverage the voluntaristic mechanisms of power realization, utility optimization, ideal calibration, and norm conformity in the functionalist framework. Power rests on resources and strengths, evolving from motivation by dispositions, needs, and goals. Utility stems from gain and hinges on achievement, success, and other rewards. Ideals sit in personal beliefs, orientations, and values. Norms are people's ideals and practices. For resilience, power has derived from agreeableness, conscientiousness, coping, emotional intelligence, emotional stability, extraversion, learning, mentoring received, organizational membership, prevention, purposiveness, self-esteem, sensation seeking, social support received, supportive services received, and wealth (Armstrong et al. 2011; Buikstra et al. 2010; Cherry et al. 2023; Corbin and Hall 2019; Jones and d'Errico 2019; Jones and Jetten 2011; Lock et al. 2020; McKay et al. 2018; Notter et al. 2008; Yu and Zhang 2007). Conversely, power for resilience dissipates due to neuroticism and trauma (Cherry et al. 2023; Yu and Zhang 2007). Utility attracting resilience has built on balance experienced and optimism (Buikstra et al. 2010; Cantor et al. 2002). Ideals calibrating or rationalizing resilience have hinged on future orientation, religiosity, social orientation, and values for affiliation or connectedness (Cherry et al.

2023; Chua et al. 2019; Lou et al. 2018). Norms assimilating resilience have stemmed from social adaptability, innovation, and safety (Jones and d'Errico 2019; Buikstra et al. 2010). Herein, resilience embodies or requires power such as assets, capability, resources, and strength, utility such as returns, ideals such as well-being, and norms such as social construction (Berger 2015; Schwarz 2018; Truebridge 2016; Van Haaften et al. 2004; White 2014; Zheng et al. 2020). Essentially, resilience, including feeling, action, and belief, is a voluntaristic action, which capitalizes on power, utility, ideals, and norms (Prilleltensky 2012; Ungar 2012; Zautra et al. 2010).

## *Kindness*

Kindness as a prosocial practice is likely to facilitate resilience (Coffey et al. 2023). To achieve the fulfillment function, kindness has rested on power constituted by agreeableness, education, empathy, friendliness, generativity, honesty and humility, income, intelligence, openness, perceptiveness, reciprocity, responsibility, skill, sociability, and social class (Bierhoff 2002; Foschi and Lauriola 2014; Greitemeyer et al. 2006; Hersberger-Langloh et al. 2022; Oliveira et al. 2021; Rossi 2004; Thielmann et al. 2020; Van de Vyver and Abrams 2018). Conversely, kindness has shrunk by countervailing power stemming from greed, impulsivity, narcissism, and psychopathy (Thielmann et al. 2020). Based on such power, kindness engenders power, utility, ideals, and norms for raising resilience.

Power driving resilience enhanced by kindness originates from forgiveness (Music 2014). Forgiveness has elevated serenity, trust, and well-being to maintain resilience (Choi and David 2012; Connors et al. 1999; Shimai et al. 2006). Moreover, kindness has consolidated competence, flexibility, protection, responsibility, restraint, self-efficacy, social attachment, social support received, and well-being to buttress resilience (Bond and Kwan 2000; Dinic and Bodroza 2021; Hui and Kogan 2018a, b; Jutengren and Medin 2019; Lee and Xiao 1998; Na and Paternoster 2019; Shahzalal and Adnan 2022; Yao and Enright 2019). Responsibility underpins sustainability (Shamir 2008). Well-being has included connectedness and meaningfulness as opposed to loneliness and negative emotion (Marsh and Dik 2021; Nelson-Coffey et al. 2023). Competence has enabled identity achievement, intimacy, and relationship satisfaction, as opposed to anxiety, to raise resilience (Adams 1985). Flexibility has buttressed life satisfaction and self-esteem as opposed to distress to enable resilience (Jen et al. 2019). Protection has uplifted self enhancement to safeguard resilience (Erickson and Feldstein 2007). Restraint has fostered well-being, including health and life satisfaction as opposed to anger and depression, to boost resilience (Cundiff et al. 2015; Etezadi and Pushkar 2013; Orlowski and Wicker 2015; Rose 2000; Xi and Hwang 2011). Self-efficacy has sustained well-being, including happiness, health, joy, and life satisfaction to facilitate resilience (Borgonovi 2008; Caprara and Steca 2005; Judge et al. 2002; Landmann and Rohmann 2020). Social attachment has raised life satisfaction to rationalize resilience (Zdrenka et al. 2015). Social support received has upheld well-being, including control, health, positive emotion and pleasure, purposiveness, relational quality, satisfaction with life, housing, and leisure, self-determination, self-efficacy, self-esteem, and social well-being, to activate resilience (George and Park 2013; Glendinning et al. 2003; Granzin and Haggard 2000; Holliman et al. 2021; Lincoln et al. 2003; Logan and Cobb 2013; Pierce and Quiroz 2018; Schwarzer and Knoll 2007; Vilhjalmsson and Thorlindsson 1998; Wen et al. 2010; Williams and Galliher 2006; Xi and Hwang 2011). Notably, social support received has boosted resilience (Cherry et al. 2018). Conversely, kindness has dampened delinquency, dysfunction, impulsivity, playfulness, and violence, thus sustaining power for resilience (Avlund et al. 2004; Hample 2018; Ma et al. 2011; Mesch 2009). Dysfunction has eroded health, satisfaction with housing, leisure, and life, and self-efficacy, thus hampering resilience (Distante 2013; Gastil 2000; Granzin and Haggard 2000). Conversely, dysfunction has distress, thus undermining resilience (Phongsavan et al. 2006). Impulsivity has revealed aggressiveness, antisociality, avoidance, neuroticism, and psychoticism as opposed to empathy and perspective-taking, thus eroding resilience (Hample 2018). Likewise, playfulness has reflected aggressiveness and violence, antisociality, impulsivity, and psychoticism as opposed to empathy, thus hindering resilience (Hample 2018; Huesmann and Kirwil 2007). Playfulness is also symptomatic for addiction, depression, gambling, schizophrenia, and other disorders to vitiate resilience (Berger et al. 2018).

Utility attracting resilience secured by kindness has covered achievement and success, autonomy granted, benefits and rewards, hope, liking and popularity experienced, safety experienced, and warmth received (Adongo et al. 2019; Bergin 2014; Bond and Kwan 2000; Dallago et al. 2009; Layous et al. 2012; Marsh and Dik 2021; Mestre et al. 2019; Padilla-Walker et al. 2018). Autonomy has sustained well-being, including life satisfaction, mastery, relational quality and relatedness, and vitality as opposed to anxiety and depression, thus advancing resilience (Delhey 2010; Hui et al. 2013; Ross and Drentea 1998; Schwartz and Melech 2000; Sheldon and Bettencourt 2002; Sieber et al. 2019; Weinstein and Ryan 2010). Benefit received has elevated well-being, including satisfaction as opposed to anger, anxiety, and depression, to boost resilience (Helgeson et al. 2006; Wells et al. 1999; Wong and Lam 2016). Popularity has uplifted positive affect and self-esteem and reduced negative affect, thus buttressing resilience (Reich et al. 2018). Saftethy has safeguarded well-being, including health and satisfaction with the country, neighborhood, and life, and diminished fear, hence championing resilience (Chen et al. 2008; Chiricos et al. 2000; Cummins et al. 2003; Frey et al. 2007; Parkes et al. 2002; Jones et al. 2014). Warmth experienced has reflected relationship quality to sustain resilience (Chen and Kaplan 2001).

Ideals rationalizing resilience upheld by kindness cherish fairness (Music 2014). Fairness in practice has reflected education, networking, and trust to facilitate resilience (Hauser et al. 2016). Moreover, kindness has strengthened religiosity and work value as ideals to rationalize resilience (Marsh and Dik 2021). Religiosity has sustained well-being, including adjustment, flourishing, health, mastery, positive affect, relationship quality, satisfaction with democracy, police, finance, and life, self-esteem, and socioemotional well-being to lift resilience (Dy-Liacco et al. 2009; Flouri and Buchanan 2002; Helliwell and Putnam 2005; Kwak et al. 2010; Marx

2014; Meulemann 2010; Moschis and Ong 2011; Ng and Fisher 2016; Schieman 2001; Skerkat and Ellison 1999; Van Praag et al. 2010; Wuthnow 2004). Conversely, religiosity has dampened depression, fear, and loneliness, thus sustaining resilience (Ellison et al. 2001; V. Hui et al. 2007; Lauder et al. 2006). Work value has reflected financial satisfaction to induce resilience (Kiecolt 2003). Conversely, kindness counters hedonism as an ideal impeding resilience (Twenge et al. 2007). Hedonism has reflected irreligiousness to hamper resilience (Devos et al. 2002).

Norms assimilating resilience exposed by kindness popularize social caring, recognition, respect, and responsibility (Glenn 2000). These norms have built trust to enhance resilience (Mutz and Reeves 2005).

## *Hardening*

Hardening is likely to achieve resilience through working hard, concentrating, learning, and other self-affirming deeds. Grounded on stoicism, hardening wields challenge, commitment, confidence, control, power, prevention and protection, and rationality (Butler et al. 2022; Ireland 2021; Pangallo et al. 2015; Perry et al. 2013; Siisiainen 2019; Zhang 2006). Conversely, hardening eschews escape, laziness, softness, tolerance, and yielding (Bjornskov et al. 2013; Brusting and Postmes 2002; Koomen and van der Pligt 2016; Siisiainen 2019). Hardening draws power by adhering to justice, law, rule, and truth or realism to assert its righteousness (Zhang 2006). The basis for hardening on rationality is functional for adaptation to optimize utility in confronting life (Zhang 2006). Hardening is thus a rational response to harassment and victimization experienced to optimize benefit, gain, or utility as opposed to cost or loss (Butler et al. 2022). As such, hardening has advanced success and well-being as opposed to anxiety to muster power, utility, and ideals to drive, attract, and rationalize resilience (Beasley et al. 2003; Greeff and van der Merwe 2004; DeNeve and Cooper 1998).

Stoicism, as the foundation for hardening, is likely to generate power, utility, ideals, and norms to engender resilience. Such engendering relies on the voluntaristic mechanisms of power realization, utility optimization, ideal calibration, and norm conformity in analytical functionalism.

Power instilled by stoicism to drive resilience rests on battling, choice, delay, dignity, dutifulness or obligation, education, exercise and preparation, masculinity, internality or self control and self-containment, invincibility, knowledge, mindfulness, physical strength, planning, rationality and reasoning, and self-direction (Holowchak 2008; Martin 2016; Mitsis 2003). Battling has unfolded competence and self-enhancement value to sustain resilience (Guan et al. 2010). Choice has generated well-being, including satisfaction with life and the neighborhood, to boost resilience (Abbott and Sapsford 2006; Day 2013; Helliwell et al. 2010). Delay reflects time availability for resilience (Wypych et al. 2018). Dignity has upheld well-being, including adjustment, happiness, health, positive affect, satisfaction with appearance, and work to enable resilience (Barnard and Curry 2011; Frederick et al. 2016;

Hull et al. 2008; Judge et al. 2002; Williams et al. 1992). Masculinity embraces choice, control, invulnerability, and reasoning to maintain resilience (Courtenay 2000; Nelson 2015). Mindfulness has raised well-being, including life satisfaction and positive affect as opposed to depression, to facilitate resilience (Andrade et al. 2019; Klussman et al. 2020; Linares et al. 2016). Planning has benefitted from achievement, health, and optimism to secure resilience (Hellevik and Settersten 2013; Poynton et al. 2015). Preparation has enabled acceptance to uphold resilience (Curry et al. 2015). Rationality has eroded anxiety, depression, disorders, and self-defeating, thus safeguarding resilience (DiGiuseppe et al. 2017). Self-control has upheld self-esteem and eroded anxiety, depression, and vulnerability to facilitate resilience (Armstrong et al. 2011; Langenderfer and Shimp 2001; Marchetti et al. 2018). Self-direction has arisen from harm avoidance to safeguard resilience (Richter et al. 2002). Conversely, stoicism prohibits anxiety or fear, desire, and emotionality as power distracting resilience (Holowchak 2008; Martin 2016). Desire contradicts self-cultivation and self-control, thus eroding resilience (Choi 2012). Emotionality has bred strain, thus worsening resilience (Hintsanen et al. 2011).

Ideals preached by stoicism to rationalize resilience embrace acceptance, calmness and equanimity, conservation, cosmopolitanism, endurance, heroism, honor, indifference, kindness, magnanimity, naturalism or harmony, perfectionism, poverty or hardship, rehabilitation, self-love, self-preservation, self-sufficiency, silence, simplicity, truthfulness, and welcoming (Holowchak 2008; Martin 2016). Cosmopolitanism valorizes activity, practicality, and reflection, as opposed to hedonism (Holowchak 2008). Additionally, cosmopolitanism has fostered social trust to empower resilience (Freitag 2003). Cosmopolitanism also aligns with stoicism to sustain resilience (Bray 2013; Held 2010). Furthermore, cosmopolitanism valorizes harm avoidance, resolution or problem-solving, and sustainability to secure resilience (Baildon and Alviar-Martin 2020; Bray 2013). Hardship has incubated self-transcendence to achieve resilience (Reeskens and Vandecasteele 2017). Heroism has stemmed from self-evaluation, comprising control, emotional stability, self-efficacy, and self-esteem (Hannah et al. 2007). Naturalism maintains joy and peacefulness to achieve resilience (Hocksmann 2004; Moeller 2004). Perfectionism accentuates self-esteem to sustain resilience (Grzegorek et al. 2004). Self-love has buttressed equanimity, happiness, and positive affect and diminished anger, anxiety, catastrophizing, distress, and self-rumination to maintain resilience (Barnard and Curry 2011; Sirois et al. 2015). Truthfulness has championed well-being, including autonomy and self-determination, growth, life satisfaction, mastery, positive affect, purposiveness, relationship quality, self-acceptance, self-actualization, self-esteem, and vitality as opposed to strain and stress, to lift resilience (Kernis and Goldman 2006). Conversely, stoicism dismisses convenience or inactivity, easiness, leisure, and pleasure as ideals, thus safeguarding resilience (Holowchak 2008). The ideal for leisure has declined by job satisfaction to erode resilience (Snir and Harpaz 2002). Hedonism, or the ideal of pleasure, has bred depression and diminished self-esteem, thus impairing resilience (Bjarnason 2009).

Commitment applies to a career, communication, destination, discourse, identity, and role (Agronick and Duncan 1998; Demerath 2012; Guerrero 2015; Patwardhan et al. 2019; Xu et al. 2018). In practice, commitment signifies fidelity, importance, intention, liking, love, and predictability regarding work (Agronick and Duncan 1998; Buunk and Dijkstra 2006; Fang et al. 2019; Guerrero 2015; Huang et al. 2018; Xu et al. 2018). Commitment can sustain resilience by providing power, utility, ideals, and norms to activate power realization, utility optimization, ideal calibration, and norm conformity for achieving the requisite functions of analytical functionalism.

Power raised by commitment to drive resilience has rested on emotional intelligence, empathy, exploration, intrinsic motivation, mindedness or mindfulness, and socioeconomic status, including education (Agronick and Duncan 1998; Hagan et al. 1996; Seaton and Beaumont 2008; Ferssizidis et al. 2010). Emotional intelligence has advanced well-being, including adaptation, happiness, health, optimism, life satisfaction, positive mood, relationship quality and relatedness, and self-esteem to sustain resilience (Ciarrochi et al. 2000; Kluemper 2008; Matthews et al. 2012; Mayer et al. 2004; Schutte et al. 2002). Conversely, emotional intelligence has erased depression, distress, and symptoms to maintain resilience (Goldenberg et al. 2006; Mayer et al. 2008). Empathy has boosted communication quality and intimacy to secure resilience (Redmond 2018). Exploration has developed self-efficacy to empower resilience (Harre 2007). Intrinsic motivation has reflected competence and meaningfulness to enable resilience (Gonzalez-Cutre et al. 2016; Morgan and Robinson 2013). Mindfulness has raised life satisfaction and positive affect and lessened depression (Andrade et al. 2019; Klussman et al. 2020; Linares et al. 2016). Socioeconomic status has upgraded health, interaction quality, life satisfaction, self-confidence, self-esteem, and general well-being and reduced distress and strain to champion resilience (Al-krenawi et al. 2011; Caplan and Schooler 2007; Molana and Adams 2019; Staudinger et al. 1999). Commitment rises by autonomy and self-determination, goal-setting, interest, investment, learning, matching experienced, responsiveness, self-efficacy, security experienced, social support received, and trust to generate power to drive resilience (Buunk and Dijkstra 2006; Ferry et al. 2000; Lawler et al. 2016; Lent 2013; Ogolsky and Monk 2018; Theiss 2018; Zhang et al. 2019). Goal-setting has supported life satisfaction and self-evaluation to secure resilience (Frazier et al. 2007; Stutzer 2004). Investment has built social capital to enhance resilience (Hlasny and Lee 2020). Learning has elevated well-being, including life satisfaction and self-efficacy, to facilitate resilience (Denver and Hands 1990; Minnaert and Janssen 1992; Richards 2016). Matching experienced has engendered well-being to underpin resilience (Chuang 2005). Responsiveness reflects tolerance to enable resilience (Peplak and Malti 2022). Security experienced has sustained well-being, including health, life satisfaction, and neighborhood quality and satisfaction as opposed to fear to lift resilience (Chen et al. 2008; Chiricos et al. 2000; Frey et al. 2007; Olson et al. 2016; Parkes et al. 2002; Jones et al. 2014). Trust has sustained health and survival, thus raising resilience (Barefoot et al. 1998). Furthermore, commitment has escalated by adaptability, agreeableness, capacity, dutifulness, education, entrepreneurship, extraversion, flexibility, human and social capital, income, openness, self-esteem, skill, attachment, bonding, closeness, and relatedness to furnish power to drive resilience (Agronick and Duncan 1998; Chen and Dwyer 2018; Child and Nikolova 2020; Creed and Patton 2003; Ellison et al. 2014;

Erez et al. 2008; Felker and Gianecchini 2015; Flouri and Buchanan 2002; Labrecque 2014; Nikolayenko 2014; Piatak 2016; Rogers and Creed 2011; Schmitt-Rodermund 2004; Sheldon and Bettencourt 2002; Urbanaviciute et al. 2016). Agreeableness has escalated growth, life satisfaction, mastery, purposefulness, relatedness, and self-acceptance to secure resilience (Hounkpatin et al. 2015). Entrepreneurship has reflected self-efficacy to enable resilience (Atitsogbe et al. 2019). Extraversion has raised well-being, including positive affect, autonomy, growth, mastery, mattering, purposefulness, relatedness, satisfaction, self-acceptance, self-determination, self-efficacy, and self-esteem to uplift resilience (Flett 2018; Hounkpatin et al. 2015; Ingledew et al. 2004; Li et al. 2017; Quilty et al. 2006; Rasmussen et al. 2018; Richards 2016; Tiwari et al. 2021). Flexibility has sustained life satisfaction and self-esteem and eroded distress to maintain resilience (Jen et al. 2019). Openness has buttressed well-being, including autonomy, growth, purposefulness, life satisfaction, relationship quality, self-acceptance, self-efficacy, and self-esteem to advance resilience (Hahn et al. 2013; Hounkpatin et al. 2014, 2015; Karwowski and Lebuda 2017; Marks 1996; Quilty et al. 2006). Conversely, commitment reflects low anxiety and disruption experienced, thus keeping power to drive resilience (Buunk and Dijkstra 2006; Hantula 2012; Ogolsky and Monk 2018). Moreover, commitment has indicated non-avoidance to resume power to drive resilience (Schindler et al. 2010). Avoidance has impaired well-being, including intimacy, life satisfaction, and mindfulness, thus weakening resilience (Alonso-Arbiol et al. 2007; Barber et al. 2010; Linares et al. 2016). Conversely, avoidance has bred anger, anxiety, depression, and loneliness to hamper resilience (Cheng and Cheung 2005; Kafetsio and Sideridis 2006; Linares et al. 2016).

Utility gained by commitment to attract resilience has resided in achievement (Agronick and Duncan 1998). Commitment indicates attractiveness, benefit, equity, and gain experienced to hold utility to attract resilience (Agnew and Vanderdrift 2018; Ogolsky and Monk 2018). Such utility has boosted well-being, including satisfaction, as opposed to anger and anxiety, to raise resilience (Helgeson et al. 2006; Wells et al. 1999; Wong and Lam 2016). Similarly, commitment has reflected incentive, justice, and value experienced to maintain utility to attract resilience (Brooks 1999; Piatak 2016). Justice experienced has boosted belongingness, health, life satisfaction, and self-esteem to establish resilience (Bjornskov et al. 2013; Dalbert 2001; Lucas et al. 2013; van Prooijen et al. 2008). Meanwhile, justice experienced has prevented anger and depression to enable resilience (Benson and Ritter 1990; Rothmund et al. 2014). Conversely, commitment maintains utility to attract resilience when reflecting low barriers, conflict, and crises experienced (Agnew and Vanderdrift 2018; Buunk and Dijkstra 2006; Demerath 2012; Finkel et al. 2016). Conflict experienced has bred distress and eroded satisfaction, thus impeding resilience (Lau et al. 2017; Mikula et al. 2012).

Ideals upheld by commitment to rationalize resilience have concerned self-acceptance (Agronick and Duncan 1998). Commitment reflects accommodation, cohesiveness, control, enjoyment, equilibrium experienced, justification, meaningfulness, order experienced, reconciliation, satisfaction, and stability experienced, thus maintaining ideals to rationalize resilience (Agnew and Vanderdrift 2018;

Demerath 2012; Ogolsky and Monk 2018; Rusbutt et al. 2006; Theiss 2018). Cohesiveness fosters confidence and reflects ease and education to maintain resilience (Achterberg and Houtman 2009; Soto et al. 2008; Simon and Read 2018). Justification has upheld positive affect to benefit resilience (Jost and Hunyady 2005). Order preference has reflected health to facilitate resilience (Cheung and Lai 2020). Reconciliation has reflected harmonious passion and order, security, and stability values to secure resilience (Belanger et al. 2019; Simmons 2020). Stability experienced has championed well-being, including health and life satisfaction as opposed to fear (Chen et al. 2008; Frey et al. 2007; Jones et al. 2014). Understanding has raised intimacy, satisfaction, and self-efficacy to support resilience (Mikulincer et al. 2003; Norris 2011; Rothwell et al. 2016). Likewise, commitment has grown due to understanding and work value to sustain ideals to rationalize resilience (Patwardhan et al. 2019; Thompson and Dahling 2010).

Norms buttressed by commitment to assimilate resilience have popularized acceptance, competence, and growth (Deemer et al. 2014; Romaioli et al. 2016; Schaufeli 2016). The acceptance norm has resisted depression, thus fostering resilience (Mullins and Dugan 1991). Competence, as raised by the competence norm, has buttressed well-being to advance resilience (Bjornskov 2008; Letki 2008). As raised by the growth norm, growth has reflected self-tolerance to furnish resilience (Ho and Li 2022; Sheldon and Hower-Marko 2001).

Control applies to emotion, feeling, health, and social relations to sustain resilience (Alsted and Haslund 2020; Lewis et al. 2006a; Schieman and Campbell 2001; Speer et al. 2013). Such sustenance benefits from power, utility, ideals, and norms raised by control to achieve requisite functions through power realization, utility optimization, ideal calibration, and norm conformity, respectively.

Control has raised power to drive resilience through attachment, health and its maintenance, influence, leisure activity, prevention, services received, social trust, and general well-being (Etezadi and Pushkar 2013; Keltener et al. 2008; Long and Perkins 2007; Rose 2000; Smith and Stasson 2000; Steinhardt 2012; Wu, Liu, and Wang 2010; Young et al. 2001). Health maintenance has safeguarded health and alleviated depression to sustain resilience (Myers 2008, Smith et al. 2006). Influence has upgraded mood and reduced depression to achieve resilience (Langner et al. 2012; Wojciszke and Struzynska-Kujolowicz 2007). Leisure activity has sustained life satisfaction to enable resilience (Roberts et al. 2001). Prevention has achieved social desirability to yield resilience (Lalwani et al. 2009). Services received have supported autonomy or self-determination, satisfaction, and reduced mortality, thus boosting resilience (Clemens and Wetle 1994; Davies et al. 1990; Elkan et al. 2001). Moreover, control has reflected agency, conscientiousness, education, empathy, extraversion, income, openness, power motive, religiosity, resources, social support received, and wisdom to boost power for driving resilience (Cheung and Chiu 2021; Etezadi and Pushkar 2013; Lincoln et al. 2003; Prenda and Lachman 2001; Ross and Drentea 1998; Schieman and Campbell 2001; Slagsvold and Sorensen 2008; Song and Zahedi 2005). Agency has established well-being, including autonomy, mastery, relational quality and relatedness, life satisfaction, and vitality (Delhey 2010; Downie et al.

2008; Sieber et al. 2019; Weinstein and Ryan 2010). Conversely, control has alleviated anger, conflict, depression, dysfunction, hospitalization experienced, risking, and stress experienced, thus retaining power to drive resilience (Bazargan et al. 1998; Brown 2001; Cundiff et al. 2015; Hoang et al. 2020; Khoo et al. 2021; Shaw 2005; Wickrama et al. 1995). Hospitalization has worsened health and reflected depression and disorders, thus impairing resilience (Bryant et al. 2000; Lincoln 2006; McBride et al. 2000). Control has also reflected low helplessness, neuroticism, strain, and trauma, thus maintaining power to drive resilience (Lincoln et al. 2003; Perrig et al. 1999). Helplessness has reflected depression, thus impeding resilience (Maatta and Nurmi 2007).

Control has furnished utility attracting resiliency through benefits experienced, life satisfaction, and optimism (Lewis et al. 2006a; Moore and Aweiss 2003). Moreover, control has reflected opportunity as utility to attract resilience (Lyness et al. 2012). Opportunity has reflected social inclusion, respect, and support received to buttress resilience (Wen et al. 2022).

Control has championed an ideal resting on justification to rationalize resilience (Jost 2020; Orlowski and Wicker 2015). Conversely, control has weakened the ideal or obsession concerning conspiracy to strengthen resilience (Kim and Kim 2021). The obsession has bred anxiety, thus weakening resilience (Leibovitz et al. 2021).

Control has reflected the norm for stability to assimilate resilience (Lefrancois et al. 2017). The norm has sustained well-being, including health, and life satisfaction, as opposed to fear, to safeguard resilience (Chen et al. 2008; Frey et al. 2007; Jones et al. 2014).

Prevention, applying to illness, infection, pandemics, risk, violence, and other happenings, is likely to preserve resilience (Flintoff et al. 2019; Frazier and Falmagro 2014; Lemay et al. 2023; Oleksy et al. 2021; Ruiter et al. 2004) Such preservation relies on power realization, utility optimization, idea calibration, and norm conformity to achieve the requisite functions of fulfillment, adaptation, latency, and integration based on analytical functionalism. Prevention thus generates power, utility, ideals, and norms conducive to resilience.

Power raised by prevention to drive resilience rests on investment and openness (Ackerman et al. 2018; Schaller and Park 2011). Prevention embraces flexibility and preservation as power bases to drive resilience (Ackerman et al. 2018; Flintoff et al. 2019). Moreover, prevention reflects responsibility to consolidate power to drive resilience (Frazier and Falmagro 2014). Prevention has also arisen from control, education, empathy, income, knowledge, and trust to generate power to drive resilience (Cheng and Ng 2006; Lee-Baggley et al. 2004; McClaran et al. 2022; Pires 2022).

Utility created by prevention to attract resilience has reflected effectiveness and confidence. Conversely, prevention has reflected low expectations for disutility from conspiracy, harm, side effects, and threats, thus safeguarding resilience (Lemay et al. 2023; McClaran et al. 2022; Pires 2022; Romer and Jamieson 2020).

Ideals upheld by prevention rationalize resilience, treasure coping, and curing (McClaran et al. 2022). Such ideals underlie coping and curing to uphold well-being to scaffold resilience (Corbin and Hall 2019; McClaran et al. 2022). Such well-being has included growth, health, intimacy, satisfaction, self-efficacy, and environmental and relational quality (Chow et al. 2014; Gattino et al. 2015; Lau et al. 2012; Paez et al. 2007; Wills 1997). Conversely, well-being has involved low depression, distress, and fear (Frazier et al. 2005; Krulichova 2019; Wills 1997).

The norm promoted by prevention to assimilate resilience concerns management (Cullen and Jonson 2017). That is, one's prevention prompts or requires other people's management norm. The norm collectively raises competence, efficiency, and productivity in sustaining resilience (Kemshall 2002).

Protection, including avoidance, defense, and other ways of hardening, addresses pandemics, risks, violence, and other assaults to reduce their harm, given their unpreventability (Ireland 2021; Warner et al. 2022). As such, protection can elevate resilience through power realization, utility optimization, ideal calibration, and norm conformity mechanisms to achieve requisite functions specified in analytical functionalism. These mechanisms operate with power, utility, ideals, and norms furnished by protection.

Power reflected by protection to drive resilience has derived from analytical assessment or rationality, coping, education, empathy, health maintenance, information and its seeking, knowledge, religiosity, self-efficacy, and self-organization (Bish and Michie 2010; Chen et al. 2021; Dinic and Bodroza 2021; Gonzalez-Castro et al. 2021; Ireland 2021; Nudelman et al. 2021; Pang et al. 2022; Stevens and Hassett 2007; Zarzeczna et al. 2023). Health maintenance has boosted health and reduced depression to establish resilience (Myers 2008; Smith et al. 2006). Rationality has eroded anxiety, depression, and dependence to uphold resilience (DiGiuseppe et al. 2017). Self-organization maintains or predisposes resilience (Hudson 2000).

Utility reflected by protection to attract resilience has concerned confidence or trust, concern or consideration, effectiveness or efficacy, and growth or improvability belief regarding protection (Bish and Michie 2010; Ireland 2021; Juanchich et al. 2021; Scholz and Freund 2021; Warner et al. 2022; Zhang and Kou 2022). Growth or improvability belief has reflected openness to raise resilience (Furnham et al. 2003). Conversely, protection has arisen from low conspiracy belief, cost, difficulty, and risk regarding protection, thus sustaining utility and attracting resilience (Hinssen and Dohle 2023; Ireland 2021; Juanchich et al. 2021; Scholz and Freund 2021). Conspiracy belief reflects abnormality, ambiguity experienced, danger felt, deviance, disorder, disruption felt, extremism, ignorance, irrationality, loss experienced, militancy, paranoia, pathology, phobia, social exclusion experienced, stigma experienced, threat experienced, and vulnerability to jeopardize resilience (Atkinson and Dewitt 2019; Difonzo 2019; Freeman et al. 2022; Grodzicka and Harambam 2021; Guan and Yang 2020; Harambam and Aupers 2015; Leibovitz et al. 2021; Stojanov and Halberstadt 2019; Sunstein and Vermeule 2009; Uscinski 2019). Ambiguity experienced and ignorance stem from anxiety to distract resilience (Theiss 2018). Danger felt has diminished well-being (Requena 2003). Extremism has reflected anomie, anxiety, self-uncertainty, and uncertainty to erode resilience (Hogg et al. 2010; Koehler and Fiebig 2019; Stankov et al. 2018). Loss experienced has bred anger and depression to negate resilience (Wells et al. 1999). Pathology has dampened resilience and other aspects of well-being, including health, life satisfaction, safety, security, and vitality

(Carrieri 2012; Jones and d'Errico 2019; Magnani and Zhu 2018; van Dijk et al. 2008). Stigma experienced has revealed mental health problems to obstruct resilience (Golberstein et al. 2008). Threat experienced has diminished well-being, including meaningfulness as opposed to anxiety, depression, fear, and hate (Edwards and Arnon 2021; MacLeod 2017; Moore and Shepherd 2006; O'Neill and Evans 1999; Rothschild and Keefer 2022; Schmid and Muldoon 2015). Conspiracy belief involves distrust to disturb resilience. Moreover, conspiracy belief has engendered anxiety, distrust, and incompliance to hamper resilience (Freeman et al. 2022; Leibovitz et al. 2021). Conspiracy belief has also arisen from anxiety, negative emotion, and powerlessness, thus impeding resilience (Kim and Kim 2021; van Prooijen 2017). Powerlessness has unfolded dissatisfaction to impair resilience (Armstrong-Stassen 2001). Conversely, conspiracy belief has reflected low well-being, including control and self-esteem, thus hindering resilience (Freeman et al. 2022; Kim and Kim 2021; Swami et al. 2011).

Ideals reflected by protection to rationalize resilience have embraced activeness and future orientation (Bish and Michie 2010; Zhang and Kou 2022). Activeness as an ideal has reflected satisfaction to calibrate resilience (Kiecolt 2003). Future orientation has underpinned resilience, life satisfaction, and general well-being (Lou et al. 2018; MacLeod 2017).

The norm reflected by protection to assimilate resilience has popularized protection (Bish and Michie 2010; Chen et al. 2021; Guo et al. 2023; Ireland 2021). Protection assimilated by the norm has reflected self-efficacy to facilitate resilience (Guo et al. 2023).

Rationality is likely to enable resilience with its excellent and virtuous qualities of abstraction, analysis, coherence, conceptualizing, consciousness, deliberation, extensive thinking, instrumentality and pragmatism, intentionality, logical thinking, systematic thinking, and unbiasedness (Domeier 2018; Epstein et al. 1996; Lambie 2008; Schafer 2015; Zezelj and Lazarevic 2019). These qualities furnish power, utility, ideals, and norms to achieve fulfillment, adaptation, latency, and integration functions to buttress resilience. Such achievement applies the voluntaristic mechanisms of power realization, utility optimization, ideal calibration, and norm conformity in analytical functionalism.

Power raised by rationality to drive resilience has encompassed comprehensibility, powerfulness, and teachability (Mallard 2020). Comprehensibility builds on education to enable resilience (Achterberg and Houtman 2009). Rationality also lifts resolution or problem-solving to exert power to drive resilience (Phye 1997). Similarly, rationality has buttressed conflict resolution, conscientiousness, constructive thinking, coping, extraversion, favorability, health, and self-regulation to maintain power to drive resilience (Epstein et al. 1996; Jokic and Puric 2021; Pacini and Epstein 1999). Favorability has reflected gratitude and satisfaction as opposed to anxiety and strain to boost resilience (Costello et al. 2019; Wood et al. 2005; Lu et al. 2016). Rationality reflects self-efficacy to yield power to drive resilience (Allen et al. 2009). Furthermore, rationality has reflected attachment and security, control, education, earnings, ego strength, and openness to accrue power for driving resilience (Barnes and Vulcano 1982; Epstein et al. 1996; Larrick et al. 1993). Conversely, rationality has dampened aggressiveness, antisociality, anxiety and fear, avoidance, dependence, depression, disorders, neuroticism, punitiveness, and self-defeating, thus maintaining power to drive resilience (Barnes and Vulcano 1982; DiGiuseppe et al. 2017; Pacini and Epstein 1999). Avoidance has dampened well-being, including intimacy, mindfulness, and satisfaction, as opposed to anger, anxiety, depression, distress, and loneliness, to block resilience (Alonso-Arbiol et al. 2007; Barber et al. 2010; Cheng and Cheung 2005; Linares et al. 2016; Littleton et al. 2007; Kafetsio and Sideridis 2006). Punitiveness has reflected fear, outrage, and worry to impede resilience (Carlsmith and Darley 2008; Cohen et al. 2006; Kafetsio and Sideridis 2006). Rationality has also reflected low vulnerability, thus holding power to drive resilience (Allen et al. 2009).

Utility enhanced by rationality to attract resilience involves success (Larrick et al. 1993). Rationality has also championed achievement, belief about meaningfulness, and trust to generate utility to attract resilience (Jokic and Puric 2021; Pacini and Epstein 1999). Such utility has fostered happiness, health, life satisfaction, and positive affect as opposed to depression and negative affect (Steger et al. 2009; Svebak et al. 2004). Furthermore, rationality reflects efficacy and reward experienced as opposed to cost experienced to maintain utility to attract resilience (Allen et al. 2009). Rationality has also reflected effectiveness experienced to uphold utility for attracting resilience (Claidiere et al. 2017).

## *Softening*

Softening realizes the life tactic of reconciliation (Giri 2011). It encompasses attracting, befriending, compensating, cooperating, communicating and dialoguing, educating or teaching, empathizing, equalizing or condescending, following or humility, harmonizing, levering or nudging, negotiating, participating, perspective-changing or reframing, rehabilitating or healing, relaxing, rewarding, supporting, and trusting (Edney 2012; Greene 1991; Koomen and van der Pligt 2016; Sui 2011; Wansink and van Itterum 2012; Zhang 2006). As such, softening applies charisma, gentleness, humanism, humbleness and humility, intimacy, leeway, maturity, openness, rapport, referents, substantiveness, warmth and concern, and win–win and mutual benefit (Greene 1991; Sui 2011). Conversely, softening eschews controlling or manipulating, revealing, speculating, and struggling (Greene 1991; Sui 2011). Herein, softening forgoes authority, desperation, and rigidity (Greene 1991; Sui 2011).

Attracting is likely to heighten resilience with the voluntaristic mechanisms of power realization, utility optimization, ideal calibration, and norm conformity in analytical functionalism. Power reflected in attracting rests on sensitivity to drive resilience (Noller et al. 2001). Utility engendered by attracting offers benefits demanded or expected by others to attract their support to maintain resilience (Burgoon et al. 2010). Ideals hailed by attracting emphasize social performance to establish social identity and responsibility for rationalizing resilience (Backhaus et al. 2002). Norms underlying attracting appeals to the culture to assimilate resilience (Burgoon et al. 2010).

Befriending features acceptance, providing, sharing, supporting, trusting, and understanding (Carbery and Buhrmester 1998; Koerner 2018). With these qualities, befriending activates power, utility, ideals, and norms to induce resilience through the voluntaristic mechanisms of analytical functionalism.

Power generated by befriending has afforded belongingness, enjoyment, gratitude, happiness, intimacy, prosociality, reassurance experienced, self-esteem, self-expansion, social integration, and social trust to drive resilience (Burgess et al. 2006; Carbery and Buhrmester 1998; Falci and McNeely 2009; Foschi and Lauriola 2014; Grunebaum 2003; Koerner 2018; Rotkirch 2014; Turner et al. 2007). Belongingness has prevented negative emotion and stress to enhance resilience (Nelson-Coffey et al. 2023). Gratitude has raised positive affect and dampened negative affect to achieve resilience (Bernabe-Valero et al. 2021). Moreover, befriending demonstrates power in acceptance, appreciation, cheerfulness, community building, cooperation, empathy, entertaining, openness, recreation, sensitivity, social networks or capital, and understanding to empower resilience (Austin et al. 2005; de Vries and Megathlin 2009; Grunebaum 2003; Sharabany 1994; Tsai 2006; Walker 1995). Openness has sustained well-being, including autonomy, growth, purposefulness, relationship quality, life satisfaction, self-acceptance, self-efficacy, and self-esteem, as opposed to hostility to enhance resilience (Hahn et al. 2013; Hounkpatin et al. 2015; Karwowski and Lebuda 2017; Marks 1996; Quilty et al. 2006; Webster et al. 2014). Recreation has elevated life satisfaction to boost resilience (Roberts et al. 2001). Self-expansion upholds self-esteem to facilitate resilience (Schindler et al. 2015). Moreover, self-expansion has buttressed attachment and love and reduced depression and negative affect to safeguard resilience (McIntyre et al. 2023; Sivami 2016; Xin et al. 2017). Sensitivity has advanced attachment quality to lift resilience (Grossman et al. 2002). Befriending has also reflected power based on attachment, education, health, homeownership, income, and intelligence and emotional intelligence to facilitate resilience (Austin et al. 2005; Child and Nikolova 2020; DeScioli and Kurzban 2009; Sharabany 1994; Tsai 2006; Volker and Flap 2007). Homeownership has raised health, morale, family and neighborhood quality, and financial, housing, life, and neighborhood satisfaction as opposed to depression, distress, and fear to strengthen resilience (Congdon 2010; Harris 2001; Lee et al. 2022; Mirowsky and Ross 1999; Montazer 2022; Roy and Chaudhuri 2008; Wulfhorst and Kranich 1999; Yu and Chiu 2016; Zheng et al. 2020). Conversely, befriending has dampened isolation experienced, loneliness, and neglect experienced, thus maintaining power to drive resilience (Guroglu et al. 2007; Xu et al. 2004; Zysberg 2012). Isolation experienced has bred negative mood and deprived life satisfaction, thus hindering resilience (Lin et al. 2013; Williams et al. 2000). Neglect experienced has stemmed from dissatisfaction, thus eroding resilience (Thomas and Au 2002). Befriending has reflected low anxiety, depression, and manipulation experienced to retain power to drive resilience (Palacios et al. 2019; van Zalk et al. 2010; Parade et al. 2010). Manipulation experienced has fomented distress to undermine resilience (Overall et al. 2020).

Utility maintained by befriending enables acceptance, affirmation, agreement and consensus, benefit, dignity, popularity, security, similarity, satisfaction with health, leisure, life, and work, and social harmony experienced to attract resilience (Bagwell and Schmidt 2011; Burgess et al. 2006; Campbell and Russo 2003; Espelage et al. 2007; Grunebaum 2003; Koerner 2018; Park 2012; Rose 2002; Rubin et al. 2008). Similarity experienced has diminished depression, thus sustaining resilience (Riad and Norris 1992). Social harmony experienced has reflected satisfaction with the economy, family, governance, mutual support, progress, and work to boost resilience (Ho and Chan 2009). Befriending also reflects expected gain and responsiveness experienced to generate utility to attract resilience (Parade et al. 2010; Volker and Flap 2007). Responsiveness experienced has raised adaptation, life satisfaction, positive emotion, and relationship evaluation to advance resilience (Algoe and Zhaoyang 2016). Conversely, befriending has reflected low uncertainty experienced, thus dismissing disutility against resilience (Noack 1999). Uncertainty experienced has hampered commitment, coping, intimacy, resolution, and satisfaction, thus eroding resilience (Theiss 2018).

Ideals championed by befriending have reflected acceptance and self-regulation to rationalize resilience (Eberl 2020; Lang and Carstensen 2002; Piercy 2000). Self-regulation has boosted self-esteem and diminished anxiety and depression to champion resilience (Marchetti et al. 2018).

Norms highlighted by befriending have featured similarity, popularity, and warmth to assimilate resilience (Brouwer and Engels 2022; Kokkinos and Hatzinikolaou 2011; Mouw and Entwisle 2006). Popularity has safeguarded belongingness, positive affect, and self-esteem and diminished negative affect to escalate resilience (Reich et al. 2018).

Compensating, meaning covering the loss, generates power, utility, ideals, and norms to sustain resilience with the voluntaristic mechanisms of analytical functionalism. The loss can apply to oneself or others.

Power enhanced by compensating has developed from creativity, religiosity, social integration, and well-being to drive resilience (Dacey and Lennon 1998; Forsyth 2003; Frazier et al. 2007, Roberto and Husser 2007). Creativity has fostered well being, including meaningfulness, to enhance resilience (Diener et al. 2009; Turner 2013). Notably, compensating has raised resilience directly (Roberto and Husser 2007). Compensating has also involved activeness, attachment and relating, education, and intimacy to muster power to drive resilience (Busseri et al. 2006; Greenwood and Long 2011; Jaeger 2012; Waanders et al. 2007; Zimmermann and Bingenheimer 2002). Intimacy has sustained purposiveness, relationship satisfaction, and self-efficacy and dampened anxiety to facilitate resilience (Arseth et al. 2009; Chou 2000; Hand et al. 2013; Henderson et al. 2009). Moreover, compensating has also reflected cognitive reserve and control to maintain power to drive resilience (Frankenmolen et al. 2018; Heckhausen 2002). Cognitive reserve has eroded depression to maintain resilience (Feinstein and Bynner 2006). Conversely, compensating lowers stress to restore power to drive resilience (Flook and Fuligni 2008). Furthermore, compensating has reduced depression (Steverink and Lindenberg 2006).

Utility engendered by compensating for the loss involves achievement to attract resilience (Crosnoe et al. 2002). Achievement has boosted development, health, life quality, satisfaction, self-efficacy, and self-esteem to raise resilience (Cook et al. 2002; Donnellan et al. 2005; Murray 2009; Tompson and Dass 2000; Xiao et al. 2009). Conversely, achievement has diminished alienation, depression, distress, and internalizing problems, thus safeguarding resilience (Fredricks and Eccles 2005; Masten et al. 2005; Menard and Mose 1984; Piko et al. 2006).

Cooperating involves conciliation and investing (Ohbuchi et al. 1999; Sanderson 2001). Eventually, cooperating is rewarding (Brewer 1996). Conversely, cooperating opposes abusing, conflicting, differentiating, offending, dominating, excluding, exploiting, fighting, and revolting (Brewer 1996; Sanderson 2001). Cooperating is likely to foster resilience by generating power, utility, ideals, and norms to activate power realization, utility optimization, ideals calibration, and norm conformity for achieving requisite functions stipulated in analytical functionalism.

Power produced by cooperating has engaged attachment and trustworthiness to drive resilience (Gerbasi and Cook 2008; Tak 2017). Moreover, cooperating reflects agreement, education, and social embeddedness to afford power to drive resilience (Nahapiet 2009; Sanderson 2001). Cooperating has also established power from community involvement, identity achievement, social integration, and trust to drive resilience (Bonaiuto et al. 2008; Groves et al. 2000; Lepkowski and Couper 2002; Zhang and Zhou 2018). Community involvement has elevated well-being, including mastery and self-efficacy to enable resilience (Harter and Arora 2010; Ohmer 2007; Peterson and Huphey 2004). Identity achievement has eroded anxiety and depression, thus sustaining resilience (Cast 2004). Furthermore, cooperating has risen with complementarity or orientation to matching with others, knowledge, perspective-taking, prosociality, social capital, social orientation, and social support received to offer power to drive resilience (Haesevoets et al. 2015; Hample 2018; Lepkowski and Couper 2002; Miao et al. 2018; Shewark et al. 2022). Complementarity has lifted well-being to foster resilience (Chuang 2005). Perspective-taking has enhanced communication quality and intimacy to facilitate resilience (Redmond 2018). Social orientation has championed relationship quality to boost resilience (Jorgensen and Nelson 2018). Conversely, cooperating has prevented arguing or quarreling as counteractive power to distract resilience (Hample 2018). Cooperating also reflects low alienation, conflict, deprivation, and domination to maintain power to drive resilience (Sanderson 2001). Arguing has fomented dissatisfaction and distress to impede resilience (Lau et al. 2017; Mikula et al. 2012). Furthermore, cooperating has reflected low antisociality, psychoticism, and stress, which have debilitated power for or generated power against resilience (Hample 2018; Hoang et al. 2020). Psychoticism means disorders as opposed to agreeableness, conscientiousness, and openness to impede resilience (Village and Francis 2010).

Utility reflecting cooperating emphasizes achievement, ease, fitness, friendliness, gain, incentive, justice, likability, payoff, popularity, recognition received, satisfaction, similarity, and trustworthiness concerning work or others to attract resilience (Bereczkei et al. 2010; Brewer 1996; de Bruyn and van den Boom 2005; Onwuegbuzie et al. 2001; Heckathorn 2001; Mark 2018; Sanderson 2001a; Van Lange et al.

2014; Yamagishi et al. 2005; Zhang and Zhou 2018). Ease experienced has activated studying to develop resilience (van de Ven et al. 2011). Justice has included distributive and procedural justice (Zhang and Zhou 2018). Experience of justice has raised belongingness, health, life satisfaction, and self-esteem and diminished anger and depression to buttress resilience (Benson and Ritter 1990; Bjornskov et al. 2013; Dalbert 2001; Lucas et al. 2013; Rothmund et al. 2014; van Prooijen et al. 2008). Popularity experienced has elevated belongingness, positive affect, and self-esteem and reduced negative affect to enhance resilience (Reich et al. 2018). Similarity experienced has reduced depression, thus sustaining resilience (Riad and Norris 1992). Cooperating has also reflected complementarity or fit experienced as utility to attract resilience (Brewer 1996). Such experience has been salutary and reduced anxiety to enhance resilience (Namini et al. 2010).

Cooperating has reflected ideals for altruism to sustain resilience (Van Lange et al. 2014). Altruism has raised well-being, including connectedness, hope, life satisfaction, meaningfulness, and self-efficacy, as opposed to loneliness and negative emotion to sustain resilience (Caprara and Steca 2005; Marsh and Dik 2021; Nelson-Coffey et al. 2023; Raposa et al. 2016; Yao and Enright 2019). Conversely, cooperating has reflected ideals or obsessions for aggressiveness, competition, inferiority, masochism, and nihilism to undermine resilience (Van Lange et al. 2014). Competition has eroded interest and enjoyment, thus resisting resilience (Frederick-Recascino and Schuster-Smith 2003).

Norms reflected by cooperating have popularized positive affect and mood to assimilate resilience (Barsade et al. 2000; Sy and Cote 2005). Such norms raise personal affect and mood positively through spillover (Turner 2007). Positive affect or mood fosters resilience (Fredrickson and Losada 2005).

Communicating includes advising, asking, complimenting, disclosing, encouraging, greeting, inspiring, persuasion, reflecting, sharing, and supporting (Chon and Park 2021; Bodie and MacGeorge 2015; Mirivel 2014; Rees 2023; Walton 2007). It builds on cooperation, deliberation, empathy, explicitness, interaction, interest, information seeking, listening, openness, regard, respect, and spontaneity (Baumeister et al. 2013; Dillard 2015; Gasiorek and Aune 2021; Mirivel 2014; Sanders 2009; Stoker 2020; Walton 2007). Communicating is meritorious for emancipation and negotiation for postmodernity (Baxter and Asbury 2015). It also fulfills equality and sensitivity and denounces domination and oppression (Wood 2015). Such fulfillment fosters power, utility, ideals, and norms to engender resilience through power realization, utility optimization, ideal calibration, and norm conformity to achieve the required functions stipulated in analytical functionalism.

Power shown by communication to drive resilience evolves from accommodation, affiliation, autonomy, collaboration or cooperation, credibility presented, empathy, equality and equity presented, flexibility, information sought, openness, self-awareness, self-management, and togetherness (Burgoon et al. 2010; Gasiorek and Aune 2021; Fuchs 2020; Klyukanov 2021; Kumkale et al. 2010; McLaren and Solomon 2015; Mirivel 2014; Pressgrove et al. 2020; Wood 2015; Zhao 2008). Accommodation includes adaptation, approval, comprehension, convergency, inclusion, liking, matching, relating, and similarity maintenance to foster resilience (Gasiorek and Aune 2021; Giles and Soliz 2015). Moreover, accommodation has reflected just world belief, perspective-taking, and trust to maintain resilience (Lipkus and Bissonette 1998). Affiliating has reduced stress, thus safeguarding resilience (Nelson-Coffey et al. 2023). Empathy and perspective-taking have facilitated communication quality and intimacy and prevented resentment to keep resilience (Redmond 2018). Equality presented has dwindled anxiety, thus buttressing resilience (Schwartz and Melech 2000). Flexibility has enabled commitment to guarantee resilience (Agronick and Duncan 1998). Information is the basis for meaningfulness to champion resilience (Allan et al. 2016). Self-awareness has raised meaningfulness, positive affect, and self-clarity to maintain resilience (Klussman et al. 2020). Self-management has boosted health and dampened depression, thus lifting resilience (Czajkowski et al. 1998; Hill-Briggs et al. 2005). Togetherness has eroded depression and negative affect, thus safeguarding resilience (McIntyre et al. 2023; Stanton et al. 2020). Consequently, communication is conducive to emancipation experienced to drive resilience (Baxter and Asbury 2015). Emancipation experienced has advanced well-being, including health, life satisfaction, and self-esteem, as opposed to depression and symptoms to warrant resilience (Gehring 2013; Glendinning et al. 2003; Haller and Hadler 2006). Communicating has also raised interest, knowledge, leadership, social capital, cohesion, solidarity, and trust, and well-being to furnish power to drive resilience (Austin and Pinkleton 1999; Gross 1995; Kahneman et al. 2010; Lee and Chan 2016; McClurg 2006; Narayan and Cassidy 2001; Rothstein and Uslaner 2005). Interest has fostered satisfaction and self-efficacy to facilitate resilience (Gilman 2001; Wen and Cui 2014). Knowledge has buttressed self-efficacy to enable resilience (Rostosky et al. 2008). Similarly, leadership has secured self-efficacy to afford resilience (Shah and Scheufele 2006). Social capital has boosted well-being, including flourishing, happiness, health, life satisfaction, and pride, as opposed to depression and distress to champion resilience (Chua et al. 2021; Congdon 2010; Yetim and Yetim 2014). Furthermore, communicating arises from adaptation, closeness, intimacy, and social integration to consolidate power to drive resilience (Burgoon et al. 2010; Keeting 2016; Littlejohn et al. 2017; Mirivel 2014). Communicating has also stemmed from attachment or its security to muster power to drive resilience (Alonso-Arbiol et al. 2007). Conversely, communicating has dampened depression, thus retaining power to drive resilience (Simon and Lively 2010).

Utility exhibited by communicating to attract resilience involves distinctiveness (Littlejohn et al. 2017). Distinctiveness experienced indicates identity achievement (Scott 2015). Identity achieved has advanced happiness, self-efficacy, and self-esteem and has erased anxiety, thus safeguarding resilience (Cast 2004). Moreover, communication has boosted positive affect and evaluation received, relationship quality, and self-enhancement as utility to induce resilience (Burgoon et al. 2010; Mirivel 2014; Tsfati et al. 2009). Positive affect and evaluation received have induced belongingness, positive affect, and self-esteem to secure resilience (Reich et al. 2018). Self-enhancement has reflected attachment and social support received to raise resilience (Hermanto et al. 2017; Ledoux et al. 2010).

Ideals involved in communicating to rationalize resilience highlight acceptance, agreement and consensus, compromise, forgiveness, harmony, resolution, and tolerance (Burgoon et al. 2010; Kelley et al. 2019; Klyukanov 2021; Kumkale et al. 2010; Littlejohn et al. 2017). Compromise has arisen from openness to buttress resilience (Rosler et al. 2018). Resolution has benefitted from harmonious passion to sustain resilience (Belanger et al. 2019). Furthermore, communicating has enabled ideals concerning assimilation, meaningfulness, and satisfaction to rationalize resilience (Baumeister et al. 2013; Knies 2012; Littlejohn et al. 2017). Assimilation has fostered self-esteem to enhance resilience (Greenman and Xie 2008).

Norms sustaining communicating have emphasized adaptation and learning to assimilate resilience (Wang and Sun 2008). Such norms determine personal adaptation and learning to uphold resilience (Jurik et al. 2014; Littlejohn et al. 2017). Learning has escalated well-being, including life satisfaction and self-efficacy, to advance resilience (Denver and Hands 1990; Minnaert and Janssen 1992; Richards 2016).

Educating functions to control and enhance efficacy and knowledge to enhance management and rationality (O'Neill 2012). Inherently, educating involves adjusting, analyzing, applying, assessing and evaluating, challenging, clarifying, collaborating, discerning, disciplining, discovering, empathizing, empowering, expecting, explaining, exploring and prospecting, feeding back and responding, guiding, helping, listening, mediating, modeling, monitoring, motivating, presenting, questioning, reflecting, reinforcing, researching, reviewing, sharing, summarizing, transmitting, and understanding (Bachkirova and Cox 2007; Booth 2003; Camerino et al. 2019; Estes and Mintz 2016; Feldman et al. 2015; Ingleby and Tummons 2012; Karpov 2014). By contrast, educating eschews violence (Sinha 2013). Educating thus is likely to sustain resilience through enhancing power, utility, ideals, and norms to build on power realization, utility optimization, ideal calibration, and norm conformity in analytical functionalism.

Power created by educating to drive resilience evolves from empathy, friendliness, influence, and motivation (Estes and Mintz 2016; Karpov 2014; Saldana et al. 2021; Sinha 2013). Empathy has raised communication quality and intimacy and diminished discontent to achieve resilience (Redmond 2018). Friendliness has elevated life satisfaction to attract resilience (Selim 2008). Influence and motivation are, respectively, the manifestation and base of power to drive resilience. Furthermore, educating has consolidated collaboration, innovation, responsibility, and self-efficacy to muster power to drive resilience (Buric and Mornar 2023; Decuyper et al. 2023; Feldman et al. 2015; Lanermann and Konig 2016; Peciuliauskiene et al. 2023; Sinha 2013). Collaboration has lifted life satisfaction to enhance resilience (Park et al. 2015). Innovation has boosted meaningfulness to sustain resilience (Turner 2013). Educating has also reflected training to sustain power to drive resilience (Camerino et al. 2019). Training has upgraded adjustment, comfort, coherence, cohesiveness, competence, emotional well-being, growth, hope, identity, purposiveness, self-efficacy, self-esteem, thriving, and transcendence to advance resilience (Ashby et al. 2018; Davidson et al. 2012; Duan and Bu 2019; Esbensen and Osgood 1999; Feldman and Dreher 2012; Moote et al. 1999; Ou et al. 2019; Umino and Dammeyer

2018; Youniss and Yates 1997). Meanwhile, training has diminished anger, anxiety, burnout, depression, hostility, loneliness, paranoia, and symptoms to secure resilience (Breso et al. 2011; Duan and Bu 2019; Moote et al. 1999; Strepparava et al. 2016). Conversely, educating has diminished confusion experienced, distress, and stress to retain power to drive resilience (Mevarech and Maskit 2015; Mordeno et al. 2023). Confusion experienced has fomented tension and reduced confidence, intimacy, and satisfaction to disrupt resilience (Theiss 2018).

Utility raised by educating to attract resilience has resided in security experienced (Gursimsek and Goregenli 2005; Mevarech and Maskit 2015). Security experienced has enhanced well-being, including health, neighborhood quality, and satisfaction with the country, life, and neighborhood as opposed to fear to warrant resilience (Chiricos et al. 2000; Cummins et al. 2003; Frey et al. 2007; Olson et al. 2016; Parkes et al. 2002; Ziersch et al. 2005).

Ideals emphasized in educating to rationalize resilience concern acceptance, adjustment, collaboration, intimacy, mediation, openness, self-regulation, sharing, and togetherness (Bachkirova and Cox 2007; Camerino et al. 2019; Estes and Mintz 2016; Karpov 2014; Sinha 2013). Mediation has manifested control, emotional stability, and solidarity to secure resilience (Kalish 2008; Ng et al. 2004). Sharing has boosted well-being, including connectedness, hope, life satisfaction, meaningfulness, and self-efficacy, as opposed to negative emotion and loneliness to elevate resilience (Marsh and Dik 2021; Nelson-Coffey et al. 2023; Raposa et al. 2016; Yao and Enright 2019). Togetherness has dismissed depression and negative affect to secure resilience (McIntyre et al. 2023; Stanton et al. 2020). Moreover, educating has fostered conformity and justification as ideals to rationalize resilience (Gursimsek and Goregenli 2005). Conformity sustains well-being, including adaptation and pleasantness as opposed to anxiety to maintain resilience (de Courville Nicol 2011; Littlejohn et al. 2017; Stavrova 2014; Turner 2006). Justification has fostered positive affect to furnish resilience (Jost and Hunyady 2005).

Empathizing realizes humanity in sharing ideas about target people in social interaction (Ferguson et al. 2020; Ishii and Watanabe 2023; Trauernicht et al. 2021). Essentially, empathizing hinges on attention, communication, compassion, mirroring, perspective-taking, and reconstruction regarding target people's ideas (Eagly et al. 2004; Ferguson et al. 2020; Halevy et al. 2019; Manassis 2017). Empathizing also involves the experiences of communion and contagion (Ferguson et al. 2020; Nagurney 2007). Conversely, empathizing dismisses egocentrism, denigrating others, and self-preoccupation (Manassis 2017; Redmond 2018). Empathizing is thus likely to underpin resilience by raising power, utility, ideals, and norms regarding their realization, optimization, calibration, and conformity based on analytical functionalism.

Power generated by empathizing to drive resilience has arisen from commitment, cooperation, religiosity, spirituality, and trust (Ishii and Watanabe 2023; Manassis 2017; Momonoki and Ishii 2023; Stern and Cassidy 2018). Commitment has facilitated self-acceptance to secure resilience (Agronick and Duncan 1998). Furthermore, empathizing reflects attachment, care received, closeness, group identification, and sharing experienced to lift power to drive resilience (Ferguson et al. 2020; Hofelich and Preston 2014; Manassis 2017; Ziv 2019). Care received has fostered functionality and satisfaction to sustain resilience (Caro and Blank 1988; Davies et al. 1990). Group identification has enhanced control to enable resilience (Fischer et al. 2007). Sharing received has raised well-being, including control, emotional well-being, health, pleasure, purposefulness, relational quality, satisfaction, self-determination, self-efficacy, self-esteem, and social well-being to facilitate resilience (George and Park 2013; Glendinning et al. 2003; Gorman et al. 2010; Granzin and Haggard 2000; Holliman et al. 2021; Lincoln et al. 2003; Logan and Cobb 2013; Pierce and Quiroz 2018; Schwarzer and Knoll 2007; Vilhjalmsson and Thorlindsson 1998; Williams and Galliher 2006; Xi and Hwang 2011). Empathizing has stemmed from agreeableness, attachment or security, education, morality, positive affect, prosociality, religiosity, and self-regulation capacity to secure power to drive resilience (Hudson and Brandenberger 2022; Juhl et al. 2020a; Keyes 2002; Mestre et al. 2018; Stern and Cassidy 2018; Troyer and Greitemeyer 2018; Ziv 2019). Morality has sustained satisfaction and eroded anxiety to boost resilience (Conzo et al. 2017; Stets et al. 2008). Conversely, empathizing weakens narcissism to restore power to drive resilience (Manassis 2017). Narcissism has bred aggression, depression, dissatisfaction, and misbehavior to impair resilience (Tracy et al. 2009). Empathizing has also diminished avoidance, disorders, and substance abuse or doping, thus maintaining power to drive resilience (Allen-Collinson 2011; Manassis 2017). Avoidance has weakened well-being, including intimacy, mindfulness, and satisfaction, to foster resilience (Alonso-Arbiol et al. 2007; Barber et al. 2010; Linares et al. 2016). Conversely, avoidance has bred anxiety, depression, and loneliness to disrupt resilience (Cheng and Cheung 2005; Kafetsio and Sideridis 2006; Linares et al. 2016). Doping has engendered depression, thus jeopardizing resilience (Kendler et al. 2006). Additionally, empathizing has reflected low burnout and negative affectivity to retain power to drive resilience (Trauernicht et al. 2021; Troyer and Greitemeyer 2018). Burnout has eroded satisfaction, thus undermining resilience (Boamah et al. 2022).

Utility based on empathizing to attract resilience has reflected incentive and justice experienced and satisfaction (Ferguson et al. 2020; Hudson and Brandenberger 2022). Justice experienced has enhanced belongingness, health, life satisfaction, and self esteem and dampened anger and depression to lift resilience (Benson and Ritter 1990; Dalbert 2001; Liao et al. 2005; Lucas et al. 2013; Rothmund et al. 2014; van Prooijen et al. 2008). Conversely, empathizing has reduced threats experienced as disutility to discourage resilience (Momonoki and Ishii 2023). Threats experienced have raised anxiety or fear and depression and reduced relationship quality to impede resilience (Jackson et al. 2006; Moore and Shepherd 2006; O'Neill and Evans 1999).

Ideals raised by empathizing engage civility, communication quality, intimacy, and justification to rationalize resilience (Fett et al. 2014; Keyes 2002; Redmond 2018; Manassis 2017; Vieira 2015). Civility has boosted well-being, including physical and mental health, to activate resilience (Tsai et al. 2018). Moreover, empathizing has enhanced confidence as an ideal to rationalize resilience (Cooper 2011). Communication quality has raised control and satisfaction and reduced uncertainty to facilitate resilience (Bordia et al. 2004). Empathizing has rested on acceptance and dominance as ideals to rationalize resilience (Eagly et al. 2004; Stern and Cassidy

2018). Dominance has fostered well-being, including health and life satisfaction as opposed to anger and depression, to elevate resilience (Cundiff et al. 2015; Etezadi and Pushkar 2013; Orlowski and Wicker 2015; Rose 2000; Xi and Hwang 2011). Conversely, empathizing has reflected avoidance of fighting or violence, hostility, and self-preoccupation as ideals contradicting resilience (Manassis 2017; Stern and Cassidy 2018). Hostility has bred anger, anxiety, irrationality, and sadness to impede resilience (Vandervoort 2006). Self-preoccupation has engendered anxiety to undermine resilience (Da Costa Bizarro Morais et al. 2019).

Norms based on empathizing to assimilate resilience have popularized empathy (Miklikowska et al. 2022). The norm for empathy has assimilated empathy (Miklikowska et al. 2022).

Equalizing, leveling, or condescending respects people's cohesion, equality, exchange, fairness or justice, plurality, and rights (Kekes 2003; Ramsay 1997; Sabbagh 2002; Thye et al. 2008; Wolff 2011). Essentially, equalizing manifests compassion, cooperation, and sharing (Hirose 2015; Moss 2014). Conversely, equalizing dismisses discrimination, gap, hierarchy, and status (Castillo 2011; Ridgeway 2001; Sidanius et al. 2001; Wolff 2011). Crucially, equalizing tends to be a norm or normative (Bauer et al. 2014). Equalizing is likely to advance resilience by raising power, utility, ideals, and norms to apply the voluntaristic mechanisms of power realization, utility optimization, ideal calibration, and norm conformity, respectively for functional achievement couched in analytical functionalism.

Power indicated by equalizing to drive resilience stems from cooperation, empathy, and social association (Lucas and Kteily 2018; Moss 2014; Scruton 2014). Social association has facilitated resilience, self-confidence, and self-esteem (Liu and Ngai 2019; Pascarella and Terenzini 2005). Equalizing benefits from education and social class to provide power to drive resilience (Lewin et al. 2003; Yucel 2015). Social class has sustained well-being, including financial adequacy, health, hope, and satisfaction, as opposed to depression to advance resilience (Burke 2008; Davis and Davenport 1999; Haller and Hadler 2006; Hadjar and Samuel 2015; Peterson and Seligman 2004; Yamaoka 2008). Moreover, equalizing has stemmed from openness, religiosity, and socioeconomic status, including income and occupational prestige, to furnish power to drive resilience (Jost et al. 2003; Saunders and Wong 2012; Nagayoshi and Sato 2014; Papadakis 1993; Thorisdottir et al. 2007; Zumbrunnen and Gangl 2008). Socioeconomic status has safeguarded health, interaction quality, life satisfaction, self-confidence, self-esteem, and subjective well-being to maintain resilience (Al-krenawi et al. 2011; Caplan and Schooler 2007; Molana and Adams 2019; Staudinger et al. 1999). Conversely, equalizing has diminished anxiety and social pressure experienced, thus maintaining power to drive resilience (Schuster et al. 2023; Schwartz and Melech 2000). Social pressure has heightened burnout, depression, powerlessness, and somatic complaints and eroded health and self-esteem, thus impairing resilience (Furnham 1997; Gerber et al. 2010; Wan et al. 2023).

Equalizing has diminished harm perceived to sustain utility attracting resilience (Lucas and Kteily 2018). Harm perceived has bred anger, fear, and sadness to disrupt resilience (Landmann and Rohmann 2020).

Ideals reflected by equalizing have involved contentment and self-direction value to rationalize resilience (Schwartz et al. 2014; Steinhardt et al. 2018). Self-direction has fostered well-being, including energy, health, mastery, meaningfulness, positive affect, pride, satisfaction, self-efficacy, and work quality as opposed to burnout to enhance resilience (Anderson-Connolly 2002; Au and Cheung 2004; De Moortel et al. 2015; Erickson 2008; Gahlawat et al. 2019; Garcia et al. 2017; Hodson 1996; Martela and Riekki 2018; Peeters and Rutte 2005; Schieman 2002; Schieman and Narisada 2014; Yoon 2001). Conversely, equalizing has reduced radicalism as an ideal or obsession, thus safeguarding resilience (Lauriola et al. 2015). Radicalism has stemmed from anomie, alienation, anxiety, meaning loss, and uncertainty or self-uncertainty to erode resilience (Hogg et al. 2010; Koehler and Fiebig 2019; Plutzer 1987; Stankov et al. 2018).

Following as a manifestation of humility realizes self-effacing rather than self-enhancement (Chen et al. 2009). Essentially, following demonstrates acceptance, impartiality, openness, respect, self-reflection, and tolerance as opposed to greed (Bowes and Tasimi 2022; Bowes et al. 2022; O'Connor et al. 2022; Smith 2024). In the youth, following furthermore exhibits altruism, fairness, self-regulation, and other virtues (Guo et al. 2023; Wiltshire et al. 2014; Yu et al. 2021). Following by the youth also upholds appreciation, emotion regulation, and other-orientation (Paine et al. 2016). Hence, following is likely to foster resilience by providing power, utility, ideals, and norms to activate power realization, utility optimization, ideal calibration, and norm conformation to achieve the requisite functioning specified in analytical functionalism.

Power enhanced by following to drive resilience stems from awareness and self-awareness, flexibility, learning, prosociality, self-reflection, self-regulation and emotion regulation, and teachability (Bowes and Tasimi 2022; Kondili et al. 2022; Lehmann et al. 2023; Paine et al. 2016; Peng 2022; Wiltshire et al. 2014). Awareness has championed intimacy, savings, and self-efficacy to enable resilience (Mikulincer et al. 2003; Rothwell et al. 2016). Self-awareness or self-reflection has fostered positive affect, meaningfulness, and self-clarity as opposed to negative affect to induce resilience (Adler and Fegley 2005; Klussman et al. 2020). Flexibility has raised life satisfaction and self-esteem and diminished distress to buttress resilience (Jen et al. 2019). Learning has boosted well-being, including life satisfaction and self-efficacy, to sustain resilience (Armstrong et al. 2011; Denver and Hands 1990; Minnaert and Janssen 1992; Richards 2016). Self-regulation has escalated self-esteem and dampened anxiety and depression to maintain resilience (Marchetti et al. 2018). Furthermore, following has fostered connectedness, empathy, innovation, knowledge, morality, perspective-taking, religiosity, responsibility, self-differentiation, and well-being to muster power to drive resilience (Angelis and Pensini 2024; Bowes and Tasimi 2022; Choe et al. 2023; Guo et al. 2023; Krumrei-Mancuso 2017; Paine et al. 2016; Peng 2022; Van Tongeren et al. 2023). Connectedness has afforded well-being, including flourishing, happiness, health, life satisfaction, and pride, as opposed to depression and distress, to champion resilience (Chua et al. 2021; Congdon 2010;

Yetim and Yetim 2014). Innovation has boosted well-being, including meaningfulness, to elevate resilience (Diener et al. 2009; Turner 2013). Empathy or perspective-taking has sustained intimacy and communication quality to safeguard resilience (Redmond 2018). Morality has raised life satisfaction to rationalize resilience (Conzo et al. 2017). Self-differentiation has raised intercultural competence to facilitate resilience (Paine et al. 2016). Moreover, self-differentiation represents autonomy, openness, prosociality, self-construction, and self-regulation to enable resilience (Wiltshire et al. 2014). Following has arisen from agreeableness, conscientiousness, extraversion, self-development, self-differentiation, and training to furnish power to drive resilience (Bowes et al. 2022; Kondili et al. 2022; MacDonell and Willoughby 2020; Sandage et al. 2017). Self-development comprises idealization, stability, and transparency about the self (Sandage et al. 2017). Essentially, self-development has reflected self-esteem to maintain resilience (DeMarree and Rios 2014). Training has facilitated adjustment, coherence, cohesiveness, comfort, competence, emotional well-being, growth, hope, purposefulness, self-efficacy, self-esteem thriving, and transcendence to boost resilience (Ashby et al. 2018; Davidson et al. 2012; Duan and Bu 2019; Esbensen and Osgood 1999; Feldman and Dreher 2012; Ou et al. 2019; Umino and Dammeyer 2018; Yates and Youniss 1996b; Youniss and Yates 1997). Meanwhile, training has prevented anger, anxiety, burnout, depression, hostility, loneliness, paranoia, and symptoms, thus safeguarding resilience (Breso et al. 2011; Duan and Bu 2019; Moote et al. 1999; Strepparava et al. 2016). Conversely, following has reduced aggression, anxiety, disorders, and negative affect, thus maintaining power to drive resilience (Lee and Ashton 2012; Levidi et al. 2024; Muris et al. 2022). Disorders have eroded well-being to impede resilience (Jans-Beken 2019). Following has also reflected low aggression and impulsivity to retain power to drive resilience (MacDonell and Willoughby 2020). Impulsivity has fomented anxiety and depression and diminished self-esteem to impair resilience (Armstrong et al. 2011; Marchetti et al. 2018).

Ideals maintained by following to rationalize resilience rest on acceptance, agreement, appreciation, collaboration, openness, regard, respect, supportiveness, tolerance, and transcendence (Bowes and Tasimi 2022; Kondili et al. 2022; Lubis and Sianipar 2022; Paine et al. 2016; Peng 2022; Smith 2024). Supportiveness has boosted well-being, including connectedness, hope, meaningfulness, life satisfaction, and self-efficacy to enable resilience (Marsh and Dik 2021; Nelson-Coffey et al. 2023; Raposa et al. 2016; Yao and Enright 2019). Conversely, supportiveness has reduced negative emotion and loneliness, thus safeguarding resilience (Nelson-Coffey et al. 2023). Transcendence has raised life satisfaction and meaningfulness and has dampened anxiety, depression, and stress to sustain resilience (Fishbein et al. 2020). Following has also elevated altruism, benevolence value, cooperation, egalitarianism, evaluation for others, favor for protection, generosity, kindness motive, prevention, tolerance, trust, and universalism to sustain ideals for rationalizing resilience (Exline and Hill 2012; Hilbig et al. 2013; Krumrei-Mancuso 2017; Krumrei-Mancuso and Newman 2021; Preston and Khan 2024; Ryu et al. 2023). Moreover, following has reflected self-forgiveness to sustain ideals for rationalizing resilience (Wiltshire et al. 2014). Forgiveness has been salutary, thus championing resilience (Shimai et al.

2006). Conversely, following denounces egocentrism and greed to uphold ideals to rationalize resilience (Lubis and Sianipar 2022; O'Connor et al. 2022; Plohl and Musil 2023). Egocentrism has bred anxiety to disturb resilience (Da Costa Bizarro Morais et al. 2019). Furthermore, following has impeded conspiracy, paranormal, and pseudo-scientific beliefs, criminal preference, delinquency, disliking for the outgroup or xenophobia, disruption, polarization or extremism, prejudice, stigmatizing, and valuation for money, power, and sex to retain ideals to rationalize resilience (Bowes and Tasimi 2022; Lee et al. 2013; Levidi et al. 2024; Oh et al. 2011; Rullo et al. 2022; Schmitt and Huynh 2024; Sgambati and Ayduk 2023; Wiltshire et al. 2014). Conspiracy belief has incurred anxiety to erode resilience (Leibovitz et al. 2021). Paranormal and pseudo-scientific beliefs have reflected self-diffidence to undermine resilience (Teovanovic et al. 2021). Crime or delinquency has eroded life satisfaction, mastery, relationship quality, self-efficacy, and self-esteem to weaken resilience (Chung and Elias 1996; Keijsers et al. 2011; Shek 2005). Conversely, crime or delinquency has raised distress and strain to hinder resilience (Hay 2003; Shek 2005). Xenophobia has weakened life quality to disrupt resilience (Ishii 2009). Extremism has bred violence to impair resilience (Pauwels and De Waele 2014). Prejudice or stigmatizing has eroded self-esteem to jeopardize resilience (Crocker and Garcia 2010). Valuation for money or mammonism has reflected disagreement and failure to weaken resilience (Lee et al. 2013; Power and Khmelkov 1999). Similarly, valuation on power has reflected low agreeableness and humility to attenuate resilience (Lee et al. 2013). Valuation for sex has lessened attachment security to hamper resilience (Dunkel et al. 2016).

Harmonizing is virtuous, notably predicated on the Chinese philosophies of naturalism and scholarism (Ip 2014; Liu et al. 2018). Essentially, harmonizing features adjustment, attuning, balancing, fitting, interconnecting, ordering, stabilizing, and being coherent, flexible, interdependent, mindful, peaceful, safe, selflessness, and transcendent (Arat and Kerelian 2019; Kjell et al. 2016). Conversely, harmonizing eliminates conflict and self-centeredness (Arat and Kerelian 2019; Kjell et al. 2016). As such, harmonizing can apply power, utility, ideals, and norms to power realization, utility optimization, ideal calibration, and norm conformity to enrich resilience following analytical functionalism.

Power sustained by harmonizing to drive resilience rests on coherence, connectedness, fitness, friendship, mindfulness, productivity, vitality, and well being (Arat and Kerelian 2019; Kjell et al. 2016; Liu 2008; Zhang 2006). Coherence raises confidence to enhance resilience (Simon and Read 2018). Fitness has elevated health, morale, and satisfaction and impeded anxiety, depression, and strain to enable resilience (Li 2006; Pereyra-Rojas et al. 2017; Sutherland and Fogarty 1995; Xie 1996). Vitality reflects resiliency as the dispositional power to drive resilience (Garg and Sarkar 2020). Harmonizing also demonstrates cleanliness, cohesiveness, and education to lift power to drive resilience (Ip 2014; Liu 2008). Cleanliness has facilitated attachment to enable resilience (Long and Perkins 2007). Cohesiveness has enhanced adjustment, hope, and life satisfaction and diminished depression to facilitate resilience (Araya et al. 2006; Dittman and Goebel 2010; James and Hunsley 1995; Paez et al. 2015). Moreover, harmonizing has raised enthusiasm and responsibility to secure power to drive resilience (Braithwaite and Ahmed 2005; Toth-Kiraly et al. 2021). Enthusiasm is a basis for resilience and resolution (Bakshi and Joshi 2014). Responsibility has incubated self-efficacy to enable resilience (Braun-Lewensohn 2016). Harmonizing has also built on education, family relationship quality, and social class to generate power to drive resilience (Yi et al. 2004; Lewin et al. 2003). Family relationship quality has furnished social support received and diminished problems, thus sustaining resilience (Nelis et al. 2006; Rook and Ituarte 1999). Conversely, harmonizing prevents corruption or dysfunction, thus retaining power to drive resilience (Ip 2014). Corruption has hurt health, satisfaction, and self-efficcay and triggered distress to disrupt resilience (Distante 2013; Gastil 2000; Michalos et al. 2000; Phongsavan et al. 2006). Harmonizing has also reduced depression, thus maintaining the power to drive resilience (Liu et al. 2023).

Utility created by harmonizing to attract resilience arises from justice, order, peacefulness, and safety experienced (Kjell et al. 2016; Zhang 2006). Justice experienced has raised belongingness, health, life satisfaction, and self-esteem and diminished anger and depression to maintain resilience (Benson and Ritter 1990; Bjornskov et al. 2013; Dalbert 2001; Lucas et al. 2013; Rothmund et al. 2014; van Prooijen et al. 2008). Order experienced has dampened anxiety to facilitate resilience (Schwartz and Melech 2000). Peacefulness experienced has boosted well-being, including life satisfaction and positive affect as opposed to depression, to raise resilience (Andrade et al. 2019; Klussman et al. 2020; Linares et al. 2016). Safety experienced has escalated well-being, including health and life satisfaction as opposed to fear, to advance resilience (Chen et al. 2008; Frey et al. 2007; Jones et al. 2014). Conversely, harmonizing prevents conflict experienced, thus retaining utility to attract resilience (Arat and Kerelian 2019). Conflict has provoked distress and eroded satisfaction, thus impeding resilience (Lau et al. 2017; Mikula et al. 2012).

Ideals raised by harmonizing to rationalize resilience emphasize adjustment, attunement, balance, control, flexibility, stability, and transcendence (Kjell et al. 2016). Balance has fostered confidence to achieve resilience (Simon and Read 2018). Control has boosted well-being, including health and life satisfaction, as opposed to anger and depression, to maintain resilience (Etezadi and Pushkar 2013. Heidemeier and Staudinger 2012; Rose 2000; Xi and Hwang 2011). Flexibility has sustained life satisfaction and self-esteem and inhibited distress to foster resilience (Jen et al. 2019). The ideal for stability has buttressed stability (Zumbrunnen and Gangl 2008). Stability has raised resilience and relational quality (Lock et al. 2020; Ross et al. 2000). Transcendence has fostered life satisfaction and meaningfulness and dampened anxiety, depression, and stress to buttress resilience (Fishbein et al. 2020). Harmonizing also demonstrates ideals for benevolence, caring, compromise, dialogue, diversity, environmentalism, equality, fairness, familism, forgiving, inclusiveness, love, morality, pluralism, respect, restraint, sharing, socialism, sustainability, and sympathy to rationalize resilience (Chan et al. 2014; Ip 2014; Liu 2008; Zhang 2006). Benevolence has reduced anxiety and negative affect and sustained life satisfaction, positive affect, and resilience (Howard and Alipour 2014; Kim et al. 2018; Muris et al. 2010). Caring or its valuation reflects well-being to advance resilience (Peterson and Klohnen 1995). Compromising builds on happiness as opposed to anger to sustain resilience (Thompson et al. 2004). Dialogue has fostered well-being, including meaningfulness and life satisfaction as opposed to depression, to lift resilience (Baumeister et al. 2013; Kahneman et al. 2010; Knies 2012; Simon and Lively 2010). Diversity as an ideal has arisen from low distress to maintain resilience (Persell 1997). Environmentalism has boosted environmental quality to foster resilience (Loukopoulos et al. 2005). Equality valuation or egalitarianism has diminished anxiety to sustain resilience (Schwartz and Melech 2000). Fairness as an ideal incubates flourishing to enable resilience (Williams 2008). Familism has built on health and financial satisfaction to maintain resilience (Kiecolt 2003; Valarino et al. 2018). Forgiving as an ideal has been salutary to facilitate resilience (Shimai et al. 2006). Inclusiveness as an ideal has reflected the low threat experienced to champion resilience (Raijman et al. 2008). Loving has stood on relational quality to elevate resilience (Nosko et al. 2011). Morality has enhanced satisfaction and dampened anger to facilitate resilience (Conzo et al. 2017; Stets et al. 2008). Pluralism emphasizes tolerance to champion resilience (Galston 2005). Respect has fostered identity to afford resilience (Renger and Reese 2017). Restraint has enhanced self-esteem and dampened anxiety and depression to foster resilience (Armstrong et al. 2011; Marchetti et al. 2018). Sharing has raised relatedness to facilitated resilience (Torlo and Lomi 2017). Socialism as an ideal means morality and responsibility to champion resilience (Collier 2001; Scruton 2014). Sustainability as an ideal has built on well-being, including control, connectedness, health, identity, pride, satisfaction, and self-efficacy, to boost resilience (Adeola 2000; Heath and Gifford 2006; Heinen 2016; Nicolai et al. 2022; Siu and Xiao 2015; Taneja and Ali 2021). Sympathy incorporates tolerance to achieve resilience (Peplak and Malti 2022). Remarkably, harmonizing has boosted accommodating and dedication as ideals to rationalize resilience (Lim 2009; Gan and Cheung 2010). Dedication has enhanced self-efficacy and self-esteem to enable resilience (Bakker et al. 2008). Harmonizing also reflects the ideals of Confucianism or scholarism and Daoism or naturalism to rationalize resilience (Liu et al. 2018). Confucianism or scholarism has raised life satisfaction and vitality to enhance resilience (Lin et al. 2021). Daoism upholds receptivity and tolerance to achieve resilience (Brooks 2020, Fang 2003). Conversely, harmonizing resists competition and discrimination as ideals against resilience (Ip 2014; Zhang 2006). Competition rests on anxiety and stress, thus disrupting resilience (Pierce and White 2006). Discriminating reflects identity inadequacy and threats received to undermine resilience (Tusicisny 2017).

Harmonizing has arisen from the norm of harmonizing to assimilate resilience (Lu and Kao 2002; Yi et al. 2004). Moreover, the norm of harmonizing has built on norms for cohesion and tolerance as opposed to conflict (Ho and Chan 2009; Wong and Shik 2011). Negotiation is a way of conflict resolution through communication (Kapoutsis et al. 2017). Essentially, negotiation proceeds with accommodation, agreement, assimilation, attack, bargaining, bluffing, concession, cooperation, flexibility, logrolling, manipulation, persuasion, promise, questioning, prediction or uncertainty reduction, summarizing, and threatening (Carrell and Heavrin 2008; Elfenbein 2013; Lewicki and Polin 2023; Rudd and Hughes 2020). Negotiation is an exemplar of softening in wielding soft power, including charisma, compensation, cooperation, empathy, friendship, gentleness, humanness, humility, openness, patience, rapport, reward, self-discipline, support, trust, warmth, and win–win benefit (Greene 1991). Conversely, negotiation withholds hard power, including authority, bribing, certainty, control, rigidity, and struggle (Greene 1991). Negotiation is likely to elevate resilience by providing power, utility, ideals, and norms to activate the voluntaristic mechanisms of analytical functionalism.

Power maintained by negotiation to drive resilience stems from charisma, empathy, expertise, gentleness, humility, humor, openness, patience, rationality, self-discipline, and warmth (Carrell and Heavrin 2008; Greene 1991; Koning and van Dijk 2013; Rudd and Hughes 2020). Humility has fostered connectedness and gratitude to facilitate resilience (Angelis and Pensini 2024; Krumrei-Mancuso 2017). Humor has sustained mental health, pleasure, and satisfaction and has diminished fear to maintain resilience (Dynel and Poppi 2018; Martin 2007; Svebak et al. 2004). Openness has raised well-being, including autonomy, growth, life satisfaction, purposefulness, relationship quality, self-acceptance, self-efficacy, and self-esteem, as opposed to hostility to boost resilience (Hahn et al. 2013; Hounkpatin et al. 2015; Karwowski and Lebuda 2017; Marks 1996; Quilty et al. 2006; Webster et al. 2014). Patience has reduced negative affect to enable resilience (Mehmood et al. 2020). Rationality has dampened anxiety, depression, and fear to retain resilience (Barnes and Vulcano 1982; DiGiuseppe et al. 2017). Self-discipline has arisen from self-esteem to facilitate resilience (Kokkinos and Hatzinikolaou 2011). Warmth involves tolerance to rationalize resilience (Peplak and Malti 2022). Essentially, negotiation has sustained enjoyment and social trust to generate power to drive resilience (Kono and Ito 2021; Barrera 2007). Social trust has fostered health and survival to sustain resilience (Barefoot et al. 1998). Negotiation has also arisen from social support received to drive resilience (Garcia-Ruiz et al. 2013). Social support received has raised resilience and general well-being, including control, emotional well-being, health, pleasure, purposiveness, relational quality, satisfaction, self-determination, self-efficacy, self-esteem, and social well-being, as opposed to anger, anxiety, depression, distress, and symptoms (Besser and Priel 2008; Cherry et al. 2018; George and Park 2013; Glendinning et al. 2003; Gorman et al. 2010; Holliman et al. 2021; Kafetsio and Sideridis 2006; Lee and Robbins 1998; Lincoln et al. 2003; Logan and Cobb 2013; Lowe et al. 2009; Pierce and Quiroz 2018; Schwarzer and Knoll 2007; Vilhjalmsson and Thorlindsson 1998; Williams and Galliher 2006; Xi and Hwang 2011). Conversely, negotiation has stemmed from low sadness to drive resilience (Kapoutsis et al. 2017).

Utility sustained by negotiation to attract resilience resides in benefit or gain and optimism (Carrell and Heavrin 2008; Elfenbein 2013). Benefit has boosted well-being, including satisfaction, as opposed to anger, anxiety, and depression, to uplift resilience (Helgeson et al. 2006; Wells et al. 1999; Wong and Lam 2016). Optimism is a basis for resilience (Mak et al. 2019).

Ideals displayed by negotiation to rationalize resilience espouse accommodation, agreement, adaptation, attunement, collaboration, compromise, flexibility, harmonizing, justice, reciprocity, and suppressing negativity (Aslani et al. 2013; Carrell and

Heavrin 2008; Fang 1999; Kono and Ito 2021; McMains and Mullins 2010; Rudd and Hughes 2020). Adaptation and flexibility are resilient manifestations (Maltby et al. 2019). Accommodation or attunement has been conducive to intimacy as well-being to lift resilience under dependency (Shoss and Kueny 2022). Agreement has sustained well-being to enhance resilience (Cheung and Leung 2011). Collaboration has escalated life satisfaction to rationalize resilience (Park et al. 2015). Compromise rests on happiness as opposed to anger to facilitate resilience (Thompson et al. 2004). Harmony reflects relationship quality to buttress resilience (Yi et al. 2004). The ideal for justice realizes flourishing to enable resilience (Williams 2008). Reciprocity has facilitated adaptation as opposed to illness to create resilience (Yamaoka 2008; Yeh et al. 2013). Suppression has retained forgiveness and positive emotion as opposed to sadness to boost resilience (van Oyen Witvliet et al. 2011).

Norms upheld by negotiation to assimilate resilience favor fairness, honesty, and reciprocity (Carrell and Heavrin 2008). Fairness upholds flourishing to generate resilience (Williams 2008). Honesty has reflected happiness to sustain resilience (Medai and Noussair 2021). Reciprocity has enabled adaptation as opposed to illness to achieve resilience (Yamaoka 2008; Yeh et al. 2013).

Participation involves collaboration, connection, influence, meeting, sharing, and social integration (Heckscher 2015; Kerrissey and Schofer 2013; Yetim and Yetim 2014). To resilience, participation is likely to contribute power, utility, ideals, and norms to achieve the requisite functions of fulfillment, adaptation, latency, and integration posited in analytical functionalism.

Power generated by participation to drive resilience accrues from association, collaboration, connection, order, religiosity, responsibility, and social capital (Heckscher 2015; Saegert and Winkel 2004; Stolle and Micheletti 2013; Yetim and Yetim 2014). Order has reflected health to enhance resilience (Cheung and Lai 2020). Responsibility particularly concerns resolution and has provided energy to champion resilience (Garcia et al. 2017; Stolle and Micheletti 2013). Moreover, participation reflects sufficiency to enable resilience (Notter et al. 2008). Sufficiency has been salutary, including enhancing life satisfaction, positive affect, self-determination, and vitality (Chen et al. 2015; Cordeiro et al. 2015; Sheldon and Krieger 2007). Participation has also fostered well-being, including mastery and self-efficacy to gather power to drive resilience (Harter and Arora 2010; Ohmer 2007; Peterson and Hughey 2004). Furthermore, participation has secured power by raising collective effectiveness, cooperation, empowerment experienced, friendship, knowledge, and social capital, integration, networking, and trust to enable resilience (Bolland and McCallum 2002; Christens et al. 2011; Groves et al. 2000; Molitor et al. 2011; Ohmer 2007; Opp 1989; Rochelle 2015). Collective effectiveness has raised social well-being and reduced anomia to champion resilience (Sani et al. 2008). Likewise, participation has stemmed from education, employment, empowerment experienced, homeownership, income, knowledge, organizational membership, self-efficacy, and social capital to furnish power to drive resilience (Broadbent and Papadopoulos 2011; Dorff 2017; Ghimire 2021a; Gotzsche-Astrup 2020; Hooghe 2003; Huber et al. 2022; Hunter et al. 2013). Empowerment experienced has boosted well-being, including satisfaction and self-efficacy to advance resilience (Biron and Samberger 2010;

Kulik 2007). Organizational membership has reduced negative emotion and stress to sustain resilience (Nelson-Coffey et al. 2023). Participation has also benefitted from agreeableness, openness, resources, skill, and religiosity to provide power to drive resilience (Gotzsche-Astrup 2020; Huber et al. 2022; Stolle and Micheletti 2013; Verba et al. 2004). Conversely, participation retains the power to drive resilience by impeding competition experienced, distraction experienced, narcissism or self-indulgence, and threat experienced (Borbath et al. 2021; Heckscher 2015). Competition has invoked crime, depression, deviance, hostility, radicalism, and violence as opposed to tolerance to impede resilience (Busch 2009; Kaplan et al. 2013; Messner et al. 2013; Mintz et al. 2022; Passini and Morselli 2015; Terhune and Matusitz 2016; White et al. 2015). Distraction experienced has elevated anxiety, fatigue, and regret to block resilience (Cotterill 2017). Narcissism has fomented depression and loneliness and eroded relationship satisfaction to impair resilience (Sedikides et al. 2004; Tracy et al. 2009).

Utility from participation reflects destigmatization to attract resilience (Notter et al. 2008). Moreover, participation reflects utility based on benefit, easiness, friendship, justice, material incentive, reward, and solidarity experienced to attract resilience (Gross 1995; Lawrence and Daniels 1997; Mintz et al. 2022; Opp 1989; Pattie et al. 2004). Friendship has stemmed from health and satisfaction with health, leisure, and life as opposed to fear to buttress resilience (Child and Nikolova 2020; Eberl 2020; Sampson 1991). Justice experienced has championed belonginess, health, life satisfaction, and self-esteem and diminished anger and depression to foster resilience (Benson and Ritter 1990; Bjornskov et al. 2013; Dalbert 2001; Lucas et al. 2013; Rothmund et al. 2014; van Prooijen et al. 2008). Solidarity experienced has eroded depression, thus upholding resilience (Mullins and Dugan 1991). Conversely, participation has arisen from low cost to attract resilience (Seyd and Whiteley 1992).

Ideals fostered by participation to rationalize resilience hail independence, integrity or self-discipline, openness, stability, tolerance, and understanding (Heckscher 2015). Independence has sustained health and mastery to foster resilience (Lu and Kao 2002; Roy and Chaudhuri 2008). Integrity or self-discipline has maintained self-esteem and impeded anxiety and depression to champion resilience (Armstrong et al. 2011; Marchetti et al. 2018). Openness has enhanced well-being, including autonomy, growth, life satisfaction, purposefulness, relationship quality, self-acceptance, self-efficacy, and self-esteem, as oppoed to hostility to boost resilience (Hahn et al. 2013; Hounknatin et al. 2014; Karwowski and Lebuda 2017; Marks 1996; Quilty et al. 2006; Webster et al. 2014). Stability has enhanced resilience and relational quality and reduced anxiety (Lock et al. 2020; Ross et al. 2000). Understanding has raised intimacy, satisfaction, and self-efficacy to underpin resilience (Mikulincer et al. 2003; Norris 2011; Rothwell et al. 2016). Participation has boosted life satisfaction to secure ideals to rationalize resilience (Appleton and Song 2008). Likewise, participation has benefitted from satisfaction and value on health to rationalize resilience (Price et al. 2006; Xu 2007). Health value has arisen from health to facilitate resilience (Whynes and Sach 2007). Conversely, participation lessens alienation or anomie as an obsession that contradicts resilience (Heckscher

2015). Alienation or anomia has raised depression and inhibited self-esteem to impair resilience (Bjarnason 2009).

Norms underlying participation to assimilate resilience popularize agency, ease, efficacy, participation, power, stability, and trust as opposed to crime (Bolland and McCallum 2002; Broadbent and Papadopoulos 2011; Bruch et al. 2010; Gamson 1992; Kang and Kwak 2003; Saegert and Winkel 2004; Uslaner and Brown 2005). Agency assimilated has buttressed well-being, including autonomy, life satisfaction, mastery, relational quality, relatedness, and vitality, as opposed to anxiety and depression to strengthen resilience (Delhey 2010; Hui et al. 2013; Schieman and Plickert 2008; Schwartz and Melech 2000; Sheldon and Bettencourt 2002; Sieber et al. 2019; Weinstein and Ryan 2010). Reframing or perspective-changing involves moralizing and resolving to achieve a match in life (Feinberg and Willer 2019). Essentially, reframing represents coping, empathy, framing, health maintenance, mindfulness, and therapy (Carrell and Heavrin 2008; Feldman and Kuyken 2019; Ferreira et al. 2021; Gattino et al. 2015; Heyman and Slep 2007; Rudd and Hughes 2020). Reframing also benefits from Buddhism (Andrade et al. 2019; Feldman and Kuyken 2019). With these properties, reframing is likely to achieve resilience through furnishing power, utility, ideals, and norms to activate voluntaristic mechanisms to realize analytical functionalism.

Power generated by reframing to drive resilience stems from attentiveness, awareness, clarity, discernment, intentionality, mindfulness, and wisdom (Andrade et al. 2019; Feldman and Kuyken 2019). Attentiveness has stemmed from well-being, including positive affect, to facilitate resilience (Kitayama 1997). Awareness has fostered intimacy, satisfaction, and self-efficacy to enable resilience (Rothwell et al. 2016; Mikulincer et al. 2003; Norris 2011). Intentionality has secured life satisfaction and self-esteem to buttress resilience (Frazier et al. 2007; Stutzer 2004). Mindfulness has sustained well-being, including intimacy and life satisfaction as opposed to depression, to foster resilience (Karremans et al. 2017; Klussman et al. 2020; Linares et al. 2016). Wisdom has raised well-being, including autonomy, coherence, maturity, meaningfulness, purposefulness, life satisfaction, and self-efficacy to effectuate resilience (Diener et al. 2009; Greene and Brown 2009, Mickler and Staudinger 2008; Webster 2010). Moreover, reframing has secured adjustment, growth, and environmental and relationship quality to afford power to drive resilience (Samios and Baran 2018; SunWolf 2008). Reframing has also reflected self-compassion to maintain power to drive resilience (Munroe et al. 2022). Self-compassion has lifted equanimity, happiness, and positive affect and has dampened anger, anxiety, depression, distress, negative affect, and self-rumination to induce resilience (Barnard and Curry 2011; Sirois et al. 2015). Conversely, reframing dismisses ignorance, thus mustering power to drive resilience (Feldman and Kuyken 2019). Ignorance has bred risking to impair resilience (Van Tongeren et al. 2023).

Ideals enhanced by reframing to rationalize resilience prize befriending, caring, compassion or kindness, contentment, equanimity, generosity, gratitude, joy or gladness, honoring, liberation, patience, presentness, and understanding (Andrade et al. 2019; Feldman and Kuyken 2019). Befriending has sustained belongingness and self-esteem as opposed to loneliness to secure resilience (Falci and McNeely 2009;

Wu and Wong 2013; Zysberg 2012). Caring reflects safety and security to advance resilience (Collins et al. 2011). Reframing has also enabled life satisfaction as an ideal to rationalize resilience (Samios and Baran 2018. Conversely, reframing erodes covetousness, craving, fear, harming, harshness, self-aggrandizing, struggle, suffering, and worry or catastrophizing as ideals or obsessions stifling resilience (Andrade et al. 2019; Feldman and Kuyken 2019). Rehabilitating or healing maintains continence, decency, fairness, happiness or conviviality, hygiene, kindness, love, modesty, peace, perseverance, purposiveness, social relation, and trust (Oh and Park 2023; Vahhab et al. 2024; Zarean and Latifi 2022). Practically, rehabilitating unfolds in brain functioning, homeopathy, meditation, prayer, relaxation, reminiscence, revision, ritual, soothing, and understanding (Johnston 2010; Vahhab et al. 2024; Zarean and Latifi 2022). Rehabilitating can proceed with devices, furniture, and potting (Oh and Park 2023). Essentially, rehabilitating represents deradicalization, justice, positivity, and therapy (Sukabdi 2019; Vahhab et al. 2024; Zarean and Latifi 2022). Rehabilitating is likely to foster resilience by generating power, utility, ideals, and norms to activate the voluntaristic mechanisms of analytical functionalism.

Power facilitated by rehabilitating to drive resilience rests on brain functioning, hygiene, meditation, prayer, purposiveness, relatedness, relaxation, reminiscence, social trust, and understanding (Oh and Park 2023; Vahhab et al. 2024; Zarean and Latifi 2022). Brain functioning has prevented depression, thus buttressing resilience (Feinstein and Bynner 2006). Hygiene has fostered health and impeded depression to enable resilience (Smith et al. 2006; Myers 2008). Meditation has advanced compassion or self-compassion and mindfulness and dwindled depression to foster resilience (Galante et al. 2014). Prayer has elevated well-being, including adjustment, flourishing, health, mastery, positive affect, relationship quality, satisfaction with democracy, finance, life, and police, self-esteem, and socioemotional well-being, to uplift resilience (Dy-Liacco et al. 2009; Flouri and Buchanan 2002; Helliwell and Putnam 2005; Kwak et al. 2010; Marx 2014; Meulemann 2010; Ng and Fisher 2016; Schieman 2001; Moschis and Ong 2011; Skerkat and Ellison 1999; Van Praag et al. 2010; Wuthnow 2004). Relaxation has raised sleep quality and dismissed anxiety to facilitate resilience (Hudetz et al. 2004; Li et al. 2016). Reminiscence has diminished depression to enable resilience (Bohlmeijer et al. 2005). Social trust has facilitated health and survival to support resilience (Barefoot et al. 1998). Understanding has fostered intimacy, satisfaction, and self-efficacy to facilitate resilience (Mikulincer et al. 2003; Norris 2011; Rothwell et al. 2016). Conversely, rehabilitating reduces the desire, expectation, and rivalry to retain the power to drive resilience (Johnston 2010). Desire and expectation have impeded satisfaction, thus weakening resilience (Nickerson et al. 2007). The rivalry has bred hostility and eroded tolerance, thus impairing resilience (Mintz et al. 2022; Passini and Morselli 2015).

Ideals upheld by rehabilitating to rationalize resilience cherish continence, Christianity, decency, fairness, happiness, kindness, liberty, love, modesty, peace, perseverance, revision, and stoicism (Dean 2020; Holowchak 2008; Johnston 2010; Vahhab et al. 2024), Continence has enhanced self-esteem and reduced anxiety and depression to sustain resilience (Armstrong et al. 2011; Marchetti et al. 2018). Christian, gospel, spiritual, or transcendental rehabilitating extols community, faith, and forgiveness as opposed to sacrifice to enable resilience (Johnston 2010). Decency has boosted well-being, including physical and mental health, to activate resilience (Tsai et al. 2018). The ideal for fairness has raised resilience and other well-being components (Diener et al. 2009; Pyszkowska 2020). Kindness has dampened stress and lifted well-being, including connectedness and life satisfaction, as opposed to loneliness and negative emotion (Curry et al. 2018; Nelson-Coffey et al. 2023). Liberty as an ideal has stemmed from growth to buttress resilience (Helson and Srivastava 2001). Love has enhanced toleration as opposed to strictness to champion resilience (Seabach 2017). Modesty has fostered connectedness and gratitude to advance resilience (Angelis and Pensini 2024; Krumrei-Mancuso 2017). Pease has rested on harmonious passion to underlie resilience (Belanger et al. 2019). Perseverance remarkably signifies resilience (Mak et al. 2019). Furthermore, perseverance raised well-being, notably including pleasure, to boost resilience (Boyes et al. 2017; Goodman et al. 2017). Revision has elevated well-being, including growth, environmental quality, and life satisfaction to facilitate resilience (Munroe et al. 2022; Samios and Baran 2018; Wrosch et al. 2000). Stoicism espouses resilience (Alrofiai et al. 2020; Owen 2023). Furthermore, stoicism exalts acceptance, calmness, endurance, flourishing, fullness, hardiness or unyielding, harmony, immunity, invincibility, magnanimity, order, peace, self-preservation, self-sufficiency, serenity, and tranquillity to champion resilience (Alrofiai et al. 2020; Case et al. 2011; Cooney 2000; Holowchak 2008; Hordern 2013; Martın 2016; Primoratz 1999; Sandoval 2017; Siisiainen 2019; Soccio 2004; Taylor 2002). Conversely, rehabilitating dampens radicalism to maintain the ideal to rationalize resilience (Sukabdi 2019). Radicalism reflects anomie, alienation, or inadequacy, anxiety, meaninglessness, and uncertainty or self-uncertainty, thus undermining resilience (Hogg et al. 2010; Koehler and Fiebig 2019; Stankov et al. 2018). Rehabilitating has arisen from low racism to secure the ideal for resilience (Burton et al. 2021). Racism has eroded life quality, thus disrupting resilience (Ishii 2009).

Relaxing features breathing, imaginating, muscle progressing, and yoga (Ghoncheh and Smith 2004; Heyman and Slep 2007). As such, relaxing rests on mutual reinforcement between mind and muscle (Cotterill 2017). Relaxing counts as ethical, hygenic, pastoral, recreational, and therapeutic (Chumbler et al. 2000; Engle and Kasser 2005; Smith 1991; Minnebo 2006; Zeidner and Matthews 2011). Essentially, relaxing manifests resilience (Ramasubramanian 2017). Relaxing is likely to boost resilience by installing power, utility, ideals, and norms for running voluntaristic mechanisms to achieve functioning, as stipulated by analytical functionalism.

Power generated by relaxing to drive resilience rests on awareness, creativity, defense, disengagement, joy, rest or refreshment, and well-being (Ghoncheh and Smith 2004; Mikulincer and Shaver 2014; Smith and Karmin 2002). Awareness has facilitated intimacy, satisfaction, and self-efficacy to enable resilience (Mikulincer et al. 2003; Norris 2011; Rothwell et al. 2016). Creativity has boosted well-being, notably including meaningfulness, to induce resilience (Diener et al. 2009; Turner 2013). Defense has benefitted from self-efficacy to sustain resilience (Guo et al. 2023). Disengagement has raised health to furnish resilience (Wrosch et al. 2005).

Resting enables refueling or recharging conducive to resilience (Schumann et al. 2022). Moreover, relaxing has enhanced performance, prevention, skill, and sleep quality to demonstrate or secure power to drive resilience (Botoin and Griffin 2003; Conlin et al. 2021; Hoover et al. 2022; Li et al. 2016). Performance has reflected self-determination, self-efficacy, and the sense of community to boost resilience (Asoodar et al. 2014; Moller et al. 2006; Yashima 2010). Prevention has benefitted from self-efficacy to enable resilience (McMahon et al. 2015). Skill has underpinned self-efficacy to buttress resilience (Larson et al. 1990). Relaxing counts as coping and leisure to retain power to drive resilience (Frydenberg 2008; Eccles and Barber 1999). Remarkably, coping has achieved resilience (Corbin and Hall 2019). Moreover, coping has propped growth, health, intimacy, quality in environment and relationship, satisfaction, self-efficacy, and general well-being to escalate resilience (Chow et al. 2014; Gattino et al. 2015; Lau et al. 2012; Paez et al. 2007; Veenstra et al. 2005; Wills 1997). Meanwhile, coping has reduced depression, distress, and fear, thus upholding resilience (Krulichova 2019; Littleton et al. 2007; Wills 1997). Leisure has attenuated anxiety, thus enabling resilience (Da Costa Bizarro Morais et al. 2019). Conversely, relaxing reduces anxiety, psychopathology, and stress to restore power to drive resilience (Davies and Bhugra 2004; Hudetz et al. 2004; Zeidner and Matthews 2011). Relaxing has also prevented fatigue, thus retaining power to drive resilience (Hoover et al. 2022). Fatigue has reflected stress to impede resilience (Hoover et al. 2022). Accordingly, stress has eroded well-being, including eudaimonia, health, positive affect, quality of life, neighborhood, and relationships, and satisfaction with life and neighbors, thus jeopardizing resilience (Baumeister et al. 2013; Greenberg 1999; Jackson et al. 2006; Mathis et al. 2016; Parkes et al. 2002; Shrira 2012; Su et al. 2021; Zotti et al. 2016).

Utility posed by relaxing to attract resilience hinges on experiences of boundlessness or liberty, ease, and peace (Ghoncheh and Smith 2004). Liberty has lifted well-being, including health, life satisfaction, and self-esteem as opposed to depression and symptoms to advance resilience (Gehring 2013; Glendinning et al. 2003; Haller and Hadler 2006). Ease experienced has attracted well-being to trigger resilience (Baumeister et al. 2013). Peace experienced has fostered life satisfaction and impeded depression to maintain resilience (Smith et al. 2016). Moreover, relaxing reflects experiences of caring and therapy as utility to attract resilience (Engle and Kasser 2005; Zeidner and Matthews 2011). Essentially, caring received enhanced resilience (Cherry et al. 2018). Moreover, caring received has boosted well-being, including control, emotional well-being, health, pleasure, purposiveness, relational quality, satisfaction with housing, leisure, and life, self-determination, self-efficacy, self-esteem, and social well-being to sustain resilience (George and Park 2013; Glendinning et al. 2003; Granzin and Haggard 2000; Holliman et al. 2021; Kafetsio and Sideridis 2006; Lincoln et al. 2003; Logan and Cobb 2013; Schwarzer and Knoll 2007; Vilhjalmsson and Thorlindsson 1998; Wen et al. 2010; Williams and Galliher 2006; Xi and Hwang 2011). Conversely, caring received has diminished anger, anxiety, depression, distress, and symptoms, thus facilitating resilience (Glendinning et al. 2003; Hwang et al. 2007; Lee and Robbins 1998; Pierce and Quiroz 2018). Therapy has raised well-being or life quality, including health and intimacy as opposed to anxiety, depression, and disturbance, thus sustaining resilience (Boulton et al. 2001; Erford et al. 2011; Goertz-Dorten et al. 2017; Lintz et al. 2019; Lucas 2012; Murphy et al. 2017).

Ideals incubated by relaxing to rationalize resilience emphasize flow, gratification, hedonism, hygiene, innocence, love, optimism, playfulness, quietude, thankfulness, and transcendence (Baas et al. 2008; Chumbler et al. 2000; Ghoncheh and Smith 2004; Ramasubramanian 2017; Roy 2009; Wansink and van Itterum 2012). Flow or engrossment involves control and reward to enable resilience (Greene et al. 2013; Kowal and Fortier 1999; Weber et al. 2017). Moreover, flow has boosted competence, motivation, and relatedness to safetuard resilience (Kowal and Fortier 1999). Hedonism has bred well-being, including life satisfaction to sustain resilience (Datler et al. 2013; Joshanloo and Jarden 2016). Hygiene has maintained health and diminished depression to uplift resilience (Smith et al. 2006; Myers 2008). Innocence or honesty has rested on happiness to advance resilience (Medai and Noussair 2021). Love has championed meaningfulness to enhance resilience (Damasio and Koller 2015). Playfulness has championed connectedness and self-efficacy and dismissed helpfulness to enhance resilience (Clifford et al. 2023; White 2024). Quietitude safeguards harmony, meaningfulness, love, and peace as opposed to conflict to secure resilience (Valle 2019). Thankfulness has raised positive affect and diminished negative affect to buttress resilience (Bernabe-Valero et al. 2021).

Rewarding, generosity, or giving generally includes contribution and gifting (Godoy et al. 2007; Molm 1997). Essentially, rewarding manifests charity orientation, cohesion, fraternity, intimacy, morality, prosociality, social interest, and welfare provision (Apinunmahakul and Devlin 2008; de Beer and Kostere 2009; Gino and Galinsky 2012; Ruggiero 2020; Stagnaro et al. 2017). Moreover, rewarding represents a strength and virtue (Carson 2000; Wilcox and Dew 2016). Rewarding is necessary to meet or realize interdependency, reciprocity, and trust (Phan et al. 2009). Furthermore, rewarding is virtuous according to Buddhism, Catholicism, Jainism, and legalism (Fierke 2022; Martin 2012; Thomas 1997; Zhang 2018). More broadly, rewarding underpins civil society, community reproduction, and exchange (Phan et al. 2009; Werbner 1996). Rewarding is likely to champion resilience by generating power, utility, ideals, and norms to achieve the requisite functions of fulfillment, adaptation, integration, and latency premised on analytical functionalism.

Power underlying rewarding to drive resilience has stemmed from agreeableness, income, majority status, relational quality, responsiveness, and reward power (Degenne et al. 2004; Godoy et al. 2007; Lemay et al. 2007; Li et al. 2024; Molm 1997; Phan et al. 2009). Agreeableness has fostered growth, life satisfaction, mastery, purposefulness, relatedness, and self-acceptance to buttress resilience (Hounkpatin et al. 2015). Income has afforded well-being, including adaptation, adequacy, belongingness, control, eudaemonia, health, mastery, power, quality of life, satisfaction, self-efficacy, self-esteem, and social well-being to sustain resilience (Anciaes et al. 2017; Carpiano 2008; Corcoran et al. 2011; Ross and Mirowsky 1989; Sengupta and Sibley 2019; Son and Wilson 2012; Wang and VanderWeele 2011; Yeh et al. 2013; Zimmerman and Reyna 2013). Meanwhile, income has dampened anomia, depression, distress, fear or anxiety, loneliness, and stagnation, thus furnishing resilience

(Clarke et al. 2011; Hou et al. 2015; McClendon 1991; Ng et al. 2006; Rijken and Groenewegen 2008). Majority status has sustained life quality and diminished distress and fatigue to enable resilience (Verschuur et al. 2010). Responsiveness has maintained well-being to drive resilience (Jasielska 2020). Rewarding raises spirituality and well-being to furnish power to drive resilience (Day 2010; Marcus 2014). Moreover, rewarding has reflected socializing to mobilize power to drive resilience (Phan et al. 2009). Socializing has reduced negative emotion and stress to safeguard resilience (Nelson-Coffey et al. 2023). Conversely, rewarding has diminished stress experienced, thus retaining power to drive resilience (Lazar and Eisenberger 2022). Rewarding also reduces violence to maintain power to drive resilience (Messner et al. 2008). Violence has bred depression, thus disturbing resilience (Wright et al. 2015).

Utility underlying rewarding to attract resilience has rested on the reduction in punishment experienced (Molm 1997). Punishment received has dampened distress, thus impeding resilience (Zalewski et al. 2017).

Ideals associated with rewarding to rationalize resilience emphasize Buddhism extolling advancement, altruism, befriending, benevolence, broadmindedness, caring, compassion, contentment, deliverance, diligence, effort, emptiness or nothingness, enlightenment, equanimity or peace, gratitude, honoring, integrity, joy or gladness, kindness, liberation, lightness, loving, love, meditation, mindfulness, orderliness, pacifying or peacefulness, patience, poise, presentness, putdown, quietness, reframing, relief, responsibility, temperance or restraint, tolerance, toughness, transcendence, understanding, usualizing, vigor, and wisdom (Feldman and Kuyken 2019; Fierke 2022; Guo 2018; Keown 2001; Narvaez 2014; Qin 2013; Thomas 1997; Wei 2015). Advancement has rested on self-evaluation to furnish resilience (Kanmeyer-Mueller and Judge 2007). Altruism has raised well-being, including connectedness, hope, life satisfaction, meaningfulness, and self-efficacy (Marsh and Dik 2021; Nelson-Coffey et al. 2023; Raposa et al. 2016; Yao and Enright 2019). Meanwhile, altruism has eroded loneliness and negative emotion (Nelson-Coffey et al. 2023). Befriending or friendliness has secured belongingness and self-esteem as opposed to loneliness to achieve resilience (Falci and McNeely 2009; Wu and Wong 2013; Zysberg 2012). Benevolence has stemmed from low depression to uphold resilience (Mancini et al. 2011). Broadmindeness comprises emptying, forgiveness, and self-acceptance as opposed to venting (Qin 2013). The ideal for caring has buttressed caring (Sarasa 2008). Caring has maintained mental clarity to boost resilience (Naruse et al. 2020). The ideal for compassion activates compassion (Clobert et al. 2015). Compassion has sustained well-being to drive resilience (Jasielska 2020). Diligence covers confession, flexibility, forbearance, and self-examination as opposed to flaunting (Qin 2013). Diligence registers conscientiousness and creativity to enable resilience (Nevarez 2011; Yu and Zhang 2007). Effort has prevented depression to maintain resilience (Barnes and Vulcano 1982; Wrosch et al. 2005). Emptiness reflects low resilience (Elfers et al. 2024). Enlightenment has reduced anxiety, depression, and fear to raise resilience (DiGiuseppe et al. 2017). Equanimity has fostered life satisfaction and reduced depression to advance resilience (Smith et al. 2016). Gratitude has boosted positive emotion as opposed to negative affect to achieve resilience (Bernabe-Valero et al. 2021). Kindness encompasses forgiveness, self-examination, and tolerance as opposed to gossiping and nitpicking (Qin 2013). As such, kindness has fostered connectedness, life satisfaction, and well-being in general as opposed to negative emotion, loneliness, and stress to buttress resilience (Curry et al. 2018; Nelson-Coffey et al. 2023). Liberation has promoted well-being, including health, life satisfaction, and self-esteem, as opposed to depression and symptoms to secure resilience (Glendinning et al. 2003; Haller and Hadler 2006). Loving has secured meaningfulness to buttress resilience (Damasio and Koller 2015). Meditation concerns gentleness, persistence, and transcendence as opposed to illusion (Qin 2013). As such, meditation has sustained compassion and mindfulness as opposed to depression to foster resilience (Galante et al. 2014). Mindfulness has raised well-being, including life satisfaction, and positive affect as opposed to depression to advance resilience (Klussman et al. 2020; Linares et al. 2016). Orderliness embeds mindfulness, persistence, and solidness as opposed to suspicion (Qin 2013). Essentially, orderliness has arisen from health to facilitate resilience (Cheung and Lai 2020). Pacifying upholds calmness, coolness, lightness, quietude, and surrendering (Qin 2013). Patience has dampened negative affect to maintain resilience (Mehmood et al. 2020). Poise has maintained life satisfaction and dampened anxiety and depression to lift resilience (Grzywacz and Bass 2003; Landolfi et al. 2021). Presentness treasures brightness, optimism, self-understanding, and surrendering as opposed to worry (Qin 2013). Reframing has sustained well-being, including adjustment, environmental quality, growth, peace, and life satisfaction as opposed to depression to enable resilience (Ferreira et al. 2021; Gattino et al. 2015; Munroe et al. 2022; Samios and Baran 2018; Sikka et al. 2023; Wrosch et al. 2000). Responsibility underlies energy and sustainability to secure resilience (Garcia et al. 2017; Shamir 2008). Temperance has enhanced self-esteem as opposed to anxiety and depression to lift resilience (Armstrong et al. 2011). Transcendence has raised life satisfaction and meaningfulness and impeded anxiety, depression, and stress to facilitate resilience (Fishbein et al. 2020). Understanding has enhanced intimacy, satisfaction, and self-efficacy to secure resilience (Mikulincer et al. 2003; Norris 2011; Rothwell et al. 2016). Usualizing champion diligence, equality, and fatalism (Qin 2013). Vigor has enhanced satisfaction and reduced depression and symptoms to maintain resilience (Adrian et al. 2018; Rose 2003). Wisdom has championed well-being, including coherence, meaningfulness, purposefulness, life satisfaction, self-efficacy, and self-understanding to induce resilience (Baumeister et al. 2013; Camp 1989; Diener et al. 2009; Takahashi and Overton 2002; Webster 2010). Moreover, rewarding embodies Daoist ideals highlighting adaptation, fearlessness, indifference, roundedness, and transcendence to rationalize resilience (Wang 1999; Zhu 2003). Rewarding also champions Jainist ideals favoring agreeableness, altruism or kindheartedness, calmness, forgiveness, humility, livability, moderation, and temperance (Thomas 1997). Forgiveness has advanced well being to induce resilience (Shimai et al. 2006). Humility has fostered connectedness and gratitude to lift resilience (Angelis and Pensini 2024; Krumrei-Mancuso 2017). Furthermore, rewarding honors legalist ideals hailing adaptation or fitting, appreciating, broadmindedness or magnanimity, calmness, correction or self-correcting, easygoing, empowerment, moderation, optimization, peace, perseverance, popularity, preservation, prevention, quietness, security, self-reliance, and understanding (Zhang 2005, 2018). Correction has maintained well-being, including adjustment, environmental quality, growth, life satisfaction, and peace as opposed to depression to enable resilience (Ferreira et al. 2021; Gattino et al. 2015; Munroe et al. 2022; Samios and Baran 2018; Sikka et al. 2023; Wrosch et al. 2000). Empowerment experienced has raised self-efficacy to drive resilience (Gullan et al. 2013). Perseverance has facilitated well-being, including pleasure, to sustained resilience (Boyes et al. 2017; Goodman et al. 2017). Popularity has maintained belongingness, positive affect, and self-esteem as opposed to negative affect to advance resilience (Reich et al. 2018). Self-reliance has lifted mastery to furnish resilience (Lu and Kao 2002). Conversely, rewarding maintains Buddhist ideals against anger, covetousness or greed, craving, desire, fear, harming, harshness, pain, self-aggrandizing, slanderousness, struggle, suffering, violence, and worry, resistance, or catastrophizing to rationalize resilience (Feldman and Kuyken 2019; Fierke 2022; Garner 1994). Harming has fomented depression to dampen resilience (Wright et al. 2015). Self-aggrandizing has bred depression, thus weakening resilience (Tracy et al. 2009). Struggling has impaired well-being, including life and marital satisfaction to block resilience (Mikula et al. 2012; Pomerleau et al. 2020; Richards 2016). Rewarding also holds the ideal against risking to rationalize resilience (Zhang 2005). Risking has eroded health, thus impeding resilience (Wickrama et al. 1995).

Norms underlying rewarding to assimilate resilience have opposed inequality and punishment (Li et al. 2024; Molm 1997). The norm of inequality has represented strain to resist resilience (Kyriacou 2020). Punishing as assimilated has increased depression, thus impairing resilience (Watt and Stewart 2003).

Supporting represents prosociality likening altruism, beneficience, collectivism, generosity, helpfulness, and kindness (Luria et al. 2019; Wang et al. 2021). Ideologically, supporting rests on Christianity, Confucianism or scholarism, and religion in general (Chen et al. 2022; Drezner 2013; Music 2014). Supporting is crucial for caring, citizenship, contracting, decency, fairness, humanity, loyalty, patience, religiousness, socializing, trust, and well-being (Dovidio et al. 2006; Glenn 2000; Hawley 2014; Mastain 2007; Music 2014; Twenge et al. 2007). The ethic of care maintains relatedness and responsibility and eliminates oppression (Featherstone and Morris 2012; Fine 2007). Caring additionally embodies acceptance, community, equality, protection, and respect (Fine 2007; Hartley and Watson 2012; Peng 2012). Furthermore, caring constitutes social capital (Chan 2009). Citizenship is essential for the commonweal, confidence, democracy, dignity, hope, justice, peace, and relatedness (Jennings and Russell 2019; White 2006). Contracting realizes rationality and mutuality or mutual recognition (Pincione and Teson 2006). Decency has boosted well-being, including physical and mental health, to activate resilience (Tsai et al. 2018). Fairness is relevant to acceptability or legitimacy, contracting, coping, religiosity, and sociotropy (Campbell 2010; Furnham 2003; Gibson 2008; Hafer and Sutton 2016). Humanity realizes education, enlightenment, and socialization (Loptson 2001). Loyalty is integral to governance and morality (Fan et al. 2022b). Patience is functional to achievement and tolerance (Al-Arja 2023; Mehmood et al.

2020). Religiousness furnishes belongingness, cohesiveness, discipline, education, meaningfulness, morality, pleasantness, sharing, survival, and well-being (Demerath 2002; Haidt 2012; Ishii and Watanabe 2023; Levin and Chatters 1998; Skerkat and Ellison 1999; Turner 2009). Socializing engenders flourishing (Goodman et al. 2019). Trust fosters collectivity, cooperation, democracy, fraternity, maturity, morality, organization, security, social capital, and social order (Brown et al. 2014; Newton 1999; Olivera 2015; Fine and Holyfield 1996; Pretsch and Ehrhardt-Madapathi 2018; Rahn 2008; Six 2014; Yamagishi et al. 1999). Supporting is likely to raise resilience by offering power, utility, ideas, and norms to achieve the requisite functions of fulfillment, adaptation, integration, and latency.

Power enhanced by supporting to drive resilience rests on competence, patience, religiousness, responsibility, self-determination, and trust (Dovidio et al. 2006; Glenn 2000; Hawley 2014; Twenge et al. 2007; Weinstein and Ryan 2010). Competence has raised well-being, including happiness, health, joy, and life satisfaction to lift resilience (Borgonovi 2008; Caprara and Steca 2005; Judge et al. 2002; Landmann and Rohmann 2020). Patience has enabled achievement and dwindled negative affect to safeguard resilience (Mehmood et al. 2020). Religiousness has sustained well-being, including adjustment, flourishing, health, life satisfaction, mastery, positive affect, relational quality, self-esteem, and socioemotional well-being to facilitate resilience (Chang 2009; Flouri and Buchanan 2002; Helliwell and Putnam 2005; Dy-Liacco et al. 2009; Moschis and Ong 2011; Ng and Fisher 2016; Schieman 2001; Skerkat and Ellison 1999; Wuthnow 2004). Responsibility has boosted energy to energize resilience (Garcia et al. 2017). Self-determination has lifted well-being, including life satisfaction, mastery, relatedness, relational quality, relatedness, vitality to facilitate resilience (Delhey 2010; Hui et al. 2013; Ross and Drentea 1998; Sieber et al. 2019; Weinstein and Ryan 2010). Trust or support expected has facilitated health and survival to realize resilience (Barefoot et al. 1998). Supporting has enhanced well-being, including connectedness, hope, life satisfaction, meaningfulness, and self-efficacy, as opposed to loneliness and negative emotion to generate power to drive resilience (Marsh and Dik 2021; Nelson-Coffey et al. 2023; Raposa et al. 2016; Yao and Enright 2019). Moreover, supporting has secured civility to secure power to drive resilience (Hample 2018). Civility has fostered well-being, including mental and physical health, to elevate resilience (Tsai et al. 2018). Generally, supporting reflects power to drive resilience (Collins 2004). Supporting also reflects agency or self-efficacy, agreeableness, capital, communality or belongingness, connectedness or bonding, control, empathy, forgiveness, friendship, leisure, relaxation, relief, security, social engagement or integration, socioeconomic status, education, or wealth, and others' facilitation and support to furnish power to drive resilience (Bierhoff 2002; Brown and Brown 2006; Carlo and Pierotti 2020; Chasiotis and Bender 2014; Dovidio et al. 2006; Grant and Gino 2010; Graser et al. 2016; Hawley 2014; Luria et al. 2019; Matts et al. 2009; Music 2014; Nai et al. 2018; O'Brien 2014; Thielmann et al. 2020). Agreeableness has facilitated growth, life satisfaction, mastery, purposefulness, relatedness, and self-acceptance to advance resilience (Hounkpatin et al. 2015). Capital includes cultural, human, and social forms (Luria et al. 2019). Human capital has enhanced economic well-being to enable resilience (Herd et al. 2008). Cultural capital has incubated religiousness to champion resilience (Wuthnow 2004). Social capital has fostered well-being, including flourishing, happiness, health, life satisfaction, pride, and the sense of community to safeguard resilience (Chua et al. 2021; Yetim and Yetim 2014). Belongingness, connectedness, or bonding has alleviated negative emotion and stress, thus buttressing resilience (Nelson-Coffey et al. 2023). Control has facilitated well-being, including health and life satisfaction to uplift resilience (Etezadi and Pushkar 2013; Orlowski and Wicker 2015; Rose 2000). Empathy has facilitated intimacy and communication quality to facilitate resilience (Redmond 2018). Forgiveness has advanced well-being to induce resilience (Shimai et al. 2006). Friendship has facilitated belongingness and self-esteem to enable resilience (Falci and McNeely 2009; Wu and Wong 2013). Leisure has boosted life satisfaction to induce resilience (Roberts et al. 2001). Relaxation has advanced sleep quality and erased anxiety to secure resilience (Hudetz et al. 2004; Li et al. 2016). Relief registers safety and well-being to buttress resilience (Kotler et al. 2006; Zhou 2009). Security has escalated well-being, including health and life satisfaction to raise resilience (Chen et al. 2008; Frey et al. 2007; Jones et al. 2014). Social integration has alleviated depression to secure resilience (Mullins and Dugan 1991). Socioeconomic status has enabled health, interactional quality, life satisfaction, and self-esteem to elevate resilience (Al-krenawi et al. 2011; Molana and Adams 2019; Staudinger et al. 1999). Social support received has fostered resilience (Cherry et al. 2018). Furthermore, supporting has rested on compassion, friendliness, generativity, humility, intelligence, mindfulness, openness, self-esteem, sociability, solidarity, sympathy, and transcendence to generate power to drive resilience (Berry et al. 2020; Caprara and Steca 2007; Foschi and Lauriola 2014; Kitayama and Markus 2000; Leiberg 2011; Rossi 2004; Thielmann et al. 2020; Wong and Yang 2022). Compassion has boosted well-being to induce resilience (Jasielska 2020). Generativity has built on well-being to facilitate resilience (Peterson and Klohnen 1995). Humility has fostered connectedness and gratitude to enable resilience (Angelis and Pensini 2024; Krumrei-Mancuso 2017). Intelligence has assuaged depression to maintain resilience (Feinstein and Bynner 2006). Mindfulness has raised well-being, including life satisfaction and positive affect, to champion resilience (Andrade et al. 2019; Hahn et al. 2013; Karwowski and Lebuda 2017; Klussman et al. 2020; Quilty et al. 2006). Openness has facilitated well-being, including autonomy, growth, life satisfaction, purposefulness, relational quality, self-acceptance, self-efficacy, and self-esteem to enable resilience (Hounkpatin et al. 2015; Webster et al. 2014). Sociability has enhanced well-being to buttress resilience (Bjornskov 2008). Solidarity has enabled adjustment, hope, and life satisfaction to secure resilience (Dittman and Goebel 2010; James and Hunsley 1995; Paez et al. 2015). Transcendence has fostered integrity, life satisfaction, and meaningfulness and has eroded anxiety, depression, and stress to maintain resilience (Fishbein et al. 2020; Hoshino et al. 2012). Conversely, supporting has dampened impulsivity and playfulness, thus mustering power to drive resilience (Hample 2018). Impulsivity represents neuroticism to impede resilience (Wright and DeLisi 2016). Playfulness reflects purposelessness to undermine resilience (Alexander et al. 2019).

Supporting reflects low alcoholism, anxiety or fear, avoidance, conflict, exploitation, greed, jealousy, madness or insanity, poverty, stress, and others' abusing, control, or inhibition to maintain power to drive resilience (Barber 2004; Collins and Feeney 2004; Ellingsen and Johannesson 2008; Matts et al. 2009; Music 2014; Parrott et al. 2020; Staub 2003; Thielmann et al. 2020). Alcoholism has induced illness, injury, and pathology to disrupt resilience (Brotchie et al. 2004; Haapanen-Niemi et al. 1999). Avoidance has hurt well-being, including intimacy, life satisfaction, and mindfulness to disturb resilience (Alonso-Arbiol et al. 2007; Barber et al. 2010; Basabe et al. 2002; Linares et al. 2016). Conflict has weakened well-being, including life and marital satisfaction, to hamper resilience (Baumeister et al. 2013; Mikula et al. 2012; Richards 2016). Exploiting others has impaired resilience and well-being generally (Diener et al. 2009; Pyszkowska 2020). Greed reflects dissatisfaction and psychopathy, thus hurting resilience (Hoyer et al. 2023; Mussel and Hewig 2016). Jealousy has raised fear, thus jeopardizing resilience (Felson and Outlaw 2007). Poverty has inhibited well-being and fomented strain to withhold resilience (Clark et al. 2008; Walker et al. 2010). Abusive experience has weakened well-being, including satisfaction and self-respect, to impede resilience (Graham et al. 2010; Krahe 2013; Singer et al. 2019). Control experienced has raised distress to attenuate resilience (Overall et al. 2020). Furthermore, supporting has reflected low aggressiveness, experiences of social exclusion or rejection, impulsivity, Machiavellianism, narcissism, and psychopathy, thus retaining power to drive resilience (Thielmann et al. 2020; Twenge et al. 2007). Aggressiveness has induced depression to inhibit resilience (Wright et al. 2015). Social exclusion experienced has fomented negative mood and life dissatisfaction to hinder resilience (Lin et al. 2013; Williams et al. 2000). Machiavellianism has generated abusing, controlling, and misbehavior, and inhibited relational satisfaction to block resilience (Brewer and Abell 2017; Jones and Paulhus 2009). Accordingly, Machiavellianism, which favors competition, dishonesty, distrust, flattering, and money, is antisocial, cynical, deceitful, and immoral (Gold et al. 1976; House et al. 2013; Lee et al. 2013; Muris et al. 2022). Narcissism has bred aggression, depression, Machiavellianism, misbehavior, and relational satisfaction to obstruct resilience (Tracy et al., 2009). Psychopathy has hurt well-being to displace resilience (Jans-Beken 2019).

Utility building on supporting to attract resilience involves experiences of benefit, controllability, cooperation, functions, incentive, justice, recognition, reward, sharing, and similarity or commonality (Bierhoff 2002; Carlo and Pierotti 2020; Dovidio et al. 2006; Grant and Dutton 2012; Ellingsen and Johannesson 2008; Levine et al. 2005, Matts et al. 2009; Pressgrove et al. 2020; Staub 2003; Weiner 2012). Controllability experienced has boosted health to sustain resilience (Tomich and Helgeson 2002). Cooperation experienced has engendered justice experienced to boost belongingness, health, life satisfaction, and self-esteem to establish resilience (Bjornskov et al. 2013; Dalbert 2001; Lucas et al. 2013; Shank 2012; van Prooijen et al. 2008). Functions materialize in career advancement, need fulfillment, norm conformity, protection, relatedness, self-enhancement, self-understanding, and value expression, such as that about humanitarianism (Carlo and Pierotti 2020; Matts et al. 2009; Weinstein and Ryan 2010). Justice experienced has bolstered belongingness, health, life satisfaction, and self-esteem to enable resilience (Bjornskov et al. 2013; Dalbert 2001; Lucas et al. 2013; van Prooijen et al. 2008). Similarity experienced has fostered adjustment to maintain resilience (Denson and Bowman 2015). Furthermore, supporting has arisen from experiences of affection, closeness, and gratitude to hold utility to attract resilience (Bjornberg and Ekbrand 2008; Iwai and de Franca Carvalho 2022; Maltseva 2016).

Ideals fostered by supporting to rationalize resilience favor fairness (Music 2014). The ideal for fairness has raised resilience and other well-being components (Diener et al. 2009; Pyszkowska 2020). Supporting has sustained cooperation and protection to embody ideals to rationalize resilience (Dinic and Bodroza 2021; Hample 2018). Cooperation has fostered life satisfaction to rationalize resilience (Park et al. 2015). Protection has embodied self-efficacy to enable resilience (Guo et al. 2023. Moreover, supporting has cultivated the ideal for work to rationalize resilience (Marsh and Dik 2021). Work value has advanced adaptability to secure resilience (Willner et al. 2020). Supporting also builds on the ideals of adaptation, communitarianism, egalitarianism, investment, repute, reciprocity, and satisfaction to rationalize resilience (Barber 2004; Brown and Brown 2006; Dovidio et al. 2006; Ellingsen and Johannesson 2008; Gaertner and Dovidio 2012; Van Lange and Rusbutt 2012; Weinstein and Ryan 2010). Adaptation realizes resilience (Maltby et al. 2016). Community involvement embraced in communitarianism has lifted well-being, including mastery and self-efficacy, to activate resilience (Harter and Arora 2010; Heckscher 2015; Ohmer 2007). Egalitarianism has diminished anxiety to sustain resilience (Schwartz and Melech 2000). Investment, following its ideal, has fostered hope, positive affect, and self-efficacy to secure resilience (Burrow et al. 2010; Yon et al. 2012). Repute, realizing its ideal, has advanced self-esteem and dampened depression to maintain resilience (Fournier 2009). Reciprocity, arising from its ideal, has fostered adaptation and prevented illness to achieve resiience (Yamaoka 2008; Yeh et al. 2013). Furthermore, supporting has arisen from ideals for autonomy, collectivism or communality, conservation, creativity, humanity or humanism, interdependence, learning, openness, responsibility, similarity, sociality, and transcendence to rationalize resilience (Bayram 2016; Butler et al. 2022; Feeney and Collins 2001; Greitemeyer et al. 2006; Heilman and Kusev 2020; Iwai and de Franca Carvalho 2022; Lemay et al. 2023; Kou et al. 2019; Maltseva 2016; Nai et al. 2018; Thielmann et al. 2020). Autonomy, based on its ideal, has propped well-being, including life satisfaction, mastery, relatedness, relational quality, and vitality to facilitate resilience (Delhey 2010; Hui et al. 2013; Ross and Drentea 1998; Sieber et al. 2019; Weinstein and Ryan 2010). Collectivism, or the ideal of commonality, has secured health and self-esteem to enable resilience (Triandis 1995). Creativity, evolving from its ideal, has underpinned well-being, notably meaningfulness, to achieve resilience (Diener et al. 2009; Turner 2013). Humanism embraces creativity, resolution, self-improvement, and vitality to facilitate resilience (Browning and Cooper 2004; Fuchs 2020; Selznick 2008; Visher 1997). Based on its value, interdependence has secured relational satisfaction to uplift resilience (Wickham and Knee 2012). Learning, standing on its value, has raised well-being, including life satisfaction and self-efficacy, to enable resilience (Denver and Hands 1990; Minnaert and Janssen 1992; Richards 2016). Openness, based on its ideal, has advanced well-being, including autonomy, growth, life satisfaction, purposefulness, relational quality, self-acceptance, self-efficacy, and self-esteem to factiliate resilience (Hahn et al. 2013; Hounkpatin et al. 2015; Karwowski and Lebuda 2017; Marks 1996; Quilty et al. 2006; Webster et al. 2014). Building on its ideal, responsibility has secured pleasantness or positive affect to factiliate resilience (Karuza et al. 1990). Similarity maintained for its ideal has reduced depression, thus sustaining resilience (Riad and Norris 1992). Sociality, as upheld by its ideal, has fostered well-being, including happiness, love, satisfaction, self-efficacy, self-esteem, and social well-being, to enhance resilience (Bada and Medve-Balint 2017; Denissen et al. 2008; Galperin and Haselton 2010; Guillen et al. 2011; Mazziotta et al. 2011; Meulemann 2010; Reeskens and Vandecasteele 2017). Transcendence, evolving from its ideal, has enhanced meaningfulness and eroded anxiety, depression, and stress to maintain resilience (Fishbein et al. 2020). Conversely, supporting stems from ideals against avoidance, competition, egoism or selfishness, risking, suicide, and xenophobia to rationalize resilience (Barber 2004; Collins and Feeney 2004; Feeney and Collins 2001; Music 2014; Nicholas et al. 2020; Straume and Odeen 2010; Wade-Benzoni and Tost 2009). Competition has eroded interest and enjoyment and fomented gloating to impede resilience (Frederick-Recascino and Schuster-Smith 2003; Hareli and Weiner 2002). Egoism or selfishness has bred anxiety to obstruct resilience (Da Costa Bizarro Morais et al. 2019). Risking has impaired health, thus disabling resilience (Wickrama et al. 1995). Suicide or its attempt has engendered anxiety to prevent resilience (Cheng et al. 2017). Xenophobia has worsened life quality to hinder resilience (Klein et al. 1998).

Norms realized by supporting to assimilate resilience popularize citizenship, communality, empathy, effectiveness, individualism, supporting, and uplifting (Batson et al. 1995; Hersberger-Langloh et al. 2022; Lemay et al. 2023; Luria et al. 2019; North et al. 2004; Steg and de Groot 2010; Welzel 2013). Based on its norm, citizenship has sustained well-being or life quality, including mental and physical health, to boost resilience (Tsai et al. 2018). Thanks to its norm, commonality has reduced negative emotion and stress, thus maintaining resilience (Nelson-Coffey et al. 2023). Building on its norm, empathy has reduced discontent and resentment and maintained intimacy and communication quality to facilitate resilience (Redmond 2018). Effectiveness perceived lessens anger and blaming to enable resilience (Evans 2013). Individualism as a social norm has fostered pleasantness to afford resilience (Basabe et al. 2002). Uplifting experience has boosted life satisfaction and positive affect to furnish resilience (Maybery et al. 2006). Conversely, supporting reflects norms against annoyance, avoidance, crime, harassment, and violence, thus assimilating resilience (Butler et al. 2022; Luria et al. 2019; Music 2014; North et al. 2004; Zhong 2010).

Trust encompasses affection, caring, commitment, cooperativeness, investment, kindness, and morality (Bellemare and Kroger 2007; Habibis et al. 2016; Paraskevopoulos 2010; Rahn 2008; Viklund and Sjoberg 2008; Wang et al. 2016). Conceptually, trust represents expectation, positivity, resourcefulness, risking, social capital, and social intelligence (Mingo and Faggiano 2020; Paraskevopoulos 2010; Six 2014; Sundquist and Yang 2007; van Swol 2003). Conversely, trust surrenders caution and rationality (Miller and Mitamura 2003; Newton 1999). Ideologically or intrinsically, trust stands on communitarianism, egalitarianism, and socialism (Abascal 2015; Brown et al. 2014; Volker and Flap 1997). Instrumentally or extrinsically, trust shoulders collectivity, cooperation, cost-saving, democracy, fraternity, emancipation, maturity, morality, organization, security, social capital, and social order (Brown et al. 2014; Falkenberg 1998; Fine and Holyfield 1996; Olivera 2015; Pretsch and Ehrhardt-Madapathi 2018; Rahn 2008; Six 2014; Yamagishi et al. 1999). Furthermore, trust is likely to enable resilience by facilitating power, utility, ideals, and norms to achieve functions dictated by analytical functionalism.

Power enhanced by trust to drive resilience arises from collectivity, cooperation, maturity, morality, organization, and social capital (Brown et al. 2014; Fine and Holyfield 1996; Six 2014). Trust has buttressed competence, friendship, health, governance, identity achievement, morality, security, self-esteem, social attachment, survival, and vitality to muster power to drive resilience (Barefoot et al. 1998; Burke and Stets 1999; Crystal and DeBell 2002; Hoegh and Bourgeois 2002; King 2007; Meeus et al. 2002). Moreover, trust rises with information received, investment, knowledge, openness, social attachment or social support received, and wealth to accrue power to drive resilience (Buskens and Raub 2013; Carter 2016; Kramer 1999; Mewes et al. 2021; Sato 2002; Volker and Flap 1997). Trust has also emanated from activism, agreeableness, autonomy, civility, control, education, friendship, functionality, happiness, health, intimacy, morality, openness, organizational membership, prestige, pride, religiosity, self-efficacy, sociability, social capital or integration, social class, social support received, and general well-being to consolidate power to drive resilience (Almakaeva et al. 2018; Cais, Torrente, and Bolancé. 2021; Child and Nikolova 2020; Freitag 2003b; Freitag and Bauer 2016; Halvorsen 2007; Huhe 2014; Kende et al. 2022; Newton 1999; Rahn 2008; Ross and Jang 2000; Sabatini and Sarracino 2019; Steinhardt 2012; Stolle and Harell 2013; ten Brinke and Keltner 2020; Uslaner 2002; van Ingen and Bekkers 2015; Zanin et al. 2013). Conversely, trust saves costs to retain power to drive resilience (Falkenberg 1998). Trust also prevents competition to retain power to drive resilience (Dinesen and Sonderskov 2015). Moreover, trust has diminished alcoholism, depression, and doping to keep power to drive resilience (Dufur et al. 2013; Wu et al. 2010). Furthermore, trust reflects low ostracism and stress experienced to maintain power to drive resiience (Carter 2016). Trust has also arisen from low discrimination experienced, disorder experienced, distress, fear, hardship experienced, obesity, problems experienced, stress experienced, unemployment, and victimization experienced to retain power to drive resilience (Burke and Stets 1999; Cais et al. 2021; Marschall and Stolle 2004; Mewes et al. 2021; Olivera 2015; Ross and Mirowsky 2009; Uslaner 2002; Williams et al. 1999; Zanin 2017).

Utility derived from trust to attract resilience involves benefits, cooperation, incentive, justice, safety, security, sharing, and understandability experienced (Adongo et al. 2019; Chiricos et al. 2000; Elsbach and Elofson 2000; Kramer 1999; McKnight and Chervany 2006; Pretsch and Ehrhardt-Madapathi 2018; Ross and LaCroix 1996; Sato 2002; Yamagishi et al. 1999). Safety or security experienced has boosted well-being, including health, life satisfaction, and neighborhood quality, as opposed to fear, to induce resilience (Chen et al. 2008; Frey et al. 2007; Olson et al. 2016; Jones et al. 2014). Understandability experienced registers order to reflect health to secure resilience (Cheung and Lai 2020; Raab 2019). Trust has also stemmed from equality experienced and life quality and reciprocity expected to secure utility to attract resilience (Barrera 2007; Uslaner 2002; Yamagishi et al. 1998). Equality experienced denotes freedom from deprivation and strain, thus safeguarding resilience (Kyriacou 2020). Reciprocity experienced has stemmed from low loneliness to maintain resilience (Espvall and Dellgran 2010). Conversely, trust reflects the absence of arrest, crisis, and risk experienced to maintain utility for resilience (Carter 2016; Kirk 2009; Paraskevopoulos 2010). Crises experienced have diminished well-being, including health, pleasure, positive affect, life quality, and life satisfaction, thus worsening resilience (Mathis et al. 2016; Mroczek 2004; Raposa et al. 2016; Shrira 2012; Su et al. 2021; Zotti et al. 2016). Risk experienced has inhibited achievement, happiness, life satisfaction, positive affect, and self-determination to dampen resilience (Schoon 2006; Schwartz and Melech 2000; Shippee 2012; Zotti et al. 2016).

Ideals raised by trust to rationalize resilience emphasize fraternity, friendliness, or reciprocation, and self-confidence (Newton 1999; Taylor-Gooby 2005). Trust has fostered an inclusive orientation to champion an ideal to rationalize resilience (Delhey et al. 2011). Inclusiveness has reflected the low threat experienced to champion resilience (Raijman et al. 2008). Furthermore, trust reflects ideals concerning egalitarianism, individualism, persistence, satisfaction, and social similarity to rationalize resilience (Carter 2016; Delhey and Newton 2005; Dinesen 2012; Gundelach and Manatschal 2017; Steinhardt 2012). Egalitarianism has reduced anxiety to sustain resilience (Schwartz and Melech 2000). Individualism has reflected pride to prop resilience (Suhay 2015). Satisfaction has covered democracy, economy, finance, life, public affairs, and volunteering (Almakaeva et al. 2018; Cais, Torrente, and Bolancé. 2021; Jung and Kwon 2011; Shao et al. 2021; Sun and Wang 2012). Similarity has reduced depression to afford resilience (Riad and Norris 1992). Furthermore, trust has rested on acceptance, cosmopolitanism, future orientation, permissiveness, and tolerance to furnish ideals to rationalize resilience (Freitag 2003; Uslaner 2002; Williams et al. 1999). Cosmopolitan has fostered appreciation, pleasantness, and self-esteem to maintain resilience (Gonzalez-Jimenez 2016; Chen et al. 2016). Future orientation has boosted well-being, including resilience and life satisfaction (Lou et al. 2018; MacLeod 2017). Permissiveness or tolerance has uplifted well-being, including health and satisfaction (Appleton and Song 2008; Napier and Jost 2008; Stafford et al. 2005). Trust has also built on ideals for consideration, moderation, social integration, and work to rationalize resilience (Goodman 2015; McCabe 2012; Rothstein and Uslaner 2005; Uslaner 2002). Consideration can foster morality to enable life satisfaction and diminish anger to safeguard resilience (Conzo et al. 2017; Thomas 1997; Stets et al. 2008). Moderation has evolved from self-compassion as opposed to apprehension to bolster resilience (Hernandez et al. 2002; Pyszkowska and Ronnlund 2021). Social integration has eroded depression to bolster resilience (Mullins and Dugan 1991). Working has fostered health and mastery to facilitate resilience (Borgonovi 2008; Schieman and Plickert 2008). Conversely, trust has reflected low cynicism to maintain ideals to rationalize resilience (Uslaner 2002).

Cynicism has reflected low life satisfaction and self-efficacy to impede resilience (Moreno-Jimenez and Villodres 2010; Schmuck et al. 2022). Trust has also reduced an ideal for risk to safeguard resilience (Ng 2016). Risking has damaged health to impair resilience (Wickrama et al. 1995).

Norms reflected in trust to assimilate resilience enforce morality and social integration (Gundelach and Manatschal 2017; Steinhardt 2012). Morality exposure fosters autonomy, compassion, competence, courage, flourishing, intimacy, love, and relatedness to enable resilience (Corrigan et al. 2012; Narvaez 2008). Trust has also evolved from norms for cosmopolitanism, development, equality, fairness, life quality, Protestantism, satisfaction, social cohesiveness, and trust to assimilate resilience (Almakaeva et al. 2018; Huhe 2014; Norris and Inglehart 2009; Su et al. 2019; Vera-Toscano et al. 2013; Uslaner 2002; Uslaner and Brown 2005). Societal development fosters success to induce resilience (Schneider 2006). Societal fairness has enhanced belongingness, health, life satisfaction, and self-esteem to underpin resilience (Bjornskov et al. 2013; Dalbert 2001; Lucas et al. 2013; van Prooijen et al. 2008). The norm for Protestantism has sustained well-being (Inglehart and Klingemann 2000). The satisfaction norm has induced satisfaction to induce resilience (Kulik 2006; Rampichini and D'Andrea 1998). Societal cohesiveness has boosted well-being, including health, neighborhood quality, and satisfaction with life and neighborhood as opposed to distress (Cramm et al. 2012; Fujisawa et al. 2009; Gary et al. 2007; Olson et al. 2016; Sampson 1991; Wen et al. 2010). Societal trust has assimilated trust (Uslaner 2002). Conversely, trust has reflected norms against crime and risk to assimilate resilience (Snijders and Keren 1999; Zanin 2017). Societal crime has eroded well-being, including health and satisfaction with life and the neighborhood to impede resilience (Jang et al. 2018; Manning et al. 2016; Parkes et al. 2002; Stafford et al. 2005).

## *Hardening and Softening*

Hardening and softening integrated is likely to deliver an extra contribution to resilience beyond the separate contributions of hardening and softening. This extra contribution lies in the complementarity between hardening and softening and the adaptative or flexible use of hardening and softening. Complementary emerges as the synergy of apparently contradictory tactics, hardening, and softening to enhance effectiveness (Campbell et al. 2008; Hornsey et al. 2018). Essentially, complementarity features compensation, correspondence, exchange, reinforcing, repetition, supplementarity, and synergy (Deeg 2007; Riley et al. 2011; Sadler et al. 2011; Svara 2001; Ya 2011). Adaptability or flexibility means using suitable tactics to tackle different problems to optimize effectiveness (Pyszkowska 2020). Essentially, adaptability enables achievement, control, coping, and regulation (Cabras and Mondo 2018; Hirschi and Vondracek 2009; Mehrabian 2000; Nelson and Padilla-Walker 2013). Such complementarity and flexibility realize their contributions through the voluntaristic mechanisms of power realization, utility optimization, ideal calibration, and norm conformity identified in analytical functionalism. These mechanisms entail generating power, utility, ideals, and norms from complementarity and adaptability or flexibility.

Complementarity has enhanced attachment, comfort, and cooperation to incubate power to drive resilience (Brewer 1996; Chuang 2005; Tiedens and Fragale 2003; Tsaur et al. 2014). Attachment has buttressed life satisfaction to enable resilience (Zdrenka et al. 2015). Cooperation has raised life satisfaction to secure resilience (Park et al. 2015). Similarly, complementarity generally upholds adjustment, fit or congruence, and well-being to brew power for driving resilience (Markey et al. 2003; Namini et al. 2010; Steel et al. 2012). Moreover, complementarity stands on harmony, integration, self-verification, and synergy to afford power to drive resilience (Campbell et al. 2008; Evans 1996; Fang 2003). Harmony has cultivated life satisfaction and dampened depression to maintain resilience (Yang 2016). Integration has advanced life satisfaction and dismissed anxiety and depression to afford resilience (Landolfi et al. 2021; Yang 2016). Self-verification has prevented distress to uphold resilience (Burke and Stets 1999). Conversely, complementarity dampens anxiety and conflict, thus retaining power to drive resilience (Namini et al. 2010; Rick et al. 2006). Conflict has impeded well-being, including satisfaction, to dismiss resilience (Baumeister et al. 2013; Richards 2016).

Complementarity raises quality experienced and satisfaction as utility to attract resilience (Hornsey et al. 2018). Alternatively, complementarity engenders moderation and satisfaction as ideals to rationalize resilience (Brennan et al. 2001. Moderation underlies quality and well-being to enable resilience (SunWolf 2008; Webster et al. 2014). Furthermore, complementarity realizes ideals for stabilizing to rationalize resilience (Deeg 2007). Stabilizing has maintained resilience and quality and eroded anxiety (Lock et al. 2020; Ross et al. 2000).

Adaptability has maintained commitment, interest, motivation, optimism, partnership, relational quality, socioeconomic status, and well-being to afford power to drive resilience (Frazier et al. 2007; Ginevra et al. 2016, 2018; Mitchell 2005; Nelson and Padilla-Walker 2013; Schoon 2006; Urbanaviciute et al. 2016). Commitment has sustained self-acceptance and relieved depression to foster resilience (Agronick and Duncan 1998; Wrosch et al. 2005). Interest has raised satisfaction and self-efficacy to secure resilience (Li and Wu 2013; Su, Lee, and Borah 2021). Motivation has underlain satisfaction to induce resilience (Ferssizidis et al. 2010). Optimism has enhanced positive affect to enable resilience (Shanahan et al. 2020). Partnership has built on power to drive resilience (Mitchell 2005). Socioeconomic status has sustained health, interactional quality, life satisfaction, self-confidence, self-esteem, and well-being generally to raise resilience (Al-krenawi et al. 2011; Caplan and Schooler 2007; Molana and Adams 2019; Staudinger et al. 1999). Besides, adaptability facilitates coordination, mastery, and self-esteem to consolidate power to drive resilience (Sargent-Cox et al. 2015; Silbereisen and Wiesner 2002; Widegren 1997). Coordination reflects adaptation, thus buttressing resilience (Widegren 1997). Adaptability also represents agency or control, brain or cognitive functioning, continuity, dominance, familiarity, insightfulness, integrality or loss prevention, morality, prospectiveness or planfulness, self-esteem, social support received, and wisdom to secure power to drive resilience (Hoare 2002; Kirkpatrick et al. 2002; Kozbelt et al. 2010; Narvaez 2014; Sanderson 2001; Shorthose and Maycroft 2017; Sidanius and Kurzban 2013). Agency has enhanced well-being, including autonomy, mastery, life satisfaction, relatedness, relational quality, and vitality (Delhey 2010; Hui et al. 2013; Ross and Drentea 1998; Sieber et al. 2019; Weinstein and Ryan 2010). Cognitive functioning has safeguarded resilience, happiness, health, satisfaction, and self-efficacy as opposed to depression and risk (Curtis et al. 2005; Jopp and Rott 2006; Khalaila 2016; Sawyer and Allman 2010; Sereny 2011). Continuity has raised resilience and relational quality and reduced anxiety (Lock et al. 2020; Ross et al. 2000). Dominance has boosted well-being, including health and life satisfaction (Etezadi and Pushkar 2013; Orlowski and Wicker 2015; Rose 2000). Familiarity has sustained satisfaction and self-efficacy to facilitate resilience (Norris 2011; Rothwell et al. 2016). Insightfulness encompasses acuity, mastery, and responsibility (Hoare 2002). Remarkably, insightfulness can maintain resilience and diminish distress (Baucom et al. 2018; Falon et al. 2021). Morality emphasizes actuality, equalizing, life-affirming, and mutuality as opposed to blaming (Hoare 2002). Loss prevention has upheld positive affect and life satisfaction and has dampened anger and depression to sustain resilience (Boyce et al. 2013; Steverink and Lindenberg 2006; Wells et al. 1999). Morality has satisfied life and reduced anxiety to maintain resilience (Conzo et al. 2017; Stets et al. 2008). Prospectiveness has built on health to develop resilience (Hellevik and Settersten 2013). Social support received has maintained well-being, including resilience, control, health, pleasure, purposefulness, relational quality, satisfaction, self-determination, self-efficacy, self-esteem, and social well-being (Cherry et al. 2018; George and Park 2013; Glendinning et al. 2003; Gorman et al. 2010; Holliman et al. 2021; Lincoln et al. 2003; Logan and Cobb 2013; Pierce and Quiroz 2018; Schwarzer and Knoll 2007; Williams and Galliher 2006; Xi and Hwang 2011). Wisdom features competence, confidence, emulation, and fitness (Hoare 2002). As such, wisdom has enhanced well-being, including coherence, maturity, meaningfulness, purposefulness, life satisfaction, self-efficacy, and self-understanding, to secure resilience (Baumeister et al. 2013; Camp 1989; Diener et al. 2009; Mickler and Staudinger 2008; Takahashi and Overton 2002; Webster 2010). Furthermore, adaptability features control, coping, flourishing, freedom, growth, meditation, presentness or mindfulness, rationality, religiosity, resistance, security or stability, self-control or self-discipline, and self-esteem to secure power to drive resilience (Cabras and Mondo 2018; Larsen 2018 l; Manroveli et al. 2007; McCullars et al. 2021; Nelson and Padilla-Walker 2013; Yang 1998; Zhang and Wang 2011). Coping has raised resilience, environmental and relational quality, growth, health, intimacy, satisfaction, and self-efficacy (Cherry et al. 2023; Chow et al. 2014; Gattino et al. 2015; Lau et al. 2012; Paez et al. 2007; Veenstra et al. 2005; Wills 1997). Freedom has enhanced well-being, including health, life satisfaction, and self-esteem, to boost resilience (Gehring 2013; Glendinning et al. 2003; Haller and Hadler 2006). Meditation has raised compassion or self-compassion and mindfulness and eroded depression to maintain resilience (Galante et al. 2014). Mindfulness has raised well-being, including positive affect and life satisfaction (Andrade et al. 2019; Klussman et al. 2020). Rationality has inhibited anxiety, depression, and fear to maintain resilience (Barnes and Vulcano 1982; DiGiuseppe et al. 2017). Religiosity has sustained well-being, including adjustment, flourishing, health, mastery, positive affect, relational quality, satisfaction, self-esteem, and socioemotional well-being, to advance resilience (Dy-Liacco et al. 2009; Helliwell and Putnam 2005; Flouri and Buchanan 2002; Meulemann 2010; Moschis and Ong 2011; Ng and Fisher 2016; Schieman 2001; Skerkat and Ellison 1999; Wuthnow 2004). Resistance underlies resilience (Rutter 2012). Security has safeguarded well-being, including health, neighborhood quality, and satisfaction, to escalate resilience (Chen et al. 2008; Frey et al. 2007; Jones et al. 2014). Self-control has maintained self-esteem and reduced anxiety and depression to enable resilience (Armstrong et al. 2011; Marchetti et al. 2018). Adaptability also rests on received competence, motivation, knowledge, learning, proactive personality or proactivity, and receptivity as power or its sources to drive resilience (Littlejohn et al. 2017; Tolentino et al. 2014; Wyman 2003). Knowledge has championed intimacy, satisfaction, and self-efficacy to boost resilience (Mikulincer et al. 2003; Norris 2011; Rothwell et al. 2016). Learning gained has enhanced self-efficacy to secure resilience (Byars-Winston and Rogers 2019). Proactivity reflects coping and protection to enable resilience (Seaton and Beaumont 2008; Shaw et al. 2023). Receptivity has sustained health, life satisfaction, and social trust to enhance resilience (Appleton and Song 2008; Stafford et al. 2005; Uslaner 2002). Furthermore, adaptability reflects agreeableness, creativity, cultural capital, emotional intelligence, openness, positive development or maturity, and wisdom to furnish power to drive resilience (Di Fabio et al. 2015; Draper and Holman 2005; Edgerton et al. 2008; Guerra and Bradshaw 2008; Sternberg 2004; Wang et al. 2017). Agreeableness has maintained growth, mastery, purposefulness, life satisfaction, relatedness, and self-acceptance to enable resilience (Hounkpatin et al. 2015). Creativity has sustained well-being, notably meaningfulness, to buttress resilience (Diener et al. 2009; Turner 2013). Cultural capital has enhanced religiosity to secure resilience (Wuthnow 2004). Emotional intelligence has facilitated well-being, including adaptation, happiness, health, life satisfaction, positive mood, relatedness, relational quality, and self-esteem to enhance resilience (Ciarrochi et al. 2000; Kluemper 2008; Matthews et al. 2012; Mayer et al. 2001; Schutte et al. 2002). Openness has secured well-being, including autonomy, growth, life satisfaction, purposefulness, relational quality, self-acceptance, self-efficacy, and self-esteem, to champion resilience (Hahn et al. 2013; Hounkpatin et al. 2014; Karwowski and Lebuda 2017; Marks 1996; Quilty et al. 2006; Webster et al. 2014). Moreover, adaptability has benefitted from agreeableness, conscientiousness, coping, education, ego strength, enjoyment, friendship, identity achieved, income, intelligence, language proficiency, optimism, positive mood, problem-solving skill, social class, social attachment, spiritual well-being, and training to maintain power to drive resilience (Aspinwall and Taylor 1992; Burgess et al. 2006; Hickman et al. 2000; Kneipp et al. 2009; Lee and Lee 2020; Liu and Chen 2010; Pratt and Matsuba 2018; Samios and Baran 2018; Simonton and Garn 2020; Stoynoff 1997; Tolentino et al. 2014; Yeh et al. 2013; Wintre and Yaffe 2000). Conscientiousness has raised attachment, autonomy, life satisfaction, mastery, purposefulness, and self-acceptance to secure resilience (Fraley et al. 2011; Hounkpatin et al. 2015). Education has sustained well-being, including health, identity, life quality and satisfaction, mastery, self-efficacy, self-esteem, and youthfulness to engender resilience (Cerin and Leslie 2008; Corcoran et al. 2011; James and Amato 2013; Pakulshi and Tranter 2000; Stavrova and Ehlebracht 2018; van Praag and Frijters 1999; Whyte and Gao 2009; Yienprugsawan et al. 2010). Ego strength has boosted well-being, including authenticity, flow, mastery, and satisfaction to furnish resilience (Bakker and Geurts 2004; Huber et al. 2020; Matsuo 2020; Nifadkar and Bauer 2016). Friendship has built on health, satisfaction, and fearlessness to sustain resilience (Child and Nikolova 2020; Eberl 2020; Sampson 1991). Identity achieved has advanced happiness, self-efficacy, and self-esteem and erased anxiety, thus safeguarding resilience (Cast 2004). Income has afforded well-being, including adaptation, adequacy, belongingness, control, eudaemonia, health, mastery, power, quality of life, satisfaction, self-efficacy, self-esteem, and social well-being to sustain resilience (Anciaes et al. 2017; Carpiano 2008; Corcoran et al. 2011; Ross and Mirowsky 1989; Sengupta and Sibley 2019; Son and Wilson 2012; Wang and VanderWeele 2011; Yeh et al. 2013; Zimmerman and Reyna 2013). Intelligence has assuaged depression to maintain resilience (Feinstein and Bynner 2006). Language proficiency has secured relational quality and satisfaction to boost resilience (Lancee and Dronkers 2011; Van Praag et al. 2010). Optimism has enhanced positive affect to enable resilience (Shanahan et al. 2020). Problem-solving skill has buttressed self-efficacy to enable resilience (Larson et al. 1990). Social class has sustained well-being, including financial adequacy, health, hope, and satisfaction, as opposed to depression to advance resilience (Burke 2008; Davis and Davenport 1999; Haller and Hadler 2006; Hadjar and Samuel 2015; Peterson and Seligman 2004; Yamaoka 2008). Social attachment has enabled compassion, health, intimacy, and life satisfaction to sustain resilience (Alonso-Arbiol et al. 2007; Headey et al. 2001; Mikulincer et al. 2005; Zdrenka et al. 2015). Training has upgraded adjustment, comfort, coherence, cohesiveness, competence, emotional well-being, growth, hope, identity, purposiveness, self-efficacy, self-esteem, thriving, and transcendence to advance resilience (Ashby et al. 2018; Davidson et al. 2012; Duan and Bu 2019; Esbensen and Osgood 1999; Feldman and Dreher 2012; Moote et al. 1999; Ou et al. 2019; Umino and Dammeyer 2018; Youniss and Yates 1997). Conservely, adaptability represents low conflict experienced, control experienced, narcissism, and pressure received, thus retaining power to drive resilience (Donnellan et al. 2009; Hoare 2002; Scharf and Levy 2015). Conflict has provoked distress and eroded satisfaction, thus impeding resilience (Lau et al. 2017; Mikula et al. 2012). Control or pressure experienced has raised distress to attenuate resilience (Overall et al. 2020). Narcissism has activated aggression, depression, misbehavior, and relational dissatisfaction, thus eroding resilience (Tracy et al. 2009). Adaptability has also benefitted from low disruption experienced, gang association, neuroticism, stress experienced, and tension experienced to muster power to drive resilience (Cadwallader and Cairns 2002; Gfellner and Cordoba 2017; Gutman et al. 2005; Hickman et al. 2000). Disruption experienced has been dissatisfying to erode resilience (Downey and Ainsworth-Darnell 2002). Stress experienced has dampened well-being, including health, life quality, positive affect, and satisfaction as opposed to depression and distress, to impede resilience (Baumeister et al. 2013. Mathis et al. 2016; Raposa et al. 2016;

Shrira 2012; Snyder et al. 2020; Zotti et al. 2016). Adaptability also precludes alienation, defectiveness, dependence, depression, disconnection, doping, floundering, limitation, shamefulness, mistrust, other-directedness or passivity, and vulnerability, thus keeping power to drive resilience (McCullars et al. 2021; Nelson and Padilla-Walker 2013). Alienation experienced has fomented feelings of depression, guilt, internalizing, loneliness, negative emotion, resentment, and stupidity to disturb resilience (Sommer et al. 2001; Tani and Schneider 1997; Witkow 2005). Defectiveness has eroded functionality, health and mental health, knowledge, optimism, security, vitality, and general well-being, thus disempowering resilience (Benitez-Silva et al. 2010; Carrieri 2012; Korkeila et al. 2004; Price et al. 2006; van Dijk et al. 2008). Dependence has weakened coping and health, thus eroding resilience (Bekker et al. 2011; Roy and Chaudhuri 2008). Disconnection has eroded well-being, including community, flourishing, health, identity, life satisfaction, and pride, thus obstructing resilience (Chua et al. 2021; Yetim and Yetim 2014). Doping has engendered depression, thus jeopardizing resilience (Kendler et al. 2006). Floundering has impaired well-being, including life and marital satisfaction, to block resilience (Mikula et al. 2012; Pomerleau et al. 2020; Richards 2016). Limitation has eroded health, satisfaction with housing, leisure, and life, and self-efficacy, thus hampering resilience (Distante 2013; Gastil 2000; Granzin and Haggard 2000). Mistrust has impeded health and survival, thus dampening resilience (Barefoot et al. 1998). Passivity reflects low commitment, thus unable to drive resilience (Guerrero 2015). Shamefulness reflects distress to impede resilience (Lively 2017). Vulnerability has eroded mattering and self-efficacy to obstruct resilience (Flett 2018; Kim et al. 2016).

Adaptability has facilitated success experienced as utility to attract resilience (Mehrabian 2000). Success has benefitted from happiness and relaxation to enhance resilience (Lyubomirsky et al. 2005; Mehrabian 2000). Moreover, adaptability enhances desirability, likability, or positivity experienced to maintain utility to attract resilience (Floyd 2019; Gifford 2011). Desirability, likability, or positivity experienced or popularity has uplifted positive affect and self-esteem and reduced negative affect, thus buttressing resilience (Reich et al. 2018). Adaptability also represents or builds on acceptance experienced or popularity, consensus experienced, controllability expected, reciprocity expected, and responsiveness experienced as utility to attract resilience (Martin et al. 1999; Narvaez 2014; Simonton and Garn 2020; Trang and Yates 2020; Wyman 2003). Consensus experienced has buttressed emotional well-being, meaningfulness, and relatedness to secure resilience (Heshmati and Oravecz 2022). Controllability expected has boosted well-being, including health and life satisfaction as opposed to anger and depression, to maintain resilience (Etezadi and Pushkar 2013; Heidemeier and Staudinger 2012; Rose 2000; Xi and Hwang 2011). Reciprocity experienced has stemmed from low loneliness to maintain resilience (Espvall and Dellgran 2010). Responsiveness experienced has raised adaptation, life satisfaction, positive emotion, and relational quality to secure resilience (Algoe and Zhaoyang 2016). Likewise, adaptability has benefitted from resolution experienced to maintain utility to attract resilience (Pratt and Matsuba 2018). Resolution has stood on autonomy, competence, and self-confidence as opposed to depression to maintain resilience (Levesque-Bristol et al. 2011; Siu and Shek 2005).

Furthermore, adaptability involves achievement and peace experienced as utility to attract resilience (Hirschi and Vondracek 2009). Achievement has fostered health, life quality, satisfaction, self-efficacy, and self-esteem as opposed to alienation, depression, and distress to uphold resilience (Donnellan et al. 2005; Fredricks and Eccles 2005; Menard and Mose 1984; Murray 2009; Piko et al. 2006; Tompson and Dass 2000; Xiao et al. 2009). Peace experienced has fostered life satisfaction and has impeded depression to maintain resilience (Smith et al. 2016). Conversely, adaptability disengages from crisis and failure, thus retaining utility to attract resilience (Cui et al. 2022; Larsen 2018; McCullars et al. 2021). The crisis experienced has weakened well-being, including health and life satisfaction, to hurt resilience (Baumeister et al. 2013; Mathis et al. 2016; Zotti et al. 2016). Failure has reflected low happiness and relaxation, thus disrupting resilience (Lyubomirsky et al. 2005; Mehrabian 2000). Adaptability has also reflected low risk experienced, thus maintaining utility to attract resilience (Schoon 2006). Risk experienced has inhibited achievement, happiness, life satisfaction, positive affect, and self-determination to dampen resilience (Schoon 2006; Schwartz and Melech 2000; Shippee 2012; Zotti et al. 2016).

Adaptability has escalated compliance, learning, the future, and satisfaction as ideals to rationalize resilience (Ginevra et al. 2016; James and Hunsley 1995; Nelson and Padilla-Walker 2013; Tolentino et al. 2014). The ideal for compliance has buttressed compliance (Van Damme 2017). Compliance has furnished achievement and its pressure, mastery-goal setting, social closeness and support received, and tolerance to benefit resilience (Feldman 2003; Jiang et al. 2015; Magnuson et al. 2006). The ideal for learning has induced learning (Hagger and Hamilton 2018). Learning has elevated well-being, including life satisfaction and self-efficacy to facilitate resilience (Denver and Hands 1990; Minnaert and Janssen 1992; Richards 2016). The ideal for the future has furnished resilience and life satisfaction (Lou et al. 2018; MacLeod 2017). Moreover, adaptability maintains caring, habituation, integration, and the set point or stability as ideals to rationalize resilience (Cummins et al. 2009; Hoare 2002; Richards 2016). The ideal for caring has buttressed caring (Sarasa 2008). Caring has maintained mental clarity to boost resilience (Naruse et al. 2020). The ideal for habituation has secured habituation (Bennett and Bennett 2004). Habituation has maintained satisfaction as opposed to discord to induce resilience (Chow et al. 2014; James and Hunsley 1995). Integration within the mind is inherently idealistic (Kulin and Seymer 2014). Essentially, integration underlies confidence to achieve resilience (Simon and Read 2018). The ideal for stability has buttressed stability (Zumbrunnen and Gangl 2008). Stability has raised resilience and relational quality (Lock et al. 2020; Ross et al. 2000). Adaptability also features ideals for calmness, compassion, equality, justice, self-acceptance, and sublimation to rationalize resilience (Larsen 2018; Vaillant 1977; Zhang and Wang 2011). The ideal for compassion activates compassion (Clobert et al. 2015). Calmness has prevented depression to sustain resilience (Hamm et al. 2021). Compassion has sustained well-being to drive resilience (Jasielska 2020). The ideal for equality or egalitarianism has diminished anxiety to sustain resilience (Schwartz and Melech 2000). Meanwhile, the ideal for justice realizes flourishing to enable resilience (Williams 2008). The ideal for self-acceptance has incubated self-acceptance (Pelham and Swann 1989). Self-acceptance has buttressed well-being, including adjustment, affect, happiness, health, positive affect, and satisfaction, as opposed to depression, distress, negative affect, and strain, to induce resilience (Barnard and Curry 2011; Frederick et al. 2016; Hull et al. 2008; Judge et al. 2002; Tracy et al. 2009; Williams et al. 1992). Sublimation means transforming weaknesses into pleasure (Vaillant 1977). As such, sublimation can buttress well-being, notably pleasure, to enable resilience (Marcus 2014; Turner 2006). Furthermore, adaptability reflects individualism as an ideal to rationalize resilience (Fouad and Bynner 2008). Individualism has bolstered well-being, including life satisfaction and self-efficacy, to enable resilience (Kim et al. 2016; Oishi 2000; Veenhoven 1998). Adaptability has also built on ideals for communion, deliberation, exploration, moderation, performance, preparation, prosociality, strategizing, and work to rationalize resilience (Autin et al. 2017; Cui et al. 2022; Guroglu et al. 2007; Izzo et al. 1999; Martin et al. 2017; Mei et al. 2021; Petress 1995; Pratt and Matsuba 2018; Stoynoff 1997). Communion has advanced connectedness and diminished negative emotions and stress to uplift resilience (Nelson-Coffey et al. 2023). Deliberation has prevented aggression, anxiety, avoidance, depression, and disorders to maintain resilience (DiGiuseppe et al. 2017). Exploration has developed self-efficacy to empower resilience (Harre 2007). Moderation has evolved from self-compassion as opposed to apprehension to bolster resilience (Hernandez et al. 2002; Pyszkowska and Ronnlund 2021). Performance has reflected self-determination, self-efficacy, and the sense of community to boost resilience (Asoodar et al. 2014; Moller et al. 2006; Yashima 2010). Preparation has enabled acceptance to uphold resilience (Curry et al. 2015). The prosocial ideal underlies prosociality (Maltseva 2016). Prosociality has elevated well-being, including connectedness, hope, life satisfaction, meaningfulness, and self-efficacy to boost resilience (Marsh and Dik 2021; Nelson-Coffey et al. 2023; Raposa et al. 2016; Yao and Enright 2019). Strategizing has raised well-being, including autonomy, coherence, maturity, meaningfulness, purposefulness, life satisfaction, and self-efficacy (Diener et al. 2009; Greene and Brown 2009; Mickler and Staudinger 2008; Webster 2010). The ideal for work has championed working (Marsh and Dik 2021). Working has advanced health and mastery to secure resilience (Borgonovi 2008; Schieman and Plickert 2008). Conversely, adaptability weakens aspiration, cynicism, isolation, and rejection as ideals against resilience (Hoare 2002; Watkins 2016). Aspiration has impaired life satisfaction, thus undermining resilience (Nickerson et al. 2007). Cynicism has reflected low life satisfaction and self-efficacy to impede resilience (Moreno-Jimenez and Villodres 2010; Schmuck et al. 2022). Self-isolation has eroded self-esteem, thus dampening resilience (Young and Bagley 1982). The ideal for rejection underlies rejection (North and Fiske 2013). Rejecting has weakened belongingness and confidence, thus impeding resilience (Juanchich et al. 2018). Furthermore, adaptability opposes aggression, blaming, catastrophizing, pessimism, rumination, self-sacrifice, and subjugation as ideals against resilience (McCullars et al. 2021; Sanchez-Perez et al. 2018; Zsido et al. 2021). The ideal for aggression has fomented aggression (Markowitz 2001). Aggression or violence has bred depression, thus disturbing resilience (Wright et al. 2015). Blaming has reflected conflict perception and distress as opposed to compromise to impede resilience (Bagci and Celebi 2017; Recchia and Howe 2010; Wayment et al. 2010). Catastrophizing dismisses resilience and has eroded well-being to weaken resilience (Alschuler et al. 2016). Adaptability has also diminished violence as an ideal against resilience (Han and Grogan-Kaylor 2012).

Adaptability has sustained norms for adjustment to assimilate resilience (James and Hunsley 1995). Moreover, adaptability has built on norms for achievement, involvement, reciprocity, and security to assimilate resilience (Sacker et al. 2002; Scharf and Levy 2015; Wintre and Yaffe 2000). The norm for achievement has assimilated achievement (Cullen and Jacob 2009; Gremmen et al. 2017; Teachman 1996). Achievement has fostered health, life quality, satisfaction, self-efficacy, and self-esteem as opposed to alienation, depression, and distress to uphold resilience (Donnellan et al. 2005; Fredricks and Eccles 2005; Menard and Mose 1984; Murray 2009; Piko et al. 2006; Tompson and Dass 2000; Xiao et al. 2009). The norm of involvement has assimilated involvement (Wong et al. 2018). Involvement has facilitated self-acceptance to secure resilience (Agronick and Duncan 1998). The norm for reciprocity has induced reciprocity (Avalos 2019). Reciprocity has facilitated adaptation as opposed to illness to create resilience (Yamaoka 2008; Yeh et al. 2013). The norm for security has fostered security (Gaitan-Rossi and Shen 2018). Security has escalated well-being, including health and life satisfaction to raise resilience (Chen et al. 2008; Frey et al. 2007; Jones et al. 2014). Conversely, adaptability arises from norms against conflict, disruption, distress, and harshness to assimilate resilience (Donnellan et al. 2009; Shumow et al. 1998; Martin et al. 2017). The norm for conflict has bred conflict (Amato and Chendle 2005). Conflict has weakened well-being, including life and marital satisfaction, to hamper resilience (Baumeister et al. 2013; Mikula et al. 2012; Richards 2016). The norm for disruption has fueled disruption (Zimmermann and Bingenheimer 2002). Disruption has undermined resilience and relational quality and has fomented anxiety, depression, distress, and dysfunction (Brensilver et al. 2011; Davis et al. 2002; Graber et al. 2016; Khamis 2006; Zalewski et al. 2017). The norm for distress has brewed distress (Cheung and Leung 2011). Distress can inhibit resilience (Park 2017).

Flexibility has generated commitment and self-esteem to sustain power to drive resilience (Agronick and Duncan 1998). Commitment has advanced self-acceptance and diminished depression to sustain resilience (Agronick and Duncan 1998; Wrosch et al. 2005). Moreover, flexibility displays power residing in coping, creativity, health, presentness, and other resources to drive resilience (Agronick and Duncan 1998; Kato 2015; Pyszkowska 2020; Pyszkowska and Ronnlund 2021). Coping has sustained resilience, health, intimacy, quality in environment and relationship, satisfaction, self-efficacy, and well-being generally (Cherry et al. 2023; Chow et al. 2014; Gattino et al. 2015; Lau et al. 2012; Veenstra et al. 2005; Wills 1997). Meanwhile, coping has reduced depression, distress, and fear to maintain resilience (Littleton et al. 2007; Krulichova 2019; Wills 1997). Creativity has boosted well-being, notably meaningfulness, to induce resilience (Diener et al. 2009; Turner 2013). Presentness is a manifestation of mindfulness (Feldman and Kuyken 2019). Mindfulness has sustained well-being, including life satisfaction and positive affect, to champion resilience (Andrade et al. 2019; Klussman et al. 2020). Flexibility has built on agreeableness, conscientiousness, emotional intelligence, enjoyment, extraversion, honesty or humility, openness, and self-esteem to generate power to drive resilience (Pyszkowska 2020; Simonton and Garn 2020; Tett and Wang 2005). Agreeableness has enabled growth, life satisfaction, mastery, purposefulness, relatedness, and self-acceptance to elevate resilience (Hounkpatin et al. 2015). Conscientiousness has secured autonomy, growth, life satisfaction, mastery, purposefulness, relatedness, and self-acceptance to activate resilience (Hounkpatin et al. 2015). Emotional intelligence has relevantly covered attention, empathy, reasoning, and recognition (Tett and Wang 2005). As such, emotional intelligence has escalated well-being, including adaptation, happiness, health, life satisfaction, optimism, positive mood, relatedness, relational quality, and self-esteem to safeguard resilience (Ciarrochi et al. 2000; Kluemper 2008; Matthews et al. 2012; Mayer et al. 2004; Schutte et al. 2002). Extraversion has raised well-being, including autonomy, growth, mastery, positive affect, purposefulness, relatedness, satisfaction, self-acceptnce, self-determination, self-efficacy, and self-esteem to facilitate resilience (Hounkpatin et al. 2015; Ingledew et al. 2004; Quilty et al. 2006; Rasmussen et al. 2018; Richards 2016; Tiwari et al. 2021). Honesty has prevented distress and fear to safeguard resilience (Ellis and Renouf 2018; Weinberg et al. 2021). Humility has enabled connectedness to facilitate resilience (Angelis and Pensini 2024). Openness has advanced well-being, including autonomy, growth, life satisfaction, purposefulness, relational quality, self-acceptance, self-efficacy, and self-esteem to boost resilience (Hahn et al. 2013; Hounknatin et al. 2014; Karwowski and Lebuda 2017; Marks 1996; Webster et al. 2014). Conversely, flexibility has reduced depression, distress, and threat experienced, thus maintaining power to drive resilience (Hudetz et al. 2004; Jen et al. 2019; Kato 2015; Quilty et al. 2006). Threat experienced had eroded relational quality and raised anxiety and depression to obstruct resilience (Jackson et al. 2006; Moore and Shepherd 2006; O'Neill and Evans 1999). Flexibility has also stemmed from low emotionality, including anxiety and sentimentality, to retain power to drive resilience (Pyszkowska 2020). Emotionality has dampened well-being, including autonomy, growth, health, positive affect, purposefulness, relatedness, relational quality, satisfaction, self-acceptance, self-compassion, and self-determination, to impede resilience (Anusic et al. 2014; Austin et al. 2005; Hounkpatin et al. 2015; Ingledew et al. 2004; Marks 1996; Pfattheicher et al. 2017; Richards 2016; Webster et al. 2014).

Flexibility has sustained utility from control expectancy to attract resilience (Simonton and Garn 2020). Control experienced has sustained well-being, including autonomy, life satisfaction, mastery, relatedness, relational quality, and vitality, to secure resilience (Delhey 2010; Hui et al. 2013; Ross and Drentea 1998; Sieber et al. 2019; Weinstein and Ryan 2010). Flexibility arises from utility or value expected to attract resilience (Simonton and Garn 2020). Furthermore, flexibility has developed from reciprocity expected to attract resilience (Jen et al. 2019). Reciprocity experienced has reflected low loneliness to enable resilience (Espvall and Dellgran 2010).

Flexibility has raised adaptation, disclosure, and life satisfaction as ideals to rationalize resilience (Hrehorciuc-Caragea and White 2017; Jen et al. 2019; Pyszkowska

2020). Disclosure has reflected self-esteem to enable resilience (Hollenbaugh and Ferris 2015). Moreover, flexibility realizes acceptance and staying or persistence as ideals to rationalize resilience (Pyszkowska 2020; Pyszkowska and Ronnlund 2021). Persistence has sustained well-being, notably pleasure, to facilitate resilience (Boyes et al. 2017; Goodman et al. 2017).

## *Westernization*

Westernization foregrounds consumerism, globalism, individualism, materialism, and Protestantism (Fu and Chiu 2007; Ma 2019; Narvaez 2014; Zhou 2008). More specifically, Westernization embraces control, democracy, detachment, entertainment, escape, freedom, knowledge, mastery, safety, standardization, status, tolerance, and unconventionality (Csanyi et al. 2023; Hodge 2018; Janion 2020; Narvaez 2014). Notably, Westernization hails its domination or hegemony (Hodge 2018; Kenny et al. 2013). Conversely, Westernization downplays collectivism, environmentalism, government, harmony, and solidarity (Fu and Chiu 2007; Kenny et al. 2013; Ma 2019). Westernization maintains civilization, industrialization, and religion, specifically Christianity (Kenny et al. 2013; Ma 2019). As such, Westernization is likely to foster resilience by generating power, utility or incentive, ideals, and norms to run the deterministic and voluntaristic mechanisms of analytical functionalism. Whereas these deterministic mechanisms comprise empowering, incentivizing, normalizing or standardizing, and framing or signifying, voluntaristic mechanisms encompass power realization, utility optimization, ideal calibration, and norm conformity.

Power reflected by Westernization to boost resilience has resided in competence and religiosity (Guan et al. 2010). Religiosity has sustained well-being, including adjustment, flourishing, health, mastery, positive affect, relational quality, satisfaction, self-esteem, and socioemotional well-being to enable resilience (Behr 2010; Dy-Liacco et al. 2009; Flouri and Buchanan 2002; Helliwell and Putnam 2005; Moschis and Ong 2011; Ng and Fisher 2016; Schieman 2001; Skerkat and Ellison 1999; Wuthnow 2004). Conversely, religiosity has diminished depression, fear, and loneliness to maintain resilience (Ellison et al. 2001; Hui et al. 2007; Lauder et al. 2006).

Ideals embraced by Westernization to rationalize resilience accentuate achievement, consumerism, controlling or mastery, domination, freedom, individualism, knowledge, Protestantism, safety, self-determination, and tolerance (AlShebali et al. 2021; Csanyi et al. 2023; Ma 2019; Narvaez 2014; Zhou 2008). The ideal for achievement has propelled achievement (Mehrabian 2000). As such, achievement reflects happiness and relaxation to arrod resilience (Lyubomirsky et al. 2005; Mehrabian 2000). The ideal for control has motivated controlling, domination, or mastery (Cheung and Chiu 2021). Consumerism represents demand, empowerment, hedonism, and rationality (Behr 2010; Guillen-Royo 2008; Himes 2007). Essentially, consumerism emphasizes expressionism, materialism, neoliberalism, privatization, self-direction, and self-help (Cherrier 2010; Stevenson et al. 2008; Yngfalk 2016;

Zukin and Maguire 2004). As such, consumerism maintains or builds on belongingness, income, independence, knowledgeability, safety or security, self-determination, and solidarity among consumers to facilitate resilience (Behr 2010; Stehr 2008). Controlling, domination, or mastery, in turn, has championed well-being, including health and life satisfaction as opposed to anger (Etezadi and Pushkar 2013; Cundiff et al. 2015; Orlowski and Wicker 2015; Rose 2000). The ideal for freedom or liberalism has rested on growth to induce resilience (Helson and Srivastava 2001). Individualism has evolved from pride to activate resilience (Suhay 2015). The ideal or interest is the basis for knowledge (Hutchings 2003). Knowledge has sustained satisfaction and self-efficacy to facilitate resilience (Norris 2011; Rothwell et al. 2016). Protestantism has alleviated negative emotionality to lift resilience (Kim and Cohen 2017). The ideal for safety has developed from health to enable resilience (Cheung and Lai 2020). Self-determination has built on its value (Waterman et al. 2003). Eventually, self-determination has sustained well-being, including life satisfaction, mastery, relatedness, relational quality, and vitality as opposed to anxiety and depression to enable resilience (Delhey 2010; Hui et al. 2013; Ross and Drentea 1998; Schwartz and Melech 2000; Sheldon and Bettencourt 2002; Sieber et al. 2019; Weinstein and Ryan 2010).

## *Socializing*

Socializing manifests assurance, closeness, disclosure, networking, openness, positivity, sharing, and understanding to others (Hampton 2007; Kayabol et al. 2022). Essentially, socializing represents flourishing (Goodman et al. 2017). Socializing is crucially valuable for resilience (Chua et al. 2019). The value lies in generating power, utility, ideals, and norms to activate the voluntaristic mechanisms of analytical functionalism.

Power enhanced by socializing to drive resilience has rested on connectedness (Nelson-Coffey et al. 2023). Moreover, socializing enhances belongingness and its need, identity, self-esteem, and social inclusion experienced to muster power to drive resilience (Baumeister and Leary 1995; Malloy 2018). Meanwhile, socializing has stemmed from happiness, mindfulness, self-esteem, and self-expansion to establish power to drive resilience (Flett 2018; Ledbetter et al. 2013). Self-expansion has reduced depression and negative affect to enhance resilience (McIntyre et al. 2023; Stanton et al. 2020). Conversely, socializing diminished negative emotion and stress to retain power to drive resilience (Nelson-Coffey et al. 2023). Moreover, socializing prevents anxiety, divorce, and social undermining experienced, thus holding power to drive resilience (Baumeister and Leary 1995). Divorce has reflected low family, life and marital satisfaction, health, self-efficacy, and self-worth, thus facilitating resilience (Burch 2020; Cast and Burke 2002; Fan and Lui 2004; Yang and Yen 2012). Socializing has also reflected low stress to retain power for driving resilience (Flett 2018).

Utility acquired by socializing to attract resilience has involved positive experiences (Nelson-Coffey et al. 2023). Positive experiences have raised life satisfaction and positive affect to raise resilience (Maybery et al. 2006). Socializing has also arisen from equity, popularity, and success experienced to create resilience (Ledbetter et al. 2013). Equity experienced has fostered belongingness, health, life satisfaction, and self-esteem as opposed to anger and depression to maintain resilience (Benson and Ritter 1990; Bjornskov et al. 2013; Dalbert 2001; Lucas et al. 2013; Rothmund et al. 2014; van Prooijen et al. 2008). Popularity experienced has sustained belongingness, positive affect, and self-esteem as opposed to negative affect to secure resilience (Reich et al. 2018). Success has benefitted from happiness and relaxation to enhance resilience (Lyubomirsky et al. 2005; Mehrabian 2000).

Ideals developed by socializing to rationalize resilience emphasize agreement (Felmlee and Sinclair 2018). Socializing also embraces ideals for openness, positivity, sharing, and understanding to rationalize resilience (Kayabol et al. 2022). Openness has facilitated well-being, including autonomy, growth, life satisfaction, purposefulness, relational quality, self-acceptance, self-efficacy, and self-esteem to induce resilience (Hahn et al. 2013; Hounknatin et al. 2014; Karwowski and Lebuda 2017; Quilty et al. 2006). Positive thinking has sustained positive affect and survival to enable resilience (Clarke et al. 2000; Shanahan et al. 2020). Sharing has reduced stress to maintain resilience (Lazar and Eisenberger 2022). The ideal for sharing has reflected social attachment to enhance resilience (Erez et al. 2008). Furthermore, socializing reflects life satisfaction and self-acceptance to maintain ideals for rationalizing resilience (Gountas et al. 2012; Kayabol et al. 2022; Utz and Breuer 2017).

## Religious Practice

Religious practice features religious attending, caring, chanting, coping, dining, forgiving, praying, reading, ritualizing, studying, and tutoring (Katz-Gerro and Shavit 1998; Lehmann and Gorsuch 2017; Marks 2004; Myers 2014; Simpson et al. 2008; Upenieks 2022; Wuthnow 2004). Such practice realizes altruism, authoritarianism, belongingness, commitment, community, faith, groupism, inculcation, morality, ritualism, sacredness, sacrifice, self-control, sharing, sociality, solidarity, spirituality, strictness, and transcendence (Donnelly 2013; Franks et al. 2013; Harris et al. 2018; Kalkstein and Tower 2009; Kay et al. 2008; Leung et al. 2002; Lichterman 2012; Lloyd et al. 2022; Peifer 2010; Petrovic et al. 2020). For the youth, religious practice additionally characterizes identity, meaningfulness, modeling, networking, skills for community, coping, and leadership, and socialization or learning (De Haan and Schulenberg 1997; King and Roeser 2009; Mayrl and Uecker 2011; Regnerus 2003). Religious practice builds on aesthetics, communitarianism, cosmology, divinity, existentialism, functionalism, miracle, morality, naturalness, solidarity, and traditionalism (Grayling 2013; Haddorff 2000; Perlin 2011; Segal 1989; von Stuckrad 2013). Existentialism relevantly hails awe or reverence, commonality, freedom, humility, love, meaningfulness, and surrendering (Friedman 1992). Religious practice is crucial for belongingness, discipline, education, meaningfulness, morality, social evolution, solidarity or unity, survival, and well-being (De Graaf 2013; Ishii and Watanabe 2023; Turner 2009; Werbner 2010). Social evolution concerns adaptiveness, binding, coherence, control, ethics or morality, and sharing (De Graaf 2013; Demerath 2002; Haidt 2012). For the youth, religious practice is additionally relevant to development or thriving, identity, motivation, resources or capital, and sociality (Heaven and Ciarrochi 2007; King and Roeser 2009). As such, religious practice is likely to nurture resilience by creating power, utility, ideals, and norms to apply the voluntaristic mechanisms of power realization, utility optimization, ideal calibration, and norm conformity in analytical functionalism.

Power raised by religious practice to drive resilience arises from adaptiveness, belongingness, controlling, discipline, education, meaningfulness, morality, positive emotion, social cohesiveness, solidarity or unity, spiritual relatedness, and well-being (Demerath 2002; Ishii and Watanabe 2023; Levin and Chatters 1998; Medvedovski and Allison 2017; Skerkat and Ellison 1999; Turner 2009; Werbner 2010). Controlling has enhanced well-being, including health and life satisfaction, as opposed to anger and depression to enable resilience (Etezadi and Pushkar 2013; Cundiff et al. 2015; Orlowski and Wicker 2015; Rose 2000; Xi and Hwang 2011). Discipline has strengthened well-being, notably self-esteem, to induce resilience (Armstrong et al. 2011; Diener and Fujita 1995). Education has sustained well-being, including health, identity, life quality and satisfaction, mastery, self-efficacy, self-esteem, and youthfulness to engender resilience (Cerin and Leslie 2008; Corcoran et al. 2011; James and Amato 2013; Pakulshi and Tranter 2000; Stavrova and Ehlebracht 2018; van Praag and Frijters 1999; Whyte and Gao 2009; Yienprugsawan et al. 2010). Morality has enabled life satisfaction and diminished anger to safeguard resilience (Conzo et al. 2017; Stets et al. 2008). Social cohesiveness, solidarity, or unity has raised hope and life satisfaction and diminished depression to generate resilience (Araya et al. 2006; Dittman and Goebel 2010; Paez et al. 2015). Spirituality has enhanced meaningfulness to facilitate resilience (George and Park 2013). Religious practice also strengthens the ego and trust to consolidate power to drive resilience (Forsyth 2003). Ego strength has boosted well-being, including authenticity, flow, mastery, and satisfaction to furnish resilience (Bakker and Geurts 2004; Huber et al. 2020; Matsuo 2020; Nifadkar and Bauer 2016). Trust has promoted health and survival to secure resilience (Barefoot et al. 1998). Furthermore, religious practice involves community or congregation, coping, divine relatedness, maturity, and social attachment and integration to secure power to drive resilience (Marsh and Dik 2021; Shorey et al. 2018; Tenorio and Lo 2011; Upenieks 2022; Wollschleger 2012). Community involvement has enhanced well-being, including mastery and self-efficacy, to enable resilience (Harter and Arora 2010; Ohmer 2007). Coping has strengthened resilience, growth, and health. intimacy, life quality, satisfaction, and self-efficacy (Cherry et al. 2023; Chow et al. 2014; Gattino et al. 2015; Lau et al. 2012; Paez et al. 2007; Veenstra et al 2005; Wills 1997). Maturity has developed from self-compassion and self-tolerance to strengthen resilience (Ho and Li 2022; Munroe et al. 2022). Social attachment has enabled compassion, health, intimacy, and life satisfaction to sustain resilience

(Alonso-Arbiol et al. 2007; Headey et al. 2001; Mikulincer et al. 2005; Zdrenka et al. 2015). Social integration has impeded depression to enable resilience (Mullins and Dugan 1991). Religious practice has also buttressed adjustment, civility, coping, empathy, friendship, health and its maintenance, mastery, organizational membership, positive affect, relational quality, self-esteem, social capital, socioemotional well-being, and trust in institutions and others to secure power to drive resilience (Dy-Liacco et al. 2009; Flouri and Buchanan 2002; Chang 2009; Hakhverdian and Mayne 2012; Helliwell and Putnam 2005; Keyes 2002; Moschis and Ong 2011; Myers 2008; Perks and Haan 2011; Saroglou and Anciaux 2004; Schieman 2001; Skerkat and Ellison 1999; Wuthnow 2004; Zanin 2017). Civility has built on satisfaction to induce resilience (Ho and Chan 2009). Empathy has enhanced intimacy and reduced discontent and resentment to elevate resilience (Redmond 2018). Friendship has built on health, satisfaction, and fearlessness to sustain resilience (Child and Nikolova 2020; Eberl 2020; Sampson 1991). Health maintenance has improved health and prevented depression to secure resilience (Smith et al. 2006; Myers 2008). Organizational membership has advanced well-being, notably health, to sustain resilience (Tsai et al. 2018). Social capital has enhanced well-being, including community, flourishing, health, identity, life satisfaction, and pride to prop resilience (Chua et al. 2021; Yetim and Yetim 2014). Furthermore, religious practice reflects power based on energy and sympathy to drive resilience (Wollschleger 2012). Religious practice has similarly evolved from agreeableness, conscientiousness, defense, education, income, openness, passion, prosociality, and social desirability to drive resilience (Corstange and York 2018; Datler et al. 2013; Ghimire 2021a; Marsh and Dik 2021; Rip et al. 2012; Saucier and Skrzypinska 2006; Sedikides and Gebauer 2010). Agreeableness has enabled growth, life satisfaction, mastery, purposefulness, relatedness, and self-acceptance to raise resilience (Hounkpatin et al. 2015). Conscientiousness has raised autonomy, growth, life satisfaction, mastery, purposefulness, relatedness, and self-acceptance to enable resilience (Hounkpatin et al. 2015). Defense has built on self-efficacy to facilitate resilience (Guo et al. 2023). Income has sustained and power well-being, including adaptation, belongingness, control, eudaimonia, financial adequacy, health, life quality and satisfaction, mastery, self-efficacy, self-esteem, and social well-being to foster resilience (Anciaes et al. 2017; Corcoran et al. 2011; Frijters et al. 2012; Hofstetter et al. 1999; Lelli 2008; Prenda and Lachman 2001; Sengupta and Sibley 2019; Ross and Mirowsky 1989; Son and Wilson 2012; Wang and VanderWeele 2011; Wen et al. 2010; Yeh et al. 2013). Passion has sustained health and pride to buttress resilience (Vallerand 2015). Prosociality has elevated well-being, including connectedness, hope, life satisfaction, meaningfulness, and self-efficacy to boost resilience (Marsh and Dik 2021; Nelson-Coffey et al. 2023; Raposa et al. 2016; Yao and Enright 2019). Social desirability has escalated gratitude and dampened anxiety and depression to maintain resilience (Ben-Zur 2002; Burroughs and Rindfleisch 2002; Krumrei-Mancuso 2017). Conversely, religious practice has prevented or reduced depression, crime or deviance, doping, eccentricity, fear, illness, loneliness, poverty, suicide, thus retaining power to drive resilience (Duberstein et al. 2004; Ellison et al. 2001; Hatch 2007; Hui et al. 2007; Lauder et al. 2006; Muennig et al. 2013; Saucier and Skrzypinska 2006; Skerkat and Ellison 1999; Urbatsch 2014).

Utility generated by religious practice to attract resilience involves social inclusion experienced (Pfeifer 2019). Social inclusion experienced enhances resilience and has dampened depression (Mullins and Dugan 1991; Pinkerten and Dolan 2007). Religious practice increased social responsiveness expected to secure utility to attract resilience (Tang 2014). Responsiveness experienced has raised adaptation, life satisfaction, positive emotion, and relational quality to secure resilience (Algoe and Zhaoyang 2016). Furthermore, religious practice has rested on purposiveness expected to hold utility to attract resilience (Marsh and Dik 2021). Purposiveness has advanced happiness, health, life satisfaction, and positive affect and has lessened depression and negative affect to induce resilience (Steger et al. 2009; Tomich and Helgeson 2002).

Ideals cultivated by religious practice to rationalize resilience accentuate binding, coherence, health maintenance, sharing, and survival (De Graaf 2013; Haidt 2012; Ishii and Watanabe 2023; Levin and Chatters 1998). The ideal for binding has consolidated social binding (Granzin and Olsen 1998). Social binding has enhanced hope and life satisfaction to maintain resilience (Dittman and Goebel 2010; Paez et al. 2015). The ideal of coherence can underlie coherence (Kawakami et al. 2017). Coherence fosters confidence to achieve resilience (Simon and Read 2018). The ideal for health maintenance has motivated health maintenance (McCarthy et al. 2017; McEachan et al. 2016). Health maintenance has safeguarded health and reduced depression to enable resilience (Smith et al. 2006; Myers 2008). The ideal of sharing has buttressed sharing (Becker and Clement 2006; Xia and Yang 2020). Sharing has reduced stress, thus maintaining resilience (Lazar and Eisenberger 2022). Survival builds on resilience (Barber et al. 2010). Furthermore, religious practice enhances ideals regarding existentialism and survival (Donahue 1985; Koole et al. 2010). Existentialism builds on intuition, spirituality, and self-understanding to achieve actualization, meaningfulness, responsibility, self-consciousness, and self-regulation or inner dictatorship (Forsyth 2003; Koole et al. 2010). Essentially, existentialism pursues courage, endurance, and transcendence and dismisses anxiety, fear, helplessness, and neuroticism to maintain resilience (Addad 1987; Hoffman et al. 2016; Lyng 2012; Strenger 2011; Temple and Gall 2018; van Deurzen 2021). Courage has sustained resilience, life satisfaction, and positive affect, and diminished anxiety and negative effect (Baptist et al. 2015; Howard and Alipour 2014; Kim et al. 2018; Muris et al. 2010). Religious practice also involves ideals regarding acceptance, caring, compassion, ethics, forgiveness, humanitarianism, individualism, love, and maturity to rationalize resilience (Ager and Ager 2011; Dy-Liacco et al. 2009; Myers 2014; Pedersen 2018; Simpson et al. 2008; Tenorio and Lo 2011). Compassion has enhanced well-being to facilitate resilience (Jasielska 2020). Ethicalness has advanced emotional development, friendship quality, identity, and relatedness to enhance resilience (Crocetti et al. 2018; Markiewicz et al. 2001; Matsuba and Walker 2004). Forgiveness upholds adaptation for underlying resilience (Sandage and Williamson 2005). Humanitarianism has built on connectedness and humility to facilitate resilience (Angelis and Pensini 2024). Individualism treasures agency, autonomy, privatization, reflexivity, self-actualization, and voluntarism (O'Brien 2015). The ideal of love has engendered love (McFarland et al. 2013). Love has fostered meaningfulness to enable resilience (Damasio and Koller 2015). Maturity has upheld success to furnish resilience (Spengler et al. 2018). Christian religious practice particularly realizes ideals for caring, compassion, dignity, hospitality, humanitarianism, and universality as opposed to oppression (Horell 2014; Paterson 2018). Religious practice has also advanced forgiveness, optimism, tolerance, and satisfaction with democracy, finance, life, and police to secure ideals for rationalizing resilience (Furnham 1997; Gibson 2013; Kwak et al. 2010; Marx 2014; Ng and Fisher 2016; Ravanera et al. 2003; Van Praag et al. 2010; Wuthnow 2004). Furthermore, religious practice has raised ideals for civility, cohesion, compliance, conformity, generativity, helping, morality, and recourse to rationalize resilience (Brown and Ferris 2007; Devos et al. 2002; Marien and Hooghe 2011; Sullivan 2001; Weisberg 2005; Wink and Dillon 2003; Wuthnow 2004). Civility has sustained well-being or life quality, including mental and physical health, to boost resilience (Tsai et al. 2018). Compliance or conformity can raise well-being, including adaptation and pleasantness as opposed to anxiety, to induce resilience (de Courville Nicol 2011; Littlejohn et al. 2017; Stavrova 2014; Turner 2006). Generativity has manifested well-being to facilitate resilience (Peterson and Klohnen 1995). The ideal for helping has sustained helping (Feeney and Collins 2001; Yao and Enright 2019; Wade-Benzoni and Tost 2009). Helping has boosted well-being, including connectedness, hope, life satisfaction, meaningfulness, and self-efficacy, to elevate resilience (Marsh and Dik 2021; Nelson-Coffey et al. 2023; Raposa et al. 2016). Recourse has alleviated distress to uphold resilience (Tracey et al. 1986). Religious practice has also stood on empathizing, hedonism, self-enhancement, social concern, and transcendence to maintain ideals for rationalizing resilience (Datler et al. 2013; Ishii and Watanabe 2023; Saucier and Skrzypinska 2006). The ideal for empathizing has consolidated empathy (Mestre et al. 2018). Empathy has raised intimacy and communication quality to enhance resilience (Redmond 2018). Hedonism has underpinned well-being, notably life satisfaction, to advance resilience (Datler et al. 2013; Joshanloo and Jarden 2016). Self-enhancement fosters self-esteem to induce resilience (Spencer-Rodgers et al. 2009). Social concern has sustained relational quality to raise resilience (Jorgensen and Nelson 2018). Transcendence has boosted life satisfaction and meaningfulness and reduced anxiety, depression, and stress to uplift resilience (Fishbein et al. 2020). Conversely, religious practice establishes ideals against suicide to rationalize resilience (Upenieks 2022). Suicidal ideation has bred anxiety to erode resilience (Cheng et al. 2017). Religious practice has also resisted ideals for protesting and struggling to rationalize resilience (Corstange and York 2018; Skerkat 1998). The ideal for protesting or struggling has buttressed protesting or struggling (Aytac and Stokes 2019; Hwang and Kim 2015). Protesting or struggling has fomented anger and worry and dampened hope to impede resilience (Boehnke and Wong 2011; Landmann and Rohmann 2020; Paez et al. 2015).

Norms exposed by religious practice to assimilate resilience popularize religiosity, liking, and self-esteem (Baker and Smith 2009; Ysseldyk et al. 2012). Religious practice has also sustained norms for harmony and security to assimilate resilience (Clemence 2001; Urbatsch 2014). The norm for liking can assimilate liking (Marcus et al. 2000). Liking represents hedonism and positive affect to uphold resilience

(Alves et al. 2016; Pe et al. 2016). The norm for self-esteem can generate self-esteem to induce resilience (Hegtvedt and Parris 2014; Mruk 2006).

## *Pet Engagement*

Pet engagement involves accompanying, admiring, anthropomorphizing, attachment, caring, comforting, confiding, exercising, loving, owning, and spending concerning pets, typically cats or dogs (Blouin 2012; Kerns et al. 2016; Knight and Edwards 2008; McNicholas and Collis 2001; Parslow et al. 2005; White et al. 2022; Wood et al. 2005). Such engagement represents a tie such as that with family and functions as a social catalyst, lubricant, or ice breaker and for distraction and therapy (Arkow 2013; Knight and Edwards 2008; Marsa-Sambola et al. 2017; White et al. 2022; Wood et al. 2015). Such therapy can heal the deficit or disorders regarding nature (Arkow 2013). Pet engagement is likely to benefit resilience by generating power, utility, ideals, and norms to activate voluntaristic mechanisms dictated by analytical functionalism.

Power enhanced by pet engagement to drive resilience has evolved from conscientiousness, coping, executive functioning, happiness or cheerfulness, knowledge of neighbors, pain relief, persistence, relaxation, self-efficacy, sociability, and social attachment (Bennett et al. 2015; Branson et al. 2016; Herrald et al. 2002; Kerns et al. 2016; Parslow et al. 2005; White et al. 2022; Wood et al. 2015). Conscientiousness has propped autonomy, life satisfaction, mastery, purposefulness, relatedness, and self-acceptance and has diminished avoidance and anxiety to secure resilience (Fraley et al. 2011; Hounkpatin et al. 2015). Coping has raised resilience, environmental and relational quality, growth, health, intimacy, satisfaction, and self-efficacy (Cherry et al. 2023; Chow et al. 2014; Gattino et al. 2015; Lau et al. 2012; Paez et al. 2007; Veenstra et al. 2005; Wills 1997). Executive functioning has benefitted from socioeconomic status to drive resilience (Ursache et al. 2015). Friendship quality has reflected intimacy and relational quality as opposed to anxiety and loneliness to maintain resilience (Lee 2018; Li et al. 2018; Parade et al. 2010; Wang et al. 2020). Neighbor knowledge constitutes neighboring (Lee et al. 1991). Neighboring has raised the sense of community and well-being to resilience (Farrell et al. 2004). Pain relief represents well-being, thus maintaining resilience (McCormack and Feeney 2015). Persistence has sustained well-being, notably pleasure, to facilitate resilience (Boyes et al. 2017; Goodman et al. 2017). Relaxation has raised sleep quality and dismissed anxiety to facilitate resilience (Hudetz et al. 2004; Li et al. 2016). Self-efficacy has raised life quality, satisfaction, self-esteem, and general well-being to safeguard resilience (Forgeard and Benson 2019; Luszczynska and Gutierrez-Dona 2005). Sociability has enhanced well-being to buttress resilience (Bjornskov 2008). Social attachment has enabled compassion, health, intimacy, and life satisfaction to sustain resilience (Alonso-Arbiol et al. 2007; Headey et al. 2001; Mikulincer et al. 2005; Zdrenka et al. 2015). Moreover, pet engagement has reflected civic engagement, co-residence, employment, knowledge in general, proactivity, and social support received to form power to drive resilience (Cheung and Kam 2018; Parslow et al. 2005; Wood et al. 2005). Civic engagement has incubated conflict resolution, education, happiness, health, income, individualism, life satisfaction, security normativity, social attachment, capital, integration, trust, tolerance, and general well-being to advance resilience (Coffe and Geys 2007; Goren 2005; Growiec and Growiec 2010; Kroll 2011; Li and Walder 2001; Myers 1999; Pena-Lopez and Sanchez-Santos 2016; Posel and Casale 2011; Tak 2017; Tang 2011; Wallace and Pichler 2009; Welzel 2013; van Ingen and Bekkers 2015; Vincens et al. 2018). Co-residence has enhanced health, life satisfaction, and sleep quality and has dampened depression and distress to boost resilience (Lofors and Sundquist 2007; Oshio and Kan 2019; Gu et al. 2010; Richards 2016). Proactivity reflects coping and protection to enable resilience (Seaton and Beaumont 2008; Shaw et al. 2023). Conversely, pet engagement has diminished anxiety, conflict experienced, depression, and detachment, thus maintaining power to drive resilience (Bennett et al. 2015; Kerns et al. 2016). Conflict has provoked distress and eroded satisfaction, thus impeding resilience (Lau et al. 2017; Mikula et al. 2012). Detachment has bred conflict to worsen resilience (Debus et al. 2019). Moreover, pet engagement has reflected low loneliness, thus retaining power to drive resilience (Wood et al. 2005).

The ideal maintained by pet engagement to rationalize resilience concerns life satisfaction and medication or healing (Bennett et al. 2015; Parslow et al. 2005). Medication has built on mental and physical health to sustain resilience (Fielding et al. 1995). Alternatively, pet engagement has maintained friendship quality as utility to attract resilience (Branson et al. 2016).

## *Experience-Based Coping*

Experience-based coping means coping based on working or other life experiences (Shirzadifard et al. 2018). Such coping conjoins experientiality and coping. Experientiality involves gut feelings, instincts, and intuition (Shirzadifard et al. 2018). It operates rapidly through association, automaticity, heuristics, imagination, implicitness, mysticism, narrative, naturalness, and preconsciousness (Epstein et al. 1996; Pacini and Epstein 1999). Meanwhile, coping represents lasting planned effort (Kleinke 2007). The crux of such coping is self-reflection to engender self-insight about coping and stress and their appraisal and reappraisal to achieve resilience (Falon et al. 2021). This insight covers evaluation, planning, reappraisal, self-awareness, and trigger to response (Falon et al. 2021). Experience-based coping is thus an experientially based effort operating intuitively and rapidly. It applies experience through self-reflection and self-insight to coping. This coping is likely to uplift resilience through experientiality, self-reflection, and coping generally. The uplifting hinges on affording power, utility, ideals, and norms to run voluntaristic mechanisms to achieve functioning based on analytical functionalism.

Experientiality has raised power to drive resilience through agreeableness, extraversion, favorability, noticing, openness, self-regulation, and trust (Jokic and

Puric 2021). Conversely, experientiality has prevented neuroticism to retain power to drive resilience (Pacini and Epstein 1999).

Experientiality has championed ideals to rationalize resilience concerning meaningfulness (Pacini and Epstein 1999),

Self-reflection or simply reflection involves or aligns with agency, reflectivity, self-connection, self-consciousness, self-description, self-evaluation, self-recognition, self-talk, and theorizing about mind (Klussman et al. 2020; Morin 2011; van Seggelen-Damen and van Dam 2016). It registers a capacity, competence, consciousness, learning, performance, processing, reasoning, and skill (Amodeo and Collins 2007; Ashby et al. 2014; Ewart et al. 2002; Gillespie 2018; Holowchak 2008; Morin 2011; Qin 2013; Wilson and Kelly 2010). As such, it generates power, utility, ideals, and norms for boosting resilience by applying the voluntaristic mechanisms of analytical functionalism. Essentially, self-reflection registers resilience (Brodsky and Cattaneo 2013; Nemeth and Olivier 2017; Yamamoto et al. 2023). Hence, self-reflection has evolved from resilience (Cowden and Meyer-Weitz 2016). Alternatively, self-reflection builds resilience (Crane et al. 2019).

Power unfolded by self-reflection to drive resilience rests on adulthood, eudaimonia or flourishing, identity, learning, openness, reasoning, religiosity, virtuousness, and wisdom (Haslam et al. 2011; Holowchak 2008; Konig and Gluck 2013; MacLeod 2015; Mirivel 2014; Qin 2013; Salagame 2014; Shek 2010). Adulthood features adaptation, autonomy, dignity, equilibrium, integrity, love, mastery, self-esteem, transcendence, as opposed to illness to induce resilience (Arnett et al. 2011; Clark et al. 2011; Eneau 2008; Hoare 2002; Kramer 2003; Manners and Durkin 2000; Stevens-Long and Michaud 2003; Wapner and Demick 2003), Moreover, adulthood has sustained health to enable resilience (Battersby and Phillips 2016). Identity has secured happiness, love, self-efficacy, and self-esteem and has diminished anxiety and depression to facilitate resilience (Cast 2004). Learning has elevated well-being, including life satisfaction and self-efficacy, to furnish resilience (Denver and Hands 1990; Minnaert and Janssen 1992; Richards 2016). Openness has buttressed well-being, including autonomy, growth, purposefulness, life satisfaction, relationship quality, self-acceptance, self-efficacy, and self-esteem to advance resilience (Hahn et al. 2013; Hounkpatin et al. 2014, 2015; Karwowski and Lebuda 2017; Marks 1996; Quilty et al. 2006). Reasoning has dampened aggressiveness, anxiety, dependence, depression, disorders, and self-defeating, thus upholding resilience (DiGiuseppe et al. 2017; Karuza et al. 1990). Religiosity has buttressed coping, friendship, forgiveness, harmony perceived, health maintenance, institutional and social trust, optimism, social capital, well-being to raise resilience (Chang 2009; Clemence 2001; Furnham 1997; Hakhverdian and Mayne 2012; Myers 2008; Saroglou and Anciaux 2004; Wuthnow 2004; Zanin 2017). Virtuousness has sustained satisfaction and eroded anxiety to boost resilience (Conzo et al. 2017; Stets et al. 2008). Wisdom has raised well-being, including autonomy, coherence, maturity, meaningfulness, purposefulness, life satisfaction, and self-efficacy to effectuate resilience (Diener et al. 2009; Greene and Brown 2009; Mickler and Staudinger 2008; Webster 2010). To the youth, self-reflection additionally registers citizenship, commitment, consciousness, creativity, criticalness, deliberation, discipline, growth, intelligence, performance, self-control, and skill to evolve power to drive resilience (Alt 2015; Chen and Lin 2018; Ewart et al. 2002; Geboers et al. 2015; Gonzalez et al. 2020; Nucci 2006; Pascarella and Terenzini 2005; Wang 1997; Zhang and Sternberg 2012; Youniss and Yates 1997; Wilson and Kelly 2010). Citizenship has fostered well-being, including mental and physical health, to elevate resilience (Tsai et al. 2018). Commitment has sustained self-acceptance and relieved depression to foster resilience (Agronick and Duncan 1998; Wrosch et al. 2005). Consciousness has enhanced meaningfulness to facilitate resilience (George and Park 2013). Creativity has sustained meaningfulness to frame resilience (Turner 2013). Criticalness has fostered identity achievement to procure resilience (Adams and Ryan 2000). Deliberation has prevented aggression, anxiety, avoidance, depression, and disorders to maintain resilience (DiGiuseppe et al. 2017). Discipline has strengthened well-being, notably self-esteem, to induce resilience (Armstrong et al. 2011; Diener and Fujita 1995). Growth has developed from self-compassion and self-tolerance to strengthen resilience (Ho and Li 2022; Munroe et al. 2022). Intelligence has enhanced social capital and diminished criminality and depression, thus facilitating resilience (Cornwall 2009; Feinstein and Bynner 2006). Performance has reflected self-determination, self-efficacy, and the sense of community to boost resilience (Asoodar et al. 2014; Moller et al. 2006; Yashima 2010). Self-control has maintained self-esteem and reduced anxiety and depression to enable resilience (Armstrong et al. 2011; Marchetti et al. 2018). Skill has underpinned self-efficacy to buttress resilience (Larson et al. 1990). Self-reflection buttresses employment, identity, meaningfulness, morality, selfhood, survival, and well-being to drive resilience (Falk 2018; Gibbs 2014; Greenberg and Pascual-Leone 2001; Mahler 2011; Mansfield 2000; Scott 2015). Employment has secured well-being, including growth, health, mastery, purposiveness, relatedness, satisfaction, self-acceptance, and self-efficacy, to maintain resilience (Carrieri 2012; Corcoran et al. 2011; Distante 2013; Ryff et al. 2004). Conversely, employment has diminished depression, distress, dysfunction, loneliness, powerlessness, and psychosis, thus sustaining resilience (Goldberg and Perry-Jenkins 2004; Keyes 2002; Koromeckyj-Cox et al. 2007; Lofors and Sundquist 2007; Myer et al. 2008; Ross and Mirowsky 2009). Meaningfulness has buttressed aspiration, engagement, happiness, health, life satisfaction, and positive affect to sustain resilience (Morgan and Robinson 2013; Steger et al. 2009). Morality has sustained satisfaction and eroded anxiety to boost resilience (Conzo et al. 2017; Stets et al. 2008). Selfhood has maintained life satisfaction, positive affect, purposiveness, and self-actualization to afford resilience (Dy-Liacco et al. 2009). Survival or its expectancy reflects resilience (Barber et al. 2010). To the youth, self-reflection additionally raises citizenship and criticalness to secure power to drive resilience (Burke et al. 2017; Maypole and Davies 2001). Likewise, self-reflection has raised well-being, including meaningfulness, positive affect, self-clarify, and self-insight, as opposed to negative effect to incubate power to drive resilience (Cowden and Meyer-Weitz 2016; Elliott and Coker 2008; Klussman et al. 2020). Self-clarify has upheld identity and impeded depression and dissociation, including absorption and depersonalization, to maintain resilience (Ickes et al. 2012; Lassri et al. 2023). Self-insight has raised resilience, autonomy, growth, life satisfaction, mastery, purposefulness, relatedness, and self-acceptance and has dampened anxiety (Harrington and Loffredo 2010; Ungar et al. 2005). Furthermore, self-insight has benefitted from resilience and low stress (Cowden and Meyer-Weitz 2016). To the youth, self-reflection has additionally elevated adjustment, elaboration, growth, self-awareness, self-esteem, and working to drive resilience (Comunian and Gielen 2006; Harrington and Loffredo 2010; Simsek 2013; Ran et al. 2023). Elaboration has prevented aggression, anxiety, avoidance, depression, and disorders to maintain resilience (DiGiuseppe et al. 2017). Self-awareness has raised meaningfulness, positive affect, and self-clarity to maintain resilience (Klussman et al. 2020). Working has advanced health and mastery to secure resilience (Borgonovi 2008; Schieman and Plickert 2008). Self-reflection has also reflected authenticity. perspective-taking, and self-efficacy as power to drive resilience (Gillespie 2007; Klussman et al. 2020; Cowden and Meyer-Weitz 2016). Authenticity has maintained autonomy, eudaimonic well-being, growth, hedonic well-being, identity integration, life satisfaction, positive affect, mastery, mindfulness, purposiveness, relational quality, self-acceptance, self-clarity, self-esteem, self-determination, and vitality to escalate resilience (Kernis and Goldman 2006). Conversely, authenticity has diminished strain and stress to secure resilience (Kernis and Goldman 2006). Perspective-taking has installed social trust to empower resilience (Fett et al. 2014). Self-efficacy has raised life quality, satisfaction, self-esteem, and general well-being to safeguard resilience (Forgeard and Benson 2019; Luszczynska and Gutierrez-Dona 2005). Conversely, self-reflection has also reduced anxiety and depression to retain power to drive resilience (Simsek 2013).

Utility achieved by self-reflection to attract resilience transpires in gain experienced (Schunk 2020). Gain experienced has raised well-being, including satisfaction as opposed to anger, anxiety, and depression, to foster resilience (Helgeson et al. 2006; Wells et al. 1999; Wong and Lam 2016).

Ideals underlying self-reflection to rationalize resilience emphasize balance, dialecticism, egalitarianism, gratitude, humanism, normativeness, realism, and self-affirmation (Frazer 1999; McKie et al. 1998; Selznick 2008; Sternberg 2014; Walsh 2014; Watkins 2016). Balance has fostered confidence to achieve resilience (Simon and Read 2018). Dialecticism has sustained creativity and reflected independence to facilitate resilience (Church et al. 2012; Yang et al. 2010). Creativity has sustained meaningfulness to enable resilience (Turner 2013). Independence has sustained health and mastery to foster resilience (Lu and Kao 2002; Roy and Chaudhuri 2008). Egalitarianism has dampened anxiety to maintain resilience (Schwartz and Melech 2000). Gratitude as positive affect has boosted other positive affect and diminished negative affect to secure resilience (Bernabe-Valero et al. 2021). Humanism embraces creativity, resolution, self-improvement, and vitality to facilitate resilience (Browning and Cooper 2004; Fuchs 2020; Selznick 2008; Visher 1997). Normativity has furnished achievement and its pressure, mastery-goal setting, social closeness and support received, and tolerance to benefit resilience (Feldman 2003; Jiang et al. 2015; Magnuson et al. 2006). Realism favors security to furnish resilience (Bell 2010). Self-affirmation has developed from its ideal (Zucker and Bay-Cheng 2021). As such, self-affirmation has fostered self-regard to secure resilience (Schneider and Weber 2020). Self-reflection sustains satisfaction as an ideal to rationalize resilience (Falk

2018). To the youth, self-reflection additionally registers Confucianism, pluralism, pragmatism, and socialism to brew ideals to rationalize resilience (Baxter Magolda 2004; Dishon 2018; Wang et al. 1998; Zhu 2003). Confucianism or scholarism has enhanced life satisfaction and vitality to induce resilience (Lin et al. 2021). Pluralism embraces or induces adjustment, agency, autonomy, compromise and tradeoff, deliberation, diversity, experimentation, individualism, innovation, liberty, openness, peace, receptiveness, respect, self-discipline, and tolerance to consolidate resilience (Connolly 2005; Galston 2005; Herman 2021; Moffitt 2018). Pragmatism hails adaptation, creativity, education, flexibility, tolerance, and understanding to induce resilience. (Ray 2004). Socialism (or its ideal) accentuates autonomy to secure resilience (Panitch 2008). Moreover, self-reflection involves acceptance, alignment, and justification as ideals to rationalize resilience (Brugman 2006; Klussman et al. 2020). Alignment has sustained well-being to enhance resilience (Cheung and Leung 2011). Justification has upheld positive affect to benefit resilience (Jost and Hunyady 2005). Self-reflection has enhanced reciprocity and self-enhancement to embody ideals to drive resilience (McFarland et al. 2007; Vandermeer et al. 2019). Reciprocity has arisen from its ideal (Rodrigo-Gonzalez et al. 2019). As such, reciprocity has facilitated adaptation as opposed to illness to create resilience (Yamaoka 2008; Yeh et al. 2013). Self-enhancement stands on its ideal (Marshall 2001). Given the standing, self-enhancement has reflected attachment and social support received to raise resilience (Hermanto et al. 2017; Ledoux et al. 2010). Conversely, self-reflection has reflected low self-deception as an ideal to obstruct resilience (Shane and Peterson 2004). Self-reflection also lessens deviance as an ideal refuting resilience (Kaplan et al. 2013). Self-deception characterizes low conscientiousness to impair attachment, autonomy, life satisfaction, mastery, purposefulness, and self-acceptance weaken resilience (Fraley et al. 2011; Hounkpatin et al. 2015; Mullet et al. 2005). Deviance stands on its ideal (Morgan 2021). As such, deviance has eroded health, thus impairing resilience (Backman and Nilsson 2011).

Coping generally represents sustained efforts at adaptation and regulation in response to stress (Kleinke 2007; Morimoto et al. 2014); Weinstein et al. 2009). Variously, coping features activeness, approach, avoidance, and buffering to focus on problems and emotions behaviorally and cognitively and personally and interpersonally (Chwyl et al. 2021; Johnson et al. 2013; Kleinke 2007; Rodebaugh and Heimberg 2008). Notably, coping has advanced resilience (Cherry et al. 2023; McKay et al. 2018). Coping is likely to achieve resilience by furnishing power, utility, ideals, and norms to leverage the voluntaristic mechanisms of analytical functionalism.

Power enhanced by coping to drive resilience evolves from adjustment, enjoyment, environmental quality, experientiality, growth, health, helpfulness, intimacy, motivation, relational quality, responsibility, self-efficacy, and well-being generally (Chow et al. 2014; Coifman et al. 2007; Gattino et al. 2015; Gurung et al. 2023; Lefcourt et al. 1997; Marcks and Woods 2007; Pollio et al. 1997; Paez et al. 2007; Zvi and Cohen-Louck 2023; Wills 1997). Helpfulness or the urge to help has elevated well-being, including connectedness, hope, life satisfaction, meaningfulness, and self-efficacy to boost resilience (Marsh and Dik 2021; Nelson-Coffey et al. 2023; Raposa et al. 2016; Yao and Enright 2019). Motivation has underlain satisfaction to induce resilience (Ferssizidis et al. 2010). Intimacy has sustained purposiveness, relationship satisfaction, and self-efficacy and has dampened anxiety to facilitate resilience (Arseth et al. 2009; Chou 2000; Hand et al. 2013; Henderson et al. 2009). Responsibility has advanced wisdom to facilitate resilience (Spengler et al. 2018). Coping exercises concentration, creativity, engagement, exercising, flexibility, humor, investment, intimacy, meaningfulness, meditation, optimism, planning, rationality, recourse, spirituality, and working to assume power to drive resilience (Kleinke 2007; Major and Townsend 2010; Pargament 1997; Rodebaugh and Heimberg 2008; Sutherland and Rehman 2018; Tam and Ip 2017; Wyer and Abbarracin 2014). Concentration has raised self-efficacy and self-esteem to advance resilience (Bakker et al. 2008). Creativity has boosted well-being, notably including meaningfulness, to induce resilience (Diener et al. 2009; Turner 2013). Exercising has sustained well-being, thus empowering resilience (Sargent-Cox et al. 2015). Flexibility has buttressed life satisfaction and self-esteem as opposed to distress to enable resilience (Jen et al. 2019). Humor has sustained mental health, pleasure, satisfaction, and diminished fear to maintain resilience (Dynel and Poppi 2018; Martin 2007; Svebak et al. 2004). Investment has strengthened social capital to facilitate resilience (Hlasny and Lee 2020). Meaningfulness has buttressed aspiration, engagement, happiness, health, life satisfaction, and positive affect to sustain resilience (Morgan and Robinson 2013; Steger et al. 2009). Meditation has advanced compassion or self-compassion and mindfulness and dwindled depression to foster resilience (Galante et al. 2014). Optimism has enhanced positive affect to enable resilience (Shanahan et al. 2020). Planning has reflected achievement, education, health, and optimism to afford resilience (Hellevik and Settersten 2013; Poynton et al. 2015). Rationality has eroded anxiety, depression, disorders, and self-defeating, thus safeguarding resilience (DiGiuseppe et al. 2017). Recourse has alleviated distress to uphold resilience (Tracey et al. 1986). Spirituality has sustained forgiveness, joy, and general well-being to foster resilience (Mullet et al. 2005; Saroglou and Anciaux 2004; Seidlitz et al. 2002). Working has fostered health and mastery to facilitate resilience (Borgonovi 2008; Schieman and Plickert 2008). Alternatively, coping has stemmed from activation, competence, education, dominance, emotional intelligence, extraversion, identity commitment, learning, monitoring, openness, perseverance, positive affect, religiosity, and social support received to secure power to drive resilience (Artuch-Garde et al. 2017; Celso et al. 2003; Chan 2008; Kim et al. 2023; Pargament 1997; Prelow et al. 2006; Rodebaugh and Heimberg 2008; Seaton and Beaumont 2008; Tam and Ip 2017). Activation has boosted self-esteem and diminished anxiety and depression to champion resilience (Marchetti et al. 2018). Dominance has fostered well-being, including health and life satisfaction as opposed to anger and depression, to elevate resilience (Cundiff et al. 2015; Etezadi and Pushkar 2013; Orlowski and Wicker 2015; Rose 2000; Xi and Hwang 2011). Emotional intelligence has facilitated well-being, including adaptation, happiness, health, life satisfaction, positive mood, relatedness, relational quality, and self-esteem to enhance resilience (Ciarrochi et al. 2000; Kluemper 2008; Matthews et al. 2012; Mayer et al. 2004; Schutte et al. 2002). Extraversion has raised well-being, including autonomy, growth, mastery, positive affect, purposefulness, relatedness, satisfaction, self-acceptance, self-determination, self-efficacy, and self-esteem to facilitate resilience (Hounkpatin et al. 2015; Ingledew et al. 2004; Quilty et al. 2006; Rasmussen et al. 2018; Richards 2016; Tiwari et al. 2021). Identity commitment has secured happiness, love, self-efficacy, and self-esteem and has diminished anxiety and depression to facilitate resilience (Cast 2004). Learning or lessons learned has facilitated self-efficacy as power to drive resilience (Byars-Winston and Rogers 2019). Monitoring stems from a commitment to furnish power to drive resilience (Tokunaga 2016). Openness has buttressed well-being, including autonomy, growth, purposefulness, life satisfaction, relationship quality, self-acceptance, self-efficacy, and self-esteem to advance resilience (Hahn et al. 2013; Hounkpatin et al. 2015; Karwowski and Lebuda 2017; Marks 1996; Quilty et al. 2006). Perseverance has facilitated well-being, including pleasure, to sustained resilience (Boyes et al. 2017; Goodman et al. 2017). Religiosity has sustained well-being, including adjustment, flourishing, health, mastery, positive affect, relational quality, satisfaction, self-esteem, and socioemotional well-being, to advance resilience (Dy-Liacco et al. 2009; Helliwell and Putnam 2005; Flouri and Buchanan 2002; Meulemann 2010; Moschis and Ong 2011; Ng and Fisher 2016; Schieman 2001; Skerkat and Ellison 1999; Wuthnow 2004). Social support received has upheld well-being, including control, health, positive emotion and pleasure, purposiveness, relational quality, satisfaction with life, housing, and leisure, self-determination, self-efficacy, self-esteem, and social well-being, to activate resilience (George and Park 2013; Glendinning et al. 2003; Granzin and Haggard 2000; Holliman et al. 2021; Lincoln et al. 2003; Logan and Cobb 2013; Pierce and Quiroz 2018; Schwarzer and Knoll 2007; Vilhjalmsson and Thorlindsson 1998; Wen et al. 2010; Williams and Galliher 2006; Xi and Hwang 2011). Notably, social support received has boosted resilience (Cherry et al. 2018). Moreover, coping rests on commitment and resources as power to drive resilience (Kelly and Steed 2004; Lewis et al. 2006b). Commitment has sustained self-acceptance and relieved depression to foster resilience (Agronick and Duncan 1998; Wrosch et al. 2005). Resources have maintained well-being and diminished depression to foster resilience (Cutrona et al. 2000; Galate et al. 2016). Conversely, coping has arisen from low anxiety, avoidance, and neuroticism to retain power to drive resilience (Rodebaugh and Heimberg 2008; Seaton and Beaumont 2008). Avoidance has impaired coping and well-being, including mindfulness and satisfaction, to hinder resilience (Barber et al. 2010; Basabe et al. 2002; Linares et al. 2016; Seaton and Beaumont 2008). Conversely, avoidance has fomented anger, anxiety, depression, and loneliness (Cheng and Cheung 2005; Kafetsio and Sideridis 2006; Linares et al. 2016), Stigmatization experienced has stemmed from phobia to weaken resilience (Yao et al. 2021). Neuroticism has worsened well-being, including autonomy, growth, health, positive affect, purposefulness, relatedness, satisfaction, self-acceptance, self-compassion, and self-determination, to resist resilience (Anusic et al. 2014; Hounkpatin et al. 2015; Ingledew et al. 2004; Pfattheicher et al. 2017; Richards 2016; Webster et al. 2014). Coping has also reduced aggressiveness, conflict, depression, distress, and fear to secure power to drive resilience (Chow et al. 2014; Erickson and Feldstein 2007; Krulichova 2019; Littleton et al. 2007; Wills 1997). Aggressiveness has bred depression, thus disturbing resilience (Wright et al. 2015). Conflict has provoked distress and eroded satisfaction, thus impeding resilience (Lau et al. 2017; Mikula et al. 2012).

Utility maximization constitutes coping to attract resilience (Wyer and Abbarracin 2014). Specifically, coping has secured benefits and success experienced as utility to attract resilience (Gurung et al. 2023; Mehrabian 2000). Benefit has boosted well-being, including satisfaction, as opposed to anger, anxiety, and depression to uplift resilience (Helgeson et al. 2006; Wells et al. 1999; Wong and Lam 2016). Success has benefitted from happiness and relaxation to enhance resilience (Lyubomirsky et al. 2005; Mehrabian 2000). Coping has also arisen from malleability expected or experienced to hold utility to attract resilience (Kneeland and Dovidio 2019). Expected malleability has sustained resilience, adjustment, confidence, health, satisfaction, and self-efficacy and diminished anxiety (Aitcheson et al. 2017; Aspinwall and Taylor 1992; Bernard 1997; Chang et al. 2011; Muenks et al. 2021; Sheridan et al. 2015). Conversely, coping has reduced problems that are expected to attract resilience (Sutherland and Rehman 2018). Problems have worsened well-being, including financial well-being, health, and satisfaction as opposed to distress, to impair resilience (Carrieri 2012; Gary et al. 2007; van Praag and Ferrer-I-Carbonell 2004; van Praag and Frijters 1999). Coping has also arisen from low barriers and risk experienced to attract resilience (Byars-Winston and Fouad 2008; Prelow et al. 2006). Barriers have reduced hygiene to impair health and foment depression to erode resilience (Clark and Janevic 2013; Smith et al. 2006; Myers 2008). Risk experienced has inhibited achievement, happiness, life satisfaction, positive affect, and self-determination to dampen resilience (Schoon 2006; Schwartz and Melech 2000; Shippee 2012; Zotti et al. 2016).

Ideals maintained by coping to rationalize resilience emphasize acceptance, compliance, control, forgiveness, protection, rationalization, reconciliation, reparation or amendment, resolution, satisfaction, and self-enhancement (Erickson and Feldstein 2007; Gattino et al. 2015; Johnson et al. 2013; Kleinke 2007; Lau et al. 2012; Major and Townsend 2010; Pollio et al. 1997; Twardawski et al. 2021). The ideal for compliance has buttressed compliance (Van Damme 2017). Compliance has furnished achievement and its pressure, mastery-goal setting, social closeness and support received, and tolerance to benefit resilience (Feldman 2003; Jiang et al. 2015; Magnuson et al. 2006). The ideal for control has motivated controlling, domination, or mastery (Cheung and Chiu 2021). Forgiveness rests on its ideal (Sandage and Williamson 2005). As such, forgiveness has elevated serenity, trust, and well-being to maintain resilience (Choi and David 2012; Connors et al. 1999; Shimai et al. 2006). Protection arises from its ideal (Gonzalez-Castro et al. 2021). As such, protection has uplifted self-enhancement to safeguard resilience (Erickson and Feldstein 2007). Rationalization reflects self-esteem to maintain resilience (Mruk 2019). Reconciliation or resolution rests on its ideal (Simmons 2020). As such, reconciliation or resolution has benefitted from harmonious passion to sustain resilience (Belanger et al. 2019). Reparation characterizes caring (Featherstone and Morris 2012). Caring has rested on its ideal (Sarasa 2008). As such, caring has maintained mental clarity to boost resilience (Naruse et al. 2020). The ideal for self-enhancement buttress self-enhancement (Marshall 2001). Self-enhancement has reflected attachment and social support received to raise resilience (Hermanto et al. 2017; Ledoux et al. 2010). Coping has stemmed from ideals for cure, growth, relational satisfaction, self-compassion, and self-direction to rationalize resilience (Chwyl et al. 2021; Dai et al. 2015; Johnson et al. 2013; McClaran et al. 2022; Sutherland and Rehman 2018). The ideal for care has buttressed caring (Sarasa 2008). Growth has developed from self-compassion and self-tolerance to strengthen resilience (Ho and Li 2022; Munroe et al. 2022). Self-compassion hinges on its ideal (Chwyl et al. 2021). As such, self-compassion has lifted equanimity, happiness, and positive affect and has dampened anger, anxiety, depression, distress, negative affect, and self-rumination to induce resilience (Barnard and Curry 2011; Sirois et al. 2015). Self-direction has rested on its ideal (Gagne and Deci 2005). As such, self-direction has arisen from harm avoidance to safeguard resilience (Richter et al. 2002).

Norms enhancing coping to assimilate resilience have popularized adaptability, cohesion, and coping effectiveness (Kelly and Steed 2004; Ma et al. 2022). Adaptability evolves from assimilation (Bennett and Bennett 2004). As such, adaptability safeguards resilience (Charles and Carstensen 2009; Pangallo et al. 2015). Moreover, adaptability reflects resilience (Maltby et al. 2016). The norm for cohesion has assimilated cohesion (Volker et al. 2007). Cohesion has buttressed hope and life satisfaction and eroded depression to maintain resilience (Araya et al. 2006; Dittman and Goebel 2010; Paez et al. 2015). Conversely, coping has arisen from the norm for low stress to assimilate resilience (Landau et al. 1998). The norm for stress has popularized stress (Walen and Lachman 2016). Stress has eroded well-being, including eudaimonia, health, positive affect, quality of life, neighborhood, and relationships, and satisfaction with life and neighbors, thus jeopardizing resilience (Baumeister et al. 2013; Greenberg 1999; Jackson et al. 2006; Mathis et al. 2016; Parkes et al. 2002; Shrira 2012; Su et al. 2021; Zotti et al. 2016).

## Original Findings

Nine practical factors are supposed to raise the Chinese person's resilience felt, behaved, and/or believed (see Table 6.1). Among them, kindness, hardening, softening, Westernization, and experience-based coping significantly contributed to resilience. Kindness also indicated significant contributions to resilience action and belief. By contrast, the interaction between hardening and softening delivered significant inverse effects on resilience felt. Meanwhile, socializing, religious practice, and pet engagement did not exhibit significant effects on resilience felt.

| |
|---|
| Socializing, past 3 months ($\alpha = 0.637$; Chuang et al. 2016) |
| Being kind to people |
| Traveling with companions |
| Helping others |

(continued)

(continued)

| |
|---|
| Volunteering |
| Hardening, past 3 months ($\alpha = 0.715$) |
| Doing your part |
| Working hard to enrich yourself |
| Concentrating on things |
| Supporting yourself |
| Trusting yourself |
| Learning to be positive |
| Doing things to the end |
| Experiencing your own strong vitality |
| Experiencing the meaning of working hard to survive |
| (Not) Feeling you wasting time |
| Being respected |
| Softening, past 3 months ($\alpha = 0.769$) |
| Being considerate of others |
| Looking at things more openly |
| Forgiving others |
| Experiencing money as an external object |
| Experiencing that people always have birth, old age, sickness, and death |
| Experiencing the fate of life and death |
| Taking it easy |
| Feeling natural dominance in the dark |
| Thinking for the better |
| Experiencing life as a dream |
| Knowing satisfaction |
| Religious practice, past 3 months ($\alpha = 0.873$; Piedmont 2012) |
| Praying for god's blessing |
| Feeling god giving you wisdom |
| Reading or chanting Sutras |
| Feeling God loving you |
| Committing yourself to God |
| Pet engagement, past 3 months ($\alpha = 0.850$) |
| Caring for pets |
| Spending time on pets |
| Accompanying pets |
| Watching pets |
| Experience-based coping, past 6 months ($\alpha = 0.799$; Shirzadifard et al. 2018) |
| Using working experience to overcome adversity |

(continued)

(continued)

| |
|---|
| Using experience other than work to overcome adversity |
| Overcoming adversity with past hard life experience |
| Westernization, past 6 months ($\alpha = 0.674$; Detenber et al. 2013) |
| Appreciating European and American art, such as painting and music |
| Watching European and American TV programs or films |
| Having tried or hoped to visit Europe and America |
| Agreeing with European and American cultures, such as customs and habits |

## *Resilience Feeling*

Specifically, kindness exhibited a significant weak positive effect on resilience in general and particularly in the elder ($\beta = 0.081$ and 0.107, see Table 6.2). Nevertheless, the positive effect was not significant on the resilience of the youth or mid-age person ($\beta = 0.090$ and 0.028).

In the elder, experience-based coping, Westernization, hardening, and softening displayed significant positive effects on resilience, particularly when weighted by Westernization to represent findings in the West ($\beta = 0.201$, 124, 0.472 and 0.287, see Table 6.3) Meanwhile, the interaction between hardening and softening exhibited a significant weak negative effect on resilience ($\beta = -0.103$). That is, while the separate effects of hardening and softening on resilience were positive, their joint effect was negative.

On inferred resilience or adjustment under adversity, kindness did not show a significant effect. The nonsignificance appeared to the young, mid-age, and older persons (Table 6.4).

In the elder, hardening indicated a significant weak inverse effect on inferred resilience based on data not weighted for Westernization ($\beta = -0.095$, see Table 6.5). That is, the effect was significant only in the Hong Kong Chinese context. Meanwhile, experienced-based coping and other factors did not unfold significant effects on inferred resilience.

## *Adjustment and Depression*

On adjustment, kindness did not present a significant effect. The effect was nonsignificant on the adjustment of the younger, mid-age person, or elder (Table 6.6).

In the elder, depression evidenced significant negative effects from experience-based coping, Westernization, hardening, socializing, hardening, softening, and the interaction between hardening and softening, with data not weighted by Westernization ($\beta = -0.099$ to $-0.309$, see Table 6.7). With data weighted by Westernization,

**Table 6.1** Practical effects on resilience

| Practice | Expected | Currently found | | |
|---|---|---|---|---|
| | | Feeling | Action | Belief |
| Kindness | + | + | + | + |
| Hardening | + | + | | |
| Softening | + | + | | |
| Hardening × softening | + | – | | |
| Westernization | + | + | | |
| Socializing | + | 0 | | |
| Religious practice | + | 0 | | |
| Pet engagement | + | 0 | | |
| Experience-based coping | + | + | | |

*Note* + positive effect; – negative effect; ? mixed effects; 0 no effect

**Table 6.2** Standardized effects on resilience (service dataset)

| Predictor | Youth | Mid-age | Elder | All |
|---|---|---|---|---|
| Kindness | 0.090 | 0.028 | 0.107* | 0.081** |
| $R^2$ | 0.265 | 0.426 | 0.188 | 0.254 |

*Note* Regression analysis controlled for background characteristics and experiences
*$p < 0.05$, **$p < 0.01$

**Table 6.3** Standardized effects on resilience (elder dataset)

| Predictor | Unweighted | Weighted by westernization |
|---|---|---|
| Experience-based coping | 0.235** | 0.201** |
| Westernization | 0.111 | 0.124* |
| $R^2$ | 0.176 | 0.112 |
| Socializing | – 0.012 | 0.039 |
| Pet engagement | 0.036 | 0.045 |
| Religious practice | 0.005 | – 0.017 |
| Hardening | 0.355*** | 0.472*** |
| Softening | 0.343*** | 0.287*** |
| Hardening × Softening | – 0.022 | – 0.103* |
| $R^2$ | 0.380 | 0.353 |

*Note* Regression analysis controlled for background characteristics and experiences
*$p < 0.05$, **$p < 0.01$, ***$p < 0.001$

**Table 6.4** Standardized effects on inferred resilience (service dataset)

| Predictor | Youth | Mid-age | Elder | All |
|---|---|---|---|---|
| Kindness | 0.027 | – 0.002 | 0.051 | 0.019 |
| $R^2$ | 0.805 | 0.719 | 0.666 | 0.724 |

*Note* Regression analysis controlled for background characteristics and experiences

**Table 6.5** Standardized effects on inferred resilience (elder dataset)

| Predictor | Unweighted | Weighted by westernization |
|---|---|---|
| Experience-based coping | – 0.037 | – 0.030 |
| Westernization | 0.018 | 0.032 |
| $R^2$ | 0.717 | 0.710 |
| Socializing | – 0.023 | – 0.025 |
| Pet engagement | – 0.013 | – 0.016 |
| Religious practice | – 0.021 | 0.027 |
| Hardening | – 0.095* | – 0.042 |
| Softening | 0.002 | – 0.024 |
| Hardening × softening | – 0.004 | – 0.022 |
| $R^2$ | 0.724 | 0.714 |

*Note* Regression analysis controlled for background characteristics and experiences
*$p < 0.05$

**Table 6.6** Standardized effects on adjustment (service dataset)

| Predictor | Youth | Mid-age | Elder | All |
|---|---|---|---|---|
| Kindness | 0.029 | 0.031 | 0.041 | 0.046 |
| $R^2$ | 0.304 | 0.501 | 0.364 | 0.405 |

*Note* Regression analysis controlled for background characteristics and experiences

the effects of Westernization and socializing were nonsignificant, indicating that they were nonsignificant in the Westernized context. Meanwhile, the effects of experience-based coping, hardening, softening, and their interaction remained significant with data weighted by Westernization ($\beta = -0.097$ to $-0.405$, see Table 6.7).

## *Resilience Action*

On resilience learning, kindness did not deliver a significant effect. The effect was nonsignificant on the resilience learning of the younger, mid-age person, or elder (Table 6.8).

**Table 6.7** Standardized effects on depression (elder dataset)

| Predictor | Unweighted | Weighted by westernization |
|---|---|---|
| Experience-based coping | – 0.155* | – 0.181** |
| Westernization | – 0.142* | – 0.055 |
| $R^2$ | 0.151 | 0.178 |
| Socializing | – 0.130* | – 0.024 |
| Pet engagement | – 0.018 | – 0.081 |
| Religious practice | 0.018 | 0.078 |
| Hardening | – 0.218** | – 0.405*** |
| Softening | – 0.309*** | – 0.162* |
| Hardening × softening | – 0.099* | – 0.097# |
| $R^2$ | 0.298 | 0.360 |

*Note* Regression analysis controlled for background characteristics and experiences
#$p < 0.10$, *$p < 0.05$, **$p < 0.01$, ***$p < 0.001$

**Table 6.8** Standardized effects on resilience learning (service dataset)

| Predictor | Youth | Mid-age | Elder | All |
|---|---|---|---|---|
| Kindness | 0.056 | 0.053 | 0.049 | 0.070 |
| $R^2$ | 0.180 | 0.319 | 0.220 | 0.175 |

*Note* Regression analysis controlled for background characteristics and experiences

On resilience handling, kindness demonstrated a significant weak positive effect ($\beta = 0.203$, see Table 6.9). The effect was significantly positive on the resilience handling of the younger, mid-age person, or elder ($\beta = 0.129$ to 0.236).

On self-awareness as a resilience action, kindness demonstrated a significant weak positive effect ($\beta = 0.210$, see Table 6.10). The effect was significantly positive on the self-awareness of the younger, mid-age person, or elder ($\beta = 0.132$ to 0.220).

**Table 6.9** Standardized effects on resilience handling (service dataset)

| Predictor | Youth | Mid-age | Elder | All |
|---|---|---|---|---|
| Kindness | 0.236*** | 0.205*** | 0.129** | 0.203*** |
| $R^2$ | 0.382 | 0.506 | 0.383 | 0.475 |

*Note* Regression analysis controlled for background characteristics and experiences
**$p < 0.01$, ***$p < 0.001$

**Table 6.10** Standardized effects on self-awareness (service dataset)

| Predictor | Youth | Mid-age | Elder | All |
|---|---|---|---|---|
| Kindness | $0.132^{**}$ | $0.209^{***}$ | $0.220^{***}$ | $0.210^{***}$ |
| $R^2$ | 0.266 | 0.456 | 0.292 | 0.310 |

*Note* Regression analysis controlled for background characteristics and experiences
$^{*}p < 0.05$, $^{**}p < 0.01$, $^{***}p < 0.001$

**Table 6.11** Standardized effects on resilience belief (service dataset)

| Predictor | Youth | Mid-age | Elder | All |
|---|---|---|---|---|
| Kindness | $0.219^{***}$ | $0.280^{***}$ | $0.163^{***}$ | $0.227^{***}$ |
| $R^2$ | 0.339 | 0.494 | 0.424 | 0.492 |

*Note* Regression analysis controlled for background characteristics and experiences
$^{*}p < 0.05$, $^{**}p < 0.01$, $^{***}p < 0.001$

**Table 6.12** Standardized effects on benevolent world belief (service dataset)

| Predictor | Youth | Mid-age | Elder | All |
|---|---|---|---|---|
| Kindness | 0.056 | $0.107^{*}$ | $0.121^{**}$ | $0.089^{**}$ |
| $R^2$ | 0.311 | 0.508 | 0.413 | 0.486 |

*Note* Regression analysis controlled for background characteristics and experiences
$^{*}p < 0.05$, $^{**}p < 0.01$, $^{***}p < 0.001$

## *Resilience Belief*

On resilience belief, kindness demonstrated a significant weak positive effect ($\beta$ = 0.227, see Table 6.9). The effect was significantly positive on the resilience belief of the younger, mid-age person, or elder ($\beta$ = 0.163 to 0.280) (Table 6.11).

On benevolenet world belief as resilience belief, kindness demonstrated a significant slight positive effect ($\beta$ = 0.089, see Table 6.9). The effect was significantly positive on the resilience handling of the mid-age person or elder ($\beta$ = 0.107 to 0.121). Nevertheless, the effect was nonsignificant on the youth's belief (Table 6.12).

## *Effects not Supporting the Hypotheses*

Four of the nine factors displayed effects on resilience feeling that did not support the hypotheses (see Table 6.1). These effects were the significant inverse effect of (1) the interaction between hardening and softening and the nonsignificant effects of (2) socializing, (3) religious practice, and (4) pet engagement. These effects suggested inverse effects offsetting or even outstripping the hypothesized positive effects.

## Combination of Hardening and Softening

The interaction or combination of hardening and softening generated an inverse effect on resilience to reflect competition, conflict, contradiction, or jamming between hardening and softening. Essentially, hardening and softening are contradictory to each other. That is, concentrating and toiling in hardening contradict easygoing, forgiving, and tolerating in softening. Contradiction and its associates are likely to impair resilience through breeding power, utility, ideals, and norms against resilience with the voluntaristic mechanisms of analytical functionalism.

Contradiction represents competition and polarization and contradicts softness or softening (Greene 1991; LaMothe 2012). It features anger, anxiety or fear, argument, discord, disquiet, dissonance, doubt, hostility, protesting, struggle, and violence (Bar-Tal and Halperin 2013; Baucom and Atkins 2013; Busby and Chiu 2017; Dew et al. 2012; Guerrero 2013; LaMothe 2012; Nail et al. 2004; Saxton and Benson 2006; Upenieks 2022; Wilt et al. 2017). These natures and features engender power, utility, ideals, and norms against resilience.

Power raised by contradiction to distract or weaken resilience rests on depression, difficulty, and hostility (Guerrero 2013; Turner 2013). Difficulty or disability has incurred distress and dampened health, life satisfaction, and self-efficacy, thus eroding resilience (Distante 2013; Gastil 2000; Michalos et al. 2000; Phongsavan et al. 2006). Hostility has provoked anger, anxiety, and sadness to impede resilience (Vandervoort 2006). Moreover, contradiction has also raised depression, distress, suicide, and violence to impede power for driving resilience (Dutton et al. 2016; Gutierrez et al. 2017; Farrington 2007). Attempted suicide has induced anxiety to obstruct resilience (Cheng et al. 2017). Violence has bred depression, thus disturbing resilience (Wright et al. 2015). Contradiction involves anger, anxiety or fear, disquiet, and vulnerability to dampen power sustaining resilience (Dew et al. 2012; Guerrero 2013; LaMothe 2012; Saxton and Benson 2006). Disquiet dismisses meaningfulness and peacefulness, thus jeopardizing resilience (Valle 2019). Vulnerability has eroded mattering and self-efficacy to obstruct resilience (Flett 2018; Kim et al. 2016). Contradiction stems from anxiety, closed-mindedness, deprivation, grievance, and reliance to weaken power for driving resilience (Dorjee 2013; Fisher et al. 2013; LaMothe 2012; Rick et al. 2006; Turner 2013). Closed-mindedness has impeded well-being, including autonomy, growth, life satisfaction, purposefulness, relational quality, self-acceptance, self-efficacy, and self-esteem to disrupt resilience (Hahn et al. 2013; Hounknatin et al. 2014; Karwowski and Lebuda 2017; Marks 1996; Webster et al. 2014). Deprivation has dampened social trust and general well-being, thus impeding resilience (Clark et al. 2008; Layte et al. 2000; Stephens et al. 2014). Grievance has bred anger, impulsivity, and worry to defuse resilience action (Boehnke and Wong 2011; Landmann and Rohmann 2020; Vestergren et al. 2017). Reliance has weakened coping and health, thus eroding resilience (Bekker et al. 2011; Roy and Chaudhuri 2008). Furthermore, contradiction has arisen from frustration, neuroticism, sickness, and strain to reduce power for driving resilience (Espvall and Dellgran 2010; Lincoln et al. 2003; Vanhee et al. 2018; Wilt et al. 2017). Frustration has incurred avoiding and withholding to impair resilience (Vanhee et al. 2018). Neuroticism has worsened well-being, including autonomy, growth, health, positive affect, purposefulness, relatedness, satisfaction, self-acceptance, self-compassion, and self-determination, to resist resilience (Anusic et al. 2014; Hounkpatin et al. 2015; Ingledew et al. 2004; Pfattheicher et al. 2017; Richards 2016; Webster et al. 2014). Sickness has eroded functionality, health and mental health, knowledge, optimism, security, vitality, and general well-being, thus disempowering resilience (Benitez-Silva et al. 2010; Carrieri 2012; Korkeila et al. 2004; Price et al. 2006; van Dijk et al. 2008). Conversely, contradiction impairs adjustment, collaboration, creativity, and social integration to withdraw power that maintains resilience (Turner 2013). Collaboration has lifted life satisfaction to enhance resilience (Park et al. 2015). Creativity has boosted well-being, notably including meaningfulness, to induce resilience (Diener et al. 2009; Turner 2013). Social integration has eroded depression to bolster resilience (Mullins and Dugan 1991). Contradiction has impaired well-being, including life satisfaction and spiritual well-being, thus lowering power to drive resilience (Baumeister et al. 2013; Richards 2016; Wilt et al. 2017). Moreover, contradiction has reduced trust, thus dampening power for driving resilience (Kunovich and Hodson 1999). Trust has fostered health and survival to sustain resilience (Barefoot et al. 1998). Besides, contradiction reflects low bonding, cognitive complexity or intelligence, compassion, cultural capital, empathy, forgiveness, gratitude, hospitality, humility, meditation, morality, peacefulness, reverence, security, self-esteem, skill, social support received, softness or softening, sufficiency, and togetherness, thus undermining power to drive resilience (Baucom and Atkins 2013; Brubaker 2015; Caughlin et al. 2013; Greene 1991; LaMothe 2012; Maoz 2018; Rick et al. 2006; Nail et al. 2004; Roloff and Wright 2013). Compassion has sustained well-being to drive resilience (Jasielska 2020). Cognitive complexity has assuaged depression to maintain resilience (Feinstein and Bynner 2006). Cultural capital has enhanced religiosity to secure resilience (Wuthnow 2004). Empathy has enhanced intimacy and reduced discontent and resentment to elevate resilience (Redmond 2018). Forgiveness has elevated serenity, trust, and well-being to maintain resilience (Choi and David 2012; Connors et al. 1999; Shimai et al. 2006). Gratitude has raised positive affect and dampened negative affect to achieve resilience (Bernabe-Valero et al. 2021). Hospitality has elevated life satisfaction to rationalize resilience (Selim 2008). Humility has fostered connectedness and gratitude to facilitate resilience (Angelis and Pensini 2024; Krumrei-Mancuso 2017). Meditation has advanced compassion or self-compassion and mindfulness and dwindled depression to foster resilience (Galante et al. 2014). Morality has satisfied the life and reduced anxiety to maintain resilience (Conzo et al. 2017; Stets et al. 2008). Peacefulness has maintained life satisfaction and attenuated depression to buttress resilience (Yang 2016). Reverence has fostered identity to afford resilience (Renger and Reese 2017). Security has escalated well-being, including health and life satisfaction to raise resilience (Chen et al. 2008; Frey et al. 2007; Jones et al. 2014). Skill has underpinned self-efficacy to buttress resilience (Larson et al. 1990). Social support received has upheld well-being, including control, health, positive emotion and pleasure, purposiveness, relational quality, satisfaction with life, housing, and leisure, self-determination, self-efficacy, self-esteem, and social well-being, to activate resilience (George and Park 2013; Glendinning et al. 2003; Granzin and Haggard 2000; Holliman et al. 2021; Lincoln et al. 2003; Logan and Cobb 2013; Pierce and Quiroz 2018; Schwarzer and Knoll 2007; Vilhjalmsson and Thorlindsson 1998; Wen et al. 2010; Williams and Galliher 2006; Xi and Hwang 2011). Notably, social support received has boosted resilience (Cherry et al. 2018). To uphold resilience, softness characterizes reconciliation to achieve well-being, including control, mastery, and self-efficacy (Giri 2011; Levesque et al. 2023; Ross and Drentea 1998; Van Haaften et al. 2004). Sufficiency has been salutary, including enhancing life satisfaction, positive affect, self-determination, and vitality (Chen et al. 2015; Cordeiro et al. 2015; Sheldon and Krieger 2007). Togetherness has eroded depression and negative affect, thus safeguarding resilience (McIntyre et al. 2023; Stanton et al. 2020). Contradiction has also arisen from low agreeableness, conscientiousness, relational quality, and self-esteem and its collective form to defuse power for driving resilience (Bar-Tal and Halperin 2013; Nail et al. 2004; Simpson et al. 2008; Wilt et al. 2017). Agreeableness has fostered growth, life satisfaction, mastery, purposefulness, relatedness, and self-acceptance to buttress resilience (Hounkpatin et al. 2015). Conscientiousness has raised attachment, autonomy, life satisfaction, mastery, purposefulness, and self-acceptance to secure resilience (Fraley et al. 2011; Hounkpatin et al. 2015).

Disutility raised by contradiction to discourage resilience covers crowdedness (Chan 1999). Crowdedness has raised depression to impede resilience (Riad and Norris 1992). Contradiction reflects exclusion or rejection, inequality, negativity, pressure, and threat experienced to lessen utility for attracting resilience (Bar-Tal and Halperin 2013; Brewer 2012; Fisher et al. 2013; Guerrero 2013; LaMothe 2012; Rick et al. 2006). Rejection experienced has raised negative mood and eroded life satisfaction to attenuate resilience (Lin et al. 2013; Williams et al. 2000). Societal inequality has escalated anxiety and mortality risk and has dampened health, satisfaction, and well-being in general to impede resilience (Kawachi et al. 1997; Kim and Kawachi 2007; Meulemann 2010; Oshio and Kobayashi 2010; Schwartz and Melech 2000). Negativity has eroded well-being, including meaningfulness and satisfaction, to hinder resilience (Baumeister et al. 2013; Goodman et al. 2017; Sun et al. 2013). Pressure experienced has heightened burnout, depression, powerlessness, and somatic complaint, and eroded health and self-esteem, thus impairing resilience (Furnham 1997; Gerber et al. 2010; Wan et al. 2023). Threat experienced has fomented anxiety, avoidance, conflict, depression, fear, and hate to disrupt resilience (Edwards and Arnon 2021; MacLeod 2017; Moore and Shepherd 2006; O'Neill and Evans 1999; Rick et al. 2006; Ruiter et al. 2003). Furthermore, contradiction has arisen from disagreement, hardship, stress, trauma, and victimization experienced to uphold disutility against resilience (Dew et al. 2012, Espvall and Dellgran 2010; Lincoln et al. 2003; Pomerleau et al. 2020). Disagreement experienced has eroded meaningfulness, positive emotion, and relatedness to obstruct resilience (Heshmati and Oravecz 2022). Hardship experienced has incubated self-transcendence to achieve resilience (Reeskens and Vandecasteele 2017). Stress or trauma experienced has dampened well-being, including health, life quality, positive affect, and satisfaction as opposed to depression and distress, to impede resilience (Baumeister et al.

2013. Mathis et al. 2016; Raposa et al. 2016; Shrira 2012; Snyder et al. 2020; Zotti et al. 2016). Vcitimization experienced has induced anxiety, depression, distress, fear, helplessness, neuroticism, powerlessness, and symptoms to weaken power for resilience (Krahe 2013; Krulichova 2019; Lincoln et al. 2003; Lineres 2004; Ross and Mirowsky 2009; Wager 2012). Meanwhile, victimization experienced has impaired safety experienced and self-respect or self-worth to erode resilience (Fernandes 2018; Krahe 2013). Conversely, contradiction has dampened harmony experienced, thus withdrawing utility to attract resilience (Wong and Shik 2011). Harmony experienced has reflected satisfaction with the economy, family, governance, mutual support, progress, and work to boost resilience (Ho and Chan 2009). Contradiction stems from low caring, investment, love, social legitimacy, understanding, and validation experienced to dismiss utility to attract resilience (Bar-Tal and Halperin 2013; Baucom and Atkins 2013; Jeffries 2000). Caring experienced has boosted well-being, including control, emotional well-being, health, pleasure, purposiveness, relational quality, satisfaction with housing, leisure, and life, self-determination, self-efficacy, self-esteem, and social well-being to sustain resilience (George and Park 2013; Glendinning et al. 2003; Granzin and Haggard 2000; Holliman et al. 2021; Kafetsio and Sideridis 2006; Lincoln et al. 2003; Logan and Cobb 2013; Schwarzer and Knoll 2007; Vilhjalmsson and Thorlindsson 1998; Wen et al. 2010; Williams and Galliher 2006; Xi and Hwang 2011). Investment has strengthened social capital to facilitate resilience (Hlasny and Lee 2020). Legitimacy perceived has reflected satisfaction to uphold resilience (Johnson 2015). Love experienced can erode depression, thus maintaining resilience (Busch 2009). Understanding or validation experienced has facilitated adaptation, positive emotion, forgiveness, and life satisfaction to induce resilience (Algoe and Zhaoyang 2016; Brik et al. 2023). Similarly, contradction has arisen from low equality and justice experienced to dismiss resilience (Mikula et al. 2012; Ruppanner 2010). Justice experienced has sustained belongingness, health, life satisfaction, and self-esteem and eroded anger and depression, thus safeguarding resilience (Bjornskov et al. 2013; Dalbert 2001; Lucas et al. 2013; Rothmund et al. 2014; van Prooijen et al. 2008).

Ideals nurtured by contradiction to counter resilience accentuate argument, blaming, discrimination, dominating, polarization, prejudice, protesting, struggle, and violence (Bar-Tal and Halperin 2013; Baucom and Atkins 2013; Busby and Chiu 2017; Dew et al. 2012; Guerrero 2013; Koomen and van der Pligt 2016; LaMothe 2012; Lutgen-Sandvik and Fletcher 2013; Saxton and Benson 2006; Upenieks 2022). Argument has sprung from the ideal for aggression breed depression and stress to dampen resilience (Grych and Kinsfogel 2010; Muradwij and Allwood 2022). Blaming has reflected conflict perception and distress as opposed to compromise to impede resilience (Bagci and Celebi 2017; Recchia and Howe 2010; Wayment et al. 2010). The ideal for discriminating underlies discriminating (North and Fiske 2013). Discriminating has weakened belongingness and confidence, thus impeding resilience (Juanchich et al. 2018). Dominating has relied on its ideal (Cheung and Chiu 2021). As such, dominating has bred depression and dampened well-being generally to impair resilience (Lincoln et al. 2003; Van Haaften et al. 2004). Contradiction also dismisses compassion to attenuate the ideal for rationalizing resilience

(LaMothe 2012; Pomerleau et al. 2020). Compassion has enhanced well-being to facilitate resilience (Jasielska 2020). Contradiction stems from ideals or concerns about comparison, conflict, dissimilarity, distinctiveness, favoritism, minority status, negativity, self-maintenance, self-serving, and social derogation, devaluation, and discrepancy to challenge resilience (Ellemers and Haslam 2012; Fisher et al. 2013; Kim 2013; Koltko-Rivera 2004; Kreidie and Monroe 2002; Miles 2015; Rick et al. 2006; Ruppanner 2010). Comparison has developed from its ideal (Buunk and Gibbons 2006). As such, comparison has bred negative affect and dampened self-esteem to worsen resilience (Fujita 2008). Conflict has arisen from its ideal (Ohbuchi et al. 1999). As such, conflict has provoked distress and eroded satisfaction, thus impeding resilience (Lau et al. 2017; Mikula et al. 2012). Dissimilarity, distinctiveness, or discrepancy has raised depression to hinder resilience (Riad and Norris 1992). Favoritism can arise from conflict to impede resilience (Malloy 2018). Minority status has dampened life quality to hurt resilience (Verschuur et al. 2010). Negativity has eroded well-being, including meaningfulness and satisfaction, to hinder resilience (Baumeister et al. 2013; Goodman et al. 2017; Sun et al. 2013). Self-maintenance, self-serving, or its basis of egoism has created anxiety to hamper resilience (Da Costa Bizarro Morais et al. 2019). Social derogation or devaluation has evolved from its ideal (Ludigdo and Mashuric 2021). As such, social derogation or devaluation has reflected low self-esteem, thus jeopardizing resilience (Chen et al. 2022). Furthermore, contradiction has emanated from ideals for equality or egalitarianism, hostility, power, and resources, thus dispelling resilience (Ohbuchi et al. 1999; Ruppanner 2010). Egalitarianism has reflected low belongingness and satisfaction to impede resilience (Kangas 2003; Suchweh 2012). Hostility has incurred anger, anxiety, and sadness to impede resilience (Vandervoort 2006). Power has created a positive mood and dampened depression to build resilience (Langner et al. 2012; Wojciszke and Struzynska-Kujolowicz 2007). Conversely, contradiction reflects low ideals about acceptance, accommodation, accountability, balance, caring, commonality, complexity, conservatism, cooperation, discipline, fairness, humanizing or humanitarianism, reconciliation, retreating, similarity, tolerance, and transcendence, thus refuting resilience (Huddy 2004; Kim 2013; LaMothe 2012; Maoz 2018; Miles 2015; Ruppanner 2010; Rick et al. 2006). Accountability has advanced wisdom to facilitate resilience (Spengler et al. 2018). Balance has fostered confidence to achieve resilience (Simon and Read 2018). The ideal for caring has stemmed from well-being to induce resilience (Peterson and Klohnen 1995). The ideal for commonality has raised relatedness to facilitated resilience (Torlo and Lomi 2017). The ideal for complexity reflects optimality to maintain resilience (Brewer and Pierce 2005). Conservatism stems from enlightenment and rationality to enable resilience (Scruton 2014). Cooperation has thrived on its ideal (Haesevoets et al. 2015). As such, cooperation has fostered life satisfaction to rationalize resilience (Park et al. 2015). Discipline has strengthened well-being, notably self-esteem, to induce resilience (Armstrong et al. 2011; Diener and Fujita 1995). The ideal for fairness has raised resilience and other well-being components (Diener et al. 2009; Pyszkowska 2020). Humanitarianism has stood on connectedness and humility to facilitate resilience (Angelis and Pensini 2024). Reconciliation has reflected harmonious passion and order, security, and stability values to secure resilience (Belanger et al. 2019; Simmons 2020).Retreating has bred distress to hamper resilience (Frazier et al. 2005). Similarity has reduced depression to afford resilience (Riad and Norris 1992). Transcendence has boosted life satisfaction and meaningfulness and reduced anxiety, depression, and stress to uplift resilience (Fishbein et al. 2020). Furthermore, contradiction has arisen from low ideals for coping and identity, thus refuting resilience (Ohbuchi et al. 1999). Coping has raised resilience, environmental and relational quality, growth, health, intimacy, satisfaction, and self-efficacy (Cherry et al. 2023; Chow et al. 2014; Gattino et al. 2015; Lau et al. 2012; Paez et al. 2007; Veenstra et al. 2005; Wills 1997). Identity has secured happiness, love, self-efficacy, and self-esteem and diminished anxiety and depression to facilitate resilience (Cast 2004).

Norms underlying contradiction to reject resilience have popularized conflict, discord, discrimination, egalitarianism, frustration, loss, and tension (Amato and Chendle 2005; Busby and Chiu 2017; Ruppanner 2010; Sorens 2011; Vanhee et al. 2018). Conflict or discord has emerged from its norm (Sorens 2011). Eventually, conflict has provoked distress and eroded satisfaction, thus impeding resilience (Lau et al. 2017; Mikula et al. 2012). Discriminating has emerged from its norm (McDougall et al. 2004). Eventually, discriminating has weakened belongingness and confidence, thus impeding resilience (Juanchich et al. 2018). Conversely, contradiction has arisen from the norm against collectivism to expel resilience (Ohbuchi et al. 1999). Collectivism has grown from its norm (Sabatier and Lannegrand-Willems 2005). Eventually, collectivism has safeguarded health, intimacy, and self-esteem to boost resilience (Kemp 2007; Triandis 1995).

## Socializing

Socializing is likely to generate an inverse effect on resilience to neutralize its positive effect on resilience. This inverse effect is likely to arise from the unstructured, unguarded, or unconventional form of socializing (Yuan and McNeeley 2018). As such, socializing breeds power, utility, ideals, and norms against resilience by the voluntaristic mechanisms of power realization, utility optimization, ideal calibration, and norm conformity in analytical functionalism.

Power reduced by socializing to drive resilience stems from guardianship or monitoring received (Benson and Simpson 2018). Guardianship or monitoring received has fostered identity achievement to facilitate resilience (Marcia 1980).

Disutility elevated by socializing to discourage resilience has rested on stress and victimization experienced (Hanish et al. 2007). Stress experienced has dampened well-being, including health, life quality, positive affect, and satisfaction as opposed to depression and distress, to impede resilience (Baumeister et al. 2013. Mathis et al. 2016; Raposa et al. 2016; Shrira 2012; Snyder et al. 2020; Zotti et al. 2016). Victimization experienced has impaired safety experienced and self-respect or self-worth to erode resilience (Fernandes 2018; Krahe 2013). Conversely, socializing has reduced achievement and warmth received as utility to attract resilience (Boccio et al. 2023; Gaunt 2011 Rosenbaum and Rochford 2008). Achievement has fostered health, life quality, satisfaction, self-efficacy, and self-esteem as opposed to alienation, depression, and distress to uphold resilience (Donnellan et al. 2005; Fredricks and Eccles 2005; Menard and Mose 1984; Murray 2009; Piko et al. 2006; Tompson and Dass 2000; Xiao et al. 2009). Warmth experienced has reflected relationship quality to sustain resilience (Chen and Kaplan 2001).

Ideals or obsessions raised by socializing to discredit resilience cherish crime or delinquency, disaffection or dissatisfaction, doping, and violence (Hanish et al. 2007; Hoffmann 2023; Leimberg and Lehmann 2022; Thomas and McGloin 2013). The ideal for crime, delinquency, or violence has originated from anger and contempt as opposed to self-efficacy to impair resilience (Tausch et al. 2011). Furthermore, the ideal has rationalized crime or delinquency (Tanner-Smith et al. 2013). Crime or delinquency has eroded life satisfaction, mastery, relationship quality, self-efficacy, and self-esteem to weaken resilience (Chung and Elias 1996; Keijsers et al. 2011; Shek 2005). The ideal for doping has buttressed doping (Leimberg and Lehmann 2022). Doping has engendered depression, thus jeopardizing resilience (Kendler et al. 2006). The ideal for violence has rationalized violence (Muluk et al. 2013). Violence has bred depression, thus disturbing resilience (Wright et al. 2015). Conversely, socializing has eroded the prosocial ideal to hinder resilience (Brandenberger and Bowman 2015). The prosocial ideal has elevated well-being, including connectedness, hope, life satisfaction, meaningfulness, and self-efficacy to boost resilience (Marsh and Dik 2021; Nelson-Coffey et al. 2023; Raposa et al. 2016; Yao and Enright 2019).

The norm registered by socializing to dissimilate resilience has popularized delinquency (Yuan and McNeeley 2018). Delinquency has grown from its norm (Hoffmann 2023). Eventually, delinquency has jeopardized achievement, coping, education, mastery, life satisfaction, relational quality, self-efficacy, self-esteem, social attachment, and social capital in the youth to impede resilience (Carroll et al. 2009; Chung and Elias 1996; Compas et al. 1988; Fasang et al. 2014; Gault-Sherman 2012; Shek 2005).

## Religious Practice

Religious practice is likely to introduce an inverse effect to offset its positive effect on resilience. The inverse effect is likely to stem from the extremist, pathological, reliant, and sacrificing properties of religious practice (Ager and Ager 2011; Harris et al. 2018; Rip et al. 2012; Rivera 2018). Moreover, the inverse effect can echo the impacts of religious practice on anxiety, irrationality, and violence (Muluk et al. 2013; Thorson 1998; Turner 2009). The effect is likely to unfold in power, utility, ideals, and norms engendered by religious practice to run the voluntaristic mechanisms of analytical functionalism.

Power for resilience diminished by religious practice has rested on humor and well-being, including satisfaction with the neighborhood (Ayalon et al. 1993;

Michalos et al. 2005; Saraglou 2004).Humor has buttressed resilience (Ungar et al. 2005). Religious practice reflects inadequate enlightenment experienced, thus impeding power to drive resilience (Forsyth 2003). Enlightenment received has reduced anxiety, depression, and fear to raise resilience (DiGiuseppe et al. 2017). Furthermore, religious practice has reflected inadequate education, health, income, openness, social class, and trust, thus impairing resilience (Fjellvang 2011; Immerzeel and van Tubergen 2013; Kunovich and Hodson 1999; Medvedovski and Allison 2017; Saucier and Skrzypinska 2006; Yuchtman-Yaar 2002). Education has sustained well-being, including health, identity, life quality and satisfaction, mastery, self-efficacy, self-esteem, and youthfulness to engender resilience (Cerin and Leslie 2008; Corcoran et al. 2011; James and Amato 2013; Pakulshi and Tranter 2000; Stavrova and Ehlebracht 2018; van Praag and Frijters 1999; Whyte and Gao 2009; Yienprugsawan et al. 2010). Income has afforded well-being, including adaptation, adequacy, belongingness, control, eudaemonia, health, mastery, power, quality of life, satisfaction, self-efficacy, self-esteem, and social well-being to sustain resilience (Anciaes et al. 2017; Carpiano 2008; Corcoran et al. 2011; Ross and Mirowsky 1989; Sengupta and Sibley 2019; Son and Wilson 2012; Wang and VanderWeele 2011; Yeh et al. 2013; Zimmerman and Reyna 2013). Openness has facilitated well-being, including autonomy, growth, life satisfaction, purposefulness, relational quality, self-acceptance, self-efficacy, and self-esteem to enable resilience (Hounkpatin et al. 2015; Webster et al. 2014). Social class has sustained well-being, including financial adequacy, health, hope, and satisfaction, as opposed to depression to advance resilience (Burke 2008; Davis and Davenport 1999; Haller and Hadler 2006; Hadjar and Samuel 2015; Peterson and Seligman 2004; Yamaoka 2008). Trust has promoted health and survival to secure resilience (Barefoot et al. 1998). Conversely, religious practice breeds anxiety, cognitive simplicity, irrationality, pathology, and reliance to reduce power for driving resilience (Harris et al. 2018; Muluk et al. 2013; Rivera 2018; Thorson 1998). Cognitive simplicity has elevated depression to hinder resilience (Feinstein and Bynner 2006). Irrationality has bred anxiety, depression, disorders, and self-defeating, thus diminishing resilience (DiGiuseppe et al. 2017). Pathology has dampened resilience and other aspects of well-being, including health, life satisfaction, safety, security, and vitality (Carrieri 2012; Jones and d'Errico 2019; Magnani and Zhu 2018; van Dijk et al. 2008). Reliance has weakened coping and health, thus eroding resilience (Bekker et al. 2011; Roy and Chaudhuri 2008). Religious practice has also increased fear, illness, narcissism, psychopathy, and social distance experienced, thus reducing power to drive resilience (Aghababaei et al. 2016; Lee et al. 2023; Pedahzur and Canetti-Nisim 2004; Yamaoka 2008). Illness has eroded functionality, health and mental health, knowledge, optimism, security, vitality, and general well-being, thus disempowering resilience (Benitez-Silva et al. 2010; Carrieri 2012; Korkeila et al. 2004; Price et al. 2006; van Dijk et al. 2008). Narcissism has activated aggression, depression, misbehavior, and relational dissatisfaction, thus eroding resilience (Tracy et al. 2009). Psychopathy has hurt well-being to displace resilience (Jans-Beken 2019). Social distance reflects a resource deficit to hurt resilience (Van Hook 2002). Religious practice also reflects alienation, death instinct, dependency, helplessness, hostility, improvishment, neuroticism, insecurity, and trauma experienced to erode power to drive resilience (Browning and Cooper 2004; Forsyth 2003; Gutierrez et al. 2017; Shorey et al. 2018). Alienation experienced has fomented feelings of depression, guilt, internalizing, loneliness, negative emotion, resentment, and stupidity to disturb resilience (Sommer et al. 2001; Tani and Schneider 1997; Witkow 2005). Dependency has raised illness and suicide and eroded health and mastery, thus shaking resilience (Bornstein 2012; Lu and Kao 2002; Roy and Chaudhuri 2008). Hostility has incurred anger, anxiety, and sadness to impede resilience (Vandervoort 2006). Impoverishment has inhibited well-being and fomented strain to withhold resilience (Clark et al. 2008; Walker et al. 2010). Neuroticism has worsened well-being, including autonomy, growth, health, positive affect, purposefulness, relatedness, satisfaction, self-acceptance, self-compassion, and self-determination, to resist resilience (Anusic et al. 2014; Hounkpatin et al. 2015; Ingledew et al. 2004; Pfattheicher et al. 2017; Richards 2016; Webster et al. 2014). Insecurity has diminished well-being, including health and life satisfaction to block resilience (Chen et al. 2008; Frey et al. 2007; Jones et al. 2014). Trauma has incurred complaints, depression, and distress to suppress resilience (Balsam et al. 2011; Fischer et al. 2016).

Disutility to resist resilience embodied by religiousness rests on conflict experienced as disutility (Davidson 2008). Conflict has fomented distress, suicide, and violence to weaken resilience (Dutton et al. 2016; Farrington 2018; Li and Leung 2012). Moreover, religious practice has elevated marginalization experience as disutility to discourage resilience (Wuthnow 2004). Marginalization experienced has installed negative mood and diminished life satisfaction, thus impairing resilience (Lin et al. 2013; Williams et al. 2000). Religious practice also reflects repression, social exclusion, status inconsistency or deprivation, stress, terror, and war experienced as distutility to deter resilience (Miller 1995; Forsyth 2003; Immerzeel and van Tubergen 2013; Kay et al. 2008; Sasaki 1979; Schaafsma and Williams 2012). Deprivation experienced has dampened social trust and general well-being, thus impeding resilience (Clark et al. 2008; Layte et al. 2000; Stephens et al. 2014). Repression experienced has fomented protesting to riase anger and discontent to disrupt resilience (Aytac and Stokes 2019; Landmann and Rohmann 2020). Stress experienced has dampened well-being, including health, life quality, positive affect, and satisfaction as opposed to depression and distress, to impede resilience (Baumeister et al. 2013. Mathis et al. 2016; Raposa et al. 2016; Shrira 2012; Snyder et al. 2020; Zotti et al. 2016). Victimization, terror, or war experienced has impaired safety experienced and self respect or self-worth to erode resilience (Fernandes 2018; Krahe 2013). Conversely, religious practice has reduced achievement experienced as utility to attract resilience (Zeon 1987). Achievement has fostered health, life quality, satisfaction, self-efficacy, and self-esteem as opposed to alienation, depression, and distress to uphold resilience (Donnellan et al. 2005; Fredricks and Eccles 2005; Menard and Mose 1984; Murray 2009; Piko et al. 2006; Tompson and Dass 2000; Xiao et al. 2009).

Ideals for rationalizing resilience eroded by religious practice have accentuated comfort, control, freedom, hedonism, individualism, studying, survival, and tolerance (Coffe and Geys 2007; Devos et al. 2002; Moore and Aweiss 2003; Saucier and Skrzypinska 2006; Shmueli 1999; Wuthnow 2004). Controlling has stemmed from its ideal. Eventually, controlling has enhanced well-being, including health and life satisfaction as opposed to anger and depression to enable resilience (Etezadi and Pushkar 2013; Cundiff et al. 2015; Orlowski and Wicker 2015; Rose 2000; Xi and Hwang 2011). The ideal for freedom or liberalism has rested on growth to induce resilience (Helson and Srivastava 2001). Hedonism has underpinned well-being, notably life satisfaction, to advance resilience (Datler et al. 2013; Joshanloo and Jarden 2016). Individualism has fostered self-enhancement (Church 2010). Self-enhancement has dampened depression (Bang et al. 2020). The ideal for studying has boosted achievement to engage resilience (Liu and Yu 2016). Survival can hinge on resiliency and has benefitted from coping (Barber et al. 2010; Fawzy et al. 2001). Sacrificing has evolved from its ideal (Kleine et al. 2009). As such, sacrificing has stemmed relational quality to uphold resilience (Degenne et al. 2004). Religious practice elevates ideals regarding extremism, sacrificing, and violence to dispel resilience (Ager and Ager 2011; Muluk et al. 2013; Rip et al. 2012). Extremism has reflected anomie, anxiety, self-uncertainty, and uncertainty to erode resilience (Hogg et al. 2010; Koehler and Fiebig 2019; Stankov et al. 2018). The ideal for violence has rationalized violence (Muluk et al. 2013). Violence has bred depression, thus disturbing resilience (Wright et al. 2015). Moreover, religious practice has bred ideals for discriminating, protesting, and radicalism to hinder resilience (Forman 2001; Norris 2002; Pedahzur and Canetti-Nisim 2004). The ideal for discriminating underlies discriminating (North and Fiske 2013). Discriminating has weakened belongingness and confidence, thus impeding resilience (Juanchich et al. 2018). The ideal for protesting has constituted protesting (Hwang and Kim 2015). Protesting has invoked anger and worry to counter resilience feeling (Boehnke and Wong 2011; Landmann and Rohmann 2020). Radicalism has bred distrust, protesting, and violence to erode resilience (Levi and Strker 2000; Pauwels and De Waele 2014). Religious practice has also reflected the ideal for hatred to dispute resilience (Rip et al. 2012). The ideal for hatred has reflected anomie, anxiety, self-uncertainty, and uncertainty to erode resilience (Hogg et al. 2010; Koehler and Fiebig 2019; Stankov et al. 2018).

Norms for assimilating resilience diminished by religious practice have popularized functioning and security (Coffe and Geys 2007; Ma et al. 2009). The norm for functioning has reduced anxiety and depression to maintain resilience (He et al. 2022). Moreover, the norm for functioning perceived has reflected happiness and satisfaction to sustain resilience (Ma et al. 2009; Smith and Hamon 2012). The norm for functioning has also buttressed functioning (Li and Chung 2008). Functioning has escalated satisfaction to induce resilience (Granzin and Haggard 2000). Conversely, religious practice has reflected norms for disaster or trauma to dissimilate resilience (Rivera 2018). The norm for trauma has bred trauma (Human et al. 2016). Trauma has caused complaints, depression, and distress to suppress resilience (Balsam et al. 2011; Fischer et al. 2016).

## Pet Engagement

Pet engagement is likely to engender an inverse effect to offset its positive effect on resilience. The inverse effect tends to rely on the voluntaristic mechanisms of power realization and utility optimization in analytical functionalism.

Power based on education and health has been deficient in the case of pet engagement, thus weakening resilience (Branson et al. 2016). Education has sustained well-being, including health, identity, life quality and satisfaction, mastery, self-efficacy, self-esteem, and youthfulness to engender resilience (Cerin and Leslie 2008; Corcoran et al. 2011; James and Amato 2013; Pakulshi and Tranter 2000; Stavrova and Ehlebracht 2018; van Praag and Frijters 1999; Whyte and Gao 2009; Yienprugsawan et al. 2010). Pet engagement has bred depression to weaken power, thus hurting resilience (Branson et al. 2016). Furthermore, pet engagement has stemmed from inadequate power due to loneliness, living alone, and the empty nest and single parenting received in the family to impede resilience (Blouin 2012; Krause-Parello and Gulick 2013; Sundquist and Yang 2007; Walsh 2009). Living alone has bred depression and distress and eroded health, life satisfaction, and sleep quality to dampen resilience (Gu et al. 2010; Kirmanoglu and Baslevent 2014; Lofors and Sundquist 2007; Oshio and Kan 2019). Single parenting received has created disorders and problems to hamper resilience (Franz et al. 2003).

Disutilty for resilience reflected by pet engagement has resided in loss and stress experienced (Krause-Parello and Gulick 2013; Walsh 2009). Loss has incurred anger and depression and diminished income and marital satisfaction to dampen resilience (Boyce et al. 2013; Mehlsen et al. 2003; Wells et al. 1999). Stress has eroded well-being, including eudaimonia, health, positive affect, quality of life, neighborhood, and relationships, and satisfaction with life and neighbors, thus jeopardizing resilience (Baumeister et al. 2013; Greenberg 1999; Jackson et al. 2006; Mathis et al. 2016; Parkes et al. 2002; Shrira 2012; Su et al. 2021; Zotti et al. 2016).

An ideal lacking in pet engagement is that for coping (Branson et al. 2016). Remarkably, coping has achieved resilience (Corbin and Hall 2019). Moreover, coping has propped growth, health, intimacy, quality in environment and relationship, satisfaction, self-efficacy, and general well-being to escalate resilience (Chow et al. 2014; Gattino et al. 2015; Lau et al. 2012; Paez et al. 2007; Veenstra et al. 2005; Wills 1997).

# Chapter 7
# Social Capital Bases for Resilience

**Abstract** This chapter attempts to elaborate on the social, deterministic influence on resilience. Accordingly, the social factors concerned are social capital and empowerment. Social capital arises from two sources, associations (e.g., parental associations) and friends, which comprises structural (i.e., relational), functional (e.g., aid), and substantive or resource (e.g., wealth) forms in the sources. In addition, extraversion is a personal factor in registering the voluntaristic mechanism of power realization. Analysis of survey data on people with visual disabilities revealed that associational social capital, friend structural social capital, friend functional social capital, and friend social capital integrated significantly sustained resilience. This sustenance demonstrates the deterministic mechanism of empowering. However, empowerment did not significantly elevate resilience, thus tempering support for the deterministic mechanism of empowering. By contrast, friend substantive social capital significantly negatively affected resilience. This effect reveals the deterministic mechanism of incentivizing, such that friends' resources devalue and discourage the personal development of resilience. In addition, extraversion displayed a significant positive effect on resilience. This effect reflects the voluntaristic mechanism of power realization. Overall, social or deterministic factors, as well as the personal factor of extraversion, influence resilience. Deterministic factors do not replace personal factors, which maintain their unique contributions.

Social capital is likely to be the basis for resilience, like that for well-being (Yetim and Yetim 2014). This likelihood happens as resilience constitutes well-being (Van Haaften et al. 2004). Social capital refers to capital that is accessible socially through social relations (Grootaert and van Bastelaer 2002; Ostrom 2009). Capital means convertible, durable, enduring, and indestructible resources (Chen et al. 2015; Robison and Ritchie 2010; Waldstrom et al. 2008). Resources as substantive elements include education, power, prestige, skill, status, and wealth (Van Der Gaag and Snijders 2005). Social relations, channels, or networks include the family, relatives, friends, neighbors, associations or organizations, and community (Woolcock and Narayan 2000). These channels can be binding, bonding, bridging, bracing, and linking, depending on intimacy and similarity (Navarra et al. 2018; Widmer 2006).

 
C. K. Cheung, *Resilience Process and Its Personal and Social Bases*,
https://doi.org/10.1007/978-981-97-7391-6_7

Accordingly, the family represents binding, close friends represent bonding, other friends represent bridging, neighbors represent bracing, and resourceful brokers represent linking (Hawkins and Mauer 2012; Rydin and Holman 2004; Widmer 2006). Binding in the family means close-knit and unsocial, outside the social proper (Coleman et al. 2022; Widmer 2006). Bonding is close, communicative, supportive, homogeneous, nearby, and strong (Coleman et al. 2022; Hawkins and Mauer 2012). Bridging involves diversity or heterogeneity, exchange, and outlying (Brisson 2009; Coleman et al. 2022; Paraskevopoulos 2010). Bracing and linking hive from bridging but less close than bridging proper (Rydin and Holman 2004; Williams and Pocock 2010). Bracing features commonality and scaffolding (Rydin and Holman 2004). Linking denotes enabling, influential or powerful, integrative, and rewarding (Hawkins and Mauer 2012; Navarra et al. 2018; Woolcock 1998; Wuthnow 2004). Meanwhile, accessibility entails social or transmission capability (Robison and Ritchie 2010; van Deth 2003). Such capability hinges on structure or networking and function or norms (Bassani 2007; Mele 2010; Torsvik 2000). Structure includes closeness or strength, density or closure, homogeneity, and multiplexity or multiple ways of connection (Bassani 2007; Mele 2010; Volker and Flap 2001). Function comprises reciprocity and trust (Fukuyama 2001; Miao et al. 2018).

Social capital features access to resources, agency, activation of help, associability, attention, banking, cohesion or inclusion, collective action and efficacy, communication, community, control, embeddedness, cooperation, empowerment, engagement, familiarity, friendship, giving or investment and drawing, helping and helpfulness, integration or linkage, interaction or participation, meeting, membership, obligation, opportunity, safety, sharing, sociability, support, sympathy, togetherness, trustworthiness, and volunteering or volunteerism (Baptista et al. 2021; Benton 2016; Campbell et al. 2008; Chang 2009; De Silva et al. 2006; Harpham et al. 2002; Hofferth et al. 1999; Jones and Woolcock 2010; Lindstrom 2006; Murayama et al. 2019; Narayan and Cassidy 2001; Nieminen et al. 2008; Offe and Fuchs 2002; Poortinga 2012; Portes 2000; Robison et al. 2002; Savelkoul et al. 2011; Son 2013; Sun and Stewart 2007; Woolcock 1998; Wuthnow 2002). Agency comprises reciprocity and trust (Thomson 2005). Resources refer to their extensivity, range, and reachability (Son 2013).

Regardless of its contribution to resilience, social capital is inherently vital because of its grounds on communitarianism, economics, pragmatism, rationalism, recognition or popular desire, social bonding or control, social cohesion or connectedness, and structuralism (Carpiano 2008; Ecclestone and Field 2003; Farr 2004; Flap and Volker 2013; Onyx and Bullen 2000; Ozbay 2008; Robison and Ritchie 2010). Communitarianism highlights commonality, morality, sharing, and solidarity (Onyx and Bullen 2000; Portes and Vickstrom 2011). Economics favors exchange, externality, productivity, and sustainability as opposed to cost and poverty (Robison and Ritchie 2010; Svendsen and Svendsen 2003). Pragmatism emphasizes sympathy (Farr 2004). Rationalism treasures evidence and logic (Ecclestone and Field 2003). Social bonding treasures attachment, belief, commitment, and involvement (Ozbay 2008). Structuralism concentrates on structure and relationships (Flap and Volker 2013).

Social capital is instrumentally vital for its contribution to resilience (Bottrell 2009). Besides, social capital is instrumentally vital in facilitating achievement or success, civicness, collective decision and action, community, democracy, exchange, other capital forms, prosociality or altruism, reproduction, resolution, social control, social support, solidarity, transfer, and well-being or welfare (Aldridge and Halpern 2002; Benton 2016; Ferguson 2006; Fuchs et al. 2001; Gray 2009; Holliday and Tam 2001; Krippner and Alvarez 2007; Laser and Leibowitz 2009; Narayan and Cassidy 2001; Oinas et al. 2020; Putnam 2002; Savage and Kanazawa 2004; Torsvik 2000; Vorhaus 2014; Woolcock 2010). Conversely, social capital reduces cost, loneliness, and opportunism (Gray 2009; Grootaert and van Bastelaer 2002; Torsvik 2000).

## Existing Knowledge

The contribution of social capital to resilience unfolds from social capital generally, friendship, associational or organizational involvement, social trust, and reciprocity. Unlike the family, they represent the social proper in social capital (Chen et al. 2015; Murayama et al. 2019; Paraskevopoulos 2010). By contrast, the family identifies the binding, private, unsocial form of social capital (Coleman et al. 2022; Edwards 2004; Son 2013; Widmer 2006).

### *Social Capital*

Social capital raises resilience (Bottrell 2009). This raising directly benefits from access to power, including assets, capability, coordination, energy, facilitation, organization, resources, and sympathy or support received through social capital (Chen et al. 2015; Robison and Ritchie 2010; Woolcock 1998). Essentially, capital including human, economic, and other forms accessible from social relations is power (Krishna and Uphoff 2002). Alternatively, social capital represents a norm or expectation to sustain life, thus guiding resilience (Robison and Ritchie 2010). As such, power can activate resilience through the voluntaristic mechanism of power realization in analytical functionalism. Furthermore, the raising indirectly benefits from the voluntaristic mechanisms of power realization, utility optimization, ideal calibration, and norm conformity in analytical functionalism. These mechanisms apply power, utility, ideals, and norms generated by social capital. Power includes or stems from capability, energy, goals, dispositions, identity, motives, needs, personality, and resources (Munch 1987, 1988). Utility includes benefits, ease, and gain from outside or the environment. Ideals include or unfold in actions, beliefs, cultures, ideas, ideologies, lifestyles, meanings, practices, and values. Norms are socially prevalent or prescriptive power, utility, or ideals.

Power for driving resilience can evolve from capital or assets of various forms, agency, attachment, attention or focusing, authenticity, civility, clarity, closeness, commitment, convoys, empowerment received, insight, knowledge, lovability, meaningfulness, morality, positive emotion, openness, optimism, relaxation, realization, resources or their conservation, responsibility, security, self-affirmation, self-awareness or its capacitgy, self-efficacy, self-reflection, self-regulation, self-worth, sharing experienced, skill, support received, virtue, and zest (Afifi et al. 2016; Bowen et al. 2013; Brodsky and Cattaneo 2013; Cocking 2017; Dwivedi 2017; Falon et al. 2021; Crane et al. 2019; Gallo et al. 2004; Gilligan 2009; Hassija and Cloitre 2014; Jayawardana et al. 2019; Kent and Davis 2010; Lerner et al. 2012; Matusitz 2017; Metzl and Morrell 2008; Mikulincer and Shaver 2014; Schwager and Rothermund 2014; Shaver and Mikulincer 2012; Sherman and Cohen 2006; Tugade and Fredrickson 2004; Van Vliet 2008). Self-regulation comprises affective processing, emotion regulation, and selective attention (Schwager and Rothermund 2014). Affective processing highlights positivity and reasoning, including problem-focusing and wishful thinking (Schwager and Rothermund 2014). Emotion regulation comprises attentional development, cognitive change, response modulation, and situational selection and modifying (Boden et al. 2014). Selective attention comprises distracting, loosening, focusing, opening, shielding, and tightening (Schwager and Rothermund 2014). Virtue comprises beauty or excellence appreciation, flourishing, gratitude, hope, humor, spirituality, and wisdom (Dwivedi 2017). Furthermore, resilience has beneftted from power based on agreeableness, balance experienced, boldness, conscientiousness, emotional intelligence, emotional stability, extraversin, honesty-humility, learning, mentoring received, organizational membership, purposiveness, religiosity, self-esteem, sensation seeking, and socioeconomic status (Armstrong et al. 2011; Buikstra et al. 2010; Cantor et al. 2002; Cherry et al. 2023; Jones and Jetten 2011; Lock et al. 2020; McKay et al. 2018; Notter et al. 2008; Ntontis et al. 2023; Yu and Zhang 2007). Conversely, power for driving resilience can weaken due to distress (Shaver and Mikulincer 2012). Moreover, power for driving resilience has declined because of emotionality, neuroticism, and trauma experienced (Cherry et al. 2023; Pyszkowska 2020). Hence, resilience registers or stands on the power of well-being, including adequacy, autonomy, belongingness, control, development, gratitude, health and mental health, hope or hopefulness, identity, independence, intimacy, mastery, meaningfulness, mindfulness, positive affect, purposiveness, relatedness, relational quality, satisfaction, self-awareness or self-insight, self-efficacy, self-esteem, self-understanding, and sleep quality (Artuch-Garde et al. 2017; Bucknell et al. 2024; Buikstra et al. 2010; Coholic 2011; Cann and Collette 2014; Dubovska et al. 2017; Gibbons et al. 2014; Goins et al. 2012; Kaye-Tzadok and Davidson-Arad 2017; Masten et al. 2009; Silk et al. 2007; Svetina 2014; Theron et al. 2011; Ungar et al. 2005; Van Haaften et al. 2004; Visaria et al. 2023; Ye et al. 2021; von Soest et al. 2010; Yu and Zhang 2007; Wong and Chui 2017). Conversely, resilience falls by the powerlessness of ill-being, including anxiety, depression, loneliness, and stress (Kaye-Tzadok and Davidson-Arad 2017; Visaria et al. 2023; Walker and Longmire-Avital 2013).

Utility for attracting resilience can reside in fit or congruence, opportunity, and valuation experienced (Gilligan 2009; Matusitz 2017; Ungar 2012). Conversely, disutility for discouraging resilience has involved stress experienced (Ntontis et al. 2023).

Ideals for rationalizing resilience can accentuate cognitive reappraisal or restructuring, coping, development, existence, the future, interaction, meaning-making, negotiation, participation, relationships, solidarity or helping, solutions, and storytelling or restorying (Alrofiai et al. 2020; Cocking 2017; Crane et al. 2019; Falon et al. 2021; Gallo et al. 2004; Matusitz 2017; Metzl and Morrell 2008; Park 2017; Park and Slattery 2014; Prilleltensky 2012; Ungar 2012) Moreover, resilience has benefitted from ideals for affiliation or connectedness, charity, culture, and protection (Cherry et al. 2018; Chua et al. 2019; Corbin and Hall 2019; Notter et al. 2008).

Norms for assimilating resilience can popularize aiming, challenge, commitment, communication, flexibility, growth or its potential, hardiness, identity, interconnectedness, meaningfulness, morality, normalcy, positive emotion, resource identification, and transformation (Batone 2017; Buzzanell 2010; Simon et al. 2005). Furthermore, resilience has benefitted from norms for adaptability, authenticity, awareness, balance, consumption, innovation, safety, and transparency (Batone 2017; Buikstra et al. 2010; Jones and d'Errico 2019). Conversely, resilience has receded by norms for illness (Jones and d'Errico 2019).

Power reflected by social capital to drive resilience stems from bonding or attachment, collective wisdom, community, connectedness, control received, coordination or organization received, investment received, morality, nobility, responsibility, social integration, solidarity or consociation, and trustworthiness (Brisson and Usher 2005; Chen et al. 2015; De Silva et al. 2006; Carpiano 2008; Kadushin 2004; Onyx and Bullen 2000; Ozbay 2008; Paraskevopoulos 2010; Sabet and Khaksar 2022; Siisiainen 2003; Williams and Pocock 2010; Woolcock 1998). Bonding or attachment has mitigated stress and negative emotion, thus upholding resilience (Nelson-Coffey et al. 2023). Wisdom has raised well-being, including autonomy, coherence, maturity, meaningfulness, purposefulness, life satisfaction, and self-efficacy to effectuate resilience (Diener et al. 2009; Greene and Brown 2009; Mickler and Staudinger 2008; Webster 2010). The sense of community has strengthened rewards to induce resilience (Nelson-Coffey et al. 2023). Connectedness has mitigated stress and negative emotion, thus upholding resilience (Nelson-Coffey et al. 2023). Control, coordination, or organization received has maintained the sense of community and diminished fatigue to enable resilience (Overall et al. 2020). Morality has sustained satisfaction and eroded anxiety to boost resilience (Conzo et al. 2017; Stets et al. 2008). Nobility has enhanced trust to facilitate resilience (Jost et al. 2003). Responsibility has incubated self efficacy to enable resilience (Braun-Lewensohn 2016). Social integration has eroded depression to bolster resilience (Mullins and Dugan 1991). Solidarity has enabled adjustment, hope, and life satisfaction to secure resilience (Dittman and Goebel 2010; James and Hunsley 1995; Paez et al. 2015). Trustworthiness has stemmed from positive experience, social status, and trust to induce resilience (Barrera 2007; Cook and Cheshire 2013; Kuwabara 2015). Social capital raises credibility, information received, prosocial motivation, resources, social control and support received, social status, and well-being to secure power to drive resilience (Benton 2016; Brisson and Usher 2005; Putnam 2002;

Torsvik 2000; Vorhaus 2014). Credibility has maintained autonomy, eudaimonic well-being, growth, hedonic well-being, identity integration, life satisfaction, positive affect, mastery, mindfulness, purposiveness, relational quality, self-acceptance, self-clarity, self-esteem, self-determination, and vitality to escalate resilience (Kernis and Goldman 2006). Information received has elevated well-being, including life satisfaction and self-efficacy, to furnish resilience (Denver and Hands 1990; Minnaert and Janssen 1992; Richards 2016). Prosocial motivation has elevated well-being, including connectedness, hope, life satisfaction, meaningfulness, and self-efficacy to boost resilience (Marsh and Dik 2021; Nelson-Coffey et al. 2023; Raposa et al. 2016; Yao and Enright 2019). Social support received has upheld resilience and well-being, including control, health, positive emotion and pleasure, purposiveness, relational quality, satisfaction with life, housing, and leisure, self-determination, self-efficacy, self-esteem, and social well-being, to activate resilience (Cherry et al. 2018; George and Park 2013; Glendinning et al. 2003; Granzin and Haggard 2000; Holliman et al. 2021; Lincoln et al. 2003; Logan and Cobb 2013; Pierce and Quiroz 2018; Schwarzer and Knoll 2007; Vilhjalmsson and Thorlindsson 1998; Wen et al. 2010; Williams and Galliher 2006; Xi and Hwang 2011). Social status has sustained coping, health, interaction quality, life satisfaction, self-esteem, and general well-being to secure resilience (Al-krenawi et al. 2011; Caplan and Schooler 2007; Molana and Adams 2019; Staudinger et al. 1999). Social capital has raised income or earnings, knowledge, religiosity, social support received, socioeconomic status, and well-being to afford power to boost resilience (Brunie 2009; Chua et al. 2021; Cross and Lin 2008; Pena-Lopez and Sanchez-Santos 2016; Yetim and Yetim 2014; Wuthnow 2004). Income has afforded well-being, including adaptation, adequacy, belongingness, control, eudaemonia, health, mastery, power, quality of life, satisfaction, self-efficacy, self-esteem, and social well-being to sustain resilience (Anciaes et al. 2017; Carpiano 2008; Corcoran et al. 2011; Ross and Mirowsky 1989; Sengupta and Sibley 2019; Son and Wilson 2012; Wang and VanderWeele 2011; Yeh et al. 2013; Zimmerman and Reyna 2013). Knowledge has underlain power, prevention, protection, satisfaction, self-efficacy, spirituality, tolerance, economic resources, and social resources and trust to facilitate resilience (Chang and Hsu 2016; Cheng and Ng 2006; Ertz et al. 2021; Mutz and Mondak 2006; Norris 2011; Nunkoo 2015; Pattie et al. 2004; Bish and Michie 2010; Rothwell et al. 2016). Religiosity has buttressed coping, friendship, forgiveness, harmony perceived, health maintenance, institutional and social trust, optimism, social capital, and well-being to raise resilience (Chang 2009; Clemence 2001; Furnham 1997; Hakhverdian and Mayne 2012; Myers 2008; Saroglou and Anciaux 2004; Wuthnow 2004; Zanin 2017). Well-being has included belongingness or the sense of community, flourishing, happiness, health, identity, life satisfaction, and pride as opposed to depression and distress (Chua et al. 2021; Congdon 2010; Phongsavan et al. 2006; Yetim and Yetim 2014). Social capital can involve advice, empowerment, enforcement, help, resources and support received, belongingness or companionship, controllability, credibility, embeddedness or fit, influence, and legitimacy experienced, mastery, meaningfulness, purposiveness, self-esteem, and virtue as power to drive resilience (Centola and Macy 2007; Flap and Volker 2013; Holtom et al. 2006; Huxhold et al. 2022; Paraskevopoulos 2010). Belongingness has strengthened rewards to induce resilience (Nelson-Coffey et al. 2023). Controllability or mastery has raised well-being, including happiness, neighborhood quality, life satisfaction, and physical and mental health, as opposed to depression, to induce resilience (Greenberg 1999; Helson and Srivastava 2001; Hwang et al. 2007; Judge et al. 2002; Lever et al. 2005; Sargent-Cox et al. 2015). Empowerment received has boosted well-being, including satisfaction and self-efficacy to advance resilience (Biron and Samberger 2010; Kulik 2007). Influence has upgraded mood and reduced depression to achieve resilience (Langner et al. 2012; Wojciszke and Struzynska-Kujolowicz 2007). Meaningfulness has buttressed aspiration, engagement, happiness, health, life satisfaction, and positive affect to sustain resilience (Morgan and Robinson 2013; Steger et al. 2009). Purposiveness has advanced happiness, health, life satisfaction, and positive affect and has lessened depression and negative affect to induce resilience (Steger et al. 2009; Tomich and Helgeson 2002). Virtuehas sustained satisfaction and eroded anxiety to boost resilience (Conzo et al. 2017; Stets et al. 2008). Social capital has benefitted from attachment, assets or wealth, coresidence, development received, education, extraversion, facilities accessible, functioning or functionality, health, income, interest, leadership, openness, organizational membership, religiosity, skill, social class, strengths, support received, and volunteering or service-learning to gather power to drive resilience (Aldridge and Halpern 2002; Angelusz and Tardos 2001; Chang 2009; Cheng et al. 2019; Curley 2010; Cornwall 2009; Eriksson and Emmelin 2013; Islam et al. 2006; Hlasny and Lee 2020; Murayama et al. 2019; Navarra et al. 2018; Scheufele and Shah 2000; Tulin et al. 2018; Wuthnow 2004). Coresidence has sustained health, life satisfaction, and sleep quality and diminished depression and distress to safeguard resilience (Gu et al. 2010; Lofors and Sundquist 2007; Oshio and Kan 2019; Richards 2016; Sundquist and Yang 2007). Development received has upgraded adjustment, comfort, coherence, cohesiveness, competence, emotional well-being, growth, hope, identity, purposiveness, self-efficacy, self-esteem, thriving, and transcendence to advance resilience (Ashby et al. 2018; Davidson et al. 2012; Duan and Bu 2019; Esbensen and Osgood 1999; Feldman and Dreher 2012; Moote et al. 1999; Ou et al. 2019; Umino and Dammeyer 2018; Youniss and Yates 1997). Education has sustained well-being, including health, identity, life quality and satisfaction, mastery, self-efficacy, self-esteem, and youthfulness to engender resilience (Cerin and Leslie 2008; Corcoran et al. 2011; James and Amato 2013; Pakulski and Tranter 2000; Stavrova and Ehlebracht 2018; van Praag and Frijters 1999; Whyte and Gao 2009; Yienprugsawan et al. 2010). Extraversion has raised well-being, including autonomy, growth, mastery, positive affect, purposefulness, relatedness, satisfaction, self-acceptance, self-determination, self-efficacy, and self-esteem to facilitate resilience (Hounkpatin et al. 2015; Ingledew et al. 2004; Quilty et al. 2006; Rasmussen et al. 2018; Richards 2016; Tiwari et al. 2021). Facilities have promoted need fulfillment to achieve resilience (Molana and Adams 2019). Functioning has escalated satisfaction to induce resilience (Granzin and Haggard 2000). Interest has fostered satisfaction and self-efficacy to facilitate resilience (Gilman 2001; Wen and Cui 2014). Leadership has secured self-efficacy to afford resilience (Shah and Scheufele 2006). Openness has raised well-being, including autonomy, growth, life satisfaction, purposefulness, relationship quality, self-acceptance, self-efficacy, and self-esteem, as opposed to hostility to boost resilience (Hahn et al. 2013; Hounkpatin et al. 2015; Karwowski and Lebuda 2017; Marks 1996; Quilty et al. 2006; Webster et al. 2014). Organizational membership has reduced negative emotion and stress to sustain resilience (Nelson-Coffey et al. 2023). Skill has underpinned self-efficacy to buttress resilience (Larson et al. 1990). Social class has sustained well-being, including financial adequacy, health, hope, and satisfaction, as opposed to depression to advance resilience (Burke 2008; Davis and Davenport 1999; Haller and Hadler 2006; Hadjar and Samuel 2015; Peterson and Seligman 2004; Yamaoka 2008). Strengths have sustained satisfaction and reduced fear to safeguard resilience (Liu, Messner, Zhang, and Zhuo 2009; Peterson and Seligman 2004). Volunteering has raised well-being, including health, life satisfaction, mastery, morale, positive affect, and self-esteem as opposed to depression, loneliness, and mortality, to enhance resilience (Borgonovi 2008; Gillath et al. 2005; Li and Ferraro 2006; Midlarsky and Kahana 1994; Oman et al. 1999; Thoits and Hewitt 2001; Zotti et al. 2016). Social capital can benefit from group identity and social cohesion experienced to afford power to drive resilience (Kramer 2009; Savelkoul et al. 2014). Identity has secured happiness, love, self-efficacy, and self-esteem and has diminished anxiety and depression to facilitate resilience (Cast 2004). Cohesion has buttressed hope and life satisfaction and eroded depression to maintain resilience (Araya et al. 2006; Dittman and Goebel 2010; Paez et al. 2015). Conversely, social capital has reflected low anxiety, depression, distress, migration or migrant status, limitations, and loneliness, thus retaining power to drive resilience (Cheng et al. 2019; Erickson 2004; Hlasny and Lee 2020; Webber and Huxley 2007). Migration has eroded well-being, including health and life satisfaction, thus diminishing power for deriving resilience (Ambrey and Fleming 2014; Islam et al. 2006). Limitations have dampened health, satisfaction with housing, leisure, and life, and self-efficacy, thus hampering resilience (Distante 2013; Gastil 2000; Granzin and Haggard 2000).

Utility revealed by social capital to attract resilience lies in equality experienced and recognition received (Latham 2000; Robison and Ritchie 2010). Equality experienced has sustained health, homeownership, life satisfaction, self-direction, social capital, and trust to raise resilience (Bond and Lun 2014; Kim and Kawachi 2007; Martin 2000; Meulemann 2010; Nilson 1981; Oishi et al. 2011; Portes and Vickstrom 2011). Recognition received has uplifted positive affect and self-esteem and reduced negative affect, thus buttressing resilience (Reich et al. 2018). Social capital generates benefits, goods, and reinforcement received as a utility to attract resilience (Brisson and Usher 2005; Coleman 1988; Vorhaus 2014). Reinforcement received has raised well-being, including satisfaction, to boost resilience (Helgeson et al. 2006; Wong and Lam 2016). Social capital can involve rewards received as utility to attract resilience (Baptista et al. 2021). Social capital has raised achievement, community evaluation, instititonal trust, safety, and success to secure utility to attract resilience (Furstenberg and Hughes 1995; McNeal 1999; Narayan and Cassidy 2001; Whitham 2012). Achievement or success has fostered health, life quality, satisfaction, self-efficacy, and self-esteem as opposed to alienation, depression, and distress to uphold resilience (Donnellan et al. 2005; Fredricks and Eccles 2005; Menard and Mose 1984; Murray 2009; Piko et al. 2006; Tompson and Dass 2000; Xiao et al. 2009).

Community evaluation has reflected mastery to enhance resilience (Greenberg 1999). Institutional trust has reflected health and satisfaction to buttress resilience (Chi et al. 2021; Mingo and Faggiano 2020). Safety has maintained achievement, life quality, mental health, and sufficiency experienced to foster resilience (Crume et al. 2019). Social capital has reflected fulfillment experienced, leisure experienced, neighborhood quality and safety, and satisfaction as utility to attract resilience (Cummins et al. 2003; Curley 2010; Glover et al. 2005; Hlasny and Lee 2020; Kleinhans et al. 2007; Yetim and Yetim 2014). Fulfillment has covered education, social, health, and other basic needs (Yetim and Yetim 2014). As such, fulfillment has sustained positive affect, self-esteem, and vitality, and reduced anxiety and negative affect to maintain resilience (Patrick et al. 2007). Leisure has attenuated anxiety, thus enabling resilience (Da Costa Bizarro Morais et al. 2019). Conversely, social capital involves low cost, thus retaining utility to attract resilience (Svendsen and Svendsen 2003). Social capital has benefitted from low limitedness, threat, and victimization experienced, thus sustaining utility to attract resilience (Hansen-Nord et al. 2014; Hepper et al. 2020; Savelkoul et al. 2015). Limitation has eroded health, satisfaction with housing, leisure, and life, and self-efficacy, thus hampering resilience (Distante 2013; Gastil 2000; Granzin and Haggard 2000). Threat experienced has fomented anxiety, avoidance, conflict, depression, fear, and hate to disrupt resilience (Edwards and Arnon 2021; MacLeod 2017; Moore and Shepherd 2006; O'Neill and Evans 1999; Rick et al. 2006; Ruiter et al. 2003). Victimization experienced has impaired safety experienced and self-respect or self-worth to erode resilience (Fernandes 2018; Krahe 2013).

Ideals underlying social capital to rationalize resilience highlight communitarianism or commonality, cooperation, exchange, fairness, and sympathy (Farr 2004; Onyx and Bullen 2000; Woolcock 1998). Communitarianism has fostered attachment and collective efficacy experienced to boost resilience (Long and Perkins 2007; Perkins and Long 2002). Cooperation has thrived on its ideal (Haesevoets et al. 2015). As such, cooperation has fostered life satisfaction to rationalize resilience (Park et al. 2015). Exchange has facilitated well-being, including interest or excitement, intimacy, pleasure, relational quality, and satisfaction as opposed to distress and jealousy, to induce resilience (Afifi et al. 2015; Blieszner 1993; Levitt and Cici-Gokaltun 2011; Stafford 2015; Thye et al. 2008). The ideal for fairness has raised resilience and other well-being components (Diener et al. 2009; Pyszkowska 2020). The ideal for sympathy has buttressed caring (Sarasa 2008). Social capital nurtures reproduction as ideals to rationalize resilience (Savage and Kanazawa 2004). The ideal for reproduction has manifested well-being to facilitate resilience (Peterson and Klohnen 1995). Social capital has advanced ideals for charity, civic engagement, community involvement, recourse, and volunteering to rationalize resilience (Bekkers et al. 2008; Broadbent and Papadopoulos 2011; Brown and Ferris 2007; Su and Feng 2013). The ideal for charity has underpinned the practice of charity (Bednall et al. 2013). Eventually, charity has enhanced well-being, notably including life satisfaction (Chang 2009; Helliwell et al. 2010). Civic engagement has stood on its ideal (Peterson and Maiden 1993). As such, civic engagement has incubated conflict resolution, education, happiness, health, income, individualism, life satisfaction, security normativity, social attachment, capital, integration, trust, tolerance, and general well-being to advance resilience (Coffe and Geys 2007; Goren 2005; Growiec and Growiec 2010; Kroll 2011; Li and Walder 2001; Myers 1999; Pena-Lopez and Sanchez-Santos 2016; Posel and Casale 2011; Tak 2017; Tang 2011; Wallace and Pichler 2009; Welzel 2013; van Ingen and Bekkers 2015; Vincens et al. 2018). Community involvement has elevated well-being, including mastery and self-efficacy to enable resilience (Harter and Arora 2010; Ohmer 2007; Peterson and Huphey 2004). Volunteering has grown from its ideal (Barr et al. 2005). Eventually, volunteering has raised well-being, including health, life satisfaction, mastery, morale, positive affect, and self-esteem as opposed to depression, loneliness, and mortality, to buttress resilience (Borgonovi 2008; Gillath et al. 2005; Li and Ferraro 2006; Midlarsky and Kahana 1994; Oman et al. 1999; Thoits and Hewitt 2001; Zotti et al. 2016). Social capital can involve ideals for exchange to rationalize resilience (Huxhold et al. 2022). Social capital has evolved from ideals for brokering or mediation, communication, donation, and social integration to rationalize resilience (Chang 2009; Halevy et al. 2019; Murayama et al. 2019). Brokering or mediating has strengthened agreeableness, empathy, morality, and openness and dampened agitation to safeguard resilience (Halevy et al. 2019). Communication has boosted positive affect and evaluation received, relationship quality, and self-enhancement as utility to induce resilience (Burgoon et al. 2010; Mirivel 2014; Tsfati et al. 2009). The ideal for donation has propped donation (Vallerand et al. 1992). Eventually, donation has reflected well-being, including control, feeling good, gratitude, happiness, joy, satisfaction, and self-efficacy as opposed to anxiety and guilt, to brew resilience (Bednall et al. 2013; Bekkers 2008; Eayrs and Ellis 1990; Liu and Hao 2017; Mussen 1982; Piliavin and Callero 1991; Wang and Graddy 2008). The ideal for social integration propels social integration (Luo and Kao 2001). Social integration has lessened depression and suicide, thus safeguarding resilience (Duberstein et al. 2004; Mullins and Dugan 1991). Conversely, social capital has benefitted from the ideal against mobility or migration to maintain resilience (Aldridge and Halpern 2002). The ideal for migration or mobility has bolstered migration or mobility (Abrams et al. 1999). Migration or mobility has eroded well-being, including health and life satisfaction, thus diminishing power for deriving resilience (Ambrey and Fleming 2014; Islam et al. 2006). Social capital can rise with ideals against materialism and selfishness (Cattell 2004). Materialism has eroded well-being or life quality, including happiness, health, life satisfaction, positive affect, and self-appraisal as opposed to anxiety, to undermine resilience (Kasser 2016; Lane 2000; Roberts and Clement 2007). Selfishness has bred anxiety to obstruct resilience (Da Costa Bizarro Morais et al. 2019). Social capital has suppressed ideals for suicide and violence, thus rationalizing resilience (Lewinsohn et al. 1994; Pulkkinen et al. 2009). Suicide has evolved from its ideal (Till et al. 2013). Attempted suicide has induced anxiety to obstruct resilience (Cheng et al. 2017). The ideal for violence has rationalized violence (Muluk et al. 2013). Violence has bred depression, thus disturbing resilience (Wright et al. 2015).

Norms reflected by social capital have demonstrated health, individualism, religiosity, and safety to assimilate resilience (Allik and Realo 2004; Curley 2010; Hlasny and Lee 2020; Portes and Vickstrom 2011). Individualism has grown from its norm

(Welzel 2013). As such, individualism has bolstered well-being, including life satisfaction and self-efficacy, to enable resilience (Kim et al. 2016; Oishi 2000; Veenhoven 1998). Religiosity has developed from its norm (Pollack and Pickel 2007; Stavrova and Siegers 2014). Eventually, religiosity has sustained well-being, including adjustment, flourishing, health, mastery, positive affect, relational quality, satisfaction, self-esteem, and socioemotional well-being, to advance resilience (Dy-Liacco et al. 2009; Helliwell and Putnam 2005; Flouri and Buchanan 2002; Meulemann 2010; Moschis and Ong 2011; Ng and Fisher 2016; Schieman 2001; Skerkat and Ellison 1999; Wuthnow 2004). Similarly, social capital has enhanced the norm for health to assimilate resilience (Portes and Vickstrom 2011). Social capital can benefit from norms for continuity and resolution to assimilate resilience (Cattell 2004; Wong 2008). Continuity has proceeded based on normative influence (Suhay 2015). Continuity has raised resilience and relational quality and reduced anxiety (Lock et al. 2020; Ross et al. 2000). Resolution evolves through normative influence (Munch 1989). Eventually, resolution has stood on autonomy, competence, and self-confidence as opposed to depression to maintain resilience (Levesque-Bristol et al. 2011; Siu and Shek 2005). Conversely, social capital has emerged from norms against deprivation, mobility, and pressure, thus assimilating resilience (Blackshaw and Long 2005; Laurence 2011). The norm for deprivation has diminished well-being, including happiness and positive emotion as opposed to depression, negative emotion, and normlessness, to weaken resilience (Hackman et al. 2019; Pei and Kim 2017; Ross and Mirowsky 2009; van Praag and Frijters 1999). Moreover, the norm for deprivation has engendered deprivation (Whelan and Maitre 2013). Deprivation experienced has fomented anxiety, fear, and sadness to block resilience (Landmann and Rohmann 2020). The norm for mobility or instability has worsened relational quality, thus impairing resilience (Ross et al. 2000). Pressure grows from its norm (Carr and Umberson 2013). Eventually, pressure experienced has raised distress to disturb resilience (Overall et al. 2020). Social capital can reflect the norm against diversity to assimilate resilience (Savelkoul et al. 2014). The norm for diversity has hurt survival, thus jeopardizing resilience (Nettle 2000).

## *Social Trust*

Social trust or interpersonal trust covers acquaintances, bonding and bridging network members, the community or neighborhood, friends, immigrants, people known, minority people, neighbors, the outgroup, partners, religious fellows, strangers, and workers (Adongo et al. 2019; Freitag and Bauer 2016; Cao et al. 2015; Flanagan 2003; Halvorsen 2007; Hoogervorst et al. 2015; Hu 2013; Lancee and Dronkers 2011; Lundasen et al. 2013; Putnam 2007; Steinhardt and Delhey 2020; Welch et al. 2007). Hence, social trust does not cover institutions, including business, government, police, medicine, and science. Essentially, trust means an expectation for help, support, or fair or favorable treatment, including cooperation and favors returned (Bellemare and Kroger 2007; Mingo and Faggiano 2020; Rahn 2008). Social trust is part of social capital or resources (Six 2014). Social trust is likely to elevate resilience by affording power, utility, ideals, and norms to leverage the voluntaristic mechanisms of power realization, utility optimization, ideal calibration, and norm conformity to fulfill analytical functionalism.

Power maintained by social trust to drive resilience has arisen from attachment, care received, citizenship, commitment, competence, friendship, health, identity, morality, security, self-esteem, survival, and vitality (Barefoot et al. 1998; Burke and Stets 1999; Crystal and DeBell 2002; Hoegh and Bourgeois 2002; King 2007; King and Furrow 2004; Meeus et al. 2002; Nucci 2006). Attachment has buttressed life satisfaction to enable resilience (Zdrenka et al. 2015). Care received has fostered functionality and satisfaction to sustain resilience (Caro and Blank 1988; Davies et al. 1990). Civility has boosted well-being, including physical and mental health, to activate resilience (Tsai et al. 2018). Commitment has sustained self-acceptance and relieved depression to foster resilience (Agronick and Duncan 1998; Wrosch et al. 2005). Competence has enabled identity achievement, intimacy, and relationship satisfaction as opposed to anxiety to raise resilience (Adams 1985). Friendship has stemmed from health and satisfaction with health, leisure, and life as opposed to fear to buttress resilience (Child and Nikolova 2020; Eberl 2020; Sampson 1991). Morality has satisfied life and reduced anxiety to maintain resilience (Conzo et al. 2017; Stets et al. 2008). Social trust develops from maturity and virtue to secure power to drive resilience (Brown et al. 2014; Laroche et al. 2019). Maturity has developed from self-compassion and self-tolerance to strengthen resilience (Ho and Li 2022; Munroe et al. 2022). Virtue has sustained satisfaction and eroded anxiety to boost resilience (Conzo et al. 2017; Stets et al. 2008). Social trust has arisen from agreeableness, autonomy, civility, education, endowments, homeownership, interest, knowledge, language proficiency, moderateness, openness, organizational membership, power, religiosity, sociability, social support received, well-being or wellness, and work motivation to drive resilience (Abascal 2015; Almakaeva et al. 2018; Barrera 2007; Cais, Torrente, and Bolancé. 2021; Fridberg and Kangas 2008b; Halvorsen 2007; Houser and Xiao 2015; Huhe 2014; Lancee and Dronkers 2011; McCabe 2012; Navarra et al. 2018; Pattie et al. 2004; Sabatini and Sarracino 2019; Uslaner 2002; van Ingen and Bekkers 2015). Agreeableness has fostered growth, life satisfaction, mastery, purposefulness, relatedness, and self-acceptance to buttress resilience (Hounkpatin et al. 2015). Autonomy has raised well-being, including energy, health, mastery, meaningfulness, positive affect, pride, satisfaction, self-efficacy, and self-esteem, to boost resilience (Au and Cheung 2004; De Moortel et al. 2015; Erickson 2008; Garcia et al. 2017; Gahlawat et al. 2019; Hodson 1996; Martela and Riekki 2018; Schieman 2002; Schieman and Narisada 2014; Yoon 2001). Education has sustained well-being, including health, identity, life quality and satisfaction, mastery, self-efficacy, self-esteem, and youthfulness to engender resilience (Cerin and Leslie 2008; Corcoran et al. 2011; James and Amato 2013; Pakulshi and Tranter 2000; Stavrova and Ehlebracht 2018; van Praag and Frijters 1999; Whyte and Gao 2009; Yienprugsawan et al. 2010). Homeownership has raised health, morale, family and neighborhood quality, and financial, housing, life, and neighborhood satisfaction as opposed to depression, distress, and fear to strengthen resilience (Congdon

2010; Harris 2001; Lee et al. 2022; Mirowsky and Ross 1999; Montazer 2022; Roy and Chaudhuri 2008; Wulfhorst and Kranich 1999; Yu and Chiu 2016; Zheng et al. 2020). Interest has fostered satisfaction and self-efficacy to facilitate resilience (Gilman 2001; Wen and Cui 2014). Knowledge has championed intimacy, satisfaction, and self-efficacy to boost resilience (Mikulincer et al. 2003; Norris 2011; Rothwell et al. 2016). Language proficiency has secured relational quality and satisfaction to boost resilience (Lancee and Dronkers 2011; Van Praag et al. 2010). Moderateness has evolved from self-compassion as opposed to apprehension to bolster resilience (Hernandez et al. 2002; Pyszkowska and Ronnlund 2021). Openness has advanced well-being, including autonomy, growth, life satisfaction, purposefulness, relational quality, self-acceptance, self-efficacy, and self-esteem to boost resilience (Hahn et al. 2013; Hounknatin et al. 2014; Karwowski and Lebuda 2017; Marks 1996; Webster et al. 2014). Organizational membership has advanced well-being, notably health, to sustain resilience (Tsai et al. 2018). Religiosity has buttressed coping, friendship, forgiveness, harmony perceived, health maintenance, institutional and social trust, optimism, social capital, well-being to raise resilience (Chang 2009; Clemence 2001; Furnham 1997; Hakhverdian and Mayne 2012; Myers 2008; Saroglou and Anciaux 2004; Wuthnow 2004; Zanin 2017). Sociability has furthermore maintained belongingness, creativity, education, friendship quality, relationship satisfaction, and security to gather power to drive resilience (Anderson-Butcher et al. 2008; Collins and van Dulmen 2006; Ghayas and Malik 2013; Hintsanen et al. 2011; Larson et al. 2007). Social support received has raised resilience and general well-being, including control, emotional well-being, health, pleasure, purposiveness, relational quality, satisfaction, self-determination, self-efficacy, self-esteem, and social well-being, as opposed to anger, anxiety, depression, distress, and symptoms (Besser and Priel 2008; Cherry et al. 2018; George and Park 2013; Glendinning et al. 2003; Gorman et al. 2010; Holliman et al. 2021; Kafetsio and Sideridis 2006; Lee and Robbins 1998; Lincoln et al. 2003; Logan and Cobb 2013; Lowe et al. 2009; Pierce and Quiroz 2018; Schwarzer and Knoll 2007; Vilhjalmsson and Thorlindsson 1998; Williams and Galliher 2006; Xi and Hwang 2011). Well-being has included control, happiness, health, intimacy, pride, self-efficacy, and self-trust as opposed to distress and fear (Burke and Stets 1999; Child and Nikolova 2020; Hu 2013; Huhe 2014; Rahn 2008; Steinhardt 2012; Uslaner 2002; Wuthnow 2004). Work motivation has reflected satisfaction to induce resilience (Kiecolt 2003). To the youth, social trust can benefitt from stability to provide power to drive resilience (Stefaniak et al. 2017). Stability has enhanced resilience and relational quality and has reduced anxiety (Lock et al. 2020; Ross et al. 2000). Conversely, social trust has prevented depression, thus retaining power to drive resilience (Wu et al. 2010). Social trust has arisen from low dysfunction or limitation and welfare dependency to maintain power to drive resilience (Hyggen 2006; Zanin et al. 2013). Dysfunction has eroded health, satisfaction with housing, leisure, and life, and self-efficacy, thus hampering resilience (Distante 2013; Gastil 2000; Granzin and Haggard 2000). Dependency has raised illness and suicide and eroded health and mastery, thus shaking resilience (Bornstein 2012; Lu and Kao 2002; Roy and Chaudhuri 2008).

Utility generated by social trust to attract resilience has evolved from services and others' trustworthiness and usefulness (Vera-Toscano et al. 2013; Wang et al. 2016; Yamagishi 1999).Trustworthiness has stemmed from positive experience, social status, and trust to induce resilience (Barrera 2007; Cook and Cheshire 2013; Kuwabara 2015). Usefulness appraised reflects liking to generate pleasure to build resilience (Bock et al. 2021; Thompson 2006). Social trust raises cooperation received and satisfaction to register utility to attract resilience (Laroche et al. 2019; Six 2014). Social trust arises from emancipation or freedom, order, security, reciprocation, and success experienced or received to maintain utility to attract resilience (Laroche et al. 2019; Newton 1999; Rahn 2008; Yamagishi et al. 1999). Freedom has enabled well-being, including health, life satisfaction, and self-esteem, as opposed to depression and symptoms to facilitate resilience action (Abbott et al. 2011; Glendinning et al. 2003; Haller and Hadler 2006). Order experienced has dampened anxiety to facilitate resilience (Schwartz and Melech 2000). Security experienced has boosted well-being, including health, life satisfaction, and neighborhood quality, as opposed to fear, to induce resilience (Chen et al. 2008; Frey et al. 2007; Olson et al. 2016; Jones et al. 2014). Reciprocity experienced has stemmed from low loneliness to maintain resilience (Espvall and Dellgran 2010). Success experienced has fostered health, life quality, satisfaction, self-efficacy, and self-esteem as opposed to alienation, depression, and distress to uphold resilience (Donnellan et al. 2005; Fredricks and Eccles 2005; Menard and Mose 1984; Murray 2009; Piko et al. 2006; Tompson and Dass 2000; Xiao et al. 2009). Social trust has benefitted from altruism, closeness or relatedness, friendship or friendliness, functionality, life quality, repute, satisfaction, security, similarity, sincerity, and understandability experienced or received to afford utility to attract resilience (Barrera 2007; Eisingerich and Bell 2008; Elsbach and Elofson 2000; Hoogervorst et al. 2015; Kas et al. 2022; Molm et al. 2007; Rothstein and Uslaner 2005; Shao et al. 2021; Volker and Flap 1997). Altruism has raised well-being, including connectedness, hope, life satisfaction, meaningfulness, and self-efficacy as opposed to loneliness and negative emotion to sustain resilience (Caprara and Steca 2005; Marsh and Dik 2021; Nelson-Coffey et al. 2023; Raposa et al. 2016; Yao and Enright 2019). Closeness has facilitated humor and social support received to lift resilience (Martin et al. 2003). Friendship has fostered gratitude to boost resilience (Rotkirch 2014). Functionality has boosted satisfaction with housing, leisure, and life to induce resilience (Granzin and Haggard 2000; Michalos et al. 2000). Repute has raised morale to sustain resilience (Wulfhorst and Kranich 1999). Security experienced has boosted well-being, including health, life satisfaction, and neighborhood quality, as opposed to fear, to induce resilience (Chen et al. 2008; Frey et al. 2007; Olson et al. 2016; Jones et al. 2014). Similarity experienced has reduced depression to afford resilience (Riad and Norris 1992). Sincerity registers intimacy to uphold resilience (Grunebaum 2003). Understandability experienced registers order to reflect health to secure resilience (Cheung and Lai 2020; Raab 2019). Social trust rests on equality, incentive, reciprocity, responsiveness, and windfalls expected or experienced to secure utility to attract resilience (Glaeser et al. 2000; Pattie et al. 2004; Uslaner 2002). Equality experienced has sustained health, homeownership, life satisfaction, self-direction, social capital, and trust to raise resilience (Bond and Lun 2014; Kim and Kawachi 2007; Martin 2000; Meulemann 2010; Nilson 1981; Oishi et al. 2011; Portes and Vickstrom 2011). Responsiveness experienced has raised adaptation, life satisfaction, positive emotion, and relationship evaluation to advance resilience (Algoe and Zhaoyang 2016). Windfalls manifest income to boost resilience (Manning et al. 2016). To the youth, social trust has additionally rested on utility in attractiveness, endowments, positivity, and returning experienced to attract resilience (Kuwabara 2015; Rodrigo-Gonzalez et al. 2021; Wang et al. 2016). Attractiveness or positivity experienced has reduced depression and negative affect to champion resilience (McIntyre et al. 2023; Stanton et al. 2020). Social trust can spring from credibility, safety, and verification experienced or received to secure utility to attract resilience (Burke and Stets 2009; Jung and Kwon 2011; Sato 2002). Conversely, social trust has prevented disutility in arrest experience to discourage resilience (Kirk 2009). Arrest experienced has reflected depression and distress and can reduce opportunities received to obstruct resilience (Ferguson et al. 2011; Kurtz 2008; Ward et al. 2014). Social trust reduces the cost experienced to maintain utility to attract resilience (Falkenberg 1998). The cost experienced has bred anger and depression to negate resilience (Wells et al. 1999). Social trust has ensued from low discrimination, hardship, inequality, punishment, risk, stress, and victimization experienced to reap utility to assimilate resilience (Alesina and La Ferrara 2002; Cais et al. 2021; Lindstrom and Rosvall 2015; Olivera 2015; Rodrigo-Gonzalez et al. 2019; Sun and Wang 2012). Discrimination experienced has raised anomie, depression, distress, and loneliness and has eroded life satisfaction, self-determination, and self-esteem to dampen resilience (Carr and Friedman 2005; Kachanoff et al. 2019; Kirmanoglu and Baslevent 2014; Pachankis et al. 2020; Schnittker 2020; Yang 2019). Hardship experienced has incubated self-transcendence to achieve resilience (Reeskens and Vandecasteele 2017). Inequality experienced has escalated anxiety and mortality risk and dampened health, satisfaction, and well-being in general to impede resilience (Kawachi et al. 1997; Kim and Kawachi 2007; Meulemann 2010; Oshio and Kobayashi 2010; Schwartz and Melech 2000). Punishment received has dampened distress, thus impeding resilience (Zalewski et al. 2017). Risk experienced has inhibited achievement, happiness, life satisfaction, positive affect, and self-determination to dampen resilience (Schoon 2006; Schwartz and Melech 2000; Shippee 2012; Zotti et al. 2016). Stress experienced has dampened well-being, including health, life quality, positive affect, and satisfaction as opposed to depression and distress, to impede resilience (Baumeister et al. 2013. Mathis et al. 2016; Raposa et al. 2016; Shrira 2012; Snyder et al. 2020; Zotti et al. 2016). Victimization experienced has impaired safety experienced and self-respect or self-worth to erode resilience (Fernandes 2018; Krahe 2013). Social trust can advance through low competition, conflict, and threat experienced to keep utility for attracting resilience (Dinesen and Sonderskov 2015). Competition experienced has dampened life satisfaction and fomented depression to jeopardize resilience (Yang 2016). Conflict experienced has bred distress and eroded satisfaction, thus impeding resilience (Lau et al. 2017; Mikula et al. 2012). Threat experienced has diminished well-being, including meaningfulness as opposed to anxiety, depression, fear, and hate (Edwards and Arnon 2021; MacLeod 2017; Moore and Shepherd 2006; O'Neill and Evans 1999; Rothschild and Keefer 2022; Schmid and Muldoon 2015).

Ideals upheld by social trust to rationalize resilience have hailed civic norms, governance, institutions, social inclusion, and volunteering or volunteerism (Crystal and DeBell 2002; Delhey et al. 2011; Marzana et al. 2012). Norm conformity can evolve from its ideal (Klingle 2004). Eventually, norm conformity has furnished achievement and its pressure, mastery-goal setting, social closeness and support received, and tolerance to benefit resilience (Feldman 2003; Jiang et al. 2015; Magnuson et al. 2006). Governance or management has rested on its ideal (Crystal and DeBell 2002). Eventually, governance or management has underpinned life satisfaction and self-efficacy to enable resilience (Corcoran et al. 2011; Rampichini and D'Andrea 1998). Institutionalism can enhance opportunities and resources to facilitate resilience (Kegler et al. 2005; Livingstone et al. 2007). Social inclusion has rested on its ideal (Guan et al. 2009). Eventually, social inclusion can enhance passion and self-esteem to buttress resilience (Allman 2013; Tomlinson et al. 2018). Volunteerism has raised well-being, including health, life satisfaction, mastery, morale, positive affect, and self-esteem as opposed to depression, loneliness, and mortality (Borgonovi 2008; Gillath et al. 2005; Li and Ferraro 2006; Midlarsky and Kahana 1994; Oman et al. 1999; Thoits and Hewitt 2001; Zotti et al. 2016). Social trust involves ideals for investment and kindness to rationalize resilience (Bellemare and Kroger 2007; Habibis et al. 2016). The ideal for investment has underpinned investment (Croy et al. 2010). Investment has strengthened financial and life satisfaction and well-being generally to facilitate resilience (Gehring 2013; Ram 2009; Tharp et al. 2020). Kindness has rested on its ideal (Maltseva 2016). Eventually, kindness has dampened stress and lifted well-being, including connectedness and life satisfaction, as opposed to loneliness and negative emotion (Curry et al. 2018; Nelson-Coffey et al. 2023). Social trust has rested on ideals for acceptance, permissiveness, or tolerance, charity or donation, civic engagement, consideration, contact or interaction, cosmopolitanism, curiosity, emancipation or liberalism, future-looking, negotiation, risk aversion, transaction, and voluntarism to rationalize resilience (Almakaeva et al. 2018; Barrera 2007; Bushen and Raub 2002; Freitag 2003; Fridberg and Kangas 2008b; Kas et al. 2022; Kende et al. 2022; Uslaner 2002; Rahn 2008; Rothstein and Uslaner 2005; Smith 1997; Williams et al. 1999). To the youth, social trust has additionally arisen from ideals for trust, exchange, security to rationalize resilience (Bidmon 2017; Kuwabara 2011; Viklund and Sjoberg 2008). The ideal for charity has underpinned the practice of charity (Bednall et al. 2013). Eventually, charity has enhanced well-being, including life satisfaction (Chang 2009; Helliwell et al. 2010). Civic engagement has stood on its ideal (Peterson and Maiden 1993). As such, civic engagement has incubated conflict resolution, education, happiness, health, income, individualism, life satisfaction, security normativity, social attachment, capital, integration, trust, tolerance, and general well-being to advance resilience (Coffe and Geys 2007; Goren 2005; Growiec and Growiec 2010; Kroll 2011; Li and Walder 2001; Myers 1999; Pena-Lopez and Sanchez-Santos 2016; Posel and Casale 2011; Tak 2017; Tang 2011; Wallace and Pichler 2009; Welzel 2013; van Ingen and Bekkers 2015; Vincens et al. 2018). Consideration can raise morality and reduce crime and violence to uplift resilience (Gottfredson 2018; Thomas 1997). The ideal for contact has propped contact (Bagozzi and Lee 2002). Contact has raised well-being, including happiness, health, life satisfaction, love, self-efficacy, self-esteem, and social well-being as opposed to anxiety and boredom, to facilitate resilience (Crisp and Turner 2012; Denissen et al. 2008; Edara 2021; Galperin and Haselton 2010; Guillen et al. 2011; Mayer 2017; Mazziotta et al. 2011; Meulemann 2010; Reeskens and Vandecasteele 2017). Cosmopolitanism has facilitated pleasantness and self-esteem to champion resilience (Chen et al. 2016; Gonzalez-Jimenez 2016). Curiosity has facilitated flow and creativity to enable resilience (Schutte and Malouff 2020). The ideal of future looking has upheld resilience, life satisfaction, and well-being generally (Lou et al. 2018; MacLeod 2017). The ideal for emancipation spells liberalism (Zhang 2022). Liberalism has rested on growth to induce resilience (Helson and Srivastava 2001). Negotiation has raised enjoyment to induce resilience (Kono and Ito 2021). Risk aversion or prevention has evolved from its ideal (Cheng and Ng 2006; Pires 2022). As such, risk aversion or prevention has rested on control to enable resilience (Cheng and Ng 2006). Transaction or exchange has unfolded from its ideal (Cropanzano and Mitchell 2005). Eventually, transaction or exchange has facilitated well-being, including interest or excitement, intimacy, pleasure, relational quality, and satisfaction as opposed to distress and jealousy, to induce resilience (Afifi et al. 2015; Blieszner 1993; Levitt and Cici-Gokaltun 2011; Stafford 2015; Thye et al. 2008). Voluntarism has propped well-being to enable resilience (Liu 2010). Social trust can rise with ideals for learning, satisficing, sharing, and universalism or cosmopolitanism to rationalize resilience (Buskens and Raub 2013; Kramer 2006; McKnight and Chervany 2006; Steinhardt 2012). The ideal for learning has induced learning (Hagger and Hamilton 2018). Learning has elevated well-being, including life satisfaction and self-efficacy, to facilitate resilience (Denver and Hands 1990; Minnaert and Janssen 1992; Richards 2016). Satisficing has impeded rumination to maintain life satisfaction and positive affect to sustain resilience (Newman and Nezlek 2019; Vargova et al. 2020). The ideal for sharing has reflected social attachment to enhance resilience (Erez et al. 2008). Conversely, social trust has eroded ideals for alcoholism, cynicism, doping, dropout, ostracism, and risking to sustain resilience (Dufur et al. 2013; Kirk 2009; Ng 2016; Shao et al. 2021; Uslaner 2002). Alcoholism has caused aggression, illness, injury, and pathology to impede resilience (Brotchie et al. 2004; Haapanen-Niemi et al. 1999). Cynicism has reflected low life satisfaction and self-efficacy to impede resilience (Moreno-Jimenez and Villodres 2010; Schmuck et al. 2022). The ideal for doping has buttressed doping (Leimberg and Lehmann 2022). Doping has engendered depression, thus jeopardizing resilience (Kendler et al. 2006). Dropout has depended on its ideal (Perez et al. 2014). As such, dropout has reflected dissatisfaction to impede resilience (Barry and Okun 2011). Ostracism has eroded belongingness and confidence to impair resilience (Juanchich et al. 2018). Risking can rest on its ideal (Breakwell 2007). Eventually, risking has weakened health and raised crime and violence, thus blocking resilience (Farrington 2018; Pulkkinen et al. 2009; Wickrama et al. 1995).

Norms underlying social trust have popularized trust, cohesiveness, communication, coresidence, cosmopolitanism, development, education, effectiveness, equality, fairness or justice, homeownership, homogeneity, income, prosperity, or wealth, liberalism, life quality, modernization, organizational membership, satisfaction, transparency, and trustworthiness to assimilate resilience (Alesina and La Ferrara 2002; Delhey and Newton 2005; Fridberg and Kangas 2008b; Geys 2012; Gundelach and Manatschal 2017; Guisan 2009; Hu 2013; Halvorsen 2007; Huhe 2014; Macias 2015; Marschall and Stolle 2004; McCabe 2012; Norris and Inglehart 2009; Rahn 2008; Sabatini and Sarracino 2019; Steinhardt and Delhey 2020; Sun and Wang 2012; Su et al. 2019; Uslaner 2002; Uslaner and Brown 2005; Vera-Toscano et al. 2013). Cohesiveness has stood on its norm (Heckathorn and Rosenstein 2002; Volker et al. 2007). Eventually, cohesiveness has enhanced adjustment, hope, and life satisfaction and diminished depression to facilitate resilience (Araya et al. 2006; Dittman and Goebel 2010; James and Hunsley 1995; Paez et al. 2015). Communication can be susceptible to its norm (Burgoon et al. 2010). As such, communication has boosted positive affect and evaluation received, relationship quality, and self-enhancement as utility to induce resilience (Burgoon et al. 2010; Mirivel 2014; Tsfati et al. 2009). Coresidence has sustained health, life satisfaction, and sleep quality and diminished depression and distress to safeguard resilience (Gu et al. 2010; Lofors and Sundquist 2007; Oshio and Kan 2019; Richards 2016; Sundquist and Yang 2007). Cosmopolitanism can depend on its norm (Cunliffe 2020). As such, cosmopolitanism has facilitated pleasantness and self-esteem to champion resilience (Chen et al. 2016; Gonzalez-Jimenez 2016). The norm for development can foster development (Thomas 2001). Development has facilitated success experienced to attract resilience (Spengler et al. 2018). The norm for education has enhanced education (Andersson 2004). Education has sustained well-being, including health, identity, life quality and satisfaction, mastery, self-efficacy, self-esteem, and youthfulness to engender resilience (Cerin and Leslie 2008; Corcoran et al. 2011; James and Amato 2013; Pakulshi and Tranter 2000; Stavrova and Ehlebracht 2018; van Praag and Frijters 1999; Whyte and Gao 2009; Yienprugsawan et al. 2010). The norm for effectiveness has raised social well-being and reduced anomia to champion resilience (Sani et al. 2008).The norm for equality has sustained health, homeownership, life satisfaction, self-direction, social capital, and trust to raise resilience (Bond and Lun 2014; Kim and Kawachi 2007; Martin 2000; Meulemann 2010; Nilson 1981; Oishi et al. 2011; Portes and Vickstrom 2011). The norm for fairness has enhanced belongingness, health, life satisfaction, and self-esteem to underpin resilience (Bjornskov et al. 2013; Dalbert 2001; Lucas et al. 2013; van Prooijen et al. 2008). The norm for homeownership has propelled homeownership (Henretta 1987). Homeownership has raised health, morale, family and neighborhood quality, and financial, housing, life, and neighborhood satisfaction as opposed to depression, distress, and fear to strengthen resilience (Congdon 2010; Harris 2001; Lee et al. 2022; Mirowsky and Ross 1999; Montazer 2022; Roy and Chaudhuri 2008; Wulfhorst and Kranich 1999; Yu and Chiu 2016; Zheng et al. 2020). Homogeneity can raise life satisfaction to induce resilience (Seder and Oishi 2009). The norm for income has raised income (Zhou 2019). Income has afforded well-being, including adaptation, adequacy, belongingness, control, eudaemonia, health, mastery, power, quality of life, satisfaction, self-efficacy, self-esteem, and social well-being to sustain resilience

(Anciaes et al. 2017; Carpiano 2008; Corcoran et al. 2011; Ross and Mirowsky 1989; Sengupta and Sibley 2019; Son and Wilson 2012; Wang and VanderWeele 2011; Yeh et al. 2013; Zimmerman and Reyna 2013). Liberalism has developed from its norm (Welzel 2013). Eventually, liberalism has rested on growth to induce resilience (Helson and Srivastava 2001). The norm for modernization has buttressed autonomy to enable resilience (Delhey 2010). Organizational membership has rested on its norm (Pavlova and Silbereisen 2015). As such, organizational membership has raised outcome expectancy and reduced stress, thus boosting resilience (Nelson-Coffey et al. 2023). The norm for satisfaction has boosted satisfaction to induce resilience (Castles 2000). The norm for transparent raises social integration to facilitate resilience (Erkkila 2012). Trustworthiness has stemmed from positive experiences and social status to induce resilience (Barrera 2007; Cook and Cheshire 2013; Kuwabara 2015). To the youth, social trust has additionally grown from norms for openness and solidarity (Flanagan and Stout 2010; Loxbo 2018). Openness has raised well-being, including autonomy, growth, life satisfaction, purposefulness, relationship quality, self-acceptance, self-efficacy, and self-esteem as opposed to hostility to boost resilience (Hahn et al. 2013; Hounkpatin et al. 2015; Karwowski and Lebuda 2017; Marks 1996; Quilty et al. 2006; Webster et al. 2014). The norm for solidarity has boosted well-being, including health, neighborhood quality, and satisfaction as opposed to depression and distress to facilitate resilience (Cramm et al. 2012; Fujisawa et al. 2009; Gary et al. 2007; Olson et al. 2016; Wen et al. 2010; Wright et al. 2015). Social trust can benefit from the norm for social integration or solidarity to assimilate resilience (Gundelach and Manatschal 2017). Conversely, social trust has rested on norms against corruption, crime, disorder, discrimination, diversity or fragmentation, doping, fundamentalism, inequality, problems, risk, stress, and unemployment to assimilate resilience (Hyggen 2006; Lundasen et al. 2013; Marschall and Stolle 2004; Richey 2010; Ross and Mirowsky 2009; Uslaner 2002; Uslaner and Brown 2005; Williams et al. 1999; Yu and Chiu 2016; Zanin 2017; Zanin et al. 2013). The norm for corruption has diminished well-being, including satisfaction, to inhibit resilience (Helliwell et al. 2010; Veenhoven 2005). The norm for crime has eroded well-being, including health and satisfaction as opposed to death and fear, to impede resilience (Hummelsheim et al. 2011; Jang et al. 2018; Kennedy et al. 1998; Manning et al. 2016; Stafford et al. 2005). The norm for disorder has weakened well-being, including happiness and positive emotion, as opposed to depression and normlessness, to impair resilience (Hackman et al. 2019; Pei and Kim 2017; Ross and Mirowsky 2009; van Praag and Frijters 1999). Discrimination can arise from its norm (Crandall and Beasley 2001). Eventually, discrimination experienced has raised anomie, depression, distress, and loneliness, and eroded life satisfaction, self-determination, and self-esteem to dampen resilience (Carr and Friedman 2005; Kachanoff et al. 2019; Kirmanoglu and Baslevent 2014; Pachankis et al. 2020; Schnittker 2020; Yang 2019). The norm for diversity has hurt survival, thus jeopardizing resilience (Nettle 2000). The norm for doping has engendered doping (McVicar and Polanski 2014). Doping has engendered depression, thus jeopardizing resilience (Kendler et al. 2006). Fundamentalism has dampened tolerance to impede resilience (Goodwin et al. 2004). The norm for inequality has hurt well-being, including health, satisfaction, and sympathy as opposed to anxiety and death, to jeopardize resilience (Hitlin and Harkness 2018; Oshio and Kobayashi 2010; Kawachi et al. 1997; Kim and Kawachi 2007; Meulemann 2010; Schwartz and Melech 2000). The norm for problems has hurt well-being, including financial well-being, health, and satisfaction as opposed to distress, to impair resilience (Carrieri 2012; Gary et al. 2007; van Praag and Ferrer-I-Carbonell 2004; van Praag and Frijters 1999). The norm for risk has eroded adjustment, positive affect, happiness, life satisfaction, and self-determination and fomented depression, fear or anxiety, negative affect, and sadness to undermine resilience (Prelow et al. 2004; Schoon 2006; Schwartz and Melech 2000; Shippee 2012; Vuori 2015; Zotti et al. 2016). The norm for stress has assimilated stress (Walen and Lachman 2016). Stress has eroded well-being, including eudaimonia, health, positive affect, quality of life, neighborhood, and relationships, and satisfaction with life and neighbors, thus jeopardizing resilience (Baumeister et al. 2013; Greenberg 1999; Jackson et al. 2006; Mathis et al. 2016; Parkes et al. 2002; Shrira 2012; Su et al. 2021; Zotti et al. 2016). The norm for unemployment has bred disability, emotional problems, and illness to cripple resilience (Benitez-Silva et al. 2010).

## *Reciprocity Experienced*

Reciprocity experienced is the functional component of social capital (Mbiba et al. 2019; Yu et al. 2019). The experience also registers love received (Burston 1991). This experience is likely to foster resilience by affording power, utility, ideals, and norms to leverage the voluntaristic mechanisms of power realization, utility optimization, ideal calibration, and norm conformity to complete functioning based on analytical functionalism.

Power raised by reciprocity experienced to drive resilience has stemmed from adjustment, friendship, gratitude, motivation, relatedness, and religiosity (Adams and Miller 2022; Brouwer and Engels 2022; Cheadle and Schwadel 2012; Liu et al. 2021; Torlo and Lomi 2017; Wintre and Yaffe 2000). Friendship has fostered gratitude to boost resilience (Rotkirch 2014). Religiosity has sustained well-being, including adjustment, flourishing, health, mastery, positive affect, relational quality, satisfaction, self-esteem, and socioemotional well-being, to advance resilience (Dy-Liacco et al. 2009; Helliwell and Putnam 2005; Flouri and Buchanan 2002; Meulemann 2010; Moschis and Ong 2011; Ng and Fisher 2016; Schieman 2001; Skerkat and Ellison 1999; Wuthnow 2004). Reciprocity experienced can raise pleasure to secure power to drive resilience (Jiang et al. 2022). Conversely, reciprocity experienced has prevented death to maintain power to drive resilience (Lochner et al. 2003). Reciprocity experienced has reflected low loneliness and unemployment to retain power to drive resilience (Espvall and Dellgran 2010). Unemployment has weakened well-being, including financial adequacy, health, mastery, positive affect, satisfaction, and transcendence as opposed to anxiety and depression, to maintain resilience (Anusic et al. 2014; Hraba et al. 2001; Lelli 2008; Lofors and Sundquist 2007; Reeskens and Vandecasteele 2017; Schieman 2001).

Utility secured by reciprocity experienced to attract resilience has featured satisfaction (Liu et al. 2021). Reciprocity experienced upholds love experienced as utility to attract resilience (Burston 1991). Love experienced can erode depression, thus maintaining resilience (Busch 2009). Reciprocity experienced can upgrade friendship and relational quality, harmony, and social integration experienced as utility to attract resilience (Lawler 2002; Martin et al. 1999; Molm 2008; Stafford 2015). Friendship quality has reflected intimacy and relational quality as opposed to anxiety and loneliness to maintain resilience (Lee 2018; Li et al. 2018; Parade et al. 2010; Wang et al. 2020). Harmony experienced has cultivated life satisfaction and dampened depression to maintain resilience (Yang 2016). Social integration experienced has impeded depression to enable resilience (Mullins and Dugan 1991).

Ideals enhanced by reciprocity experienced to rationalize resilience have prized reciprocity, affiliating, civic engagement, consumption, giving, helping, homophily, liking, proactivity, prosociality, recourse, and social interaction (Adams and Miller 2022; Avalos 2019; Brouwer and Engels 2022; Dovidio et al. 2006; Gui et al. 2020; Linden-Andersen et al. 2009; Malloy 2018; Mbiba et al. 2019; Pratkanis and Turner 1996; Stadtfeld and Pentland 2015). Affiliating has reduced stress, thus safeguarding resilience (Nelson-Coffey et al. 2023). Civic engagement has stood on its ideal (Peterson and Maiden 1993). As such, civic engagement has incubated conflict resolution, education, happiness, health, income, individualism, life satisfaction, security normativity, social attachment, capital, integration, trust, tolerance, and general well-being to advance resilience (Coffe and Geys 2007; Goren 2005; Growiec and Growiec 2010; Kroll 2011; Li and Walder 2001; Myers 1999; Pena-Lopez and Sanchez-Santos 2016; Posel and Casale 2011; Tak 2017; Tang 2011; Wallace and Pichler 2009; Welzel 2013; van Ingen and Bekkers 2015; Vincens et al. 2018). The ideal for consumption has sustained consumption (Xu et al. 2004). Eventually, consumption can erect identity to advance resilience (McDonald and Wearing 2013). Giving can maintain spirituality and well-being and reduce violence, thus securing resilience (Day 2010, Messner et al. 2008, Turner 2013). The ideal for helping has sustained helping (Feeney and Collins 2001; Yao and Enright 2019; Wade-Benzoni and Tost 2009). Helping has boosted well-being, including connectedness, hope, life satisfaction, meaningfulness, and self-efficacy, to elevate resilience (Marsh and Dik 2021; Nelson-Coffey et al. 2023; Raposa et al. 2016). Recourse has alleviated distress to uphold resilience (Tracey et al. 1986). Homphily or similarity has reduced depression to afford resilience (Riad and Norris 1992). Liking has generated pleasure to build resilience (Thompson 2006). Proactivity represents coping, protection, and power to enable resilience (Greene 1991; Seaton and Beaumont 2008, Shaw et al. 2023). Recourse has rested on its ideal (Heffren and Hausdorf 2016). Eventually, recourse has alleviated distress to uphold resilience (Tracey et al. 1986). The ideal for social interaction has propped contact (Bagozzi and Lee 2002). Social interaction has raised well-being, including happiness, health, life satisfaction, love, self-efficacy, self-esteem, and social well-being as opposed to anxiety and boredom, to facilitate resilience (Crisp and Turner 2012; Denissen et al. 2008; Edara 2021; Galperin and

Haselton 2010; Guillen et al. 2011; Mayer 2017; Mazziotta et al. 2011; Meulemann 2010; Reeskens and Vandecasteele 2017). Resilience experienced can boost ideals for cooperation and visiting to rationalize resilience (Capistrano and Weaver 2017; Nahapiet 2009). Cooperation has thrived on its ideal (Haesevoets et al. 2015). As such, cooperation has fostered life satisfaction to rationalize resilience (Park et al. 2015). Visiting has originated from its ideal, evaluation, or preference (Ertz et al. 2021). Eventually, visiting has enhanced life satisfaction to facilitate resilience (Winkelmann 2009). Conversely, reciprocity experienced has reduced the ideal for discriminating, thus rationalizing resilience (Tusicisny 2017). Discriminating has emerged from its norm (McDougall et al. 2004). Eventually, discriminating has weakened belongingness and confidence, thus impeding resilience (Juanchich et al. 2018).

## *Associational Involvement*

Associational involvement is a component of social capital or civic engagement (Palmer et al. 2011; Wang and Graddy 2008). Such involvement embraces belongingness, interest, leisure activity, membership, programming, and tying or networking concerning associations (Bagherior et al. 2009; Cotterell 2007; Jacobs et al. 2009; Palmer-Rubin et al. 2021; Wetterbeng 2007). The involvement is likely to facilitate resilience by offering power, utility, ideals, and norms to run the voluntaristic mechanisms of power realization, utility optimization, ideal calibration, and norm conformity to complete the function posited in analytical functionalism.

Power generated by associational involvement to drive resilience has rested on attachment, civility, happiness, health, knowledge, skill, support received, and trust (Geys 2012; Guillen et al. 2011; Hansen et al. 2003; Pattie et al. 2004; Tak 2017; Thoits and Hewitt 2001; Wetterbeng 2007). Attachment has buttressed life satisfaction to enable resilience (Zdrenka et al. 2015). Civility has boosted well-being, including physical and mental health, to activate resilience (Tsai et al. 2018). Knowledge has championed intimacy, satisfaction, and self-efficacy to boost resilience (Mikulincer et al. 2003; Norris 2011; Rothwell et al. 2016). Skill comprises cognitive skill, emotion regulation, physical skill, and teamwork and social skill (Hansen et al. 2003). Social skill comprises that concerning feedback, group processes, and leadership (Hansen et al. 2003). Skill has underpinned self-efficacy to buttress resilience (Larson et al. 1990). Social support received has fostered resilience (Cherry et al. 2018). Furthermore, supporting has rested on compassion, friendliness, generativity, humility, intelligence, mindfulness, openness, self-esteem, sociability, solidarity, sympathy, and transcendence to generate power to drive resilience (Berry et al. 2020; Caprara and Steca 2007; Foschi and Lauriola 2014; Kitayama and Markus 2000; Leiberg 2011; Rossi 2004; Thielmann et al. 2020; Wong and Yang 2022). Trust has sustained health and survival, thus raising resilience (Barefoot et al. 1998). Associational involvement affords power, including that based on learning and networking, to drive resilience (Cotterell 2007; Delgado and Staples 2008; Quinn 1995). Such power stems from advocacy, collaboration, consultation, informing, partnership, and therapy (Delgado and Staples 2008). Learning gained has facilitated well-being, including life satisfaction and self-efficacy as opposed to death, to enhance resilience (Denver and Hands 1990; Minnaert and Janssen 1992; Mirowsky and Ross 2000; Richards 2016). Networking has boosted well-being, including flourishing, happiness, health, life satisfaction, and pride as opposed to depression and distress to champion resilience (Chua et al. 2021; Congdon 2010; Yetim and Yetim 2014). Associational involvement can stem from encouragement received to boost power to drive resilience (Larson 1994). Encouragement is a component of social support (Frost 2007). Associational involvement has realized education as power to drive resilienve (Nussio 2019). Education has sustained well-being, including health, identity, life quality and satisfaction, mastery, self-efficacy, self-esteem, and youthfulness to engender resilience (Cerin and Leslie 2008; Corcoran et al. 2011; James and Amato 2013; Pakulshi and Tranter 2000; Stavrova and Ehlebracht 2018; van Praag and Frijters 1999; Whyte and Gao 2009; Yienprugsawan et al. 2010). Associational involvement embraces belongingness, empowerment received, interest, and leadership experienced to give power to drive resilience (Delgado and Staples 2008; Jacobs et al. 2009; Quinn 1995). Belongingness has strengthened rewards to induce resilience (Nelson-Coffey et al. 2023). Empowerment, including facilitating, helping, and supporting, facilitates resilience, choice, partnership, relating, resource acquisition, and success (Delgado and Staples 2008). Empowerment received has boosted well-being, including satisfaction and self-efficacy to advance resilience (Biron and Samberger 2010; Kulik 2007). Association involvement reflects agency or initiative-taking to maintain power to drive resilience (Dworkin et al. 2003). Agency has maintained mastery, relational quality, satisfaction, and vitality to facilitate resilience (Delhey 2010; Hui et al. 2013; Ross and Drentea 1998; Sieber et al. 2019).

Utility given by associational involvement to attract resilience has transpired in life satisfaction and social integration (Myers 1999; Thoits and Hewitt 2001). Social integration has prevented depression and suicide to buttress resilience (Duberstein et al. 2004; Mullins and Dugan 1991). Associational involvement provides community and leisure experience as utility to attract resilience (Cotterell 2007; Delgado and Staples 2008). The sense of community has strengthened rewards to induce resilience (Nelson-Coffey et al. 2023). Leisure has attenuated anxiety, thus enabling resilience (Da Costa Bizarro Morais et al. 2019). Associational involvement can stem from beneficiary status, benefits, public goods, respect, services, and subsidies received to secure utility to attract resilience (Bagherior et al. 2009; Palmer-Rubin et al. 2021; Sturmer et al. 2008). Benefits received have elevated well-being, including satisfaction as opposed to anger, anxiety, and depression, to boost resilience (Helgeson et al. 2006; Wells et al. 1999; Wong and Lam 2016). Respect received has rested on education and health to generate power to drive resilience action (Malat 2001). Services received have supported autonomy or self-determination, satisfaction, and reduced mortality, thus boosting resilience (Clemens and Wetle 1994; Davies et al. 1990; Elkan et al. 2001). Conversely, associational involvement has reduced costs and stress experienced to maintain utility to attract resilience (Hansen et al. 2003). The cost experienced has bred anger and depression to negate resilience (Wells et al. 1999). Stress experienced has dampened well-being, including health, life quality, positive affect, and satisfaction as opposed to depression and distress, to impede resilience (Baumeister et al. 2013. Mathis et al. 2016; Raposa et al. 2016; Shrira 2012; Snyder et al. 2020; Zotti et al. 2016). Associational involvement has arisen from low risk experienced to retain utility to attract resilience (Quinn 1995). Associational involvement can arise free of coercion to maintain utility for attracting resilience (Bagherior et al. 2009). Risk experienced has inhibited achievement, happiness, life satisfaction, positive affect, and self-determination to dampen resilience (Schoon 2006; Schwartz and Melech 2000; Shippee 2012; Zotti et al. 2016). Coercion experienced has bred alienation, distress, externalizing behavior, failure, relationship problems, and violence to contradict resilience (Antunes et al. 2014; Xing et al. 2011; Woodward and Fergusson 1999; Zalewski et al. 2017).

Ideals advanced by associational involvement accentuate charity, choice, civic or community engagement or participation, civility, cohesion, donation, identity work, initiative-taking, prosociality, and socialism (Boiney and Paletz 1991; Bowman et al. 2015; Chan 2014; Christens et al. 2016; Gilberbloom and Markham 1995; Hansen et al. 2003; Palmer et al. 2011; Quinn 1995; Sokolowski 1996; Wang and Graddy 2008). The ideal for charity has underpinned the practice of charity (Bednall et al. 2013). Eventually, charity has enhanced well-being, including life satisfaction (Chang 2009; Helliwell et al. 2010). Choice is a manifestation of liberalism (Patall et al. 2008). As such, choice has buttressed competence, effort and performance, life and neighborhood satisfaction, motivation, and self-determination to safeguard resilience (Day 2013; Gagne and Deci 2005; Helliwell et al. 2010; Patall et al. 2008). Civic engagement has stood on its ideal (Peterson and Maiden 1993). As such, civic engagement has incubated conflict resolution, education, happiness, health, income, individualism, life satisfaction, security normativity, social attachment, capital, integration, trust, tolerance, and general well-being to advance resilience (Coffe and Geys 2007; Goren 2005; Growiec and Growiec 2010; Kroll 2011; Li and Walder 2001; Myers 1999; Pena-Lopez and Sanchez-Santos 2016; Posel and Casale 2011; Tak 2017; Tang 2011; Wallace and Pichler 2009; Welzel 2013; van Ingen and Bekkers 2015; Vincens et al. 2018). Community participation rests on communitarianism (Heckscher 2015). As such, community participation has elevated well-being, including mastery and self-efficacy to enable resilience (Harter and Arora 2010; Ohmer 2007; Peterson and Huphey 2004). Civility has evolved from its ideal (Peterson and Maiden 1993). As such, civility has fostered well-being, including mental and physical health, to elevate resilience (Tsai et al. 2018). Cohesion has developed from its ideal (Granzin and Olsen 1998). As such, cohesion has buttressed hope and life satisfaction and eroded depression to maintain resilience (Araya et al. 2006; Dittman and Goebel 2010; Paez et al. 2015). The ideal for donation has propped donation (Vallerand et al. 1992). Eventually, donation has reflected well-being, including control, feeling good, gratitude, happiness, joy, satisfaction, and self-efficacy as opposed to anxiety and guilt, to brew resilience (Bednall et al. 2013; Bekkers 2008; Eayrs and Ellis 1990; Liu and Hao 2017; Mussen 1982; Piliavin and Callero 1991; Wang and Graddy 2008). Identity work comprises exploration and reflection (Hansen et al. 2003). Identity exploration has hinged on its ideal (Cote and Levine 1988a). ISuch exploration develops identity (Crocetti et al. 2010). Identity has secured happiness, love, self-efficacy, and self-esteem and has diminished anxiety and depression to facilitate resilience (Cast 2004). Initiative-taking covers goal setting, effort, problem-solving or resolution, and time management (Hansen et al. 2003). Essentially, initiative-taking represents coping, protection, and power to enable resilience (Greene 1991; Seaton and Beaumont 2008; Shaw et al. 2023). The prosocial ideal underlies prosociality (Maltseva 2016). Prosociality has elevated well-being, including connectedness, hope, life satisfaction, meaningfulness, and self-efficacy to boost resilience (Marsh and Dik 2021; Nelson-Coffey et al. 2023; Raposa et al. 2016; Yao and Enright 2019). Socialism maintains harmony, love, morality, relationality or cohesion, responsibility, and toegetherness to champion resilience (Collier 2001; Lin 2017; Liu 2008; Scruton 2014; Sturm 1998). Associational involvement has fostered the ideal for respect to rationalize resilience (Sturmer et al. 2008). Respect has fostered identity to afford resilience (Renger and Reese 2017). Associational involvement reflects the ideal for accountability to rationalize resilience (Quinn 1995). Accountability has developed from its ideal (Killian and Ganong 2002). As such, accountability has advanced wisdom to facilitate resilience (Spengler et al. 2018). Conversely, associational involvement has reduced ideals for alcoholism and cheating (Ozbay 2008). Alcoholism has caused aggression, illness, injury, and pathology to impede resilience (Brotchie et al. 2004; Haapanen-Niemi et al. 1999). Cheating has brewed from its ideal (Rawwas et al. 2004). As such, cheating has raised the cost experienced to discourage resilience (Thielmann and Hilbig 2019).

Norms enhanced by associational involvement to assimilate resilience emphasize prosociality (Hansen et al. 2003). The norm for prosociality has developed prosociality. Prosociality has elevated well-being, including connectedness, hope, life satisfaction, meaningfulness, and self-efficacy to boost resilience (Marsh and Dik 2021; Nelson-Coffey et al. 2023; Raposa et al. 2016; Yao and Enright 2019). Associational involvement has benefitted from norms for control and prestige to assimilate resilience (Bowman et al. 2015). Control has boosted well-being, including health and life satisfaction as opposed to anger and depression, to maintain resilience (Etezadi and Pushkar 2013. Heidemeier and Staudinger 2012; Rose 2000; Xi and Hwang 2011). Conversely, associational involvement has diminished the norm for corruption to maintain resilience (Morris and Klesner 2010; Uslaner and Brown 2005; Williams et al. 1999; Yu and Chiu 2016; Zanin 2017; Zanin et al. 2013). The norm for corruption has diminished well-being, including satisfaction, to inhibit resilience (Helliwell et al. 2010; Veenhoven 2005).

## *Friendship*

Friendship is integral to social capital (Wuthnow 2002). Essentially, friendship signifies acceptance, affirmation, association, attachment, confluence, enjoyment, equality, equilibration, familiarity, influence, intimacy or closeness, investment, nonkinship, reciprocity, reconciliation, security, selection, self-expansion, sharing, similarity, social integration, social fulfillment or provision, support, trust, understanding, and voluntariness (Adler and Adler 1998; Chow and Ng 2004; Eberl 2020; Houldcroft et al. 2014; Koerner 2018; Light and Dishion 2007; Myers 1999; Pellegrini and Blatchford 2000; Rook and Ituarte 1999; Rose 2002; Rubin et al. 2008; Seibert and Kerns 2009; Turner et al. 2007; Wakimoto and Fujihara 2004). Social fulfillment or provision covers advice, affection, aid, alliances, companionship, counseling, disclosure, guidance, nurturance, and reassurance (Carbery and Buhrmester 1998). Friendship features acceptance, affection, appreciation, assistance, benevolence, companionship, commitment, communication, community, contact, cooperation, disclosure, empathy, entrusting, fusion, interdependence, intimacy, love, loyalty, networking, pleasure or entertaining, presence, privileges, respect, sharing, sociality, solidarity, trust, and understanding (Albeck and Kaydar 2002; Austin et al. 2005; Bucher 2013; de Vries and Megathlin 2009; Filip et al. 2006; Grunebaum 2003; Koerner 2018; Policarpo 2015; Sharabany 1994; Tsai 2006). Affection unfolds in care and compatibility (de Vries and Megathlin 2009). Intimacy displays attachment or connection, assistance or support, cheerfulness or sweetness, commonability, communication or discussion, communion, confiding, disclosure or self-revelation, criticism, desire, emotions, empathy, exclusiveness or preference, feedback, frankness or spontaneity, giving or sharing, happiness, inclination, knowing, listening, loyalty, openness, reciprocity, reception, sensitivity, sincerity, sympathy, trust, trustworthiness, unburdening, understanding, and uprightness (Grunebaum 2003; Sharabany 1994). To the youth, friendship additionally involves concern, equality, forgiving, influence, integration, motivation, mutuality, provision, reliability, and similarity (Asher and Weeks 2018; Bagwell and Schmidt 2011; Chang et al. 2012; Cotterell 2007; Massengale et al. 2017; Williams and Eberhardt 2008). In the elder, friendship additionally emphasizes identity and recourse (Hawthorne 2006; Moen et al. 2000). With these, friendship is likely to uphold resilience by providing power, utility, ideals, and norms using the voluntaristic mechanisms of analytical functionalism.

Power raised by friendship to drive resilience has rested on attachment, religiosity, resources, social desirability, trust, and well-being (Baker and Smith 2009; Keillor et al. 2001; Mesch and Manor 1998; Gudmundsdottir 2013; Kende et al. 2022; Palmer et al. 2011). Well-being has included health as opposed to anxiety and loneliness (Binder et al. 2012; Cichy et al. 2007; Raymo 2015). Attachment has buttressed life satisfaction to enable resilience (Zdrenka et al. 2015). Religiosity has buttressed coping, friendship, forgiveness, harmony perceived, health maintenance, institutional and social trust, optimism, social capital, and well-being to raise resilience (Chang 2009; Clemence 2001; Furnham 1997; Hakhverdian and Mayne 2012; Myers 2008; Saroglou and Anciaux 2004; Wuthnow 2004; Zanin 2017). Social desirability has escalated gratitude and dampened anxiety and depression to maintain resilience (Ben-Zur 2002; Burroughs and Rindfleisch 2002; Krumrei-Mancuso 2017). Trust has fostered health and survival to sustain resilience (Barefoot et al. 1998). Friendship involves commitment, cheerfulness, happiness, or pleasure, cooperation need, community experienced, and assistance or support, care, and sharing received to afford power to drive resilience (de Vries and Megathlin 2009; Grunebaum 2003; Tsai 2006). Commitment has sustained self-acceptance and relieved depression to foster resilience (Agronick and Duncan 1998; Wrosch et al. 2005). Cooperation has raised life satisfaction to secure resilience (Park et al. 2015). Assistance or social support received has upheld resilience and well-being, including control, health, positive emotion and pleasure, purposiveness, relational quality, satisfaction with life, housing, and leisure, self-determination, self-efficacy, self-esteem, and social well-being, to activate resilience (Cherry et al. 2018; George and Park 2013; Glendinning et al. 2003; Granzin and Haggard 2000; Holliman et al. 2021; Lincoln et al. 2003; Logan and Cobb 2013; Pierce and Quiroz 2018; Schwarzer and Knoll 2007; Vilhjalmsson and Thorlindsson 1998; Wen et al. 2010; Williams and Galliher 2006; Xi and Hwang 2011). Care received has fostered functionality and satisfaction to sustain resilience (Caro and Blank 1988; Davies et al. 1990). Community experienced has elevated well-being, including mastery and self-efficacy to enable resilience (Harter and Arora 2010; Ohmer 2007; Peterson and Huphey 2004). Sharing received has raised well-being, including control, emotional well-being, health, pleasure, purposefulness, relational quality, satisfaction, self-determination, self-efficacy, self-esteem, and social well-being to facilitate resilience (George and Park 2013; Glendinning et al. 2003; Gorman et al. 2010; Granzin and Haggard 2000; Holliman et al. 2021; Lincoln et al. 2003; Logan and Cobb 2013; Pierce and Quiroz 2018; Schwarzer and Knoll 2007; Vilhjalmsson and Thorlindsson 1998; Williams and Galliher 2006; Xi and Hwang 2011). Friendship has hinged on emotional intelligence, education, health, homeownership, and income to afford power to drive resilience (Austin et al. 2005; Child and Nikolova 2020; Tsai 2006). Emotional intelligence has facilitated well-being, including adaptation, happiness, health, life satisfaction, positive mood, relatedness, relational quality, and self-esteem to enhance resilience (Ciarrochi et al. 2000; Kluemper 2008; Matthews et al. 2012; Mayer et al. 2004; Schutte et al. 2002). Education has sustained well-being, including health, identity, life quality and satisfaction, mastery, self-efficacy, self-esteem, and youthfulness to engender resilience (Cerin and Leslie 2008; Corcoran et al. 2011; James and Amato 2013; Pakulshi and Tranter 2000; Stavrova and Ehlebracht 2018; van Praag and Frijters 1999; Whyte and Gao 2009; Yienprugsawan et al. 2010). Homeownership has raised health, morale, family and neighborhood quality, and financial, housing, life, and neighborhood satisfaction as opposed to depression, distress, and fear to strengthen resilience (Congdon 2010; Harris 2001; Lee et al. 2022; Mirowsky and Ross 1999; Montazer 2022; Roy and Chaudhuri 2008; Wulfhorst and Kranich 1999; Yu and Chiu 2016; Zheng et al. 2020). Income has afforded well-being, including adaptation, adequacy, belongingness, control, eudaemonia, health, mastery, power, quality of life, satisfaction, self-efficacy, self-esteem, and social well-being to sustain resilience (Anciaes et al. 2017; Carpiano 2008; Corcoran et al. 2011; Ross and Mirowsky 1989; Sengupta and Sibley 2019; Son and Wilson 2012; Wang and VanderWeele 2011; Yeh et al. 2013, Zimmerman and Reyna 2013). Liberalism has developed from its norm (Welzel 2013). Conversely, friendship precludes conflict or protest need and jealousy to retain power to drive resilience (Grunebaum 2003). Protesting has provoked anger and discontent to erode resilience (Landmann and Rohmann 2020). Jealousy has raised fear, thus jeopardizing resilience (Felson and Outlaw 2007). Friendship has reflected low fear to maintain power to drive resilience (Sampson 1991).

Utility given by friendship to attract resilience has unfolded in reciprocity expected, satisfaction, and social integration experienced (Gundert and Hohendanner 2015; Orlowski and Wicker 2015; Rotkirch 2014). Reciprocity expected has reflected low loneliness to enable resilience (Espvall and Dellgran 2010). Social integration experienced has impeded depression to enable resilience (Mullins and Dugan 1991). Friendship manifests acceptance, appreciation, autonomy, benevolence, communion, compatibility, dignity, empathy, equality, intimacy, love, openness or reception, respect, sympathy, and understanding experienced as utility to attract resilience (de Vries and Megathlin 2009; Grunebaum 2003; Sharabany 1994). Acceptance experienced has diminished depression, thus sustaining power to drive resilience (Mullins and Dugan 1991). Appreciation experienced has reflected satisfaction to induce resilience (Pfister et al. 2020). Autonomy has raised well-being, including energy, health, mastery, meaningfulness, positive affect, pride, satisfaction, self-efficacy, and self-esteem, to boost resilience (Au and Cheung 2004; De Moortel et al. 2015; Erickson 2008; Garcia et al. 2017; Gahlawat et al. 2019; Hodson 1996; Martela and Riekki 2018; Schieman 2002; Schieman and Narisada 2014; Yoon 2001). Benevolence has reduced anxiety and negative affect and sustained life satisfaction, positive affect, and resilience (Howard and Alipour 2014; Kim et al. 2018; Muris et al. 2010). Communion experienced has impeded depression to enable resilience (Mullins and Dugan 1991). Compatibility experienced has raised health, identity, morale, and satisfaction and diminished anxiety, depression, and strain to boost resilience (Li 2006; Pereyra-Rojas et al. 2017; Sutherland and Fogarty 1995; Xie 1996). Dignity experienced has upheld well-being, including adjustment, happiness, health, positive affect, and satisfaction with appearance and work to enable resilience (Barnard and Curry 2011; Frederick et al. 2016; Hull et al. 2008; Judge et al. 2002; Williams et al. 1992). Empathy has facilitated intimacy and communication quality to facilitate resilience (Redmond 2018). Equality experienced denotes freedom from deprivation and strain, thus safeguarding resilience (Kyriacou 2020). Intimacy experienced has sustained purposiveness, relationship satisfaction, and self-efficacy and dampened anxiety to facilitate resilience (Arseth et al. 2009; Chou 2000; Hand et al. 2013; Henderson et al. 2009). Love received can reduce depression to secure resilience (Busch 2009). Openness has facilitated well-being, including autonomy, growth, life satisfaction, purposefulness, relational quality, self-acceptance, self-efficacy, and self-esteem to enable resilience (Hounkpatin et al. 2015; Webster et al. 2014). Respect received raises well-being to sustain resilience (Fingerman et al. 2011). Sympathy or understanding received has boosted adaptation, positive emotion, forgiveness, and life satisfaction to maintain resilience (Algoe and Zhaoyang 2016; Brik et al. 2023). Conversely, friendship has eroded threat experienced to uphold utility to attract resilience (Schneider 2007). Threat experienced has fomented anxiety, avoidance, conflict, depression, fear, and hate to disrupt resilience (Edwards and Arnon 2021; MacLeod 2017; Moore and Shepherd 2006; O'Neill and Evans 1999; Rick et al. 2006; Ruiter et al. 2003). Friendship precludes burdening and comparison and competition experienced to maintain utility to attract resilience (Grunebaum 2003). Burden experienced has heightened burnout, depression, powerlessness, and somatic complaint, and eroded health and self-esteem, thus impairing resilience (Furnham 1997; Gerber et al. 2010; Wan et al. 2023). Competition experienced has dampened life satisfaction and fomented depression to jeopardize resilience (Yang 2016). Friendship has developed from low war experience to secure utility to attract resilience (Child and Nikolova 2020). War experienced has bred depression, fear, and stress to undermine resilience (Goodrum et al. 2020; Tang et al. 2020). Friendship can benefit from relational quality to sustain utility to attract resilience (Sharabany 1994).

Ideals maintained by friendship to rationalize resilience have prized cohesion, compliance, donation, gratitude, tolerance, and volunteering (Corcoran 2013; Opp 2001; Rotkirch 2014; Sampson 1991; Tang 2006; Wise and Driskell 2017). Cohesion has developed from its ideal (Granzin and Olsen 1998). As such, cohesion has buttressed hope and life satisfaction and eroded depression to maintain resilience (Araya et al. 2006; Dittman and Goebel 2010; Paez et al. 2015). The ideal for compliance has buttressed compliance (Van Damme 2017). Compliance has furnished achievement and its pressure, mastery-goal setting, social closeness and support received, and tolerance to benefit resilience (Feldman 2003; Jiang et al. 2015; Magnuson et al. 2006). The ideal for donation has propped donation (Vallerand et al. 1992). Eventually, donation has reflected well-being, including control, feeling good, gratitude, happiness, joy, satisfaction, and self-efficacy as opposed to anxiety and guilt, to brew resilience (Bednall et al. 2013; Bekkers 2008; Eayrs and Ellis 1990; Liu and Hao 2017; Mussen 1982; Piliavin and Callero 1991; Wang and Graddy 2008). The ideal for gratitude has buttressed gratitude (Algoe and Haidt 2009). Gratitude has raised positive affect and dampened negative affect to achieve resilience (Bernabe-Valero et al. 2021). Volunteering has grown from its ideal (Barr et al. 2005). Eventually, volunteering has raised well-being, including health, life satisfaction, mastery, morale, positive affect, and self-esteem as opposed to depression, loneliness, and mortality, to buttress resilience (Borgonovi 2008; Gillath et al. 2005; Li and Ferraro 2006; Midlarsky and Kahana 1994; Oman et al. 1999; Thoits and Hewitt 2001; Zotti et al. 2016). Friendship can foster the prosocial ideal to rationalize resilience (Bierhoff 2002). The prosocial ideal underlies prosociality (Maltseva 2016). Prosociality has elevated well-being, including connectedness, hope, life satisfaction, meaningfulness, and self-efficacy to boost resilience (Marsh and Dik 2021; Nelson-Coffey et al. 2023; Raposa et al. 2016; Yao and Enright 2019). Friendship holds ideals for communication, duty, equality, goodwill, and sharing to rationalize resilience (Grunebaum 2003). Communication has boosted positive affect and evaluation received, relationship quality, and self-enhancement as utility to induce resilience (Burgoon et al. 2010; Mirivel 2014; Tsfati et al. 2009). Friendship has realized ideals for civic participation, helping, and socializing to rationalize resilience (Benton 2016; Eberl 2020). Civic participation has evolved from its ideal (Peterson and Maiden 1993). As such, civic participation has fostered well-being, including mental and physical health, to elevate resilience (Tsai et al. 2018). The ideal for helping has sustained helping (Feeney and Collins 2001; Yao and Enright 2019; Wade-Benzoni and Tost 2009). Helping has boosted well-being, including connectedness, hope, life satisfaction, meaningfulness, and self-efficacy, to elevate resilience (Marsh and Dik 2021; Nelson-Coffey et al. 2023; Raposa et al. 2016). Socializing has hinged on its ideal (Chen et al. 2009). Eventually, socializing has reduced negative emotions and stress to safeguard resilience (Nelson-Coffey et al. 2023). Friendship can stem from ideals for investment and self-enhancement to rationalize resilience (Turner et al. 2007; Volker and Flap 2007). The ideal for investment has underpinned investment (Croy et al. 2010). Investment has strengthened financial and life satisfaction and well-being generally to facilitate resilience (Gehring 2013; Ram 2009; Tharp et al. 2020). Self-enhancement stands on its ideal (Marshall 2001). Given the standing, self-enhancement has reflected attachment and social support received to raise resilience (Hermanto et al. 2017; Ledoux et al. 2010). Conversely, friendship has dismissed ideals of egoism and racism to rationalize resilience (Kitts 2003; Meeusen et al. 2013). Egoism has bred anxiety to impair resilience (Da Costa Bizarro Morais et al. 2019). Racism has diminished life quality to hamper resilience (Ishii 2009).

Norms responsible for friendship to assimilate resilience have highlighted balance, popularity, reciprocity, sameness or similarity, stability, and warmth (Brouwer and Engels 2022; Kokkinos and Hatzinikolaou 2011; Mouw and Entwisle 2006; Palacios et al. 2019; Sampson 1991). Balance has developed from its norm (He et al. 2014). As such, balance has fostered confidence to achieve resilience (Simon and Read 2018). Popularity has benefitted from its norm (Lei 2004). Eventually, popularity has uplifted positive affect and self-esteem and reduced negative affect, thus buttressing resilience (Reich et al. 2018). The norm for reciprocity has induced reciprocity (Avalos 2019. Reciprocity has facilitated adaptation as opposed to illness to create resilience (Yamaoka 2008; Yeh et al. 2013). Similarity has arisen from its norm (Wakimoto and Fujihara 2004). As such, similarity has reduced depression to afford resilience (Riad and Norris 1992). The norm for stability has sustained relational quality to enhance resilience (Ross et al. 2000). Warmth has benefitted from its norm (Haberkern and Szydlik 2010). As such, warmth has maintained mental clarity to boost resilience (Naruse et al. 2020). Conversely, friendship has developed from the norm against diversity to assimilate resilience (Mouw and Entwisle 2006). The norm for diversity has hurt survival, thus jeopardizing resilience (Nettle 2000).

## *Combinations of Social Capital Components*

The combinations of social capital components are likely to generate extra contributions to resilience beyond those by the components separately due to complementarity based on coordination among the components. Complementarity means fitting, matching, or integrating to achieve completeness, which is extraordinarily powerful (Van Vianen et al. 2008). Inherently, complementarity registers cooperation, harmony, stability, supermodularity, and synergy (Campbell et al. 2008; Deeg 2007; Fang 2003; Johnson and Johnson 2005). Synergy comprises compensation and coordination (Riley et al. 2011). These structural bases and components generate power to activate the power realization mechanism in analytical functionalism for fulfillment or goal attainment.

Power raised by complementarity has rested on cooperation, integration, and quality enhanced (Brewer 1996; Tsaur et al. 2014). Cooperation reflects balance, empowerment, and order to enhance power (Breton 2004; Burt 2009; Lawler et al. 2014). Balance can reduce discrepancy to maintain power (Adkins and Premeaux 2019). Order has reflected continuity and stability to afford power (Arts et al. 1999). Continuity or stability reflects strength or power (Von Culin et al. 2014). Complementarity reflects harmony and stability to generate power (Deeg 2007; Fang 2003). Harmony manifests cohesiveness, diversity, fitting, inclusiveness, and order as opposed to competition, conflict, and corruption to evolve power (Chan et al. 2014; Ip 2014; Zhang 2006). Cohesiveness or inclusiveness exhibits or reflects diversity, empowerment, exchange, fitting, fulfillment, and sharing to enhance power (Green and Janmaat 2011; Loewy 1993; Miranti and Evans 2019; Paez et al. 2015; Schiefer and van der Noll 2017; Sturm 1998; Turner and Maryanski 2005). Diversity reflects low competition, deprivation, and opposition to secure power (Gimpel and Lay 2008; King et al. 2010). Exchange can achieve integration and reflect resourcefulness to raise power (Brinberg and Castell 1982; Skopek et al. 2011). Integration involves or registers resourcefulness as opposed to distancing to uphold power (Frei et al. 2009; Wilson and Musick 1997). Fitting encompasses fulfilling and supplying to raise power (Chuang et al. 2016). Sharing reflects fitting to maintain power (Becker and Clement 2006). Compensation involves or can reflect balance or equilibrium, coherence, maintenance or stability, and unity to secure power (Muuss 1996; Proulx and Heine 2006). Complementarity activates compensation, coordination, exchange, reinforcing, and supplementarity to generate power (Riley et al. 2011; Sadler et al. 2011; Svara 2001). Coordination characterizes, has raised, or has reflected efficacy, empowerment, exchange, and integration to hold power (Abu Bakar and Sheer 2013; Breton 2004; Fiske 2000; Henson 2001). Efficacy maintains or reflects capacity and functioning as power (John 2001; Quinn et al. 2010; Schmid 2022). Complementarity can uphold complexity or systematicity to boost power (Patton and McMahon 2021). Complexity embraces or has enhanced efficacy, holism, and integration to uphold power (Byrne 1998; Little et al. 2003; Luskin 1990). Conversely, complementarity can prevent conflict, thus retaining power (Rick et al. 2006; Shewark et al. 2022). Conflict involves or can reflect competition, deprivation, discord, imbalance, insecurity, limitedness, and loss as opposed to balance, compatibility, cohesion, flexibility, and resourcefulness to weaken power (Baucom and Atkins 2013; De Carlo et al. 2019; Fenwick and Tausig 2001; Fisher et al. 2013; Gronlund and Oun 2010; Qiu and Fan 2015; Reese et al. 2019; Willis et al. 2008). Competition reflects insecurity, instability, and separation, as opposed to cohesion to diminish power (Borsenberger et al. 2016; Music 2014; Pierce and White 2006; Sui 2011). Flexibility reflects resourcefulness as power (Pyszkowska 2020).

Complementarity among components structurally entails interdependence among the components for fulfilling matching to achieve completeness (Chernikova et al. 2017). Interdependence embraces bonding, concordance, cooperation, coordination, exchange, harmony, inclusiveness, and relatedness as opposed to competition, conflict, discordance, individuation, opposition, and rejection (Harb and Smith 2008; Johnson and Johnson 2005; Schunk et al. 2023; Wickham and Knee 2012). Bonding or relatedness benefits from reciprocity, sharing, similarity, support received, tie multiplexity and strength, and trust (Jackson et al. 2006; Ledbetter 2015; Logan and Cobb 2013; Sharma 2003; Stafford 2015). Cooperation has developed or can develop from social capital and its embeddedness, reciprocity, and trust (Miao et al. 2018; Nahapiet 2009). Harmony can hinge and has hinged on cohesion and exchange (Ho and Chan 2009; Lawler 2002). Moreover, cooperation can arise or has arisen from commonality, sharing, similarity, and trust (Brewer 1996; Gaertnel et al. 1999; Lawler et al. 2014; Zhang and Zhou 2018). Coordination has benefitted from networking, solidarity, support received, and trust (Miao et al. 2018; Ng et al. 2004). Harmony has benefitted from relational quality (Yi et al. 2004). Inclusiveness can develop or has developed from social capital, including support received and volunteering (Garcia and Herrero 2004; Isham et al. 2006; Stolz 2011). Bonding, cohesion, commonality, exchange, networking, relational quality, reciprocity, sharing, similarity, solidarity, support received, tie multiplexity and strength, and trust characterize social capital (Baptista et al. 2021; Coleman et al. 2022; Grootaert and van Bastelaer 2002; Harpham et al. 2002; Lochner et al. 1999; Paraskevopoulos 2010; Robison and Ritchie 2010; Tulin et al. 2018; van Deth 2003). Conversely, competition can develop from separation and low cooperation (Pierce and White 2006). Conflict or discordance has declined by commonality, cooperation, exchange, similarity, support received, togetherness, and trust (Baucom and Atkins 2013; Maoz 2018; Molm et al. 2007). Opposition or rejection has arisen from mistrust (Ross and Mirowsky 2009). Commonality, cooperation, exchange, similarity, support received, togetherness, and trust, as opposed to individuation, mistrust, and separation, indicate social capital (Geys and Murdoch 2010; Lochner et al. 1999; Murayama et al. 2019; Narayan and Cassidy 2001; Paraskevopoulos 2010; Tulin et al. 2018). Eventually, interdependence breeds attraction and supporting (Johnson and Johnson 2005). Attraction or liking has arisen from friendship and trust (Kende et al. 2022; Lu et al. 2016). Supporting can benefit from social capital, similarity, support received, and trust (Collins and Feeney 2004; Luria et al. 2019; Maltseva 2016; Thielmann et al. 2020). Friendship, similarity, support received, and trust embody social capital (Murayama et al. 2019; Rivera 2018; Tulin et al. 2018; Wuthnow 2002). Hence, social capital components can underpin interdependence and complementarity.

Interdependence also brings structure or a power base to achieve complementarity by activating the power realization mechanism in analytical functionalism. Such structure or power furnished by interdependence rests on attachment, coordination, holism, integrity, and interaction among interdependent components (Feldman and Kuyken 2019; Heckscher 2015; Irwin 2016; Li 2018; Wickham and Knee 2012). Attachment embraces or reflects or can generate benefit, integration, and resolution to embody complementarity (Rippl et al. 2010; Scannell and Gifford 2017; Shemmings 2006). Coordination reflects adaptation and integration to demonstrate complementarity (Fiske 2000; Widegren 1997). Holism registers enlightenment and wisdom to afford the power of complementarity (Knight and Johnson 2011; Thin 2012). Integrity has sustained friend support, life quality, and satisfaction and reduced depression and suicide to maintain resilience (McIntosh et al. 1994; Miner 1995; Mullins and Dugan 1991; Steinkamp and Kelly 1987). Interaction can achieve alignment, balance, bridging or resolution, and merging to register complementarity (Sandstrom et al. 2014; Vezzali et al. 2014). Power generated by interdependence can also evolve from cooperation, harmony, inclusion, and regulation (Atkinson 2012; Brewer 1996; Leung et al. 2005; Uskul et al. 2004). Cooperation can facilitate achievement, completion, and resolution, as opposed to conflict to realize complementarity (Johnson and Johnson 2005). Harmony indicates adjustment, balance, fitness, and holism as opposed to conflict to manifest complementarity (Kjell et al. 2016). Inclusion facilitates or registers reconciliation, resourcefulness, resurrection, and supportiveness to signify complementarity (Giri 2011; Koramaz 2014; Wilson and Musick 1997; Zamperini et al. 2020).

Coordination or management is pivotal for interdependence to achieve complementarity (Heckscher 2015; Johnson and Johnson 2005). Such achievement hinges on power generated by coordination to leverage the power realization mechanism in analytical functionalism. This power functions for adapting, balancing, integrating, receiving or accepting, relating or connecting, and understanding components to constitute complementarity (Amir and Auslander 2003; Burt 2009; Fiske 2000; Kalish 2008; Thomas 1999; Widegren 1997). Coordination applies to the components of a network or system (Dess and Sauerwald 2014; Paakkanen et al. 2021). A network or system is social capital, whose structure is a network (Chua et al. 2021; Woolcock 1998).

## Original Findings

Four components of social capital suggested four main effects, six two-way interaction effects, one three-way interaction effect, and one four-way interaction effect on resilience in the Chinese adult's resilience (see Table 7.1). These four components were associational structural social capital, friend substantive social capital, friend structural social capital, and friend functional social capital. The three-way interaction covered the three friend social capital components, whereas the four-way interaction covered all four components, including associational and friend social capital. Interaction among social capital components meant combining or integrating the components to engender complementarity or synergistic effects.

Associations and friends were two channels of social capital. For friend social capital, substantive, structural, and functional components referred to substantive resources, structural networking, and functional activities, respectively. Structural networking comprised closeness, density, and homogeneity, whereas functional activities worked under trust and reciprocity. Trust meant unconditional support received, whereas reciprocity meant support received conditional on support provided.

**Table 7.1** Social capital effects on resilience

| Social capital | Expected | Currently found |
|---|---|---|
| Associational structural | + | + |
| Friend substantive | + | − |
| Friend structural | + | + |
| Friend functional | + | − |
| Friend substantive × structural | + | + |
| Friend substantive × functional | + | 0 |
| Friend structural × functional | + | 0 |
| Associational × friend substantive | + | 0 |
| Associational × friend structural | + | 0 |
| Association × friend functional | + | 0 |
| Friend substantive × structural × functional | + | + |
| Associational × friend substantive × structural × functional | + | 0 |

*Note* + positive effect; − negative effect; ? mixed effects; 0 no effect

| *Variable* |
|---|
| Resilience, recent month ($\alpha = 0.630$) |
| Having the ability to face adversity |
| Facing difficulties positively |
| Rolling with punches |
| Keeping calm in the face of pressure |
| (not) Feeling anxious when under pressure |
| (not) Having difficulty recovering from setbacks |
| Associational structural social capital, past half-year ($\alpha = 0.802$) |
| Having close ties with groups |
| Participating in group activities |
| Participating in group activities |
| Friend substantive social capital, past half-year ($\alpha = 0.724$) |
| Your friends being knowledgeable |
| Your friends having financial resources |
| Your friends having social status |
| *Friend structural social capital* |
| Friend social capital closeness, past half-year ($\alpha = 0.774$) |
| Having close ties with friends |
| Having interaction with friends |
| Having a long relationship with friends |

(continued)

(continued)

| |
|---|
| Having a long relationship with friends |
| Friend social capital density, past half-year ($\alpha = 0.681$) |
| Your friends knowing each other |
| Taking part in activities with your friends |
| Friend social capital homogeneity, past half-year ($\alpha = 0.643$) |
| Having the same background as friends |
| Having the same interests as friends |
| *Friend functional social capital* |
| Friend functional social capital, past half-year ($\alpha = 0.793$) |
| Your friends repaying you |
| Your friends (not) ignoring the help that you gave them |
| Your friends helping you unconditionally |
| Your friends (not) ignoring you |

## Predicting Resilience

Three of the four social capital components in the past half-year presented significant positive effects on resilience in the recent month. Accordingly, the effects of associational structural social capital, friend structural social capital, and friend functional social capital on resilience were significantly positive ($\beta = 0.126, - 0.211$, see Table 8.1). These effects aligned with the expectation. However, the effect of friend substantive social capital on resilience was significantly negative ($\beta = - 0.175$). This effect contradicted the expectation (Table 7.2).

In addition to the main effects, only one of the six two-way interaction effects, stemming from combining friend substantive and structural social capital, was significantly positive on resilience ($\beta = 0.194$, see Table 8.1). The other two-way interaction effects were nonsignificant.

The three way interaction effect was significantly positive based on the combination of the three components of friend social capital ($\beta = 0.128$, see Table 8.1). However, based on the combination of the social capital components of associations and friends, the four-way interaction effect was nonsignificant.

## Social Capital Effects

Friend substantive or resource social capital alone did not contribute to resilience. Instead, combining friend substantive social capital and friend structural social capital, and additionally friend functional social capital contributed to resilience.

**Table 7.2** Standardized effects of social capital on resilience (visual impairment dataset)

| Predictor | Resilience |
|---|---|
| Associational structural | 0.145* |
| Friend substantive | – 0.175** |
| Friend structural | 0.211** |
| Friend functional | 0.126# |
| Empowerment | – 0.071 |
| Extraversion | 0.119* |
| $R^2$ | 0.397 |
| Friend substantive × structural | 0.194* |
| Friend substantive × functional | – 0.037 |
| Friend structural × functional | – 0.043 |
| Associational × friend substantive | – 0.067 |
| Associational × friend structural | 0.052 |
| Association × friend functional | – 0.116 |
| $R^2$ | 0.410 |
| Friend substantive × structural × functional | 0.128* |
| $R^2$ | 0.414 |
| Associational × friend substantive × structural × functional | – 0.006 |
| $R^2$ | 0.414 |

*Note* Regression analysis controlled for background characteristics, empowerment, and personality
$^{\#}p < 0.10$, $^{*}p < 0.05$, $^{**}p < 0.01$, $^{***}p < 0.001$

That is, the contribution of friend substantive social capital depended on the combination with friend structural capital. Instead, the main effect of friend substantive on resilience was negative, probably revealing the effect of social comparison or jealousy.

Social comparison can diminish well-being (Locke 2003). Notably, social comparison has raised negative effects and reduced self-esteem to jeopardize resilience (Fujita 2008). More crucially, social comparison can make friend resources as referential resources to weaken relative resources. That is, when friend or referential resources are higher, one's relative resources are lower. This social comparison effect dampens resilience through the utility optimization mechanism in analytical functionalism. Meanwhile, friend resources are influential (Adler and Adler 1998). Social comparison also involves jealousy (Crusius et al. 2021). Herein, friend resources would be a power base to foment jealousy through the power realization mechanism.

Jealousy is likely to weaken resilience by diminishing well-being. Accordingly, jealousy has provoked fear (Felson and Outlaw 2007). Essentially, jealousy is a negative affect, debilitating to reduce power for the power realization mechanism (Pfeiffer and Wong 1989). Jealousy can also reflect conflict, dependency, and poverty to restrain power to drive resilience (Buunk 1991; Felson and Outlaw 2007; Firestone et al. 2006). Moreover, jealousy has evoked ideals for aggression and violence to hamper resilience (Felson and Outlaw 2007). Jealousy has furthermore bred injury to lower utility for resilience (Felson and Outlaw 2007).

The inverse effect of friend substance social capital on resilience nevertheless reveals the dark side of social capital. As such, social capital can diminish power, utility, and ideals for resilience. Such diminishment would offset some contribution of social capital.

Power to drive resilience dampened by social capital has involved creativity and knowledge (Burt 2004; Lee 2009). Creativity has sustained happiness, meaningfulness, positive mood, satisfaction, and general well-being (Henderson 2004; Tavares 2016; Schneck 2014). Well-being as a power source has included health and job and life satisfaction as opposed to anxiety, burnout, and distress (Clark et al. 2013; Dust et al. 2020; Moen et al. 2013; Xie 1996). Knowledge has buttressed self-efficacy to enable resilience (Rostosky et al. 2008). Social capital can downplay agency and thinking quality or critical thinking as power to drive resilience (Morrow 1999; Rovio et al. 2009). Agency has maintained mastery, relational quality, satisfaction, and vitality to facilitate resilience (Delhey 2010; Hui et al. 2013; Ross and Drentea 1998; Sieber et al. 2019). Thinking quality or critical thinking has fostered identity achievement to support resilience (Adams and Ryan 2000). Social capital has reflected low care and closeness received, education, and relative income as power to drive resilience (Chang 2009; Cornwall 2009; Eberl 2020). Care received has fostered functionality and satisfaction to sustain resilience (Caro and Blank 1988; Davies et al. 1990). Closeness experienced has invited social support to buttress resilience (Gant et al. 1999).

Utility to attract resilience reduced by social capital has rested on community or organization evaluation and life satisfaction because of the strain imposed by social capital (Abbott and Sapsford 2006; Yuan 2016; Crowe 2010). Community evaluation has reflected mastery to enhance resilience (Greenberg 1999). Social capital can also limit freedom as utility to attract resilience (Ozbay 2008). Freedom has enabled well-being, including health, life satisfaction, and self-esteem, as opposed to depression and symptoms to facilitate resilience action (Abbott et al. 2011, Glendinning et al. 2003; Haller and Hadler 2006). Conversely, social capital has bred victimization experienced to weaken utility for attracting resilience (Hansen-Nord et al. 2014). Victimization experienced has impaired safety experienced and self-respect or self-worth to erode resilience (Fernandes 2018; Krahe 2013). Social capital can be a disgrace or disutility to discourage resilience (Wetterberg 2007).

An ideal to rationalize resilience eroded by social capital has concerned innovation (Clark 2004a). Innovation has evolved from its ideal (Stutchbury 2022). Eventually, innovation has reflected satisfaction and self-efficacy to prop resilience (Wang et al. 2013).

More specifically, friendship as a constituent of social capital can impair resilience by weakening power, utility, ideals, and norms for resilience. This weakening disrupts the voluntaristic mechanisms of power realization, utility optimization, ideal calibration, and norm conformity concerning functioning. The disabling would offset some contribution of friend social capital.

Power to drive resilience reduced by or inversely related to friendship stems from education, family bonding and quality, identity, income, religiosity, social closeness, wealth, and various resources (Bagwell and Schmidt 2011; Cheadle and Schwadel 2012; Cornwell 2011; Franzen and Hangartner 2006; Kornienko et al. 2016; Mesch 2002; Oh 2003; Rook and Ituarte 1999; Treas 2011). Education has sustained well-being, including health, identity, life quality and satisfaction, mastery, self-efficacy, self-esteem, and youthfulness to engender resilience (Cerin and Leslie 2008; Corcoran et al. 2011; James and Amato 2013; Pakulshi and Tranter 2000; Stavrova and Ehlebracht 2018; van Praag and Frijters 1999; Whyte and Gao 2009; Yienprugsawan et al. 2010). Family bonding has nurtured well-being, including identity, life satisfaction, meaningfulness, self-clarity, and self-esteem (Fosco and Lydon-Staley 2020; Nemeth and Bernath 2022; Watson and Protinsky 1988; Xiang et al. 2020). Identity has secured happiness, love, self-efficacy, and self-esteem and has diminished anxiety and depression to facilitate resilience (Cast 2004). Income has afforded well-being, including adaptation, adequacy, belongingness, control, eudaemonia, health, mastery, power, quality of life, satisfaction, self-efficacy, self-esteem, and social well-being to sustain resilience (Anciaes et al. 2017; Carpiano 2008; Corcoran et al. 2011; Ross and Mirowsky 1989; Sengupta and Sibley 2019; Son and Wilson 2012; Wang and VanderWeele 2011; Yeh et al. 2013; Zimmerman and Reyna 2013). Religiosity has buttressed coping, friendship, forgiveness, harmony perceived, health maintenance, institutional and social trust, optimism, social capital, and well-being to raise resilience (Chang 2009; Clemence 2001; Furnham 1997; Hakhverdian and Mayne 2012; Myers 2008; Saroglou and Anciaux 2004; Wuthnow 2004; Zanin 2017). Social closeness has facilitated humor and social support received to lift resilience (Martin et al. 2003). Wealth has reduced depression to maintain power to drive resilience (Zhang and Hayward 2001). Conversely, friendship has reflected depression to weaken power to drive resilience (van Rijsewijk et al. 2016).

Utility to attract resilience suffering in friendship has involved popularity (Palacios et al. 2019). Possibly, deficiency in popularity has promoted friend making. Anyhow, popularity has fostered positive affect and self-esteem to elevate resilience (Reich et al. 2018). Friendship is costly, thus dampening utility to attract resilience (Espelage et al. 2007). Moreover, friendship can grow as a response to social rejection, which represents disutility for resilience (Brown et al. 2009; van Rijsewijk et al. 2016). Social rejection experienced has raised a negative mood and eroded life satisfaction to attenuate resilience (Lin et al. 2013; Williams et al. 2000).

Ideals countering resilience raised by friendship can uphold crime and protesting (Fahmy 2006; Haynie and Kreager 2013). The ideal for crime has rationalized crime (Tanner-Smith et al. 2013). Crime has eroded life satisfaction, mastery, relationship quality, self-efficacy, and self-esteem to weaken resilience (Chung and Elias 1996; Keijsers et al. 2011; Shek 2005). The ideal for protesting has constituted protesting (Hwang and Kim 2015). Protesting has invoked anger and worry to counter resilience feeling (Boehnke and Wong 2011; Landmann and Rohmann 2020). Friendship has eroded the ideal for the family or familism or familialism to impede resilience (Lang and Carstensen 2002). Familism or familialism has rested on health and financial satisfaction to afford resilience (Kiecolt 2003; Valarino et al. 2018).

Norms impeding resilience underlying friendship have registered low development and resources (Sampson 1991). That is, friendship has risen when societal development or resources have been low. The norm for development has fostered health to facilitate resilience (Hadden et al. 2003).

Whereas the three-way interaction combining friend substantive, structural, and functional social capital yielded a significant positive effect on resilience, two-way interactions not combining friend substantive and structural social capital did not. Hence, combining friend substantive and structural social capital was pivotal to engender a joint contribution. This combination registers the static or stable manifestation of social capital, not depending on the dynamic and labile functional form. Such stability functions as a power base for complementarity (Deeg 2007).

By contrast, interactions combining association and friend social capital did not evidence significant effects on resilience. This null effect reveals that associational and friend social capital are independent, incompatible, and unmatched, thus failing to achieve complementarity. That is, interdependency, compability, and matching buttress complementarity (Chernikova et al. 2017; Van Vianen et al. 2008).

In all, social capital evidenced positive main and interaction or joint effects on resilience. The main effects emanated from associational and friend channels, covering their functional, substantive, and structural components. Meanwhile, the joint effects stemmed from the two-way combination of friend substantive and structural social capital and the three-way combination of friend functional, substantive, and structural social capital. The interaction effects embodied the contribution of complementarity among social capital components from the friend channel. This complementarity illustrates the effective contribution of substantive resources through the stable structure and active function. Essentially, the complementarity property of social capital is demonstrable (Robison and Ritchie 2010). Notably, friend substantive social capital alone was counterproductive. It became contributory by the static support of friend structural social capital. This support illustrates the transmission capability integral to social capital (Robison and Ritchie 2010). By contrast, the functional and structural components were contributory when working individually. Notably, the static structure was helpful, showing the contribution of the mere presence of friends. All the contributions benefit from the direct provision of power and indirect provision of utility, ideals, and norms by social capital to achieve functioning based on analytical functionalism.

# Chapter 8
# Developmental Conditions for Resilience

**Abstract** This chapter additionally focuses on a survey of 3564 junior secondary school pupils in the Chinese cities of Hong Kong, Macau, and Guangzhou to clarify the impacts of developmental conditions on resilience. Such conditions include individual sports, collective sports, sports coaching, adventuring, volunteering, religious activity, carnival activity, musical activity, and ritualistic and nation-related activity. They contribute to resilience through the voluntaristic mechanism of power realization, following empowerment through individual or collective activity. Such power includes physical, spiritual, and social ones buttressed by religion and the nation, reflecting coaching and nurturing generally. They provide disciplining, training, and support to confront difficulties to develop resilience. As such, the developmental effect of such practices starts with social or collective empowerment, notably involving rituals. Nevertheless, the effectiveness of such practices hinges on their fostering of voluntarism or self-determination to raise personal power to realize the voluntaristic mechanism. The fostering, in turn, benefits from the assimilation of social norms according to the voluntaristic mechanism of norm conformity. As such, ritualistic activity can inculcate the religious and national norms of resilience. Furthermore, nation-related activity is more normative and empowering for resilience in Guangzhou than in Macau and Hong Kong.

Development conditions, including personality, empowerment, sport, coaching, other activities, belongingness, and distress, are likely to shape resilience. The other activities cover adventuring, carnival, musical, nation-related, religious, ritualistic, and volunteering. Herein, development means growth and maturity featuring attractiveness, autonomy, conformity, identity, and sociotrophy, as opposed to doping, psychopathology, and rebellion (Browning and Cooper 2004; Hale 1999; Hendry and Kloep 2012). Meanwhile, resilience is an aim, criterion, or focus for development, including that through activation, affordance or provisioning, blessing, gratification, reinforcing, therapy, and training (Cornum et al. 2011; Kent and Davis 2010; Kelley et al. 2019; Sandler 2001; Ungar 2011). Notably, resilience stands on empowerment, health, personality, and other practices as developmental indicators (Brodsky and Cattaneo 2013; Leigert and Reutter 2005; Pyszkowska 2020; Rutter 2012). Resilience

 
C. K. Cheung, *Resilience Process and Its Personal and Social Bases*,
https://doi.org/10.1007/978-981-97-7391-6_8

also essentially functions as a critical mass based on development (Balsas 2017). This function means that resilience can only work with enough development. Similarly, resilience grows with age, indicating the developmental nature of resilience (Charles and Carstensen 2009). Resilience also means growth and is dynamic, thus subject to development (Bowers et al. 2017; Truebridge 2016). Crucially, resilience is an outcome, implying its amenability to development (Crane et al. 2019). Resilience also embraces or rests on such developmental features as construction, education, investment, and learning (Garrett 2016; Kent and Davis 2010; Solomon and Roloff 2018; Taylor and Distelberg 2016).

The development of resilience hinges on power, utility, ideals, and norms to activate voluntaristic mechanisms stipulated in analytical functionalism. Power covers agency, arousal, authority, capability, commitment, competence or proficiency, dispositions, goals, health, identity, income, knowledge, mastery, motivation or motive, need, potency, resources, responsibility, skill, social position, social relationships, and structure (Dolinski 2016; Goldner et al. 2019; Haugaard 2020; Hofstetter et al. 1999; Munch 1987; Reed 2013). Utility covers benefit, gain, reward, and satisfaction expected or experienced. Ideals cover or transpire in attitudes, beliefs, habits, ideas, ideologies, orientations, practices, and values (Munch 1987; Trebilcock 2014). Norms cover power, utility, and ideals from the social, society, or others (Munch 1987). Power fuels the voluntaristic mechanism of power realization to drive action. Utility is the currency for the voluntaristic mechanism of utility optimization to attract action. Ideals are the currency for the voluntaristic mechanism of ideal calibration to rationalize action. Norms are the currency for the voluntaristic mechanism of norm conformity to assimilate action.

## Existing Knowledge

Through voluntaristic mechanisms, resilience develops from power, utility, ideals, and norms. Power, utility, ideals, and norms can arise from empowerment, conscientiousness, extraversion, emotional stability as opposed to neuroticism and distress, belongingness, and various activities. These activities include adventuring, carnival, musical, nation-related, ritualistic, volunteering, and sport and its coaching.

Power driving resilience has stemmed from the states of coherence, gratitude, health, purposeiveness, self-compassion, self-esteem, and strength (Alvarez and Pinto 2023; Buikstra et al. 2010; Elfers et al. 2024; Eshel et al. 2017; Harvey and Boynton 2021). These states indicate that well-being is a basis for resilience (Van Haaften et al. 2004). Moreover, resilience has developed from the dispositional or state power of agreeableness, conscientiousness, emotional intelligence, and emotional stability as opposed to neuroticism, extraversion, honesty-humility, openness, optimism, and sensation-seeking (Armstrong et al. 2011; Buikstra et al. 2010; McKay et al. 2018; Pyszkowska 2020; Yu and Zhang 2007). Conscientiousness has included diligence and forgiveness (Pyszkowska 2020). Resilience has furthermore developed from the sociodemographic power of age, organizational membership, and socioeconomic status as opposed to minority status (Cherry et al. 2023; Elfers et al. 2024; Jones and Jetten 2011; Ntontis et al. 2023). Additionally, resilience has developed from power received from societal infrastructure, mentoring, resources, services, and support (Buikstra et al. 2010; Cherry et al. 2023; Notter et al. 2008; Sawyers et al. 2020). In the youth, power driving resilience has additionally stemmed from the states of adaptation, aspiration for mastery, attachment or bonding, autonomy, belongingness, competence, control, enjoyment or joy, eudaimonia, health, hope or hopefulness, independence, mastery, meaningfulness, mindfulness, motivation for achievement, positive affect, purposiveness, relatedness, relational quality, self-awareness or insight, self-efficacy, sleep quality, sufficiency (Alrabai and Alamer 2022; Artuch-Garde et al. 2017; Jones and Lafreniere 2014; Kaye-Tzadok and Davidson-Arad 2017; Masten et al. 2009; Scales et al. 2000; Silk et al. 2007; Ungar et al. 2005; Villasana et al. 2017; von Soest et al. 2010; Wang et al. 2022; Yang and Oka 2022; Ye et al. 2021; Zolkoski and Bullock 2012). Resilience has thrived on the developmental power of trust, autonomy, initiative, industry, identity, and intimacy (Svetina 2014). Furthermore, resilience has developed from power based on calming, connectedness, friendship and its quality, parenting quality, social capital, social integration, and stimulation experienced, (Armstrong et al. 2005; Graber et al. 2016; Li et al. 2018; Masten 2014; Sattler and Font 2018; Villasana et al. 2017; Wong and Chui 2017). Parenting quality has covered aid, esteem, and resolution (Graber et al. 2016). Resilience has also grown from the dispositional power of adaptability, appealingness or attractiveness, assertiveness, cognitive capacity, competitiveness, cooperativeness, courage, creativity, criticalness, curiosity, easiness, empathy, evocativeness, maturity, novelty seeking, perseverance, persistence, power or powerfulness, problem-solving ability or skill, prosociality, reflexivity, religiosity or spirituality, responsiveness, security, self-directedness, self-regulation, talent, tenacity, transcendence, and virtue (Alessandri et al. 2014; Annalakshmi and Abeer 2011; Artuch-Garde et al. 2017; Baptist et al. 2015; Chen et al. 2018; Kim et al. 2013; Manglos-Weber and Avelis 2019; Masten et al. 2009; Qouta et al. 2007; Scales et al. 2000; Shibue and Kasai 2014; Ungar et al. 2005; Wang et al. 2022; van Aken 1994; Xing et al. 2024; Zolkoski and Bullock 2012). Reflexivity has covered discipline, justice, progress, and providence (Manglos-Weber and Avelis 2019). Religiosity or spirituality raises resilience through attachment or lateness, gifting, growth, morality, purposiveness, counseling, reward, and social support received (Crawford et al. 2005). Virtue has included commitment, courage, integrity, transcendence, and wisdom (Kim et al. 2018). Conversely, resilience has suffered from power lost from ambiguity, anxiety, avoidance, boredom, disability, emotional reactivity, fear, negative affect, and resistance (Alrabai and Alamer 2022; Armfield et al. 2021; Cann and Collette 2014; Low and Chong 2024; Pitzer and Skinner 2017; Scales et al. 2000; Shibue and Kasai 2014; Wang et al. 2022; Yang and Oka 2022).

Utility attracting resilience has resided in the experiences of balance and satisfaction with life and study (Cantor et al. 2002; Dou et al. 2023; Wong and Chui 2017). Conversely, resilience has suffered from of disutility of abuse, stress or stressors, and trauma experienced (Cherry et al. 2023; Sobeck et al. 2020; Yu et al. 2022). In the youth, utility attracting resilience has concerned the experiences of achievement, art, cooperation, food, opportunity, recreation, safety, and expectancy about caring, study, and skill (Hartley 2013; Kim 2015; Kwarikunda et al. 2023; Masten 2014; Ungar et al. 2005; von Essen and Martensson 2017; Wang et al. 2022). Conversely, resilience has declined due to disutility in bullying, danger, difficulty, discrimination, and maltreatment experienced (Hong et al. 2018; Ungar et al. 2005; Wang et al. 2022).

Ideals rationalizing resilience has covered such attitudes as beliefs in resilience, religion and safety, focus on relationships, identification with the social, obligation on prevention, and values on affiliation and connectedness (Alvarez and Pinto 2023; Cherry et al. 2023; Chua et al. 2019; Lou et al. 2018; Ntontis et al. 2023; Truebridge 2016). Resilience has also thrived on ideals manifested in the practices of coping, cultural or ceremonial activity, learning, and protection (Buikstra et al. 2010; Corbin and Hall 2019; Notter et al. 2008). Coping has included humor, problem-focused, and religious coping (Cherry et al. 2018; McKay et al. 2018). In the youth, ideals rationalizing resilience additionally favor community, constructiveness, Daoism, effort, expressiveness, growth, initiative, involvement, justice, managing emotions, metacognition, learning, planning, reflection, regulation or self-regulation, schooling, sporting, striving, and transition (Alrabai and Alamer 2022; Griciute 2015; Jones and Lafreniere 2014; Kwarikunda et al. 2023; Sattler and Font 2018; Seaton and Beaumont 2015; Ungar et al. 2005; Wang et al. 2022; Wu et al. 2011; Zeng et al. 2016), Metacongiion has included assessing, remembering, summarizing, and understanding (Wang et al. 2022). Regulation has included planning, reappraisal, and suppression (Mouatsou and Koutra 2023). Striving has covered generativity, growth, independence, and positivity (Seaton and Beaumont 2015). Conversely, resilience has diminished with ideals for absence or withdrawal, abusing or doping, and aggression (Shure and Aberson 2012; Ungar et al. 2005; Ye et al. 2021).

Norms assimilating resilience have concerned social functioning and innovation (Buikstra et al. 2010; Dou et al. 2023). In the youth, resilience has grown from social norms for adaptability, appealingness or attractiveness, coherence, collaboration, collectivism, competence, development, easiness, economic stability, education, expressiveness, faith, flexibility, functioning, interest, involvement, meaningfulness, monitoring, organization, passage or adulthood, participation, problem-solving skill, prosociality, resourcefulness, rule abidance, self-efficacy, self-regulation skill, stimulation, socioeconomic status, success, supportiveness, talent, and warmth (Aitcheson et al. 2017; Dou et al. 2023; Graber et al. 2016; Haverfield and Theiss 2017; Kim-Cohen et al. 2004; Masten et al. 2009; Sosa and Gomez 2012; Stoiber and Gettinger 2011; Ungar et al. 2005; von Soest et al. 2010; Wang et al. 2022; Wu et al. 2011). Conversely, resilience has eroded due to social norms for conflict, control, and failure (Haverfield and Theiss 2017; Ungar et al. 2005).

### *Empowerment*

Empowerment registers well-being, particularly social quality (Peterson 1999; Phillips 2006). It involves power, helping, support, and training (Anderson 2010; Baily 2014; Hollander 2018; Stanton-Salazar 2011). Empowerment also implies choice, justice, leadership, and relatedness (Cooper et al. 2013; Praszkier 2018; Sturm 1998; Winstock and Eisikovits 2003). Essentially, empowerment involves or enhances activeness, autonomy, awareness, bridging, capacitation, caring, community, competence, conscience, control, creativity, decision, development, diversity, employability, health, information, knowledge, mastery, positivity, resources, respect, responsibility, skill, space, status, strength, and voicing (Albuquerque et al. 2017; Evers 2009; Fischer et al. 2022; Heward et al. 2007; Phillips 2006; Praszkier 2018; Tracy 2002; Wildemeersch 2014; Zimmerman 1995). Empowerment can raise resilience (Metzl and Morrell 2008; Thompson 2006). Moreover, empowerment is likely to foster resilience through enabling power, utility, ideals, and norms to activate the voluntaristic mechanisms of analytical functionalism to achieve functioning.

Power has risen with empowerment to drive resilience (Grealish et al. 2017; Lin et al. 2021). Moreover, empowerment has elevated well-being, including development, mastery, recovery, and self-efficacy, as power to drive resilience (Berkowitz et al. 2006; Grealish et al. 2017; Gullan et al. 2013). Empowerment has fostered leadership as power to drive resilience (Gullan et al. 2013). Leadership has secured self-efficacy to afford resilience (Shah and Scheufele 2006). Empowrment nurtures citizenship as power to drive resilience (Le Bosse et al. 1998). Citizenship has fostered well-being, including mental and physical health, to elevate resilience (Tsai et al. 2018). Empowerment can raise ability, self-worth, and zest to secure power to drive resilience (Metzl and Morrell 2008). Furthermore, empowerment involves activeness and virtuousness to secure power to drive resilience (Evers 2009; Zhang 2005). Virtuousness has sustained satisfaction and eroded anxiety to boost resilience (Conzo et al. 2017; Stets et al. 2008). Empowerment reflects choice, education received, mentoring received, relatedness, self-help, social quality, support received, training, and well-being to engage power to drive resilinece (Baily 2014; Hollander 2018; Killick 2018; Liang et al. 2008; Phillips 2006; Stanton-Salazar 2011; Sturm 1998; Winstock and Eisikovits 2003), Choice has buttressed competence, effort and performance, life and neighborhood satisfaction, motivation, and self-determination to safeguard resilience (Day 2013; Gagne and Deci 2005; Helliwell et al. 2010; Patall et al. 2008). Education has sustained well-being, including health, identity, life quality and satisfaction, mastery, self-efficacy, self-esteem, and youthfulness to engender resilience (Cerin and Leslie 2008, Corcoran et al. 2011; James and Amato 2013; Pakulshi and Tranter 2000; Stavrova and Ehlebracht 2018; van Praag and Frijters 1999; Whyte and Gao 2009; Yiengprugsawan et al. 2010). Mentoring received has secured resilience, certainty, confidence, and self-efficacy (Ogbuanya and Chukwuedo 2017; Stoeger et al. 2019; Ungar et al. 2005). Self-help has elevated confidence, enthusiasm, functioning, positive affect, power, satisfaction, self-esteem, and skill to uplift resilience (Anderson-Butcher et al. 2004; Cameron 2002; Hatzidimitriadou 2002; Kelly et al.

2019; Kondo and Wada 2009; Schiff and Bargal 2000). Social support received has facilitated creativity to secure resilience (Chen et al. 2022). Training has upgraded adjustment, comfort, coherence, cohesiveness, competence, emotional well-being, growth, hope, identity, purposiveness, self-efficacy, self-esteem, thriving, and transcendence to advance resilience (Ashby et al. 2018; Davidson et al. 2012; Duan and Bu 2019; Esbensen and Osgood 1999; Feldman and Dreher 2012; Moote et al. 1999; Ou et al. 2019; Umino and Dammeyer 2018; Youniss and Yates 1997). Empowerment has reflected curiosity to provide power to drive resilience (Kaczmarek et al. 2014). Curiosity has facilitated flow and creativity to enable resilience (Schutte and Malouff 2020). Empowerment involves affiliation, autonomy, commitment, community, competence or skillfulness, confidence, conscientiousness, creativity, criticalness, development, employability, enlightening experienced, facilitation received, gratitude, health, hope, identity, knowledge, mastery, placation or therapy received, resourcefulness, responsibility, self-esteem, spirituality, social status, and strength to maintain power to drive resilience (Albuquerque et al. 2017; Checkoway 1998; Delgado and Staples 2008; Ekholm and Sol 2019; Fischer et al. 2022; Heward et al. 2007; Itzhaky and York 2000; Kaczmarek et al. 2014; Mallick and Watts 2008; McWhirter 1994; Miller and Van Ness Sheppard 2014; Phillips 2006; Praszkier 2018; Wildemeersch 2014; Zimmerman 1995). Affiliation has strengthened rewards to induce resilience (Nelson-Coffey et al. 2023). Autonomy has sustained well-being, including life satisfaction, mastery, relational quality and relatedness, and vitality as opposed to anxiety and depression, thus advancing resilience (Delhey 2010; Hui et al. 2013; Ross and Drentea 1998; Schwartz and Melech 2000; Sheldon and Bettencourt 2002; Sieber et al. 2019; Weinstein and Ryan 2010). Commitment has sustained self-acceptance and relieved depression to foster resilience (Agronick and Duncan 1998; Wrosch et al. 2005). The sense of community has strengthened rewards to induce resilience (Nelson-Coffey et al. 2023). Competence has enabled identity achievement, intimacy, and relationship satisfaction, as opposed to anxiety, to raise resilience (Adams 1985). Conscientiousness has raised attachment, autonomy, life satisfaction, mastery, purposefulness, and self-acceptance to secure resilience (Fraley et al. 2011; Hounkpatin et al. 2015). Creativity has boosted well-being, notably meaningfulness, to induce resilience (Diener et al. 2009; Turner 2013). Criticalness has fostered identity achievement to procure resilience (Adams and Ryan 2000). Development has buttressed success to induce resilience (Spengler et al. 2018). Employability has reflected self-efficacy and self-evaluation to boost resilience (Atitsogbe et al. 2019; Creed and Gagliardi 2015). Enlightenment has eroded anxiety, depression, disorders, and self-defeating, thus safeguarding resilience (DiGiuseppe et al. 2017). Facilitation received has reflected support received to drive resilience (Demerouti et al. 2013). Gratitude has raised positive affect and dampened negative affect to achieve resilience (Bernabe-Valero et al. 2021). Knowledge has championed intimacy, satisfaction, and self-efficacy to boost resilience (Mikulincer et al. 2003; Norris 2011; Rothwell et al. 2016). Responsibility has advanced wisdom to facilitate resilience (Spengler et al. 2018). Spirituality has sustained forgiveness, joy, and general well-being to foster resilience (Mullet et al. 2005; Saroglou and Anciaux 2004; Seidlitz et al. 2002). Social status has sustained coping, health, interaction quality, life satisfaction, self-esteem, and general well-being to secure resilience (Al-krenawi et al. 2011; Caplan and Schooler 2007; Molana and Adams 2019; Staudinger et al. 1999). Therapy received has raised well-being or life quality, including health and intimacy as opposed to anxiety, depression, and disturbance, thus sustaining resilience (Boulton et al. 2001; Erford et al. 2011; Goertz-Dorten et al. 2017; Lintz et al. 2019; Lucas 2012; Murphy et al. 2017). Conversely, empowerment has reflected low depression, thus retaining power to drive resilience (Kaczmarek et al. 2014).

Utility enhanced by empowerment to attract resilience has resided in fulfillment and life satisfaction (Fischer et al. 2022; Lin et al. 2021). Empowerment can raise success experienced as utility to attract resilience (Tracy 2002). Success experienced has fostered health, life quality, satisfaction, self-efficacy, and self-esteem as opposed to alienation, depression, and distress to uphold resilience (Donnellan et al. 2005; Fredricks and Eccles 2005; Menard and Mose 1984; Murray 2009; Piko et al. 2006; Tompson and Dass 2000; Xiao et al. 2009). Empowerment indicates justice experienced to secure utility to attract resilience (Cooper et al. 2013). Justice experienced has lifted positive mood, life satisfaction, and self-esteem to sustain resilience (Dalbert 2001). Empowerment involves achievement, emancipation, positivity, respect, and social integration experienced as utility to attract resilience (Albuquerque et al. 2017; McWhirter 1994; Phillips 2006). Achievement has fostered health, life quality, satisfaction, self-efficacy, and self-esteem as opposed to alienation, depression, and distress to uphold resilience (Donnellan et al. 2005; Fredricks and Eccles 2005; Menard and Mose 1984; Murray 2009; Piko et al. 2006; Tompson and Dass 2000; Xiao et al. 2009). Emancipation has advanced well-being, including health, life satisfaction, and self-esteem, as opposed to depression and symptoms to warrant resilience (Gehring 2013; Glendinning et al. 2003; Haller and Hadler 2006). Positivity experienced has reduced depression and negative affect to champion resilience (McIntyre et al. 2023; Stanton et al. 2020). Respect received has secured identity to drive resilience (Renger and Reese 2017). Social integration has eroded depression to bolster resilience (Mullins and Dugan 1991). Conversely, empowerment has assuaged victimization experienced to retain utility to attract resilience (Hollander 2018). Victimization experienced has impaired safety experienced and self-respect or self-worth to erode resilience (Fernandes 2018; Krahe 2013). Empowerment dampens oppression experienced to maintain utility to attact resilience (Stanton-Salazar 2011). Oppression experienced can weaken pleasure, thus impeding resilience. Empowerment involves ideals against blaming to secure resilience (McWhirter 1994). Blaming has fomented anger, fear, and sadness and eroded joy and love to impair resilience (Nezlek et al. 2008).

Ideals upheld by empowerment to rationalize resilience have hailed civility, community involvement, donation, the future, prosociality, resolution, self-direction, and volunteering (Bond and Lun 2014; Fischer et al. 2022; Hunter et al. 2013; Klucarova and He 2021; Lakin and Mahoney 2006; Mahajna 2017b; Thulin et al. 2022). Civility has boosted well-being, including physical and mental health, to activate resilience (Tsai et al. 2018). Community involvement stands on communitarianism (Heckscher 2015). As scuh, community involvement has enhanced well-being, including mastery and self-efficacy, to enable resilience (Harter and Arora 2010;

Ohmer 2007). The ideal for donation has propped donation (Vallerand et al. 1992). Eventually, donation has reflected well-being, including control, feeling good, gratitude, happiness, joy, satisfaction, and self-efficacy as opposed to anxiety and guilt, to brew resilience (Bednall et al. 2013; Bekkers 2008; Eayrs and Ellis 1990; Liu and Hao 2017; Mussen 1982; Piliavin and Callero 1991; Wang and Graddy 2008). Future orientation has fostered control and social trust to facilitate resilience (Prenda and Lachman 2001; Uslaner 2002). Prosociality has evolved from its ideal (Maltseva 2016). Eventually, prosociality has elevated well-being, including connectedness, hope, life satisfaction, meaningfulness, and self-efficacy to boost resilience (Marsh and Dik 2021; Nelson-Coffey et al. 2023; Raposa et al. 2016; Yao and Enright 2019). Resolution rests on its ideal (Simmons 2020). As such, resolution has benefitted from harmonious passion to sustain resilience (Belanger et al. 2019). Self-direction has rested on its ideal (Gagne and Deci 2005). As such, self-direction has arisen from harm avoidance to safeguard resilience (Richter et al. 2002). Volunteering has grown from its ideal (Barr et al. 2005). Eventually, volunteering has raised well-being, including health, life satisfaction, mastery, morale, positive affect, and self-esteem as opposed to depression, loneliness, and mortality, to buttress resilience (Borgonovi 2008; Gillath et al. 2005; Li and Ferraro 2006; Midlarsky and Kahana 1994; Oman et al. 1999; Thoits and Hewitt 2001; Zotti et al. 2016). Empowerment fosters ideals for civic engagement and institutionalism to rationalize resilience (Lowndes and Roberts 2013; Speer and Hughey 1995). Civic engagement has stood on its ideal (Peterson and Maiden 1993). As such, civic engagement has incubated conflict resolution, education, happiness, health, income, individualism, life satisfaction, security normativity, social attachment, capital, integration, trust, tolerance, and general well-being to advance resilience (Coffe and Geys 2007; Goren 2005; Growiec and Growiec 2010; Kroll 2011; Li and Walder 2001; Myers 1999; Pena-Lopez and Sanchez-Santos 2016; Posel and Casale 2011; Tak 2017; Tang 2011; Wallace and Pichler 2009; Welzel 2013; van Ingen and Bekkers 2015; Vincens et al. 2018). Institutionalism has benefitted health and well-being generally to facilitate resilience (Klein 2013; Sulemana 2015; Mayer 2017). Empowement involves ideals for bridging, caring, conformity, control, culture, goal-setting, and learning to rationalize resilience (Ekholm and Sol 2019; Hewitt 1995; Kegler and Wyatt 2003; Praszkier 2018; Tracy 2002; Walkner and Finney 1999; Zimmerman 1995). Bridging has strengthened agreeableness, empathy, morality, and openness and has dampened agitation to safeguard resilience (Halevy et al. 2019).The ideal for caring has buttressed caring (Sarasa 2008). Caring has maintained mental clarity to boost resilience (Naruse et al. 2020). Conformity has rested on its ideal (Lalot et al. 2022). As such, conformity has furnished achievement and its pressure, mastery-goal setting, social closeness and support received, and tolerance to benefit resilience (Feldman 2003; Jiang et al. 2015; Magnuson et al. 2006). Control has boosted well-being, including health and life satisfaction, as opposed to anger and depression, to maintain resilience (Etezadi and Pushkar 2013. Heidemeier and Staudinger 2012; Rose 2000; Xi and Hwang 2011). Cultural activity has fostered resilience and life satisfaction (Corbin and Hall 2019; Roberts et al. 2001). Goal-setting has supported life satisfaction and self-evaluation to secure resilience (Frazier et al. 2007; Stutzer 2004). Investment has built social capital to enhance resilience (Hlasny and Lee 2020). The ideal for learning has induced learning (Hagger and Hamilton 2018). Learning has elevated well-being, including life satisfaction and self-efficacy, to facilitate resilience (Denver and Hands 1990; Minnaert and Janssen 1992; Richards 2016). Conversely, empowerment can weaken ideals for conspiracism and doping to sustain resilience (Mallick 2007; van Prooijenn 2019). Conspiracism has fomented anxiety to hinder resilience (Leibovitz et al. 2021). Furthermore, conspiracism reflects abnormality, ambiguity experienced, danger felt, deviance, disorder, disruption felt, extremism, ignorance, irrationality, loss experienced, militancy, paranoia, pathology, phobia, social exclusion experienced, stigma experienced, threat experienced, and vulnerability to jeopardize resilience (Atkinson and Dewitt 2019; Difonzo 2019; Freeman et al. 2022; Grodzicka and Harambam 2021; Guan and Yang 2020; Harambam and Aupers 2015; Leibovitz et al. 2021; Stojanov and Halberstadt 2019; Sunstein and Vermeule 2009; Uscinski 2019). The ideal for doping has buttressed doping (Leimberg and Lehmann 2022). Doping has engendered depression, thus jeopardizing resilience (Kendler et al. 2006).

## *Belongingness*

Belongingness embraces closeness to and connection with a target collectivity (Holt-Lunstad 2022; Hampton 2007). Essentially, belongingness characterizes flourishing and motivation (Goodman et al. 2019; Ye and Wallace 2014). Belongingness value has remarkably boosted resilience (Chua et al. 2019). Furthermore, belongingness is likely to buttress resilience by providing power, utility, ideals, and norms to achieve functioning through the voluntaristic mechanisms of analytical functionalism.

Power generated by belongingness to drive resilience stems from well-being, including connectedness and meaningfulness (Baumeister et al. 2013; Nelson-Coffey et al. 2023). Belongingness has buttressed friendship to acquire power to drive resilience (Eberl 2020). Friendship has fostered gratitude to boost resilience (Rotkirch 2014). Belongingness sustains identity, self esteem, and prosociality as dispositional power to drive resilience (Dovidio et al. 2006; Malloy 2018). Prosociality has elevated well-being, including connectedness, hope, life satisfaction, meaningfulness, and self-efficacy to boost resilience (Marsh and Dik 2021; Nelson-Coffey et al. 2023; Raposa et al. 2016; Yao and Enright 2019). Belongingness involves social closeness, connection, and recourse to consolidate power to drive resilience (Hampton 2007; Holt-Lunstad 2022; Kayabol et al. 2022). Social closeness or connection has facilitated humor and social support received to lift resilience (Martin et al. 2003). Recourse has alleviated distress, thus safeguarding resilience (Tracey et al. 1986). Belongingness has benefitted from happiness, health, mindfulness, popularity, religiosity, self-acceptance, social interaction ability, and support received to consolidate power to drive resilience (Amit and Bar-Lev 2015; Carella et al. 2021; Flett 2018; Gountas et al. 2012; Hughes 2011; Stadtfeld and Pentland 2015). Popularity has uplifted positive affect and self-esteem and reduced negative affect, thus buttressing resilience (Reich et al. 2018). Religiosity has sustained well-being, including adjustment, flourishing, health, mastery, positive affect, relationship quality, satisfaction with democracy, police, finance, and life, self-esteem, and socioemotional well-being to lift resilience (Dy-Liacco et al. 2009; Flouri and Buchanan 2002; Helliwell and Putnam 2005; Kwak et al. 2010; Marx 2014; Meulemann 2010; Moschis and Ong 2011; Ng and Fisher 2016; Schieman 2001; Skerkat and Ellison 1999; Van Praag et al. 2010; Wuthnow 2004). Self-acceptance has buttressed well-being, including adjustment, affect, happiness, health, positive affect, and satisfaction, as opposed to depression, distress, negative affect, and strain, to induce resilience (Barnard and Curry 2011; Frederick et al. 2016; Hull et al. 2008; Judge et al. 2002; Tracy et al. 2009; Williams et al. 1992). Social interaction ability has enhanced well-being to buttress resilience (Bjornskov 2008). Social support received has maintained well-being, including resilience, control, health, pleasure, purposefulness, relational quality, satisfaction, self-determination, self-efficacy, self-esteem, and social well-being (Cherry et al. 2018; George and Park 2013; Glendinning et al. 2003; Gorman et al. 2010; Holliman et al. 2021; Lincoln et al. 2003; Logan and Cobb 2013; Pierce and Quiroz 2018; Schwarzer and Knoll 2007; Williams and Galliher 2006; Xi and Hwang 2011). Conversely, belongingness has dampened negative emotion and strain to retain power to drive resilience (Nelson-Coffey et al. 2023). Belongingness can prevent anxiety, thus holding power to drive resilience (Baumeister and Leary 1995). Similarly, belongingness has arisen from low depression and sadness to maintain power to drive resilience (Flett 2018).

Utility achieved by belongingness to attract resilience has resided in life satisfaction and positive outcomes experienced (Magnani and Zhu 2018; Nelson-Coffey et al. 2023). Belongingness involves assurance or certainty experienced to uphold utility to attract resilience (Kayabol et al. 2022). Assurance has reduced risk perceived to attract resilience (Schulz 2014). Belongingness has benefitted from equity and success experienced to secure utility to attract resilience (Gountas et al. 2012; Ledbetter et al. 2013). Equity experienced has fostered belongingness, health, life satisfaction, and self-esteem as opposed to anger and depression to maintain resilience (Benson and Ritter 1990; Bjornskov et al. 2013; Dalbert 2001; Lucas et al. 2013; Rothmund et al. 2014; van Prooijen et al. 2008). Success experienced has fostered health, life quality, satisfaction, self-efficacy, and self-esteem as opposed to alienation, depression, and distress to uphold resilience (Donnellan et al. 2005; Fredricks and Eccles 2005; Menard and Mose 1984; Murray 2009; Piko et al. 2006; Tompson and Dass 2000; Xiao et al. 2009). Conversely, belongingness has arisen from low conflict and stress experienced to sustain utility to attract resilience (Flett 2018; Hughes 2011). Conflict experienced has bred distress and eroded satisfaction, thus impeding resilience (Lau et al. 2017; Mikula et al. 2012). Stress experienced has dampened well-being, including health, life quality, positive affect, and satisfaction as opposed to depression and distress, to impede resilience (Baumeister et al. 2013. Mathis et al. 2016; Raposa et al. 2016; Shrira 2012; Snyder et al. 2020; Zotti et al. 2016). Belongingness has sprung from the ideal for including others to rationalize resilience (Ledbetter et al. 2013). Inclusiveness has reflected the low threat experienced to champion resilience (Raijman et al. 2008). Conversely, belongingness has benefitted from the ideal against extremism to rationalize resilience (Leighton et al. 2020). Extremism has reflected anomie, anxiety, self-uncertainty, and uncertainty to erode resilience (Hogg et al. 2010; Koehler and Fiebig 2019; Stankov et al. 2018).

The norm underlying belongingness to assimilate resilience has popularized socioeconomic status (He and Fischer 2020). The norm for socioeconomic status has raised education, health, life satisfaction, knowledge, relationship quality, self-efficacy, social trust, and value for independence to facilitate resilience (Baldacci et al. 2003; Bonini 2008; Fjellvang 2011; Fridberg and Kangas 2008; Miller 2015; Norris 2011; Traunmuller 2011).

## *Conscientiousness*

Conscientiousness embraces conforming or norm following, aimfulness, cautiousness, control, conventionality, decisiveness, industriousness, normativity, orderliness or organization, patience or delaying gratification, planning or playfulness, reliability or dependability, task orientation, tenaciousness, and virtuousness (Bogg 2008; Roberts et al. 2009). Conversely, conscientiousness dismisses carelessness, impulsivity, indecisiveness, laziness, and sloppiness (Roberts et al. 2009). Conscientiousness has buttressed resilience (Plouffe et al. 2020; Yu and Zhang 2007). The raising reflects the direct contribution of power based on the power realization mechanism. Furthermore, the raising is likely to benefit from power, utility, ideals, and norms generated or reflected in conscientiousness to reinforce power realization, utility optimization, ideal calibration, and norm conformity mechanisms essential in analytical functionalism.

Power generated by conscientiousness to drive resilience has evolved from well-being, including adjustment, autonomy or self-determination, competence, forgiveness, growth, health, mastery, purposefulness, relatedness or relational quality, self-acceptance, self-compassion, and self-esteem (Bogg et al. 2008; Fan et al. 2021; Hounkpatin et al. 2015; Ingledew et al. 2004; Keightley et al. 2006; Mullet et al. 2005; Pratt and Matsuba 2018; Pyszkowska 2020). Autonomy has sustained well-being, including life satisfaction, mastery, relational quality and relatedness, and vitality as opposed to anxiety and depression, thus advancing resilience (Delhey 2010; Hui et al. 2013; Ross and Drentea 1998; Schwartz and Melech 2000; Sheldon and Bettencourt 2002; Sieber et al. 2019; Weinstein and Ryan 2010). Competence has raised well being, including happiness, health, joy, and life satisfaction to lift resilience (Borgonovi 2008; Caprara and Steca 2005; Judge et al. 2002; Landmann and Rohmann 2020). Patience has enabled achievement and dwindled negative affect to safeguard resilience (Mehmood et al. 2020). Forgiveness has elevated serenity, trust, and well-being to maintain resilience (Choi and David 2012; Connors et al. 1999; Shimai et al. 2006). Growth has developed from self-compassion and self-tolerance to strengthen resilience (Ho and Li 2022; Munroe et al. 2022). Mastery has raised well-being, including happiness, neighborhood quality, life satisfaction, and physical and mental health as opposed to depression, to induce resilience (Greenberg

1999; Helson and Srivastava 2001; Hwang et al. 2007; Judge et al. 2002; Lever et al. 2005; Sargent-Cox et al. 2015). Purposefulness has raised such power as aspiration (Morgan and Robinson 2013). Relatedness is a basis for stability (Fingerman et al. 2011). Self-compassion has lifted equanimity, happiness, and positive affect and has dampened anger, anxiety, depression, distress, negative affect, and self-rumination to induce resilience (Barnard and Curry 2011; Sirois et al. 2015). Conscientiousness has also raised dispositional power in attachment security, creativity, courage, emotional intelligence, prosocial motivation, prudence, rationality, responsibility, and spirituality to drive resilience (Beutler and Gudmunson 2012; Carver 1997; Chen 2016; Hannah et al. 2007; Howard and Alipour 2014; MacDonald 2000; Mullet et al. 2005; Pacini and Epstein 1999; Siegling et al. 2012). Attachment security has buttressed life satisfaction to enable resilience (Zdrenka et al. 2015). Creativity has sustained well-being, notably meaningfulness, to buttress resilience (Diener et al. 2009; Turner 2013). Courage has sustained resilience, life satisfaction, and positive affect, and diminished anxiety and negative effect (Baptist et al. 2015; Howard and Alipour 2014; Kim et al. 2018; Muris et al. 2010). Emotional intelligence has facilitated well-being, including adaptation, happiness, health, life satisfaction, positive mood, relatedness, relational quality, and self-esteem to enhance resilience (Ciarrochi et al. 2000; Kluemper 2008; Matthews et al. 2012; Mayer et al. 2004; Schutte et al. 2002). Prosocial motivation has elevated well-being, including connectedness, hope, life satisfaction, meaningfulness, and self-efficacy to boost resilience (Marsh and Dik 2021; Nelson-Coffey et al. 2023; Raposa et al. 2016; Yao and Enright 2019). Prudence has upheld self-compassion to induce resilience (Pyszkowska 2020). Rationality has prevented aggression, anxiety, avoidance, depression, and disorders (DiGiuseppe et al. 2017). Responsibility has advanced wisdom to facilitate resilience (Spengler et al. 2018). Spirituality has enhanced meaningfulness to facilitate resilience (George and Park 2013). Conscientiousness has benefitted from agreeableness to secure dispositional power to drive resilience (Stober 2001). Agreeableness has enabled growth, life satisfaction, mastery, purposefulness, relatedness, and self-acceptance to raise resilience (Hounkpatin et al. 2015). Conversely, conscientiousness has eroded anxiety, depression, distress, hate, impulsivity, and negativity, thus retaining power to drive resilience (Becker et al. 1997; Lee and Ashton 2012; Li et al. 2017; Quilty et al. 2006; Wilt et al. 2017). Conscientiousness reflects low psychoticisim to sustain dispositional power to drive resilience (Village and Francis 2010). Psychoticism consolidates disorders characterized by hostility and toughness as opposed to responsiveness, sympathy, and trust (Village and Francis 2010). As such, psychoticism has dampened well-being, including self-determination, to impede resilience (Furnham and Cheng 2000; Ingledew et al. 2004). Conscientiousness can diminish loneliness, thus retaining power to drive resilience (Cacioppo and Hawkley 2009). Conscientious involves conventionality or normativity, dependability or reliability, decisiveness, and industriousness or tenaciousness as power to drive resilience (Bogg 2008; Roberts et al. 2009; Wright and DeLisi 2016). Conventionality has sustained life satisfaction, marital quality, and meaningfulness to safeguard resilience (Damasio and Koller 2015; Datler et al. 2013; Greenstein 1996). Dependability has stemmed from positive experience, social status, and trust to induce resilience (Barrera 2007; Cook and Cheshire 2013; Kuwabara 2015).

Utility secured by conscientiousness to attract resilience has included achievement or success, fairness, growth, friendship, love, safety, security expected or experienced, and life satisfaction (Becker et al. 1997; Fehr and Broughton 2001; Furnham et al. 2003; Hounkpatin et al. 2015; Homant 2013; Steca et al. 2017; van de Ven et al. 2011; Wolfradt and Dalbert 2003). Achievement has fostered health, life quality, satisfaction, self-efficacy, and self-esteem as opposed to alienation, depression, and distress to uphold resilience (Donnellan et al. 2005; Fredricks and Eccles 2005; Menard and Mose 1984; Murray 2009; Piko et al. 2006; Tompson and Dass 2000; Xiao et al. 2009). Fairness experienced has lifted positive mood, life satisfaction, and self-esteem to sustain resilience (Dalbert 2001). Growth experienced developed from self-compassion and self-tolerance to strengthen resilience (Ho and Li 2022; Munroe et al. 2022). Friendship has fostered gratitude to boost resilience (Rotkirch 2014). Love experienced can enhance influence and reduce depression to facilitate resilience (Busch 2009; Engelstad 2009). Safety or security experienced has escalated well-being, including health and life satisfaction as opposed to fear, to advance resilience (Chen et al. 2008; Frey et al. 2007; Jones et al. 2014). Conversely, conscientiousness has reduced conflict, exclusion, and transgression experienced, thus maintaining utility to attract resilience (Chapman and Hayslip 2005; Maltby et al. 2019; Wilt et al. 2017). Conflict experienced has bred distress and eroded satisfaction, thus impeding resilience (Lau et al. 2017; Mikula et al. 2012). Exclusion experienced has fomented negative mood and life dissatisfaction to hinder resilience (Lin et al. 2013; Williams et al. 2000). Transgression experienced has impaired safety experienced and self-respect or self-worth to erode resilience (Fernandes 2018; Krahe 2013).

Ideals raised by conscientiousness to rationalize resilience have embraced compliance or conformity, control, conventionality, order, patience, prevention, prosociality, studying, and volunteering (Bekkers 2005; Conroy and Visser 2016; Crede et al. 2010; Howard and Alipour 2014; Maltby et al. 2019; Mondak and Hurwitz 2012; Schnitker 2012; Twardawski et al. 2021). The ideal for compliance has buttressed compliance (Van Damme 2017). Compliance has furnished achievement and its pressure, mastery-goal setting, social closeness and support received, and tolerance to benefit resilience (Feldman 2003; Jiang et al. 2015; Magnuson et al. 2006). Control has boosted well-being, including health and life satisfaction as opposed to anger and depression, to maintain resilience (Etezadi and Pushkar 2013. Heidemeier and Staudinger 2012; Rose 2000; Xi and Hwang 2011). Conventionality has sustained life satisfaction, marital quality, and meaningfulness to safeguard resilience (Damasio and Koller 2015; Datler et al. 2013; Greenstein 1996). The ideal for order has stemmed from health to enable resilience (Cheung and Lai 2020). Patience has dampened negative affect to maintain resilience (Mehmood et al. 2020). Conscientiousness embodies ideals for achievement, adulthood or maturity, broadmindedness, constructiveness, and integrity to rationalize resilience (Ackerman and Wolman 2007; Caprara and Vecchione 2013; Curtis and Wee 2021; Sirgy 2012; Wang 2012). The ideal for achievement has enhanced meaningfulness, thus boosting resilience (Damasio and

Koller 2015). Adulthood or maturity has developed from self-compassion and self-tolerance to strengthen resilience (Ho and Li 2022; Munroe et al. 2022). Broadmindedness reflects wisdom to raise well-being, including autonomy, coherence, maturity, meaningfulness, purposefulness, life satisfaction, and self-efficacy to effectuate resilience (Diener et al. 2009; Greene and Brown 2009; Kramer 2000; Mickler and Staudinger 2008; Webster 2010). Contructiveness has fostered well-being to induce resilience (Katz and Esptein 1991). Integrity has sustained friend support, life quality, and satisfaction, and reduced depression and suicide to maintain resilience (McIntosh et al. 1994; Miner 1995; Mullins and Dugan 1991; Steinkamp and Kelly 1987). Conscientiousness stems from Protestantism as an ideal to rationalize resilience (Lane 2000). Protestantism has alleviated negative emotionality to lift resilience (Kim and Cohen 2017). Conscientiousness involves ideals for deliberation, goal-setting, persistence, planning, self-discipline, striving, and task orientation to rationalize resilience (Hannah et al. 2007; Roberts et al. 2009; Wright and DeLisi 2016). Deliberation has rested on its ideal (Acosta and Hsu 2014). As such, deliberation has prevented aggression, anxiety, avoidance, depression, and disorders to maintain resilience (DiGiuseppe et al. 2017). Goal-setting has supported life satisfaction and self-evaluation to secure resilience (Frazier et al. 2007; Stutzer 2004). Patience has reduced negative affect to enable resilience (Mehmood et al. 2020). Persistence has sustained well-being, notably pleasure, to facilitate resilience (Boyes et al. 2017; Goodman et al. 2017). Planning has reflected achievement, education, health, and optimism to afford resilience (Hellevik and Settersten 2013; Poynton et al. 2015). Self-discipline has arisen from self-esteem to facilitate resilience (Kokkinos and Hatzinikolaou 2011). Striving has sustained self-acceptance and relieved depression to foster resilience (Agronick and Duncan 1998; Wrosch et al. 2005). Task orientation has arisen from competence and meaningfulness to strengthen resilience (Gonzalez-Cutre et al. 2016; Morgan and Robinson 2013). Conversely, conscientiousness has upheld ideals against abusing in drinking and doping, deviance, risking, sexuality, and violence, thus sustaining resilience (Conroy and Visser 2016; de la Haye et al. 2015; Howard and Alipour 2014; Lee et al. 2013; Van Heel et al. 2019; Wright and DeLisi 2016; Zhang 2008). The ideal for abusing has buttressed abusing (Leimberg and Lehmann 2022). Abusing has engendered depression, thus jeopardizing resilience (Kendler et al. 2006). Deviance stands on its ideal (Morgan 2021). As such, deviance has eroded health, thus impairing resilience (Backman and Nilsson 2011). Risking can rest on its ideal (Breakwell 2007). Eventually, risking has weakened health and raised crime and violence, thus blocking resilience (Farrington 2018; Pulkkinen et al. 2009; Wickrama et al. 1995). Sexuality has engendered stress to dampen resilience (Ein-Dor and Hirschberger 2012). The ideal for violence has originated from anger and contempt as opposed to self-efficacy to impair resilience (Tausch et al. 2011).

The norm buttressed by conscientiousness to assimilate resilience has popularized justice (Nudelman 2013). The norm for justice has boosted prosperity to secure resilience (Rindermann 2008). Conversely, conscientiousness has dampened the norm for delinquency, thus sustaining resilience (Kendler et al. 2015). Delinquency has grown from its norm (Hoffmann 2023). Eventually, delinquency has jeopardized achievement, coping, education, mastery, life satisfaction, relational quality, self-efficacy, self-esteem, social attachment, and social capital in the youth to impede resilience (Carroll et al. 2009; Chung and Elias 1996; Compas et al. 1988; Fasang et al. 2014; Gault-Sherman 2012; Shek 2005).

## *Extraversion*

Extraversion is a personality trait for achievement, activity, ambition, assertiveness, boldness, enthusiasm, expressiveness, liveliness, positivity, potency, sociability, and social closeness (Foschi and Lauriola 2014; Witt and Revelle 200). Remarkably, extraversion has buttressed resilience (Plouffe et al. 2020). Extraversion is also likely to boost resilience by generating power, utility, ideals, and norms to leverage the voluntaristic mechanisms of analytical functionalism.

Power generated by extraversion to drive resilience has stemmed from well-being, including positive affect, autonomy or self-determination, growth, mastery, mattering, purposefulness, relatedness, self-acceptance, self-efficacy, and self-esteem (Hounkpatin et al. 2015; Ingledew et al. 2004; Li et al. 2017; Quilty et al. 2006; Rasmussen et al. 2018; Tiwari et al. 2021). Extraversion has also raised alliances, attachment, control, courage, creativity, criticalness, employability, intelligence and emotional intelligence, humor, motivation, uplift experience, social capital, spirituality, and support received to maintain power to drive resilience (Bishop 2015; Fraley et al. 2011; Howard and Alipour 2014; Raty et al. 2020; Leybman et al. 2011; Tulin et al. 2018; MacDonald and Friedman 2002; Maybery et al. 2006; Prenda and Lachman 2001; Savicki et al. 2004; Schbley and McCauley 2005; Vernon et al. 2008; Wang et al. 2017; Webster et al. 2014). Alliances have raised health and satisfaction to maintain resilience (Fuertes et al. 2017). Attachment has buttressed life satisfaction to enable resilience (Zdrenka et al. 2015). Control has boosted well-being, including health and life satisfaction as opposed to anger and depression, to maintain resilience (Etezadi and Pushkar 2013. Heidemeier and Staudinger 2012; Rose 2000; Xi and Hwang 2011). Courage has sustained resilience, life satisfaction, and positive affect and has diminished anxiety and negative affect (Baptist et al. 2015; Howard and Alipour 2014; Kim et al. 2018; Muris et al. 2010). Creativity has fostered well-being, including meaningfulness, to enhance resilience (Diener et al. 2009; Turner 2013). Criticalness has fostered identity achievement to procure resilience (Adams and Ryan 2000). Employability has reflected self-efficacy and self-evaluation to boost resilience (Atitsogbe et al. 2019; Creed and Gagliardi 2015). Intelligence has enhanced social capital and diminished criminality and depression, thus facilitating resilience (Cornwall 2009; Feinstein and Bynner 2006). Emotional intelligence has facilitated well-being, including adaptation, happiness, health, life satisfaction, positive mood, relatedness, relational quality, and self-esteem to enhance resilience (Ciarrochi et al. 2000; Kluemper 2008; Matthews et al. 2012; Mayer et al. 2004; Schutte et al. 2002). Humor has sustained mental health, pleasure, and satisfaction and has diminished fear to maintain resilience (Dynel and Poppi 2018; Martin

2007; Svebak et al. 2004). Motivation has covered career, education, prosociality, and understanding (Cassidy and Lynn 1991; Erez et al. 2008; Howard and Alipour 2014). As such, motivation has underlain satisfaction to induce resilience (Ferssizidis et al. 2010). Uplift experience has boosted joy, life satisfaction, love, and positive affect and has dampened anger to facilitate resilience (Maybery et al. 2006; Nezlek et al. 2008). Social capital has enhanced well-being, including community, flourishing, health, identity, life satisfaction, and pride to prop resilience (Chua et al. 2021; Yetim and Yetim 2014). Spirituality has sustained forgiveness, joy, and general well-being to foster resilience (Mullet et al. 2005; Saroglou and Anciaux 2004; Seidlitz et al. 2002). Social support received has upheld well-being, including control, health, positive emotion and pleasure, purposiveness, relational quality, satisfaction with life, housing, and leisure, self-determination, self-efficacy, self-esteem, and social well-being, to activate resilience (George and Park 2013; Glendinning et al. 2003; Granzin and Haggard 2000; Holliman et al. 2021; Lincoln et al. 2003; Logan and Cobb 2013; Pierce and Quiroz 2018; Schwarzer and Knoll 2007; Vilhjalmsson and Thorlindsson 1998; Wen et al. 2010; Williams and Galliher 2006; Xi and Hwang 2011). Conversely, extraversion has dampened anxiety, depression, disorders, distress, and hostility to maintain power to drive resilience (Becker et al. 1997; Eggert et al. 2007; Hounkpatin et al. 2015; Kim 2017; Weinberg et al. 2021).

Utility upheld by extraversion to attract resilience has resided in satisfaction, security, and success experienced (Becker et al. 1997; Colbert et al. 2012; Li et al. 2017). Security experienced has boosted well-being, including health, life satisfaction, and neighborhood quality, as opposed to fear, to induce resilience (Chen et al. 2008; Frey et al. 2007; Olson et al. 2016; Jones et al. 2014). Success experienced has fostered health, life quality, satisfaction, self-efficacy, and self-esteem as opposed to alienation, depression, and distress to uphold resilience (Donnellan et al. 2005; Fredricks and Eccles 2005; Menard and Mose 1984; Murray 2009; Piko et al. 2006; Tompson and Dass 2000; Xiao et al. 2009). Conversely, extraversion has reduced exclusion and stress experienced to maintain utility for attracting resilience (Maltby et al. 2019; Weinberg et al. 2021). Exclusion experienced has fomented negative mood and life dissatisfaction to hinder resilience (Lin et al. 2013; Williams et al. 2000). Stress experienced has dampened well-being, including health, life quality, positive affect, and satisfaction as opposed to depression and distress, to impede resilience (Baumeister et al. 2013. Mathis et al. 2016; Raposa et al. 2016; Shrira 2012; Snyder et al. 2020; Zotti et al. 2016).

Ideals raised by extraversion to rationalize resilience have treasured career, civic engagement, donation, humor, nationalism, prosociality, rationality, self-direction, socializing or sociality, and volunteering (Bekkers 2010; Celso et al. 2003; Erez et al. 2008; Howard and Alipour 2014; Kreber 1998; Omoto et al. 2010; Petrides et al. 2007; Rogers and Creed 2011; Schbley and McCauley 2005; Ward and Forney 2020). Civic engagement has stood on its ideal (Peterson and Maiden 1993). As such, civic engagement has incubated conflict resolution, education, happiness, health, income, individualism, life satisfaction, security normativity, social attachment, capital, integration, trust, tolerance, and general well-being to advance resilience (Coffe and Geys 2007; Goren 2005; Growiec and Growiec 2010; Kroll 2011; Li and Walder

2001; Myers 1999; Pena-Lopez and Sanchez-Santos 2016; Posel and Casale 2011; Tak 2017; Tang 2011; Wallace and Pichler 2009; Welzel 2013; van Ingen and Bekkers 2015; Vincens et al. 2018). The ideal for donation has propped donation (Vallerand et al. 1992). Eventually, donation has reflected well-being, including control, feeling good, gratitude, happiness, joy, satisfaction, and self-efficacy as opposed to anxiety and guilt, to brew resilience (Bednall et al. 2013; Bekkers 2008; Eayrs and Ellis 1990; Liu and Hao 2017; Mussen 1982; Piliavin and Callero 1991; Wang and Graddy 2008). Nationalism has raised well-being, including life satisfaction, to enable resilience (Lalot et al. 2023; Chang and Kang 2018). Extraversion has stemmed from dialecticism as the ideal to rationalize resilience (Spencer-Rodgers et al. 2009). Dialecticism has sustained creativity and reflected independence to facilitate resilience (Church et al. 2012; Yang et al. 2010). Conversely, extraversion has dampened the ideal for delinquency to maintain resilience (Morizot and Le Blanc 2007). The ideal for delinquency has bred delinquency (Hati et al. 2019). Delinquency has jeopardized achievement, coping, education, mastery, life satisfaction, relational quality, self-efficacy, self-esteem, social attachment, and social capital in the youth to impede resilience (Carroll et al. 2009; Chung and Elias 1996; Compas et al. 1988; Fasang et al. 2014; Gault-Sherman 2012; Shek 2005).

The norm underlying extraversion for assimilating resilience has popularized religiosity (van Hemert et al. 2002). The norm for religiosity has enforced religiosity (Stavrova and Siegers 2014). Religiosity has buttressed coping, friendship, forgiveness, harmony perceived, health maintenance, institutional and social trust, optimism, social capital, and well-being to raise resilience (Chang 2009; Clemence 2001; Furnham 1997; Hakhverdian and Mayne 2012; Myers 2008; Saroglou and Anciaux 2004; Wuthnow 2004; Zanin 2017). Conversely, extraversion has dampened norms for danger to assimilate resilience (Sibley and Duckitt 2009). The norm for risk has eroded adjustment, positive affect, happiness, life satisfaction, and self-determination and fomented depression, fear or anxiety, negative affect, and sadness to undermine resilience (Prelow et al. 2004; Schoon 2006; Schwartz and Melech 2000; Shippee 2012; Vuori 2015; Zotti et al. 2016).

## *Neuroticism*

Neuroticism, the opposite of emotional stability, is a personality trait characterizing negative affectivity (Baay et al. 2014; Ormel et al. 2004). Essentially, neuroticism features dispositional anxiety, depression, emotionality, irrationality, neediness, reactivity to stress, and shyness (Denissen et al., 2009; Village and Francis, 2010). Functionally, neuroticism connects to psychopathology (Ormel et al. 2004). Remarkably, neuroticism has impaired resilience (Campbell-Sills et al. 2006). Moreover, neuroticism is likely to erode resilience by reducing power, utility, ideals, and norms to drive, attract, rationalize, and assimilate resilience through the voluntaristic mechanisms of analytical functionalism.

Power to drive resilience weekend by neuroticism has rested on well-being, including autonomy or self-determination, existential well-being, growth, health, positive affect, purposiveness, relatedness, relational quality, self-acceptance, and self-compassion (Anusic et al. 2014; Finggerman et al. 2008; Hounkpatin et al. 2015; Ingledew et al. 2004; MacDonald and Friedman 2002; Marks 1996; Pfattheicher et al. 2017; Webster et al. 2014). Existential well-being covers attachment or security, authenticity, consciousness, freedom, love, reason, and responsibility (Burston 1991; Cox 2012; Quackenbush et al. 2016; Slaby and Stephan 2008). Attachment has buttressed life satisfaction to enable resilience (Zdrenka et al. 2015). Security has escalated intimacy and satisfaction and eroded anger, anxiety, loneliness, and regret to raise resilience (Alonso-Arbiol et al. 2007; Buelow et al. 1996; Gillath et al. 2005; Kafetsio and Sideridis 2006; Lavy et al. 2010). Authenticity has maintained autonomy, eudaimonic well-being, growth, hedonic well-being, identity integration, life satisfaction, positive affect, mastery, mindfulness, purposiveness, relational quality, self-acceptance, self-clarity, self-esteem, self-determination, and vitality to escalate resilience (Kernis and Goldman 2006). Consciousness has enhanced meaningfulness to facilitate resilience (George and Park 2013). Freedom has enabled well-being, including health, life satisfaction, and self-esteem, as opposed to depression and symptoms to facilitate resilience action (Abbott et al. 2011; Glendinning et al. 2003; Haller and Hadler 2006). Love has enhanced toleration as opposed to strictness to champion resilience (Seabach 2017). Reason or rationality has inhibited anxiety, depression, and fear to maintain resilience (Barnes and Vulcano 1982; DiGiuseppe et al. 2017). Responsibility has advanced wisdom to facilitate resilience (Spengler et al. 2018). Neuroticism has eroded control, forgiveness, intelligence, self-enhancement, and spirituality as dispositional power to drive resilience (Lincoln et al. 2003; Mullet et al. 2005; Schaie 2013; Vernon et al. 2008). Control has boosted well-being, including health and life satisfaction, as opposed to anger and depression, to maintain resilience (Etezadi and Pushkar 2013. Heidemeier and Staudinger 2012; Rose 2000; Xi and Hwang 2011). Forgiveness has elevated serenity, trust, and well-being to maintain resilience (Choi and David 2012; Connors et al. 1999; Shimai et al. 2006). Intelligence has assuaged depression to maintain resilience (Feinstein and Bynner 2006). Self-enhancement has reflected attachment and social support received to raise resilience (Hermanto et al. 2017; Ledoux et al. 2010). Spirituality has sustained forgiveness, joy, and general well-being to foster resilience (Mullet et al. 2005; Saroglou and Anciaux 2004; Seidlitz et al. 2002). Conversely, neuroticism has reduced power for driving resilience by raising aggressiveness, anxiety, body decline, depression, hostility, loneliness, self-defeating, and superstitiusness (Hounkpatin et al. 2015; Maltby et al. 2016; Melton 2016; Neto and Barros 2003; Rossi 2004a; Vernon et al. 2008; Wiseman and Watt 2004). Aggressiveness reflects panic (Petrou and Kandylis 2016). Self-defeating has induced anxiety to obstruct resilience (Cheng et al. 2017). Superstitiousness has impaired life satisfaction, thus undermining resilience (Wiseman and Watt 2004). Neuroticism underlies psychopathology, thus weakening power for driving resilience (Ormel et al.

2004). Psychopathology has impaired well-being, thus obstructing resilience (Jans-Beken 2019). Neuroticism embodies negative affectivity to dampen power for driving resilience (Ormel et al. 2004).

Utility for attracting resilience diminished by neuroticism has emanated from satisfaction, success, and uplift experienced (Maybery et al. 2006; Steca et al. 2017). Satisfaction has covered appearance, friendship, life, and weight (Austin et al. 2005; Frederick et al. 2016; Richards 2016). Success has buttressed acceptance or tolerance, development, education, health, income, life quality, satisfaction, self-efficacy or competence, self-esteem, and social support received to induce resilience (Cook et al. 2002; Donnellan et al. 2005; Gibbs et al. 2015; Mackinnon 2012; Morgan and Streb 2001; Murray 2009; Pabilonic 2001; Tompson and Dass 2000; Xiao et al. 2009). Uplift experience has raised life satisfaction and positive affect to safeguard resilience (Maybery et al. 2006). Conversely, neuroticism has raised financial and interpersonal problems, stress, and trauma as disutility disincentivizing resilience (Lincoln et al. 2003). Problems have worsened well-being, including financial well-being, health, and satisfaction as opposed to distress, to impair resilience (Carrieri 2012; Gary et al. 2007; van Praag and Ferrer-I-Carbonell 2004; van Praag and Frijters 1999). Stress has eroded well-being, including eudaimonia, health, positive affect, quality of life, neighborhood, and relationships, and satisfaction with life and neighbors, thus jeopardizing resilience (Baumeister et al. 2013; Greenberg 1999; Jackson et al. 2006; Mathis et al. 2016; Parkes et al. 2002; Shrira 2012; Su et al. 2021; Zotti et al. 2016). Trauma has raised depression, disability, distress, memory loss, substance abuse, and suicide (Dutton et al. 2016; Grzywacz and Almeida 2008; Lantz et al. 2005; Lowe et al. 2009; Lupien et al. 2009; Snyder et al. 2020).

Ideals for rationalizing resilience dampened by neuroticism have emphasized civic engagement, coordination, planning, socializing, and volunteering (Bekkers 2005; Kalish 2008; Prenda and Lachman 2001; Ward and Forney 2020). Civic engagement has stood on its ideal (Peterson and Maiden 1993). As such, civic engagement has incubated conflict resolution, education, happiness, health, income, individualism, life satisfaction, security normativity, social attachment, capital, integration, trust, tolerance, and general well-being to advance resilience (Coffe and Geys 2007; Goren 2005; Growiec and Growiec 2010; Kroll 2011; Li and Walder 2001; Myers 1999; Pena-Lopez and Sanchez-Santos 2016; Posel and Casale 2011; Tak 2017; Tang 2011; Wallace and Pichler 2009; Welzel 2013; van Ingen and Bekkers 2015; Vincens et al. 2018). Coordination has developed from its ideal (Michael et al. 2020). Furthermore, coordination has benefitted from networking, solidarity, support received, and trust (Miao et al. 2018; Ng et al. 2004). Planning has reflected achievement, education, health, and optimism to afford resilience (Hellevik and Settersten 2013; Poynton et al. 2015). Socializing has hinged on its ideal (Chen et al. 2009). Eventually, socializing has reduced negative emotions and stress to safeguard resilience (Nelson-Coffey et al. 2023). Volunteering has grown from its ideal (Barr et al. 2005). Eventually, volunteering has raised well-being, including health, life satisfaction, mastery, morale, positive affect, and self-esteem as opposed to depression, loneliness, and mortality, to buttress resilience (Borgonovi 2008; Gillath et al. 2005; Li and Ferraro 2006; Midlarsky and Kahana 1994; Oman et al. 1999; Thoits and Hewitt 2001; Zotti et al.

2016). Conversely, neuroticism has bred comparison, crime, and revenge as ideals to hinder resilience (Pulkkinen et al. 2009; Mullet et al. 2005; Fujita 2008). Comparison has developed from its ideal (Buunk and Gibbons 2006). As such, comparison has bred negative affect and dampened self-esteem to worsen resilience (Fujita 2008). The ideal for crime has rationalized crime (Tanner-Smith et al. 2013). Crime has eroded life satisfaction, mastery, relationship quality, self-efficacy, and self-esteem to weaken resilience (Chung and Elias 1996; Keijsers et al. 2011; Shek 2005). Revenge has bred distress, negative affect, and symptoms to hamper resilience (Barcaccia et al. 2022b; Strelan et al. 2020).

Norms enhanced by neuroticism to discourage resilience have highlighted competition and risk (Breakwell 2007; Sibley and Duckitt 2009). The norm for competition has bred crime, hostility, and violence, and erased tolerance to impair resilience (Messner et al. 2013; Mintz et al. 2022; Passini and Morselli 2015). The norm for risk has eroded adjustment, positive affect, happiness, life satisfaction, and self-determination and fomented depression, fear or anxiety, negative affect, and sadness to undermine resilience (Prelow et al. 2004; Schoon 2006; Schwartz and Melech 2000; Shippee 2012; Vuori 2015; Zotti et al. 2016).

## *Distress*

Distress as a manifestation of neuroticism indicates development (Village and Francis 2010). Inherently, distress is negative affect registering avoidance (Oltean et al. 2022; Stevens et al. 2018). Distress features anger, anxiety, depression, dissatisfaction, frustration, grief, isolation, misadjustment, pain, sadness, shame, stress, sorrow, unpleasantness, and other symptoms (Abu-Raiya et al. 2015; Carreno et al. 2021; Carver and Scheier 2016; Cochrane 2018; Holloway et al. 2017; Becchetta 2010; Franks 2003; Lee 2016; Lively 2017; Ntontis et al. 2023; Pachankis et al. 2020; Pomerleau et al. 2020; Stevens et al. 2018). Distress has dampened resilience (Tett and Wang 2005). Such dampening can happen when distress withdraws power, utility, ideals, and norms to disrupt voluntaristic mechanisms emphasized in analytical functionalism.

Power to drive resilience weakened by distress has rested on creativity, health, social capital, and social trust (Baas et al. 2008; Bassani 2008; Burke and Stets 1999; Webber and Huxley 2007). Creativity has boosted well-being, notably meaningfulness, to induce resilience (Diener et al. 2009; Turner 2013). Social capital has enhanced well-being, including community, flourishing, health, identity, life satisfaction, and pride to prop resilience (Chua et al. 2021; Yetim and Yetim 2014). Social capital has enhanced well-being, including community, flourishing, health, identity, life satisfaction, and pride to prop resilience (Chua et al. 2021; Yetim and Yetim 2014). Social trust has fostered health and survival to sustain resilience (Barefoot et al. 1998). Distress has sprung from inadequate strength, agreeableness, conscientiousness, extraversion, education, gratitude, homeownership, honesty-humility, income, living standards, positivity, religiosity, self-compassion, social capital, social class, and social support experienced or received, thus eroding power to drive resilience

(Behler et al. 2019; Chan et al. 2022; Frank et al. 2014; Ferreira et al. 2021; Li et al. 2017; Lowe et al. 2009; Martinez-Marti and Ruch 2017; Montazer 2022; Oltean et al. 2022; Pitonak et al. 2023; Sirois et al. 2015; Weinberg et al. 2021). Strength has prevented fear and fostered satisfaction to drive resilience (Liu, Messner, Zhang, and Zhuo 2009; Peterson and Seligman 2004). Agreeableness has raised attachment and its security to enable resilience (Carver 1997). Conscientiousness has raised attachment, autonomy, life satisfaction, mastery, purposefulness, and self-acceptance to secure resilience (Fraley et al. 2011; Hounkpatin et al. 2015). Extraversion has raised well-being, including autonomy, growth, mastery, positive affect, purposefulness, relatedness, satisfaction, self-acceptance, self-determination, self-efficacy, and self-esteem to facilitate resilience (Hounkpatin et al. 2015; Ingledew et al. 2004; Quilty et al. 2006; Rasmussen et al. 2018; Richards 2016; Tiwari et al. 2021). Education has sustained well-being, including health, identity, life quality and satisfaction, mastery, self-efficacy, self-esteem, and youthfulness to engender resilience (Cerin and Leslie 2008; Corcoran et al. 2011; James and Amato 2013; Pakulshi and Tranter 2000; Stavrova and Ehlebracht 2018; van Praag and Frijters 1999; Whyte and Gao 2009; Yienprugsawan et al. 2010). Gratitude has raised positive affect and dampened negative affect to achieve resilience (Bernabe-Valero et al. 2021). Homeownership has raised health, morale, family and neighborhood quality, and financial, housing, life, and neighborhood satisfaction as opposed to depression, distress, and fear to strengthen resilience (Congdon 2010; Harris 2001; Lee et al. 2022; Mirowsky and Ross 1999; Montazer 2022; Roy and Chaudhuri 2008; Wulfhorst and Kranich 1999; Yu and Chiu 2016; Zheng et al. 2020). Honesty has reflected happiness to sustain resilience (Medai and Noussair 2021). Income has afforded well-being, including adaptation, adequacy, belongingness, control, eudaemonia, health, mastery, power, quality of life, satisfaction, self-efficacy, self-esteem, and social well-being to sustain resilience (Anciaes et al. 2017; Carpiano 2008; Corcoran et al. 2011; Ross and Mirowsky 1989; Sengupta and Sibley 2019; Son and Wilson 2012; Wang and VanderWeele 2011; Yeh et al. 2013; Zimmerman and Reyna 2013). Positivity has buttressed benefits experienced, coping, curability, and survival to enable resilience (Clarke et al. 2000; Nes and Segerstrom 2006). Religiosity has buttressed coping, friendship, forgiveness, harmony perceived, health maintenance, institutional and social trust, optimism, social capital, and well-being to raise resilience (Chang 2009; Clemence 2001; Furnham 1997; Hakhverdian and Mayne 2012; Myers 2008; Saroglou and Anciaux 2004; Wuthnow 2004; Zanin 2017). Self compassion has lifted equanimity, happiness, and positive affect and dampened anger, anxiety, depression, distress, negative affect, and self-rumination to induce resilience (Barnard and Curry 2011; Sirois et al. 2015). Social class has sustained well-being, including financial adequacy, health, hope, and satisfaction, as opposed to depression to advance resilience (Burke 2008; Davis and Davenport 1999; Haller and Hadler 2006; Hadjar and Samuel 2015; Peterson and Seligman 2004; Yamaoka 2008). Social support received has upheld resilience and well-being, including control, health, positive emotion and pleasure, purposiveness, relational quality, satisfaction with life, housing, and leisure, self-determination, self-efficacy, self-esteem, and social well-being, to activate resilience (Cherry et al. 2018; George and Park 2013;

Glendinning et al. 2003; Granzin and Haggard 2000; Holliman et al. 2021; Lincoln et al. 2003; Logan and Cobb 2013; Pierce and Quiroz 2018; Schwarzer and Knoll 2007; Vilhjalmsson and Thorlindsson 1998; Wen et al. 2010; Williams and Galliher 2006; Xi and Hwang 2011). Distress can arise from inadequate altruism, attachment, intrinsic motivation, learning, nurturing experienced, resources, and security to constrain power that drives resilience (Hobfoll 1998; Janoff-Bulman 1992; Jarvis 2004; Ferssizidis et al. 2010; Kafetsio and Sideridis 2006). Altruism has raised well-being, including connectedness, hope, life satisfaction, meaningfulness, and self-efficacy, as opposed to loneliness and negative emotion to sustain resilience (Caprara and Steca 2005; Marsh and Dik 2021; Nelson-Coffey et al. 2023; Raposa et al. 2016; Yao and Enright 2019).Attachment has buttressed life satisfaction to enable resilience (Zdrenka et al. 2015). Intrinsic motivation has reflected competence and meaningfulness to enable resilience (Gonzalez-Cutre et al. 2016; Morgan and Robinson 2013). Learning has elevated well-being, including life satisfaction and self-efficacy, to facilitate resilience (Denver and Hands 1990; Minnaert and Janssen 1992; Richards 2016). Nurturing received has boosted well-being, including control, emotional well-being, health, pleasure, purposiveness, relational quality, satisfaction with housing, leisure, and life, self-determination, self-efficacy, self-esteem, and social well-being to sustain resilience (George and Park 2013; Glendinning et al. 2003; Granzin and Haggard 2000; Holliman et al. 2021; Kafetsio and Sideridis 2006; Lincoln et al. 2003; Logan and Cobb 2013; Schwarzer and Knoll 2007; Vilhjalmsson and Thorlindsson 1998; Wen et al. 2010; Williams and Galliher 2006; Xi and Hwang 2011). Security has escalated well-being, including health and life satisfaction to raise resilience (Chen et al. 2008; Frey et al. 2007; Jones et al. 2014). Conversely, distress has raised dependency, substance abuse, and suicide to erode power that drives resilience (Abrutyna and Mueller 2014; Benitez-Silva et al. 2010; Bentler et al. 2002). Dependency has raised illness and suicide and eroded health and mastery, thus shaking resilience (Bornstein 2012; Lu and Kao 2002; Roy and Chaudhuri 2008). Substance abuse has engendered depression, thus jeopardizing resilience (Kendler et al. 2006). Attempted suicide has induced anxiety to obstruct resilience (Cheng et al. 2017). Distress has stemmed from powerlessness, dysfunction, emotionality or reactivity, extrinsic motivation, illness, insecurity, insomnia, neuroticism, psychopathology, rejection sensitivity, and revenge motivation, thus impairing power to drive resilience (Barcaccia et al. 2022b; Boyes et al. 2017; Carreno et al. 2021; Ferssizidis et al. 2010; Green et al. 2014; Lau et al. 2021; Li et al. 2017; Pachankis et al. 2020; Phongsavan et al. 2006; Ross and Mirowsky 2009; Weinberg et al. 2021). Powerlessness has unfolded dissatisfaction to impair resilience (Armstrong-Stassen 2001). Emotionality or reactivity has dampened well-being, including autonomy, growth, health, positive affect, purposefulness, relatedness, relational quality, satisfaction, self-acceptance, self-compassion, and self-determination, to impede resilience (Anusic et al. 2014; Austin et al. 2005; Hounkpatin et al. 2015; Ingledew et al. 2004; Marks 1996; Pfattheicher et al. 2017; Richards 2016; Webster et al. 2014). Extrinsic motivation has created negative affect and reduced achievement to obstruct resilience (Walls and Little 2005). Illness has eroded functionality, health and mental health, knowledge, optimism, security, vitality, and general well-being, thus disempowering resilience

(Benitez-Silva et al. 2010; Carrieri 2012; Korkeila et al. 2004; Price et al. 2006; van Dijk et al. 2008). Insecurity has diminished well-being, including health and life satisfaction, to block resilience (Chen et al. 2008; Frey et al. 2007; Jones et al. 2014). Insomnia has bred negativity to undermine resilience (Dubar et al. 2021). Neuroticism has worsened well-being including autonomy, growth, health, positive affect, purposeness, relatedness, satisfaction, self-acceptance, self-compassion, and self-determination, to resist resilience (Anusic et al. 2014; Hounkpatin et al. 2015; Ingledew et al. 2004; Pfattheicher et al. 2017; Richards 2016; Webster et al. 2014). Psychopathology has impaired well-being, thus obstructing resilience (Jans-Beken 2019). Rejection sensitivity has eroded self-efficacy and generated anxiety to inhibit resilience (Wu et al. 2022). Revenge motivation has bred negative affect and symptoms to hamper resilience (Barcaccia et al. 2022b; Strelan et al. 2020). Distress can arise from inferiority and uncertainty to indicate powerlessness to erode resilience (Jarvis 2004; Quick et al. 2001). Inferiority has triggered anxiety and fear to impede resilience (Li et al. 2023). Uncertainty has raised diffidence, dissatisfaction, and tension to jeopardize resilience (Theiss 2018).

Utility to attract resilience cut by distress has highlighted achievement and popularity (Baskin et al. 2014; Dougherty 2006). Achievement has fostered health, life quality, satisfaction, self-efficacy, and self-esteem as opposed to alienation, depression, and distress to uphold resilience (Donnellan et al. 2005; Fredricks and Eccles 2005; Menard and Mose 1984; Murray 2009; Piko et al. 2006; Tompson and Dass 2000; Xiao et al. 2009). Popularity has uplifted positive affect and self-esteem and reduced negative affect, thus buttressing resilience (Reich et al. 2018). Distress has emerged from inadequate benefit, gratitude, and unfairness received, thus dampening utility to attract resilience (Holmstrom et al. 2021; Oltean et al. 2022; Schulz et al. 2000; Zheng et al. 2020b). Gratitude has raised positive affect and dampened negative affect to achieve resilience (Bernabe-Valero et al. 2021). Unfairness experienced has eroded positive mood, life satisfaction, and self-esteem, thus jeopardizing resilience (Dalbert 2001). Distress can arise from inadequate gain, thus reducing utility to attract resilience (Hobfoll 1998). Gain received has raised well-being, including satisfaction as opposed to anger, anxiety, and depression, to foster resilience (Helgeson et al. 2006; Wells et al. 1999; Wong and Lam 2016). Conversely, distress has fomented conflict, problems, stress, trauma, and victimization experienced to reduce utility for attracting resilience (Doane et al. 2013; Gutman et al. 2005; McMunn et al. 2001; Schreck et al. 2007). Conflict experienced has bred distress and eroded satisfaction, thus impeding resilience (Lau et al. 2017; Mikula et al. 2012). Problems experienced have worsened well-being, including financial well-being, health, and satisfaction as opposed to distress, to impair resilience (Carrieri 2012; Gary et al. 2007; van Praag and Ferrer-I-Carbonell 2004; van Praag and Frijters 1999). Stress or trauma experienced has dampened well-being, including health, life quality, positive affect, and satisfaction as opposed to depression and distress, to impede resilience (Baumeister et al. 2013. Mathis et al. 2016; Raposa et al. 2016; Shrira 2012; Snyder et al. 2020; Zotti et al. 2016). Victimization experienced has impaired safety experienced and self-respect or self-worth to erode resilience (Fernandes 2018; Krahe 2013). Distress has arisen from conflict, cost, danger, deprivation, discrimination, hardship, harm, problems, stress, shaming received, terrorism or war experienced, and victimization experienced, thus impairing utility to attract resilience (Ahnquist et al. 2012; Becchetta 2010; Carreno et al. 2021; Creed and Evans 2002; Eshel et al. 2017; Lau et al. 2017; Montazer 2022; Pachankis et al. 2020; Pomerleau et al. 2020; Starrin et al. 2009; Wager 2012). Distress can arise from consensus experienced, discrepancy from ideals, inequity, loss, rivalry, and victimization experienced as disutility against resilience (Carver and Scheier 2016; Jarvis 2004; Lively 2017; Lowe et al. 2009; White et al. 2015).

Ideals to rationalize resilience erased by distress have treasured morality and sports (Wentzel et al. 2004). Distress has arisen from ideals against commitment, endurance, family, friendship, helping, and religion to discourage resilience (Abu-Raiya et al. 2015; Hall et al. 2022; Yasuma et al. 2019). Conversely, distress has fomented ideals for blaming, compartmentalization or isolation, delinquency, externalizing, resistance, retaliation, and sexuality (Amiot et al. 2017; Broidy 2001; Fauth et al. 2007; Kelley et al. 2011; Pulkkinen et al. 2009; South et al. 2005; Wayment et al. 2010). Distress has hinged on ideals for alcoholism, attacking, avoidance, restraint, struggle to refute resilience (Abu-Raiya et al. 2015; Ferreira et al. 2021; Martinez-Marti and Ruch 2017; Oshio and Kan 2019; Pomerleau et al. 2020).

Norms against resilience underlying distress have generalized distress, discrimination, problems, spending, strain, and stress (Amiot et al. 2017; Cheung and Leung 2011; Gary et al. 2007; Haslam et al. 2004; Oshio and Kan 2019; Pierce and Quiroz 2018; Walen and Lachman 2016). Distress can grow with norms for error and mortality to discourage resilience (Franks 2003; Skyttner 2005). Conversely, distress has risen with norms against cohesion and income (Gary et al. 2007; Lau et al. 2021).

## *Adventuring*

Adventuring or risking means acting under uncertainty (Thielmann et al. 2020). This act embodies masculinity, openness, and youth (Huyck and Gutmann 2006; Mitchell et al. 2001). Adventuring features alcoholism, camping, experimenting, libertinism, recklessness, and sexuality as opposed to protection (Koegl and Day 2019; Morokoff et al. 2009; Morris and Orton-Johnson 2024; Oliver 2006; Taubman-Ben-Ari and Findler 2003; Tyson et al. 2014; Van Tongeren et al. 2023). As such, adventuring is likely to impede resilience by eroding power, utility, ideals, and norms to achieve functioning through voluntaristic mechanisms dictated by analytical functionalism.

Power to drive resilience dampened by adventuring has emanated from health and religiosity (Uecker et al. 2007; Wickrama et al. 1995). Religiosity has buttressed coping, friendship, forgiveness, harmony perceived, health maintenance, institutional and social trust, optimism, social capital, and well-being to raise resilience (Chang 2009; Clemence 2001; Furnham 1997; Hakhverdian and Mayne 2012; Myers 2008; Saroglou and Anciaux 2004; Wuthnow 2004; Zanin 2017). Adventuring has arisen from low agreeableness, assertiveness, conscientiousness, development, education, maturity, self-control, self-efficacy, self-esteem, social bonding, social desirability, support received, and understanding thus weakening power for driving resilience (de Jong et al. 2012; Dodge and Jaccard 2002; Fang et al. 2019; Goldman and Peleg 2010; Hamilton 2010; Howard and Alipour 2014; Koegl and Day 2019; Morokoff et al. 2009; Olivari et al. 2018; Shaw et al. 2014; Vermeersch et al. 2011; Wilczenski and Coomey 2007). Agreeableness has enabled growth, life satisfaction, mastery, purposefulness, relatedness, and self-acceptance to raise resilience (Hounkpatin et al. 2015). Conscientiousness has raised autonomy, growth, life satisfaction, mastery, purposefulness, relatedness, and self-acceptance to enable resilience (Hounkpatin et al. 2015). Defense has built on self-efficacy to facilitate resilience (Guo et al. 2023). Development has facilitated success experienced to attract resilience (Spengler et al. 2018). Education has sustained well-being, including health, identity, life quality and satisfaction, mastery, self-efficacy, self-esteem, and youthfulness to engender resilience (Cerin and Leslie 2008; Corcoran et al. 2011; James and Amato 2013; Pakulshi and Tranter 2000; Stavrova and Ehlebracht 2018; van Praag and Frijters 1999; Whyte and Gao 2009; Yienprugsawan et al. 2010). Maturity has developed from self-compassion and self-tolerance to strengthen resilience (Ho and Li 2022; Munroe et al. 2022). Social attachment has enabled compassion, health, intimacy, and life satisfaction to sustain resilience (Alonso-Arbiol et al. 2007; Headey et al. 2001; Mikulincer et al. 2005; Zdrenka et al. 2015). Self-control has maintained self-esteem and reduced anxiety and depression to enable resilience (Armstrong et al. 2011; Marchetti et al. 2018). Social bonding has mitigated stress and negative emotion, thus upholding resilience (Nelson-Coffey et al. 2023). Social desirability has escalated gratitude and dampened anxiety and depression to maintain resilience (Ben-Zur 2002; Burroughs and Rindfleisch 2002; Krumrei-Mancuso 2017). Trust has fostered health and survival to sustain resilience (Barefoot et al. 1998). Social support received has maintained well-being, including resilience, control, health, pleasure, purposefulness, relational quality, satisfaction, self-determination, self-efficacy, self-esteem, and social well-being (Cherry et al. 2018; George and Park 2013; Glendinning et al. 2003; Gorman et al. 2010; Holliman et al. 2021; Lincoln et al. 2003; Logan and Cobb 2013; Pierce and Quiroz 2018; Schwarzer and Knoll 2007; Williams and Galliher 2006; Xi and Hwang 2011). Understanding has raised intimacy, satisfaction, and self-efficacy to support resilience (Mikulincer et al. 2003; Norris 2011; Rothwell et al. 2016). Adventuring reflects low adaptiveness or adaptability, controllability or self-control, learning, rationality, reflexivity, and positive mood as power to drive resilience (Chuang and Lin 2007; Lawy 2002; Lyng et al. 2009; Masters and Hayes 2020; Parker and Stanworth 2005; Reyna and Farley 2006; Zhang et al. 2010). Learning has escalated well being, including life satisfaction and self-efficacy, to advance resilience (Denver and Hands 1990; Minnaert and Janssen 1992; Richards 2016). Rationality covers comparison, identity building, and learning (Lawy 2002). As such, rationality has dampened anxiety, depression, and fear to retain resilience (Barnes and Vulcano 1982; DiGiuseppe et al. 2017). Reflectivity has sustained well-being, including meaningfulness, to boost resilience (Baumeister et al. 2013; Michaeli et al. 2022). Adventuring can arise from low competence, conventionality, pleasantness, and security, thus weakening power for driving resilience (Dahlback 2003; Reyna and Farley 2006; Simons et al. 2016). Competence covers instrumentality, insusceptibility, recourse, and resolution (Reyna and Farley 2006). Conventionality has nurtured life satisfaction, marital quality, and meaningfulness to induce resilience (Datler et al. 2013; Damasio and Koller 2015; Greenstein 1996). Security has escalated intimacy and satisfaction and eroded anger, anxiety, loneliness, and regret to raise resilience (Alonso-Arbiol et al. 2007; Buelow et al. 1996; Gillath et al. 2005; Kafetsio and Sideridis 2006; Lavy et al. 2010). Conversely, adventuring has risen from depression, ignorance, negative affect, rebelliousness, and sensation-seeking, thus undermining power to drive resilience (Chuang and Lin 2007; Crone and van Duijvenvoorde 2021; Morokoff et al. 2009; Ongen 2007; Van Tongeren et al. 2023). Rebelliousness has fomented arousal and distress to hinder resilience (Hatcher et al. 2018; Magnuson et al. 2006). Sensation-seeking has incurred doping to engender depression, thus jeopardizing resilience (Ball 1995; Kendler et al. 2006). Adventruing breeds hate to reduce power for driving resilience (Hawdon et al. 2019). Adventuring involves aggressiveness, alcoholism, disorders, infection, intoxication, recklessness, and suicidality to reduce power for driving resilience (Bouffard and Rice 2011; Koegl and Day 2019; Miller-Day 2004; Taubman-Ben-Ari and Findler 2003; Vermeersch et al. 2011; Yue et al. 2020). Aggressiveness has induced depression to inhibit resilience (Wright et al. 2015). Alcoholism has caused aggression, illness, injury, and pathology to impede resilience (Brotchie et al. 2004; Haapanen-Niemi et al. 1999). Disorders have eroded well-being to impede resilience (Jans-Beken 2019). Ignorance has arisen from dissatisfaction to forestall resilience (Noack et al. 2001). Infection has eroded functionality, health and mental health, knowledge, optimism, security, vitality, and general well-being, thus disempowering resilience (Benitez-Silva et al. 2010; Carrieri 2012; Korkeila et al. 2004; Price et al. 2006; van Dijk et al. 2008). Intoxication has caused aggression, illness, injury, and pathology to impede resilience (Brotchie et al. 2004; Haapanen-Niemi et al. 1999). Recklessness reflects risking to weaken health and raise crime and violence, thus blocking resilience (Farrington 2018; Pulkkinen et al. 2009; Taubman-Ben-Ari and Findler 2003; Wickrama et al. 1995). Suicidality has induced anxiety to obstruct resilience (Cheng et al. 2017). Adventuring has stemmed from doping, minority status, and neuroticism to weaken power for driving resilience (Koegl and Day 2019; Zhang et al. 2010). Doping has engendered depression, thus jeopardizing resilience (Kendler et al. 2006). Minority status has dampened life quality to hurt resilience (Verschuur et al. 2010). Neuroticism has worsened well-being, including autonomy, growth, health, positive affect, purposefulness, relatedness, satisfaction, self-acceptance, self-compassion, and self-determination, to resist resilience (Anusic et al. 2014; Hounkpatin et al. 2015; Ingledew et al. 2004; Pfattheicher et al. 2017; Richards 2016; Webster et al. 2014). Adventuring arises from a cognitive deficit, emotionality, hypersensitivity, meaninglessness, negative mood, resentment, and uncertainty to weaken power for driving resilience (Chuang and Lin 2007; Defoe et al. 2015; Howard and Alipour 2014; Lyng et al. 2009; Parker and Stanworth 2005). Adventuring can grow from anxiety and impulsivity, thus weakening power to drive resilience (Vermeersch et al. 2011). Cognitive deficit or low intelligence has impeded social capital and diminished criminality and depression, thus facilitating resilience (Cornwall 2009; Feinstein and Bynner 2006). Emotionality has dampened well-being, including autonomy, growth, health, positive affect, purposefulness, relatedness, relational quality, satisfaction, self-acceptance, self-compassion, and self-determination, to hamper resilience (Anusic et al. 2014; Austin et al. 2005; Hounkpatin et al. 2015; Ingledew et al. 2004; Marks 1996; Pfattheicher et al. 2017; Richards 2016; Webster et al. 2014). Sensitivity has bred anger, anxiety, depression, and shyness and weakened self-efficacy to hinder resilience (Chen et al. 2023; Cuadrado et al. 2015; Wu et al. 2022). Uncertainty has arisen from dissatisfaction to forestall resilience (Noack et al. 2001).

Utility to attract resilience falling by adventuring has concerned controllability experienced and relational satisfaction (Dodge and Jaccard 2002; Wickrama et al. 1995). Controllability experienced has boosted well-being, including health and life satisfaction as opposed to anger and depression, to maintain resilience (Etezadi and Pushkar 2013. Heidemeier and Staudinger 2012; Rose 2000; Xi and Hwang 2011). Adventuring reflects low gain and opportunity experienced as disutility to disincentivize resilience (Levy 2013). Gain experienced has raised well-being, including satisfaction as opposed to anger, anxiety, and depression, to foster resilience (Helgeson et al. 2006; Wells et al. 1999; Wong and Lam 2016). Opportunity experienced has reflected social inclusion, respect, and supported received to buttress resilience (Wen et al. 2022). Conversely, adventuring has risen from abuse, mortality, and negativity awareness or experienced to compromise utility for attracting resilience (Jessop et al. 2008; Morokoff et al. 2009; Xie and Wang 2003). Abuse experienced has impaired safety experienced and self-respect or self-worth to erode resilience (Fernandes 2018; Krahe 2013). Mortality awareness has fomented fear to impede resilience (McManus 2017). Adventuring reflects difficulty, failure, loss, mortality, social exclusion, and threat experienced to impair utility for attracting resilience (Jessop et al. 2008; Levy 2013; Muenks et al. 2021; Parker and Stanworth 2005; Peruzzi 2014). Adventuring can evolve from frustration, harm, and harshness experienced to erode utility for attracting resilience (Finnerty-Myers 2011; Simons et al. 2016; Vermeersch et al. 2011). Difficulty experienced has dampened well-being, including health, life quality, positive affect, and satisfaction as opposed to depression and distress, to impede resilience (Baumeister et al. 2013. Mathis et al. 2016; Raposa et al. 2016; Shrira 2012; Snyder et al. 2020; Zotti et al. 2016). Failure experienced has reflected low happiness and relaxation, thus disrupting resilience (Lyubomirsky et al. 2005; Mehrabian 2000). Loss experienced has bred anger and depression to negate resilience (Wells et al. 1999). Social exclusion experienced has fomented negative mood and life dissatisfaction to hinder resilience (Lin et al. 2013; Williams et al. 2000). Threat experienced has fomented anxiety, avoidance, conflict, depression, fear, and hate to disrupt resilience (Edwards and Arnon 2021; MacLeod 2017; Moore and Shepherd 2006; O'Neill and Evans 1999; Rick et al. 2006; Ruiter et al. 2003).

Ideals for rationaling resilience reduced by adventuring have emphasized compliance, health, and prevention (Chan et al. 2024; Steffen and Cheng 2022; Umeh 2004). The ideal for compliance has buttressed compliance (Van Damme 2017). Compliance has furnished achievement and its pressure, mastery-goal setting, social closeness and support received, and tolerance to benefit resilience (Feldman 2003; Jiang et al. 2015; Magnuson et al. 2006). Health value has arisen from health to facilitate resilience (Whynes and Sach 2007). The ideal for prevention has buttressed prevention (Pires 2022). Prevention has benefitted from control and self-efficacy to enable resilience (Cheng and Ng 2006; McMahon et al. 2015). Adventuring contests legalism as an ideal to rationalize resilience (Zhang 2005). Legalism reduces panic and reflects identity and development to boost resilience (Cohn and White 1990; Drinkard et al. 2017; Shek et al. 2022a). Adventuring has stemmed from low ideals for calculation or deliberation, consideration, education, responsibility, and work, thus discouraging resilience (Axinn et al. 1999; Dodge and Jaccard 2002; Kloep et al. 2009); Vaughan et al. 2019). Calculation, consideration, or deliberation has established meaningfulness to facilitate resilience (Baumeister et al. 2013). The ideal for responsibility has upheld responsibility (Shahzalal and Adnan 2022). Responsibility has incubated self-efficacy to enable resilience (Braun-Lewensohn 2016). Work value has reflected financial satisfaction to induce resilience (Kiecolt 2003). Adventuring can rise from ideals against tolerance, thus dispelling resilience (Miller-Day 2004). Tolerance has sustained health, life satisfaction, and social trust to enhance resilience (Appleton and Song 2008; Stafford et al. 2005; Uslaner 2002). Adventuring involves an ideal against protection to discourage resilience (Morokoff et al. 2009). Protection arises from its ideal (Gonzalez-Castro et al. 2021). As such, protection has uplifted self-enhancement to safeguard resilience (Erickson and Feldstein 2007). Adventuring emerges from an ideal against sociality, thus rejecting resilience (Lyng et al. 2009). The social ideal has championed relationship quality to boost resilience (Jorgensen and Nelson 2018). Conversely, adventuring has fostered ideals for crime and violence to refute resilience (Farrington 2018; Pulkkinen et al. 2009). The ideal for crime has rationalized crime (Tanner-Smith et al. 2013). Crime has eroded life satisfaction, mastery, relationship quality, self-efficacy, and self-esteem to weaken resilience (Chung and Elias 1996; Keijsers et al. 2011; Shek 2005). The ideal for violence has originated from anger and contempt as opposed to self-efficacy to impair resilience (Tausch et al. 2011). Adventuring embodies the ideal for militancy to dispel resilience (Zhang 2018). The ideal for militancy has rationalized militancy (Hwang and Kim 2015). Militancy has triggered anger and worry to dampen resilience (Boehnke and Wong 2011; Landmann and Rohmann 2020). Adventuring involves ideals for disconnection and escapism to dissuade resilience (Morris and Orton-Johnson 2024). Disconnection has eroded well-being, including community, flourishing, health, identity, life satisfaction, and pride, thus obstructing resilience (Chua et al. 2021; Yetim and Yetim 2014). Escapism has inhibited well-being to impede resilience (Kaczmarek and Drążkowski 2014). Adventuring has stemmed from hedonism as an ideal to impede resilience (Kloep et al. 2009). Hedonism has bred depression, shoplifting, substance abuse, and suicide and lowered self-esteem, thus impeding resilience (Bjarnason 2009). Adventuring springs from cynicism, nihilism, and skepticism as ideals against resilience (Lyng et al. 2009). Cynicism has reflected low life satisfaction and self-efficacy to impede resilience (Moreno-Jimenez and Villodres 2010; Schmuck et al. 2022). Nihliism has fomented depression and negative affect and dampened life satiscation, meaningfulness, positive affect, and purposeiveness to hinder resilience (Forsythe and Mongrain 2023). Skepticism can engender tension and erode intimacy and satisfaction to impede resilience (Theiss 2018).

Norms underlying adventuring have discounted cautiousness, control, and warmth to dispel resilience (Grasmick et al. 1996; Morrissey 2008; Nelson et al. 2015). Cautiousness has upheld self-compassion to induce resilience (Pyszkowska 2020). Control has evolved from its norm (Usher and Pajares 2006). Eventually, control has uplifted health maintenance, optimism, power, prevention, social trust, and well-being to elevate resilience (Cheng and Ng 2006; Etezadi and Pushkar 2013; Keltener et al. 2008; Moore and Aweiss 2003; Smith and Stasson 2000; Steinhardt 2012). The norm for warmth has reflected relationship quality to sustain resilience (Chen and Kaplan 2001). Adventuring has arisen from norms against education and income to discourage resilience (Baril et al. 2007; Vandell et al. 2020). The norm for education has enhanced education (Andersson 2004). Education has sustained well-being, including health, identity, life quality and satisfaction, mastery, self-efficacy, self-esteem, and youthfulness to engender resilience (Cerin and Leslie 2008; Corcoran et al. 2011; James and Amato 2013; Pakulshi and Tranter 2000; Stavrova and Ehlebracht 2018; van Praag and Frijters 1999; Whyte and Gao 2009; Yienprugsawan et al. 2010). The norm for income has raised income (Zhou 2019). Income has afforded well-being, including adaptation, adequacy, belongingness, control, eudaemonia, health, mastery, power, quality of life, satisfaction, self-efficacy, self-esteem, and social well-being to sustain resilience (Anciaes et al. 2017; Carpiano 2008; Corcoran et al. 2011; Ross and Mirowsky 1989; Sengupta and Sibley 2019; Son and Wilson 2012; Wang and VanderWeele 2011; Yeh et al. 2013; Zimmerman and Reyna 2013). Conversely, adventuring arises from norms for deviance and risk to discourage resilience (Lawy 2002; Simons et al. 2016). The norm of deviance has assimilated deviance (Kobayashi et al. 2019). Eventually, deviance has eroded health, thus impairing resilience (Backman and Nilsson 2011). The norm for risk perceived has eroded adjustment, happiness, life satisfaction, positive affect, self-determination and sustained anxiety and fear, depression, negative affect, and sadness, thus undermining resilience (Prelow et al. 2004; Schoon 2006; Schwartz and Melech 2000; Shippee 2012; Vuori 2015). Adventuring has sprung from norms for conflict, poverty, suicidality, and violence to deter resilience (Baril et al. 2007; Hagan and Foster 2001; Harding 2003). The norm for conflict has bred conflict (Amato and Chendle 2005). Conflict has weakened well-being, including life and marital satisfaction, to hamper resilience (Baumeister et al. 2013; Mikula et al. 2012; Richards 2016). The norm of poverty has underlain poverty (Dekkers 2008). Poverty has inhibited well-being and fomented strain to withhold resilience (Clark et al. 2008; Walker et al. 2010). The norm of suicidality has assimilated suicidality (Zimmerman 1992). Suicidality has induced anxiety to obstruct resilience (Cheng et al. 2017). The norm for violence has degraded neighborhood quality to jeopardize resilience (Sampson and Raudenbush 2004).

## *Carnival Activity*

Carnival activity is recreational activity characterized by bodily involvement, celebration, freedom, indulgence, intoxication, performance, sexuality, and spectacle as opposed to submissiveness, creativity, hierarchy, and restriction (Halnon 2006; Wadds et al. 2022). Particularly, carnival activity features grotesqueness characterized by disgusting, exaggeration, and obscenity as opposed to morality (Halnon 2006). Nevertheless, carnival activity, reflecting recreational activity, may sustain resilience by generating power, utility, ideals, and norms to achieve functioning based on analytical voluntarism.

Power generated by recreational activity to drive resilience stems from flow or absorption, life quality, and social integration experienced (Steinkamp and Kelly 1987; Walker et al. 1998). Flow has boosted competence, motivation, and relatedness to safeguard resilience (Kowal and Fortier 1999). Social integration has eroded depression to bolster resilience (Mullins and Dugan 1991). Recreational activity can promote choice, community, freedom, health, responsibility, self-development, social capital, solidarity, spontaneity experienced, and well-being generally to secure power to drive resilience (Arai and Pedlar 1997; Kuentzel 2000; Rojek 2005; Tink et al. 2020). Choice experienced has buttressed competence, effort and performance, life and neighborhood satisfaction, motivation, and self-determination to safeguard resilience (Day 2013; Gagne and Deci 2005; Helliwell et al. 2010; Patall et al. 2008). The sense of community has strengthened rewards to induce resilience (Nelson-Coffey et al. 2023). Freedom has enabled well-being, including health, life satisfaction, and self-esteem, as opposed to depression and symptoms to facilitate resilience action (Abbott et al. 2011; Glendinning et al. 2003; Haller and Hadler 2006). Responsibility has advanced wisdom to facilitate resilience (Spengler et al. 2018). Self-development has reflected self-esteem to maintain resilience (DeMarree and Rios 2014). Social capital has fostered well-being, including flourishing, happiness, health, life satisfaction, pride, and the sense of community to safeguard resilience (Chua et al. 2021; Yetim and Yetim 2014). Solidarity has enabled adjustment, hope, and life satisfaction to secure resilience (Dittman and Goebel 2010; James and Hunsley 1995; Paez et al. 2015). Spontaneity has furnished self-efficacy to drive resilience (Davelaar et al. 2008). Recreational activity involves affiliation, agency, flexibility, identity, intimacy, inspiration experienced, pleasure or ecstasy, self-realization to sustain power for driving resilience (Blackshaw 2017; Kyle and Chick 2004; Rojek 2005). Agency has maintained mastery, relational quality, satisfaction, and vitality to facilitate resilience (Delhey 2010; Hui et al. 2013; Ross and Drentea 1998; Sieber et al. 2019). Affiliation has strengthened rewards to induce resilience (Nelson-Coffey et al. 2023). Flexibility has buttressed life satisfaction and self-esteem as opposed to distress to enable resilience (Jen et al. 2019). Identity has secured happiness, love, self-efficacy, and self-esteem and has diminished anxiety and depression to facilitate resilience (Cast 2004). Inspiration has raised meaningfulness, positive affect, and well-being to induce resilience (Ji et al. 2021; Thrash et al. 2010). Intimacy has sustained purposiveness, relationship satisfaction, and self-efficacy and has dampened anxiety to facilitate resilience (Arseth et al. 2009; Chou 2000; Hand et al. 2013; Henderson et al. 2009). Recreational activity has built on attachment, competence, control, and education to supply power to drive resilience (Laverie and Arnett 2000; Lawton et al. 2002; Wu, Liu, and Wang 2010). Attachment has buttressed life satisfaction to enable resilience (Zdrenka et al. 2015). Competence has enabled identity achievement, intimacy, and relationship satisfaction, as opposed to anxiety, to raise resilience (Adams 1985). Control has boosted well-being, including health and life satisfaction, as opposed to anger and depression, to maintain resilience (Etezadi and Pushkar 2013; Heidemeier and Staudinger 2012; Rose 2000; Xi and Hwang 2011). Education has sustained well-being, including health, identity, life quality and satisfaction, mastery, self-efficacy, self-esteem, and youthfulness to engender resilience (Cerin and Leslie 2008; Corcoran et al. 2011; James and Amato 2013; Pakulshi and Tranter 2000; Stavrova and Ehlebracht 2018; van Praag and Frijters 1999; Whyte and Gao 2009; Yienprugsawan et al. 2010).

Utility offered by recreational activity to attract resilience has rested on benefit or gain expeirnced, leisure, and life satisfaction (Ragheb and Griffith 1982; Roberts 2004; Roberts et al. 2001; Russell 1990). The former has covered achievement, control, independence, leading, learning, self-development, sharing, socializing, stress relief, and teaching (Searle et al. 1998). Achievement has fostered health, life quality, satisfaction, self-efficacy, and self-esteem as opposed to alienation, depression, and distress to uphold resilience (Donnellan et al. 2005; Fredricks and Eccles 2005; Menard and Mose 1984; Murray 2009; Piko et al. 2006; Tompson and Dass 2000; Xiao et al. 2009). Independence has sustained health and mastery to foster resilience (Lu and Kao 2002; Roy and Chaudhuri 2008). Leading has secured self-efficacy to afford resilience (Shah and Scheufele 2006). Learning has elevated well-being, including life satisfaction and self-efficacy, to facilitate resilience (Denver and Hands 1990; Minnaert and Janssen 1992; Richards 2016). Self-development has reflected self-esteem to maintain resilience (DeMarree and Rios 2014). Sharing has reduced stress, thus maintaining resilience (Lazar and Eisenberger 2022). Socializing has reduced negative emotion and stress to safeguard resilience (Nelson-Coffey et al. 2023). Stress relief has restored well-being, including eudaimonia, health, positive affect, quality of life, neighborhood, and relationships, and satisfaction with life and neighbors, thus facilitating resilience (Baumeister et al. 2013; Greenberg 1999; Jackson et al. 2006; Mathis et al. 2016, Parkes et al. 2002; Shrira 2012; Su et al. 2021; Zotti et al. 2016). Teaching has secured self-efficacy to advance resilience (Lam et al. 2023). Recreational activity can foster equality, reward, and warmth experienced as utility to attract resilience (Blackshaw 2017; Rojek 2005; Tink et al. 2020). Equality experienced has sustained health, homeownership, life satisfaction, self-direction, social capital, and trust to raise resilience (Bond and Lun 2014; Kim and Kawachi 2007; Martin 2000; Meulemann 2010; Nilson 1981; Oishi et al. 2011; Portes and Vickstrom 2011). Warmth experienced has reflected relationship quality to sustain resilience (Chen and Kaplan 2001). Conversely, recreational activity involves low control or domination experienced to maintain utility to attract resilience (Blackshaw 2017). Control experienced has raised distress to attenuate resilience (Overall et al. 2020).

The ideal involved in recreational activity to rationalize resilience is self-discipline (Blackshaw 2017). Self-discipline has built on its ideal (Pintrich et al. 2001). Eventually, self-discipline has arisen from self-esteem to facilitate resilience (Kokkinos and Hatzinikolaou 2011). Recreational activity reflects ideals for coping and social involvement to rationalize resilience. (Frydenberg 2008; Laverie and Arnett 2000). Coping has evolved from its ideal (McClaran et al. 2022). Eventually, coping has raised resilience, environmental and relational quality, growth, health, intimacy, satisfaction, and self-efficacy (Cherry et al. 2023; Chow et al. 2014; Gattino et al. 2015; Lau et al. 2012; Paez et al. 2007; Veenstra et al. 2005; Wills 1997). Social involvement has facilitated self-acceptance to secure resilience (Agronick and Duncan 1998).

Norms reflected by recreational activity favor cohesion and education to assimilate resilience (Cradock et al. 2009). The norm for cohesion has assimilated cohesion (Volker et al. 2007). Cohesion has buttressed hope and life satisfaction and eroded depression to maintain resilience (Araya et al. 2006; Dittman and Goebel 2010; Paez et al. 2015). The norm for education has enhanced education (Andersson 2004). Education has sustained well-being, including health, identity, life quality and satisfaction, mastery, self-efficacy, self-esteem, and youthfulness to engender resilience (Cerin and Leslie 2008; Corcoran et al. 2011; James and Amato 2013; Pakulshi and Tranter 2000; Stavrova and Ehlebracht 2018; van Praag and Frijters 1999; Whyte and Gao 2009; Yienprugsawan et al. 2010).

## *Musical Activity*

Musical activity is artistic activity that creates an atmosphere of harmony for communication and expression (Alain et al. 2019; Palmer and Griscom 2013; Sun et al. 2024; Yang et al. 2022). Essentially, musical activity features ease, harmony, order, rhythm, and tempo (Wong 2012). Musical activity is likely to induce resilience by furnishing power, utility, ideals, and norms to leverage the voluntaristic mechanism to achieve functioning emphasized in analytical functionalism.

Power enhanced by musical activity to drive resilience has stemmed from well-being, including connectedness, emotional well-being, energy or vigor, relational quality, and self-esteem (Clements-Cortes 2017; Fu and Tu 2023; Rose-Krasnor et al. 2005; Swarbrick and Vuoskoski 2023; Wallace and Harwood 2018; Yang et al. 2022). Connectedness has afforded well-being, including flourishing, happiness, health, life satisfaction, and pride, as opposed to depression and distress, to champion resilience (Chua et al. 2021; Congdon 2010; Yetim and Yetim 2014). Vigor has enhanced satisfaction and reduced depression and symptoms to maintain resilience (Adrian et al. 2018; Rose 2003). Musical activity has facilitated empathy, friendship, functionality, and intelligence to uphold power to drive resilience (Broh 2002; Hanna-Pladdy and MacKay 2011; Wallace and Harwood 2018). Empathy has facilitated intimacy and communication quality to facilitate resilience (Redmond 2018). Friendship has built on health, satisfaction, and fearlessness to sustain resilience (Child and Nikolova 2020; Eberl 2020; Sampson 1991). Functionality has boosted satisfaction with housing, leisure, and life to induce resilience (Granzin and Haggard 2000; Michalos et al. 2000). Musical activity functions to achieve autonomy, freedom, harmony, and serenity to secure power to drive resilience (Griffin et al. 2018; Lin 1988). Autonomy has raised well-being, including energy, health, mastery, meaningfulness, positive affect, pride, satisfaction, self-efficacy, and self-esteem, to boost resilience (Au and Cheung 2004; De Moortel et al. 2015; Erickson 2008; Garcia et al. 2017; Gahlawat et al. 2019; Hodson 1996; Martela and Riekki 2018; Schieman 2002; Schieman and Narisada 2014; Yoon 2001). Freedom has enabled well-being, including health, life satisfaction, and self-esteem, as opposed to depression and symptoms to facilitate resilience action (Abbott et al. 2011; Glendinning et al. 2003; Haller and Hadler 2006). Harmony or serenity has afforded life satisfaction and dampened depression to maintain resilience (Yang 2016). Musical activity embodies transcendence to uphold power to drive resilience (TenHouten 2017). Transcendence has maintained life satisfaction and meaningfulness and impeded anxiety, depression, and stress to enhance resilience (Fishbein et al. 2020). Musical activity has benefitted from education and verbal ability to furnish power to drive resilience (Jankovic and Bogaerts 2021; Van Eijck 2001). Education has sustained well-being, including health, identity, life quality and satisfaction, mastery, self-efficacy, self-esteem, and youthfulness to engender resilience (Cerin and Leslie 2008; Corcoran et al. 2011; James and Amato 2013; Pakulshi and Tranter 2000; Stavrova and Ehlebracht 2018; van Praag and Frijters 1999; Whyte and Gao 2009; Yienprugsawan et al. 2010). Musical activity can hinge on social class to afford power to drive resilience (Haynes and Nowak 2021). Social class has sustained well-being, including financial adequacy, health, hope, and satisfaction, as opposed to depression to advance resilience (Burke 2008; Davis and Davenport 1999; Haller and Hadler 2006; Hadjar and Samuel 2015; Peterson and Seligman 2004; Yamaoka 2008). Verbal ability has enabled self-efficacy to dirve resilience (Soller et al. 2017). Conversely, musical activity prevents dementia, thus retaining power to drive resilience (Bright 1992). Dementia obstructs satisfaction, thus preventing resilience (Henry and Capitman 1995).

Utility generated by musical activity to attract resilience has resided in achievement (Broh 2002). Achievement has fostered health, life quality, satisfaction, self-efficacy, and self-esteem as opposed to alienation, depression, and distress to uphold resilience (Donnellan et al. 2005; Fredricks and Eccles 2005; Menard and Mose 1984; Murray 2009; Piko et al. 2006; Tompson and Dass 2000; Xiao et al. 2009). Musical activity can heighten similarity experienced to attract resilience. Similarity experienced has diminished depression (Tan et al. 2010), thus sustaining resilience (Riad and Norris 1992).

Ideals facilitated by musical activity to rationalize resilience have emphasized coordination, empathy, and studying (Broh 2002; Colverson et al. 2021; Wallace and Harwood 2018). Music activity can facilitate ideals for continuation and sharing to rationalize resilience (Tan et al. 2010). Coordination has developed from its ideal (Michael et al. 2020). Furthermore, coordination has benefitted from networking, solidarity, support received, and trust (Miao et al. 2018; Ng et al. 2004). The ideal for empathizing has consolidated empathy (Mestre et al. 2018). Empathy has raised intimacy and communication quality to enhance resilience (Redmond 2018). The ideal for studying has boosted achievement to engage resilience (Liu and Yu 2016). Conversely, musical activity has eroded ideals for delinquency and violence to rationalize resilience (Krahe 2013; Rose-Krasnor et al. 2005). The ideal of delinquency has bred delinquency (Hati et al. 2019). Delinquency has jeopardized achievement, coping, education, mastery, life satisfaction, relational quality, self-efficacy, self-esteem, social attachment, and social capital in the youth to impede resilience (Carroll et al. 2009; Chung and Elias 1996; Compas et al. 1988; Fasang et al. 2014; Gault-Sherman 2012; Shek 2005). The ideal for violence has bred depression and stress in the youth (Muradwij and Allwood 2022).

## *Nation-Related Activity*

Nation-related activity functions to build nationalism (Kuah-Pearce and Fong 2010). Nationalism represents conservatism to hail the nation and its culture, ethnicity, history, language, religion, sovereignty, and/or territory (Gao et al. 2021; Moore 2010; Katartzi 2018; Smith 2010; Wiltgren 2014). Essentially, nationalism embodies activeness, anti-foreignness, competition, dominance, hegemony, idealization, particularism, racism, self-determination, struggling, success, and superiority or supremacy (Federico et al. 2023; Moore 2010; Pinto et al. 2020; Ozkirimli 2005; Tartakovsky 2011; Whigham 2019; Wiltgren 2014). Nationalism features authoritarianism, belongingness, chauvinism, communiutarianism, contractarianism, differentiation or division, fanaticism, fascism, glorification, historicism, imperialism, institutionalization, militarism or warfare, nativism, patriotism, pleasure based on influence and reputation, pride, racism, sacrifice, symbolism, terrorism, threat sensitivity, tribalism, xenophobia, we-ness, and values on attachment, autonomy or independence, commonness, government or regulation, homogeneity, leadership, legitimacy, loyalty,, order, purity, sovereignty, unity, and voting (Baldwin et al. 2018; Blank 2003; Coenders and Scheepers 2003; Fuchs 2020; Fukuyama 2018; Moore 2001; Ozkirimli 2005; Smith 2010; Sutherland 2012; Thomas 2002; Vadher and Barrett 2009; Yack 2012). Communitarian nationalism hails culture, ethnicity, the family, harmony, history, morality, and socialization (Thomas 2002). Contractarian nationalism highlights succor and balance between duty and rights (Thomas 2002). Conversely, nationalism rejects colonialism, equality, globalization or globalism, individualism, and liberalism (Fuchs 2020; Massey et al. 2003; Wang 2006). Nation-related activity in securing nationalism is likely to boost resilience by providing power, utility, ideals, and norms to sustain functioning, as predicated on analytical functionalism.

Power afforded by nationalism to drive resilience has arisen from attachment, identity, knowledge, religiousness, and well-being (Huddy and Khatib 2007; Kunovich and Hodson 1999; Lalot et al. 2023; Rippl et al. 2010; Ziemes et al. 2019). Attachment has buttressed life satisfaction to enable resilience (Zdrenka et al. 2015). Identity has secured happiness, love, self-efficacy, and self-esteem and has diminished anxiety and depression to facilitate resilience (Cast 2004). Knowledge has underlain power, prevention, protection, satisfaction, self-efficacy, spirituality, tolerance, economic resources, and social resources and trust to facilitate resilience (Bish and Michie 2010; Chang and Hsu 2016; Cheng and Ng 2006; Ertz et al. 2021; Mutz and Mondak 2006; Norris 2011; Nunkoo 2015; Pattie et al. 2004; Rothwell et al. 2016). Religiousness has sustained well-being, including adjustment, flourishing, health, life satisfaction, mastery, positive affect, relational quality, self-esteem, and socioemotional well-being to facilitate resilience (Chang 2009; Dy-Liacco et al. 2009; Flouri and Buchanan 2002; Helliwell and Putnam 2005; Moschis and Ong 2011; Ng and Fisher 2016; Schieman 2001; Skerkat and Ellison 1999; Wuthnow 2004). Nationalism secures citizenship, civic engagement, community, development, liberation, and social trust to accrue power to drive resilience. (Brubaker 2004; Fukuyama 2018b; Moore 2001; Osborne et al. 2017; Ozkirimli 2005; Umana-Taylor et al. 2020). Citizenship has fostered well-being, including mental and physical health, to elevate resilience (Tsai et al. 2018). Civic engagement has incubated conflict resolution, education, happiness, health, income, individualism, life satisfaction, security normativity, social attachment, capital, integration, trust, tolerance, and general well-being to advance resilience (Coffe and Geys 2007; Goren 2005; Growiec and Growiec 2010; Kroll 2011; Li and Walder 2001; Myers 1999; Pena-Lopez and Sanchez-Santos 2016; Posel and Casale 2011; Tak 2017; Tang 2011; Wallace and Pichler 2009; Welzel 2013; van Ingen and Bekkers 2015; Vincens et al. 2018). The sense of community has strengthened rewards to induce resilience (Nelson-Coffey et al. 2023). Development has facilitated success experienced to attract resilience (Spengler et al. 2018). Liberation has lifted well-being, including health, life satisfaction, and self-esteem, as opposed to depression and symptoms to advance resilience (Gehring 2013; Glendinning et al. 2003; Haller and Hadler 2006). Social trust has fostered health and survival to sustain resilience (Barefoot et al. 1998). Nationalism can enhance self-esteem to secure power to drive resilience (Tartakovsky 2011). Nationalism registers the power of flourishing, fulfillment, and ritual to drive resilience (Dekker et al. 2003; Ozkirimli 2005; Whigham 2019). Ritual involvement has sustained well-being, including health, intimacy, and pleasure (Crespo et al. 2008; Rossner and Meher 2014; Yang and Wang 2023). Nationalism evolves from social integration to secure power to drive resilience (Brubaker 2004). Social integration has eroded depression to bolster resilience (Mullins and Dugan 1991). Nationalism features belongingness, commonness, loyalty, pleasure, and pride to muster power to drive resilience (Blank 2003; Fuchs 2020; Ozkirimli 2005; Sutherland 2012; Yack 2012). Belongingness has strengthened rewards to induce resilience (Nelson-Coffey et al. 2023). Commonness has eroded depression and negative affect, thus safeguarding resilience (McIntyre et al. 2023; Stanton et al. 2020). Loyalty has facilitated self-acceptance to secure resilience (Agronick and Duncan 1998). Nationalism has developed from curiosity, emotional stability, encouragement received, extraversion, homeownership, income and family income, and self-control as power to drive resilience (Blank 2003; Fairbrother 2003; Lee 2020; Norris and Inglehart 2009; Schbley and McCauley 2005; Steinhardt et al. 2018). Nationalism can benefit from power, notably based on advantaged status, motivation for meaning, and need for superiority to drive resilience (Finell and Liebkind 2010; Jang et al. 2022; van Tilburg and Lgou 2011). Curiosity has facilitated flow and creativity to enable resilience (Schutte and Malouff 2020). Emotional stability has buttressed control, forgiveness, intelligence, spirituality, success, uplift experience, and well-being to raise resilience (Hounknatin et al. 2014; Lincoln et al. 2003; Maltby et al. 2016; Maybery et al. 2006; Mullet et al. 2005; Schaie 2013; Steca et al. 2017). Encouragement received has boosted well-being, including development, identity, recovery, and self-efficacy to buttress resilience (Berkowitz et al. 2006; Grealish et al. 2017; Gullan et al. 2013). Extraversion has shaped autonomy and self-determination, coping, emotional intelligence, growth, humor, mastery, positive affect, purposefulness, relatedness, satisfaction with appearance, life, and weight, security experienced, self-acceptance, self-efficacy, social support received, spirituality, and uplift experience to facilitate resilience (Anusic et al. 2014; Becker et al. 1997; Bishop 2015; Celso et al. 2003; Frederick et al. 2016; Hounkpatin et al. 2015; Ingledew et al. 2004; Judge et al. 2002; MacDonald and Friedman 2002; Matthews et al. 2012; Maybery et al. 2006; Quilty et al. 2006; Richards 2016; Vernon et al. 2008). Homeownership has raised health, morale, family and neighborhood quality, and financial, housing, life, and neighborhood satisfaction as opposed to depression, distress, and fear to strengthen resilience (Congdon 2010; Harris 2001; Lee et al. 2022; Mirowsky and Ross 1999; Montazer 2022; Roy and Chaudhuri 2008; Wulfhorst and Kranich 1999; Yu and Chiu 2016; Zheng et al. 2020). Income has afforded well-being, including adaptation, adequacy, belongingness, control, eudaemonia, health, mastery, power, quality of life, satisfaction, self-efficacy, self-esteem, and social well-being to sustain resilience (Anciaes et al. 2017; Carpiano 2008; Corcoran et al. 2011; Ross and Mirowsky 1989; Sengupta and Sibley 2019; Son and Wilson 2012; Wang and VanderWeele 2011; Yeh et al. 2013; Zimmerman and Reyna 2013). Family income has enabled financial adequacy, health and mental health, identity, the living standard, mastery, neighborhood quality, satisfaction, self-efficacy, and self-esteem, as opposed to mortality and strain to boost resilience (Ambrey and Fleming 2014; Becchetta 2010; Cerin and Leslie 2008; Kunovich 2009; Oliver 2003; Phelan et al. 2004; Powdthavee 2009; Thoits and Hewitt 2001; Whyte and Gao 2009; Woldoff and Ovadia 2009). Self-control has eroded anxiety, crime, depression, risking, victimization experienced, violence, and vulnerability, thus favoring resilience (Koegl and Day 2019; Langenderfer and Shimp 2001; Marchetti et al. 2018; Zavala and Guadalupe-Diaz 2019).

Utility generated by nationalism to attract resilience has resided in life satisfaction and popularity experienced (Chang and Kang 2018; Umana-Taylor et al. 2020). Nationalism affords fairness or justice and recognition experienced as utility to attract resilience (Moore 2001; Ozkirimli 2005). Fairness or justice experienced has lifted positive mood, life satisfaction, and self-esteem to sustain resilience (Dalbert 2001). Recognition experienced has uplifted positive affect and self-esteem and reduced negative affect, thus buttressing resilience (Reich et al. 2018). Nationalism can reflect security and success experienced as utility to attract resilience (Lee 2020; Wiltgren 2014). Security experienced has boosted well-being, including health, life satisfaction, and neighborhood quality, as opposed to fear, to induce resilience (Chen et al. 2008; Frey et al. 2007; Olson et al. 2016; Jones et al. 2014). Success experienced has fostered health, life quality, satisfaction, self-efficacy, and self-esteem as opposed to alienation, depression, and distress to uphold resilience (Donnellan et al. 2005; Fredricks and Eccles 2005; Menard and Mose 1984; Murray 2009; Piko et al. 2006; Tompson and Dass 2000; Xiao et al. 2009). Conversely, nationalism can arise from low discrimination experienced to retain utility to attract resilience (Fleischmann et al. 2019). Discrimination experienced has raised anomie, depression, distress, and loneliness and has eroded life satisfaction, self-determination, and self-esteem to dampen resilience (Carr and Friedman 2005; Kachanoff et al. 2019; Kirmanoglu and Baslevent 2014; Pachankis et al. 2020; Schnittker 2020; Yang 2019).

Ideals cultivated by nationalism to rationalize resilience have highlighted donation, government trust, inclusion or inclusiveness, patriotism, prosociality, and system justification (Chen 2012; Jost 2020; Osborne et al. 2017; Pinto et al. 2020; Stevenson and Manning 2010). The ideal for donation has propped donation (Vallerand et al. 1992). Eventually, donation has reflected well-being, including control, feeling good, gratitude, happiness, joy, satisfaction, and self-efficacy as opposed to anxiety and guilt, to brew resilience (Bednall et al. 2013; Bekkers 2008; Eayrs and Ellis 1990; Liu and Hao 2017; Mussen 1982; Piliavin and Callero 1991; Wang and Graddy 2008). Identity work comprises exploration and reflection (Hansen et al. 2003). Government trust has induced life and political satisfaction and neighborhood quality to safeguard resilience (Abbott et al. 2011; Greenberg 1999; van Ryzin et al. 2004). Inclusiveness can boost loving, passion, and self-esteem to advance resilience (Allman 2013; Aron et al. 2006; Tomlinson et al. 2018). Patriotism has reflected relational quality and satisfaction to sustain resilience (Lu, Cai, Zheng, Hu, and Song 2018; Opp 2005). The prosocial ideal underlies prosociality (Maltseva 2016). Prosociality has elevated well-being, including connectedness, hope, life satisfaction, meaningfulness, and self-efficacy to boost resilience (Marsh and Dik 2021; Nelson-Coffey et al. 2023; Raposa et al. 2016; Yao and Enright 2019). System justification has upheld positive affect to benefit resilience (Jost and Hunyady 2005). Nationalism stands on ideals for communitarianism and continuity to rationalize resilience (Costelloe 2014; Mayall 2003). Communitarianism has fostered attachment and collective efficacy experienced to boost resilience (Long and Perkins 2007; Perkins and Long 2002). The ideal for continuity has buttressed stability (Zumbrunnen and Gangl 2008). Continuity has raised resilience and relational quality (Lock et al. 2020; Ross et al. 2000). Nationalism embodies ideals for activeness, conservatism, and culture to rationalize resilience (Gao et al. 2021; Moore 2010). Activeness has raised satisfaction to attract resilience (Bonk 2016). Conservatism underlies happiness and meaningfulness to enhance resilience (Dutton and Rayner-Hilles 2022). Cultural activity has boosted life satisfaction to maintain resilience (Roberts et al. 2001). Nationalism benefits from ideals for bonding, choice, and solidarity to rationalize resilience (Moore 2001; Ozkirimli 2005). Bonding has mitigated stress and negative emotion, thus upholding resilience (Nelson-Coffey et al. 2023). Choice rests on its ideal (Patall et al. 2008). As such, choice has buttressed competence, effort and performance, life and neighborhood satisfaction, motivation, and self-determination to safeguard resilience (Day 2013; Gagne and Deci 2005; Helliwell et al. 2010; Patall et al. 2008). Solidarity arises from its ideal (Crow 2002). As such, solidarity has enabled adjustment, hope, and life satisfaction to secure resilience (Dittman and Goebel 2010; James and Hunsley 1995; Paez et al. 2015). Nationalism features ideals for harmony, morality, sharing, and similarity to rationalize resilience (Kim 2018; Smith 2010; Sant and Hanley 2018). Harmony has cultivated life satisfaction and dampened depression to maintain resilience (Yang 2016). Morality has developed from its ideal (Van Kenhove et al. 2003). Consequently, morality has enabled life satisfaction and diminished anger to safeguard resilience (Conzo et al. 2017; Stets et al. 2008). The ideal for sharing has buttressed sharing (Becker and Clement 2006; Xia and Yang 2020). Sharing has reduced stress, thus maintaining resilience (Lazar and Eisenberger 2022). Similarity has strengthened due to its ideal (Granzin and Olsen 1998). As such, similarity has reduced depression to afford resilience (Riad and Norris 1992). Nationalism has arisen from ideals for acceptance, malleability, religion, security, and sport to rationalize resilience (Fleischmann and Phalet 2018; Hong et al. 2006; Lee 2020; Vargas-Salfate et al. 2020). Acceptance has championed well-being, including health, life satisfaction, and social trust to facilitate resilience (Appleton and Song 2008; Stafford et al. 2005; Uslaner 2002). Malleability rests on its ideal (Pyszkowska 2020). As such, malleability has buttressed life satisfaction and self-esteem as opposed to distress to enable resilience (Jen et al. 2019). The ideal for religion has sustained well-being, including adjustment, flourishing, health, mastery, positive affect, relationship quality, satisfaction with democracy, police, finance, and life, self-esteem, and socioemotional well-being to lift resilience (Dy-Liacco et al. 2009; Flouri and Buchanan 2002; Helliwell and Putnam 2005; Kwak et al. 2010; Marx 2014; Meulemann 2010; Moschis and Ong 2011; Ng and Fisher 2016; Schieman 2001; Skerkat and Ellison 1999; Van Praag et al. 2010; Wuthnow 2004). Security has escalated intimacy and satisfaction and eroded anger, anxiety, loneliness, and regret to raise resilience (Alonso-Arbiol et al. 2007; Buelow et al. 1996; Gillath et al. 2005; Kafetsio and Sideridis 2006; Lavy et al. 2010). Sporting has contributed to health, income, and social capital and has reduced depression (Growiec and Growiec 2010; Kunovich and Hudson 1999; Lee 2020; Luschen et al. 1996; Meeus 2019). Conversely, nationalism has withheld ideals for extremism and protesting to maintain resilience (Flanagan and Lee 2000; Yu et al. 2023; Miglietta et al. 2018). Extremism has reflected anomie, anxiety, self-uncertainty, and uncertainty to erode resilience (Hogg et al. 2010; Koehler and Fiebig 2019; Stankov et al. 2018). The ideal for protesting has constituted protesting (Hwang and Kim 2015). Protesting has invoked anger and worry to counter resilience feeling (Boehnke and Wong 2011; Landmann and Rohmann 2020). Nationalism has emerged from the ideal against skepticism to rationalize resilience (Fairbrother 2003). Skepticism can engender tension and erode intimacy and satisfaction to impede resilience (Theiss 2018).

The norm sustained by nationalism has popularized nationalism to assimilate resilience (Karasawa 2003). Hence, nationalism can reinforce itself and its contribution to resilience. Moreover, nationalism maintains norms for achievement, safety, and security to assimilate resilience (Fukuyama 2018b; Ozkirimli 2005). The norm for achievement has assimilated achievement (Cullen and Jacob 2009; Gremmen et al. 2017; Teachman 1996). Achievement has fostered health, life quality, satisfaction, self-efficacy, and self-esteem as opposed to alienation, depression, and distress to uphold resilience (Donnellan et al. 2005; Fredricks and Eccles 2005; Menard and Mose 1984; Murray 2009; Piko et al. 2006; Tompson and Dass 2000; Xiao et al. 2009). The safety norm has escalated well-being, including health and life satisfaction as opposed to fear, to advance resilience (Chen et al. 2008; Frey et al. 2007; Jones et al. 2014). The security norm has boosted well-being, including health, life satisfaction, and neighborhood quality, as opposed to fear, to induce resilience (Chen et al. 2008; Frey et al. 2007; Olson et al. 2016; Jones et al. 2014). Nationalism has stood on norms for acceptance, fitness or congruence, malleability, maintenance, and social status to assimilate resilience (Gharaei et al. 2018; Fleischmann and Phalet 2018; Lee 2020). The acceptance norm has diminished depression, thus sustaining power to drive resilience (Mullins and Dugan 1991). The fitness norm has sustained health, life satisfaction, morale, and power to raise resilience (Li 2006; Pereyra-Rojas et al. 2017; Xie 1996). Malleability has been susceptible to its norm (Karwowski et al. 2020). Eventually, malleability has raised well-being and reduced helplessness to sustain resilience (Ortner and Pennekamp 2020; Pyszkowska and Ronnlund 2021). Maintenance can hinge on its norm (Demerath 2012). Eventually, maintenance has sustained self-acceptance and relieved depression to foster resilience (Agronick and Duncan 1998; Wrosch et al. 2005). The social status norm has boosted achievement to secure resilience (Furstenberg et al. 1999). Nationalism can benefit from the norm for friendliness to assimilate resilience (Stevenson and Muldoon 2010). Friendliness has benefitted from its norm (Mouw and Entwisle 2006). Eventually, friendliness has elevated life satisfaction to attract resilience (Selim 2008). Conversely, nationalism has arisen from the norm against stress (Gharaei et al. 2018). The stress norm has dampened well-being, including health, life quality, positive affect, and satisfaction as opposed to depression and distress, to impede resilience (Baumeister et al. 2013. Mathis et al. 2016; Raposa et al. 2016; Shrira 2012; Snyder et al. 2020; Zotti et al. 2016).

## *Ritual Activity*

Ritual activity characterizes activity that is communicative, compulsory, functioning, identificatory, intentional, interactional, moralistic, normatizing, orchestrated, orderly, regulatory, repetitive, and symbolic (Boyer and Lienard 2006; de Lira and de Morais 2020; Fararo and Doreian 1998; Izenstart and Ebata 2016; Mangion 2011; Schjoedt et al. 2013b; Strenger 2011; Turner 2021; Yang and Wang 2023; Zhang 2003). Essentially, ritual activity features or requires attention or focus, authority and deference, celebration, collectivity, composure, culture, deindividuation, explicitness, extraordinariness, fasting, formality, gifting, logos, meditation, music, nationalism, parading, propriety, religion, responsibility, rhythm, rigidity, sincerity, spectacle, sport, stereotypy, tradition, togetherness, and unity (Annalakshmi and Abeer 2011; Dekker et al. 2003; Boyer and Lienard 2006; Costa 2013;

Brown 2011; Marshall 2002; Xygalatas et al. 2021; Raab 2019; Schjoedt et al. 2013). Togetherness upholds immediacy, similarity, and social facilitation (Marshall 2002). Ritual activity aims to achieve passage, safety, and security and prevents crises and death (Boyer and Lienard 2006; Kwan 2007; McManus 2017). Remarkably, ritual activity reflects resilience (Annalakshmi and Abeer 2011). Moreover, ritual activity is likely to boost resilience by generating power, utility, ideals, and norms to run voluntaristic mechanisms to achieve functioning stipulated in analytical functionalism.

Power secured by ritual activity to drive resilience has stemmed from well-being, including health, intimacy, and pleasure (Rossner and Meher 2014; Turner 2007; Yang and Wang 2023). Ritual activity has fostered attachment, motivation, optimism, and trust to maintain power to drive resilience (Collins 2004; Mazumdar and Mazumdar 2004; Xygalatas et al. 2021). Attachment has raised life satisfaction to rationalize resilience (Zdrenka et al. 2015). Motivation has underlain satisfaction to induce resilience (Ferssizidis et al. 2010). Optimism has enhanced positive affect to enable resilience (Shanahan et al. 2020). Trust has promoted health and survival to secure resilience (Barefoot et al. 1998). Ritual raises belongingness, collective action, ecstasy, energy, loyalty, meaningfulness, stability, and unity or togetherness to muster power to drive resilience (Bulbulia et al. 2013; Hobson et al. 2017; Izenstart and Ebata 2016; Schjoedt et al. 2013; Yang and Wang 2023). Belongingness has strengthened rewards to induce resilience (Nelson-Coffey et al. 2023). Collective action has secure well-being, covering autonomy, coherence, flow, growth, hope, identity, life satisfaction, mastery, meaningfulness, positive affect, relatedness, self-acceptance, self-actualization, self-efficacy, self-esteem, social contribution, and vitality to facilitate resilience (Becker et al. 2011; Klar and Kasser 2009; Landmann and Rohmann 2020; Opp 1989; Paez et al. 2015; Vestergren et al. 2017). Loyalty has facilitated self-acceptance to secure resilience (Agronick and Duncan 1998). Stability has enhanced resilience and relational quality and has reduced anxiety (Lock et al. 2020; Ross et al. 2000). Unity has attenuated depression and negative affect to maintain resilience (McIntyre et al. 2023; Stanton et al. 2020). Ritual activity can benefit functioning, relational quality, and survival to consolidate power to drive resilience (McClemon 2013; Smith and Hamon 2012; SunWolf 2008). Functioning has escalated satisfaction to induce resilience (Granzin and Haggard 2000). Ritual activity registers education, morality or virtuousness, and social capital to offer power to drive resilience (Liu 2004; Mayer 2003; Tse 2007; Zhang 2003). Education has sustained well-being, including health, identity, life quality and satisfaction, mastery, self-efficacy, self-esteem, and youthfulness to engender resilience (Cerin and Leslie 2008; Corcoran et al. 2011; James and Amato 2013; Pakulshi and Tranter 2000; Stavrova and Ehlebracht 2018; van Praag and Frijters 1999; Whyte and Gao 2009; Yienprugsawan et al. 2010). Morality has sustained satisfaction and eroded anxiety to boost resilience (Conzo et al. 2017; Stets et al. 2008). Social capital has raised income or earnings, knowledge, religiosity, social support received, socioeconomic status, and well-being to afford power to boost resilience (Brunie 2009; Chua et al. 2021; Cross and Lin 2008; Pena-Lopez and Sanchez-Santos 2016; Yetim and Yetim 2014; Wuthnow 2004). Ritual activity involves meditation, music, proactiveness, responsibility, and sincerity to procure power to drive resilience (Guo 2018; Marshall 2002; Wong 2012; Raab 2019; Tian et al. 2018). Meditation has advanced compassion or self-compassion and mindfulness and dwindled depression to foster resilience (Galante et al. 2014). Musical involvement has sustained well-being, including connectedness, emotional well-being, energy or vigor, relational quality, and self-esteem, to drive resilience (Clements-Cortes 2017; Fu and Tu 2023; Rose-Krasnor et al. 2005; Swarbrick and Vuoskoski 2023; Wallace and Harwood 2018; Yang et al. 2022). Proactiveness reflects coping and protection to enable resilience (Seaton and Beaumont 2008; Shaw et al. 2023). Responsibility has advanced wisdom to facilitate resilience (Spengler et al. 2018). Sincerely builds on self-esteem to facilitate resilience (Merolla 2014). Conversely, ritual activity has alleviated anxiety and poverty to secure power to drive resilience (Homer et al. 2007; Kotler et al. 2006). Poverty has inhibited well-being and fomented strain to withhold resilience (Clark et al. 2008; Walker et al. 2010).

Utility involved in ritual activity highlights safety and security to attract resilience (Boyer and Lienard 2006). Safety has maintained achievement, life quality, mental health, and sufficiency experienced to foster resilience (Crume et al. 2019). Security experienced has boosted well-being, including health, life satisfaction, and neighborhood quality, as opposed to fear, to induce resilience (Chen et al. 2008; Frey et al. 2007; Olson et al. 2016; Jones et al. 2014).

Ideals fostered by ritual activity to rationalize resilience have prized civility, cohesion, community involvement and service, cooperation, patriotism, religion, regulation, and self-control (Barnes 2005; Collins 2004; Hunter et al. 2013; Taylor et al. 2009; Tian et al. 2018; Wiltermuth and Heath 2009; Wollschleger 2012). Civility has evolved from its ideal (Peterson and Maiden 1993). As such, civility has fostered well-being, including mental and physical health, to elevate resilience (Tsai et al. 2018). Cohesion has developed from its ideal (Granzin and Olsen 1998). As such, cohesion has buttressed hope and life satisfaction and eroded depression to maintain resilience (Araya et al. 2006; Dittman and Goebel 2010; Paez et al. 2015). The ideal for community has fostered attachment and collective efficacy experienced to boost resilience (Long and Perkins 2007, Perkins and Long 2002). Cooperation has thrived on its ideal (Haesevoets et al. 2015). As such, cooperation has fostered life satisfaction to rationalize resilience (Park et al. 2015). Patriotism has reflected relational quality and satisfaction to sustain resilience (Lu et al. 2018; Opp 2005). Religiousness has evolved from its ideal (Hagger et al. 2022). Eventually, religiousness has sustained well-being, including adjustment, flourishing, health, life satisfaction, mastery, positive affect, relational quality, self-esteem, and socioemotional well-being to facilitate resilience (Chang 2009; Flouri and Buchanan 2002; Helliwell and Putnam 2005; Dy-Liacco et al. 2009; Moschis and Ong 2011; Ng and Fisher 2016; Schieman 2001; Skerkat and Ellison 1999; Wuthnow 2004). The ideal for regulation has motivated controlling, domination, or mastery (Cheung and Chiu 2021). Self-control has built on its ideal (Pintrich et al. 2001). Eventually, self-control has maintained self-esteem and reduced anxiety and depression to enable resilience (Armstrong et al. 2011; Marchetti et al. 2018). Ritual activity breeds ideals for culture and order to rationalize resilience (Schjoedt et al. 2013b; Seeman 2004). Cultural activity has fostered resilience and life satisfaction (Corbin and Hall 2019; Roberts et al. 2001). The ideal for order has stemmed from health to enable resilience (Cheung and Lai 2020). Ritual activity can induce the ideal for compliance (Turner 1988). The ideal for compliance has buttressed compliance (Van Damme 2017). Compliance has furnished achievement and its pressure, mastery-goal setting, social closeness and support received, and tolerance to benefit resilience (Feldman 2003; Jiang et al. 2015; Magnuson et al. 2006). Ritual activity embodies ideals for continuity, control, rehabilitation, repetition, and self-cultivation to rationalize resilience (Izenstart and Ebata 2016; Johnston 2010; Mangion 2011; Wang 2012; Yang and Wang 2023). The ideal for continuity or repetition has buttressed stability (Zumbrunnen and Gangl 2008). Continuity or repetition has raised resilience and relational quality (Lock et al. 2020; Ross et al. 2000). The ideal for control has motivated controlling, domination, or mastery (Cheung and Chiu 2021). The ideal for rehabilitation reflects stoicism (Holowchak 2008). Self-cultivation has uplifted resilience (Svetina 2014). Stoicism honors accepting, calmness or equanimity, conservation, controlling, dignity, enduring, invincibility, magnanimity, rehabilitation, resolve, self-control, self-direction, self-love, self-preservation, self-sufficiency, and simplicity to boost resilience (Holowchak 2008; Martin 2016; Mitsis 2003). Persistence has sustained well-being, notably pleasure, to facilitate resilience (Boyes et al. 2017; Goodman et al. 2017). Ritual activity involves ideals for gifting, nationalism, propriety, and sport to rationalize resilience (Boyer and Lienard 2006; Brown 2011; Dekker et al. 2003; Tian et al. 2018; Xygalatas et al. 2021). Nationalism has raised well-being, including life satisfaction, to enable resilience (Lalot et al. 2023; Chang and Kang 2018). Gifting has raised life satisfaction and meaningfulness to induce resilience (d'Astous and Mouakhar-Klouz 2022; Puente-Diaz and Cavazos-Arroyo 2021). The ideal for sporting has propped sporting (Jaf et al. 2021). Propriety reflects ritual activity to raise life satisfaction and diminish anger to safeguard resilience to facilitate resilience (Conzo et al. 2017; Stets et al. 2008). Sporting has contributed to health, income, and social capital and reduced depression (Growiec and Growiec 2010; Kunovich and Hudson 1999; Lee 2020; Luschen et al. 1996; Meeus 2019). Conversely, ritual activity can dampen the ideal for protest to rationalize resilience (Buechler 2011). The ideal for protesting has constituted protesting (Hwang and Kim 2015). Protesting has evoked anger and worry to counter resilience feeling (Boehnke and Wong 2011; Landmann and Rohmann 2020).

The norm established by ritual activity can popularize wellness to assimilate resilience (Paez et al. 2007). The norm of wellness has buttressed well-being, including health and life satisfaction, to uplift resilience (Basabe et al. 2002; Eikemo et al. 2008; Meulemann 2010).

## *Sporting*

Sporting is competition, exercising, or gaming that is physically skillful, planned, structured, and repetitive (Biddle et al. 2015; Frederick-Recascino and Schuster-Smith 2003; McFee 2004). More generally, sporting represents civic engagement and training, reflecting modernization (Bekkers et al. 2008; Durbin 2020; Njoh 2009). Sporting features or upholds business, dignity, equality or non-discrimination, formality or rule-following, friendship, globaltiy or boundarylessness, health or hygiene, nationalism, peace, and spectatorship (Allison 2001; Beesley and Chalip 2011; Beyer 2006; McFee 2004; Moscoso-Sanchez et al. 2015; Njoh 2009; Roche 2002). Remarkably, sporting has propped resilience (Griciute 2015). Sporting is also likely to nurture resilience by enhancing power, utility, ideals, and norms to leverage voluntaristic mechanisms accentuated in analytical functionalism.

Power boosted by sporting to drive resilience has stemmed from control, education, enjoyment or interest, gratitude, health, income, knowledge, leadership, optimism, organizational membership, self-esteem, social attachment, social capital, social integration, social trust, and well-being (Apinunmahakul and Devlin 2008; Bang et al. 2020; Frederick-Recascino and Schuster-Smith 2003; Growiec and Growiec 2010; Lee 2020; Oberle et al. 2019; Pascarella and Terenzini 2005; Reitan and Stenberg 2019; Rose-Krasnor et al. 2005; Snyder and Spreitzer 1992; Sukys et al. 2015; Zanin 2017). Control has uplifted health maintenance, optimism, power, prevention, social trust, and well-being to elevate resilience (Cheng and Ng 2006; Etezadi and Pushkar 2013; Keltener et al. 2008; Moore and Aweiss 2003; Smith and Stasson 2000; Steinhardt 2012). Education has sustained well-being, including health, identity, life quality and satisfaction, mastery, self-efficacy, self-esteem, and youthfulness to engender resilience (Cerin and Leslie 2008; Corcoran et al. 2011; James and Amato 2013; Pakulshi and Tranter 2000; Stavrova and Ehlebracht 2018; van Praag and Frijters 1999; Whyte and Gao 2009). Interest has fostered satisfaction and self-efficacy to facilitate resilience (Gilman 2001; Wen and Cui 2014). Gratitude has raised positive affect and dampened negative affect to achieve resilience (Bernabe-Valero et al. 2021). Income has afforded well-being, including adaptation, adequacy, belongingness, control, eudaemonia, health, mastery, power, quality of life, satisfaction, self-efficacy, self-esteem, and social well-being to sustain resilience (Anciaes et al. 2017; Carpiano 2008; Corcoran et al. 2011; Ross and Mirowsky 1989; Sengupta and Sibley 2019; Son and Wilson 2012; Wang and VanderWeele 2011; Yeh et al. 2013; Zimmerman and Reyna 2013). Knowledge has championed intimacy, satisfaction, and self-efficacy to boost resilience (Mikulincer et al. 2003, Norris 2011; Rothwell et al. 2016). Leadership has secured self-efficacy to afford resilience (Shah and Scheufele 2006). Optimism has enhanced positive affect to enable resilience (Shanahan et al. 2020). Organizational membership has raised outcome expectancy and reduced stress, thus boosting resilience (Nelson-Coffey et al. 2023). Social attachment has raised life satisfaction to rationalize resilience (Zdrenka et al. 2015). Social capital has boosted well-being, including flourishing, happiness, health, life satisfaction, and pride as opposed to depression and distress to champion resilience

(Chua et al. 2021; Congdon 2010; Yetim and Yetim 2014). Social integration has eroded depression to bolster resilience (Mullins and Dugan 1991). Social trust has fostered health and survival to sustain resilience (Barefoot et al. 1998). Well-being has covered resilience, health, self-determination, and self-esteem (Broh 2002; Griciute 2015; Mechanic and Hansell 1987). Self-determination has maintained commitment, effectiveness, and performance to boost resilience (Delhey 2010; Gagne and Deci 2005; Hui et al. 2013; Weinstein and Ryan 2010). Sporting enhances discipline, fitness, friendship, identity, self-confidence, self-efficacy, social inclusion experienced, teamwork, and virtuousness to secure power to drive resilience (Griciute 2015; Eccles and Barber 1999; Graupensperger et al. 2021; Jaeger 2004; Kavussanu and Roberts 2001; Koehler 2017; Tink et al. 2020). Discipline has strengthened well-being, notably self-esteem, to induce resilience (Armstrong et al. 2011; Diener and Fujita 1995). Fitness has elevated health, morale, and satisfaction and has impeded anxiety, depression, and strain to enable resilience (Li 2006; Pereyra-Rojas et al. 2017; Sutherland and Fogarty 1995; Xie 1996). Friendship has stemmed from health and satisfaction with health, leisure, and life as opposed to fear to buttress resilience (Child and Nikolova 2020; Eberl 2020; Sampson 1991). Identity has secured happiness, love, self-efficacy, and self-esteem and has diminished anxiety and depression to facilitate resilience (Cast 2004). Social inclusion experienced enhances resilience and has dampened depression (Mullins and Dugan 1991; Pinkerten and Dolan 2007). Teamwork has enhanced capability use to maintain resilience (Steijn 2001). Virtuousness has sustained satisfaction and eroded anxiety to boost resilience (Conzo et al. 2017; Stets et al. 2008). Sporting would achieve hardworking, loyalty, prestige, superiority, and toughness to muster power to drive resilience (Moscoso-Sanchez et al. 2015; Shor and Yonay 2010; Shakib and Dunbar 2002; Shields and Bredemeier 2005; Stevenson et al. 2008). Hardworking or diligence has bolstered meaningfulness and mindfulness and diminished depression to enable resilience (Galla et al. 2020; Kleiman et al. 2013; Liu et al. 2022). Loyalty has facilitated self-acceptance to secure resilience (Agronick and Duncan 1998). Prestige has sustained coping, health, interaction quality, life satisfaction, self-esteem, and general well-being to secure resilience (Al-krenawi et al. 2011; Caplan and Schooler 2007; Molana and Adams 2019; Staudinger et al. 1999). Superiority has upheld mindfulness and self-esteem to drive resilience (Vonk and Visser 2021). Sporting involves development, dignity, enjoying, excitement, flow, friendship, health, recourse, security, skill, and social closeness to furnish power to drive resilience (Beyer 2006; Hendry et al. 1993; Moscoso-Sanchez et al. 2015; Roche 2002; Stafford 2000; Vilhjalmsson and Thorlindsson 1998; Willig 2012). Development has facilitated success experienced to attract resilience (Spengler et al. 2018). Dignity has upheld well-being, including adjustment, happiness, health, positive affect, and satisfaction with appearance and work to enable resilience (Barnard and Curry 2011; Frederick et al. 2016; Hull et al. 2008; Judge et al. 2002; Williams et al. 1992). Flow has boosted competence, motivation, and relatedness to safeguard resilience (Kowal and Fortier 1999). Recourse has alleviated distress, thus safeguarding resilience (Tracey et al. 1986). Security has escalated well-being, including health and life satisfaction to raise resilience (Chen et al. 2008; Frey et al. 2007; Jones et al. 2014). Skill has underpinned self-efficacy to buttress resilience (Larson et al. 1990). Social closeness has facilitated humor and social support received to lift resilience (Martin et al. 2003). Sporting represents activeness, encouragement received, energy, patience, self-determination, and training to afford power to drive resilience (Durbin 2020; Eccles and Barber 1999; Ntoumanis et al. 2009; Tinsley and Levers 2007; Spreitzer 1994). Activeness has raised satisfaction to attract resilience (Bonk 2016). Encouragement received has boosted well-being, including development, identity, recovery, and self-efficacy to buttress resilience (Berkowitz et al. 2006; Grealish et al. 2017; Gullan et al. 2013). Patience has reduced negative affect to enable resilience (Mehmood et al. 2020). Training has upgraded adjustment, comfort, coherence, cohesiveness, competence, emotional well-being, growth, hope, identity, purposiveness, self-efficacy, self-esteem, thriving, and transcendence to advance resilience (Ashby et al. 2018; Davidson et al. 2012; Duan and Bu 2019; Esbensen and Osgood 1999; Feldman and Dreher 2012; Moote et al. 1999; Ou et al. 2019; Umino and Dammeyer 2018; Youniss and Yates 1997). Sporting has stood on cognitive ability, emotional well-being, recreational experience, sociability, social support received, and socioeconomic status, including education and social class, to secure power to drive resilience (Cradock et al. 2009; Scherger 2009; Spreitzer 1994; Thrasher et al. 2004; Vilhjalmsson and Thorlindsson 1998). Cognitive ability has enhanced social capital and diminished criminality and depression, thus facilitating resilience (Cornwall 2009; Feinstein and Bynner 2006). Recreational experience has fostered life satisfaction to induce resilience (Roberts et al. 2001). Sociability has enhanced well-being to buttress resilience (Bjornskov 2008). Social support received has boosted resilience (Cherry et al. 2018). Socioeconomic status has upgraded health, interaction quality, life satisfaction, self-confidence, self-esteem, and general well-being and reduced distress and strain to champion resilience (Al-krenawi et al. 2011; Caplan and Schooler 2007; Molana and Adams 2019; Staudinger et al. 1999). Conversely, sporting has diminished anxiety, depression, and stress to retain power to drive resilience (Baron 2007; Bang et al. 2024; Oberle et al. 2019). Sporting has emerged from low disability to maintain power to drive resilience (Scherger 2009). Disability has incurred distress and dampened health, life satisfaction, and self-efficacy, thus eroding resilience (Distante 2013; Gastil 2000; Michalos et al. 2000; Phongsavan et al. 2006).

Utility delivered by sporting to attract resilience has covered achievement, body and life satisfaction, and popularity (Gomez-Baya et al. 2019; Marsh 1993; Morris and Kaljl 2006; Winkelmann 2009). Popularity has uplifted positive affect and self-esteem and reduced negative affect, thus buttressing resilience (Reich et al. 2018). Sporting provides acceptance experienced, entertainment, structure, and understanding experienced as utility to attract resilience (Eitle and Eitle 2002; Jaeger 2004; Koehler 2017). Acceptance experienced has diminished depression, thus sustaining power to drive resilience (Mullins and Dugan 1991). Entertainment has generalized to well-being to facilitate resilience (Fekete et al. 2024). Structure experienced has reflected health to enhance resilience (Cheung and Lai 2020). Understanding received has boosted adaptation, positive emotion, forgiveness, and life satisfaction to maintain resilience (Algoe and Zhaoyang 2016; Brik et al. 2023). Sporting would secure achievement and profitability as utility to attract resilience (Darnell 2012; Hovden 2012). Achievement has fostered health, life quality, satisfaction, self-efficacy, and self-esteem as opposed to alienation, depression, and distress to uphold resilience (Donnellan et al. 2005; Fredricks and Eccles 2005; Menard and Mose 1984; Murray 2009; Piko et al. 2006; Tompson and Dass 2000; Xiao et al. 2009). Profitability experienced has elevated well-being, including satisfaction as opposed to anger, anxiety, and depression, to boost resilience (Helgeson et al. 2006; Wells et al. 1999; Wong and Lam 2016). Conversely, sporting relieves frustration and pressure, thus maintaining utility to attract resilience (Koehler 2017). Frustration experienced has incurred avoiding and withholding to impair resilience (Vanhee et al. 2018). Pressure experienced has heightened burnout, depression, powerlessness, and somatic complaint, and eroded health and self-esteem, thus impairing resilience (Furnham 1997; Gerber et al. 2010; Wan et al. 2023). Sporting precludes discrimination experienced to maintain utility to attract resilience (Roche 2002). Discrimination experienced has raised anomie, depression, distress, and loneliness and eroded life satisfaction, self-determination, and self-esteem to dampen resilience (Carr and Friedman 2005; Kachanoff et al. 2019; Kirmanoglu and Baslevent 2014; Pachankis et al. 2020; Schnittker 2020; Yang 2019). Sporting has arisen from low stress experienced to sustain utility to attract resilience (Seo et al. 2012). Stress experienced has dampened well-being, including health, life quality, positive affect, and satisfaction as opposed to depression and distress, to impede resilience (Baumeister et al. 2013. Mathis et al. 2016; Raposa et al. 2016; Shrira 2012; Snyder et al. 2020; Zotti et al. 2016).

Ideals inspired by sporting to rationalize resilience have embraced bonding, cohesion, conformity, learning, nutrition, prosociality, teamwork, and volunteering (Apinunmahakul and Devlin 2008; Baron 2007; Broh 2002; Osterlund and Seippel 2013; Takano and Sogon 2008; Van de Vyver and Abrams 2018). Bonding has mitigated stress and negative emotion, thus upholding resilience (Nelson-Coffey et al. 2023). Cohesion has buttressed hope and life satisfaction and eroded depression to maintain resilience (Araya et al. 2006; Dittman and Goebel 2010; Paez et al. 2015). Conformity has rested on its ideal (Lalot et al. 2022). As such, conformity has furnished achievement and its pressure, mastery-goal setting, social closeness and support received, and tolerance to benefit resilience (Feldman 2003; Jiang et al. 2015; Magnuson et al. 2006). The ideal for learning has induced learning (Hagger and Hamilton 2018). Learning has elevated well-being, including life satisfaction and self-efficacy, to facilitate resilience (Denver and Hands 1990; Minnaert and Janssen 1992; Richards 2016). Nutrition reflects and can enhance health and well-being to enable resilience (Dean 2020; Hattie et al. 2004; Van de Vliert and Postmes 2014). Moreover, nutrition reflects the ideal for health, which maintains autonomy to facilitate resilience (Arguedas 2020; Wiest et al. 2015). The prosocial ideal underlies prosociality (Maltseva 2016). Prosociality has elevated well-being, including connectedness, hope, life satisfaction, meaningfulness, and self-efficacy to boost resilience (Marsh and Dik 2021; Nelson-Coffey et al. 2023; Raposa et al. 2016; Yao and Enright 2019). Teamwork has enhanced capability use or self-actualization to maintain resilience (Steijn 2001). Volunteerism has raised well-being, including health, life satisfaction, mastery, morale, positive affect, and self-esteem as opposed to depression, loneliness, and mortality (Borgonovi 2008; Gillath et al. 2005; Li and Ferraro 2006; Midlarsky and Kahana 1994; Oman et al. 1999; Thoits and Hewitt 2001; Zotti et al. 2016). Sporting sustains ideals for fairness or fair play to rationalize resilience (Baron 2007; Shields and Bredemeier 2008). The ideal for fairness has raised resilience and other well-being components (Diener et al. 2009; Pyszkowska 2020). Sporting can reduce the ideal for crime, thus safeguarding resilience (Renel and Segev 2014). The ideal for crime has rationalized crime (Tanner-Smith et al. 2013). Crime has eroded life satisfaction, mastery, relationship quality, self-efficacy, and self-esteem to weaken resilience (Chung and Elias 1996; Keijsers et al. 2011; Shek 2005). Sporting involves ideals for career or occupations, continuation, fitness, initiation, maintenance, organization, and peace to facilitate resilience (Beyer 2006; Jaf et al. 2021; Jodl et al. 2001; Lawler et al. 2020; Prins et al. 2014; Simpkins et al. 2006). The ideal for career has advanced adaptability to secure resilience (Willner et al. 2020). The ideal for continuation has buttressed stability (Zumbrunnen and Gangl 2008). Continuation has raised resilience and relational quality (Lock et al. 2020; Ross et al. 2000). Fitness has elevated health, morale, and satisfaction and impeded anxiety, depression, and strain to enable resilience (Li 2006; Pereyra-Rojas et al. 2017; Sutherland and Fogarty 1995; Xie 1996). Initiation can advance positive affect, satisfaction, and well-being generally to enable resilience (Zacher et al. 2019). The ideal for maintenance has rationalized maintenance (Zhang et al. 2019). Maintenance has sustained self-acceptance and relieved depression to foster resilience (Agronick and Duncan 1998; Wrosch et al. 2005). Peacefulness develops from its ideal (Xu et al. 2015). Eventually, peacefulness has maintained life satisfaction and attenuated depression to buttress resilience (Yang 2016). Sporting represents ideals for civic engagement, ritual, and self-expression to rationalize resilience (Bekkers et al. 2008; Tinsley and Levers 2007; Xygalatas et al. 2021). Civic engagement has stood on its ideal (Peterson and Maiden 1993). As such, civic engagement has incubated conflict resolution, education, happiness, health, income, individualism, life satisfaction, security normativity, social attachment, capital, integration, trust, tolerance, and general well-being to advance resilience (Coffe and Geys 2007; Goren 2005; Growiec and Growiec 2010; Kroll 2011; Li and Walder 2001; Myers 1999; Pena-Lopez and Sanchez-Santos 2016; Posel and Casale 2011; Tak 2017; Tang 2011; Wallace and Pichler 2009; Welzel 2013; van Ingen and Bekkers 2015; Vincens et al. 2018). Ritual involvement follows its ideal (Reavy 2023). Eventually, ritual involvement has escalated well-being, including health, intimacy, and pleasure to drive resilience (Fiese and Hammons 2013; Rossner and Meher 2014; Yang and Wang 2023). Sporting has stemmed from the ideal for planning to rationalize resilience (Macdonald and Palfai 2008). Planning has reflected achievement, education, health, and optimism to afford resilience (Hellevik and Settersten 2013; Poynton et al. 2015). Conversely, sporting has fostered ideals against abusing alcohol and drugs, gambling, smoking, suicide, and trouble to safeguard resilience (Baron 2007; Cutler et al. 2001; Spreitzer 1994; Luschen et al. 1996; Sweeting and West 2003; Thorlindsson and Bernburg 2006). The ideal for abusing has buttressed abusing (Leimberg and Lehmann 2022). Abusing has engendered depression, thus jeopardizing resilience (Kendler et al. 2006). Gambling has raised negative feelings and suicide to erode resilience (Ladouceur et al. 1999; Peacock et al. 1999). The ideal for smoking has underlain smoking (Gunther et al. 2006). Smoking has impaired health to impede resilience (Chen et al. 2008). Suicide has evolved from its ideal (Till et al. 2013). Attempted suicide has induced anxiety to obstruct resilience (Cheng et al. 2017). Involvement in trouble has eroded hope, relational quality, and self-esteem and heightened anxiety, depression, and distress to jeopardize resilience (Gerard and Buehler 2004; Krishnakumar and Black 2003; Muris and van den Berg 2003; Prelow et al. 2004; Sanderson et al. 2016). Sporting reduces ideals for aggression or violence and radicalism, thus maintaining resilience (Ferguson and Rueda 2010; Koehler 2017). The ideal for aggression has fomented aggression (Markowitz 2001). Aggression or violence has bred depression, thus disturbing resilience (Wright et al. 2015). Radicalism has bred distrust, protesting, and violence to erode resilience (Levi and Strker 2000; Pauwels and De Waele 2014). Sporting has developed from the ideal for health to rationalize resilience (Scherger 2009). The ideal for health would warrant health to maintain resilience (Petersen 1996).

Norms underlying sporting to assimilate resilience have popularized cohesion, discipline, prosperity, socioeconomic status, and sporting (Cradock et al. 2009; Garcia et al. 2016; Johnson and Ali 2004; Umeh 2003; Takano and Sogon 2008). The norm for cohesion has assimilated cohesion (Volker et al. 2007). Cohesion has buttressed hope and life satisfaction and eroded depression to maintain resilience (Araya et al. 2006; Dittman and Goebel 2010; Paez et al. 2015). The norm of discipline has shaped discipline (Ngai et al. 2013). Discipline has strengthened well-being, notably self-esteem, to induce resilience (Armstrong et al. 2011; Diener and Fujita 1995). The norm for prosperity has maintained well-being, including health, relational quality, life satisfaction, and self-efficacy to sustain resilience (Corcoran et al. 2011; Fridberg and Kangas 2008; Helliwell et al. 2010; Inglehart 2010; Miller 2015). Socioeconomic status has encompassed education, income, and social class (Henderson et al. 2012; Simpkins et al. 2006; Spreitzer 1994). The norm for socioeconomic status has raised education, health, life satisfaction, knowledge, relationship quality, self-efficacy, social trust, and value for independence to facilitate resilience (Baldacci et al. 2003; Bonini 2008; Fjellvang 2011; Fridberg and Kangas 2008; Miller 2015; Norris 2011; Traunmuller 2011). Conversely, sporting has declined by the norm for minority status to discourage resilience (McNeal 1999). The norm for minority status has foregrounded minority status due to segregation (Daley 2009). Minority status has dampened life quality to hurt resilience (Verschuur et al. 2010).

## *Teamwork*

Teamwork is integral to team sporting as a form of sporting (Takano and Sogon 2008). Generally, teamwork reflects altruism or prosociality, collaboration, commonality, cooperation, interaction, interdependence, management or organization, and order in working with team members (Batson and Moran 1999; Bennett and Hays 2023;

Gander et al. 2020; Lawler et al. 2014; Rand 2016; Romero-Simpson 1995). Teamwork is likely to boost resilience by affording power, utility, ideals, and norms to activate voluntaristic mechanisms to upgrade functioning as aimed by analytical functionalism.

Power raised by teamwork to drive resilience has grown from attachment, commitment, morale, and trustworthiness (Gander et al. 2020; Gerbasi and Cook 2008; Gould-Williams 2005; Tak 2017). Attachment has buttressed life satisfaction to enable resilience (Zdrenka et al. 2015). Commitment has facilitated self-acceptance to secure resilience (Agronick and Duncan 1998). Morale reflects well-being and involves resilience (Kimhi et al. 2021; Peterson et al. 2008). Trustworthiness has stemmed from a positive experience, social status, and trust to induce resilience (Barrera 2007; Cook and Cheshire 2013; Kuwabara 2015). Teamwork stands on citizenship, managing, prosociality, and strength to generate power to drive resilience (Bennett and Hays 2023; Brightman and Moran 1999; Romero-Simpson 1995; Shimai et al. 2006). Citizenship has fostered well-being, including mental and physical health, to elevate resilience (Tsai et al. 2018). Managing has buttressed life satisfaction and self-efficacy to secure resilience (Corcoran et al. 2011; Rampichini and D'Andrea 1998). Prosociality has evolved from its ideal (Maltseva 2016). Eventually, prosociality has elevated well-being, including connectedness, hope, life satisfaction, meaningfulness, and self-efficacy to boost resilience (Marsh and Dik 2021; Nelson-Coffey et al. 2023; Raposa et al. 2016; Yao and Enright 2019). Teamwork involves social support received to enhance power to drive resilience (Rosenfeld and Richman 1997). Social support includes appreciation, assistance, confirmation, encouragement, listening, and sympathy (Rosenfeld and Richman 1997). Social support received has maintained well-being, including resilience, control, health, pleasure, purposefulness, relational quality, satisfaction, self-determination, self-efficacy, self-esteem, and social well-being (Cherry et al. 2018; George and Park 2013; Glendinning et al. 2003; Gorman et al. 2010; Holliman et al. 2021; Lincoln et al. 2003; Logan and Cobb 2013; Pierce and Quiroz 2018; Schwarzer and Knoll 2007; Williams and Galliher 2006; Xi and Hwang 2011). Teamwork rests on rationality to furnish power to drive resilience (Van Lange et al. 2014). Rationality has prevented aggression, anxiety, avoidance, depression, and disorders to safeguard resilience (DiGiuseppe et al. 2017). Teamwork has arisen from awe, complementarity, perspective-taking, prosociality, rationality, social capital, sociality, and trust to attain power to drive resilience (Hample 2018; Haesevoets et al. 2015; Miao et al. 2018; Penarroja et al. 2017; Shewark et al. 2022; Wu et al. 2022; Zhang and Zhou 2018). Awe has fostered resilience, happiness, and meaningfulness (Braswell and Prichard 2024; Cohen 2004; Gilmore et al. 2013). Complementarity has lifted well-being to foster resilience (Chuang 2005). Perspective-taking has installed social trust to empower resilience (Fett et al. 2014). Social capital has raised income or earnings, knowledge, religiosity, social support received, socioeconomic status, and well-being to afford power to boost resilience (Brunie 2009; Chua et al. 2021; Cross and Lin 2008; Pena-Lopez and Sanchez-Santos 2016; Yetim and Yetim 2014; Wuthnow 2004). Sociality has enhanced well-being to buttress resilience (Bjornskov 2008). Trust has sustained health and survival, thus raising resilience (Barefoot et al. 1998).

Teamwork can spring from its critical mass, complementarity, dependability or trustworthiness, education, familiarity, and similarity to furnish dispositional power to drive resilience (Brewer 1996; Oliver and Marwell 2001; Sanderson 2001; Zhang and Zhou 2018). Education has sustained well-being, including health, identity, life quality and satisfaction, mastery, self-efficacy, self-esteem, and youthfulness to engender resilience (Cerin and Leslie 2008; Corcoran et al. 2011; James and Amato 2013; Pakulshi and Tranter 2000; Stavrova and Ehlebracht 2018; van Praag and Frijters 1999; Whyte and Gao 2009; Yienprugsawan et al. 2010). Familiarity has sustained satisfaction and self-efficacy to facilitate resilience (Norris 2011; Rothwell et al. 2016). Similarity has reduced depression to afford resilience (Riad and Norris 1992). Conversely, teamwork precludes isolation or separation to maintain power to drive resilience (Steca et al. 2017). Isolation has bred a negative mood and impeded life satisfaction and reasoning to dampen resilience (Guillen et al. 2011; Lin et al. 2013; Williams et al. 2000). Teamwork has developed from low aggressiveness, antisociality, and psychoticism to retain power to drive resilience (Hample 2018). Aggressiveness has induced depression to inhibit resilience (Wright et al. 2015). Antisociality has generated violence to disrupt resilience (Kornienko et al. 2018). Psychoticism has eroded well-being, notably self-determination, to disrupt resilience (Furnham and Cheng 2000; Ingledew et al. 2004).

Utility raised by teamwork to attract resilience has resided in achievement, job and life satisfaction, and popularity (de Bruyn and van den Boom 2005; Onwuegbuzie et al. 2001; Park et al. 2015). Achievement has fostered health, life quality, satisfaction, self-efficacy, and self-esteem as opposed to alienation, depression, and distress to uphold resilience (Donnellan et al. 2005; Fredricks and Eccles 2005; Menard and Mose 1984; Murray 2009; Piko et al. 2006; Tompson and Dass 2000; Xiao et al. 2009). Popularity has uplifted positive affect and self-esteem and reduced negative affect, thus buttressing resilience (Reich et al. 2018). Utility reflected by teamwork has concerned complementarity, cooperation, justice, and recognition expected or experienced to attract resilience (Bereczkei et al. 2010; Brewer 1996; Mulford et al. 1998; Zhang and Zhou 2018). Justice experienced has boosted belongingness, health, life satisfaction, and self-esteem to establish resilience (Bjornskov et al. 2013; Dalbert 2001; Lucas et al. 2013; van Prooijen et al. 2008). Recognition experienced has uplifted positive affect and self-esteem and reduced negative affect, thus buttressing resilience (Reich et al. 2018). Teamwork can rest on satisfaction to secure utility to attract resilienve (Sanderson 2001). Conversely, teamwork has alleviated stress experienced as disutility that discourages resilience (Conti et al. 2006). Stress experienced has dampened well-being, including health, life quality, positive affect, and satisfaction as opposed to depression and distress, to impede resilience (Baumeister et al. 2013. Mathis et al. 2016; Raposa et al. 2016; Shrira 2012; Snyder et al. 2020; Zotti et al. 2016). Teamwork can stem from low alienation and deprivation experienced to maintain utility to attract resilience (Sanderson 2001). Alienation experienced has fomented feelings of depression, guilt, internalizing, loneliness, negative emotion, resentment, and stupidity to disturb resilience (Sommer et al. 2001; Tani and Schneider 1997; Witkow 2005). Deprivation experienced has dampened social trust and general well-being, thus impeding resilience (Clark et al. 2008; Layte et al. 2000; Stephens et al. 2014).

Ideals nurtured by teamwork rationalize resilience have extolled cohesion, decision, intrinsic value, morality, performance, and self-realization, capability use, or humanism (Chen and McDonald 2015; Choi et al. 2011; Hodson 2001; Gander et al. 2020; Lincoln and Kalleberg 1990; Steijn 2001). Cohesion has developed from its ideal (Granzin and Olsen 1998). As such, cohesion has buttressed hope and life satisfaction and eroded depression to maintain resilience (Araya et al. 2006; Dittman and Goebel 2010; Paez et al. 2015). Decision rests on its ideal (Cosculluela 1995). Eventually, decision has reduced stress experienced to sustain resilience (Fenwick and Tausig 1994). Intrinsic value has enhanced life satisfaction to induce resilience (Ferssizidis et al. 2010). The ideal for morality or moralism accentuates divinity, dutifulness, rule abidance, and virtuousness to insist on one's resilience belief (Garner 1994). Performance has reflected self-determination, self-efficacy, and the sense of community to boost resilience (Asoodar et al. 2014; Moller et al. 2006; Yashima 2010). Self-realization constitutes well-being to induce resilience (Meadows 2014). Moreover, humanism embraces meaningfulness, self-improvement, toleration, and vitality to facilitate resilience (Browning and Cooper 2004; Visher 1997; Waterman 2013). Teamwork manifests altruism, commonality, happiness or hedonism, interdependence, order, organization, and stoicism as ideals to rationalize resilience (Batson and Moran 1999; Gander et al. 2020; Lawler et al. 2014; Van Lange et al. 2014). Altruism has raised well-being, including connectedness, hope, life satisfaction, meaningfulness, and self-efficacy, as opposed to loneliness and negative emotion to sustain resilience (Caprara and Steca 2005; Marsh and Dik 2021; Nelson-Coffey et al. 2023; Raposa et al. 2016; Yao and Enright 2019). The ideal for commonality has raised relatedness to facilitated resilience (Torlo and Lomi 2017). Hedonism has bred well-being, including life satisfaction to sustain resilience (Datler et al. 2013; Joshanloo and Jarden 2016). Interdependence has raised relational quality to enhance resilience (Wickham and Knee 2012). The ideal for order has stemmed from health to enable resilience (Cheung and Lai 2020). Organization has sustained happiness, health, and life satisfaction and eroded depression to maintain resilience (Guillen et al. 2011; Thoits and Hewitt 2001). Stoicism embraces resilience and treasures logical thinking, reasoning, and virtuousness (Johnson and Samp 2022; Van Lange et al. 2014). Teamwork involves conciliation as an ideal to rationalize resilience (Ohbuchi et al. 1999). Conciliation has reflected harmonious passion and order, security, and stability values to secure resilience (Belanger et al. 2019; Simmons 2020). Teamwork has risen by ideals for accommodation, collectivism, community, liberalism, morality, relatedness, and social integration to rationalize resilience (Groves et al. 2000; Hample 2018; Kertzer et al. 2014; Lepkowski and Couper 2002; Ohbuchi et al. 1999; Shoss and Kueny 2022; Zhang and Zhou 2018). Accommodation has reflected just world belief, perspective-taking, and trust to maintain resilience (Lipkus and Bissonette 1998). Collectivism has safeguarded health, intimacy, and self-esteem to boost resilience (Kemp 2007; Triandis 1995). Liberalism has rested on growth to induce resilience (Helson and Srivastava 2001). Social integration develops from its ideal (Luo and Kao 2001). Eventually, social integration has lessened depression and suicide, thus safeguarding resilience (Duberstein et al. 2004; Mullins and Dugan 1991). Teamwork can emanate from agreement, reasoning, reciprocity, sharing, and social value as ideals to rationalize resilience (Perner and Esken 2015; Sanderson 2001; Van Lange et al. 2014). Agreement has sustained well-being to enhance resilience (Cheung and Leung 2011). Reasoning has dampened aggressiveness, anxiety, dependence, depression, disorders, and self-defeating, thus upholding resilience (DiGiuseppe et al. 2017; Karuza et al. 1990). Reciprocity has arisen from its ideal (Rodrigo-Gonzalez et al. 2019). As such, reciprocity has facilitated adaptation as opposed to illness to create resilience (Yamaoka 2008; Yeh et al. 2013). The ideal for sharing has reflected social attachment to enhance resilience (Erez et al. 2008). Social value prizes altruism and cooperation and discounts aggression, competition, individualism, inferiority, masochism, and nihilism (Van Lange et al. 2014). Eventually, social value has propped contact to raise well-being, including happiness, health, life satisfaction, love, self-efficacy, self-esteem, and social well-being as opposed to anxiety and boredom, to facilitate resilience (Bagozzi and Lee 2002; Crisp and Turner 2012; Denissen et al. 2008; Edara 2021; Galperin and Haselton 2010; Guillen et al. 2011; Mayer 2017; Mazziotta et al. 2011; Meulemann 2010; Reeskens and Vandecasteele 2017). Conversely, teamwork dismisses conflict, crime, domination, fighting, and revolution as ideals that refute resilience (Sanderson 2001). Conflict has rested on its ideal (Ohbuchi et al. 1999). Eventually, conflict has weakened well-being, including life and marital satisfaction, to hamper resilience (Baumeister et al. 2013; Mikula et al. 2012; Richards 2016). The ideal for crime has rationalized crime (Tanner-Smith et al. 2013). Crime has eroded life satisfaction, mastery, relationship quality, self-efficacy, and self-esteem to weaken resilience (Chung and Elias 1996; Keijsers et al. 2011; Shek 2005). Domination has evolved from its ideal (Cheung and Chiu 2021). Eventually, domination has bred depression to impair resilience (Lincoln et al. 2003). The ideal for fighting has originated from anger and contempt as opposed to self-efficacy to impair resilience (Tausch et al. 2011). The ideal for revolution has rested on reactance to oppose resilience (Traut-Mattausch et al. 2011).

‘ Norms underlying teamwork to assimilate resilience has rested on collectivism (Ohbuchi et al. 1999). Collectivism has grown from its norm (Sabatier and Lannegrand-Willems 2005). Eventually, collectivism has safeguarded health, intimacy, and self-esteem to boost resilience (Kemp 2007; Triandis 1995).

## *Coaching Received*

Coaching, typically coming with sporting, focuses on skill building through close and responsive interaction (Jones et al. 2021). Essentially, coaching develops the career, ego or self, and health (Bezner et al. 2020; Ebner et al. 2020; Gearity and Murray 2011). Coaching functions as a catalyst rather than advice, counseling, or informing (Ebner et al. 2020). The function is likely to raise resilience through consolidating power, utility, ideals, and norms to activate voluntaristic mechanisms covered in analytical functionalism.

Power boosted by coaching received to drive resilience has rested on fitness, health, self-efficacy, skill, and well-being generally (Bezner et al. 2020; Krebs et al. 2019; Theeboom et al. 2014). Fitness has elevated health, morale, and satisfaction and impeded anxiety, depression, and strain to enable resilience (Li 2006; Pereyra-Rojas et al. 2017; Sutherland and Fogarty 1995; Xie 1996). Skill has underpinned self-efficacy to buttress resilience (Larson et al. 1990). Coaching received highlight the ego or its development and health to sustain power to drive resilience (Gearity and Murray 2011). Ego development emphasizes coping, featuring flexibility, openness, resolution, responsiveness, and sensitivitiy, to enable resilience (Walker and Hennig 1999).

Ideals cultivated by coaching received to rationalize resilience have accentuated control, coping, exercising, performance, and self-regulation (Krebs et al. 2019; Pianta et al. 2017; Rakap and Balikci 2023; Theeboom et al. 2014). The ideal for control has motivated controlling, domination, or mastery (Cheung and Chiu 2021). Coping has evolved from its ideal (McClaran et al. 2022). Eventually, coping has raised resilience, environmental and relational quality, growth, health, intimacy, satisfaction, and self-efficacy (Cherry et al. 2023; Chow et al. 2014; Gattino et al. 2015; Lau et al. 2012; Paez et al. 2007; Veenstra et al. 2005; Wills 1997). The ideal for exercise has underlain exercising (Wister and Romeder 2002). Exercising has sustained well-being, thus empowering resilience (Sargent-Cox et al. 2015). Self-regulation has boosted self-esteem and diminished anxiety and depression to champion resilience (Marchetti et al. 2018).

## *Original Findings*

Existing work expects that developmental conditions buttress resilience (see Table 8.1). Herein, neuroticism and distress are negative developmental conditions expected to impede resilience. Nevertheless, an exception is that existing work expects adventuring to impair resilience. By contrast, the present findings indicated that extraversion, conscientiousness, and ritualistic activity exhibited positive effects on resilience. Conversely, the present findings showed that distress and neuroticism delivered a negative effect on resilience. However, empowerment displayed an inverse effect on resilience. No other developmental conditions manifested effects on resilience, based on statistical analysis.

| |
|---|
| *Visual impairment dataset* |
| Resilience, recent month ($\alpha = 0.630$) |
| Having the ability to face adversity |
| Facing difficulties positively |
| Rolling with punches |

(continued)

(continued)

| |
|---|
| Keeping calm in the face of pressure |
| (not) Feeling anxious when under pressure |
| (not) Having difficulty recovering from setbacks |
| Empowerment ($\alpha = 0.961$; Cheung and Ngan 2007; Gould-Williams and Davies 2005) |
| Leading ability increase, past year |
| Enhancing the ability to guide others |
| Enhancing the ability to assess performance |
| Enhancing leadership |
| Planning ability increase, past year |
| Enhancing the planning capacity |
| Enhancing the ability to organize work |
| Enhancing the ability to set goals |
| *Personality (Sibley and Duckitt 2009)* |
| Conscientiousness, all along ($\alpha = 0.498$) |
| Keeping neat |
| Handling chores instantly |
| Extraversion, all along ($\alpha = 0.648$) |
| Attending a party |
| Talking to different people |
| Neuroticism, all along ($\alpha = 0.495$) |
| Mood swinging |
| Fidgeting |
| Having ease of mind |
| *Youth dataset* |
| Resilience based on adjustment under adversity, past month ($\alpha = 0.984$) |
| Personal study |
| Getting along with family |
| Getting along with friends |
| Getting along with teachers |
| Emotion concerning the opposite sex |
| Money |
| Personal health |
| Others |
| Resilience, one year ago ($\alpha = 0.792$) |
| Being able to deal with crisis/adversity |
| Overcoming crises/adversity |
| Getting help in case of crisis/adversity |
| Distress, past month ($\alpha = 0.831$) |

(continued)

(continued)

| |
|---|
| Personal study |
| Getting along with family |
| Getting along with friends |
| Getting along with teachers |
| Emotion concerning the opposite sex |
| Money |
| Personal health |
| Others |
| Distress, one year ago ($\alpha = 0.750$) |
| Crisis/adversity bothering you |
| Duration of crisis/adversity |
| Sequels of crisis/adversity |
| Social desirability, recent month ($\alpha = 0.632$) |
| (not) lying to elders |
| (not) shouting because of anger |
| (Not) being unplanned |
| (Not) getting angry because of something bad |
| Treating disliked people politely |
| Being sure to do things right |
| Being happy most of the time |
| Listening carefully to elders' instruction |
| Individual sport, past 3 months ($\alpha = 0.695$) |
| Fitness/gymnastics |
| Running |
| Ball games |
| Water |
| Cycling |
| Jumping, throwing |
| Martial arts |
| Others |
| Team sport, past 3 months ($\alpha = 0.724$) |
| Fitness/gymnastics |
| Running |
| Ball games |
| Water |
| Cycling |
| Jumping, throwing |
| Martial arts |

(continued)

(continued)

| |
|---|
| Others |
| Coaching received, sport under guidance, past 3 months ($\alpha = 0.699$) |
| Fitness/gymnastics |
| Running |
| Ball games |
| Water |
| Cycling |
| Jumping, throwing |
| Martial arts |
| Others |
| Nation-related activity, past half-year ($\alpha = 0.491$) |
| Sport |
| Volunteering |
| Adventure/training camp |
| Religious activity |
| Carnival |
| Concert |
| Prime activity, past half-year |
| Volunteering |
| Adventure/training camp |
| Religious activity |
| Carnival |
| Concert |
| Participants |
| Ritual activity (collective sentiment), past half-year ($\alpha = 0.803$) |
| Ceremony |
| Singing, shouting, and reading together |
| Having fun together |
| Being in high spirits together |
| (not) Each doing one's own thing |
| Achieving eye alignment |
| Bodily contact |
| Achieving harmony in pace |
| (not) arguing |
| Belongingness to the nation, past year ($\alpha = 0.838$) |
| Being happy because of Chinese athletes winning gold metals |
| Volunteering for building China |
| Participating in the activities of protecting Diaoyutai |

(continued)

(continued)

| |
|---|
| (not) Recognizing China's shame |
| (not) Recognizing Chinese people's bad habits |
| (not) Meeting the Chinese people you hated |

## *Predicting Resilience*

Developmental dispositions showed expected effects on resilience. Accordingly, resilience in the recent month witnessed significant positive effects from extraversion and conscientiousness all along ($\beta = 0.120-0.157$, see Table 8.2). Conversely, resilience received significant inverse effects from neuroticism ($\beta = -0.265$). However, contrary to expectation, empowerment in the past year manifested a significant inverse effect on resilience in the recent month ($\beta = 0.140$).

Distress one year ago indicated a significant inverse effect ($\beta = -0.080$, see Table 8.3) on resilience in the past month, given the control for resilience one year ago and background characteristics. Ritualistic activity in the past six months displayed a statistically significant but practically trivial positive effect on resilience in the past month ($\beta = 0.048$).

Running sporting in the past three months manifested a significant positive effect ($\beta = 0.074$, see Table 8.3) on resilience in the past month whereas water sporting in the past three months evinced a significant inverse effect ($\beta = -0.043$) on resilience. However, running coaching received in the past three months generated a significant negative effect on resilience ($\beta = -0.072$). These findings indicated that running without receiving coaching fostered resilience.

Nation-related activity in the past six months unfolded a significant positive effect on resilience in the past month in Guangzhou, but not in Hong Kong and Macau ($\beta = 0.041$, see Table 8.3). By contrast, volunteering mostly done in the past 6 months engendered a significant inverse effect on resilience in Guangzhou only ($\beta = -0.035$).

## *Empowerment Effect*

The inverse effect of empowerment experienced on resilience indicated that this effect overshadowed the positive effect. Empowerment received might attenuate power, utility, ideals, and norms conducive to resilience, considering the analytical-functionalist framework.

Power reduced by empowerment received to inhibit resilience has stemmed from distress (Grealish et al. 2017). That is, the empowerment received has raised distress to erode power to drive resilience. This distressing effect reflected the challenge

**Table 8.1** Development effects on resilience

| Development | Expected | Currently found |
|---|---|---|
| Empowerment, past year | + | – |
| Extraversion, all along | + | + |
| Conscientiousness, all along | + | + |
| Neuroticism, all along | – | – |
| Distress, one year ago | – | – |
| Belongingness to the nation, one year ago | + | 0 |
| Nation-related activity, past 6 months | + | 0 |
| Ritualistic activity, past 6 months | + | + |
| Volunteering most, past 6 months | + | 0 |
| Adventuring most, past 6 months | – | 0 |
| Religious activity most, past 6 months | + | 0 |
| Carnival activity most, past 6 months | + | 0 |
| Musical activity most, past 6 months | + | 0 |
| Individual sport, past 3 months | + | 0 |
| Team sport, past 3 months | + | 0 |
| Coaching received, past 3 months | + | 0 |

*Note* + positive effect; – negative effect; ? mixed effects; 0 no effect

**Table 8.2** Standardized effects on resilience, recent month (visual impairment dataset)

| Predictor | Resilience |
|---|---|
| Empowerment, past year | $-0.144^{*}$ |
| Extraversion, all along | $0.120^{*}$ |
| Conscientiousness, all along | $0.157^{***}$ |
| Neuroticism, all along | $-0.265^{***}$ |
| $R^2$ | 0.477 |

*Note* Regression analysis controlled for background characteristics and social capital
$^{\#}p < 0.10$, $^{*}p < 0.05$, $^{**}p < 0.01$, $^{***}p < 0.001$

of empowerment received, such as taking responsibility for leading and planning (Cheung and Ngan 2007; Gordon 2008; Gould-Williams and Davies 2005). Empowerment received breeds narcissism to obstruct power that drives resilience (Feddes et al. 2015). Empowerment can incur overwhelming experience to dampen power that drives resilience (Snyder et al. 2018). Overwhelming experience has dampened well-being, including health, life quality, positive affect, and satisfaction as opposed to depression and distress, to impede resilience (Baumeister et al. 2013. Mathis et al. 2016; Raposa et al. 2016; Shrira 2012; Snyder et al. 2020; Zotti et al. 2016). Empowerment received reflects the lack of information, marginalized status, and powerlessness, thus losing power that drives resilience (Bartle et al. 2002; Pearrow

**Table 8.3** Standardized effects on resilience, past month ($N = 3.564$) (youth dataset)

| Predictor | All |
|---|---|
| Distress, one year ago | – 0.080*** |
| Resilience, one year ago | 0.107*** |
| Belongingness to the nation, one year ago | – 0.033 |
| $R^2$ | 0.050 |
| Nation-related activity, past 6 months | – 0.019 |
| Ritualistic activity, past 6 months | 0.048* |
| Volunteering most, past 6 months | 0.010 |
| Adventuring most, past 6 months | 0.022 |
| Religious activity most, past 6 months | – 0.012 |
| Carnival activity most, past 6 months | 0.026 |
| Musical activity most, past 6 months | – 0.003 |
| $R^2$ | 0.053 |
| Individual sport, past 3 months | 0.022 |
| Team sport, past 3 months | – 0.022 |
| Coaching received, past 3 months | – 0.032 |
| $R^2$ | 0.054 |
| Water sport, past 3 months | – 0.043* |
| Running coached, past 3 months | – 0.072** |
| Running, past 3-months | 0.074** |
| $R^2$ | 0.061 |
| Guangzhou × nation-related activity, past 6 months | 0.041* |
| Guangzhou × volunteering most, past 6 months | – 0.035* |
| $R^2$ | 0.063 |

*Note* Regression analysis controlled for background characteristics
$^{*}p < 0.05$, $^{**}p < 0.01$, $^{***}p < 0.001$

2011; Thompson and Thompson 2001). Information received has elevated well-being, including life satisfaction and self-efficacy, to furnish resilience (Denver and Hands 1990; Minnaert and Janssen 1992; Richards 2016). Marginalized status has installed negative mood and diminished life satisfaction, thus impairing resilience (Lin et al. 2013; Williams et al. 2000). Powerlessness has unfolded dissatisfaction to impair resilience (Armstrong-Stassen 2001).

Utility enhanced by empowerment received to discourage resilience has rested on social exclusion experienced (Secker et al. 2009). Accordingly, power has been threatening to others, thus triggering their exclusive response (Peruzzi 2014; Yogeeswaran and Dasgupta 2014). Social exclusion experienced has fomented a negative mood and life dissatisfaction to hinder resilience (Lin et al. 2013; Williams et al. 2000). Conversely, empowerment received can diminish justice experienced to discourage resilience (van Prooijenn 2019). Justice experienced has lifted positive mood, life satisfaction, and self-esteem to sustain resilience (Dalbert 2001). Empowerment received evolves from discrimination or oppression experienced to indicate disutility discouraging resilience (Thompson and Thompson 2001). Discrimination experienced has raised anomie, depression, distress, and loneliness and eroded life satisfaction, self-determination, and self-esteem to dampen resilience (Carr and Friedman 2005; Kachanoff et al. 2019; Kirmanoglu and Baslevent 2014; Pachankis et al. 2020; Schnittker 2020; Yang 2019).

Ideals raised by empowerment received to refute resilience have emphasized avoidance, protesting, and radicalism (Ran et al. 2023; Selvanathan and Lickel 2019). Avoidance involves disgust and prejudice (Tybur et al. 2014). As such, avoidance has impaired coping and well-being, including mindfulness and satisfaction, to hinder resilience (Barber et al. 2010; Basabe et al. 2002; Linares et al. 2016; Seaton and Beaumont 2008). The ideal for protesting has constituted protesting (Hwang and Kim 2015). Protesting has invoked anger and worry to counter resilience feeling (Boehnke and Wong 2011; Landmann and Rohmann 2020). Radicalism has bred distrust, protesting, and violence to erode resilience (Levi and Strker 2000; Pauwels and De Waele 2014). Empowerment received involves consumerism, risking, and resistance as an ideal to distract resilience (Himes 2007; Lashley 2001; Stacki and Monkman 2003). Consumerism engages hedonism and irrationality to hinder resilience (Himes 2007). Risking can rest on its ideal (Breakwell 2007). Eventually, risking has impaired health and activated criminal behavior and violence, thus weakening resilience (Farrington 2018; Pulkkinen et al. 2009; Wickrama et al. 1995). Resistance can erode solidarity and thus hope and life satisfaction to dampen resilience (Dittman and Goebel 2010; Foy et al. 2014; Paez et al. 2015). Conversely, empowerment received can dampen the ideal for cooperation to refute resilience (Sanderson 2001). Cooperation has thrived on its ideal (Haesevoets et al. 2015). As such, cooperation has fostered life satisfaction to rationalize resilience (Park et al. 2015).

Norms underlying empowerment received to dismiss resilience have rested on improvement need or inadequacy and violence (Gordon 2008; Huang-Isherwood and Pena 2021). Inadequacy has fueled helplessness and retarded self-efficacy to erode resilience (Campagna 2016). The norm for violence has degraded neighborhood quality to jeopardize resilience (Sampson and Raudenbush 2004).

## *Ritualistic Activity Effect*

Ritualistic activity showed a significant but trivial positive effect on resilience. This effect was noteworthy because most other activities did not unfold significant effects. The significant effect reflects that ritualistic activity particularly amplified the effects of power, utility, ideals, and norms for raising resilience. Such amplification is likely to hinge on such ritualistic activity natures as civilization or culture, compulsion, continuity and repetition, interaction, morality or virtue, normatizing, orchestration, and social capital (Boyer and Lienard 2006; Hobson et al. 2017; Izenstart and Ebata

2016; Liu 2004; Mayer 2003; Raphals 1992; Turner 2002, 2021; Yang and Wang 2023; Zhang 2003). Civilization is amplifying through its integration, persistence, and pervasiveness (Halas 2010; Huntington 1993; Inglehart and Baker 2000). Culture is amplifying through its contagiousness and passion (Kral 2019; Walton 2012). Continuity, persistence, and repetition are amplifying regarding resilience because they manifest resilience and strength (Rojas and Tyler 2018; Von Culin et al. 2014). Interaction is amplifying by nature and through reciprocity (Tindall and Wellman 2001; Hallett 2003). Morality or virtue is amplifying through its cultural support (Cast and Stets 2016). Normatizing is amplifying through approving and prohibiting (Massengale et al. 2017). Orchestrating is amplifying through interaction (Fiske 2000). Social capital is amplifying through its durability, reciprocity, reliability, and multiplication effect among social network members (Chen et al. 2015; Robison et al. 2002; Siisiainen 2003). The amplification is also likely to benefit from such ritualistic activity features as authoritativeness, collectivity or togetherness, deference, responsibility, religiousness, rhythm or music, and spectacles (Marshall 2002; Guo 2018; Raab 2019; Schjoedt et al. 2013). Authoritativeness is amplifying when it underlies influence (Li 2022). Collectivity or togetherness is amplifying through inducing attachment, liking, sharing, and susceptibility (Baxter and Bylund 2004; McIntyre et al. 2023; Sivami 2016; Xin et al. 2017). Deference is amplifying through attachment, identification, learning, and obsession (McCabe et al. 2016; McCutcheon et al. 2006; Onu et al. 2016; Pleiss and Feldhusen 1995). Responsibility is amplifying through commitment, compliance, conformism, morality or virtue, preemption (Dean 2004; Fasoli 2017; Kaurin 2020; Sukabdi 2019; Tomasello 2019). Religiousness is amplifying through awe or deference, commitment, faith, inculcation, legitimacy or authoritativeness, morality or virtue, sacredness, solidarity, and strictness (Donnelly 2013; Garrod and Jones 2009; Gay and Lynxwiler 2009; Harris et al. 2018; Lloyd et al. 2022; McDowell and Brown 2009; Peifer 2010), Music is amplifying through coordination and harmonizing (Palmer and Griscom 2013; Wallace and Harwood 2018). Spectacles are amplifying through inducing deference and influenceability (Haas and Gregory 2005).

Some features or nature of ritualistic activity have demonstrated their amplifying effects on power, utility, ideals, and norms. Power amplified by ritualistic activity has evolved from the activity features or natures of commitment, compulsion, culture, religiousness, social capital, solidarity, and togetherness (Engelstad 2009; Isham et al. 2006; Keltener et al. 2008; Matthewman 2011; ten Brinke and Keltner 2020; Van Voorhis et al. 2006). Culture covers aristocracy, beauty, justice, and god that are consonant with ritualistic activity (Engelstad 2009). Utility or benefit experienced amplified by ritualistic activity has benefitted from such activity features or natures as religiousness, relatedness, rhythm, and sharing (Helgeson et al. 2006; Iwanaga et al. 2020; Liu and Cai 2013; Short 2018). Ideals underlying resilience are cynicism, individualism, neoliberalism, and stoicism (Owen 2023; Schwarz 2018). Cynicism hails frugality, simplicity, and normalizing adversity (Owen 2023; Schwarz 2018). This ideal has evolved from ritualistic activity features or natures such as conservation and stability (Kirk and Papachristos 2011; Martin et al. 2018). Individualism highlights risk management (Hall and Lamont 2013). This idea has evolved from ritualistic activity features of faith or religiousness, notably Christianity (Hordern 2013; Speed et al. 2018). Neoliberalism accentuates adaptation, autonomy, rationality, and responsibility (Garrett 2016; Hall and Lamont 2013; Schwarz 2018; Tierney 2015). This ideal involves the ritualistic activity feature of responsibility (Campbell 2019). Stoicism treasures acting, perfecting, and reasoning (Owen 2023; Alrofiai et al. 2020). This ideal concerns the ritualistic activity features of compliance, religiousness, responsibility, and sociality (Akrim et al. 2021; Furnham and Robinson 2024; Holowchak 2008; Kaurin 2020). Norms underlying resilience are collectivism, commitment, and morality (Batone 2017; Wu et al. 2011). Collectivism involves or has depended on such ritualistic activity features as connectedness or relatedness, solidarity, and religiousness, particularly its fundamentalist form (Braun 2011; Oyserman et al. 2002; Realo et al. 2008; Triandis 1995). Commitment and morality are integral to ritualistic activity (Izenstart and Ebata 2016; Zhang 2003).

Alternatively, amplification has benefitted from such ritualistic activity qualities as consistency or regularity, normativity, responsibility, and social interaction (Eccles and Gootman 2002; Epstein and Boisvert 2006; Tolmatcheff et al. 2022). Consistency has been amplifying by raising acceptance (Knafo and Schwartz 2001). Regularity can enhance maturity to secure success to sustain resilience (Skinner et al. 2019; Spengler et al. 2018). Normativity has been amplifying by facilitating assertiveness and susceptibility (Hornsey et al. 2003; Unger et al. 2001). Responsibility has been assimilating by consolidating hardiness and wisdom (Butler et al. 2022; Spengler et al. 2018). Social interaction has been amplifying by uplifting self-efficacy and vividness (Crisp and Turner 2012; Mazziotta et al. 2011).

Overall, ritualistic activity is amplifying through enhancing bonding, ecstasy, energy, functioning, obsession, stability, unity, and social cohesion and interaction (Boyer and Lienard 2006; Bulbulia et al. 2013; Crow 2002; Fiske 2000; Smith and Hamon 2012; Yang and Wang 2023). Bonding is amplifying through raising collaboration (Holt-Lunstad 2022). Ecstasy is an amplified emotion for amplifying (Burnett 2012). Obsession and unity are activating, thus amplifying (McIntyre et al. 2023; St-Louis and Vallerand 2015). Unity also enables self-expansion, thus amplifying (Tomlinson et al. 2018). Stability musters strength, thus amplifying (Von Culin et al. 2014). Social cohesion facilitates growth and support reception, thus amplifying (Berger-Schmitt 2002; Paez et al. 2015). Social interaction triggers collective action and cooperation conducive to amplifying (Gaertnel et al. 1999; Sandstrom et al. 2014).

## *Running Effect*

Running was the only sporting form displaying a significant positive effect on resilience. This unique contribution may benefit from commitment and psychodiversity afforded by running (Major 2001; Watkins et al. 2022). Commitment to running has raised accomplishments, affiliation, fitness, and health to enhance resilience

(Major 2001). Psychodiversity covers conformity, distinctiveness, mastery, purposiveness, spontaneity, and sympathy (Watkins et al. 2022). Conformity encompasses dedication, planning, and preparation (Watkins et al. 2022). As such, conformity has furnished achievement and its pressure, mastery-goal setting, social closeness and support received, and tolerance to benefit resilience (Feldman 2003; Jiang et al. 2015; Magnuson et al. 2006). Distinctiveness includes adventuring, escape, and freedom (Watkins et al. 2022). As such, distinctiveness can underlie attachment, cohesion, and humor to facilitate resilience (Anton and Lawrence 2014; Ferguson and Ford 2008; Huddy 2013). Mastery consists of self-improvement as opposed to injury (Watkins et al. 2022). As such, mastery has raised well-being, including happiness, neighborhood quality, life satisfaction, and physical and mental health, as opposed to depression, to induce resilience (Greenberg 1999; Helson and Srivastava 2001; Hwang et al. 2007; Judge et al. 2002; Lever et al. 2005; Sargent-Cox et al. 2015). Purposiveness embraces finishing and self-improvement (Watkins et al. 2022). As such, purposiveness has advanced happiness, health, life satisfaction, and positive affect and lessened depression and negative affect to induce resilience (Steger et al. 2009; Tomich and Helgeson 2002). Spontaneity features excitement and nature as opposed to competitiveness (Watkins et al. 2022). As such, spontaneity has furnished self-efficacy to drive resilience (Davelaar et al. 2008). Sympathy involves community and teamwork as opposed to competitiveness (Watkins et al. 2022). As such, sympathy has sustained mental clarity and well-being generally to facilitate resilience (Jasielska 2020; Naruse et al. 2020).

## *Running Coaching Effect*

Running coaching received exhibited a slight but significant negative effect on resilience. This effect might reflect the harm of coaching generally. The harm has transpired in self-doubt increased and cohesion and well-being reduced to impair resilience (Gearity and Murray 2011; Szabo et al. 2019). Cohesion has buttressed hope and life satisfaction and eroded depression to maintain resilience (Araya et al. 2006; Dittman and Goebel 2010; Paez et al. 2015).

## *Water Sporting Effect*

Water sporting notably indicated a slight but significant inverse effect on resilience. This effect might reflect sporting harm generally. Such sporting harm has resided in aggressiveness, aggression or violence, conflict, distress, illness, and irritability (Bensimon and Bodner 2011; Carter et al. 2023; Hansen et al. 2003; Rees and Howell 1990; Wright and Fitzpatrick 2006). Aggressiveness has induced depression to inhibit resilience (Wright et al. 2015). Aggression or violence has bred depression, thus disturbing resilience (Wright et al. 2015). Conflict has weakened well-being, including life and marital satisfaction, to hamper resilience (Baumeister et al. 2013; Mikula et al. 2012; Richards 2016). Distress has dampened resilience (Tett and Wang 2005). Illness has eroded functionality, health and mental health, knowledge, optimism, security, vitality, and general well-being, thus disempowering resilience (Benitez-Silva et al. 2010; Carrieri 2012; Korkeila et al. 2004; Price et al. 2006; van Dijk et al. 2008). Irritability is inadequate openness (Draper and Holman 2005). Openness has buttressed well-being, including autonomy, growth, purposefulness, life satisfaction, relationship quality, self-acceptance, self-efficacy, and self-esteem to advance resilience (Hahn et al. 2013; Hounkpatin et al. 2015; Karwowski and Lebuda 2017; Marks 1996; Quilty et al. 2006). Conversely, sporting has eroded academic achievement or performance, academic involvement, criticalness, employability, maturity, self-control, and self-determination (Bonnard 2020; Ntoumanis et al. 2009; Pascarella et al. 1995; Rees and Howell 1990; Shields and Bredemeier 2005). Academic achievement has fostered development, health, life quality, satisfaction, self-efficacy, and self-esteem to boost resilience (Cook et al. 2002; Donnellan et al. 2005; Murray 2009; Tompson and Dass 2000; Xiao et al. 2009). Academic involvement has maintained satisfaction to induce resilience (Jones 2014). Criticalness has fostered identity achievement to procure resilience (Adams and Ryan 2000). Employability has reflected self-efficacy and self-evaluation to boost resilience (Atitsogbe et al. 2019; Creed and Gagliardi 2015). Maturity has developed from self-compassion and self-tolerance to strengthen resilience (Ho and Li 2022; Munroe et al. 2022). Self-control has maintained self-esteem and reduced anxiety and depression to enable resilience (Armstrong et al. 2011; Marchetti et al. 2018). Self-determination has maintained commitment, effectiveness, and performance to boost resilience (Delhey 2010; Gagne and Deci 2005; Hui et al. 2013; Weinstein and Ryan 2010).

## *Nation-Related Activity Effect*

Nation-related activity displayed s significant positive effect on resilience in Guangzhou but not in Hong Kong or Macau. This conditional effect suggested that nationalism, or its contribution from nation-related activity, strengthened in the Chinese mainland rather than in the outlying special administrative regions returning to China. The national context, such as the Chinese mainland, has foregrounded or intensified nationalism (Cai et al. 2020; He 2018). Moreover, the fit between the national location and nation-related activity, higher on the mainland than on the outlying, can amplify the activity effect. Accordingly, fitness has enhanced acceptance, accomplishment, commitment, compliance, engagement, involvement, power, and resilience (Brkich et al. 2002; Dennis et al. 2005; Foy et al. 2014; Guan et al. 2021; Heshmati and Oravecz 2022; Mahoney et al. 2009; Ungar et al. 2007). Alternatively, activity effectiveness has risen with activity fitness (Johnson et al. 2015).

## *Volunteering Effect*

Volunteering manifested a slight but significant negative effect of resilience in Guangzhou but not in Hong Kong or Macau. This negative effect might reflect the harm due to the incongruity between volunteering and contextual irreligiousness. Accordingly, irreligiousness has nullified the developmental effect of volunteering (Musick and Wilson 2008). Herein, Guangzhou downplayed religiousness, while Hong Kong and Macau embraced religiousness (Guan et al. 2010; Nai et al. 2020; Wu and Zhao 2017). Essentially, contextual religiousness normalizes awe, meaning-making, ritual, and universalism (Garrod and Jones 2009; McDowell and Brown 2009; van Uden and Zondag 2016). Awe or role modeling and meaningfulness have boosted the contribution of volunteering (Dong 1998; Musick and Wilson 2008). Ritual raises energy and meaningfulness, which can strengthen the volunteering contribution (Izenstart and Ebata 2016; Yang and Wang 2023). Religiousness and universalism are congruous with volunteering (Ossewaarde 2007; Penner 2002; Vermeer and Scheepers 2019). Congruity or fitness amplifies power, thus volunteering contribution (Heshmati and Oravecz 2022).

# Chapter 9
# Conclusion

**Abstract** This chapter reveals that resilience and its processes have personal and social bases simultaneously explicable by the analytical-functionalist framework. The personal bases are evident in the resilience process, with resilience belief successively generating resilience learning, resilience action, and resilience feeling. Moreover, the personal bases are demonstrable in the contributions of the practical bases of hardening and softening to resilience. Other personal factors affect resilience, including marriage, earnings, extraversion, kindness, and functional disability. Meanwhile, the social bases are evident in the influences of caring, peace, violence, pragmatism, and social exclusion experienced in society. Moreover, kindness, sociability, social inclusion, and social capital experienced interpersonally testify to the significance of social bases. The simultaneous influences of personal and social factors thus dispel the suspicion that social factors exert predominant influences on resilience and its processes. Hence, resilience is personally developable, notably through the personal practices of hardening and softening. Nevertheless, social factors such as social capital, caring, and social exclusion in society also exerted enormous influences on resilience. For the pupil, ritualistic and other social activities develop resilience. Voluntaristic and deterministic mechanisms for the functions of goal attainment, integration, and latency are, therefore, particularly influential on resilience.

Resilience as a compound of adjustment and adversity involves a process initiating exposure to resilience to nurture belief in resilience to learn and handle resilience to feel resilience eventually (Hariharan and Rana 2017). Herein, resilience learning and handling constitute resilience action. Hence, adjustment or well-being more generally is a necessary cornerstone of resilience (Van Haaften et al. 2004). Well-being represents episodic power to run the voluntaristic mechanism of power realization to build resilience (Jayawickreme et al. 2012). Generally, resilience or specifically its action embodies adapting, balancing, coping, developing, functioning, endurance, managing, meaning-making, recovering, resisting, returning, stabilizing, steeling, and strengthening (Boden et al. 2014; Bowers et al. 2017; Crafter et al. 2019; Eshel et al. 2017; Huta 2017; Prilleltensky 2012; Rutter 2012; Schwager and Rothermund

 
C. K. Cheung, *Resilience Process and Its Personal and Social Bases*,
https://doi.org/10.1007/978-981-97-7391-6_9

2014; Zautra et al. 2010). More generally, resilience is integral to continuous or normal living or surviving (Hildon et al. 2008; Supkoff et al. 2012).

The core and marker of resilience is the feeling of resilience as adjustment under adversity, meaning rebounding from perturbation due to adversity. This resilience feeling indicates a momentary reality rather than a longstanding capability, disposition, or trait. Resilience feeling turned out to stand on resilience action, including learning and handling. Such action, in turn, stood on resilience belief. Meanwhile, resilience feeling, action, and belief maintained weak positive correlations with exposure to resilience demand. These correlations register the integration function of analytical functionalism to leverage the voluntaristic mechanism to achieve norm conformity. Meanwhile, resilience belief functions to maintain latency in functionalism through the voluntaristic mechanism of ideal calibration to constitute resilience action and feeling. Resilience action, in turn, achieves the function of adaptation by the voluntaristic mechanism of utility optimization in analytical functionalism. Eventually, resilience represents the goal or power to achieve fulfillment or goal attainment function in analytical functionalism to sustain overall functioning with the voluntaristic mechanism of power realization. Resilience thus functions as empowerment to facilitate adaptation, character development, competence, confidence, coping, courage, health, life quality, and further asset and resource building (Bowers et al. 2017; Brodsky and Cattaneo 2013; Cotterill 2017; Ge et al. 2020; Leigert and Reutter 2005; Pyszkowska 2020; Ungar 2012). The essence of functionalism is to regard resilience or its process as functional in upholding personal functioning, which entails resilience.

## Functionalist Development

Besides its functioning process, resilience is developable by other personal and societal factors, working on the voluntaristic and deterministic mechanisms of analytical functionalism, respectively. Personal factors vary across persons, including backgrounds, peer conditions, practices, social capital, and developmental conditions. By contrast, societal factors originate from societal or collective sources.

Analytical-functionalist mechanisms apply power, utility, ideals, and norms to develop resilience. Power functions to drive resilience. Utility functions to attract resilience. Ideals function to rationalize resilience. Norms originating outside the person function to assimilate resilience.

Power has rested on dispositions, emotional intelligence, mentoring, services, and social support received, socioeconomic status, and well-being (Armstrong et al. 2011; Buikstra et al. 2010; Cherry et al. 2023; Notter et al. 2008; Ntontis et al. 2023). Dispositions giving power to drive resilience include agreeableness, conscientiousness, extraversion, honesty-humility, optimism, sensation seeking, and stability (Buikstra et al. 2010; Lock et al. 2020; Pyszkowska 2020; Yu and Zhang 2007). Conversely, dispositions weakening power include emotionality and neuroticism (Pyszkowska

2020; Yu and Zhang 2007). Well-being includes coherence, gratitude, health, intimacy, mastery, meaningfulness, purposiveness, relational quality, self-compassion, self-efficacy, self-esteem, and strength (Alvarez and Pinto 2023; Buikstra et al. 2010; Elfers et al. 2024; Eshel et al. 2017; Harvey and Boynton 2021; Jones and Lafreniere 2014; Masten et al. 2009; Svetina 2014). Conversely, ill-being manifesting powerlessness has included anxiety, boredom, and fear (Alrabai and Alamer 2022; Wang et al. 2022).

Utility has resided in achievement experienced, safe perceived, and satisfaction (Alvarez and Pinto 2023; Dou et al. 2023; Hartley 2013). Conversely, disutility has stemmed from abuse, stress, and trauma experienced (Cherry et al. 2023; Sobeck et al. 2020; Yu et al. 2022).

Ideals rationalizing resilience have covered resilience, affiliation, coping, culture, future orientation, learning, and social identification or orientation (Buikstra et al. 2010; Chua et al. 2019; Corbin and Hall 2019; Lee et al. 2010; Lou et al. 2018; Ntontis et al. 2023). Conversely, ideals discouraging resilience have covered aggression, doping, and externalizing (Graber et al. 2016; Shure and Aberson 2012; Ungar et al. 2005).

Norms assimilating resilience have covered resilience, abidance, adaptability, assets or wealth, coherence, collaboration, competence, flexibility, functioning, innovation, meaningfulness, prosociality, resources, safety, self-efficacy, services, stability, structure, success, supportiveness, talent, and warmth (Aitcheson et al. 2017; Buikstra et al. 2010; Dou et al. 2023; Jones and d'Errico 2019; Masten et al. 2009; Pitzer and Skinner 2017; Sawyers et al. 2020; Ungar et al. 2005). Conversely, norms rejecting resilience have covered conflict, discrimination, and illness (Wang et al. 2022; Jones and d'Errico 2019; Ungar et al. 2005).

## *Societal Conditions*

Societal factors showing positive effects on resilience were societal caring, pragmatism, and the Hong Kong context versus that of Guangzhou or Macau, whereas societal factors displaying inverse effects on resilience were societal exclusion and pragmatism (see Table 9.1). By contrast, societal inclusion, peace, and violence did not affect personal resilience.

Essentially and directly, societal care registers collective resilience as a direct deterministic mechanism to enable personal resilience (Ungar 2011). Additionally, societal care represents empowering as the indirect deterministic mechanism of analytical functionalism to raise power to run the voluntaristic mechanism. Such raised power has rested on health and neighborhood quality as opposed to distress and illness (Fujisawa et al. 2009; Gary et al. 2007; Olson et al. 2016; Wen et al. 2010). Moreover, societal care has facilitated life satisfaction and success as opposed to victimization experienced to afford utility to attract resilience through the voluntaristic mechanism of utility optimization (Cramm et al. 2012; Furstenberg and Hughes 1995; Hansen-Nord et al. 2014). This facilitation embodies empowering

**Table 9.1** Societal effects on resilience

| Predictor | Expected | Currently found |
|---|---|---|
| *Societal condition* | | |
| Caring | + | + |
| Inclusion | + | 0 |
| Exclusion | – | – |
| Peace | + | 0 |
| Violence | – | 0 |
| Pragmatism | + | – |
| Westernization | + | + |
| Guangzhou versus Hong Kong | – | – |
| Macau versus Hong Kong | – | – |
| *Personal background* | | |
| Age | + | ? |
| Female | – | – |
| Born in Hong Kong | + | + |
| Born in Mainland China | – | 0 |
| Residency | + | + |
| Education | + | – |
| Married | + | + |
| Divorced | – | 0 |
| Widowed | – | 0 |
| Living with the spouse | + | 0 |
| Living with offspring | + | 0 |
| Living with siblings | + | 0 |
| Living with parents | + | + |
| Living with other relatives | + | 0 |
| Living alone | – | 0 |
| Family size | – | – |
| Owned public housing | – | 0 |
| Rental public housing | – | – |
| Owned private housing | – | – |
| Private housing | – | 0 |
| Private flat | – | 0 |
| Rental private housing | – | – |
| Rental private room | – | 0 |
| Divided rental private flat | – | – |
| Hostel | – | 0 |
| Aged home | – | 0 |

(continued)

**Table 9.1** (continued)

| Predictor | Expected | Currently found |
|---|---|---|
| Employer | – | 0 |
| Self-employed | – | – |
| Employee | – | – |
| Both employer and employee | + | 0 |
| Managerial role | – | 0 |
| Unemployed | – | – |
| Earnings | + | + |
| Personal income | + | + |
| Family income | + | 0 |
| Family income per capita | + | + |
| Poor family | – | 0 |
| Receiving social welfare | + | + |
| Receiving social welfare formerly | + | 0 |
| Irreligious | + | 0 |
| Functional disability/visual impairment | – | – |
| Visual impairment duration | – | – |
| Adversity | – | – |
| *Peer condition* | | |
| Speaker sociability | + | + |
| Relational kindness | + | + |
| Aid received | + | + |
| Advice received | + | 0 |
| Peer functional disability | – | 0 |
| Peer adversity | – | – |
| Peer resilience demand received | + | 0 |
| Peer speaker sociability | + | – |
| Peer relational kindness | + | 0 |
| Peer aid received | + | + |
| Peer kindness | + | 0 |
| Peer resilience belief | + | – |
| Peer benevolent world belief | + | + |
| Peer resilience learning | + | + |
| Peer resilience handling | + | 0 |
| Peer self-awareness | + | 0 |
| *Practice* | | |
| Kindness | + | + |
| Hardening | + | + |

(continued)

**Table 9.1** (continued)

| Predictor | Expected | Currently found |
|---|---|---|
| Softening | + | + |
| Hardening × softening | + | – |
| Socializing | + | 0 |
| Religious practice | + | 0 |
| Pet engagement | + | 0 |
| Experience-based coping | + | + |
| *Social capital* | | |
| Associational structural | + | + |
| Friend substantive | + | – |
| Friend structural | + | + |
| Friend functional | + | – |
| Friend substantive × structural | + | + |
| Friend substantive × functional | + | 0 |
| Friend structural × functional | + | 0 |
| Associational × friend substantive | + | 0 |
| Associational × friend structural | + | 0 |
| Association × friend functional | + | 0 |
| Friend substantive × structural × functional | + | + |
| Associational × friend substantive × structural × functional | + | 0 |
| *Development* | | |
| Empowerment, past year | + | – |
| Extraversion, all along | + | + |
| Conscientiousness, all along | + | + |
| Neuroticism, all along | – | – |
| Distress, one year ago | – | – |
| Belongingness to the nation, one year ago | + | 0 |
| Nation-related activity, past 6 months | + | 0 |
| Ritualistic activity, past 6 months | + | + |
| Volunteering most, past 6 months | + | 0 |
| Adventuring most, past 6 months | – | 0 |
| Religious activity most, past 6 months | + | 0 |
| Carnival activity most, past 6 months | + | 0 |
| Musical activity most, past 6 months | + | 0 |
| Individual sport, past 3 months | + | 0 |
| Team sport, past 3 months | + | 0 |
| Coaching received, past 3 months | + | 0 |

*Note* + positive effect; – negative effect; ? mixed effects; 0 no effect as an indirect deterministic mechanism to activate the voluntaristic mechanism of utility optimization.

Societal Westernization, higher in Hong Kong than in Mainland China, features consumerism, entertainment, and neoliberalism to induce resilience (Csanyi et al. 2023; Hodge 2018; Janion 2020). The inducement involves the deterministic mechanism of framing to activate voluntaristic mechanisms. Consumerism embraces hedonism to achieve well-being to buttress resilience (Joshanloo and Jarden 2016). Entertainment is a basis for well-being to uphold resilience (Fekete et al. 2024). Neoliberalism has fostered self-affirmation as well-being to underpin resilience (Zucker and Bay-Cheng 2021).

Moreover, Westernization personally upholds ideals for controlling, individualism, mastery, self-determination, and tolerance (AlShebali et al. 2021; Ma 2019; Narvaez 2014). These ideals have fostered well-being, including life satisfaction and self-efficacy to induce resilience (Appleton and Song 2008; Delhey 2010; Etezadi and Pushkar 2013; Kim et al. 2016; Napier and Jost 2008; Orlowski and Wicker 2015; Veenhoven 1998). The fostering benefits from the voluntaristic mechanisms of power realization and utility optimization.

Hong Kong upholds resilience as an ethos to induce personal resilience (Li 2012; Vickers 2024). This inducement works through the direct and indirect deterministic mechanisms of framing. Conversely, Guangzhou is lower in Westernization, thus its framing for resilience (Yu 2014). Meanwhile, Macau has lower self-worth as an ethos to champion well-being and resilience (van Schalkwyk and Sit 2013).

Societal exclusion, as the opposite of societal care, has bred a negative mood and dissatisfaction to impede resilience (Lin et al. 2013; Williams et al. 2000). The impedance stems from the deterministic mechanisms of empowering and incentivizing to disempower and disincentivize resilience. Societal exclusion and care might crowd out societal inclusion in influencing resilience.

Societal pragmatism, dictating gaining by any means, can favor crime (Matsueda and Grigoryeva 2014). Societal crime has worsened well-being to impair resilience (Jang et al. 2018). Such worsening militates from the deterministic mechanisms of framing and incentivizing. By the framing mechanism, societal crime cultivates ill-being. Alternatively, the incentivizing mechanism generates the disutility of victimization from societal crime.

## *Personal Backgrounds*

Personal backgrounds conducive to resilience were Hong Kong native status, residency, marriage, living with parents, earnings, personal income, family income per capita, and receiving social welfare. Meanwhile, female gender, education, family size, rental public housing, owned private housing, rental private housing, divided mental private housing, self-employment, employee status, unemployment, functional disability and its duration, and adversity delivered inverse effects on resilience.

Hong Kong native status and residency embody the resilience ethos and Westernization to induce resilience (Li 2012; Vickers 2024). This inducement emanates from the voluntaristic mechanism of ideal calibration. Moreover, native status has secured well-being to facilitate resilience (Ambrey and Fleming 2014). Similarly, residency has developed well-being to enable resilience (Melzer 2011).

Marriage has raised well-being to sustain resilience (Carrieri 2012). Additionally, marriage cherishes maintenance as an ideal to rationalize resilience (Segrin and Flora 2019). This rationalization rests on the voluntaristic mechanism of ideal calibration.

Living with parents reflects closeness to parents and filiality (Yi and Lin 2009). Essentially, filiality as enduring support registers resilience (Croll 2006). Additionally, filiality champions pride to maintain resilience (Dabbagh et al. 2017).

Earnings or personal income, as a resource, has buttressed well-being to induce resilience (Wang and VanderWeele 2011). The resource functions with the voluntaristic mechanism of power realization. Furthermore, income has fostered resistance as an ideal to rationalize resilience (Lubbers et al. 2006). Such rationalization builds on the voluntaristic mechanism of ideal calibration.

Family income similarly represents a resource to afford health and mental health, mastery, neighborhood quality, satisfaction, self-efficacy, and self-esteem to prop resilience (Ambrey and Fleming 2014; Cerin and Leslie 2008; Oliver 2003; Oshio and Kobayashi 2010; Thoits and Hewitt 2001; Woldoff and Ovadia 2009). Such power or resources function with the voluntaristic mechanism of power realization.

Welfare reception has sustained well-being, including health, to enable resilience (Headey and Headey 2003; Knab et al. 2008). Nevertheless, welfare reception has also predicted illness (Grundy and Sloggett 2003). The coupling of illness and health or well-being exactly constitutes resilience. Hence, welfare reception provides conditions for resilience owing to the voluntaristic mechanism of power realization.

Female gender has weakened well-being, thus dampening resilience (Gattino et al. 2015). Essentially, female gender downplays agency and self-esteem (Fyall and Gazley 2015; Thapa et al. 2021). Female gender has also dismissed the ideal for self-enhancement to lose resilience (Daniel et al. 2022). Hence, female gender lowers the power and ideal to run the voluntaristic mechanisms of power realization and ideal calibration to sustain resilience.

Education has bred dissatisfaction and injustice and victimization experienced to undermine resilience (Chen and Davey 2009; Jasso 2015; Norris 2011; Pratt et al. 2010; Tiliouine et al. 2006; Yienprugsawan et al. 2010). These experiences represent disutility concerned in the voluntaristic mechanism of utility optimization. Specifically, education in the context of visual impairment reduced resilience, possibly because of the incongruity between education and impairment or dependency (Papastephanon 2015). Accordingly, incongruity or contradiction can dampen power to impede resilience (ten Brinke and Keltner 2020).

Family size has diminished well-being to jeopardize resilience (Luttmer 2005). Moreover, family size has discounted the ideal for health to impair resilience (Zweifel and Breyer 1997). Resilience thus suffers due to the inadequate ideal and power to run the voluntaristic mechanisms of ideal calibration and power realization.

Housing influences resilience through its quality and homeownership (Jiang et al. 2011). Housing quality has sustained well-being to facilitate resilience. Homeownership has raised family and neighborhood quality, health, and satisfaction to constitute well-being to secure resilience (Park et al. 2022; Roy and Chaudhuri 2008; Woldoff and Ovadia 2009). These influences emanate from the voluntaristic mechanism of power realization.

Social class, which is highest in the employer and lowest in the unemployed person, has maintained well-being to enable resilience (Haller and Hadler 2006). Moreover, social class has fostered the ideal for adaptation to rationalize resilience (Yeh et al. 2013). Social class thus secures resilience through the voluntaristic mechanisms of power realization and ideal calibration.

Disability has engendered depression and distress and weakened health, satisfaction, self-efficacy, and thus well-being to impede resilience (Distante 2013; Flett 2018; Gastil 2000; Granzin and Haggard 2000; Phongsavan et al. 2006). Essentially, disability means inadequate power to maintain well-being and resilience (Herd et al. 2008). Such maintenance depends on the voluntaristic mechanism of power realization.

Adversity has endangered well-being to undermine resilience (Baumeister et al. 2013). Furthermore, adversity has led to suicide to purge resilience (Dutton et al. 2016). Resilience thus suffers under adversity, following the operation of the voluntaristic mechanisms of power realization and ideal calibration.

## *Peer Conditions*

Peer conditions in speaker sociability, relational kindness, aid received, peer aid received, peer benevolent world belief, and peer resilience learning showed positive effects on resilience. Meanwhile, peer adversity, peer speaker sociability, and peer resilience belief displayed negative effects on resilience. Generally, these peer conditions manifest normative influences through the deterministic mechanism of standardizing and the voluntaristic mechanism of norm conformity to assimilate resilience, sociability, kindness, benevolent world belief, and aid received.

Peer resilience can directly induce resilience through the direct deterministic mechanism. As such, peer abidance and prosociality have sustained resilience (Masten et al. 2009). Similarly, family adaptability has buttressed resilience (Jones and d'Errico 2019). However, peer resilience belief can also discourage resilience by raising the comparison standard to reduce the relative gain from resilience according to the voluntaristic mechanism of utility optimization.

Peer aid has elevated resilience (Kwarikunda et al. 2023). This elevation builds on the deterministic mechanism of empowering and the voluntaristic mechanism of power realization.

Peer kindness has sustained resilience (Masten et al. 2009). This sustenance benefits from the deterministic mechanism of standardizing and the voluntaristic mechanisms of norm conformity and ideal calibration. Accordingly, peer kindness induces the ideal for kindness, advancing resilience (Alessandri et al. 2014).

Peer sociability has escalated resilience (Masten et al. 2009). This escalation stems from the deterministic mechanism of standardizing and the voluntaristic mechanisms of norm conformity and power realization. Accordingly, peer sociability induces sociability, which drives resilience (Pyszkowska 2020).

Peer benevolent world belief reflects the community's expectation for gain to attract resilience (Ungar et al. 2005). This attraction stands on the deterministic mechanism of standardizing and the voluntaristic mechanism of utility optimization. Accordingly, peer benevolent world belief assimilates benevolent world belief, which in turn indicates utility to attract resilience (Alvarez and Pinto 2023; Wu et al. 2011).

Peer adversity has impeded resilience (Ungar et al. 2005). This impedance evolves from the deterministic mechanism of standardizing and the voluntaristic mechanism of utility optimization. Accordingly, peer adversity generalizes adversity, disincentivizing resilience (Sobeck et al. 2020).

## *Practices*

Practices exhibiting positive effects on resilience were kindness, hardening, softening, and experience-based coping. However, combining hardening and softening generated an additional inverse effect on resilience. That is, hardening attenuated the positive effect of softening and vice versa. This attenuation reveals the competition between hardening and softening in their contribution to resilience.

Kindness has facilitated resilience (Alessandri et al. 2014). The facilitation arises from the voluntaristic mechanism of ideal calibration. Moreover, kindness has buttressed well-being, including life satisfaction to induce resilience (Nelson-Coffey et al. 2023; Raposa et al. 2016). This buttressing benefits from the voluntaristic mechanisms of power realization and utility optimization.

Hardening encompasses building commitment, confidence, power, and rationality (Pangallo et al. 2015; Perry et al. 2013; Zhang 2006). As such, hardening has strengthened well-being to advance resilience (DeNeve and Cooper 1998). For instance, commitment has raised self-acceptance to maintain resilience (Agronick and Duncan 1998). Conversely, rationality has reduced anxiety, depression, and fear to sustain resilience (Barnes and Vulcano 1982; DiGiuseppe et al. 2017). This strengthening illustrates the voluntaristic mechanism of power realization. Moreover, hardening has facilitated success to elevate resilience (Greeff and van der Merwe 2004). This facilitation evolves from the voluntaristic mechanism of utility optimization.

Softening embraces attracting, befriending, compensating or rewarding, cooperating, dialoguing, educating, empathizing, equalizing, following, harmonizing, relaxing, and trusting (Edney 2012; Greene 1991; Koomen and van der Pligt 2016; Sui 2011; Wansink and van Itterum 2012; Zhang 2006). As such, softening has boosted well-being, including adaptation, adjustment, health, intimacy, and survival to enable resilience (Barefoot et al. 1998; Littlejohn et al. 2017; Marcus 2014; Redmond 2018; Rosen et al. 2017; Stavrova 2014). This boost applies to the voluntaristic mechanism of power realization. Moreover, softening, such as relaxing, has triggered success to attract resilience (Mehrabian 2000). This triggering evolves from the voluntaristic mechanism of utility optimization.

Hardening and softening combined, however, introduced an inverse effect on resilience to reduce the positive effects of hardening and softening. This inverse effect reflects the contradiction between hardening and softening to weaken the individual effects. For instance, contradiction can erode collaboration, integration, intelligence, and thus power to impede resilience (Schaie 2013; Turner 2013). This impedance arises from the voluntaristic mechanism of power realization.

Experience-based coping combines learning and coping, enabling resilience (Buikstra et al. 2010; Corbin and Hall 2019). This enabling demonstrates the voluntaristic mechanism of ideal calibration. Besides, learning and coping have boosted well-being, including environmental and relational quality, growth, health, intimacy, satisfaction, and self-efficacy to achieve resilience (Chow et al. 2014; Gattino et al. 2015; Lau et al. 2012; Minnaert and Janssen 1992; Paez et al. 2007; Sobeck et al. 2020; Wills 1997). This boost engages the voluntaristic mechanisms of power realization and utility optimization.

## *Social Capital*

Social capital components displaying positive effects on resilience were the associational structural component, friend structural component and its combination with the friend substantive component, and additional combination with the friend functional component. However, friend substantive and functional components individually manifested inverse effects on resilience. These components thus required the friend structural component to catalyze their positive effects on resilience.

Social capital generally constitutes or can engender resilience (Jayawardana et al. 2019; Jones and d'Errico 2019). Moreover, social capital has boosted well-being, including flourishing, happiness, health, and life satisfaction, to induce resilience (Chua et al. 2021; Yetim and Yetim 2014). This boosting leverages the voluntaristic mechanisms of power realization and utility optimization.

Friend functional and substantive social capital involves reciprocity, mutual trust, and resources through social networking (Chen et al. 2015; Murayama et al. 2019; Tulin et al. 2018). Mutual trust or reciprocity, including retaliation experienced, has generated hate, substance abuse, and violence to erode resilience (de la Haye et al. 2015; Lorant and Nicaise 2015; Palacios et al. 2019; Shin et al. 2019). Substance abuse and violence have hampered well-being to impede resilience (Kendler et al. 2006; Wright et al. 2015). Reciprocity experience can also stimulate protesting to obstruct resilience (Brock and Carrigan 2015). Protesting has obstructed well-being to erode resilience (Landmann and Rohmann 2020). Social network resources have reduced satisfaction and social support received and increased obesity, protesting, victimization experienced, and violence to impair resilience (Farrington 2007; Hurlbert et al. 2000; Marmot and Fuhrer 2004; Norris 2011; Oliver 2003; Yip et al. 2007; Zhang et al. 2007). Social support received has advanced well-being to maintain resilience. Obesity, protesting, victimization experienced, and violence have dampened well-being, including health, intimacy, satisfaction, and self-esteem, to impede resilience (Carr and Friedman 2005; Graham et al. 2010; Hanson et al. 2010; Kahneman et al. 2010; Krahe 2013; Landmann and Rohmann 2020; Wright et al. 2015). These impacts involve the voluntaristic mechanisms of power realization, utility optimization, and ideal calibration.

Nevertheless, the impacts of friend functional and substantive social capital on resilience turned from negative to positive with increasing friend structural social capital. That is, friend structural social capital reduced the negative impacts of friend functional and substantive social capital and increased their positive impacts. In other words, friend structural social capital diminished the contrast or jealousy effects of friend functional and substantive social capital and heightened their assimilation or sharing effects. The contrast or jealousy effect occurs when others' resources discount one's relative resources, whereas the assimilation or sharing effect arises when others' resources add to one's resources. Whereas the former follows the voluntaristic mechanism of utility optimization, the latter leverages the voluntaristic mechanism of power realization. Accordingly, the bonding structure prevents contrasting and jealousy and enables assimilation and sharing or pooling (Chia 2021; Firestone et al. 2006).

## *Developmental Conditions*

Developmental conditions with positive effects on resilience were extraversion, conscientiousness, and ritualistic activity. Meanwhile, empowerment, neuroticism, and distress were developmental conditions displaying inverse effects on resilience. Nevertheless, most activities, including coaching received, musical activity, and sporting, did not manifest effects on resilience.

Extraversion has underlain well-being, including autonomy, growth, mastery, mattering, positive affect, purposefulness, relatedness, satisfaction, self-acceptance, self-determination, self-efficacy, and self-esteem, to champion resilience (Anusic et al. 2014; Flett 2018; Hounkpatin et al. 2015; Ingledew et al. 2004; Quilty et al. 2006; Rasmussen et al. 2018; Richards 2016; Tiwari et al. 2021). This championing benefits from the voluntaristic mechanisms of power realization and utility optimization.

Conscientiousness has enhanced resilience (Yu and Zhang 2007). Besides, conscientiousness has fostered well-being, including autonomy, competence, growth, health, life satisfaction, mastery, purposefulness, relatedness, relational quality, positive affect, self-acceptance, self-compassion, self-determination, self-efficacy, self-esteem, and survival, to induce resilience (Bowes et al. 2022; Hounkpatin et al.

2015; Ingledew et al. 2004; Judge et al. 2002; Keightley et al. 2006; Li et al. 2017; Maltby et al. 2019; Marks 1996; McCrae and Terracciano 2008; Pyszkowska 2020; Quilty et al. 2006; Richards 2016; Tiwari et al. 2021). The inducement rests on the voluntaristic mechanisms of power realization and utility optimization.

Ritualistic activity has maintained well-being, including health, intimacy, and pleasure, to enable resilience (Crespo et al. 2008; Fiese and Hammons 2013; Rossner and Meher 2014; Yang and Wang 2023). Such enablement builds on the voluntaristic mechanism of power realization.

Empowerment based on deciding, leading, and planning has triggered protesting, radicalism, and social exclusion experienced to impede resilience (Secker et al. 2009; Selvanathan and Lickel 2019). This impedance withdraws ideals and utility to run the voluntaristic mechanisms of ideal calibration and utility optimization to facilitate resilience. Conversely, empowerment can lessen cooperation to hinder resilience (Sanderson 2001). This hindrance stems from losing the ideal to rationalize resilience through the voluntaristic mechanism of ideal calibration.

Neuroticism has eroded well-being, including autonomy, growth, health, positive affect, purposefulness, relatedness, relational quality, satisfaction, self-acceptance, self-compassion, and self-determination, to undermine resilience (Anusic et al. 2014; Austin et al. 2005; Hounknatin et al. 2015; Ingledew et al. 2004; Marks 1996; Pfattheicher et al. 2017). This undermining embodied the voluntaristic mechanisms of power realization and utility optimization.

## *Mechanic Development*

Functionalistic development encompassing power, utility, ideals, and norms as forces is explicable by applying mechanics to psychosocial dynamics. Accordingly, the four modes of forces generalize to psychosocial mechanic force on the product of mass and acceleration or velocity transmitted at an angle through a directional vector (Ambrose 2002; Bahr and Passerinin 1998, Cheung 2013, Dzendolet 1999). Thus, the impact of a force depends on its vector, angle, direction, or tropicity. As such, when resilience impact is the direct impact of concern, an oblige impact shows an angle, correlation, or cosine with resilience. Hence, a direct positive impact on resilience can come from prior resilience as a force, whereas an oblige positive impact can emanate from a factor compatible with, correlated with, or like resilience, such as adjustment or well-being. Conversely, a direct negative impact can stem from a factor contradicting resilience, whereas an oblige negative impact can spring from a factor incompatible, negatively correlated with, or unlike resilience, for example, distress or ill-being. Meanwhile, the impact also depends on the mass or intensity and acceleration or velocity constituting the force, For instance, kissing is stronger than blinking as mass to show intimacy intensity. The acceleration or velocity of a force indicates its contact depth, intensity, duration, frequency, or, more generally, relevance. An inverse of contact is distance. Hence, impact is higher when distance is shorter or frequency or relevance is higher. For instance, the resilience impact of one's prior resilience is higher than that of a friend's resilience as one is closer to oneself than a friend. Psychosocial mechanics is thus a more general theoretical lens covering analytical functionalism to warrant the effects of predictors found. Essentially, psychosocial mechanics takes power, utility, ideals, and norms as currencies or vehicles to transmit forces to create impacts.

Resilience represents such positive vectors as adaptation, assets or resourcefulness, buffering, capability, coping, endurance, functioning, growth, heroism, homeostasis or balance, meaningfulness, morale, order, recovery, resistance, return, self-determination, stability, steeling, strength, and well-being (Allison et al. 2017; Boden et al. 2014; Bowers et al. 2017; Berger 2015; Cohn and Fredrickson 2009; Eshel et al. 2017; Huta 2017; Lawler et al. 2009; Johnson et al. 2017; Peterson et al. 2008; Prilleltensky 2012; Rutter 2012; Schwager and Rothermund 2014; Van Haaften et al. 2004; Zautra et al. 2010; Zheng et al. 2020). Moreover, resilience encompasses such positive vectors as acceptance, activeness, adaptation, adjustment, agency, altruism or empathy, attractiveness, awareness, character, coherence, cohesion, commitment, compensation, competence, confidence, control, courage, creativity, energy, engagement, exercising, expressiveness, faith, flexibility, hardiness, health, hope, holism, humor, insight, instrumentality, intelligence, investment, learning, maintenance, maturity, moderating, nobility, optimism, patience, perseverance, persistence, prevention, proactivity, productivity, protection, purposefulness, rebounding, reconstruction, reflection, robustness, restoration, safety, self-actualization, self-regulation, self-righting, skill, spirituality, sustainability, talent, teamwork, tenacity, thoroughness, tolerance, training, transcendence, understanding, virtue or benevolence, and warmth (Alrofiai et al. 2020; Brodsky and Cattaneo 2013; Castro and Murray 2010; Connor et al. 2003; Elfers et al. 2024; Friedman and Robbins 2012; Hjemdal et al. 2015; Jayawardana et al. 2019; Kent and Davis 2010; Kelley et al. 2019; Mak et al. 2019; Metzl and Morrell 2008; Mukherjee and Kumar 2017; Nemeth and Olivier 2017; Park and Slattery 2014; Richardson 2017; Solomon and Roloff 2018; Schoon 2006; Ungar 2010; Van Vliet 2008; Yu and Zhang 2007; Xie and Wong 2021). Character comprises honesty, honor, integrity, kindness, loyalty, morality, and trustworthiness (Richardson 2017). Hardiness comprises commitment, control, and challenge (Pangallo et al. 2015). Intelligence covers choice, cohesion, empathy, humanization, perspective-taking, and uniqueness (Nemeth and Olivier 2017; Zautra 2014). Nobility comprises self-efficacy and self-esteem (Richardson 2017). Reconstruction covers onding, growth, and peace (Elfers et al. 2024). Resourcefulness covers acceptance, awareness, cognition, control, encountering, integration, and intentionality (Celinski and Allen 2017). Self-regulation covers commitment, inhibition, mobilization, reorientation, and resolution (Schwager and Rothermund 2014). The negative vectors associated with resilience are disruption, emptiness, fear, grief, loss, martyrdom, meaninglessness, risk, suicide, and terrorism (Boden et al. 2014; Elfers et al. 2024; Hariharan and Rana 2017; Kent and Davis 2010; Matusitz 2017; Nemeth and Olivier 2017). These vectors figure in the predictors of resilience.

To the youth, the additional positive vectors of resilience are adherence, agreeableness, authenticity, autonomy, caring, certainty, cheerfulness, comfort, conformity, confronting, constructiveness, cooperation, dignity or honor, discipline, equanimity, extraversion, fitness, flourishing, grit, habit, honesty, humor, identity, initiative, integrity, kindness, knowledge, love, management, mastery, motivation, normality or normal development, normalization, open-mindedness or openness, overcoming, power, prospection or future orientation, prosociality, purposiveness, reflection, relatedness, relaxation, resolution, satisfaction, self-esteem, self-expression, self-improvement, self-reliance, self-righting, sociability, support received, tolerance, trust, trustworthiness, and wisdom (Boulton and Macaulay 2022; Brooks and Brooks 2014; Callegari et al. 2016; Davis and Paster 2000; Eisenberg et al. 2002; Fredrickson and Losada 2005; Johnson et al. 2015; Joseph 1994; Kennison 2022; Kim 2015; Lee et al. 2010; Li et al. 2018; Ma et al. 2022; Ni et al. 2016; Panter-Brick 2015; Pitzer and Skinner 2017; Plouffe et al. 2020; Qouta et al. 2007; Ramasubramanian 2017; Roth and Herzberg 2017; Scales et al. 2000; Supkoff et al. 2012; Ungar 2015; Ungar et al. 2007; van Rensburg et al. 2019; Wong and Chui 2017; Wang, Zhang, and Zimmerman 2015; Wright and Masten 2015; Yamamoto et al. 2023; Yuan et al. 2024). Mastery covers acceptability, adaptability, decision, functioning, judgment, learning, optimism, resolution, and self-efficacy (Plouffe et al. 2020; Prince-Embury 2014a). Relatedness covers assertiveness, comfort, cooperation, empathy, engagement, listening, role-taking, self-control, support received, tolerance, and trust (Plouffe et al. 2020; Prince-Embury 2014a). Relaxation covers awareness, energy, flow, joy, optimism, restfulness, and transcendence (Ramasubramanian 2017). Conversely, to the youth, additional negative vectors are antisociality, avoidance, brittleness, depression, doping, hopelessness, impulsivity, neuroticism, reactivity, rigidity, stress, symptoms, and psychopathology (Brooks and Brooks 2014; Gardner et al. 2008; Haverfield and Theiss 2017; Kaplan 2012; Kaye-Tzadok and Davidson-Arad 2017; Masten 2014; Roth and Herzberg 2017; Svetina 2014; Villasana et al. 2017; Wong 2008; Wong and Chui 2017).

To the elder, the additional positive vectors of resilience are accommodating, assertiveness, balance, banding, generativity, hope, independence, living, preparation, saving, self-affirmation, staying, strategizing, and tricking (Greene et al. 2012; Hrostowski and Rehner 2012; Lou and Ng 2012; Moen et al. 2010; Morrissey 2015; Nakashima and Canda 2005; Nelson Becker 2006; Tanner 2007; Wiles et al. 2012). Conversely, additional negative vectors are anxiety, defiance, loss, surrender, and victimization experienced (Boerner et al. 2005; Halpin et al. 2017; Hrostowski and Rehner 2012; Nakashima and Canda 2005).

To the working person, the additional positive vectors of resilience are curiosity, humility, mindfulness, stamina, success, and thriving (Lin 2018; Luthans et al. 2015; McCray et al. 2016; Thompson 2023). Conversely, burnout is another negative vector (Ruiz et al. 2023).

To the client or patient, the additional positive vectors of resilience are aiming or goal setting, collaboration, determination, freedom, gentleness, goodness, gratitude, happiness, immunity, inclusiveness, justice, loyalty, normativity, pride, self-sufficiency, serenity, survival, and truthfulness (Davydov et al. 2010; Godwin et al. 2015; Hassija and Gray 2012; Hendricks and Testa 2012; Henry 2001; Hines et al. 2005; Liebenberg and Moore 2018; Mota and Matos 2015; Samuels and Pryce 2008; Veronese and Barola 2018; Woodier 2011). Conversely, additional negative vectors are alcoholism, emotionality, illness, and vulnerability (Aldwin et al. 2009; Park 2009; Rajan-Rankin 2014; Wong et al. 2018).

## *Societal Conditions*

Societal caring has its vector toward resilience involving devotion or dutifulness, empowerment, harmonizing, helping, loving, meaning maintaining, protecting, supporting, and warming (Fine 2007; Ip 2014; Tracy 2002). That is, caring is compatible with or similar to resilience in maintaining well-being. The mass of societal caring rests on its societal source.

Scoetal exclusion delivers a negative vector toward resilience through exclusion and being excluded. Exclusion involves depriving, disabling, hurting, punishing, resigning, and threatening (Allman 2013; Barry and Hullett 1998; Gallie 2004; Hammer et al. 2009; Riva et al. 2017). Being excluded involves anxiety or fear, deviance, dying, offending, poverty, risking, and unemployment (Botti and D'Ippoliti 2014; Delanty 2008; Peruzzi 2014; Stanley et al. 2011; Wacquant 2008; Zamperini et al. 2020). They are antithetical to resilience.

Societal pragmatism involves vectors incompatible with resilience, such as debate or conflict, diversity or plurality, and temporality or instability (Bromley 2004; Knight and Johnson 2011; Mahoney 2004). Conversely, societal pragmatism dismisses vectors compatible with resilience as morality, rationality, spirituality, and transcendence (Mahoney 2004; Stuhr 2003; Webb 2007).

Westernization holds such vectors compatible with resilience: control, creativity, individualism, knowledge, mastery, safety, tolerance, and work (Ma 2019; Narvaez 2014; Taplin et al. 2013; Zhou 2008). The mass of Westernization grows with industrialization (Ma 2019).

Hong Kong cultivates resilience as a direct vector toward resilience (Li 2012). Moreover, Hong Kong features such vectors compatible with resilience as autonomy or self-determination, capitalism, creativity, entertainment, flexibility, individualism, knowledge, openness, safety, self-enhancement, self-help, transcendence, wealth or affluence, and Westernization (Cartier 2008; DeGolyer 2001; Delang and Lung 2010; Estes 2002; Guan et al. 2009, 2010; Kwong and Wong 2017; Ma 2011b; Ng and Wong 1999; Park et al. 2015; Welzel 2013). Capitalism idealizes diligence, honesty, and success (Ng and Wong 1999). Individualism highlights entrepreneurship, liberty, and self-enhancement (Guan et al. 2010).

Macau displays vectors incompatible with resilience, such as confusion and fragmentation (Greenwood and Dwyer 2017; van Schalkwyk and Sit 2013). Conversely, Macau is inadequate in vectors compatible with resilience, such as belongingness and self-worth (Greenwood and Dwyer 2017; van Schalkwyk and Sit 2013).

## *Personal Backgrounds*

Residency has maintained such vectors compatible with resilience as attachment, awareness, cohesion, health, morale, supporting, volunteering, and well-being (Anton and Lawrence 2014; Hutchings 2003; Jorgensen et al. 2010; La Grange 2011; Patulny and Morris 2012; Melzer 2011; Rotolo et al. 2010; Wulfhorst and Kranich 1999). Conversely, residency has prevented vectors incompatible with resilience such as suffering (Zhang et al. 2007).

Marriage denotes such vectors compatible with resilience as agreement, assurance, attachment, caring, gratification, gratitude, love, maintenance, meaningfulness, positivity, provisioning, responsibility, understanding, warmth, and thus enjoying benefits (Carbery and Buhrmester 1998; Caughlin et al. 2018; Hartley and Watson 2012; Segrin and Flora 2019; Su et al. 2015; Turner 2005a). Conversely, marriage prohibits such vectors incompatible with resilience as arguing, conflict, and harming (Arneson 2005; Segrin and Flora 2019; Su et al. 2015).

Living with parents manifests such vectors compatible with resilience as acceptance, commitment, love, respect, and responsibility (Bawin-Legros 2001; Chin and Loh 2008; Szinovacy 1997). Moreover, such coresidence reflects helping and resourcefulness as vectors toward resilience (Chattopadhyay and Marsh 1999; Szinovacy 1997). Conversely, such co-residence reflects low disability, a vector incompatible with resilience (Lagergren 1996).

Homeownership engages such vectors compatible with resilience as resourcefulness or socioeconomic status, security, and self-reliance (Montazer 2022; Zhan et al. 2022; Zheng et al. 2020). Moreover, homeownership transmits such vectors as attachment, health, life quality, morale, prosociality, and satisfaction, which are compatible with resilience (Anton and Lawrence 2014; Degenne et al. 2004; Park et al. 2022; Roy and Chaudhuri 2008; Woldoff and Ovadia 2009; Wulfhorst and Kranich 1999). The mass of homeownership rests on its nature as critical consumption and the most important event (Henretta 1987; Park et al. 2022).

Employer status carries vectors compatible with resilience, such as activeness, admirability, charity, social capital, and social status or resourcefulness (Gerth 2011; Ma and Cheng 2010; Song and Lee 2010). More generally, social class signifies vectors compatible with resilience, such as autonomy, creativity, power, and security (Nollmann and Strasser 2007; Reicher et al. 2010; Todorova 2013).

Earnings or income indicates such vectors compatible with resilience as control, effort, self-efficacy, self-support, skill, and success (Braun et al. 2011; Gerhart and Rynes 2003; Lauder et al. 2018; Reitzle et al. 1998; Zhang and Eriksson 2010). Conversely, earnings or income precludes such a vector incompatible with resilience as loss (Gangl 2006).

Welfare reception issues such vectors compatible with resilience as guarantee, insurance, protection, safety, and security (Ansel 2014; Dean 2020; Haskins 1995; Johnston et al. 2017; Lessnoff 1986; Sotirovic 2001). Conversely, welfare reception counters vectors incompatible with resilience, such as crisis and risk (Fischer et al. 1996).

Female gender features such vectors incompatible with resilience as anxiety or fear, dependence, depression, and sacrifice. (Goldberg 1993; Hopcroft 2016; Rundman and Glick 2008). Conversely, female gender downplays such vectors compatible with resilience as achievement, agency, control, heroism, independence, instrumentality, power, status or resourcefulness, and self-esteem (Carli 2004; Diekman and Schneider 2010; Fyall and Gazley 2015; Guo et al. 2008; Irwin 2011; Rundman and Glick 2008; Thapa et al. 2021).

Education has evolved vectors incompatible with resilience, such as aspiration, deservingness, rights consciousness, and protesting (Attewell 2022; Norris 2011; Straughn and Andriot 2011; Welzel 2013). Aspiration has impaired life satisfaction and eroded relational quality, thus undermining resilience (Nickerson et al. 2007). Deservingness or rights consciousness has bred hostility to undermine resilience (Moeller et al. 2009). Conversely, education has dispelled such vectors compatible with resilience as diligence or hard work, harmony, obedience, and survival (Bullock 2021; Datler et al. 2013; Fjellvang 2011; Lu and Kao 2002). Specifically, education in the face of impairment displays can generate the vectors of contradiction and incongruity incompatible with resilience (Papastephanon 2015; ten Brinke and Keltner 2020).

Disability emits vectors incompatible with resilience, such as dependency and suffering (Bornstein 2006; White et al. 2015). Conversely, disability loses such vectors compatible with resilience as functioning, instrumentality, life quality, and self-care (Caplan and Schooler 2003; Stewart and King 1994; Vittengl et al. 2006).

Adversity evolves or involves such vectors incompatible with resilience as anxiety or worry, conflict, dependency, depression, disorders, distress, failure, hostility, loss, submissiveness, suffering, and uncontrollability (Berger 2015; Demertzis 2020; Eberhart and Hammen 2009; Garfin et al. 2015; Kleiman and Riskind 2014; Lupien et al. 2009; Mandel et al. 2018; Matthews et al. 2006; Snyder et al. 2020; Staton-Tindall et al. 2012; Vollhardt and Staub 2011). Conversely, adversity loses such vectors compatible with resilience as control and engagement (Gatersleben and Griffin 2017; Matthews et al. 2006).

## *Peer Conditions*

Peer resilience represents a vector directly conducive to resilience. Nevertheless, the impact of peer resilience is not maximal because of the peer distance or separation from oneself.

Peer aid provision represents such vectors compatible with resilience as altruism, awareness, caring, charity, collaboration, commitment, cooperation, empathy, heroism, and volunteering (Jirsaraie et al. 2019; Kafashun et al. 2017; Luria et al. 2019; Mastain 2007; Matts et al. 2009; Premo et al. 2018; Wang et al. 2021). Conversely, peer aid provision discounts such vectors incompatible with resilience as competition, loneliness, and punishment (Coyne et al. 2018; Stagnaro et al. 2017; Van Lange et al. 2012).

Peer aid reception indicates or generates such vectors compatible with resilience as attachment, belongingness, empathy, love, resourcefulness, responsiveness, security, social capital, and togetherness (Barrera 1988; Feeney and Collins 2018; Godoy et al. 2007; Holliman et al. 2021; Manassis 2017; Thoits 2011; Tomlinson et al. 2018). Moreover, peer aid involves such vectors compatible with resilience as acceptance, caring, health, openness, and prevention (Biglan 2018; Davis-Lipman et al. 2007; Glendinning et al. 2003; Marti et al. 2017; Patulny and Morris 2012). Conversely, peer aid dismisses such vectors incompatible with resilience as anomie and conflict (Helgeson 2003; Stewart 1989).

Peer adversity involves the same vectors as those of oneself. The difference is that peer adversity is farther than one's adversity from oneself. Hence, the impact of peer adversity was weaker than that of one's adversity (see Tables 3.4 and 5.3@@@).

## *Practices*

Kindness involves or represents such vectors compatible with resilience as adjustment, altruism, awareness or insight, conformity, courage, faith, forbearance, gratitude, harmony, learning, moderation, morality or virtue, quiescence, relief, tolerance, and transcendence (Bang and Zhou 2014; Barcalow 2007; Bosacki et al. 2018; Luk 2001; Peplak and Malti 2022; Wang 2004; Zhang 2003). Conversely, kindness dismisses such vectors incompatible with resilience as greed and indifference (Miller and Verhaeghen 2022; Stevenson 2011).

Hardening incorporates such vectors compatible with resilience: challenge, commitment, confidence, control, power, and rationality (Pangallo et al. 2015; Perry et al. 2013; Zhang 2006). Conversely, hardening downplays such vectors incompatible with resilience as escape, laziness, and yielding (Bjornskov et al. 2013).

Softening upholds such vectors compatible with resilience as cooperation, empathy, harmony, openness, patience, persistence, proactivity, rebailitation, relaxing, self-discipline, supporting, and warmth (Clubb and O'Connor 2019; Greene 1991; Hallsworth and Young 2010; Koomen and van der Pligt 2016; Wansink and van Itterum 2012). Conversely, softening downplays such vectors as desperation and struggle incompatible with resilience (Greene 1991; Sui 2011).

Hardening and softening combined register contradictions to display vectors incompatible with effectiveness, such as avoidance, deprivation, powerlessness, restriction, and strain (Busby and Chiu 2017; Somma et al. 2020; Turner 2013; Ward 2002). Conversely, contradiction dismisses such vectors compatible with effectiveness as collaboration, control, resourcefulness, and strength (Kivimaki 2012; Lawler et al. 2009; Lilly et al. 2011; Turner 2013).

Experience-based coping maintains vectors through learning and coping. Learning generates or involves such vectors compatible with resilience as acceptance, activeness, agency, empathy, engagement, intelligence, insight, meaningfulness, open-mindedness, reasoning, and self-regulation (Booth 2003; Bussey 2020; Clem et al. 2014; Hagger and Hamilton 2018; Mesirow 2003; Schunk and Usher

2019; Severiens and Geert 1997). Conversely, learning dismisses such a vector incompatible with resilience as impulsivity (Mesirow 2003). Coping involves such vectors compatible with resilience as activeness or proactivity, buffering or protection, control and self-control, engagement, flexibility, optimism, reparation, resolution, and responsibility (Johnson et al. 2013; Kleinke 2007; Major and Townsend 2010; Pollio et al. 1997; Seaton and Beaumont 2008; Wyer and Abbarracin 2014).

## Social Capital

Social capital as a social resource generally registers such vectors compatible with resilience as attachment, commitment, durability or stability, flexibility, morality, productivity, reliability, resourcefulness, responsibility, self-reinforcing, and sustainability (Cattell 2004; Chen et al. 2015; Onyx and Bullen 2000; Ozbay 2008; Sabet and Khaksar 2022; Robison et al. 2002; Robison and Ritchie 2010; Siisiainen 2003). Moreover, social capital involves such vectors compatible with resilience as caring, cohesion, engagement, helping or supporting, meaningfulness, power, and volunteerism (Flap and Volker 2013; Huxhold et al. 2022; Jones and Woolcock 2010; Narayan and Cassidy 2001; Poortinga 2012; Reay 2004).

Structural social capital specifically reflects such vectors compatible with resilience as agreement, collaboration, flourishing, openness, positivity, prosociality, and understanding (Dovidio et al. 2006; Felmlee and Sinclair 2018; Goodman et al. 2019; Holt-Lunstad 2022; Kayabol et al. 2022). Conversely, structural social capital dismisses such a vector incompatible with resilience as shyness (Baumeister and Leary 1995).

Structural, functional, and substantive social capital combined indicates complementarity or synergy to engage vectors compatible with effectiveness, such as exchange, fitness or congruence, harmony, and stability (Deeg 2007; Fang 2003; Namini et al. 2010; Svara 2001). Conversely, complementarity or synergy dismisses such vectors as conflict and separateness incompatible with effectiveness (Rick et al. 2006; Svara 2001).

## Developmental Conditions

Empowerment experienced, comprising leading, organizing, and planning, emits such vectors incompatible with resilience as aspiration, conflict, confusion, overwhelming experience, protesting, radicalism, rights orientation or entitlement, and stress or pressure (Badawy and Schieman 2021; Castells 2012; Kegler and Wyatt 2003; Selvanathan and Lickel 2019; Snyder et al. 2018; Thompson and Thompson 2001; Zhuang 2020). Conversely, empowerment counters such vectors compatible with resilience as caring and cooperation (Sanderson 2001; Thompson and Thompson 2001). Specifically, leading involves such vectors incompatible with resilience as aspiration, sacrifice, self-questioning, serving, and surrendering (Case et al. 2011; Conger 2011; Hanaway 2020; Wang 1997; Yeagley et al. 2010). Conversely, leading dismisses defense as a vector compatible with resilience (Hanaway 2020).

Extraversion features such vectors compatible with resilience as enthusiasm, pleasure, positivity, poise, and warmth (Batey et al. 2010; Muris et al. 2007; Sun et al. 2018). Conversely, extraversion dismisses such vectors incompatible with resilience as apprehension and shyness (Bassett et al. 2017; Draper and Holman 2005).

Conscientious reflects the resilience vector directly (Roth and Herzberg 2017). Alternatively, conscientiousness registers such vectors compatible with resilience as achievement, broadmindedness, constructiveness, maturity or adulthood, motivation, and responsibility (Ackerman and Wolman 2007; Arnett et al. 2011; Curtis and Wee 2021; Roberts et al. 2009; Sirgy 2012; Stichter 2018; Wang 2012). Moreover, conscientious embraces such vectors compatible with resilience as competence, conformity, control, deliberation, dutifulness, efficiency, industriousness or tenaciousness, order or orderliness, patience, persistence, reliability, self-control, self-discipline, striving, and virtue (Hannah et al. 2007; Roberts et al. 2009; Rocha et al. 2023; Sun et al. 2018; Wright and DeLisi 2016). Conversely, conscientiousness dismisses such vectors incompatible with resilience as laziness, messiness, and sloppiness (Draper and Holman 2005; Sun et al. 2018).

Neuroticism features such vectors incompatible with resilience as anxiety, depression, irrationality, moodiness, reactivity, volatility, and withdrawal (Denissen et al. 2009; Sun et al. 2018; Village and Francis 2010). Volatility covers anger, hostility, and impulsivity (Sun et al. 2018). Conversely, neuroticism rejects such vectors compatible with resilience as calmness and tranquility (Sun et al. 2018).

Distress and its vectors of agitation, anger, avoidance, comorbidity, death, depression, frustration, grief, groundlessness, isolation, misadjustment, pain, sadness, shame, sorrow, stress, symptoms, trauma, and unpleasantness including are incompatible with resilience (Becchetta 2010; Carreno et al. 2021; Carver and Scheier 2016; Cochrane 2018; Franks 2003; Holloway et al. 2017; Lee 2016; Lively 2017; Pachankis et al. 2020; Palker-Corell and Marcus 2004; Pomerleau et al. 2020; Ross and Mirowsky 2009; Stevens et al. 2018; Tenorio and Lo 2011; Van Tongeren et al. 2023). Conversely, distress opposes such vectors compatible with resilience as acceptance, achievement, empathy or understanding, insight, reward reception, satisfaction, security, and tolerance (Abu-Raiya et al. 2015; Baucom et al. 2018; Becchetta 2010).

Ritualistic activity reflects the resilience vector directly (Annalakshmi and Abeer 2011). Alternatively, ritualistic activity registers such vectors compatible with resilience as continuity or repetition, control, functioning, order, rehabilitation, social capital, and virtue (Boyer and Lienard 2006; Costa 2013; Izenstart and Ebata 2016; Johnston 2010; Liu 2004; Mangion 2011; Mayer 2003; Yang and Wang 2023). Moreover, ritualistic activity embraces resilient vectors such as composure, invariance, safety, and security (Boyer and Lienard 2006; Raab 2019; Schjoedt et al. 2013). Conversely, ritualistic dismisses such a vector incompatible with resilience as avoidance (Crespo et al. 2008). Meanwhile, the mass of ritualistic activity rests on its collective, compulsory, continuous or repeated, controlled, cultural or durable, everyday or pervasive, humanity-common, normatizing, orchestrated, and regular natures (Boyer and Lienard 2006; Hobson et al. 2017; Jiang 2012; Sandage and Williamson 2005; Schjoedt et al. 2013b; Tian et al. 2018; Turner 2021; Yang and Wang 2023). They constitute the strength of ritualistic activity (Kristjansson 2013; ten Brinke and Keltner 2020).

# Appendix

**Table A.1** Means and standard deviations (poverty dataset)

| Variable | Scoring | *M* | *SD* |
|---|---|---|---|
| *Resilience, recent month* | | | |
| Facing difficulties actively | 0–100 | 59.0 | 21.6 |
| (Not) Feeling anxious at the time of pressure | 0–100 | 51.5 | 23.2 |
| Keeping calm in the face of pressure | 0–100 | 54.7 | 21.6 |
| *Caring in society, past three months* | | | |
| (no) Indifference of Hong Kong people to decrepit or wounded people | 0–100 | 62.6 | 21.4 |
| Care of Hong Kong people to poor people | 0–100 | 46.3 | 23.5 |
| Care of Hong Kong people experiencing privation | 0–100 | 43.6 | 21.0 |
| Hong Kong people just taking care of themselves | 0–100 | 47.3 | 26.5 |
| Care of Hong Kong people to new arrivals | 0–100 | 46.8 | 23.5 |
| *Social exclusion in society, past three months* | | | |
| Income (in)equality in Hong Kong | 0–100 | 70.2 | 23.1 |
| Hong Kong people's (in)ability to buy private housing | 0–100 | 73.2 | 24.6 |
| (no) Disparity between the rich and the poor in Hong Kong | 0–100 | 76.2 | 24.3 |
| (no) Opportunity for Hong Kong people to get rich | 0–100 | 64.1 | 25.7 |
| Poverty in Hong Kong | 0–100 | 65.4 | 23.1 |
| *Social inclusion experienced, past three months* | | | |
| Chance to make friends with Hong Kong people | 0–100 | 49.0 | 22.4 |
| Chance to rise at work and society | 0–100 | 36.1 | 22.4 |
| (no) Barriers to your personal development in society | 0–100 | 63.3 | 23.4 |

(continued)



C. K. Cheung, *Resilience Process and Its Personal and Social Bases*,
https://doi.org/10.1007/978-981-97-7391-6

**Table A.1** (continued)

| Variable | Scoring | *M* | *SD* |
|---|---|---|---|
| *Caring received, past three months* | | | |
| Non-family care for you | 0–100 | 55.7 | 23.4 |
| Company/organizational care for you | 0–100 | 38.3 | 24.3 |
| Family care for you | 0–100 | 70.0 | 23.2 |
| *Social participation, past three months* | | | |
| Joining religious activities | 0–100 | 18.8 | 27.6 |
| Joining non-work activities held by companies and superiors | 0–100 | 27.5 | 24.1 |
| Joining activities held by community centers | 0–100 | 24.6 | 25.8 |
| Joining activities held by government | 0–100 | 19.1 | 22.2 |
| Joining extracurricular activities held by school | 0–100 | 28.4 | 25.6 |
| Joining activities of the family that were outside the home | 0–100 | 39.1 | 23.5 |
| Joining the activities of social movement organizations | 0–100 | 23.5 | 24.0 |
| Joining activities held by concern groups | 0–100 | 20.0 | 24.1 |
| Acquiescence | 0–100 | 42.6 | 5.6 |
| Personal monthly income | log(HK$) | 9.8 | 1.1 |
| Family monthly income per capita | log(HK$) | 8.2 | 1.0 |
| Living in owned private housing | 0, 100 | 0.4 | 0.5 |
| Irreligious | 0, 100 | 0.8 | 0.4 |
| Residency | Years | 37.5 | 16.5 |
| Born in Hong Kong | 0, 100 | 62.8 | 48.3 |
| Born in Mainland China | 0, 100 | 32.6 | 46.9 |
| Norn outside Hong Kong and Mainland China | 0, 100 | 4.0 | 19.5 |
| Education | Years | 10.4 | 4.5 |
| Employer | 0, 100 | 1.7 | 13.0 |
| Employee | 0, 100 | 72.5 | 44.6 |
| Both employer and employee | 0, 100 | 0.5 | 7.0 |
| Self-employed | 0, 100 | 3.3 | 18.0 |
| Unemployed | 0, 100 | 0.1 | 3.6 |
| Not working | 0, 100 | 21.8 | 41.2 |
| Family size | 0, 100 | 4.0 | 1.3 |
| Poor | 0, 100 | 25.2 | 43.4 |
| Married | 0, 100 | 69.5 | 46.1 |
| Divorced | 0, 100 | 3.9 | 19.3 |
| Widowed | 0, 100 | 2.0 | 13.9 |
| Unmarried | 0, 100 | 24.6 | 43.1 |
| Age | Years | 45.6 | 16.7 |
| Female | 0, 100 | 52.9 | 49.9 |

**Table A.2** Means and standard deviations (violence dataset)

| Variable | Scoring | *M* | *SD* |
|---|---|---|---|
| *Resilience, recent month* | | | |
| Being able to face adverse circumstances | 0–100 | 48.4 | 36.4 |
| Facing difficulties actively | 0–100 | 58.6 | 34.8 |
| Keeping calm in the face of pressure | 0–100 | 50.5 | 33.6 |
| *Peace awareness, past 2 months* | | | |
| Discussing peacefully | 0–100 | 41.6 | 30.8 |
| Discussing rationally | 0–100 | 37.7 | 30.8 |
| Being negotiable | 0–100 | 38.2 | 30.1 |
| *Violence awareness, past 2 months* | | | |
| Assaulting government facilities | 0–100 | 37.8 | 31.5 |
| Enclosing and blocking public facilities | 0–100 | 39.3 | 32.5 |
| Opposing police | 0–100 | 37.4 | 32.3 |
| Disrupting councils | 0–100 | 39.2 | 31.6 |
| Assaulting officials | 0–100 | 32.9 | 31.4 |
| *Pragmatism awareness, past 2 months* | | | |
| Paying attention to feasibility | 0–100 | 38.2 | 28.6 |
| Paying attention to adjustment to changing conditions | 0–100 | 38.6 | 28.6 |
| Suiting the remedy to the case | 0–100 | 38.3 | 28.9 |
| Stressing practicality | 0–100 | 40.4 | 27.8 |
| Acquiescence | 0–100 | 34.9 | 10.5 |
| Female | 0, 100 | 55.1 | 49.8 |
| Age | Years | 46.4 | 17.2 |
| Born in Hong Kong | 0, 100 | 61.9 | 48.6 |
| Born in Mainland China | 0, 100 | 36.5 | 48.2 |
| Born outside Hong Kong and Mainland China | 0, 100 | 1.6 | 12.4 |
| Residency | Years | 38.9 | 16.7 |
| Education | Years | 10.4 | 4.7 |
| Living in owned private housing | 0, 100 | 42.0 | 49.4 |
| Irreligious | 0, 100 | 73.0 | 44.4 |
| Employer | 0, 100 | 4.8 | 21.5 |
| Employee | 0, 100 | 82.9 | 37.7 |
| Self-employed | 0, 100 | 2.6 | 15.8 |
| Unemployed | 0, 100 | 0.5 | 7.0 |
| Not working | 0, 100 | 10.8 | 31.1 |
| Stocking holding role | 0, 100 | 0.7 | 8.1 |
| Managing role | 0, 100 | 16.6 | 37.3 |
| Decision-making role | 0, 100 | 6.6 | 24.9 |

(continued)

**Table A.2** (continued)

| Variable | Scoring | *M* | *SD* |
|---|---|---|---|
| Expert role | 0, 100 | 18.4 | 38.8 |
| No occupational ole | 0, 100 | 74.7 | 43.5 |
| Personal monthly income | log(HK$) | 8.8 | 2.0 |
| Receiving social welfare | 0, 100 | 0.9 | 9.3 |
| Adult | Persons | 3.1 | 1.2 |
| Child | Persons | 0.9 | 1.2 |
| Divorced | 0, 100 | 1.7 | 12.9 |
| Widowed | 0, 100 | 5.1 | 22.0 |
| Married | 0, 100 | 66.0 | 47.4 |
| Unmarried | 0, 100 | 27.2 | 44.5 |

**Table A.3** Weighted means (service dataset)

| Variable | Scoring | Youth | Mid-age | Elder | All |
|---|---|---|---|---|---|
| Living with the spouse | 0, 100 | 2.1 | 48.5* | 39.1* | 29.9 |
| Living with offspring | 0, 100 | 1.7 | 54.1* | 42.1* | 32.6 |
| Living with siblings | 0, 100 | 61.5* | 13.5 | 1.8 | 25.6 |
| Living with parents | 0, 100 | 92.5* | 21.6 | 0.8 | 38.3 |
| Living with other relatives | 0, 100 | 4.5 | 11.0 | 15.1* | 10.2 |
| Education | 0, 100 | 11.0* | 8.6* | 4.3 | 7.7 |
| Family size | 0, 100 | 3.8* | 3.5* | 2.3 | 3.2 |
| Public rental housing | 0, 100 | 47.6 | 56.8* | 45.7 | 50.0 |
| Owned public housing | 0, 100 | 16.9 | 15.5 | 13.0 | 15.1 |
| Private housing | 0, 100 | 32.6 | 20.7 | 40.1* | 31.1 |
| Hostel | 0, 100 | 1.4 | 3.2* | 0.2 | 1.6 |
| Divided flat | 0, 100 | 1.3 | 2.8 | 0.9 | 1.7 |
| Age | 0, 100 | 19.0 | 44.4 | 75.1* | 46.5 |
| Female | 0, 100 | 51.8 | 68.0 | 86.1* | 68.7 |
| Earnings | 0, 100 | 3.0* | 2.5* | 0.2 | 1.9 |
| Family income per capita | 0, 100 | 8.5* | 8.0 | 7.8 | 8.1 |
| Survey assisted by fellows | 0, 100 | 0.7 | 0.2 | 0.0 | 0.3 |
| Survey assisted by service workers | 0, 100 | 1.1 | 1.2 | 0.1 | 0.8 |
| Interviewed | 0, 100 | 1.5 | 2.7 | 86.0* | 30.1 |
| Self-administered survey | 0, 100 | 52.4* | 52.7* | 12.0 | 39.0 |
| Survey date | Date | 2013.8 | 2014.0 | 2014.0* | 2014.0 |
| Wave 2 | 0, 100 | 47.0 | 48.1 | 48.7 | 47.9 |
| Repeated response | 0, 100 | 4.3 | 3.5 | 8.2* | 5.3 |
| Acquiescence | 0–100 | 45.4* | 42.3* | 35.1 | 40.9 |

(continued)

**Table A.3** (continued)

| Variable | Scoring | Youth | Mid-age | Elder | All |
|---|---|---|---|---|---|
| Functional disability | 0–100 | 5.9 | 16.3* | 17.3* | 13.2 |
| Adversity | 0–100 | 22.3 | 30.1* | 20.5 | 24.3 |
| Resilience demand received | 0–100 | 53.4* | 49.5 | 42.2 | 48.4 |
| Speaker sociability | 0–100 | 54.2 | 51.6 | 65.4* | 57.1 |
| Relational kindness | 0–100 | 66.4 | 67.5 | 81.6* | 71.8 |
| Aid received | 0–100 | 57.4 | 51.4 | 60.7* | 56.5 |
| Kindness | 0–100 | 67.5 | 71.6 | 84.4* | 74.5 |
| Resilience belief | 0–100 | 62.3 | 62.0 | 75.2* | 66.5 |
| Benevolent world belief | 0–100 | 54.8 | 58.0 | 74.8* | 62.5 |
| Resilience handling | 0–100 | 58.2 | 58.7 | 70.2* | 62.4 |
| Self-awareness | 0–100 | 58.1 | 57.0 | 61.4* | 58.8 |
| Compensation | 0–100 | 54.2* | 50.8 | 48.6 | 51.2 |
| Resilience learning | 0–100 | 52.4 | 52.8 | 50.3 | 51.8 |
| Resilience | 0–100 | 54.0 | 52.6 | 56.7* | 54.4 |
| Adjustment | 0–100 | 67.2 | 65.2 | 74.0* | 68.8 |
| Inferred resilience: adjustment × adversity | 0 100 | 32.9 | 36.2* | 34.5 | 34.5 |
| Youth | 0, 100 | 100.0 | 0.0 | 0.0 | 33.4 |
| Mid-age | 0, 100 | 0.0 | 100.0 | 0.0 | 32.3 |
| Elder | 0, 100 | 0.0 | 0.0 | 100.0 | 34.3 |

* Significantly higher at $p < 0.001$

**Table A.4** Means and standard deviations (elder dataset)

| Variable | Scoring | *M* | *SD* |
|---|---|---|---|
| Resilience, recent month | 0–100 | 64.5 | 14.7 |
| Implied resilience, recent month | 0–100 | 2.8 | 3.5 |
| Depression, recent month | 0–100 | 38.1 | 10.5 |
| Socializing, past 3 months | 0–100 | 50.8 | 24.5 |
| Pet engagement, past 3 months | 0–100 | 7.9 | 19.0 |
| Religious practice, past 3 months | 0–100 | 33.0 | 31.7 |
| Hardening, past 3 months | 0–100 | 65.4 | 15.0 |
| Softening, past 3 months | 0–100 | 71.1 | 16.2 |
| Demand received, past 6 months | 0–100 | 17.6 | 18.9 |
| Experiential coping, past 6 months | 0–100 | 40.6 | 31.7 |
| Westernization, past 6 months | 0–100 | 27.0 | 23.7 |
| Adversity, before past 6 months | 0–100 | 10.8 | 17.7 |
| Functional disability, past year | 0–100 | 12.8 | 19.5 |
| Acquiescence | 0–100 | 35.3 | 9.1 |
| Living with the spouse | 0, 100 | 38.2 | 48.7 |

(continued)

**Table A.4** (continued)

| Variable | Scoring | *M* | *SD* |
|---|---|---|---|
| Living with the offspring | 0, 100 | 41.5 | 49.3 |
| Living with other relatives | 0, 100 | 0.0 | 0.0 |
| Living alone | 0, 100 | 35.9 | 48.0 |
| Education | Years | 4.3 | 4.3 |
| Personal income | ln(HK$) | 6.7 | 2.6 |
| Family income | ln(HK$) | 7.9 | 1.5 |
| Rented public housing | 0, 100 | 0.9 | 9.4 |
| Owned public housing | 0, 100 | 43.5 | 49.7 |
| Private flat | 0, 100 | 15.3 | 36.0 |
| Aged home | 0, 100 | 37.4 | 48.4 |
| Hostel | 0, 100 | 0.9 | 9.4 |
| Rented room | 0, 100 | 2.1 | 14.2 |
| Age | Years | 75.6 | 7.6 |
| Female | 0, 100 | 67.7 | 46.9 |
| Credibility | 0, 100 | 77.4 | 14.6 |
| Survey assisted by fellows | 0, 100 | 1.8 | 13.2 |
| Survey assisted by workers | 0, 100 | 0.6 | 7.7 |
| Self-administered survey | 0, 100 | 0.0 | 0.0 |
| Interviewed | 0, 100 | 100.0 | 0.0 |
| Survey month | Month | 8.2 | 1.2 |
| Depression, recent month | 0–100 | 38.1 | 10.5 |
| (Not) Living happily | 0–100 | 29.4 | 24.7 |
| Fearing | 0–100 | 16.0 | 25.6 |
| Feeling sad | 0–100 | 16.7 | 24.8 |
| Feeling lonely | 0–100 | 23.9 | 32.5 |
| Being depressed | 0–100 | 25.7 | 27.2 |
| (Not) Being in the same good mood as others | 0–100 | 36.9 | 27.8 |
| (Not) Being happy | 0–100 | 27.1 | 24.9 |
| (Not) Having confidence in the future | 0–100 | 39.6 | 30.8 |
| Resilience, recent month | 0–100 | 64.5 | 14.7 |
| Keeping calm when faced with stress | 0–100 | 49.9 | 36.1 |
| Rolling with the punches | 0–100 | 48.4 | 36.7 |
| Actively facing difficulties | 0–100 | 62.6 | 33.3 |
| Being able to face adversity | 0–100 | 62.2 | 33.0 |
| (Not) Feeling anxious when stressed | 0–100 | 74.9 | 31.6 |
| (Not) Having difficulty to recover from setbacks | 0–100 | 69.1 | 33.9 |
| (Not) Worrying under pressure | 0–100 | 70.9 | 32.7 |

(continued)

**Table A.4** (continued)

| Variable | Scoring | *M* | *SD* |
|---|---|---|---|
| (Not) Having difficulty to deal with problems | 0–100 | 78.5 | 28.4 |
| Socializing, past 3 months | 0–100 | 50.8 | 24.5 |
| Being kind to people | 0–100 | 74.6 | 22.0 |
| Traveling with companions | 0–100 | 40.9 | 36.5 |
| Helping others | 0–100 | 48.5 | 35.8 |
| Volunteering | 0–100 | 39.4 | 42.1 |
| Hardening, past 3 months | 0–100 | 65.4 | 15.0 |
| Doing your part | 0–100 | 80.9 | 23.1 |
| Working hard to enrich yourself | 0–100 | 59.3 | 37.0 |
| Concentrating on things | 0–100 | 68.1 | 30.8 |
| Supporting yourself | 0–100 | 80.1 | 23.6 |
| Trusting yourself | 0–100 | 79.4 | 24.0 |
| Learning to be positive | 0–100 | 61.1 | 32.2 |
| Doing things to the end | 0–100 | 75.3 | 25.7 |
| Experiencing your own strong vitality | 0–100 | 60.8 | 30.6 |
| Experiencing the meaning of working hard to survive | 0–100 | 60.4 | 33.4 |
| (Not) Feeling you wasting time | 0–100 | 85.3 | 25.4 |
| Being respected | 0–100 | 63.7 | 27.6 |
| Softening, past 3 months | 0–100 | 71.1 | 16.2 |
| Being considerate of others | 0–100 | 70.1 | 27.3 |
| Looking at things more openly | 0–100 | 79.1 | 23.9 |
| Forgiving others | 0–100 | 62.2 | 33.6 |
| Experiencing money as an external object | 0–100 | 74.9 | 28.8 |
| Experiencing that people always have birth, old age, sickness, and death | 0–100 | 82.4 | 24.4 |
| Experiencing the fate of life and death | 0–100 | 76.4 | 27.7 |
| Taking it easy | 0–100 | 53.3 | 39.6 |
| Feeling natural dominance in the dark | 0–100 | 69.7 | 32.7 |
| Thinking for the better | 0–100 | 72.1 | 26.3 |
| Experiencing life as a dream | 0–100 | 60.9 | 34.9 |
| Knowing satisfaction | 0–100 | 81.4 | 23.4 |
| Religious practice, past 3 months | 0–100 | 33.0 | 31.7 |
| Praying for God's blessing | 0–100 | 37.9 | 40.4 |
| Feeling God giving you wisdom | 0–100 | 34.9 | 39.5 |
| Reading or chanting Sutras | 0–100 | 18.9 | 32.8 |
| Feeling God loving you | 0–100 | 38.5 | 41.4 |
| Committing yourself to God | 0–100 | 35.0 | 40.4 |

(continued)

**Table A.4** (continued)

| Variable | Scoring | *M* | *SD* |
|---|---|---|---|
| Pet engagement, past 3 months | 0–100 | 7.9 | 19.0 |
| Caring for pets | 0–100 | 7.3 | 24.1 |
| Spending time on pets | 0–100 | 4.6 | 17.5 |
| Accompanying pets | 0–100 | 5.5 | 20.4 |
| Watching pets | 0–100 | 14.2 | 27.9 |
| Experiential coping, past 6 months | 0–100 | 40.6 | 31.7 |
| Using working experience to overcome adversity | 0–100 | 43.1 | 38.7 |
| Using experience other than work to overcome adversity | 0–100 | 35.2 | 35.3 |
| Overcoming adversity with past hard life experience | 0–100 | 43.9 | 38.7 |
| Advice received, past 6 months | 0–100 | 17.6 | 18.9 |
| Experts teaching you how to overcome adversity | 0–100 | 12.5 | 24.9 |
| Friends teaching you how to overcome adversity | 0–100 | 23.6 | 32.0 |
| Other elders teaching you how to overcome adversity | 0–100 | 21.5 | 31.0 |
| Religious people teaching you how to overcome adversity | 0–100 | 14.2 | 28.3 |
| Family members teaching you how to overcome adversity | 0–100 | 20.4 | 32.1 |
| Social workers teaching you how to overcome adversity | 0–100 | 19.8 | 32.4 |
| People in the media teaching you how to overcome adversity | 0–100 | 11.0 | 23.3 |
| Learning to cope, past 6 months | 0–100 | 19.2 | 18.4 |
| Learning how to overcome adversity through reading | 0–100 | 22.5 | 32.9 |
| Overcoming adversity for the sake of family | 0–100 | 27.1 | 34.3 |
| Westernization, past 6 months | 0–100 | 27.0 | 23.7 |
| Appreciating European and American art, such as painting and music | 0–100 | 17.2 | 28.3 |
| Watching European and American TV programs or films | 0–100 | 28.0 | 32.8 |
| Having tried or hoped to visit Europe and America | 0–100 | 24.9 | 36.1 |
| Agreeing with European and American cultures, such as customs and habits | 0–100 | 38.5 | 34.8 |
| Adversity, before past 6 months | 0–100 | 10.8 | 17.7 |
| Sickness | 0–100 | 15.9 | 30.8 |
| Family member passing away | 0–100 | 8.8 | 20.7 |
| Economic loss | 0–100 | 7.7 | 20.1 |
| Functional disability, past year | 0–100 | 12.8 | 19.5 |
| Walking up and down stairs | 0–100 | 31.8 | 46.6 |
| Bathing | 0–100 | 4.1 | 19.9 |
| Taking transportation | 0–100 | 10.0 | 30.0 |
| Shopping | 0–100 | 7.4 | 26.1 |
| Handling money | 0–100 | 3.8 | 19.2 |
| Walking half an hour | 0–100 | 19.7 | 39.8 |

**Table A.5** Means and standard deviations (elder dataset)

| Variable | *M* | *SD* |
|---|---|---|
| Depression, recent month | 38.1 | 10.5 |
| (Not) Living happily | 29.4 | 24.7 |
| Fearing | 16.0 | 25.6 |
| Feeling sad | 16.7 | 24.8 |
| Feeling lonely | 23.9 | 32.5 |
| Being depressed | 25.7 | 27.2 |
| (Not) Being in the same good mood as others | 36.9 | 27.8 |
| (Not) Being happy | 27.1 | 24.9 |
| (Not) Having confidence in the future | 39.6 | 30.8 |
| Resilience, recent month | 64.5 | 14.7 |
| Keeping calm when faced with stress | 49.9 | 36.1 |
| Rolling with the punches | 48.4 | 36.7 |
| Actively facing difficulties | 62.6 | 33.3 |
| Being able to face adversity | 62.2 | 33.0 |
| (Not) Feeling anxious when stressed | 74.9 | 31.6 |
| (Not) Having difficulty to recover from setbacks | 69.1 | 33.9 |
| (Not) Worrying under pressure | 70.9 | 32.7 |
| (Not) Having difficulty to deal with problems | 78.5 | 28.4 |
| Socializing, past 3 months | 50.8 | 24.5 |
| Being kind to people | 74.6 | 22.0 |
| Traveling with companions | 40.9 | 36.5 |
| Helping others | 48.5 | 35.8 |
| Volunteering | 39.4 | 42.1 |
| Hardening, past 3 months | 65.4 | 15.0 |
| Doing your part | 80.9 | 23.1 |
| Working hard to enrich yourself | 59.3 | 37.0 |
| Concentrating on things | 68.1 | 30.8 |
| Supporting yourself | 80.1 | 23.6 |
| Trusting yourself | 79.4 | 24.0 |
| Learning to be positive | 61.1 | 32.2 |
| Doing things to the end | 75.3 | 25.7 |
| Experiencing your own strong vitality | 60.8 | 30.6 |
| Experiencing the meaning of working hard to survive | 60.4 | 33.4 |
| (Not) Feeling you wasting time | 85.3 | 25.4 |
| Being respected | 63.7 | 27.6 |
| Softening, past 3 months | 71.1 | 16.2 |
| Being considerate of others | 70.1 | 27.3 |

(continued)

**Table A.5** (continued)

| Variable | *M* | *SD* |
|---|---|---|
| Looking at things more openly | 79.1 | 23.9 |
| Forgiving others | 62.2 | 33.6 |
| Experiencing money as an external object | 74.9 | 28.8 |
| Experiencing that people always have birth, old age, sickness, and death | 82.4 | 24.4 |
| Experiencing the fate of life and death | 76.4 | 27.7 |
| Taking it easy | 53.3 | 39.6 |
| Feeling natural dominance in the dark | 69.7 | 32.7 |
| Thinking for the better | 72.1 | 26.3 |
| Experiencing life as a dream | 60.9 | 34.9 |
| Knowing satisfaction | 81.4 | 23.4 |
| Religious practice, past 3 months | 33.0 | 31.7 |
| Praying for God's blessing | 37.9 | 40.4 |
| Feeling God giving you wisdom | 34.9 | 39.5 |
| Reading or chanting Sutras | 18.9 | 32.8 |
| Feeling God loving you | 38.5 | 41.4 |
| Committing yourself to God | 35.0 | 40.4 |
| Pet engagement, past 3 months | 7.9 | 19.0 |
| Caring for pets | 7.3 | 24.1 |
| Spending time on pets | 4.6 | 17.5 |
| Accompanying pets | 5.5 | 20.4 |
| Watching pets | 14.2 | 27.9 |
| Experiential coping, past 6 months | 40.6 | 31.7 |
| Using working experience to overcome adversity | 43.1 | 38.7 |
| Using experience other than work to overcome adversity | 35.2 | 35.3 |
| Overcoming adversity with past hard life experience | 43.9 | 38.7 |
| Advice received, past 6 months | 17.6 | 18.9 |
| Experts teaching you how to overcome adversity | 12.5 | 24.9 |
| Friends teaching you how to overcome adversity | 23.6 | 32.0 |
| Other elders teaching you how to overcome adversity | 21.5 | 31.0 |
| Religious people teaching you how to overcome adversity | 14.2 | 28.3 |
| Family members teaching you how to overcome adversity | 20.4 | 32.1 |
| Social workers teaching you how to overcome adversity | 19.8 | 32.4 |
| People in the media teaching you how to overcome adversity | 11.0 | 23.3 |
| Learning to cope, past 6 months | 19.2 | 18.4 |
| Learning how to overcome adversity through reading | 22.5 | 32.9 |
| Overcoming adversity for the sake of family | 27.1 | 34.3 |
| Westernization, past 6 months | 27.0 | 23.7 |

(continued)

**Table A.5** (continued)

| Variable | *M* | *SD* |
|---|---|---|
| Appreciating European and American art, such as painting and music | 17.2 | 28.3 |
| Watching European and American TV programs or films | 28.0 | 32.8 |
| Having tried or hoped to visit Europe and America | 24.9 | 36.1 |
| Agreeing with European and American cultures, such as customs and habits | 38.5 | 34.8 |
| Adversity, before past 6 months | 10.8 | 17.7 |
| Sickness | 15.9 | 30.8 |
| Family member passing away | 8.8 | 20.7 |
| Economic loss | 7.7 | 20.1 |
| Functional disability, past year | 12.8 | 19.5 |
| Walking up and down stairs | 31.8 | 46.6 |
| Bathing | 4.1 | 19.9 |
| Taking transportation | 10.0 | 30.0 |
| Shopping | 7.4 | 26.1 |
| Handling money | 3.8 | 19.2 |
| Walking half an hour | 19.7 | 39.8 |

**Table A.6** Means and standard deviations (visual impairment dataset)

| Variable | Scoring | *M* | *SD* |
|---|---|---|---|
| *Achievement, recent month* | 0–100 | 43.5 | 15.6 |
| Having outstanding performance | 0–100 | 33.4 | 26.0 |
| Solving problems | 0–100 | 42.9 | 27.6 |
| Putting it over | 0–100 | 32.2 | 26.4 |
| Achieving goals | 0–100 | 34.9 | 27.4 |
| (Not) Having difficulty to overcome difficulties | 0–100 | 58.8 | 26.7 |
| (Not) Having difficulty to achieve results | 0–100 | 58.7 | 26.5 |
| *Resilience, recent month* | 0–100 | 50.4 | 14.5 |
| Having ability to face adversity | 0–100 | 47.9 | 24.1 |
| Facing difficulties positively | 0–100 | 48.5 | 25.5 |
| Rolling with punches | 0–100 | 49.4 | 23.8 |
| Keeping calm in the face of pressure | 0–100 | 48.2 | 24.5 |
| (Not) Feeling anxious when under pressure | 0–100 | 49.5 | 25.4 |
| (Not) Having difficulty to recover from setbacks | 0–100 | 59.0 | 26.4 |
| *Social integration, recent month* | 0–100 | 49.4 | 17.1 |
| Being accepted by others | 0–100 | 44.3 | 27.7 |
| Getting help from others | 0–100 | 41.9 | 26.7 |
| Being recognized by others | 0–100 | 45.3 | 27.9 |
| Being invited to participate in activities | 0–100 | 41.5 | 27.0 |

(continued)

**Table A.6** (continued)

| Variable | Scoring | *M* | *SD* |
|---|---|---|---|
| Others (not) ignoring your needs | 0–100 | 62.9 | 25.7 |
| Others (not) ignoring your opinions | 0–100 | 60.3 | 25.5 |
| *Associational social capital closeness, past half year* | 0–100 | 39.1 | 22.7 |
| Having close ties with groups | 0–100 | 40.1 | 28.3 |
| Participating in group activities | 0–100 | 40.0 | 26.2 |
| Participating in group activities | 0–100 | 37.2 | 26.6 |
| *Friend substantive social capital, past half year* | 0–100 | 36.8 | 20.9 |
| Your friends being knowledgeable | 0–100 | 37.2 | 26.0 |
| Your friends having financial resources | 0–100 | 40.6 | 26.0 |
| Your friends having social status | 0–100 | 32.6 | 25.8 |
| *Friend social capital closeness, past half year* | 0–100 | 44.3 | 20.6 |
| Having close ties with friends | 0–100 | 39.3 | 27.6 |
| Having interaction with friends | 0–100 | 39.7 | 26.4 |
| Having a long relationship with friends | 0–100 | 41.1 | 26.6 |
| Having a long relationship with friends | 0–100 | 57.0 | 27.6 |
| *Friend social capital density, past half year* | 0–100 | 40.6 | 23.6 |
| Your friends knowing each other | 0–100 | 39.3 | 25.5 |
| Taking part in activities with your friends | 0–100 | 41.8 | 28.8 |
| *Friend social capital homogeneity, past half year* | 0–100 | 42.9 | 23.2 |
| Having the same background as friends | 0–100 | 42.3 | 26.8 |
| Having the same interests as friends | 0–100 | 43.5 | 27.5 |
| *Friend social capital reciprocity, past half year* | 0–100 | 38.3 | 22.1 |
| Your friends repaying you | 0–100 | 44.0 | 27.7 |
| Your friends (not) ignoring the help that you gave them | 0–100 | 32.5 | 25.5 |
| *Friend social capital trust, past half year* | 0–100 | 40.6 | 24.2 |
| Your friends helping you unconditionally | 0–100 | 44.1 | 28.1 |
| Your friends (not) ignoring you | 0–100 | 37.0 | 26.3 |
| *Friend functional social capital, past half year* | 0–100 | 39.4 | 21.1 |
| Your friends repaying you | 0–100 | 44.0 | 27.7 |
| Your friends (not) ignoring the help that you gave them | 0–100 | 32.5 | 25.5 |
| Your friends helping you unconditionally | 0–100 | 44.1 | 28.1 |
| Your friends (not) ignoring you | 0–100 | 37.0 | 26.3 |
| *Friend structural social capital, past half year* | 0–100 | 41.7 | 21.2 |
| Having the same background as friends | 0–100 | 42.3 | 26.8 |
| Having the same interests as friends | 0–100 | 43.5 | 27.5 |
| Having the same background as friends | 0–100 | 39.3 | 25.5 |
| Having the same interests as friends | 0–100 | 41.8 | 28.8 |

(continued)

**Table A.6** (continued)

| Variable | Scoring | *M* | *SD* |
|---|---|---|---|
| *Actualization ability increase, past year* | 0–100 | 25.9 | 25.5 |
| Enhancing the ability to develop abilities | 0–100 | 26.5 | 28.3 |
| Enhancing the ability to express oneself | 0–100 | 25.6 | 28.1 |
| Enhancing the ability to realize potential | 0–100 | 25.7 | 28.7 |
| *Leading ability increase, past year* | 0–100 | 25.6 | 26.3 |
| Enhancing the ability to guide others | 0–100 | 23.8 | 27.0 |
| Enhancing the ability to assess performance | 0–100 | 26.3 | 28.8 |
| Enhancing leadership | 0–100 | 26.7 | 29.1 |
| *Planning ability increase, past year* | 0–100 | 26.9 | 26.5 |
| Enhancing the planning capacity | 0–100 | 27.1 | 29.2 |
| Enhancing the ability to organize work | 0–100 | 27.3 | 29.6 |
| Enhancing the ability to set goals | 0–100 | 26.3 | 28.5 |
| *Conscientiousness, all along* | 0–100 | 47.3 | 18.8 |
| Keeping neat | 0–100 | 51.5 | 22.8 |
| Handling chores instantly | 0–100 | 43.1 | 23.3 |
| *Extraversion, all along* | 0–100 | 42.4 | 22.7 |
| Attending a party | 0–100 | 40.8 | 27.0 |
| Talking to different people | 0–100 | 44.0 | 25.9 |
| *Neuroticism, all along* | 0–100 | 44.9 | 17.9 |
| Mood swinging | 0–100 | 42.0 | 26.5 |
| Fidgeting | 0–100 | 40.6 | 26.5 |
| Having ease of mind | 0–100 | 52.2 | 23.8 |
| Rental public housing | 0, 100 | 60.8 | 48.9 |
| Owned public housing | 0, 100 | 7.1 | 25.7 |
| Rental private housing | 0, 100 | 7.9 | 27.0 |
| Owned private housing | 0, 100 | 27.7 | 44.8 |
| Non-flat | 0, 100 | 3.9 | 19.3 |
| Irreligious | 0, 100 | 80.2 | 39.9 |
| Protestant | 0, 100 | 8.7 | 28.2 |
| Catholic | 0, 100 | 2.6 | 15.8 |
| Buddhist | 0, 100 | 7.1 | 25.6 |
| Daoist | 0, 100 | 0.5 | 6.7 |
| Minority religion | 0, 100 | 1.1 | 10.2 |
| Residency | Years | 44.0 | 14.7 |
| Born in Hong Kong | 0, 100 | 46.0 | 49.9 |
| Norn in Mainland China | 0, 100 | 51.5 | 50.0 |
| Born outside Hong Kong or Mainland China | 0, 100 | 2.5 | 15.6 |

(continued)

**Table A.6** (continued)

| Variable | Scoring | *M* | *SD* |
|---|---|---|---|
| Education | Years | 8.4 | 4.4 |
| Employer | 0, 100 | 1.7 | 12.9 |
| Employee | 0, 100 | 78.4 | 41.2 |
| Both employer and employee | 0, 100 | 0.0 | 0.0 |
| Self-employed | 0, 100 | 1.9 | 13.8 |
| Unemployed | 0, 100 | 1.6 | 12.4 |
| Not working | 0, 100 | 16.5 | 37.1 |
| Family size | Persons | 3.7 | 1.1 |
| Receiving social welfare | 0, 100 | 9.9 | 29.9 |
| Receiving social welfare formerly | 0, 100 | 7.1 | 25.7 |
| Expected to receive social welfare | 0, 100 | 0.0 | 0.0 |
| Unmarried | 0, 100 | 8.3 | 27.6 |
| Married | 0, 100 | 87.4 | 33.2 |
| Divorced/separated | 0, 100 | 0.7 | 8.1 |
| Widowed | 0, 100 | 3.7 | 18.8 |
| Age | 0, 100 | 58.1 | 29.0 |
| Age 60+ | 0, 100 | 47.5 | 50.0 |
| Visual impairment duration | Years | 8.6 | 8.8 |
| Female | 0, 100 | 62.3 | 48.5 |
| Credibility | 0, 100 | 75.1 | 8.5 |
| Willingness to respond | 0, 100 | 75.0 | 9.4 |
| Family income | log(HK$) | 9.8 | 1.0 |
| Family income per capita | log(HK$) | 8.3 | 0.9 |
| Visual impairment | 0–100 | 16.8 | 20.8 |
| Acquiescence | 0–100 | 38.6 | 12.2 |
| Friend structural social capital, past half year | 0–100 | 43.0 | 19.7 |
| Empowerment, past half year | 0–100 | 26.1 | 25.0 |

**Table A.7** Means (youth dataset)

| Variable | Scoring | Hong Kong | Guangzhou | Macau | All | $\eta$ |
|---|---|---|---|---|---|---|
| *Resilience, past month* | 0–100 | 60.9 | 60.9 | 54.4 | 59.7 | 0.069 |
| Personal study | 0–100 | 62.6 | 61.9 | 57.4 | 61.4 | 0.051 |
| Getting along with family | 0–100 | 65.5 | 62.7 | 55.5 | 62.9 | 0.087 |
| Getting along with friends | 0–100 | 59.1 | 62.1 | 55.2 | 59.3 | 0.052 |
| Getting along with teachers | 0–100 | 57.1 | 57.1 | 53.0 | 56.3 | 0.036 |
| Emotion concerning the opposite sex | 0–100 | 47.0 | 42.2 | 41.9 | 44.8 | 0.055 |
| Money | 0–100 | 53.3 | 52.1 | 49.3 | 52.0 | 0.037 |
| Personal health | 0–100 | 57.4 | 54.1 | 53.2 | 55.6 | 0.042 |
| Others | 0–100 | 47.3 | 35.9 | 40.9 | 42.1 | 0.115 |
| *Distress, past month* | 0–100 | 25.3 | 20.8 | 28.6 | 24.5 | 0.131 |
| Personal study | 0–100 | 42.6 | 42.2 | 49.5 | 43.7 | 0.085 |
| Getting along with family | 0–100 | 31.1 | 24.9 | 35.0 | 29.9 | 0.116 |
| Getting along with friends | 0–100 | 26.7 | 22.2 | 26.5 | 25.3 | 0.068 |

(continued)

**Table A.7** (continued)

| Variable | Scoring | Hong Kong | Guangzhou | Macau | All | $\eta$ |
|---|---|---|---|---|---|---|
| Getting along with teachers | 0–100 | 16.5 | 17.6 | 23.0 | 18.0 | 0.087 |
| Emotion concerning the opposite sex | 0–100 | 16.8 | 12.9 | 17.5 | 15.7 | 0.068 |
| Money | 0–100 | 26.1 | 19.4 | 38.2 | 26.3 | 0.189 |
| Personal health | 0–100 | 23.6 | 20.8 | 29.1 | 23.8 | 0.091 |
| Others | 0–100 | 10.9 | 6.8 | 10.0 | 9.4 | 0.084 |
| *Social desirability, recent month* | 0–100 | 57.1 | 66.1 | 54.5 | 59.3 | 0.311 |
| (Not) Lying to elders | 0–100 | 69.5 | 79.3 | 67.6 | 72.1 | 0.204 |
| (Not) Shouting because of anger | 0–100 | 63.2 | 64.2 | 64.7 | 63.7 | 0.021 |
| (Not) Being unplanned | 0–100 | 52.7 | 58.3 | 52.9 | 54.4 | 0.093 |
| (Not) Getting angry because of something bad | 0–100 | 56.8 | 64.2 | 56.3 | 58.9 | 0.125 |
| Treating disliked people politely | 0–100 | 48.5 | 61.5 | 41.2 | 51.1 | 0.270 |
| Being sure to do things right | 0–100 | 53.5 | 61.4 | 50.6 | 55.3 | 0.163 |
| Being happy most of the time | 0–100 | 60.8 | 72.2 | 55.7 | 63.3 | 0.210 |
| Listening carefully to elders' instruction | 0–100 | 51.8 | 68.0 | 47.2 | 55.8 | 0.301 |
| *Sport, past 3 months* | Times | 5.8 | 16.0 | 5.8 | 8.8 | 0.474 |
| Fitness/gymnastics | Times | 1.1 | 4.3 | 1.6 | 2.1 | 0.416 |
| Running | Times | 1.6 | 4.4 | 1.5 | 2.4 | 0.369 |
| Ball games | Times | 2.0 | 3.0 | 1.3 | 2.2 | 0.140 |
| Water | Times | 0.4 | 0.4 | 0.3 | 0.4 | 0.035 |
| Cycling | Times | 0.4 | 2.6 | 0.5 | 1.0 | 0.299 |
| Jumping, throwing | Times | 0.5 | 2.0 | 0.7 | 1.0 | 0.254 |
| Martial arts | Times | 0.3 | 0.4 | 0.2 | 0.3 | 0.067 |
| Others | Times | 0.2 | 0.3 | 0.1 | 0.2 | 0.063 |
| *Sport, past 3 months* | Minutes | 386.0 | 503.2 | 238.3 | 391.3 | 0.297 |
| Fitness/gymnastics | Minutes | 35.5 | 86.4 | 41.6 | 51.6 | 0.229 |

(continued)

**Table A.7** (continued)

| Variable | Scoring | Hong Kong | Guangzhou | Macau | All | $\eta$ |
|---|---|---|---|---|---|---|
| Running | Minutes | 47.7 | 82.5 | 40.0 | 56.6 | 0.164 |
| Ball games | Minutes | 112.0 | 106.7 | 59.0 | 101.0 | 0.114 |
| Water | Minutes | 21.1 | 13.9 | 10.1 | 17.0 | 0.058 |
| Cycling | Minutes | 16.3 | 53.7 | 16.1 | 27.2 | 0.205 |
| Jumping, throwing | Minutes | 13.2 | 34.3 | 16.9 | 20.1 | 0.131 |
| Martial arts | Minutes | 11.7 | 11.7 | 10.6 | 11.5 | 0.007 |
| Others | Minutes | 11.8 | 9.8 | 5.0 | 9.8 | 0.042 |
| *Team sport, past 3 months* | Times | 4.1 | 8.6 | 4.0 | 5.4 | 0.245 |
| Fitness/gymnastics | Times | 0.6 | 2.3 | 1.0 | 1.2 | 0.196 |
| Running | Times | 0.9 | 2.7 | 1.1 | 1.5 | 0.207 |
| Ball games | Times | 2.0 | 2.5 | 1.6 | 2.0 | 0.070 |
| Water | Times | 0.2 | 0.2 | 0.2 | 0.2 | 0.029 |
| Cycling | Times | 0.2 | 0.8 | 0.3 | 0.4 | 0.167 |
| Jumping, throwing | Times | 0.2 | 1.1 | 0.5 | 0.5 | 0.156 |
| Martial arts | Times | 0.2 | 0.2 | 0.2 | 0.2 | 0.021 |
| Others | Times | 0.2 | 0.3 | 0.1 | 0.2 | 0.037 |
| *Sport under guidance, past 3 months* | Times | 2.6 | 5.5 | 2.6 | 3.5 | 0.195 |
| Fitness/gymnastics | Times | 0.5 | 1.3 | 0.7 | 0.8 | 0.118 |
| Running | Times | 0.6 | 1.7 | 0.6 | 0.9 | 0.195 |
| Ball games | Times | 1.0 | 1.0 | 0.6 | 0.9 | 0.049 |
| Water | Times | 0.2 | 0.4 | 0.2 | 0.3 | 0.039 |
| Cycling | Times | 0.1 | 0.5 | 0.1 | 0.2 | 0.100 |
| Jumping, throwing | Times | 0.2 | 0.8 | 0.3 | 0.4 | 0.181 |
| Martial arts | Times | 0.3 | 0.2 | 0.2 | 0.3 | 0.033 |
| Others | Times | 0.2 | 0.2 | 0.0 | 0.1 | 0.048 |
| *Nation-related activity, past half-year* | Times | 3.4 | 7.1 | 3.1 | 4.5 | 0.140 |
| Sport | Times | 1.3 | 3.7 | 1.4 | 2.0 | 0.104 |
| Volunteering | Times | 0.8 | 0.8 | 0.4 | 0.7 | 0.032 |
| Adventure/training camp | Times | 0.3 | 0.7 | 0.4 | 0.4 | 0.073 |
| Religious activity | Times | 0.8 | 0.5 | 0.4 | 0.6 | 0.039 |

(continued)

**Table A.7** (continued)

| Variable | Scoring | Hong Kong | Guangzhou | Macau | All | $\eta$ |
|---|---|---|---|---|---|---|
| Carnival | Times | 0.2 | 2.0 | 0.3 | 0.8 | 0.415 |
| Concert | Times | 0.3 | 0.8 | 0.6 | 0.5 | 0.110 |
| *Prime activity, past half-year* | 0, 100 | 33.0 | 26.0 | 28.1 | 29.9 | 0.069 |
| Volunteering | 0, 100 | 24.2 | 22.7 | 20.2 | 23.0 | 0.035 |
| Adventure/training camp | 0, 100 | 19.8 | 10.7 | 30.0 | 18.8 | 0.169 |
| Religious activity | 0, 100 | 8.0 | 0.9 | 3.1 | 4.9 | 0.149 |
| Carnival | 0, 100 | 7.6 | 32.7 | 7.0 | 15.2 | 0.325 |
| Concert | 0, 100 | 7.3 | 6.7 | 11.6 | 7.9 | 0.065 |
| Participants | Persons | 516.2 | 594.4 | 229.8 | 489.6 | 0.045 |
| *Ritual activity (collective sentiment), past half-year* | 0–100 | 56.1 | 69.3 | 53.7 | 59.7 | 0.365 |
| Ceremony | 0–100 | 39.6 | 55.3 | 34.3 | 43.4 | 0.267 |
| Singing, shouting, reading together | 0–100 | 47.2 | 69.2 | 41.6 | 52.8 | 0.346 |
| Having fun together | 0–100 | 63.8 | 86.0 | 63.7 | 70.5 | 0.360 |
| Being in high spirits together | 0–100 | 53.5 | 77.1 | 53.6 | 60.6 | 0.357 |
| (Not) Each doing one's own thing | 0–100 | 72.7 | 77.3 | 71.7 | 73.9 | 0.096 |
| Achieving eye alignment | 0–100 | 52.0 | 66.9 | 49.6 | 56.0 | 0.275 |
| Bodily contact | 0–100 | 48.8 | 47.9 | 46.5 | 48.1 | 0.030 |
| Achieving harmony in pace | 0–100 | 52.8 | 65.4 | 46.9 | 55.6 | 0.247 |
| (Not) arguing | 0–100 | 74.7 | 78.7 | 75.6 | 76.0 | 0.075 |
| *Belongingness to the nation, past year* | 0–100 | 45.6 | 57.6 | 46.7 | 49.4 | 0.299 |
| Being happy because of Chinese athletes winning gold metals | 0–100 | 58.0 | 88.1 | 55.0 | 66.4 | 0.438 |
| Volunteering for building China | 0–100 | 23.4 | 51.4 | 24.7 | 31.9 | 0.385 |
| Participating in the activities of protecting Diaoyutai | 0–100 | 12.8 | 31.7 | 13.1 | 18.4 | 0.290 |

(continued)

**Table A.7** (continued)

| Variable | Scoring | Hong Kong | Guangzhou | Macau | All | $\eta$ |
|---|---|---|---|---|---|---|
| (Not) Recognizing China's shame | 0–100 | 67.4 | 68.3 | 71.7 | 68.4 | 0.049 |
| (Not) Recognizing Chinese people's bad habits | 0–100 | 52.3 | 45.1 | 54.1 | 50.4 | 0.112 |
| (Not) Meeting the Chinese people you hated | 0 –100 | 59.9 | 60.5 | 61.9 | 60.4 | 0.022 |
| *Resilience, one year ago* | 0–100 | 53.4 | 62.7 | 48.5 | 55.3 | 0.240 |
| Being able to deal with crisis/ adversity | 0–100 | 53.9 | 61.7 | 48.5 | 55.2 | 0.180 |
| Overcoming crises/adversity | 0 –100 | 54.6 | 65.7 | 50.0 | 57.1 | 0.232 |
| Getting help in case of crisis/ adversity | 0–100 | 51.7 | 60.7 | 46.9 | 53.5 | 0.184 |
| *Distress, one year ago* | 0–100 | 39.5 | 34.1 | 39.1 | 37.8 | 0.111 |
| Crisis/adversity bothering you | 0–100 | 46.9 | 44.9 | 47.7 | 46.5 | 0.041 |
| Duration of crisis/adversity | 0–100 | 44.1 | 37.7 | 41.5 | 41.8 | 0.103 |
| Sequels of crisis/adversity | 0–100 | 27.4 | 19.5 | 28.1 | 25.2 | 0.136 |
| Acquiescence | 0 –100 | 43.5 | 49.1 | 42.5 | 45.0 | 0.314 |
| Catholicism | 0, 100 | 3.4 | 1.9 | 4.4 | 3.1 | 0.050 |
| Protestantism | 0, 100 | 45.4 | 6.1 | 19.6 | 29.4 | 0.388 |
| Buddhism | 0, 100 | 4.2 | 15.9 | 10.8 | 8.8 | 0.183 |
| Another religion | 0, 100 | 1.3 | 1.3 | 2.2 | 1.4 | 0.030 |
| Irreligious | 0, 100 | 45.7 | 74.7 | 62.8 | 57.2 | 0.260 |
| Cohabiting parents | Persons | 1.9 | 2.0 | 1.9 | 1.9 | 0.081 |
| Cohabiting elder siblings | Persons | 0.6 | 0.4 | 0.7 | 0.6 | 0.136 |
| Cohabiting younger siblings | Persons | 0.5 | 0.3 | 0.5 | 0.4 | 0.128 |
| Cohabiting others | Persons | 0.4 | 0.5 | 0.3 | 0.4 | 0.052 |
| Family member | Persons | 4.1 | 4.0 | 4.4 | 4.2 | 0.059 |

(continued)

**Table A.7** (continued)

| Variable | Scoring | Hong Kong | Guangzhou | Macau | All | $\eta$ |
|---|---|---|---|---|---|---|
| Grade complete | Grade | 7.7 | 7.9 | 7.9 | 7.8 | 0.125 |
| Father education | Grade | 8.1 | 11.2 | 5.0 | 8.5 | 0.456 |
| Mother education | Grade | 7.3 | 10.4 | 4.9 | 7.8 | 0.436 |
| Father as an employee | 0, 100 | 68.8 | 56.0 | 68.0 | 64.9 | 0.120 |
| Father as an employer | 0, 100 | 17.4 | 11.1 | 13.2 | 14.8 | 0.079 |
| Father as self-employed | 0, 100 | 8.2 | 22.7 | 11.3 | 13.1 | 0.188 |
| Father being long-term unemployed | 0, 100 | 2.1 | 4.0 | 3.0 | 2.8 | 0.052 |
| Father not working | 0, 100 | 3.6 | 6.1 | 4.5 | 4.5 | 0.053 |
| Mother as an employee | 0, 100 | 60.3 | 57.2 | 64.8 | 60.2 | 0.051 |
| Mother as an employer | 0, 100 | 6.3 | 4.8 | 5.2 | 5.7 | 0.029 |
| Mother as self-employed | 0, 100 | 3.6 | 18.6 | 7.2 | 8.7 | 0.233 |
| Mother being long-term unemployed | 0, 100 | 1.6 | 3.6 | 2.4 | 2.3 | 0.060 |
| Mother not working | 0, 100 | 28.3 | 15.7 | 20.3 | 23.1 | 0.133 |
| Age | Years | 13.7 | 14.0 | 14.6 | 14.0 | 0.204 |
| Residency in the city | Years | 12.5 | 12.9 | 12.8 | 12.7 | 0.047 |
| Female | 0, 100 | 47.4 | 52.8 | 56.9 | 50.6 | 0.075 |
| Family monthly income | HK$ | 11,181.4 | 5348.0 | 9611.8 | 8518.4 | 0.496 |
| Receiving welfare now | 0, 100 | 3.9 | 3.3 | 6.5 | 4.2 | 0.056 |
| Receiving welfare before | 0, 100 | 2.4 | 3.3 | 10.7 | 4.1 | 0.153 |
| Receiving welfare in future | 0, 100 | 1.3 | 2.0 | 4.5 | 2.1 | 0.082 |
| Never receiving welfare | 0, 100 | 91.5 | 91.0 | 78.1 | 89.0 | 0.161 |
| Month | Month | 2.9 | 3.0 | 3.1 | 3.0 | 0.274 |
| Grade 7 | 0, 100 | 28.5 | 30.6 | 39.7 | 31.0 | 0.088 |
| Grade 8 | 0, 100 | 33.4 | 36.5 | 35.2 | 34.6 | 0.029 |
| Grade 9 | 0, 100 | 38.1 | 32.9 | 25.1 | 34.3 | 0.101 |

*Note* $\eta$ over 0.10 was significant at the 0.001 level

# References


Abascal, M. 2015. "Love thy Neighbor: Ethnoracial Diversity and Trust Reexamined." *American Journal Of Sociology* 121(3):622–782.

Abbott, Pamela, and Roger Sapsford. 2006. "Life-satisfaction in Post-Soviet Russia and Ukraine." *Journal of Happiness Studies* 7:251–287.

Abbott, Pamela, Claire Wallace, and Roger Sapsford. 2011. "Surviving the Transformation: Social Quality in Central Asia and the Caucuses." *Journal of Happiness Studies* 12:199–223.

Aberg, Yvonne, and Peter Hedstrom. 2011. "Youth Unemployment: A Self-reinforcing Process?" Pp. 201–226 in *Analytical Sociology and Social Mechanisms*, edited by Pierre Demeulenaere. Cambridge, UK: Cambridge University Press.

Abrahms, Max. 2008. "What Terrorists Really Want: Terrorist Motives and Counterterrorism Strategy." *International Security* 32(4):78–105.

Abrams, Dominic, Steve Hinkle, and Melissa Tomlias. 1999. "Leaving Hong Kong? The Roles of Attitude, Subjective Norm, Perceived Control, Social Identity and Relative Deprivation." *International Journal of Intercultural Relation* 23(2):319–338.

Abu Bakar, Hassan, and Vivian C. Sheer. 2013. "The Mediating Role of Perceived Cooperative Communication in the Relationship between Interpersonal Exchange Relationships and Perceived Group Cohesion." *Management Communication Quarterly* 27(3):443–465.

Abu-Raiya, Hisham, Kenneth I. Pargament, Neal Krause, and Gail Ironson. 2015. "Robust Links between Religious/Spiritual Struggles, Psychological Distress, and Well-Being in a National Sample of American Adults." *American Journal of Orthopsychiatry* 85(6):565–75.

Achterberg, Peter, and Dick Houtman. 2009. "Ideologically Illogical? Why Do the Lower-educated Dutch Display So Little Value Coherence?" *Social Forces* 87(3):1649–1670.

Achterkamp, R., H. J. Hermens and M. M. R. Vollenbroek-Hutten. 2016. "The Influence of Vicarious Experience Provided through Mobile Technology on Self-Efficacy When Learning New Tasks." *Computers in Human Behavior* 62:327–32.

Acker, Gila M., and Dorothea Lawrence. 2009. "Social Work and Managed Care: Measuring Competence, Burnout, and Role Stress of Workers Providing Mental Health Services in a Managed Care Era." *Journal of Social Work* 9(3):269–283.

Ackerman, Joshua M., Sarah E. Hill, and Damian R. Murray. 2018. "The Behavioral Immune System: Current Concerns and Future Directions." *Social & Personality Psychology Compass* 12(2):e12371.

Ackerman, Phillip L., and Stacey D. Wolman. 2007. "Determinants and Validity of Self-estimates of Abilities and Self-concept Measures." *Journal of Experimental Psychology: Applied* 13(2):57–78.




C. K. Cheung, *Resilience Process and Its Personal and Social Bases*,
https://doi.org/10.1007/978-981-97-7391-6

Acosta, Sandra, and Hsien-Yuan Hsu. 2014. "Shared Academic Values: Testing a Model of The Association between Hong Kong Parents? and Adolescents? Perception of the General Value of Science and Scientific Literacy." *Educational Studies* 40(2):174–195.

Adams, Gerald R. 1985. "Identity and Political Socialization." *New Directions for Child Development* 30:61–77.

Adams, Gerald, and Bruce A. Ryan. 2000. "Family Relationships, Academic Environments, and Psychological Development During the University Experience: A Longitudinal Investigation." *Journal of Adolescent Research* 15(1):99–112.

Adams, Marian M. and Joan G. Miller. 2022. "The Flexible Nature of Everyday Reciprocity: Reciprocity, Helping, and Relationship Closeness." *Motivation & Emotion* 46(4):461–75.

Adams, Matthew. 2007. *Self and Social Change*. London, CA: Sage. (HM1033.A33) \d04–4.4

Addad, Moshe. 1987. "Neuroticism, Extraversion and Meaning of Life: A Comparative Study of Criminals and Non-Criminals." *Personality & Individual Differences* 8(6):879–83.

Adeola, Francis O. 2000. "Endangered Community, Enduring People: Toxic Contamination, Health, and Adaptive Responses in a Local Context." *Environment & Behavior* 32(2):209–249.

Adkins, Cheryl L., and Sonya F. Premeaux. 2019. "A Cybernetic Model of Work-Life Balance through Time." *Human Resource Management Review* 29(4):100680.

Adler, Mitchel G., and N.S. Fegley. 2005. "Appreciation: Individual Differences in Finding Value and Meaning as a Unique Predictor of Subjective Well-being." *Journal of Parenting* 73(1):79–114.

Adler, Patricia A., and Peter Adler. 1998. *Peer Power: Preadolescent Culture and Identity*. New Brunswick, NJ: Rutgers University.

Adnanes, Marian. 2007. "Social Transitions and Anomie among Post-Communist Bulgarian Youth." *Young* 15(1):49–69.

Adongo, Raymond, Seongseop Kim, and Statia Elliot. 2019. "Give and Take: A Social Exchange Perspective on Festival Stakeholder Relations." *Annals of Tourism Research* 75:42–57.

Adrian, Amanda L., Amy B. Adler, and Jonathan N. Metzler. 2018. "Vigor Predicting Health Outcomes in a High Risk Occupational Context." *Military Psychology* 30(1):54–62.

Afifi, Tamara D., Anne F. Merrill, and Sharde Davis. 2016. "The Theory of Resilience and Relational Load." *Personal Relationships* 23(4):663–83.

Ager, Alustair. and J. Ager. 2011. "Faith and the Discourse of Secular Humanitarianism." *Journal of Refugee Studies* 24(3):456–72.

Aghababaei, Naser, Faramarz Sohrabi, Hossein Eskandari, Ahmad Borjali, Noorali Farrokhi, 2016. Zhuo Job Chen. 2016. "Predicting Subjective Well-Being by Religious and Scientific Attitudes with Hope, Purpose in Life, and Death Anxiety as Mediators." *Personality & Individual Differences* 90:93–98.

Agnew, Robert S. 2007. "Strain Theory and Violent Behavior." Pp. 519–528 in *The Cambridge Handbook of Violent Behavior and Aggression*, edited by Daniel J. Flannery, Alexander T. Vazsonyi and Irwin D. Waldman. Cambridge, UK: Cambridge University Press.

Agronick, Gail S., and Lauren E. Duncan. 1998. "Personality and Social Change: Individual Differences, Life Path, and Importance Attributed to the Women's Movement." *Journal of Personality & Social Psychology* 76(6):1545–1555.

Ahadi, Stephan A., Mary K. Rothbart, and Renmin Yi. 1993. "Children's Temperament in the US and China: Similarities and Differences." *European Journal of Personality* 7:359–377.

Ahern, Melissa M., and Michael S. Hendryx. 2003. "Social Capital and Trust in Providers." *Social Science & Medicine* 57:1195–1203.

Ahmad, Fahad, and Jeffrey Monaghan. 2019. "Mapping Criminological Engagements within Radicalization Studies." *British Journal of Criminology* 59(6):1288–1308.

Ahmed, S., L. Foulkes, J. T. Leung, C. Griffin, A. Sakhardande, M. Bennett, D. L. Dunning, K. Griffiths, J. Parker, W. Kuyken, J. M. G. Williams, T. Dalgleish, and S. J. Blakemore. 2020. "Susceptibility to Prosocial and Antisocial Influence in Adolescence." *Journal of Adolescence* 84:56–68.

Ahmed, Wondimu, Alexander Minnaert, Greete van der Werf, and Hans Kuyner. 2010. "Perceived Social Support and Early Adolescents" Achievement: The Mediational Roles of Motivational Beliefs and Emotions." *Journal of Youth & Adolescence* 39:36–46.

Ahmetoglu, Gorkan, Franziska Leutner, and Tomas Chamorro-Premuzic. 2011. "EQ-nomics: Understanding the relationship between Individual Differences in Trait Emotional Intelligence and Entrepreneurship." *Personality & Individual Differences* 51:1028–1033.

Ahnquist, Johanna, Sarah P. Wamala, and Martin Lindstrom. 2012. "Social Determinants of Health: A Question of Social or Economic Capital? Interaction Effects of Socioeconomic Factors on Health Outcomes." *Social Science & Medicine* 74(6):930–939.

Aiken, Lewis. 2002. *Attitudes and Related Psychosocial Constructs: Theories, Assessment, and Research*. Thousand Oaks, CA: Sage.

Aitcheson, Rozanna J., Soleman H. Abu-Bader, Mary K. Howell, Deena Khalil, and Salman Elbedour. 2017. "Resilience in Palestinian Adolescents Living in Gaza." *Psychological Trauma: Theory, Research, Practice, & Policy* 9(1):36–43.

Aizer, Anna. 2009. "Neighborhood Violence and Urban Youth." Pp. 275–307 in *The Problems of Disadvantaged Youth: An Economic Perspective*, edited by Jonathan Gruber. Chicago, IL: University of Chicago Press.

Akkerman, Agnes. 2013. "Solidarity, Strikes, and Scabs: How Participation Norms Affect Union Members" Willingness to Strike." *Work & Occupations* 40(3):250–80.

Akrim, A., Rudianto Rudianto, and Abrar Adhani. 2021. "Interactive Effects of Stoicism and Religious Coping on Psychological Distress, Fatigue and Intercultural Communication: Muslim Health Workers in Bali." *Journal of Ethnic & Cultural Studies* 8(4):214–37.

Alain, Claude, Aline Moussard, Julia Singer, Yunjo Lee, Gavin M. Bidelman and Sylvain Moreno. 2019. "Music and Visual Art Training Modulate Brain Activity in Older Adults." *Frontiers in Neuroscience* 13:1–15.

Al-Arja, Nahida Saba. 2023. "Patience and Its Relationship to Stress Tolerance in Relation to Demographic Factors of the Medical System in Bethlehem Governorate During the Covid-19 Pandemic." *Frontiers in Psychology* 14:1059589.

Albeck, Shulamith and Dania Kaydar. 2002. "Divorced Mothers." *Journal of Divorce & Remarriage* 36(3–4):111–38.

Albuquerque, Cristina Pinto, Clara Cruz Santos, and Helena Da Silva Neves Santos Almeida. 2017. "Assessing Empowerment" as Social Development: Goal and Process." *European Journal of Social Work* 20(1):88–100.

Aldridge, Stephen, and David Halpern. 2002. *Social Capital*. Performance & Innovation Unit. London.

Aldwin, Carolyn M., Michael R. Levenson, and Linda Kelly. 2009. "Life Span Developmental Perspectives on Stress-related Growth." Pp. 87–104 in *Medical Illness and Positive Life Change: Can Crisis Lead to Psychological Personal Transformation?* edited by Crystal L. Park, Suzanne C. Lechner, Michael H. Antoni and Annette L. Stanton. Washington, DC: American Psychological Association.

Alea, Nicole, Susan Bluck, and Angelania B. Semegon. 2004. "Young and Older Adults" Experience of Emotional Experience: Do Autobiographical Narratives Tell a Different Story?" *Journal of Adult Development* 11(4):235–250.

Aleksandrowicz, Dov R. 2009. "Mastery, Aggression and Narcissism: A Contribution to Psychoanalytic Drive Theory." *Archives of Psychiatry & Psychotherapy* 2:13–21.

Alesina, Alberto, and Eliana La Ferrara. 2002. "Who Trusts Others?" *Journal of Public Economics* 85(2):207–234.

Alessandri, Guido, Bernadette Paula Luengo Kanacri, Nancy Eisenberg, Antonio Zuffiano, Michela Milioni, Michele Vecchione, and Gian Vittorio Caprara. 2014. "Prosociality During the Transition From Late Adolescence to Young Adulthood: The Role of Effortful Control and Ego-resiliency." *Personality & Social Psychology Bulletin* 40(11):1451–1465.

Alexander, Stephanie A., Katherine L. Frohlich, and Caroline Fusco. 2019. *Play, Physical Activity and Public Health: The Reframing of Children's Leisure Lives*. Abingdon, UK: Routledge.

Alexiadou, Nafsika. 2002. "Social Inclusion and Social Exclusion in England: Tensions in Education Policy." *Journal of Education Policy* 17(1):71–86.

Algoe, Sara B., and Jonathan Haidt. 2009. "Witnessing Excellence in Action: The Other-Praising Emotions of Elevation, Gratitude, and Admiration." *Journal of Positive Psychology* 4(2):105–127.

Algoe, Sara B., and Ruixue Zhaoyang. 2016. "Positive Psychology in Context: Effects of Expressing Gratitude in Ongoing Relationships Depend on Perceptions of Enactor Responsiveness." *Journal of Positive Psychology* 11(4):399–415.

Al-krenawi, Alean, John R Graham, Fakir Al Gharaibeh. 2011. "A Comparison Study of Psychological, Family Function Marital and Life Satisfactions of Polygamous and Monogamous Women in Jordan." *Community Mental Health Journal* 47(5):594–602.

Allan, Blake A., Richard P. Douglass, Ryan D. Duffy, and Ryan J. McCarty. 2016. "Meaningful Work as a Moderator of the Relation between Work Stress and Meaning in Life." *Journal of Career Assessment* 24(3):429–440.

Allan, Julie, and Alison Whybrow. 2007. "Gestalt Coaching." Pp. 133–159 in *Handbook of Coaching Psychology: A Guide for Practitioners*, edited by Stephen Palmer and Alison Whybrow. Hove, UK: Routledge.

Allemand, Mathias, Patrick L. Hill, and Regula Lehmann. 2015. "Divorce and Personality Development across Middle Adulthood." *Personal Relationships* 22(1):122–37.

Allen, Joseph P., Maryfrances R. Porter, F. Christy McFarland, and Penny Marsh. 2005. "The Two Faces of Adolescents" Success with Peers: Adolescent Popularity, Social Adaptation, and Deviant Behavior." *Child Development* 76(3):747–760.

Allen, Rebecca S. et al. 2009. "Living Well with Living Wills: Application of Protection Motivation Theory to Living Wills." *Clinical Gerontologist* 32:44–59.

Allidina, Suraiya, Nathan L. Arbuckle, and William A. Cunningham. 2019. "Considerations of Mutual Exchange in Prosocial Decision-Making." *Frontiers in Psychology* 10:1216.

Allik, Juri, and Anu Realo. 2004. "Individualism-collectivism and Social Capital." *Journal of Cross-Cultural Psychology* 35(1):29–49.

Allison, Lincoln. 2001. "The Olympic Movement and the End of the Cold War." *World Affairs* 157(2):92–97.

Allison, Scott T., George R. Goethals, and Roderick M. Kramer. 2017. "Setting the Scene: The Rise and Coalescence of Heroism Science." Pp. 1–16 in *Handbook of Heroism and Heroic Leadership*, edited by Scott t. Allison, George R. Goethals and Roderick M. Kramer. New York: Routledge.

Allman, Dan. 2013. "The Sociology of Social Inclusion." *SAGE Open* 2013:1–16.

Almakaeva, Anna, Christian Welzel, and Eduard Ponarin. 2018. "Human Empowerment and Trust in Strangers: The Multilevel Evidence." *Social Indicators Research* 139(3):923–62.

Alonso-Arbiol, Itziar, Nekane Baluerka, and Phillip R. Shaver. 2007. "A Spanish Version of the Experiences in Close Relationships (ECR) Adult Attachment Questionnaire." *Personal Relationships* 14:45–63.

Alrabai, Fakieh and Abdullah Alamer. 2022. "The Role of Learner Character Strengths and Classroom Emotions in L2 Resilience." *Frontiers in Psychology* 13:956216.

Alrofiai, Fawaz, Jessica Bellingham, and Paul S. Gibson. 2020. "Realism and Resilience: An Inquiry into the Helpfulness of Adopting an Existential Outlook." *Psychological Reports* 123(6):2173–95.

Alschuler, Kevin N., Anna L. Kratz, Dawn M. Ehde. 2016. "Resilience and Vulnerability in Individuals with Chronic Pain and Physical Disability." *Rehabilitation Psychology* 61(1):7–18.

AlShebali, Munirah, Ahmad AlHadi, and Glenn Waller. 2021. "The Impact of Ongoing Westernization on Eating Disorders and Body Image Dissatisfaction in a Sample of Undergraduate Saudi Women." *Eating & Weight Disorders* 26(6):1835–44.

Alsted, Jacob and Ditte Haslund. 2020. *Psychodynamic Organisational Theory: Key Concepts and Cases*. Abingdon, UK: Routledge.

Alt, Dorit. 2015. "Assessing the Contribution of a Constructivist Learning Environment to Academic Self-Efficacy in Higher Education." *Learning Environments Research* 18(1):47–67.

Alvarez, Mar Alcolea and Natalia Solano Pinto. 2023. "Experiential Covid-19 Factors Predicting Resilience among Spanish Adults." *BMC Psychology* 11(1):118.

Alves, Hans, Alex Koch, and Christian Unkelbach. 2016. "My Friends Are All Alike: The Relation between Liking and Perceived Similarity in Person Perception." *Journal of Experimental Social Psychology* 62:103–17.

Amato, Paul R., and Jacob Chendle. 2005. "The Long Reach of Divorce: Divorce and Child Well-being across Three Generations." *Journal of Marriage & Family* 67:191–206.

Ambrey, Christopher L., and Christopher M. Fleming. 2014. "Valuing Ecosystem Diversity in South East Queensland: A Life Satisfaction Approach." *Social Indicators Research* 115:45–65.

Ambrose, James. 2002. *Simplified Mechanics and Strength of Materials.* New York: John Wiley & Sons.

Amiot, Catherine E., Winnifred R. Louis, Sarah Bourdeau, and Oulma Maalouf. 2017. "Can Harmful Intergroup Behaviors Truly Represent the Self?: The Impact of Harmful and Prosocial Normative Behaviors on Intra-Individual Conflict and Compartmentalization." *Self & Identity* 16(6):703–31.

Amir, Varda, and Gail K. Auslander. 2003. "Inter-organizational Collaboration among Social Workers: The Case of Community Mental Health Centers and Local Social Service Departments in Israel." *British Journal of Social Work* 33(4):557–566.

Amit, Karin and Shirly Bar-Lev. 2015. "Immigrants' Sense of Belonging to the Host Country: The Role of Life Satisfaction, Language Proficiency, and Religious Motives." *Social Indicators Research* 124(3):947–61.

Anciaes, Paulo Rui, Paul James Metcalfe, and Chris Heywood. 2017. "Social Impacts of Road Traffic: Perceptions and Priorities of Local Residents." *Impact Assessment & Project Appraisal* 35(2):172–183.

Anderman, Lynley H. 2003. "Academic and Social Perceptions as Predictors of Change in Middle School Students" Sense of School Belonging." *Journal of Experimental Education* 72(1):5–22.

Anderson, Alistair R., and Claire J. Miller. 2003. "Class Matters: Human and Social Capital in the Entrepreneurial Process." *Journal of Socio-Economics* 32:17–36.

Anderson, Jon. 2010. "From Zombies to Coyotes: Environmentalism Where We Are." *Environmental Politics* 19(6):973–91.

Anderson, Sarah E., Mark T. Buntaine, Mengdi Liu, and Bing Zhang. 2019. "Non-Governmental Monitoring of Local Governments Increases Compliance with Central Mandates: A National-Scale Field Experiment in China." *American Journal of Political Science* 63(3):626–43.

Anderson, Steven G., and Mary Keegan Eamon. 2004. "Health Coverage Instability for Mothers in Working Families." *Social Work* 49(3):395–405.

Anderson-Butcher, Dawn, Aidyn L. Iachini, and Anthony J. Amorose. 2008. "Initially Reliability and Validity of the Perceived Social Competence Scale." *Research on Social Work Practice* 18(1):47–54.

Anderson-Butcher, Dawn, Angela Oliver Khairallah, and Janis Race-Bigelow. 2004. "Mutual Support Groups for Long-term Recipients of TANF." *Social Work* 49(1):131–140.

Anderson Connolly, Richard. 2002. "Is Lean Mean? Workplace Transformation and Employee Well being." *Work, Employment & Society* 16(3):389–413.

Andrade, Carla, Patricia Arriaga, and Marina Carvalho. 2019. "The Psychometric Properties of the Portuguese Version of the State Mindfulness Scale." *Mindfulness* 10(12):2661.

Andrews, Kenneth T., Kraig Beyerlein, and Tuneka Tucker Farnum. 2015. "The Legitimacy of Protest: Explaining White Southerners" Attitudes toward the Civil Rights Movement." *Social Forces* 94(3):1021–1044.

Andrews, Naomi C. Z. 2020. "Prestigious Youth Are Leaders but Central Youth Are Powerful: What Social Network Position Tells Us about Peer Relationships." *Journal of Youth & Adolescence* 49(3):631–644.

Angelis, Sophia and Pamela Pensini. 2024. "Honesty-Humility Predicts Humanitarian Prosocial Behavior via Social Connectedness: A Parallel Mediation Examining Connectedness to Community, Nation, Humanity, and Nature." *Scandinavian Journal of Psychology* 64(6):810–18.

Angelusz, Robert, and Robert Tardos. 2001. "Change and Stability in Social Network Resources: The Case of Hungary under Transformation." Pp. 297–323 in *Social Capital: Theory and Research*, edited by Nan Lin, Karen Cook, and Ronald S. Burt. New York: Aldine de Gruyter.

Angermeyer, Matthias C., Herbert Matschinger, Bruce G. Link, and Georg Schomerus. 2014. "Public Attitudes Regarding Individual and Structural Discrimination: Two Sides of the Same Coin?". *Social Science & Medicine* 103:60–66.

Annalakshmi, Narayanan and Mohammed Abeer. 2011. "Islamic Worldview, Religious Personality and Resilience among Muslim Adolescent Students in India." *Europe's Journal of Psychology* 7(4):716–738.

Armstrong, Andrew R, Roslyn F. Galligan, and Christine R. Critchley. 2011. "Emotional Intelligence and Psychological Resilience to Negative Life Events." *Personality & Individual Differences* 51(3):331–336.

Ano, Gene G., and Rin B. Vasconelles. 2005. "Religious Coping and Psychological Adjustment to Stress: A Mea-analysis." *Journal of Clinical Psychology* 61(4):461–480.

Anton, Charis E., and Carmen Lawrence. 2014. "Home is Where the Heart Is: The Effect of Place of Residence on Place Attachment and Community Participation." *Journal of Environmental Psychology* 40:451–461.

Antonakis, John, and Joerg Dietz. 2011. "Looking for Validity or Testing It? The Perils of Stepwise Regression, Extreme-score Analysis, Heteroscedasticity, and Measurement Error." *Personality & Individual Differences* 50:409–415.

Antunes, Maria Joao Lobo, and Eileen M. Ahlin. 2014. "Family Management and Youth Violence: Are Parents or Community More Salient?" *Journal of Community Psychology* 42(3):316–337.

Anusic, Ivana, Stevie C.Y. Yap, and Richard E. Lucas. 2014. "Does Personality Moderate Reaction and Adaptation to Major Life Events? Analysis of Life Satisfaction and Affect in an Australian National Sample." *Journal of Research in Personality* 51:69–77.

Apinunmahakul, Amornat, and Rose Anne Devlin. 2008. "Social Networks and Private Philanthropy." *Journal of Public Economics* 92:309–328.

Appleton, Simon, and Lina Song. 2008. "Life Satisfaction in Urban China: Components and Determinants." *World Development* 36(11):2335–2340.

Arai, Susan M., and Alison M. Pedlar. 1997. "Building Communities through Leisure: Citizen Participation in a Healthy Communities Initiative." *Journal of Leisure Research* 29(2):167–182.

Arat, Gizem and Narine N. Kerelian. 2019. "The Promotion of Socially Inclusive East Asian Society: The Hong Kong Case." *Journal of Human Rights & Social Work* 4(4):275–84.

Araya, Ricardo, Frank Dunstan, Rebecca Playle, Hollie Thomas, Stephen Palmer, and Glyn Lewis. 2006. "Perceptions of Social Capital and the Built Environment and Mental Health." *Social Science & Medicine* 62:3072–3083.

Arguedas, Amy A. Ross 2020. "Can Naughty Be Healthy? Healthism and Its Discontents in News Coverage of Orthorexia Nervosa." *Social Science & Medicine* 246:112784.

Armfield, Jason M., Lesley-Anne Ey, Carole Zufferey, Emmanuel S. Gnanamanickam, and Leonie Segal. 2021. "Educational Strengths and Functional Resilience at the Start of Primary School Following Child Maltreatment." *Child Abuse & Neglect* 122:105301.

Armon, Cheryl, and Theo Linda Dawson. 2003. "The Good Life: A Longitudinal Study of Adult Value Reasoning." Pp. 271–300 in *Handbook of Adult Development*, edited by Jack Demick and Carrie Andreoletti. New York: Kluwer Academic.

Armstrong-Stassen, Marjorie. 2001. "Reactions of Older Employees to Organizational Downsizing: The Role of Gender, Job Level, and Time." *Journal of Gerontology: Psychological Sciences* 56B(4):234–43.

Arneson, Richard J. 2005. "Joel Feinberg and the Justification of Hard Paternalism." *Legal Theory* 11(3):259–84.

Arnett, Jeffrey Jensen, Marrion Kloep, Leo B. Hendry, and Jennifer L. Tanner. 2011. *Debating Emerging Adulthood: Stage or Process?* New York: Oxford University Press. (BF724.5D43)

Aron, Arthur, Jodie L. Steele, Todd B. Kashdan, and M. A. X. Perez. 2006. "When Similars Do Not Attract: Tests of a Prediction from the Self-Expansion Model." *Personal Relationships* 13(4):387–96.

Arseth, Annie K., Jane Kroger, Monica Martinussen, and Guro Bakken. 2009. "Intimacy Status, Attachment, Separation-Individuation Patterns, and Identity Status in Female University Students." *Journal of Social & Personal Relationships* 26(5):697–712.

Arts, S.E., A. Kerkstra, J. van der Zee, and H. Huyer Abu-Saad. 1999. "Workload, Capacity for Coping and Psychological and Physical Outcomes amongst Home Help in the Netherlands." *Health & Social Care in the Community* 7(2):79–90.

Artuch-Garde, Raquel, Maria del Carmen González-Torres, Jesús de la Fuente, M. Mariano Vera, María Fernández-Cabezas, and Mireia López-García. 2017. "Relationship between Resilience and Self-regulation: A Study of Spanish Youth at Risk of Social Exclusion." *Frontiers in Psychology* 8:612.

Aryee, Samuel, Susanna Lo, and Inn-Lee Kang. 1999. "Antecedents of Early Career Stage Mentoring among Chinese Employees." *Journal of Organizational Behavior* 20:563–576.

Ashby, Kimberly M., Dana L. Collins, Janet E. Helms, and Joshua Manlove. 2018. "Let's Talk About Race: Evaluating a College Interracial Discussion Group on Race." *Journal of Multicultural Counseling & Development* 46(2):97–114.

Ashby, Mike, Hugh Shercliff, and David Cebon. 2014. *Materials: Engineering Science, Processing and Design.* Oxford, UK: Butterworth-Heinemann.

Asher, Steven R., and Molly S. Weeks. 2018. "Friendships in Childhood." Pp. 119–134 in *The Cambridge Handbook of Personal Relationships*, edited by Anita L. Vangelisti and Daniel Perlman. Cambridge, UK: Cambridge University Press.

Aslani, Soroush, Jimena Ramirez-Marin, Zhaleh Semnani-Azad, Jeanne M. Brett, and Catherine Tinsley. 2013. "The Demise of the Rational Negotiator: Emotional Forces in Conflict and Negotiation." Pp. 249–282 in *Handbook of Research on Negotiation*, edited by Mara Olekalns and Wendi L. Adair. Cheltenham, UK: Elgar.

Asoodar, Maryam, Mahmood Reza Atai, Shahin Vaezi, and Seyyedeh Susan Marandi. 2014. "Examining Effectiveness of Communities of Practice in Online English for Academic Purposes (EAP) Assessment in Virtual Classes." *Computers & Education* 70:291–300.

Aspinwall, Lisa G., and Shelley E. Taylor. 1992. "Modeling Cognitive Adaptation: A Longitudinal Investigation of the Impact of Individual Differences and Coping on College Adjustment and Performance." *Journal of Personality & Social Psychology* 63(6):989–1003.

Aspy, David N., Cheryl B. Aspy, Gene Russel, and Mack Wedel. 2000. "Carkhuff's Human Technology: A Verification and Extension of Kelly's (1997) Suggestion to Integration the Humanistic and Technical Components of Counseling." *Journal of Counseling & Development* 78:29–37.

Atchley, Robert C. 1999. *Continuity and Adaptation in Aging*: Creating Positive Experiences. Baltimore, MY: Johns Hopkins University Press.

Atitsogbe, Kobou A. et al. 2019. "Perceived Employability and Entrepreneurial Intentions across Univesity Students and Job Seekers in Togo: The Effects of Career Adaptability and Self-efficacy." *Frontiers in Psychology* 10:180.

Atkinson, Giles, Andrew Healey, and Susana Mourato. 2005. "Valuing the Costs of Violent Crime: A Stated Preference Approach." *Oxford Economic Papers* 57(4):559–585.

Atkinson, Matthew D. and Darin Dewitt. 2019. "The Politics of Disruption: Social Choice Theory and Conspiracy Theory." Pp. 122–134 in *Conspiracy Theories and the People Who Believe Them*, edited by Joseph E. Uscinski. New York, NY: Oxford University Press.

Atkinson, Mike. 2012. "Norbert Elias and the Body." Pp. 49–61 in *Routledge Handbook of Body Studies*, edited by Bryan S. Turner. Abington, UK: Routledge.

Au, Kevin, and Mike W.L. Cheung. 2004. "Intra-cultural Variation and Job Autonomy in 42 Countries." *Organization Studies* 25(8):1339–1362.

Auerbach, Randy P., Christian A. Webb, Meghan Schreck, Chad M. McWhinnie, Moon-Ho Ringo Ho, Xiongzhao Zhu and Shuqiao Yao. 2011. "Examining the Pathway through Which Intrinsic and Extrinsic Aspirations Generate Stress and Subsequent Depressive Symptoms." *Journal of Social & Clinical Psychology* 30(8):856–86.

Austin, Elizabeth J., Donald H. Saklofsko, and Vincent Egan. 2005. "Personality, Well-being and Health Correlates of Trait Emotional Intelligence." *Personality & Individual Differences* 38:547–558.

Austin, Erica Weintraub, and Bruce E. Pinkleton. 1999. "The Relation between Media Content Evaluations and Political Disaffection." *Mass Communication & Society* 2(3/4):105–122.

Autin, Kelsey L., Richard P. Douglass, Ryan D. Duffy, Jessica W. England, and Blake A. Allan. 2017. "Subjective Social Status, Work Volition, and Career Adaptability: A Longitudinal Study." *Journal of Vocational Behavior* 99:1–10.

Avalos, Lizbeth Pulido, Emilio Ribes Iñesta, Iván López Ortiz, Gloria A. Marinero Villa, and Iván Hernández Miranda. 2019. "Effects of Reciprocity Induction on Partial-Altruistic and Unequal-Asymmetric Labor Exchange Interactions." *Psychological Record* 69(1):25–37.

Avlund, Kirsten, Rikke Lund, Bjorn E. Holstein, Pernille Due, Ritva Sakari-Rantala, and Riitta-Liisa Heikkinen. 2004. "The Impact of Structural and Functional Characteristics of Social Relations as Determinants of Functional Decline." *Journal of Gerontology: Social Sciences* 59B(1):S44–S51.

Axinn, William, Jennifer S. Barber, and Arland Thornton. 1999. "Values and Beliefs as Determinants of Outcomes in Children's Lives." Pp. 118–127 in *Transitions to Adulthood in a Changing Economy: No Work, No Family, No Future?* edited by Alan Booth, Ann C. Crouter, and Michael J. Shanahan. Westport, CT: Praeger.

Ayalon, Hanna, Eliezer Ben-Rafael, and Abraham Yogev. 1993. *Community in Transition: Mobility, Integration, and Conflict*. Westport, CT: Greenwood.

Ayers, C. D., J. H. Williams, J. D. Hawkins, P. L. Peterson, R. F. Catalano, and R. D. Abbott. 1999. "Assessing Correlates of Onset, Escalation, Deescalation, and Desistance of Delinquent Behavior." *Journal of Quantitative Criminology* 15(3):277–306.

Aytac, Işık A., Bruce H. Rankin, and Arda İbikoğlu. 2015. "The Social Impact of the 2008 Global Economic Crisis on Neighborhoods, Households, and Individuals in Turkey." *Social Indicators Research* 124(1):1–19.

Aytac, S. Esdem, and Susan C. Stokes. 2019. *Why Bother? Rethinking Participation in Elections and Protests*. Cambridge, UK: Cambridge University Press.

Baas, Mathijs, Carsten K.W. de Dreu, and Bernard A. Nijstad. 2008. "A Meta-analysis of 25 Years of Mood-creativity Research: Hedonic Tone Activation or Regulatory Focus?" Psychological Bulletin 134(6):779–806.

Baay, Pieter E., Marcel A.G. van Aken, Denise T.D. de Ridder, and Tanja van der Lippe. 2014. "Understanding the Role of Social Capital In Adolescents" Big Five Personality Effects on School-to-work Transitions." *Journal of Adolescence* 37(5):739–748.

Babcicky, Philipp and Sebastian Seebauer. 2017. "The Two Faces of Social Capital in Private Flood Mitigation: Opposing Effects on Risk Perception, Self-Efficacy and Coping Capacity." *Journal of Risk Research* 20(8):1017–37.

Bachkirova, Tatiana, and Elaine Cox. 2007. "A Cognitive-developmental Approach for Coach Development." Pp. 325–350 in *Handbook of Coaching Psychology: A Guide for Practitioners*, edited by Stephen Palmer and Alison Whybrow. Hove, UK: Routledge.

Bachkirova, Tatiana. 2018. "Psychological Development in Adulthood and Coaching." Pp. 124–139 in *The Complete Handbook of Coaching*, edited by Elaine Cox, Tatiana Bachkirova, and David Clutterbuck. London, UK: SAGE.

Backman, Olof, and Anders Nilsson. 2011. "Pathways to Social Exclusion: A Life-course Study." *European Sociological Review* 27(1):107–123.

Badawy, Philip J. and Scott Schieman. 2021. "With Greater Power Comes Greater Stress? Authority, Supervisor Support, and Work-Family Strains." *Journal of Marriage & the Family* 83(1):40–56.

Baer, Judith. 2002. "Is Family Cohesion a Risk or Protection Factor During Adolescent Development?" *Journal of Marriage & Family* 64(3):668–675.

Bagci, Sabahat C. and Elif Celebi. 2017. "Cross-Group Friendships and Outgroup Attitudes among Turkish–Kurdish Ethnic Groups: Does Perceived Interethnic Conflict Moderate the Friendship-Attitude Link?" *Journal of Applied Social Psychology* 47(2):59–73.

Bagherior, Reza, A. S. Bahaman, A. S. Asnarulkhadi, and A. Shamsudain. 2009. "A Social Exchange Approach to People's Participation in Watershed Management Programs in Iran." *European Journal of Scientific Research* 34(3):428–441.

Bagozzi, Richard P., and Kyu-Hyun Lee. 2002. "Multiple Routes for Social Influence: The Role of Compliance, Internalization, and Social Identity." *Social Psychology Quarterly* 65(3):226–247.

Bagwell, Catherine L., and Michelle E. Schmidt. 2011. *Friendships in Childhood & Adolescence.* New York: Guilford.

Bahr, David B. and Eve Passerini. 1998. "Statistical Mechanics of Collective Behavior: Macro-Sociology." *Journal of Mathematical Sociology* 23(1):29–49.

Baildon, Mark and Theresa Alviar-Martin. 2020. "Taming Cosmopolitanism: The Limits of National and Neoliberal Civic Education in Two Global Cities." Asia Pacific Journal of Education 40(1):98–111.

Bailey, Richard. 2005. "Evaluating the Relationship between Physical Education, Sport and Social Inclusion." *Educational Review* 57(1):71–90.

Bailey, Sandra J., Bethany L. Letiecq, Minde Erickson, and Rebecca Koltz. 2013. "Resilient Grandparent Caregivers: Pathways to Positive Adaptation." Pp. 70–87 in *Resilient Grandparent Caregivers: A Strengths-based Perspective*, edited by Bert Hayslip, Jr. and Gregory C. Smith. New York: Routledge.

Bailly, Lionel. 2012. "Lacanian Therapy." Pp. 264–267 in T*he SAGE Handbook of Counselling and Psychotherapy*, edited by Colin Feltham and Ian Horton. London: SAGE.

Baily, Supriya. 2014. "Deconstructing Gatekeepers Discourses in the Establishment of Self-Help Groups for Women in Rural India." *Community Development Journal* 49(4):589–602.

Baim, Clark. 2012. "Psychodrama." Pp. 325–334 in *The SAGE Handbook of Counselling and Psychotherapy*, edited by Colin Feltham and Ian Horton. London: SAGE. (BF637.C6H3623)

Baker, Joseph O., and Buster G. Smith. 2009. "Growing up in Context: The Nones: Social Characteristics of the Religiously Unaffiliated." *Social Forces* 87(3):1251–1263.

Baker, Susan Gonzalez, and Marilyn Espitia. 2000. "From Latin American Immigrant to Hispanic Citizen: The Role of Social Capital in Seeking U.S. Citizenship." *Social Science Quarterly* 81(4):1053–1064.

Bakker, Arnold B., and Sabine A.E. Geurts. 2004. "Toward a Dual-process Model of Work-home Interference." *Work & Occupations* 31(3):345–366.

Bakker, Arnold B., Wilmar B. Schaufeli, Michael P. Leiter, and Toon W. Taris. 2008. "Work Engagement: An Emerging Concept." Occupational Health Psychology 22(3):187–200.

Bakshi, Anuradha J., and Jahnvee Joshi. 2014. "The Interface between Positive Youth Development and Youth Career Development: New Avenues for Career Guidance Practice." Pp. 173–201 in *Handbook of Career Development: International Perspectives*, edited by Salvatore Soresi, Laura Nota, Lea Ferrari, and Maria Cristina Ginevra. New York, NY: Springer.

Baldacci, Emanuele, Maria Teresa Guin-Siu, and Luiz de Mello. 2003. "More on the Effectiveness of Public Spending on Health Care and Education: A Covariance Structure Model." *Journal of International Development* 15:709–725.

Baldwin, Matthew, Mark H. White, and Daniel Sullivan. 2018. "Nostalgia for America's Past Can Buffer Collective Guilt." *European Journal of Social Psychology* 48(4):433–446.

Ball, Samuel A. 1995. "The Validity of an Alternative Five-factor Measure of Personality in Cocaine Abusers." *Psychological Assessment* 7(2):148–154.

Balsam, Kimberly F., Yamile Molina, Blair Beadnell, Jane Simoni, and Karina Walters. 2011. "Measuring Multiple Minority Stress: The LGBT People of Color Microaggressions Scale." *Cultural Diversity & Ethnic Minority Psychology* 17(2):163–174.

Balsas, Carlos J. L. 2017. "The Right to Walk in Cities, a Comparative Review of Macau, Lisbon and Las Vegas." *Journal of Property, Planning & Environmental Law* 9(2):123–42.

Bandura, Albert. 2012. "Social Cognitive Theory." Pp. 349–373 in *Handbook of Theories of Social Psychology* (vol. 1), edited by Paul A.M. Van Lange, Arie W. Kruglanski and E. Tory Higgins. Los Angeles, CA: SAGE.

Bang, Hyejin, Doyeon Won, and Sanghyun Park. 2020. "School Engagement, Self-Esteem, and Depression of Adolescents: The Role of Sport Participation and Volunteering Activity and Gender Differences." *Children & Youth Services Review* 113:105012.

Bang, Hyejin, Mido Chang, and Sunha Kim. 2024. "Team and Individual Sport Participation, School Belonging, and Gender Differences in Adolescent Depression." *Children & Youth Services Review* 159:107517.

Bang, Hyeyoung and Yuchun Zhou. 2014. "The Function of Wisdom Dimensions in Ego-Identity Development among Chinese University Students." *International Journal of Psychology* 49(6):434–445.

Banicki, Konrad. 2014. "Positive Psychology on Character Strengths and Virtues: A Disquieting Suggestion." *New Ideas in Psychology* 33:21–36.

Banks, Donice M. and Carl F. Weems. 2014. "Family and Peer Social Support and Their Links to Psychological Distress among Hurricane-Exposed Minority Youth." *American Journal of Orthopsychiatry* 84(4):341–52.

Bankston, Carl L., III, and Min Zhou. 2002b. "Social Capital as Process: The Meaning and Problems of a Theoretical Metaphor." *Sociological Inquiry* 72(2):285–317.

Bao, Yan, Alexandra von Stosch, Mona Park, and Ernst Pöppel. 2017. "Complementarity as Generative Principle: A Thought Pattern for Aesthetic Appreciations and Cognitive Appraisals in General." *Frontiers in Psychology* 8:727.

Baptist, Joyce, Patricia Barros, Bryan Cafferky, and Elaine Johannes. 2015. "Resilience Building among Adolescents from National Guard Families." *Journal of Adolescent Research* 30(3):306–34.

Baptista, N., José Carlos Pinho, and Helena Alves. 2021. "Examining Social Capital and Online Social Support Links: A Study in Online Health Communities Facing Treatment Uncertainty." *International Review on Public & Nonprofit Marketing* 18(1):57–94 \102–351.

Barak, Adi. 2016. "Critical Consciousness in Critical Social Work: Learning from the Theatre of the Oppressed." *British Journal of Social WORK* 46(6):1776–92.

Barbarin, Oscar A., and Linda Richter. 2001. "Economic Status, Community Danger and Psychological Problems among South African Children." *Childhood* 8(1):115–133.

Barber, Jennifer S. 2004. "Community Social Context and Individualistic Attitudes toward Marriage." *Social Psychology Quarterly* 67(3):236–256.

Barber, Larissa K., Patricia G. Bagsby, and David C. Munz. 2010. "Affect Regulation Strategies for Promoting (or Preventing) Flourishing Emotional Health." *Personality & Individual Differences* 49:663–666.

Barcaccia, Barbara, Marco Salvati, Susanna Pallini, Angelo Maria Saliani, Roberto Baiocco, and Giovanni Maria Vecchio. 2022b. "The Bitter Taste of Revenge: Negative Affect, Depression and Anxiety." *Current Psychology* 41(3):1198–203.

Barcalow, Emmett. 2007. *Moral Philosophy: Theories and Issues* (4th ed.). Belmont, CA: Thomson.

Bardeen, Joseph R., Thomas A. Fergus, and Holly K. Orcutt. 2016. "Examining the Specific Dimensions of Distress Tolerance That Prospectively Predict Perceived Stress." *Cognitive Behaviour Therapy* 46(3):1–13.

Bardo, Michael T., Thomas Kelly, Donald R. Lynam, and Richard Milich. 2003. "Basic Science and Drug Abuse Prevention: Neuroscience, Learning, and Personality Perspectives." Pp. 429–446 in *Handbook of Drug Abuse Prevention: Theory, Science, and Practice*, edited by Zili Sloboda and William J. Bukoski. New York: Kluwer Academic.

Barefoot, John C., Kimberly E. Maynard, Jean C. Beckham, Beverly H. Brummett, Karen Hooker, and Ilene C. Siegler. 1998. "Trust, Health, and Longevity." *Journal of Behavioral Medicine* 21(6):517–526.

Barge, J. Kevin, and Dorothy C. Andreas. 2013. "Communities, Conflict, and the Design of Dialogic Conversations." Pp. 609–634 in *The SAGE Handbook of Conflict Communication*, edited by John G. Oetzel and Stelle Ting-Toomey. Thousand Oaks, CA: SAGE.

Baril, Megan E., Ann C. Crouter and Susan M. McHale. 2007. "Processes Linking Adolescent Well-Being, Marital Love, and Coparenting." *Journal of Family Psychology* 21(4):645–54.

Barkan, Steven E., and Steven F. Cohn. 2005. "Why Whites Favor Spending More Money to Fight Crime: The Role of Racial Prejudice." *Social Problems* 52(2):300–314.

Barker, David C. and James D. Tinnick, III. 2006. "Competing Visions of Parental Roles and Ideological Constraint." *American Political Science Review* 100(2):249–263.

Barlow, Sally H., and Gary M. Burlingame. 2006. "Essential theory, Processes, and Procedures for Successful Group Psychotherapy: Group Cohesion as Exemplar." *Journal of Contemporary Psychotherapy* 36:107–112.

Barnard, Laura K., and John F. Curry. 2011. "Self-compassion: Conceptualizations, Correlates, and Interventions." *Review of General Psychology* 15(4):289–303.

Barnes, Gordon E., and Brent A. Vulcano. 1982. "Measuring Rationality Independent of Social Desirability." *Personality & Individual Differences* 3(3):303–309.

Barnes, Sandra L. 2005. "Black Church Culture and Community Action." *Social Forces* 84(2):967–994.

Barnes, Sandra L., and Charles Janet. 2003. "The American Dream in Poor Urban Neighborhoods: An Analysis of Home Ownership Attitudes and Behavior and Financial Saving Behavior." *Sociological Focus* 36:219–239.

Barnett, Melissa A., Laura V. Scaramella, Tricia K. Neppl, and Lenna L. Ontai, and Rand D. Conger. 2010. "Grandmother Involvement as a Protective Factor for Early Childhood Social Adjustment." *Journal of Family Psychology* 24(5):635–645.

Baron, Lois. 2007. *Contemporary Issues in Youth Sports*. New York, NY: Nova.

Barr, Jeffrey A., Nambee G. Choi, Jun E. Mutchler, and Francis G. Caro. 2005. "Caregiving and Volunteering: A Private and Public Helping Behaviors Linked?" *Journal of Gerontology: Social Sciences* 60B(5):S247–S256.

Barrera, Davide. 2007. "The Impact of Negotiated Exchange on Trust and Trustworthiness." *Social Networks* 29:508–526.

Barrera, Maru, Eshetu G. Atenafu, Lillian Sung, Ute Bartels, Fiona Schulte, Joanna Chung, Danielle Cataudella, Kelly Hancock, Laura Janzen, Amani Saleh, Douglas Strother, Andrea Downie, Shayna Zelcer, Juliette Hukin, and Dina McConnell. 2018. "A Randomized Control Intervention Trial to Improve Social Skills and Quality of Life in Pediatric Brain Tumor Survivors." *Psycho-oncology* 27(1):91–98.

Barry, Carolyn McNamara, and Allan Wigfield. 2002. "Social Perceptions of Friendship-making Ability and Perceptions of Friends' Deviant Behavior: Childhood to Adolescence." *Journal of Early Adolescence* 22(2):143–172.

Barry, Carolyn, Laura Padilla-Walker, Laura, Larry Nelson. 2012. "The Role of Mothers and Media on Emerging Adults" Religious Faith and Practices by Way of Internalization of Prosocial Values." *Journal of Adult Development* 19(2):66–78.

Barry, Chloe Y. H. and Morris A. Okun. 2011. "Application of Investment Theory to Predicting Maintenance of the Intent to Stay among Freshmen." *Journal of College Student Retention* 13(1):87–107.

Barsade, Sigal G., Andrew J. Ward, Jean D.F. Turner, and Jeffrey A. Sonnenfeld. 2000. "To Your Heart's Content: A Model of Affective Diversity in Top Management Teams." *Administrative Science Quarterly* 45(4):802–836.

Bar-Tal, Daniel and Eran Halperin. 2013. "The Psychology of Intractable Conflicts: Eruption, Escalation, and Peacemaking." Pp. 923–956 in *The Oxford Handbook of Political Psychology*, edited by Leone Huddy, David O. Sears and Jack S. Levy. New York: Oxford University Press.

Bartle, Elizabeth E., Graciela Couchonnal Edward R. Canda, and Martha D. Staker. 2002. "Empowerment as a Dynamically Developing Concept for Practice: Lessons Learned from Organizational Ethnography." *Social Work* 47(1):32–43.

Bartos, Otomar J., and Paul. Wehr. 2002. *Using Conflict Theory*. Cambridge, UK: Cambridge University Press.

Bartusch, Dawn Jeglum, and Ross L. Matsueda. 1996. "Gender, Reflected Appraisals, and Labeling: A Cross-group Test of an Interactionist Theory of Delinquency." *Social Forces* 75(1):145–177.

Bartusevicius, Henrikas. 2021. "Physical Strength Predicts Political Violence." *Evolution & Human Behavior* 42(5):423–30.

Basabe, Nekane, Dario Paez, Jose Valencia, Jose Luis Gonzalez, Bernard Rime, and Ed Diener. 2002. "Cultural Dimensions, Socioeconomic Development, Climate, and Emotional Hedonic Level." *Cognition & Emotion* 16(1):103–125.

Bask, Miia. 2005. "Welfare Problems and Social Exclusion among Immigrants in Sweden." *European Sociological Review* 21(1):73–89.

Baskin, Thomas W., Stephen M. Quintana, and Christopher D. Slaten. 2014. "Family Belongingness, Gang Friendships, and Psychological Distress in Adolescent Achievement." *Journal of Counseling & Development* 92(4):398–405.

Bass, David M., Linda S. Noelker, and Catherine A. McCarthy. 1999. "The Influence of Formal and Informal Helpers or Primary Caregivers" Perceptions of Quality of Care." *Journal of Applied Gerontology* 18(2):177–200.

Bassani, Cherylynn. 2007. "Five Dimensions of Social Capital Theory as They Pertain to Youth Studies." *Journal of Youth Studies* 10(1):17–34.

Basseches, Michael. 2003. "Adult Development and the Practice of Psychotherapy." Pp. 533–563 in *Handbook of Adult Development*, edited by Jack Demick and Carrie Andreoletti. New York: Kluwer Academic.

Bassett, Hideko Hamada, Susanne A. Denham, Nicole B. Fettig, Timothy W. Curby, Mandana Mohtasham and Nila Austin. 2017. "Temperament in the Classroom: Children Low in Surgency Are More Sensitive to Teachers" Reactions to Emotions." *International Journal of Behavioral Development* 41(1):4–14.

Batalha, Luisa, and Katherine J. Reynolds. 2013. "Gender and Personality: Beyond Gender Stereotypes to Social Identity and the Dynamics of Social Change." Pp. 165–182 in *The SAGE Handbook of Gender and Psychology*, edited by Michelle K. Ryan and Myla R. Branscombe. London, UK: SAGE.

Batone, Paul T. 2017. "Leader Influences on Resilience and Adaptability in Organizations." Pp. 355–368 in *The Routledge International Handbook of Psychosocial Resilience*, edited by Updesh Kumar. Abingdon, UK: Routledge.

Batson, C. Daniel, and Tecia Moran. 1999. "Empathy-induced Altruism in a Prisoner's Dilemma." *European Journal of Social Psychology* 29:909–924.

Batson, C. Daniel, Judy G. Batson, R. Matthew Todd, Beverly H. Brumett, Laura L. Shaw, and Carlo M.R. Aldeguer. 1995. "Empathy and the Collective Good: Caring for One of the Others in a Social Dilemma." *Journal of Personality & Social Psychology* 68(4):619–631.

Battersby, Annabel, and Lisa Phillips. 2016. "In the End It All Makes Sense Meaning in Life at Either End of the Adult Lifespan." *International Journal of Aging & Human Development* 83(2):184–204. \

Baucom, Brian R., and David C. Atkins. 2013. "Understanding Marital Distress: Polarization Processes." Pp. 145–166 in *Handbook of Family Theories: A Content-based Approach*, edited by Mark A. Fine and Frank D. Fincham. New York: Routledge.

Baucom, Donald A., Jennifer M. Belus, Susan Stanton, and Norman B. Epstein. 2018. "Treating Relationship Distress." Pp. 538–549 in *The Cambridge Handbook of Personal Relationships*, edited by Anita L. Vangelisti and Daniel Perlman. Cambridge, UK: Cambridge University Press.

Bauer, Jack J., Dan P. McAdams, and April R. Sakaeda. 2005. "Interpreting the Good Life: Growth Memories in the Lives of Mature, Happy People." *Journal of Personality & Social Psychology* 88(1):203–217.

Bauer, Michal, Alessandra Cassar, Julie Chytilová, and Joseph Henrich. 2014. "War's Enduring Effects on the Development of Egalitarian Motivations and in-Group Biases." *Psychological Science* 25(1):47–57.

Bauman, Zygmunt. 2001. "The Great War of Recognition." *Theory, Culture & Society* 18(2–3):137–150.
Baumeister, Roy F., and Mark R. Leary. 1995. "The Need to Belong: Desire for Interpersonal Attachments as a Fundamental Human Motivation." *Psychological Bulletin* 117(3):497–529.
Baumeister, Roy F., Kathleen D. Vohs, and Dianne M. Tice. 2007. "The Strength Model of Self-Control." *Current Directions in Psychological Science* 16(6):351–355.
Baumeister, Roy F., Kathleen D. Vohs, Jennifer L. Aaker, and Emily N. Garbinsky. 2013. "Some Key Differences between a Happy Life and a Meaningful Life." *Journal of Positive Psychology* 8(6):505–516.
Baumeister, Roy F., Laura Smart, and Joseph M. Boden. 1996. "Relation of Threatened Egotism to Violence and Aggression: The Dark Side of High Self-esteem." *Psychological Review* 103(1):5–33.
Bavetta, Sebastiano, Pietro Navarra, and Dario Maimone. 2014. *Freedom and the Pursuit of Happiness: An Economic and Political Perspective*. New York, NY: Cambridge University Press.
Bawin-Legros, Bernadette. 2001. "Families in Europe: A Private and Political Stake: Intimacy and Solidarity." *Current Sociology* 49(5):49–65.
Baxter Magolda, Marcia B. 2004. "Evolution of a Constructivist Conceptualization of Epistemological Reflection." *Educational Psychologist* 39(1):31–42.
Baxter, Leslie A., and Bryan Asbury. 2015. "Critical Approaches to Interpersonal Communication." Pp. 189–201 in *Engaging Theories in Interpersonal Communication: Multiple Perspectives*, edited by Dawn O. Braithwaite and Paul Schrodt. Thousand Oaks, CA: SAGE.
Baxter, Leslie A., and Carma L. Bylund. 2004. "Social Influence in Close Relationships." Pp. 317–336 in *Perspectives and Persuasion, Social Influence, and Compliance Gaining*, edited by John S. Seiter and Robert H. Gass. Boston, MA: Pearson.
Baylis, Nick. 2005. "Relationship with Reality and Its Role in the Well-being of Young Adults." Pp. 241–272 in *The Science of Well-being*, edited by Felica A. Huppert, Nick Baylis and Barry Keverne. Oxford, UK: Oxford University Press.
Bayram, A. Burcu. 2016. "Values and Prosocial Behaviour in the Global Context: Why Values Predict Public Support for Foreign Development Assistance to Developing Countries." *Journal of Human Values* 22(2):93–106.
Bazargan, Mohsen, Shahrzad Bazargan, and Richard S. Baker. 1998. "Emergency Department Utilization, Hospital Admissions, and Physician Visits among Elderly African American Persons." *Gerontologist* 38(1):25–36.
Beasley, Margaret, Ted Thompson, and John Davidson. 2003. "Resilience Response to Life Stress: The Effects of Coping Style and Cognitive Hardiness." *Personality & Individual Differences* 34:77–95.
Beaudoin, Christopher E. 2009. "Bonding and Bridging Neighborliness: An Individual-Level Study in the Context of Health." *Social Science & Medicine* 68(12):2129–2136.
Beaudoin, Christopher, and Esther Thorson. 2006. "The Social Capital of Blacks and Whites: Differing Effects of the Mass Media in the United States." *Human Communication Research* 32:157–177.
Bebber, Charles C. 1995. "Thematic Images Linking American Militancy Strikes of the 1980s and Rising U.S. Civil Violence." *Metaphor & Symbolic Activity* 10(2):139–154.
Becchetta, Leonardo. 2010. "The Money happiness Relationships in Transition Countries: Evidence from Albania." *Transition Studies Review* 17:39–62.
Beck, Ulrich, and Elisabeth Beck-Gernsheim. 2002. Individualization: Institutionalized Individualism and Its Social and Political Consequences. London: Sage.
Beck, Ulrich. 1999. *World Risk Society*. Cambridge, UK: Polity.
Beck, Ulrich. 2006. "Living in the World Risk Society." *Economy & Society* 31(3):329–345.
Becker, Jan U., and Michel Clement. 2006. "Dynamics of Illegal Participation in Peer-to-peer Networks: Why Do People Illegally Share Media Files?" *Journal of Media Economics* 19(1):7–32.

Becker, Thomas E., Robert S. Billings, Daniel M. Eveleth, and Nicole W. Gilbert. 1997. "Validity of Scores on Three Attachment Style Scales: Exploratory and Confirmatory Evidence." *Educational & Psychological Measurement* 57(3):477–493.

Bednall, Timothy C., Liliana L. Boveb, Ali Cheethamb, and Andrea L. Murray. 2013. "A Systematic Review and Meta-Analysis of Antecedents of Blood Donation Behavior and Intentions." *Social Science & Medicine* 96(13):86–94.

Beesley, Lisa G., and Laurence Chalip. 2011. "Seeing and Not Seeking to Leverage Mega-sport Events in Non-host Destinations: The Case of Shanghai and the Beijing Olympics." *Journal of Sport & Tourism* 16(4):323–344.

Beetham, David. 1985. *Max Weber and the Theory of Modern Politics*. Cambridge: Polity Press.

Behler, Rachel, Rachel Donnelly, and Debra Umberson. 2019. "Psychological Distress Transmission in Same-Sex and Different-Sex Marriages." *Journal of Health & Social Behavior* 60(1):18–35.

Behr, Rafael. 2010. "Anti-Consumerism." *Public Policy Research* 17(3):123–29.

Bekker, Marrie H.J., Judit Arends-Toth, and Marcel A. Croon. 2011. "Autonomy-Connectedness, Acculturation, and Independence-Interdependence among Various Cultural Groups in a Multicultural Society." *International Journal of Intercultural Relations* 35(3):368–376.

Bekkers, Rene, Beate Volker, Martin van der Gaag, and Henk Flap. 2008. "Social Networks of Participants in Voluntary Associations." Pp. 185–205 in *Social Capital: An International Research Program*, edited by Nan Lin and Bonnie H. Erickson. Oxford, UK: Oxford University Press.

Belanger, Jocelyn J., Birga M. Schumpe, Noemie Nociti, Manuel Moyano, Stephane Dandeneau, Pier-Eric Chamberland, and Robert J. Vallerand. 2019. "Passion and Moral Disengagement: Different Pathways to Political Activism." *Journal of Personality* 87(6):1234–1249.

Bell, Duncan. 2010. "Political Realism and the Limits of Ethics." Pp. 93–110 in *Ethics and World Politics*, edited by Duncan Bell. Oxford, UK: Oxford University Press. (JA89.E8235)

Bellah, Robert N., Richard Madson, William M. Sullivan, Ann Swidler, and Steven M. Tipton. 1985. *Habit of the Heart: Individualism and Commitment in American Life*. New York: Harper & Row.

Bellemare, Charles and Sabine Kroger. 2007. "On Representative Social Capital." *European Economic Review* 51(1):183–202.

Bellingtier, Jennifer A., Marcus Mund, and Cornelia Wrzus. 2022. "The Role of Extraversion and Neuroticism for Experiencing Stress during the Third Wave of the Covid-19 Pandemic." *Current Psychology* 42(14):12202–12.

Benda, Brent B. 2002. "A Test of Three Competing Theoretical Models of Delinquency Using Structural Equation Modeling." *Journal of Social Service Research* 29(2):55–91.

Bendixsen, Synnøve. 2018. "Differentiation of Rights in the Norwegian Welfare State: Hierarchies of Belonging and Humanitarian Exceptionalism." *Social Inclusion* 6(3):162–71.

Benitez-Silva, Hugo, Richard Disney, and Sergi Jimenez-Martin. 2010. "Disability, Capacity for Work and the Business Cycle: An International Perspective." *Economic Policy* 25(63):483–56.

Benjamins, Baureen Reindl, and Carolyn Brown. 2004. "Religion and Preventive Health Care Utilization among the Elderly." *Social Science & Medicine* 58:109–118.

Bennett, John L., and Francine Campone. 2017. "Coaching and Theories of Learning." Pp. 162–120 in *The SAGE Handbook of Coaching*, edited by Tatiana Bachkirova, Gordon Spence, and David Drake. London, UK: SAGE.

Bennett, Pauleen C., Joshua L. Trigg, Tim Godber, and Cynthia Brown. 2015. "An Experience Sampling Approach to Investigating Associations between Pet Presence and Indicators of Psychological Wellbeing and Mood in Older Australians." *Anthrozoos* 28(3):403–420.

Bennett, W. Lance, Alexandra Segerberg & Shawn Walker. 2014. "Organization in the Crowd: Peer Production In Large-Scale Networked Protests." *Information, Communication & Society* 17(2):232–260.

Bennett, W. Lance, and Alexandra Segerberg. 2012. "The Logic of Connective Action." *Information, Communication & Society* 15(5):739–768.

Benson, D.E., and Christian Ritter. 1990. "Belief in a Just World, Job Loss, and Depression." *Sociological Focus* 23(1):49–61.

Benson, Michael L., and Sally S. Simpson. 2018. *White-collar Crime: An Opportunity Perspective.* New York: NY: Routledge.

Benson, Peter L., Peter C. Scales, and Amy K. Syvertsen. 2011. "The Contribution of the Developmental Assets Framework to Positive Youth Development Theory and Practice." *Advances in Child Development & Behavior* 197–230.

Benton, Richard A. 2016. "Uniters or Dividers? Voluntary Organizations and Social Capital Acquisition." *Social Networks* 44:209–18.

Ben-Zur, Hasida. 2002. "Coping, Affect and Aging: The Roles of Mastery and Self-Esteem." *Personality & Individual Differences* 32(2):357–372.

Bereczkei, Tamas, Bela Birkas, and Zsuzsanna Kerekes. 2010. "Altruism Towards Strangers in Need: Costly Signaling in an Industrial Society." *Evolution & Human Behavior* 31(2):95–103.

Berends, Mark, David W. Grissmer, Sheila Nataraj Kirby, and Stephanie Williamson. 1999. "The Changing American Family and Student Achievement Trends." *Research in Sociology of Education & Socialization* 12:67–101.

Berger, Charles R. 2015. "Planning Theory of Communication: Goal Attainment through Communicative Action." Pp. 89–102 in *Engaging Theories in Interpersonal Communication: Multiple Perspectives*, edited by Dawn O. Braithwaite and Paul Schrodt. Thousand Oaks, CA: SAGE.

Berger, Philipp, Florian Bitsch, Henrike Bröhl, and Irina Falkenberg. 2018. "Play and Playfulness in Psychiatry: A Selective Review." *International Journal of Play* 7(2):210–25.

Berger-Schmitt, Reina. 2002. "Considering Social Cohesion in Quality of Life Assessments: Concept and Measurement." *Social Indicators Research* 58:403–428.

Bergin, Christi. 2014. "Educating Students to Be Prosocial at School." Pp. 277–301 in *Prosocial Development: A Multidimensional Approach*, edited by Laura M. Padilla-Walker and Gustavo Carlo. New York, NY: Oxford University Press.

Berkowitz, Leonard. 2012. "A Cognitive-Association Theory of Aggression." Pp. 99–117 in *Handbook of Theories of Social Psychology* (vol. 2), edited by Paul A.M. Van Lange, Arie W. Kruglanski and E. Tory Higgins. London, CA: SAGE.

Berkowitz, Marvin W., Stephen A. Sherblom, Melinda C. Bier, and Victor Battistich. 2006. "Educating for Positive Youth Development." Pp. 683–701 in *Handbook of Moral Development*, edited by Melanie Killen and Judith S. Smetana. Mahwah, NJ: Lawrence Erlbaum.

Bernabe-Valero, Gloria, José Salvador Blasco-Magraner, Remedios Aguilar-Moya, and Carmen Moret-Tatay. 2021. "The Moderation Effects of Comparative Thinking between Gratitude and Negative Affect During the Covid-19 Outbreak." *Frontiers in Psychology* 12:644323.

Bernard, Michael E. 1997. You Can Do It: How to Boost Your Child's Achievement in School. New York: Warner.

Bernard, Nathalie et al. 2017. "Executive Function, Social Emotional Learning, and Social Competence in School-aged Boys with Autism Spectrum Disorder." *Canadian Journal of Social Psychology* 32(3–4):265–281.

Bernardon, Stephanie, Kimberley A. Babb, Julie Hakim-Larson, Marcia Gragg 2011. "Loneliness, Attachment, and the Perception and Use of Social Support in University Students." *Canadian Journal of Behavioural Science* 43(1):40–51.

Berndt, Thomas J., and Keunho Keefe. 1996. "Friends" Influence on School Adjustment: A Motivational Analysis." Pp. 248–278 in Social Motivation. *Understanding Children's School Adjustment*, edited by Jeana Juvonen, and Kathryn R. Wentzel. Cambridge. Cambridge.

Bernstein, Mary. 2005. "Identity Politics." *Annual Review of Sociology* 31:47–74.

Berry, Daniel R., Jonathan P. Hoerr, Selena Cesko, Amir Alayoubi, Kevin Carpio, Hannah Zirzow, Wesley Walters, Genny Scram, Katie Rodriguez, and Vanessa Beaver. 2020. "Does Mindfulness Training without Explicit Ethics Based Instruction Promote Prosocial Behaviors? A Meta-Analysis." *Personality & Social Psychology Bulletin* 46(8):1247–1269.

Besser, Avi, and Beatriz Priel. 2008. "Attachment, Depression and Fear of Feath in Older Adults: The Roles of Neediness and Perceived Availability of Social Support." *Personality & Individual Differences* 44:1711–1725.

Betz, Diana E., Laura R. Ramsey, and Denise Sekaquaptewa. 2013. "Gender Stereotype Threat among Women and Girls." Pp. 428–449 in *The SAGE Handbook of Gender and Psychology*, edited by Michelle K. Ryan and Myla R. Branscombe. London, UK: SAGE.

Beutler, I. F., and Clinton G. Gudmunson. 2012. "New Adolescent Money Attitude Scales: Entitlement and Conscientiousness." *Journal of Financial Counseling & Planning* 23(2):18–31.

Beyer, Stefanie. 2006. "The Green Olympic Movement: Beijing 2008." *Chinese Journal of International Law* 5(2):423–440.

Bezner, Janet R., Katherine A. Franklin, Lisa K. Lloyd. and Sylvia H. Crixell. 2020. "Effect of Group Health Behaviour Change Coaching on Psychosocial Constructs Associated with Physical Activity among University Employees." *International Journal of Sport & Exercise Psychology* 18(1):93–107.

Bhochhibhoya, Shristi, Sarah B. Maness, Marshall Cheney, and Daniel Larson. 2021. "Risk Factors for Sexual Violence among College Students in Dating Relationships: An Ecological Approach." *Journal of Interpersonal Violence* 36(15–16):7722–46

Biagas, David E., Jr., and Alison J. Bianchi. 2016. "The Latin Americanization Thesis: An Expectation States Approach." *Social Forces* 94(3):1335–1358.

Biddle, Stuart. Nanette Mutrie, and Trish Gorely. 2015. *Psychology of Physical Activity: Determinants, Well-Being and Interventions*. Abingdon, UK: Routledge.

Biddulph, Sarah, and Chuanyu Xie. 2008. "Regulating Drug Dependency in China: The 2008 PRC Drug Prohibition Law." *British Journal of Criminology* 51(6):978–996.

Bidmon, Sonja. 2017. "How Does Attachment Style Influence the Brand Attachment: Brand Trust and Brand Loyalty Chain in Adolescents?" *International Journal of Advertising* 36(1):164–189.

Bierhoff, Hans-Werner. 2002. *Prosocial Behavior*. Hove, UK; Psychology

Biggart, Laura, Emma Ward, Laura Cook, and Gillian Schofield. 2017. "The Team as a Secure Base: Promoting Resilience and Competence in Child and Family Social Work." *Children & Youth Services Review* 83:119–30.

Biglan, Anthony, and Ronald Prinz. 2017. "Progress in Nurturing Human Well-Being." *Clinical Child & Family Psychology Review* 20(1):1–2.

Biglan, Anthony. 2018. "The Ultimate Goal of Prevention and the Larger Context for Translation." *Prevention Science* 19(3):328–336.

Bimrose, Jenny. 2012. "Gender." Pp. 24–29 in *The SAGE Handbook of Counselling and Psychotherapy*, edited by Colin Feltham and Ian Horton. London: SAGE

Binder, Jens F., Sam G.B. Roberts, Alistair G. Sutcliffe. 2012. "Closeness, Loneliness, Support: Core Ties and Significant Ties in Personal Communication." *Social Networks* 34:206–214.

Biron, Michal, and Peter Samberger. 2010. "The Impact of Structural Empowerment on Individual Well-being and Performance: Taking Agent Performances, Self-efficacy and Operational Constraints into Account." *Human Relations* 63(2):163–191.

Bish, Alison, and Susan Michie. 2010. "Demographic and Attitudinal Determinants of Protective Behaviors during Pandemic: A Review." *British Journal of Health Psychology* 15:797–824.

Bishop, Brian J., Sheridan J. Coakes, and Pamela N. D"Rozario. 2002. "Sense of Community in Rural Communities: A Mixed Methodological Approach." Pp. 271–290 in *Psychological Sense of Community: Research, Applications and Implications*, edited by Adrian T. Fisher, Christopher C. Sonn and Brian J. Bishop. New York: Kluwer Academic.

Bishop, Michael A. 2015. The Good Life: Unifying the Philosophy and Psychology of Well-being. New York: Oxford University Press.

Bissell-Havran, Joanna M., and Eric Loken. 2009. "The Role of Friends in Early Adolescents? Academic Self-competence and Intrinsic Value for Math and English." *Journal of Youth and Adolescence* 38(1):41–50.

Biswas-Diener, Robert, and Ed Diener. 2001. "Making the Best of a Bad Situation: Satisfaction in the Slums of Calcutta." *Social Indicators Research* 55:329–352.

Bjarnason, Thoroddur. 2009. "Anomie among European Adolescents: Conceptual and Empirical Clarification of a Multilevel Sociological Concept." *Sociological Forum* 24(1):135–161.

Bjarnegard, Elin, Karen Brounéus, and Erik Melander. 2019. "Violent Boyhoods, Masculine Honor Ideology, and Political Violence: Survey Findings from Thailand." *Journal of Interpersonal Violence* 36(15–16):7136–60.

Bjornberg, Ulla, and Hans Ekbrand. 2008. "Financial and Practical Kin Support in Sweden: Normative Guidelines and Practice." *Journal of Comparative Family Studies* 39(1):73–95.

Bjornberg, Ulla, and Mia Latta. 2007. "The Roles of the Family and the Welfare State: The Relationship between Public and Private Financial Support in Sweden." *Current Sociology* 55(3):415–445.

Bjornskov, Christian, Axel Dreher, Justina A.V. Fiskher, Jan Schnellenbach, and Kai Gehring. 2013. "Inequality and Happiness: When Perceived Social Mobility and Economic Reality Do Not Match." *Journal of Economic Behavior & Organization* 91:75–92.

Blackshaw, Tony. 2017. *Re-imaging Leisure Studies.* Abingdon, UK: Routledge.

Blank, Thomas. 2003. "Determinants of National Identity in East and West Germany: An Empirical Comparison of Theories on The Significance of Authoritarianism, Anomie, and General Self-Esteem." *Political Psychology* 24(2 SPEC.):259–288.

Bleidorn, Wiebke, Theo A. Klimstra, Jaap J. A. Denissen, Peter J. Rentfrow, Jeff Potter, and Samuel D. Gosling. 2013. "Personality Maturation around the World." *Psychological Science* 24(12):2530–40.

Blieszner, Rosemary. 1993. "Resource Exchange in the Social Networks of Elderly Women." Pp. 67–79 in *Resource Theory: Explorations and Applications*, edited by Uriel G. Foa, John Converse, Jr., Kjell Y. T¡±rnblom, and Edna B. Foa. San Diego, CA: Academic Press.

Blokker, Paul. 2018. "Democracy and Democratization: Theory and Research." Pp. 622–636 in *The SAGE Handbook of Political Sociology*, edited by William Outhwaite and Stephen Turner. London, UK: SAGE.

Bloom, John R., Pat Fobair, David Spiegel, Rick S. Cox, Anna Varghese, and Richard Hoppe. 1991. "Social Supports and the Social Well-being of Cancer Survivors." *Advances in Medical Sociology* 2:95–114.

Blouin, David D. 2012. "Understanding Relations between People and Their Pets." *Sociology Compass* 6(11):856–869.

Bluckert., Peter. 2018. "The Gestalt Approach to Coaching." Pp. 66–80 in *The Complete Handbook of Coaching*, edited by Elaine Cox, Tatiana Bachkirova, and David Clutterbuck. London, UK: SAGE.

Blum, Diane, Elizabeth Clark, Paul Jacobsen, Jimmie Holland, Mary Jo Monahan, and Patricia Doykos Duquette. 2006. "Building Community-based Short-term Psychosocial Counseling Capacity for Cancer Patients and Their Families: The Individual Cancer Assistance Network (ICAN) Model." *Social Work in Health Care* 43(4):71–83.

Boccio, Cashen M., Michelle E. Protas, Dylan B. Jackson, and Wanda E. Leal. 2023. "Virtual Socializing and Nonlinear Effects on Victimization." *Journal of Interpersonal Violence* 38(23–24):12113–34.

Bock, Dora, Veronica Thomas, Jeremy Wolter, Christina Saenger, and Pei Xu. 2021. "An Extended Reciprocity Cycle of Gratitude: How Gratitude Strengthens Existing and Initiates New Customer Relationships." *Psychology & Marketing* 38(3):564–76.

Boda, Zsolt and Gergő Medve-Balint. 2017. "How Perceptions and Personal Contact Matter: The Individual Level Determinants of Trust in Police in Hungary." *Policing & Society* 27(7):732–49.

Boden, Matthew Tyler, Madhr Kulkarni, Ashley Shurick, Marcel O. Bonn-Miller, and James J. Gross. 2014. "Responding to Trauma and Loss: An Emotion Regulation Perspective." Pp. 86–99 in *The Resilience Handbook: Approaches to Stress and Trauman*, edited by Martha Kent, Mary C. Davis and John W. Reich. New York: NY: Routledge.

Bodie, Graham D., and Erina L. MacGeorge. 2015. "Supportive Communication Theories: Dual-process Theory of Supportive Messy Outcomes and Advice Response Theory." Pp. 129–141 in *Engaging Theories in Interpersonal Communication: Multiple Perspectives*, edited by Dawn O. Braithwaite and Paul Schrodt. Thousand Oaks, CA: SAGE.

Boehnke, Klaus, and Becky Wong. 2011. "Adolescent Political Activism and Long-Term Happiness: A 21-Year Longitudinal Study on the Development of Micro- and Macrosocial Worries." *Personality & Social Psychology Bulletin* 37(3):435–47.

Boerner, Kathrin, Camille B. Wortman, and George A. Bonanno. 2005. "Resilient or at Risk? A 4-year Study of Older Adults Who Initially Showed High or Low Distress Following Conjugal Loss." *Journal of Gerontology: Psychological Sciences* 66B(2):P67–P73.

Bogg, Tim, Michelle W. Voss, Dustin Wood, and Brent W. Roberts. 2008. "A Hierarchical Investigation of Personality and Behavior: Examining Neo-Socioanalytic Models of Health-Related Outcomes." *Journal of Research in Personality* 42(1):183–207.

Bogg, Tim. 2008. "Conscientiousness, the Transtheoretical Model of Change, and Exercise: A Neo-Socioanalytic Integration of Trait and Social-Cognitive Frameworks in the Prediction of Behavior." *Journal of Personality* 76(4):775–802.

Bohlmeijer, E., M. Valenkamp, G. Westerhof, F. Smit, and P. Cuijpers. 2005. "Creative Reminiscence as an Early Intervention for Depression: Results of A Pilot Project." *Aging & Mental Health* 9(4):302–304.

Bolland, John M., and Debra Moehle McCallum. 2002. "Neighboring and Community Mobilization in High-poverty Inner City Neighborhoods." *Urban Affairs Review* 38(1):42–69.

Bollmann, Grégoire, Franciska Krings, Christian Maggiori, and Jérôme Rossier. 2015. "Differential Associations of Personal and General Just-World Beliefs with the Five-Factor and the Hexaco Models of Personality. " *Personality & Individual Differences* 87:312–19.

Bonaiuto, Marino, Antonio Aiello, Marco Perugini, Mirilia Bonnes, and Anna Parla Ercolani. 1999. "Multidimensional Perception of Residential Environment Quality and Neighbourhood Attachment in the Urban Environment." *Journal of Environmental Psychology* 19:331–352.

Bonaiuto, Marino, Elena Bilotta, Mirilia Bonnes, Manuela Ceccarelli, Helga Martorella, and Giuseppe Carrus. 2008. "Local Identity and the Role of Individual Differences in the Use of Natural Resources: The Case of Water Consumption." *Journal of Applied Social Psychology* 38(4):947–67.

Bond, Michael Harris, and Virginia S.Y. Kwan. 2000. "Decomposing a Sense of Superiority: The Differential Social Impact of Self-regard and Regard for Others." *Journal of Research in Personality* 34:537–553.

Bond, Michael Harris, and Vivian Miu-Chi Lun. 2014. "Citizen-making: The Role of National Goals for Socializing Children." *Social Science Research* 44:75–85.

Bonini, Astra N. 2008. "Cross-national Variation in Individual Life Satisfaction: Effects of National Wealth, Human Development, and Environmental Conditions." *Social Indicators Research* 87:223–236 \105–40.

Boniwell, Ilona, and Carol Kauffman. 2018. "The Positive Psychology Approach to Coaching." Pp. 158–166 in *The Complete Handbook of Coaching*, edited by Elaine Cox, Tatiana Bachkirova, and David Clutterbuck. London, UK: SAGE.

Bonk, Edyta. 2016. "The Influence of Activeness and Independence on the Quality of Life of Senior Citizens." *Polish Psychological Bulletin* 47(3):338–45.

Bonnard, Claire. 2020. "What Employability for Higher Education Students?" *Journal of Education & Work* 33(5–6):425–45.

Booker, Jordan A., and Julie C. Dunsmore. 2017. "Affective Social Competence in Adolescence: Current Findings and Future Directions." *Social Development* 26(1):3–20.

Bookwala, Jamila. 2014. "Spouse Health Status, Depressed Affect, and Resilience in Mid and Late Life: A Longitudinal Study." *Developmental Psychology* 50(4):1241–1249.

Boone, Erin M., and Bonnie J. Leadbeater. 2006. "Game on: Diminishing Risks for Depressive Symptoms in Early Adolescence through Positive Involvement in Team Spirits." *Journal of Research on Adolescence* 16(1):79–90.

Boorman, John, Eric Morris, and Joe Oliver. 2012. "Acceptance and Commitment Therapy." Pp. 281–285 in *The SAGE Handbook of Counselling and Psychotherapy*, edited by Colin Feltham and Ian Horton. London: SAGE.

Booth, Alan. 2003. *Teaching History at University: Enhancing Learning and Understanding*. London, UK: Routledge.

Borbath, Endre, Sophia Hunger, Swen Hutter and Ioana-Elena Oana. 2021. "Civic and Political Engagement during the Multifaceted COVID-19 Crisis." *Swiss Political Science Review* 27(2):311–24.

Bordia, Prashant, Elizabeth Hunt, Neil Paulsen, Dennis Tourish, and Nicholas DiFonzo. 2004. "Uncertainty during Organizational Change: Is It all about Control?" *European Journal of Work & Organizational Psychology* 13(3):345–365.

Borgonovi, Francesca. 2008. "Doing Well by Doing Good: The Relationships between Formal Volunteering and Self-reported Health and Happiness." *Social Science & Medicine* 66:2321–2334.

Bornstein, Robert F. 2006. "the Complex Relationship between Dependency and Domestic Violence: Converging Psychological Factors and Social Forces." *American Psychologist* 62(7):709–711.

Bornstein, Robert F. 2009. "Interpersonal Dependency." Pp. 82–92 in *Handbook of Individual Differences in Social Behavior*, edited by Mark R. Leary and Rick H. Hoyle. New York, NY: Guilford.

Bornstein, Robert F. 2012. "Illuminating a Neglected Clinical Issue: Societal Costs of Interpersonal Dependency and Dependent Personality Disorder." *Journal of Clinical Psychology* 68(7):766–81.

Borsenberger, Monique, Charles Fleury, and Paul Dickes. 2016. "Welfare Regimes and Social Cohesion Regimes: Do They Express the Same Values?" *European Societies* 18(3):221–44.

Bosacki, Sandra, Valentina Sitnik, Keeley Dutcher, and Victoria Talwar. 2018. "Gratitude, Social Cognition, and Well Being in Emerging Adolescents." *Journal of Genetic Psychology* 179(5):256–269.

Botoin, Gilbert J., and Kenneth W. Griffin. 2003. "Drug Abuse Prevention Curricula in Schools." Pp. 45–74 in *Handbook of Drug Abuse Prevention: Theory, Science, and Practice*, edited by Zili Sloboda and William J. Bukoski. New York: Kluwer Academic.

Botti, Fabrizio, and Carlo D'Ippoliti. 2014. "Don't Ask, Don't Tell (That You're Poor). Sexual Orientation and Social Exclusion in Italy." *Journal of Behavioral & Experimental Economics* 49:8–25.

Bottrell, Dorothy. 2009. "Dealing with Disadvantage: Resilience and the Social Capital of Young People's Networks." *Youth & Society* 40(4):476–501.

Boudreaux, Michael J. and Daniel J. Ozer. 2013. "Goal Conflict, Goal Striving, and Psychological Well-Being." *Motivation & Emotion* 37(3):433–43.

Bouffard, Jeffrey A., and Stephen K. Rice. 2011. "The Influence of the Social Bond on Self-control at the Moment of Decision: Testing Hirschi's Redefinition of Self-control." *American Journal of Criminal Justice* 36(2):138–157.

Boulianne, Shelley, Chris Tenove, and Jordan Buffie. 2022. "Complicating the Resilience Model: A Four Country Study about Misinformation." *Media & Communication* 10(3):169–82.

Boulton, Mary, Markeda Boudioni, Jean Mossman, Clare Moynihan, Geraldine Leyon, and Amanda Ramirez. 2001. "Dividing the Desolation: Clients View on the Benefits of a Cancer Counselling Service." *Psycho-Oncology* 10:124–136.

Boulton, Michael J. and Peter J. R. Macaulay. 2022. "Parenting About Challenges and Adolescents" Social Anxiety, Disrupted Classroom Concentration, and Resilience Knowledge: The Mediating Role of Authentic Self-Esteem." *Families Systems & Health* 40(3).332–42.

Bouton, Mark E., Susan Mineka, and David H. Barlow. 2001. "A Modern Learning Theory Perspective on the Etiology of Panic Disorder." *Psychological Review* 108(1):4–32.

Bowen, Gary L., James A. Martin, and Jay A. Mancini. 2013. "The Resilience of Military Families: Theoretical Perspectives." Pp. 417–436 in *Handbook of Family Theories: A Content-based Approach*, edited by Mark A. Fine and Frank D. Fincham. New York: Routledge.

Bowers, Clint, Christine Kreutzer, Janis Cannon-Bowers, and Jerry Lamb. 2017. "Team Resilience as a Second-Order Emergent State: A Theoretical Model and Research Directions." *Frontiers in Psychology* 8:1360.

Bowes, Shauna M. and Arber Tasimi. 2022. "Clarifying the Relations between Intellectual Humility and Pseudoscience Beliefs, Conspiratorial Ideation, and Susceptibility to Fake News." *Journal of Research in Personality* 98:104220.

Bowes, Shauna M., Thomas H. Costello, Caroline Lee, Stacey McElroy-Heltzel, Don E. Davis, and Scott O. Lilienfeld. 2022. "Stepping Outside the Echo Chamber: Is Intellectual Humility Associated with Less Political Myside Bias?" *Personality & Social Psychology Bulletin* 48(1):150–64.

Bowman, Nicholas, A., Julie J. Park, and Nida Denson. 2015. "Student Involvement in Ethnic Student Organizations: Examining Civic Outcomes 6 Years after Graduation." *Research in Higher Education* 56(2):127–45.

Boyce, Christopher J., Alex M. Wood, James Banks, Andrew E. Clark, and Gordon D. A. Brown. 2013. "Money, Well-Being, and Loss Aversion: Does an Income Loss Have a Greater Effect on Well-Being than an Equivalent Income Gain?" *Psychological Science* 24(12):2557–2562.

Boyd, Michael P., and Zenong Yin. 1996. "Cognitive-affective Sources of Sport Enjoyment in Adolescent Sport." *Adolescence* 31(22):383–395.

Boyer, Pascal and Pierre Lienard. 2006. "Why Ritualized Behavior? Precaution Systems and Action Parsing in Developmental, Pathological and Cultural Rituals." *Behavioral & Brain Sciences* 29(6):595–613.

Boyes, Mark E., Thea M. Carmody, Patrick J. F. Clarke, and Penelope A. Hasking. 2017. "Emotional Reactivity and Perseveration: Independent Dimensions of Trait Positive and Negative Affectivity and Differential Associations with Psychological Distress." *Personality & Individual Differences* 105:70–77.

Brackett, Marc A., Susan E. Rivers, and Sara Shiffman. 2006. "Relating Emotional Abilities to Social Functioning: A Comparison of Self-report and Performance Measures of Emotional Intelligence." *Journal of Personality & Social Psychology* 91(4):780–795.

Brackney, Barbara E., and Stuart A. Karabenick. 1995. "Psychopathology and Academic Performance: The Role of Motivation and Learning Strategies." *Journal of Counseling Psychology* 42(4):456–465.

Bradstreet, Tyler C., and Mike C. Parent. 2018. "To Be (Healthy) or Not to Be: Moderated Mediation of The Relationships between Masculine Norms, Future Orientation, Family Income, and College Men's Healthful Behaviors." *Psychology of Men & Masculinity* 19(4):500–511.

Brady, David. 2005. "The Welfare State and Relative Poverty in Rich Western Democracies, 1967–1997." *Social Forces* 83(4):1329–1364.

Braithwaite, Valerie, and Eliza Ahmed. 2005. "A Threat to Tax Morale: The Case of Australian Higher Education Policy." *Journal of Economic Psychology* 26:523–540.

Braman, Amie, and Alan J. Lambert. 2001. "Punishing Individuals for Their Infirmities: Effects of Personal Responsibility, Just-world Belief, and In-group/out-group Status." *Journal of Applied Social Psychology* 31(5):1096–1109.

Brancati, Dawn. 2016. *Democracy Protests: Origins, Features, and Significance*. Cambridge, UK: Cambridge University Press.

Brandenberger, Jay W. 2005. "College, Character, and Social Responsibility: Moral Learning through Experience." Pp. 305–334 in *Parenting the Custodial Grandchild: Implications for Clinical Practice*, edited by Bert Hayslip, Jr. and Patricia L. Kamlinski. New York: Springer.

Brandstadter, Jochen, and Bernhard Baltes-Gotz. 1990. "Personal Control over Development and Quality Life Perspectives in Adulthood." Pp. 197–223 in *Successful Aging: Perspectives from the Behavioral Sciences*, edited by Paul B. Baltes and Margret M. Baltes. Cambridge, UK: Cambridge University Press.

Branson, Sandy, Lisa Boss, Stanley Cron, and Duck-Hee Kang. 2016. "Examining Differences between Homebound Older Adult Pet Owners and Non-pet Owners in Depression, Systemic Inflammation, and Executive Function." *Anthrozoos* 29(2):323–334.

Bratter, Thomas Edward. 2003. "Confrontation Group Psychotherapy with Gifted, Dually Diagnosed, and Self-destruction Adolescents in a Residential Setting." *Group* 27(2/3):131–136.
Braun, Jerome. 2011. To Break Our Chains: Social Cohesiveness and Modern Democracy. Leiden, Netherlands: Brill.
Braun, Jerome. 2019. "The Present Relevance of Christopher Lasch's *The Culture of Narcissism* for Studying the Sociology of Morality." *American Sociologist* 50(3):414–429.
Braun-Lewensohn, Orna. 2016. "Sense of Coherence, Values, Youth Involvement, Civic Efficacy and Hope: Adolescents During Social Protest." *Social Indicators Research* 128(2):661–73.
Braunstein-Bercovitz, Hedva. 2013. "A Multidimensional Mediating Model of Perceived Resource Gain, Work-family Conflict Sources, and Burnout." *International Journal of Stress Management* 20(2):95–115.
Bray, Daniel. 2013. "Pragmatic Ethics and the Will to Believe in Cosmopolitanism." *International Theory* 5(3):446–476.
Brazier, David. 1995. Zen Therapy: Transcending the Sorrows of the Human Mind. New York: Wiley.
Breakwell, Glynis M. 2007. *The Psychology of Risk*. Cambridge, UK: Cambridge University Press.
Brendtro, Larry, and Scott Larson. 2004. "The Resilience Code: Finding Greatness in Youth." *Reclaiming Children & Youth* 12(4):194–200.
Brennan, Robert T. Rosalind Chart Barnett, and Karen C. Gareis. 2001. "When She Earns More than He Does: A Longitudinal Study of Dual-earner Couples." *Journal of Marriage & Family* 63:168–182.
Brensilver, Matthew, Sonya Negriff, Ferol E. Mennen, and Penelope K. Trickett. 2011. "Longitudinal Relations between Depressive Symptoms and Externalizing Behavior in Adolescence: Moderating Effects of Maltreatment Experience and Gender." *Journal of Clinical Child & Adolescent Psychology* 40(4):607–617.
Breso, Edgar, Wilmar B. Schaufeli, and Marisa Salanova. 2011. "Can a Self-efficacy-based Intervention Decrease Burnout, Increase Engagement, and Enhance Performance? A Quasi-experimental Study." *Higher Education* 61:339–355.
Breton, Margot. 2004. "An Empowerment Perspective." Pp. 58–75 in *Handbook of Social Work with Groups*, edited by Charles D. Garvin, Lorraine M. Gutierrez, and Maeda J. Galinsky. New York: Guilford.
Brewer, Gayle and Loren Abell. 2017. "Machiavellianism, Relationship Satisfaction, and Romantic Relationship Quality." *Europe's Journal of Psychology* 13(3):491–502.
Brewer, Marilynn B. 1996. "When Contact Is Not Enough: Social Identity and Intergroup Cooperation." *International Journal of Intercultural Relations* 20(4):291–303.
Brewer, Marilynn B. 1996. "When Contact Is Not Enough: Social Identity and Intergroup Cooperation." *International Journal of Intercultural Relations* 20(3/4):291–303.
Brewer, Marilynn B. 2012. "Optimal Distinctiveness Theory: Its History and Development." Pp. 81–98 in *Handbook of Theories of Social Psychology* (vol. 2), edited by Paul A.M. Van Lange, Arie W. Kruglanski and E. Tory Higgins. London, CA: SAGE.
Brewer, Marilynn B., and Kathleen P., Pierce. 2005. "Social Identity Complexity and Outgroup Tolerance." *Personality & Social Psychology Bulletin* 31(3):428–437.
Brezina, Timothy and Alex R. Piquero. 2007. "Moral Beliefs, Isolation from Peers, and Abstention from Delinquency." *Deviant Behavior* 28(5):433–65.
Bridoux, Denis, and Martin Weaver. 2000. "Neuro-linguistic Psychotherapy." Pp. 73 105 in *Therapeutic Perspectives on Working with Lesbian, Gay and Bisexual Clients*, edited by Dominic Davies and Charles Neal. Buckingham, UK: Open University Press.
Brigg, Morgan. 2018. "Humanitarian Symbolic Exchange: Extending Responsibility to Protect through Individual and Local Engagement." *Third World Quarterly* 39(5):838–53.
Bright, Ruth. 1992. "Music Therapy in the Management of Dementia." Pp. 162–180 in *Care-giving in Dementia: Research and Applications*, Vol. 1, edited by Gemma M.M. Jones and Bere M.L. Miesen. London: Routledge.

Brik, Tymofii, Andrew G. Livingstone, Maria Chayinska, and Evgeniya Bliznyuk. 2023. "How Feeling Understood Predicts Trust and Willingness to Forgive in the Midst of Violent Intergroup Conflict: Longitudinal Evidence from Ukraine." *Social Psychological & Personality Science.*

Brinberg, David, and Patricia Castell. [1982] 1993. "A Resource Exchange Theory Approach to Interpersonal Interactions: A Test of Foa's Theory." Pp. 41–56 in *Resource Theory: Explorations and Applications*, edited by Uriel G. Foa, John Converse, Jr., Kjell Y. Tornblom, and Edna B. Foa. San Diego, CA: Academic Press.

Brisson, Daniel S., and Charles L. Usher. 2005. "Bonding Social Capital in Low-income Neighborhoods." *Family Relations* 54:644–653.

Brisson, Daniel. 2009. "Testing the Relationship of Formal Bonding, Informal Bonding, and Formal Bridging Social Capital on Key Outcomes for Females in Low Income Neighborhoods." *Journal of Sociology & Social Welfare* 36(1):167–183.

Brkich, Mariana, Danielle Jeffs, and Sally A. Carless. 2002. "A Global Self-Report Measure of Person-Job Fit." *European Journal of Psychological Assessment* 18(1):43–51.

Broadbent, Robyn, and Theo Papadopoulos. 2011. "Getting Wired@Collingwood: An ICT Project Underpinned by Action Research." *Community Development Journal* 47(2):248–265.

Brodsky, Anne E. and Lauren Bennett Cattaneo. 2013. "A Transconceptual Model of Empowerment and Resilience: Divergence, Convergence and Interactions in Kindred Community Concepts." *American Journal of Community Psychology* 52(3–4):333–346.

Brodsky, Beth S., and Barbara Stanley. 2013. The Dialectical Behavior Therapy Primer: Hower DBT Can Inform Clinical Practice. Chichester, UK: Wiley.

Brody, David C., and Nicholas P. Lovrich. 2002. "Social Capital and Protecting the Rights of the Accused in the American States: An Investigation of the Dark Side of Social Capital." *Journal of Contemporary Criminal Justice* 18(2):115–131.

Brody, Gene H., Zolinda Stoneman, and Douglas Flor. 1995. "Linking Family Processes and Academic Competence among Rural African American Youths." *Journal of Marriage & the Family* 57:567–579.

Broh, Beckett A. 2002. "Linking Extracurricular Programming to Academic Achievement: Who Benefits and Why?" *Sociology of Education* 75(1):69–91.

Broidy, Lisa M. 2001. "A Test of General Strain Theory." *Criminology* 39(1):9–35.

Bromley, Daniel W., 2004. "Reconsidering Environmental Policy: Prescriptive Consequentialism and Volitional Pragmatism." *Environmental & Resource Economics* 28:73–99.

Bronk, Kendall Cotton, Patrick L. Hill, Daniel K. Lapsley, Tasneem L. Talib, and Holmes Finch. 2009. "Purpose, Hope, and Life Satisfaction in Three Age Groups." *Journal of Positive Psychology* 4(6):500–510.

Brooks, Ann. 2011. *Social Theory in Contemporary Asia.* Abingdon, UK: Routledge.

Brooks, Clem. 1999. "values or Views of Government? Analyzing the Ideological Sources of Public Policy Preferences." *Social Science Research* 28:137–161.

Brooks, Onel. 2020. "Finishing School, Fishing and Flourishing: Appetite, Engagement and Compliance in Daoism, Existentialism and Psychoanalysis." *European Journal of Psychotherapy & Counselling* 22(3–4):233–54.

Brooks, Robert, and Suzanne Brooks. 2014. "Creating Resilient Mindsets in Children and Adolescents: A Strength-based Approach for Clinical and Nonclinical Populations." Pp. 59–82 in *Resilience Interventions for Youth in Diverse Populations*, edited by Sandra Prince-Embury and Donald H. Saklofske. New York, NY: Springer.

Broome, Benjamin J. 2013. "Building Cultures of Peace: The Role of Intergroup Dialogue." Pp. 737–761 in *The SAGE Handbook of Conflict Communication*, edited by John G. Oetzel and Stelle Ting-Toomey. Thousand Oaks, CA: SAGE.

Brossard, Baptiste. 2019. "Why Mental Disorders Flourish and Wither: Extending the Theory of Ecological Niches." *Social Science & Medicine* 237:112445.

Brotchie, Janet, Caroline Meyer, Alex Copello, Robert Kidney, and Glenn Waller. 2004. "Cognitive Representations in Alcohol and Opiate Abuse: The Role of Core Beliefs." *British Journal of Clinical Psychology* 43:337–342.

Brouwer, Jasperina and Maaike Engels. 2022. "The Role of Prosocial Attitudes and Academic Achievement in Peer Networks in Higher Education." *European Journal of Psychology of Education* 37(2):567–84.

Brown, Christina M., Steven G. Young, Donald F. Sacco, Michael J. Bernstein, and Heather M. Claypool. 2009. "Social Inclusion Facilitates Interest in Mating." *Evolutionary Psychology* 7(1):147470490900700–27.

Brown, Graham, Barbara B. Brown, and Douglas D. Perkins. 2004. "New Housing as Neighborhood Revitalization: Place Attachment and Confidence among Residents." *Environment & Behavior* 36(6):749–775.

Brown, Jacob R. and Michael Zoorob. 2022. "Resisting Broken Windows." *Political Behavior* 44:679–703.

Brown, Jason. 2019. *Anti-oppressive Counseling and Psychotherapy: Action for Personal and Social Change.* New York, NY: Routledge.

Brown, Keith R. 2011. "Interaction Ritual Chains and the Mobilization of Conscientious Consumers." *Qualitative Sociology* 34:121–141.

Brown, Kevin M., Russell Hoye, and Matthew Nicholson. 2014. "Generating Trust? Sport and Community Participation." *Journal of Sociology* 50(4):437–457.

Brown, Ruth Christine Chanan. 2011. *The Development of the Common Factor Therapist Competence Scale for Youth Psychotherapy.* Doctoral Dissertation, Virginia Commonwealth University.

Brown, Stephanie L. and R. Michael Brown. 2006. "Target Article: Selective Investment Theory: Recasting the Functional Significance of Close Relationships." *Psychological Inquiry* 17(1):1–29.

Brown, Tony N. 2001. "Measuring Self-perceived Racial and Ethnic Discrimination in Social Surveys." *Sociological Spectrum* 21:377–392.

Browning, Don S., and Terry D. Cooper. 2004. *Religious Thought and the Modern Psychologies.* Minneapolis, MN: Fortress.

Brubaker, Rogers. 2004. "In the Name of the Nation: Reflections of Nationalism and Patriotism." *Citizenship Studies* 8(2):115–127.

Brubaker, Rogers. 2015. "Religious Dimensions of Political Conflict and Violence." *Sociological Theory* 33(1).1–19.

Bruch, Sarah K., Myra Marx Ferree, and Joe Soss. 2010. "From Policy to Polity: Democracy, Paternalism, and the Incorporation of Disadvantaged Citizens." *American Sociological Review* 75(2):205–226.

Brugman, Gerard M. 2006. "Wisdom and Aging." Pp. 445–476 in *Handbook of the Psychology of Aging*, edited by James E. Birren and K. Warner Schaie. Burlington, MA: Academic.

Brunie, Aurelie. 2009. "Meaningful Distinctions within a Concept: Relational, Collective, and Generalized Social Capital." *Social Science Research* 38:251–265.

Brusting, Suzanne, and Tom Postmes. 2002. "Social Movement Participation in the Digital Age: Predicting Offline and Online Collective Action." *Small Group Research* 33(5):525 554.

Bryant, Lucinda L., Arne Beck, and Diane L. Fairclough. 2000. "Factors that Contribute to Positive Perceived Health in an Older Population." *Journal of Aging & Health* 12(2):169–192.

Bryant-Davis, Thema. 2007. "Healing Requires Recognition: The Case for Race-Based Traumatic Stress." *Counseling Psychologist* 35(1).135–143.

Brynin, Malcolm, Alvaro Martinez Perez, and Simonetta Longhi. 2009. "How Close Are Couples?" Pp. 93–108 in *Changing Relationships*, edited by Malcolm Brynin and John Ermisch. New York. Routledge.

Bucher, Taina. 2013. "The Friendship Assemblage: Investigating Programmed Sociality on Facebook." *Television & New Media* 14(6):479–93.

Buck, Nick. 2001. "Identifying Neighbourhood Effects on Social Exclusion." *Urban Studies* 38(12):2251–2275.

Buckingham, Alan. 1999. "Is There an Underclass in Britain?" *British Journal of Sociology* 56(1):49–75.

Bucknell, Kirsten J., Maria Kangas, Eyal Karin, and Monique F. Crane. 2024. "A Randomized Controlled Trial Comparing the Effects of Self-Reflective Writing Focused on Successful and Unsuccessful Coping Experiences on Resilience." *Stress & Health* 40(2):e3311.

Buelow, George, Mark McClain, and Irene McIntosh. 1996. "A New Measure for an Important Construct: The Attachment and Object Relations Inventory." *Journal of Personality Assessment* 66(3):604–623.

Bueno de Mesuita, Bruce, James D. Morrow, Randolph Siverson, and Alastair Smith. 2002. "The Selectorate Model: A Theory of Political Institutions." Pp. 267–292 in *New Directions in Contemporary Sociological Theory*, edited by Joseph Berger and Morris Zelditch, Jr. Lanham, MY: Rowman & Littlefield.

Bufacchi, Vittorio. 2007. *Violence and Social Justice*. Houndmills, UK: Palgrave.

Buikstra, Elizabeth, Helen Ross, Christine A. King, Peter G. Baker, Desley Hegney, Kathryn McLachlan, and Cath Rogers-Clark. 2010. "The Components of Resilience-Perceptions of an Australian Rural Community." *Journal of Community Psychology* 38(8):975–91

Bulbulia, Joseph A., Dimitris Xygalatas, Uffe Schjoedt, Sabela Fondevila, Chris G. Sibley, and Ivana Konvalinka. 2013. "Images from a Jointly-Arousing Collective Ritual Reveal Affective Polarization." *Frontiers in Psychology* 4:960.

Bullock, John G. 2021. "Education and Attitudes toward Redistribution in the United States." *British Journal of Political Science* 51(3):1230–50.

Bullough, John. 2012. "Emotional Freedom Technique." Pp. 351–355 in *The SAGE Handbook of Counselling and Psychotherapy*, edited by Colin Feltham and Ian Horton. London: SAGE.

Bunge, Mario. 1996. *Finding Philosophy in Social Science*. New Haven, CT: Yale University Press.

Burch, Tyler. 2020. "All in the Family: The Link between Couple-Level Work-Family Conflict and Family Satisfaction and Its Impact on the Composition of the Family over Time." *Journal of Business & Psychology* 35(5):593–607.

Burchardt, Marian. 2013. "Faith-Based Humanitarianism: Organizational Change and Everyday Meanings in South Africa." *Sociology of Religion* 74(1):30–55.

Burger, Kaspar, and Robin Samuel. 2017. "The Role of Perceived Stress and Self-Efficacy in Young People¡¯s Life Satisfaction: A Longitudinal Study." *Journal of Youth & Adolescence* 46(1):78–90.

Burgess, Adam. 2018. "Individualization Revisited: Global Family Developments, Uncertainty and Risk." *Journal of Risk Research* 21(1):83–95.

Burgess, Kim B., Julie C. Wojslawowicz, Kenneth H. Rubin, Linda Role-Krasnor, and Cathryn Booth-LaForce. 2006. "Social Information Processing and Coping Strategies of Shy/withdrawn and Aggressive Children: Does Friendship Matter?" *Child Development* 77(2):371–383.

Burgoon, Judee K., Laura K. Guerrero, and Kory Floyd. 2010. *Nonverbal Communication*. Columbus, MA: Allyn & Bacon.

Burgoyne, Carole B., David A. Routh, and Svetlana Sidorenko-Stephenson. 1999. "Perceptions, Attributions and Policy in the Economic Domain: A Theoretical and Comparative Analysis." *International Journal of Comparative Sociology* 40(1):79–93.

Buric, Irena and Mirta Mornar. 2023. "Teacher Dispositional Affectivity, Emotional Labor, and Self-Efficacy: A Longitudinal Analysis." *Current Psychology* 42(21):18382–95.

Burke, Peter J. 2008. "Identity, Social Status and Emotion." Pp. 75–93 in *Social Structure and Emotion*, edited by Jody Clay-Warner and Dawn T. Robinson. San Diego, CA: Academic.

Burke, Peter J., and Jan E. Stets. 1999. "Trust and Commitment through Self-verification." *Social Psychology Quarterly* 62(4):347–360.

Burke, Sara E., John F. Dovidio, Marianne LaFrance, Julia M. Przedworski, Sylvia P. Perry, Sean M. Phelan, Diana J. Burgess, Rachel R. Hardeman, Mark W. Yeazel, and Michelle van Ryn. 2017. "Beyond Generalized Sexual Prejudice: Need for Closure Predicts Negative Attitudes toward Bisexual People Relative to Gay/Lesbian People." *Journal of Experimental Social Psychology* 71:145–50.

Burnett, Simon. 2012. *The Happiness Agenda: A Modern Obsession*. New York, NY: Palgrave.

Burroughs, James, and Aric Rindfleisch. 2002. "Materialism and Well-being: A Conflicting Values Perspective." *Journal of Consumer Research* 29(3):348–370.

Burrow, Anthony L. Amanda C. O'Dell, and Patrick L. Hill. 2010. "Profiles of a Developmental Asset: Youth Purpose as a Context for Hope and Well-Being." *Journal of Youth & Adolescence* 39(11):1265–1273.

Burston, Daniel. 1991. *The Legacy of Erich Fromm*. Cambridge, MA: Harvard University Press.

Burt, Ronald S. 2009. "Network Duality of Social Capital." Pp. 39–83 in *Social Capital: Reaching out, Reaching in*, edited by Viva Ona Bartkus and James H. Davis. Cheltenham, UK: Edward Elgar.

Burton, Alexander L., Francis T. Cullen, Justin T. Pickett, Velmer S. Burton, and Angela J. Thielo. 2021. "Beyond the Eternal Criminal Record: Public Support for Expungement." *Criminology & Public Policy* 20(1):123–51.

Busby, Dean M. and Lena Hsin-Yao Chiu. 2017. "Perceived Conflict Styles of Adult Children and Their Parents: What Is the Connection?" *Journal of Child & Family Studies* 26(12):3412–24.

Busch, Fredric N. 2009. "Anger and Depression." *Advances in Psychiatric Treatment* 15(4):271–278.

Bushens, vincent, and Werner Raub. 2002. "Embedded Trust: Control and Learning." *Advances in Group Processes* 19:167–202.

Buskens, Vincent, and Werner Raub. 2013. "Rational Choice Research on Social Dilemmas: Embeddedness Effects on Trust." Pp. 113–150 in *The Handbook of Rational Choice Social Research*, edited by Rafael Wittek, Tom A. H. Snijders, and Victor Nee. Stanford, CA: Stanford University Press.

Busseri, Michael A., Linda Rose-Kiasnor, Teena Willoughby, and Heather Chalmers. 2006. "A Longitudinal Examination of Breath and Intensity of Youth Activity Involvement and Successful Development." *Developmental Psychology* 42(6):1313–1326.

Bussey, Kay. 2020. "Development of Moral Disengagement: Learning to Make Wrong Right." Pp. 306–326 in *The Oxford Handbook of Moral Development: An Interdisciplinary Perspective*, edited by Lene Arnett Jensen. New York, NY: Oxford University Press.

Bussolari, Cori J., and Judith A. Goodell. 2009. "Chaos Theory as a Model for Life Transitions Counselling: Nonlinear Dynamics and Life Change." *Journal of Counseling & Development* 87:98–107.

Butler, Leah C., Amanda Graham, Bonnie S. Fisher, Billy Henson and Bradford W. Reyns. 2022. "Examining the Effect of Perceived Responsibility on Online Bystander Intervention, Target Hardening, and Inaction." *Journal of Interpersonal Violence* 37(21–22):20847–72.

Buunk, Abraham P., and Fredrick X. Gibbons. 2006. "Social Comparison Orientation: A New Perspective on Those Who Do and Those Who Don't Compare with Others." Pp. 15–32 in *Social Comparison and Social Psychology: Understanding Cognitive, Intergroup Relations, and Culture*, edited by Berge Guimond. Cambridge, UK: Cambridge University Press.

Buunk, Abrham P., and Pieternel Dijkstra. 2006. "Temptation and Threat: Extradyadic Relations and Jealousy." Pp. 533–555 in *The Cambridge Handbook of Personal Relationships*, edited by Anita L. Vangelisti and Daniel Perlman. New York: Cambridge University Press.

Buzzanell, Patrice M. 2010. "Resilience: Talking, Resisting, and Imagining New Normalcies into Being." *Journal of Communication* 60:1–14.

Byars Winston, Angela M., and Nadya A. Fouad. 2008. "Math and Science Social Cognitive Variables in College Students: Contributions of Contextual Factors in Predicting Goals." *Journal of Career Assessment* 16(4):425–440.

Byars-Winston, Angela, and Jenna Griebe Rogers. 2019. "Testing Intersectionality of Race/Ethnicity? Gender in A Social-Cognitive Career Theory Model With Science Identity." *Journal of Counseling Psychology* 66(1):30–44.

Bynner, John, and Samantha Parsons. 2002. "Social Exclusion and the Transition from School to Work: The Case of Young People Not in Education, Employment, or Training (NEET)." *Journal of Vocational Behavior* 60:289–309.

Byrne, David. 1998. Complexity Theory and the Social Sciences: An Introduction. London: Routledge.

Cabras, Cristina, and Marina Mondo. 2018. "Future Orientation as a Mediator between Career Adaptability and Life Satisfaction in University Students." *Journal of Career Development* 45(6):597–609.

Caciagli, Mario. 2003. "Christian Democracy." Pp. 165–180 in *The Cambridge History of Twentieth-century Political Thought*, edited by Terence Ball and Richard Bellamy. Cambridge, UK: Cambridge University Press.

Cacioppo, John T., and Louise C. Hawkley. 2009. "Loneliness." Pp. 227–240 in *Handbook of Individual Differences in Social Behavior*, edited by Mark R. Leary and Rick H. Hoyle. New York, NY: Guilford.

Cadwallader, Tom W., and Robert B. Cairns. 2002. "Developmental Influences and Gang Awareness among African-American Inner City Youth." *Social Development* 11(2):245–265.

Cai, Tianji, Ruoyang Tang, Hongyu Wang, and Spencer De Li. 2020. "One Country Two Systems: A Comparative Study of National Identity between Hong Kong and Macau." *Chinese Sociological Review* 54(2):107–130.

Cais, Jordi, Diego Torrente, and Catalina Bolancé. 2021. "The Effects of Economic Crisis on Trust: Paradoxes for Social Capital Theory." *Social Indicators Research* 153:173–92.

Caldas, Stephen J. and Diana G. Pounder. 1990. "Teenage Fertility and Its Social Integration Correlates: A Control Theory Explanation." *Sociological Spectrum* 10:541–560.

Callegari, Camilla, Lorenza Bert?, Melissa Lucano, Marta Ielmini, Elena Braggio, and Simone Vender. 2016. "Reliability and Validity of the Italian Version of the 14-Item Resilience Scale." *Psychology Research & Behavior Management* 9:277–284. 98–310

Calsyn, R.J., L.A. Roades, and W.D. Klinkenberg. 1998. "Using Theory to Design Needs Assessment Studies of the Elderly." *Evaluation & Program Planning* 21:277–286.

Camerino, Oleguer, Alfonso Valero-Valenzuela, Queralt Prat, David Manzano Sánchez, and Marta Castañer. 2019. "Optimizing Education: A Mixed Methods Approach Oriented to Teaching Personal and Social Responsibility (TPSR)." *Frontiers in Psychology* 10:1439.

Cameron, Gary. 2002. "Motivation to Join and Benefits from Participation in Parent Mutual Aid Organizations." *Child Welfare* 81(1):33–57.

Camp, Cameron J. 1989. "World-Knowledge Systems." Pp. 457–482 in *Everyday Cognition in Adulthood and Late Life*, edited by Leonard W. Poon, David C. Rubin, and Barbara A. Wilson. Cambridge: Cambridge University Press.

Camp, William G. 1990. "Participation in Student Activities and Achievement: A Covariance Structural Analysis." *Journal of Educational Research* 83(5):275–278.

Campagna, Grace. 2016. "Linking Crowding, Housing Inadequacy, and Perceived Housing Stress." *Journal of Environmental Psychology* 45:252–66.

Campbell, Andrea Louise. 2003. "Participatory Reactions to Policy Threats: Senior Citizens and the Defense of Social Security and Medicare." *Political Behavior* 25(1):29–49.

Campbell, Andrea, Joanne Hughes, Miles Hewstone, and Ed Cairns. 2008. "Social Capital as a Mechanism for Building a Sustainable Society in Northern Ireland." *Community Development Journal* 45(1):22–38.

Campbell, David E. 2019. "What Social Scientists Have Learned About Civic Education: A Review of the Literature." *Peabody Journal of Education* 94(1):32–47.

Campbell, Mary E., and Jennifer Eggerling-Boeck. 2006. "What about the Children? The Psychological and Social Well-being of Multiracial Adolescents." *Sociological Quarterly* 47:147–173

Campbell, Scott W., and Tracy C. Russo. 2003. "The Social construction of Mobile Telephony: An Application of the Social Influence Model to Perceptions and Uses of Mobile Phones within Personal Communication Networks." *Communication Monographs* 70(4):317–334.

Campbell, Tom. 1981. *Seven Theories of Human Society*. Oxford, UK: Clarendon. (H61.C238)

Campbell, Tom. 2010. *Justice*. Houndmills, UK: Palgrave.

Campbell-Sills, Laura, Sharon L. Cohan, and Murray B. Stein. 2006. "Relationship of Resilience to Personality, Coping, and Psychiatric Symptoms in Young Adults." *Behaviour Research & Therapy* 44(4):585–599.

Cann, Arnie and Chantal Collette. 2014. "Sense of Humor, Stable Affect, and Psychological Well-Being." *Europe's Journal of Psychology* 10(3):464–79.

Cannuscio, Carolyn C., Graham A. Colditz, Eric B. Rimm, Lisa F. Berkman, Camara P. Jones, and Ichiro Kawachi. 2004. "Employment Status, Social Ties, and Caregiver Mental Health." *Social Science & Medicine* 58:1247–1256.

Cano, Annmarie, and Dina Vivian. 2003. "Are Life Stressors Associated with Marital Violence?" *Journal of Family Psychology* 17(3):302–314.

Cantor, Nancy, Markus Kemmelmeier, Jay Basten, and Deborah A. Prentice. 2002. "Life Task Pursuit in Social Groups: Balancing Self-Exploration and Social Integration." *Self & Identity* 1(2):177–84.

Cao, Liqun, Jihong Zhao, Ling Ren, and Ruohui Zhao. 2015. "Do In-Group and Out-Group Forms of Trust Matter in Predicting Confidence in the Order Institutions? A Study of Three Culturally Distinct Countries." *International Sociology* 30(6):674–693.

Cao, Liqun, Lanying Huang, and Ivan Sun. 2016. "From Authoritarian Policing to Democratic Policing: A Case Study of Taiwan." *Policing & Society* 26(6):642–658.

Capistrano, Robert Charles, and Adam Weaver. 2017. " Host-guest Interactions between First-Generation Immigrants and Their Visiting Relatives: Social Exchange, Relations of Care and Travel." *International Journal of Culture, Tourism, & Hospitality Research* 11(3):406–420.

Caplan, Bryan. 2006. "Terrorism: The Relevance of the Rational Choice Model." *Public Choice* 128(1–2):91–107.

Caplan, Leslie J., and Carmi Schooler. 2007. "Socioeconomic Status and Financial Coping Strategies: The Mediating Role of Perceived Control." *Social Psychology Quarterly* 70(1):43–58.

Caprara, Gian Vittorio and Michele Vecchione. 2017. *Personalizing Politics and Realizing Democracy*. New York, NY: Oxford University Press.

Caprara, Gian Vittorio, and Michele Vecchione. 2013. "Personality Approaches to Political Behavior." Pp. 23–58 in *The Oxford Handbook of Political Psychology*, edited by Leone Huddy, David O. Sears and Jack S. Levy. New York: Oxford University Press.

Caprara, Gian Vittorio, and Patrizia Steca. 2005. "Self-efficacy Beliefs as Determinants of Prosocial Behavior Conducive to Life Satisfaction across Ages." *Journal of Social & Clinical Psychology* 24(2):191–217.

Caprara, Gian Vittorio, and Patrizia Steca. 2007. "Prosocial Agency: The Contribution of Values and Self-efficacy Beliefs to Prosocial Behavior across Ages." *Journal of Social & Clinical Psychology* 26(2):218–239.

Caputo, Andrea, Chiara Fregonese, and Viviana Langher. 2018. *Principles and Practices for Psychodynamic Group Career Counseling: The PICS Program*. Newcastle, UK: Cambridge Scholars.

Carbery, Julie, and Duane Buhrmester. 1998. "Friendship and Need Fulfillment during Three Phases of Young Adulthood." *Journal of Social & Personal Relationships* 15(3):393–409.

Carella, Maria, Thaís García-Pereiro, and Roberta Pace. 2021. "Subjective Well-Being, Transnational Families and Social Integration of Married Immigrants in Italy." *Social Indicators Research* 161(2–3):785–816.

Carli, Linda L. 2004. "Gender Effects on Social Influence." Pp. 133–148 in *Perspectives and Persuasion, Social Influence, and Compliance Gaining*, edited by John S. Seiter and Robert H. Gass. Boston, MA: Pearson.

Carli, Linda L., and Panuta Bukatko. 2000. "Gender, Communication, and Social Influence: A Developmental Perspective." Pp. 295–331 in *The Developmental Social Psychology of Gender*, edited by Thomas Eckes and Hannes M. Trautner. Mahwah, NJ: Lawrence Erlbaum.

Carlo, Gustoavo, George P. Knight, Camille D. Basilio, and Alexandra N. Davis. 2014. "Predicting Prosical Tendencies among Mexican American Youth: The Intersection of Cultural Values,

Social Cognitions, and Social Emotions." Pp. 242–257 in *Prosocial Development: A Multidimensional Approach,* edited by Laura M. Padilla-Walker and Gustavo Carlo. New York, NY: Oxford University Press.

Carlson, Jon, Richard E. Wutts, and Michael Maniacci. 2006. *Adlerian Therapy: Theory and Practice.* Washington, DC: American Psychological Association.

Caro, Francis G. and Arthur E. Blank. 1988. *Quality Impact of Home Care for the Elderly.* New York: Haworth Press.

Carol, Gustavo and Sarah Pierotti. 2020. "the Development of Prosocial Motives." Pp. 27–51 in *The Oxford Handbook of Moral Development: An Interdisciplinary Perspective*, edited by Lene Arnett Jensen. New York, NY: Oxford University Press.

Carpiano, Richard M. 2008. "Actual or Potential Neighborhood Resources and Access to Them: Testing Hypotheses of Social Capital for the Health of Female Caregivers." *Social Science & Medicine* 67:568–582.

Carr, Deborah, and Debra Umberson. 2013. "The Social Psychology of Stress, Health, and Coping." Pp. 465–487 in *Handbook of Social Psychology*, edited by John Delamater and Amanda Ward. Dordrecht, Netherlands: Springer.

Carr, Deborah, and Michael A. Friedman. 2005. "Is Obesity Stigmatizing? Body weight, Perceived Discrimination and Psychological Well-being in the United States." *Journal of Health & Social Behavior* 46(3):244–259.

Carrell, Michaell R., and Christina Heavrin. 2008. *Negotiating Essentials: Theory, Skills, and Practices.* Upper Saddle River, NJ: Pearson.

Carreno, David F., Nikolett Eisenbeck, José Antonio Pérez-Escobar, and José M. García-Montes. 2021. "Inner Harmony as an Essential Facet of Well-Being: A Multinational Study During the Covid-19 Pandemic." *Frontiers in Psychology* 12:648280.

Carreras, Miguel. 2018. "Why No Gender Gap in Electoral Participation? A Civic Duty Explanation." *Electoral Studies* 52:36–45.

Carrieri, Vincenzo. 2012. "Social Comparison and Subjective Well-being: Does the Health of Others Matter?" *Bulletin of Economic Research* 64(1):31–55.

Carroll, Annemaree, Stephen Houghton, Robert Wood, Kerrie Unsworth, John Hattie, Lisa Gordon, and Julie Bower. 2009. "Self-efficacy and Academic Achievement in Australian High School Students: The Mediating Effects of Academic Aspirations and Delinquency." *Journal of Adolescence* 32:797–817.

Carson, Dena C. 2013. "Perceptions of Prosocial and Delinquent Peer Behavior and the Effect on Delinquent Attitudes: A Longitudinal Study." *Journal of Climate Justice* 41:151–161.

Carson, Thomas L. 2000. *Value and the Good Life.* Notre Dame, IN: University of Notre Dame Press.

Carter, Michael J. 2016. "Microsociologies: Social Exchange, Trust, Justice, and Legitimacy." Pp. 369–386 in *Handbook of Contemporary Sociological Theory*, edited by Seth Abrutyn. Cham, Switzerland: Springer.

Cartwright, Kelly B., M. Paz Galupo, Seth D. Tyree, and Jennifer Gavin Jennings. 2009. "Reliability and Validity of the Complex Postformal Thought Questionnaire: Assessing Adults' Cognitive Development." *Journal of Adult Development* 16:183–189.

Carver, Charles S. 1997. "Adult Attachment and Personality: Converging Evidence and a New Measure." *Personality & Social Psychology Bulletin* 23(8):865–883.

Carver, Charles S., and Michael F. Scheier. 2016. "Self-regulation of Action and Affect." Pp. 3–23 in *Handbook of Self-regulation: Research, Theory, and Application*, edited by Kathleen D. Vohs and Roy F. Baumeister. New York, NY: Guilford.

Case, Peter, Robert French, and Peter Simpson. 2011. "Philosophy of Leadership." Pp. 242–254 in *The SAGE Handbook of Leadership*, edited by Alan Bryman, David Collinson, Keith Grint, Brad Jackson and Mary Uhl-Bien. London: SAGE.

Cassano, G.B., M. Mula, P. Rucci, M. Miniati, E. Frank, D.J. Kupfer, A. Oppo, S. Calugi, Maggi R. Gibbons, and A. Fagiolini. 2009. "The Structure of Lifetime Manic-hypomanic Spectrum." *Journal of Affective Disorders* 112:59–70.

Cassidy, Tony, and Richard Lynn. 1991. "Achievement Motivation, Educational Attainment, Cycles of Disadvantage, and Social Competence: Some Longitudinal Data." *British Journal of Educational Psychology* 61:1–12.
Cast, Alicia D. 2004. "Well-Being And The Transition to Parenthood: An Identity Theory Approach." *Sociological Perspectives* 47(1):55–78.
Cast, Alicia D., and Jan E. Stets. 2016. "The Self." Pp. 343–365 in *Handbook of Contemporary Sociological Theory*, edited by Seth Abrutyn. Cham, Switzerland: Springer.
Cast, Alicia D., and Peter J. Burke. 2002. "A Theory of Self-esteem." Social Forces 80(3):1041–1068.
Castells, Manuel. 2012. Networks of Outrage and Hope: Social Movements in the Internet Age. Cambridge, UK: Polity.
Castillo, Juan Carols. 2011. "Legitimacy of Inequality in Highly Unequal Context: Evidence from the Chilean Case." *Social Justice Research* 24:314–340.
Castles, Francis G. 2000. "Putting the Economy First: Or Does Postmodernization Really Matter?" *Political Studies* 48(1):38–50.
Castro, Felice Gonzalez and Kate E. Murray. 2010. "Cultural Adaptation and Resilience: Controversies, Issues, and Emerging Models." Pp. 375–403 in *Handbook of Adult Resilience*, edited by John W. Reich, Alex J. Zautra and John Stuart Hall. New York, NY: Guilford.
Catalano, Richard F., James J. Mazza, Tracy W. Harachi, Robert D. Abbott, Kevin P. Haggerty, and Charles B. Fleming. 2003. "Raising Healthy Children through Enhancing Social Development in Elementary School: Results after 1.5 Years." *Journal of School Psychology* 41:143–164.
Cattell, Vicky. 2004. "Having a Laugh and Muckerg in Together Using Social Capital to Explore Dynamics between Structure and Agency in the Context of Declining and Regenerated Neighborhood." *Sociology* 38(5):945–963.
Caughlin, John P., Anita L. Vangelisti, and Sylvia L. Mikuchi-Enyart. 2013. "Conflict in Dating and Marital Relationships." Pp. 161–185 in *The SAGE Handbook of Conflict Communication*, edited by John G. Oetzel and Stelle Ting-Toomey. Thousand Oaks, CA: SAGE.
Caughlin, John P., Ted L. Huston, and Erin C. Wehrlman. 2018. "The Affective Structure of Marriage over Time." Pp. 90–105 *The Cambridge Handbook of Personal Relationships*, edited by Anita L. Vangelisti and Daniel Perlman. Cambridge, UK: Cambridge University Press.
Celinski, Marc J., and Lyle M. Allen, III. 2017. "Universality of the Challenge-resilience-resourcefulness Model." Pp. 59–74 in *The Routledge International Handbook of Psychosocial Resilience*, edited by Updesh Kumar. Abingdon, UK: Routledge.
Celso, B.G., D.J. Ebener, and E.J. Burkhead. 2003. "Humor coping, Health Status, and Life Satisfaction among Older Adults Residing in Assisted Living Facilities." *Aging & Mental Health*.7(6):438–445.
Centola, Damon, and Michael Macy. 2007. "Complex Contagions and the Weakness of Long Ties." *American Journal of Sociology* 113(3):702–734.
Cepulic, Dominik-Borna, Giovanni A. Travaglino, Stavroula Chrona, Ena Uzelac, Alma Jeftić, Cecilia Reyna, and Marta Kowal. 2022. "Iron Fists and Velvet Gloves: Investigating the Associa tions between the Stringency of Governments" Responses to COVID-19, Stress, and Compliance in the Early Stages of the Pandemic." *British Journal of Social Psychology*.
Cerin, Ester, and Eva Leslie. 2008. "How Socio-economic Status Contributes to Participation in Leisure-time Physical Activity." *Social Science & Medicine* 66:2596–2609. Low-response
Cetin, Füsun Çuhadaroğlu, Zeynep Tüzün, Berna Pehlivantürk, Fatih Ünal, and Bahar Gökle. 2010. "Attachment Styles and Self-Image in Turkish Adolescents." *Journal of Research on Adolescence* 20(4):840–848.
Chaiwutikornwanich, Apitchaya. 2015. "Belief in the Afterlife, Death Anxiety, and Life Satisfaction of Buddhists and Christians in Thailand: Comparisons Between Different Religiosity." *Social Indicators Research* 124(3):1015–1032.
Chan, Cecilia Lai-wan, and June Mui-hing Mak. 2000. "Benefits and Drawbacks of Chinese Rituals Surrounding Care for the Dying." Pp. 255–270 in *Psychosocial Oncology and Palliative Care*

*in Hong Kong*, edited by Richard Fielding and Cecilia Lai-wan Chan. Hong Kong, China: Hong Kong University Press.

Chan, David W. 2006. "Emotional Intelligence and Components of Burnout among Chinese Secondary School Teachers in Hong Kong." *Training & Teacher Education* 22:1042–1054.

Chan, Elaine. 2014. "Are Informal Connections a Functional Alternative to Associational Life in Enhancing Social Cohesion? Findings from Hong Kong." *Social Indicators Research* 119(2):803–821.

Chan, Ho Fai, Stephanie M. Rizio, Ahmed Skali, and Benno Torgler. 2024. "Patience Predicts Attitudes toward Vaccination and Uptake of Vaccines." *Social Psychological & Personality Science*. \110–267, 110–282

Chan, Kara, and Yolanda Cheng. 2012. "Portrayal of Females in Magazine Advertisements in Hong Kong." *Journal of Asian Pacific Communication* 22(1):78–96.

Chan, Kara, Sherrill Evans, Yu-Leung Ng, Marcus Yu-Lung Chiu, and Peter J. Huxley. 2014. "A Concept Mapping Study on Social Inclusion in Hong Kong." *Social Indicators Research* 119(1):121–37.

Chan, Raymond K.H. 2006. "Risk and Its Management in Post-financial Crisis Hong Kong." *Social Policy & Administration* 40(2):215–229.

Chan, Raymond K.H. 2012. "Competence Trust, Reflexivity and Risk Management in Hong Kong." *Asian Journal of Political Science* 20(3):267–283.

Chan, Siu Ming and Hung Wong. 2022. "Housing and Subjective Well-Being in Hong Kong: A Structural Equation Model." *Applied Research in Quality of Life* 17(3):1745–66.

Chan, Siu Ming, Hung Wong, Tat Chor Au-Yeung, Xuan Huo, and Qin Gao. 2022. "Impacts of Poverty Stigma on Negative Affect among Welfare Recipients: Path Analysis on Mainland China and Hong Kong Sar." *Journal of Asian Public Policy* 15(1):145–64.

Chan, Wallace Chi Ho, and Cecilia L.W. Chan. 2011. "Acceptance of Spousal Death: The Factor of Time in Bereaved Older Adults?? Search for Meaning." *Death Studies* 35:147–162.

Chan, Ying-keung. 1999. "Density, Crowding, and Factors Intervening in Their Relationships: Evidence for a Hyper-dense Metropolis." *Social Indicators Research* 48:103–124.

Chang, Chun-Ming, and Meng-Hsiang Hsu. 2016. "Understanding the Determinants of Users" Subjective Well-Being in Social Networking Sites: An Integration of Social Capital Theory and Social Presence Theory." *Behaviour & Information Technology* 35(9):720–729.

Chang, Chun-Tuan. 2005. "The Social Impacts of the Public Welfare Lottery: An Empirical Study in Taiwan." *Modern Asia Studies* 39(1):133–153.

Chang, Edward C., Marguerite R. Bodem, Lawrence J. Sanna, and Cathryn G. Fabian. 2011. "Optimism-Pessimism and Adjustment in College Students: Is There Support for the Utility of a Domain-Specific Approach to Studying Outcome Expectancies?" *Journal of Positive Psychology* 6(5):418–28.

Chang, Han Il and Woo Chang Kang. 2018. "Why Do the Poor Oppose Income Redistribution? An Empirical Test on the Impacts of Nationalism and Fatalism." *Social Science Journal* 55(4):422–31.

Chang, Weining, Wing Keung Wong, Grace Teo, and Amy Fam. 1997. "The Motivation to Achieve in Singapore: In Search of a Core Construct." *Personality & Individual Differences* 23(5):885–895.

Chang, Wei-Wan. 2009. "Schema Adjustment in Cross-Cultural Encounters: A Study of Expatriate International Aid Service Workers." *International Journal of Intercultural Relations* 33:57–68.

Chang, Wen-Chun. 2009. "Social Capital and Subjective Happiness in Taiwan." *International Journal of Social Economics* 36(8):844–868.

Chang, Yen-Ping, Yi-Cheng Lin, and Lung Hung Chen. 2012. "Pay It Forward: Gratitude in Social Networks." *Journal of Happiness Studies* 13(5):761–781.

Chang, Ying-Hwa, Chin-Chun Yi, and Kuei-Hsiu Lin. 2008. "Kin Network and Its Effect on the Psychological Well-being of the Youth: The Case of Taiwan." *Journal of Comparative Family Studies* 39(1):19–37.

Chapman, Benjamin P., and Bert Hayslip, Jr. 2005. "Incremental Validity of a Measure of Emotional Intelligence." *Journal of Personality Assessment* 85(2):154–169.

Charles, Susan T., and Laura L. Carstensen. 2009. "Social and Emotional Aging." *Annual Review of Psychology* 61:383–409.
Charles, Susan Turk, and Laura L. Carstensen. 2008. "Unpleasant Situations Elicit Different Emotional Responses in Younger and Older Adults." *Psychology and Aging* 23(3):495–504.
Charyton, Christine, Shannon Hutchison, Lindsay Snow, Mohammed A. Rahman, and John O. Elliott. 2009. "Creativity as an Attribute of Positive Psychology: The Impact of Positive and Negative Affect on the Creative Personality." *Journal of Creativity in Mental Health* 4(1):57–66.
Chasiotis, Athanasios, and Michael Bender. 2014. "Childhood Context Explains Cultural Variance in Implicit Parenting Motivation: Results from Two Studies with Six Samples from Cameroon, Costa Rica, Germany, and PR China." *Evolutionary Psychology* 12(2):295–317.
Chattopadhyay, Arpita, and Robert Marsh. 1999. "Changes in Living Arrangement and Familial Support for the Elderly in Taiwan: 1963–1991." *Journal of Comparative Family Studies* 30(3):523–537.
Cheadle, Jacob E., and Bridget J. Goosby. 2010. "Birth Weight, Cognitive Development, and Life Chances: A Comparison of Siblings from Childhood into Early Adulthood." *Social Science Research* 39(4):570–584.
Cheadle, Jacob E., and Philip Schwadel. 2012. "The Friendship Dynamics of Religion or the Religious Dynamics of Friendship? A Social Network Analysis of Adolescents Who Attend Small Schools." *Social Science Research* 41:1198–1212.
Cheavens, Jen. 2000. "Hope and Depression: Light through the Shadows." Pp. 321–340 in *Handbook of Hope: Theory, Measures, Applications*, edited by C.R. Snyder. San Diego, CA: Academic.
Cheavens, Jennifer S., and Madison M. Guter. 2018. "Hope Therapy." Pp. 133–142 in *The Oxford Handbook of Hope*, edited by Matthew W. Gallagher and Shane J. Lopez. New York, NY: Oxford University Press.
Checkoway, Barry. 1998. "Involving Young People in Neighborhood Development." *Child Care & Youth Services Review* 20(9/10):765–795.
Chen, Beiwen, Maarten Vansteenkiste, Wim Beyers, Liesbet Boone, Edward Deci, Jolene Kaap-Deeder, Bart Duriez, Willy Lens, Lennia Matos, Athanasios Mouratidis, Richard Ryan, Kennon Sheldon, Bart Soenens, Stijn Petegem, and Joke Verstuyf. 2015. "Basic Psychological Need Satisfaction, Need Frustration, and Need Strength Across Four Cultures," *Motivation & Emotion* 39(2):216–236.
Chen, Bin-Bin. 2016. "Conscientiousness and Everyday Creativity Among Chinese Undergraduate Students." *Personality & Individual Differences* 102:56–59.
Chen, Chuan-Yu, Carla L. Storr, and James C. Anthony. 2009. "Early-onset Drug Use and Risk for Drug Dependence Problems." *Addictive Behaviors* 34(3):319–322.
Chen, Duan-Rung, Ly-Yun Chang, and Meng-Li Yang. 2008. "Gender-specific Responses to Social Determinants Associated with Self-perceived Health in Taiwan: A Multilevel Approach." *Social Science & Medicine* 69:1630–1640.
Chen, Guo-hai, and Rod A. Martin. 2007. "A Comparison of Humor Styles, Coping Humor, and Mental Health between Chinese and Canadian University Students." *Humor* 20(3):215–234.
Chen, Limei, Yirong Guo, Lynda Jiwen Song, and Bei Lyu. 2022. "From Errors to Ocbs and Creativity: A Multilevel Mediation Mechanism of Workplace Gratitude." *Current Psychology* 41(9):6170–84. doi:
Chen, Ni. 2012. "Branding National Image: The 2008 Beijing Summer Olympics, 2010 Shanghai World Expo, and 2010 Guangzhou Asian Games." *Pubic Relations Review* 38:731–745.
Chen, Ning, and Larry Dwyer. 2018. "Residents? Place Satisfaction and Place Attachment on Destination Brand-Building Behaviors: Conceptual and Empirical Differentiation." *Journal of Travel Research* 57(8):1026–1041.
Chen, Pan, and Alexander T Vazsonyi. 2013. "Future Orientation, School Contexts, and Problem Behaviors: A Multilevel Study." *Journal of Youth & Adolescence* 42(1):67–81.

Chen, Qiong, Yining Song, Yuancheng Huang, and Caina Li. 2023. "The Interactive Effects of Family Violence and Peer Support on Adolescent Depressive Symptoms: The Mediating Role of Cognitive Vulnerabilities." *Journal of Affective Disorders* 323:524–33.

Chen, Sijing, Jianwei Liu and Huamin Hu. 2021. "A Norm-Based Conditional Process Model of the Negative Impact of Optimistic Bias on Self-Protection Behaviors During the Covid-19 Pandemic in Three Chinese Cities." *Frontiers in Psychology* 12:659218.

Chen, Sylvia Xiaohua, Ben C. P. Lam, Bryant P. H. Hui, Jacky C. K. Ng, Winnie W. S. Mak, Yanjun guan, Emma E. Buchtel, Wille C.S. Tang, and Victor C.Y. Lau. 2016. "Conceptualizing Psychological Processes in Response to Globalization: Components, Antecedents, and Consequences of Global Orientations." *Journal of Personality & Social Psychology* 110(2):302–331.

Chen, Weixia, Xiaoyu Li, E. Scott Huebner, and Lili Tian. 2022. "Parent-Child Cohesion, Loneliness, and Prosocial Behavior: Longitudinal Relations in Children." *Journal of Social & Personal Relationships* 39(9):2939–63.

Chen, Xinguang, Maggie Lau, Ming Yue Kan, I. Chyun Chiang, Yih-Jin Hu, Jie Gong, Lue Li, and King-Lun Ngok. 2016. "Lifestyle and Addictive Behaviors among Chinese Adolescents in Hong Kong, Macau, Taipei, Wuhan, and Zhuhai—a First Cross-Subculture Assessment." *International Journal of Behavioral Medicine* 23(5):561–70.

Chen, Xinguang, Peigang Wang, Rhiana Wegner, Jie Gong, Xiaoyi Fang, and Linda Kaljee. 2015. "Measuring Social Capital Investment: Scale Development and Examination of Links to Social Capital and Perceived Stress." *Social Indicators Research* 120(3):669–87.

Chen, Xinjie, Hoi Yan Cheung, Xitao Fan, and Joseph Wu. 2018. "Factors Related to Resilience of Academically Gifted Students in The Chinese Cultural and Educational Environment." *Psychology in the Schools* 55(2):107–119.

Chen, Xinjie, Jinbo He, and Xitao Fan. 2020. "Applicability of the Ego-Resilience Scale (ER89) in the Chinese Cultural Context: A Validation Study." *Journal of Psychoeducational Assessment* 38(6):675–691.

Chen, Xinling, Suiqing Li, Yijie Zhang, Yuzhu Zhai, Zhixin Zhang, and Chunliang Feng. 2022. "Different Drives of Herding: An Exploratory Study of Motivations Underlying Social Conformity." *Psych Journal* 11(2):247–58.

Chen, Yang-Hsueh and Yu-Ju Lin. 2018. "Validation of the Short Self-Regulation Questionnaire for Taiwanese College Students (TSSRQ)." *Frontiers in Psychology* 9:259.

Chen, Yun Chung, and Ngai Pun. 2007. "Neoliberalization and Privatization in Hong Kong after the 1997 Financial Crisis." *China Review* 7(2):65–92.

Chen, Zeng-yin, and Howard B. Kaplan. 2001. "Intergenerational Transmission of Constructive Parenting." *Journal of Marriage & the Family* 63(1):17–31.

Chen, Zhenghui, and Gareth Davey. 2009. "Subjective Quality of Life in Zhuhai City, South China: A Public Survey Using the International Wellbeing Index." *Social Indicators Research* 91:243–258.

Cheng, Cecilia, and Aik-kwang Ng. 2006. "Psychosocial Factors Predicting SARS-Preventive Behaviors in Four Major SARS-Affected Regions." *Journal of Applied Social Psychology* 36(1):222–247.

Cheng, Cecilia, and Mike W.L. Cheung. 2005. "Psychological Responses to Outbreak of Severe Acute Respiratory Symptom: A Prospective, Multiple Time-point Study." *Journal of Personality* 73(1):261–285.

Cheng, Cecilia, Hsin-Yi Wang, Leif Sigerson, and Chor-Lam Chau. 2019. "Do the Socially Rich Get Richer? A Nuanced Perspective on Social Network Site Use and Online Social Capital Accrual." *Psychological Bulletin* 145(7):734–764.

Cheng, Cuiping and Xiting Huang. 2017. "An Exploration of Courage in Chinese Individuals." *Journal of Positive Psychology* 12(2):141–50.

Cheng, Hsiu-Lan, Helen Youngju Kim, Jason D Reynolds (Taewon Choi), Yuying Tsong, and Joel Y. Wong. 2021. "COVID-19 Anti-Asian Racism: A Tripartite Model of Collective Psychosocial Resilience." *American Psychologist* 76(4):627–642.

Cherry, K.E., Galea Sampson, Stanko Marks, and Baudoin Nezat. 2018. "Spirituality, Humor, and Resilience after Natural and Technological Disasters." *Journal of Nursing Scholarship* 50(5):492–501.

Cheng, Qijin, Tim Mh Li, Chi-Leung Kwok, Tingshao Zhu, and Paul Siu-fai Yip. 2017. "Assessing Suicide Risk and Emotional Distress in Chinese Social Media: A Text Mining and Machine Learning Study." *Journal of Medical Internet Research* 19(7):e243.

Chernikova, Marina, Calogero Lo Destro, Antonio Pierro, E. Tory Higgins, and Arie W. Kruglanski. 2017. "A Multilevel Analysis of Person-Group Regulatory-Mode Complementarity: The Moderating Role of Group-Task Interdependence." *Group Dynamics* 21(2):108–20.

Cherrier, Hélène. 2010. "Custodian Behavior: A Material Expression of Anti-Consumerism." *Consumption, Markets & Culture* 13(3):259–72.

Cherry, Katie E., Matthew R. Calamia, Emily M. Elliott, Katelyn J. McKneely, Quyen P. Nguyen, Cayman A. Loader, Luke R. Miller, Laura Sampson, and Sandro Galea. 2023. "Religiosity and Social Support Predict Resilience in Older Adults after a Flood." International Journal of Aging & Human Development 96(3):285–311.

Cheung, Adam Ka-Lok and Tuen Yi Chiu. 2021. "Husband-to-Wife Sexual Coercion in Cross-Border Marriage: A Relationship Power Perspective." *Current Sociology* 69(1):77–98.

Cheung, Chau-kiu. 2018. *Emerging Adulthood in Hong Kong: Social Forces and Civic Engagement.* Singapore: Routledge.

Cheung, Chau-kiu, and Raymond Kwok-hong Chan. 2010. "Social Capital as Exchange: Its Contribution to Morale." *Social Indicators Research* 96:205–227.

Cheung, Chau-kiu and Ping Kwong Kam. 2012. "Resiliency in Older Hong Kong Chinese: Using the Grounded Theory Approach to Reveal Social and Spiritual Conditions." *Journal of Aging Studies* 26:355 367.

Cheung, Chau-kiu and Ping Kwong Kam. 2018. "Conditions for Pets to Prevent Depression in Older Adults." *Aging & Mental Health* 22(12):1627–1633.

Cheung, Chau-kiu, and Julian Chuk-ling Lai. 2020.7. "Public Priority for Allocating Kidney Transplants." Pp. 109–136 in *A Closer Look at Social Sustainability*, edited by Chau-kiu Cheung. New York: Nova.

Cheung, Chau-kiu, and Kwan-kwok Leung. 2011.6. "Neighborhood Homogeneity and Cohesion in Sustainable Community Development." *Habitat International 35*:564–572.

Cheung, Chau-kiu, and Ngan-pun Ngai. 2004. "Humanist Approaches to Youth Development in the Summer Youth Program of Hong Kong." *Journal of Social Service Research* 31(2):1–24.

Cheung, Chau-kiu, and Raymond Man-hung Ngan. 2007.11. "Empowering for Community Integration in Hong Kong." *Journal of Developmental & Physical Disabilities* 19(4):305–322.

Cheung, Chau-kiu, and Xiao Dong Yue. 2013. "Sustaining Resilience through Local Connectedness among Sojourn Students." *Social Indicators Research* 111(3):785–800.

Cheung, Chau-kiu, and Xiao Dong Yue. 2020. *Creativity in Chinese Contexts: Sociocultural and Dispositional Analyses.* Abington, UK, Routledge.

Cheung, Cho-Yung. 2011. "How Political Accountability Undermines Public Service Elites: The Case of Hong Kong." *Journal of Contemporary China* 20(70):499–515.

Cheung, Nicole W. T. 2014. "Low Self-Control and Co-occurrence of Gambling with Substance Use and Delinquency among Chinese Adolescents." *Journal of Gambling Studies* 30(1):105–124.

Cheung, Siu-keung. 2013. "The Colonial and Postcolonial Hong Kong under Bio-political Control." *Hong Kong Journal of Social Sciences* 45:1 32.

Cheung, Yuet W., Susanne Y.P. Choi, and Adam K.L. Cheung. 2014. "Strain, Self-control, and Spousal Violence: A Study of Husband-to-Wife Violence in Hong Kong." *Violence & Victims* 29(2):280–299.

Chi, Shang-xin, Shi-xi Su, and Ying Xu. 2021. "A Comparative Study from the Perspectives of Institutionalism and Culturalism of Patient Trust and Related Influencing Factors in the Chinese Mainland and Taiwan." *China* 19(4):188–209.

Chia, Kai-Chieh. 2021. "The Identification of Ideal Social Media Influencers: Integrating the Social Capital, Social Exchange, and Social Learning Theories." *Journal of Electronic Commerce Research* 22(1):4–21.

Child, Travers Barclay and Elena Nikolova. 2020. "War and Social Attitudes." *Conflict Management & Peace Science* 37(2):152–71.

Chilton, Paul. 2004. Analysing Political Discourse: Theory and Practice. London: Routledge.

Chin, Voon Phua, and Jason Loh. 2008. "Filial Piety and Intergenerational Co-residence: The Case of Chinese Singaporeans." *Asian Journal of Social Science* 36:659–679.

Chiricos, Ted, Kathy Padgett, and Marc Gertz. 2000. "Fear, TV News, and the Reality of Crime." *Criminology* 38(3):755–785.

Chirkov, Valery, Richard M. Ryan Youngmee Kim, and Ulas Kaplan. 2003. "Differentiating Autonomy from Individualism and Independence: A Self-determination Theory Perspective on Internalization of Cultural Orientations and Well-being." *Journal of Personality & Social Psychology* 84(1):97–110.

Chishima, Yuta and Anne E. Wilson. 2021. "Conversation with a Future Self: A Letter-Exchange Exercise Enhances Student Self-Continuity, Career Planning, and Academic Thinking." *Self & Identity* 20(5):646–71.

Chiu, Rebecca L. H. 2012. "Urban Sustainability and the Urban Forms of China's Leading Mega Cities: Beijing, Shanghai and Guangzhou." *Urban Policy & Research* 30(4):359–83.

Choe, Elise J. Y., Peter J. Jankowski, Steven J. Sandage, Sarah A. Crabtree, and Laura E. Captari. 2023. "A Practice-Based Study of Cultural Humility and Well-Being among Psychotherapy Clients." *Counselling & Psychotherapy Research* 23(1):152–63.

Choi, Alex H. 2016. "The Politics of Consent in the Casino Economy." *Asian Education & Development Studies* 5(4):408–422.

Choi, Jiyoung, David W. Johnson, and Roger Johnson. 2011. "Relationships among Cooperative Learning Experiences, Social Interdependence, Children's Aggression, Victimization, and Prosocial Behaviors." *Journal of Applied Social Psychology* 41(4):976–1003.

Choi, Mihwa. 2012. "Extreme Asceticism: Confucian Practice and Riesebrodt's Religious Virtuoso." *Journal for the Scientific Study of Religion* 51(3):456–67.

Choi, Susanne Y. P., and Roman David. 2012. "Lustration Systems and Trust: Evidence from Survey Experiments in the Czech Republic, Hungary, and Poland." *American Journal of Sociology* 117(4):1172–1201.

Chon, Myoung-Gi and Hyojung Park. 2021. "Predicting Public Support for Government Actions in a Public Health Crisis: Testing Fear, Organization-Public Relationship, and Behavioral Intention in the Framework of the Situational Theory of Problem Solving." *Health Communication* 36(4):476–86.

Chong, Daniel P. L. 2014. *Debating Human Rights*. Boulder, CO: Lynne.

Chou, Kee-lee, Iris Chi, and Angela Leung. 2003. "Interest in Formal Learning among Soon-to-be-aged Adults in Hong Kong." *Educational Gerontology* 29:723–737.

Chou, Kee-Lee. 2000. "Intimacy and Psychosocial Adjustment in Hong Kong Chinese Adolescents." *Journal of Genetic Psychology* 161(2):141–151

Chouliaraki, Lilie.2013. *The Ironic Spectator: Solidarity in the Age of Post-Humanitarianism*. Cambridge, UK: Polity.

Chow, Chong Man, Duane Buhrmester, and Cin Cin Tan. 2014. "Interpersonal Coping Styles and Couple Relationship Quality: Similarity Versus Complementarity Hypotheses." *European Journal of Social Psychology* 44(2):175–186.

Chow, Irene Hau-siu, and Ignace Ng. 2004. "The Characteristics of Chinese Personal Ties (Guanxi): Evidence from Hong Kong." *Organization Studies* 25(&):1075–1093.

Chow, Peter C.Y. 2016. "Taiwan in International Economic Relations." *Orbis: A Journal of World Affairs* 60(4):531–549.

Christens, Brian D., Paul W Speer, and N. Andrew Peterson. 2011. "Social Class as Moderator of the Relationship Between (Dis)Empowering Processes and Psychological Empowerment." *Journal of Community Psychology* 39(2):170–182.

Christens, Brian D., Paul W. Speer and N. Andrew Peterson. 2016. "Assessing Community Participation: Comparing Self-Reported Participation Data with Organizational Attendance Records." *American Journal of Community Psychology* 57(3–4):415–425.

Christians, Clifford G., Theodore L. Glasser, Denis McQuail, Kaarle Nordenstreng, and Robert A. White. 2009. *Normative Theories of the Media: Journalism in Democratic Societies*. Urbana, IL: University of Illinois Press.

Christopher, John Chambers, and Robert L. Campbell. 2008. "An Interactivist-hermeneutic Metatheory for Positive Psychology." *Theory & Psychology* 18(5):675–697.

Chua, Ryan Yumin, Amudha Kadirvelu, Shajahan Yasin, Fahad Riaz Choudhry, and Miriam Sang-Ah Park. 2019. "The Cultural, Family and Community Factors for Resilience in Southeast Asian Indigenous Communities: A Systematic Review." *Journal of Community Psychology* 47(7):1750–1771.

Chua, Vincent, Gillian Koh, TanErn Ser, and Draw Shih. 2021. *Social Capital in Singapore: The Power of Network Diversity*. Singapore: Routledge.

Chuang, Shih-Chieh, and Hung-Ming Lin. 2007. "The Effect of Induced Positive and Negative Emotion and Openness-to-Feeling in Student's Consumer Decision Making." *Journal of Business & Psychology* 22(1):65–78.

Chuang, Yao-Chia. 2005. "Effects of Interaction Pattern in Family Harmony and Well-being: Test of Interpersonal Theory, Relational Models Theory, and Confucian Ethics." *Asian Journal of Social Psychology* 8:272–291.

Chui, Wing Hong, and Kevin Kwok-Yin Cheng. 2017. "Criminal Sentiments and Behaviours Among Young People in Hong Kong." *International Journal of Adolescence & Youth* 22(1):57–67.

Chumbler, Neale R., Ashley Foster, James W. Grimm, and Philip Williams. 2000. The Influence of Mid-life Adult Status and Functional Health Status on Health Lifestyles." *Research in the Sociology of Health Care* 18:249–267.

Chun, Allen. 2019. "(Post)Colonial Governance in Hong Kong and Macau: A Tale of Two Cities and Regimes." *Postcolonial Studies Culture, Politics, Economy* 22(4):413–27.

Chung, Chung-Soo. 2000. The I Ching on Man and Society: An Exploration into Its Theoretical Implications in Social Sciences. Lanham, MD: University Press of America.

Chung, HyunHee, and Maurice Elias. 1996. "Patterns of Adolescent Involvement in Problem Behaviors: Relationship to Self-efficacy, Social Competence, and Life Events." *American Journal of Community Psychology* 24(6):711–784.

Church, A. Timothy, Marcia S. Katigbak, Kenneth D. Locke, Hengsheng Zhang, Jiliang Shen, Jose de Jesus Vargas-Flores, Joselina Ibanez-Reyes, Junko Tanaka-Matsumi, Guy J. Curtis, Helena F. Cabrera, Khairul A. Mastor, Juan M. Alvarez, Fernando A. Ortiz, Jan-Yves R. Simon, and Charles M. Ching. 2012. "Need Satisfaction and Well-being: Testing Self-determinant on Theory in Eight Cultures." *Journal of Cross-Cultural Psychology* 44(4):507–534.

Church, A. Timothy. 2010. "Measurement Issues in Cross-cultural Research." Pp. 151–175 in *The SAGE Handbook of Measurement*, edited by Geoffrey Walford, Eric Tucker, and Madhu Viswanathan. London, UK: SAGE.

Chwyl, Christina, Patricia Chen, and Jamil Zaki. 2021. "Beliefs About Self-Compassion: Implications for Coping and Self-Improvement." *Personality & Social Psychology Bulletin* 47(9):1327–42.

Cialdini, Robert. 2016. *Pre-suasion. A Revolutionary Way to Influence and Persuade*. New York: NY: Simon & Schuster.

Ciarrochi, Joseph V., Amy Y.C. Chan, Peter Caputi. 2000. "A Critical Evaluation of the Emotional Intelligence Construct." *Personality & Individual Differences* 28:539–561.

Cichy, Kelly E., Karen L. Fingerman, and Eva S. Lefkowitz. 2007. "Age Differences in Types of Interpersonal Tensions." *International Journal of Aging & Human Development* 64(2):171–193.

Cicognani, Elvira, Luca Pietrantoni, Luigi Palestini, and Gabriele Prati. 2009. "Emergency Workers?? Quality of Life: The Protective Role of Sense of Community, Efficiency Belies and Coping Strategies." *Social Indicators Research* 94:449–463.

Claidiere, Nicolas, Emmanuel Trouche, and Hugo Mercier. 2017. "Argumentation and the Diffusion of Counter-Intuitive Beliefs." *Journal of Experimental Psychology* 146(7):1052–66.

Clain, Suzanne Heller. 2007. "How Living Wage Legislation Affect U.S. Poverty Rates." *Journal of Labor Research* 29:205–218.

Clare, L. 2002. "We'll Fight It as Long as We Can: Coping with the Onset of Alzheimer's Disease." *Aging & Mental Health* 6(2):139–148 \102–92.

Clark, Andrew E., Paul Frijters, and Michael A. Shields. 2008. "Relative Income Happiness and Utility: An Explanation for the Easterlin Paradox and Other Puzzles." *Journal of Economic Literature* 46(1):95–144.

Clark, Caitlin M., Eric R. Dahlen and Bonnie C. Nicholson. 2015. "The Role of Parenting in Relational Aggression and Prosocial Behavior among Emerging Adults." *Journal of Aggression, Maltreatment & Trauma* 24(2):185–202.

Clark, Cynthia M., R. Eric Landrum, and Danh T. Nguyen. 2013. "Development and Description of the Organizational Civility Scale (OCS)." *Journal of Theory Construction & Testing* 17(1):11–17.

Clark, M. Carolyn, Sharon B. Merriam, and Jennifer A. Sardlin. 2011. "The Relationship between Adult Learning and Development: Challenging Normative Assumptions." Pp. 17–38 in *The Oxford Handbook of Reciprocal Adult Development Learning*, edited by Carol Hoare, New York: Oxford University Press.

Clark, Noreen M., and Mary R. Janevic. 2013. "Individual Theories." Pp. 3–76 in *The Handbook of Health Behavior Change*, edited by Kristin A. Riekert, Judith K. Ockene and Lori Pbert. New York, NY: Springer.

Clark, Terry Nichols. 2004a. "A Political Theory of Consumption." *Research in Urban Policy* 19:19–102.

Clarke, Clifford J., and Lillian Shyu. 1991. "Spatial Economy and Integrative Labor in Turkey: An Ecological, Modernization and World-System Investigation." *Sociological Focus* 24(3):245–269.

Clarke, Philippa, Victor Marshall, James House, and Paula Lantz. 2011. "The Social Structuring of Mental Health over the Adult Life Course: Advancing Theory in the Sociology of Aging." *Social Forces* 89(4):1287–1314.

Clarke, Valerie A., Hildegarde Lovegrove, Amanda Williams & Michelle Machpherson. 2000. "Unrealistic Optimism and the Health Belief Model." *Journal of Behavioral Medicine* 23(4):367–376.

Cleaver, Frances. 2005. "The inequality of Social Capital and the Reproduction of Chronic Poverty." *World Development* 33(6):893–906.

Clemence, Alain. 2001. "Social Positioning and Social Representations." Pp. 83–95 in *Representations of the Social: Bridging Theoretical Traditions*, edited by Kay Deaux and Gina Philogene. Oxford, UK: Blackwell.

Clemens, Elizabeth, and Terrie Wetle. 1994. "Contradictions in Case Management: Client-centered Theory and Directive Practice with Frail Elderly." *Journal of Aging & Health* 6(1):70–88.

Clements-Cortes, Amy. 2017. "Artful Wellness: Attending Chamber Music Concert Reduces Pain and Increases Mood and Energy for Older Adults." *Arts in Psychotherapy* 52:41–49.

Clifford, Christopher, Ellis Paulk, Qiyang Lin, Jeanne Cadwallader, Kathy Lubbers, and Leslie D. Frazier. 2023. "Relationships among Adult Playfulness, Stress, and Coping during the COVID-19 Pandemic." *Current Psychology* 43(9):8403–12.

Clobert, Magali, Vassilis Saroglou, and Kwang-Kuo Hwang. 2015. "Buddhist Concepts as Implicitly Reducing Prejudice and Increasing Prosociality." *Personality & Social Psychology Bulletin* 41(4):513–25.

Clubb, Gordon, and Ryan O'Connor. 2019. "Understanding the Effectiveness and Desirability of De-Radicalisation: How De-Radicalisation Is Framed in the Daily Mail." *British Journal of Politics & International Relations* 21(2):349–366.

Cobb, Mark. 2001. *The Dying Soul: Spiritual Care at the End of Life*. Buckingham, UK: Open University.

Cochrane, Tom, 2018. *The Emotional Mind: A Control Theory of Affective States*. Cambridge, UK: Cambridge University Press.
Cocking, Chris. 2017. "Collective Resilience and Social Support in the Face of Adversity: Evidence from Social Psychology." Pp. 111–123 in *The Routledge International Handbook of Psychosocial Resilience*, edited by Updesh Kumar. Abingdon, UK: Routledge.
Coenders, Marcel and Peer Scheepers. 2003. "The Effect of Education on Nationalism and Ethnic Exclusionism: An International Comparison." *Political Psychology* 24:313–43.
Coffe, Hilde, and Benny Geys. 2006. "Community Heterogeneity: A Burden for the Creation of Social Capital?" *Social Science Quarterly* 87(5):1053–1072.
Coffe, Hilde, and Benny Geys. 2007. "Participation in Bridging and Bonding Associations and Civic Attitudes: Evidence from Flanders." *Voluntas* 18:385–406.
Coffey, Julia and David Farrugia. 2014. "Unpacking the Black Box: The Problem of Agency in the Sociology of Youth." *Journal of Youth Studies* 17(4):461–74.
Cohen, Dov, Etsuko Hoshino-Browne, and Angela K.Y. Leung. 2007. "Culture and the Structure of Personal Experience: Insider and Outsider Phenomenologies of the Self and Social World." *Advances in Experimental Social Psychology* 39:1–67.
Cohen, Estee Shapiro, and Kim Fromme. 2002. "Differential Determinants of Young Adult Substance Use and High-risk Sexual Behavior." *Journal of Applied Social Psychology* 32(6):1124–1150.
Cohen, Jonathan. 2004. "Parasocial Break-up from Favorite Television Characters: The Role of Attachment Styles and Relationship Intensity." *Journal of Social & Personal Relationships* 21(2):187–202.
Cohen, Joseph R., Benjamin L. Hankin, Brandon E. Gibb, Constance Hammen, Nicholas A. Hazel, Denise Ma, Shuqiao Yao, Xiong Zhao Zhu, and John R. Z. Abela. 2013. "Negative Attachment Cognitions and Emotional Distress in Mainland Chinese Adolescents: A Prospective Multi-wave Test of Vulnerability-Stress and Stress Generation Models." *Journal of Clinical Child & Adolescent Psychology* 42(4):531–544.
Cohen, LeoNora M., and Judith A. Gelbrich. 1999. "Early Childhood Interests: Seeds of Adult Creativity." Pp. 147–177 in *Investigating Creativity in Youth: Research and Methods*, edited by Anne S. Fishkin, Bonnie Cramond, and Paula Olszewski-Kubilius. Cresskill, NJ: Hampton.
Cohen-Mansfield, Jiska, and Perla Werner. 1998. "Longitudinal Changes in Behavioral Problem in Old Age: A Study in an Adult Day Care Population." *Journal of Gerontology: Medical Sciences* 51A(1):M65–M71.
Cohn, Ellen S., and Susan O. White. 1990. *Legal Socialization: A Study of Norms and Rules*. New York: Springer-Verlag.
Cohn, Michael A., and Barbara L. Fredrickson. 2009. "Positive Emotions." Pp. 13–24 in *Oxford Handbook of Positive Psychology*, edited by C. R. Synder and Shane J. Lopez. New York, NY: Oxford University Press.
Coholic, Diana A. 2011. "Exploring the Feasibility and Benefits of Arts-Based Mindfulness-Based Practices with Young People in Need: Aiming to Improve Aspects of Self-Awareness and Resilience." *Child & Youth Care Forum* 40(4):303–317.
Coie, John D., Kenneth A. Dodge, and Janis B. Kupersmidt. 1990. "Peer Group Behavior and Social Status." Pp. 17–59 in *Peer Rejection in Childhood*, edited by Steven R. Asher and John D. Coie. Cambridge, UK: Cambridge UniversityPress.
Coifman, Karin G., George A. Bonanno, Rebecca D. Ray, and James J. Gross. 2007. "Does Repressive Coping Promote Resilience? Affective-Autonomic Response Discrepancy during Bereavement." *Journal of Personality & Social Psychology* 92(4):745–758.
Colbert, Amy E., Timothy A. Judge, Daejeong Choi, and Gang Wang. 2012. "Assessing the Trait Theory of Leadership Using Self and Observer Ratings of Personality: The Mediating Role of Contributions to Group Success." *Leadership Quarterly* 23(4):670–685.
Cole, Brenda S., and Kenneth I. Pargament. 1999. "Spiritual Surrender: A Paradoxical Path to Control." Pp. 179–198 in *Integrating Spirituality into Treatment: Resources for Practitioners*, edited by William R. Miller. Washington, DC: American Psychological Association.

Cole, Elli, Shu Su, Anjolii Diaz, and Mengxi Zhang. 2022. "Social Support and Resilience among Burmese Adolescent Refugees: Examining Ethnic Identity Searching and Belonging as Moderators." *Children & Youth Services Review* 142:106647.

Coleman, Earle J. 2002. "Aesthetic Commonalities in the Ethics of Daoism and Stoicism." *Journal of Chinese Philosophy* 29(3):385–395.

Coleman, Max E., Mohit K. Manchella, Adam R. Roth, Siyun Peng, and Brea L. Perry. 2022. "What Kinds of Social Networks Protect Older Adults" Health during a Pandemic? The Tradeoff between Preventing Infection and Promoting Mental Health." *Social Networks* 70:393–402.

Collier, Andrew. 2001. *Christianity and Marxism: A Philosophical Contribution to Their Reconciliation*. London, UK: Routledge.

Collier, Gerald. 1997. "Learning Moral Commitment in Higher Education." *Journal of Moral Education* 26(1):73–83.

Collins, Nancy L., and Brooke C. Feeney. 2000. "A Safe Haven: An Attachment Theory Perspective on Support Seeking and Caregiving in Intimate Relationships." *Journal of Personality & Social Psychology* 78(6):1053–1073.

Collins, Nancy L., and Brooke C. Feeney. 2004. "Working Models of Attachment Shape Perceptions of Social Support: Evidence from Experimental and Observational Studies." *Journal of Personality & Social Psychology* 87(3):363–383 \80–177.

Collins, Nancy L., Maire B. Ford, and Brooke C. Feeney. 2011. "An Attachment-theory Perspective on Social Support in Close Relationships." Pp. 209–231 in *Handbook of Interpersonal Psychology Theory, Research, Assessment, and Therapeutic Interventions*, edited by Leonard M. Horowitz and Stephen Strack. Hoboken, NJ: Wiley.

Collins, R. Lorraine, Brian Quigley, and Kenneth E. Leonard. 2007. "Women's Physical Aggression in Bars: An Event-Based Examination of Precipitants and Predictors of Severity." *Aggressive Behavior* 33(4):304–313.

Collins, Randall. 2012a. "C-escalation and D-escalation: A Theory of the Time-dynamics of Conflict." *American Sociological Review* 77(1):1–20.

Collins, Stewart. 2004. "Young People, Alcohol and Supervision Orders." *Youth Justice* 3(3):169–82.

Collins, W. Andrew, and Manfred van Dulmen. 2006. "The Significance of Middle Childhood Peer Competence for Work and Relationships in Early Adulthood." Pp. 23–40 in *Developmental Contexts in Middle Childhood: Bridges to Adolescence and Adulthood*, edited by Aletha C. Huston and Marika N. Ripke. Cambridge, UK: Cambridge University Press.

Colverson, Aaron, Damon Lamb, Cyndi Garvan, Kok-Ben Toh, Eric Porges, Welson Tremura, and John Williamson. 2021. "Relationships between Music and Empathic Decision Making in Healthy Young Adults." *Music & Science* 4:1–11.

Compas, Bruce E., Malcarbem Vanessa L., and Karen M. Fondacaro, 1988. "Coping with stressful events in older children and young adolescents." *Journal of Consulting & Clinical Psychology* 56(3):405–411.

Comunian, Anna L., and Uwe P. Gielen. 2006. "Promoting of Moral Judgment Maturity through Stimulation of Social Role-taking and Social Reflection: An Italian Intervention Study." *Journal of Moral Education* 35(1):51–69.

Congdon, Peter. 2010. "A Multiple Indicator, Multiple Cause Method for Representing Social Capital with an Application to Psychological Distress." *Journal of Geographical Systems* 12(1):1–23.

Conger, Jay A. 2011. "Charismatic Leadership." Pp. 86–102 in *The SAGE Handbook of Leadership*, edited by Alan Bryman, David Collinson, Keith Grint, Brad Jackson and Mary Uhl-Bien. London: SAGE.

Conger, Jay A., Stephen A. Miles, and Meredith D. Ashby. 2000. "Optimizing Human Capital with a People Operating System Approach." Pp. 209–219 in *Leaders Talk Leadership*, edited by Meredith D. Ashby and Stephen A. Miles. Oxford, UK: Oxford University Press.

Conger, Rand D., Katherine Jewsbruy Conger, and Glen H. Elder, Jr. 1997. "Family Economic Hardship and Adolescent Adjustment: Mediating and Moderating Processes." Pp. 289–310 in *Consequences of Growing up Poor*, edited by Greg J. Duncan and Jeanne Brooks-Gunn. New York: Russell Sage.

Conlin, Amanda, Xinyu Hu, and Larissa K. Barber. 2021. "Comparing Relaxation Versus Mastery Microbreak Activity: A within-Task Recovery Perspective." *Psychological Reports* 124(1):248–65.

Connolly, Mary Beth, and Paul Crits-Christoph. 1999. "The Reliability and Validity of a Measure of Self-Understanding of Interpersonal Patterns." *Journal of Counseling Psychology* 46(4):472–482.

Connolly, Willliam E. 2005. *Pluralism*. Durham, NC: Duke University Press. (HM1271.C656)

Connor, Kathryn M., and Jonathan R.T. Davidson. 2003. "Development of a New Resilience Scale: The Connor-Davidson Resilience Scale (CD-RISC)." *Depression & Anxiety* 18:76-82.

Connors, Gerard J., Radka T. Toscova, and J. Scott Tonigan. 1999. "Serenity." Pp. 235–250 in *Integrating Spirituality into Treatment: Resources for Practitioners*, edited by William R. Miller. Washington, DC: American Psychological Association.

Consedine, Nathan S. 2011. "Emotion, Regulation, and Learning across the Adult Lifespan: Implications from Developmental Functionalism." Pp. 132–154 in *The Oxford Handbook of Reciprocal Adult Development Learning*, edited by Carol Hoare, New York: Oxford University Press.

Constantino, Michael J., Keely R. Wilson, and Leonard M. Horowitz, and Elizabeth C. Pinel. 2006. "The Direct and Stress-buffering Effects of Self-organization on Psychological Adjustment." *Journal of Social & Clinical Psychology* 25(3):333–360.

Conti, Robert, Jannis Angelis, Cary Cooper, Brian Faragher, and Colin Gill. 2006. "The Effects of Lean Production on Worker Job Stress." *International Journal of Operations & Production Management* 26(9):1013–38.

Conzo, Pierluigi, Arnstein Aassve, Giulia Fuochi, and Letizia Mencarini. 2017. "The Cultural Foundations of Happiness." *Journal of Economic Psychology* 62:268–83.

Cook, Karen S., and Coye Cheshire. 2013. "Social Exchange, Power, and Inequality in Networks." Pp. 185–219 in *The Handbook of Rational Choice Social Research*, edited by Rafael Wittek, Tom A. H. Snijders, and Victor Nee. Stanford, CA: Stanford University Press.

Cook, Philip J., and Michael J. Moore. 2001. "Environment and Persistence in Youthful Drinking Patterns." Pp. 375–437 in *Risky Behavior among Youth: An Economic Analysis*, edited by Jonathan Gruber. Chicago, IL: University of Chicago Press.

Cook, Thomas D., Melissa R. Herman, Meredith Phillips, and Richard A. Settersen, Jr. 2002. "Some Ways in Which Neighborhoods, Nuclear Families, Friendship Groups, and Schools Jointly Affect Changes in Early Adolescent Development." *Child Development* 73(4):1283–1309.

Cooke, Richard, and Paschal Sheeran. 2004. "Moderation of Cognition-intention and Cognition-behavior Relations: A Meta-analysis of Properties of Variables from the Theory of Planned Behavior." *British Journal of Social Psychology* 43:159–186.

Cooney, William. 2000. The Quest for Meaning: A Journey through Philosophy, the Arts, and Creative Genius. Lanham, MD: University Press of America.

Cooper, Bridget. 2011. *Empathy in Education: Engagement, Values and Achievement*. London, UK: Continuum.

Cooper, Jo, and Peter Seal. 2012. "Neuro linguistic Programming." Pp. 383–387 in *The SAGE Handbook of Counselling and Psychotherapy*, edited by Colin Feltham and Ian Horton. London: SAGE.

Cooper, Laurence D. 1999. *Rousseau, Nature, and the Problem of the Good Life*. University Park, PE: Pennsylvania State University Press.

Cooper, Laurie Ball, Elizabeth Levy Paluck, and Erin K. Fletcher. 2013. "Reducing Gender-based Violence." Pp. 359–377 in *The SAGE Handbook of Gender and Psychology*, edited by Michelle K. Ryan and Myla R. Branscombe. London, UK: SAGE.

Cooper, Maisha, Alexander H. Updegrove, Shaun L. Gabbidon, George E. Higgins, and Hillary Potter. 2021. "Examining the Effects of Race/Ethnicity and Race Relations on Public Opinion about the Overrepresentation of Black People in U.S. Prisons." *Victims & Offenders* 16(1):1–19.

Corbin, Joanne N. and J. Camille Hall. 2019. "Resettlement Post Conflict: Risk and Protective Factors and Resilience among Women in Northern Uganda." *International Social Work* 62(2):918–32.

Corcoran, Katie E. 2013. "Divine Exchanges: Applying Social Exchange Theory to Religious Behavior." *Rationality & Society* 25(3):335–369.

Corcoran, Katie E., David Pettinicchio, and Jacob T.N. Young. 2011. "The Context of Control: A Cross-national Investigation of the Link between Political Institutions Efficacy, and Collective Action." *British Journal of Social Psychology* 50:575–605.

Cordeiro, Pedro M., Maria P. Paixao, Willy Lens, Marlies Lacante, and Koen Luyckx. 2015. "Cognitive-motivational antecedents of Career Decision-Making Processes in Portuguese High School Students: A Longitudinal Study." *Journal of Vocational Behavior* 90:145–153.

Cornelis, Ilse, Alain Van Hiel, Arne Roets, and Malgorzata Kossowska. 2009. "Age Differences in Conservatism: Evidence on the Mediating Effects of Personality and Cognitive Style." *Journal of Personality* 77:51–87.

Cornell, Dewey G.., Peter J. Lovegrove, Michael W. Baly. 2014. "Invalid Survey Response Patterns Among Middle School Students." *Psychological Assessment* 26(1):277–287.

Cornum, Rhonda, Michael D. Matthews, and Martin E.P. Seligman. 2011. "Comprehensive Soldier Fitness: Building Resilience in a Challenging Institutional Context." *American Psychologist* 66(1):4–9.

Cornwall, Benjamin. 2009. "Good Health and the Bridging of Structural Holes." *Social Networks* 31:92–103.

Corrigan, Michael W., Ann Higgins-D'Alessandro, and Philip M. Brown. 2012. "Prosocial Education: A Coherent Approach to Putting Applied Theory into Action." Pp. 91–111 in *Handbook of Prosocial Education* (Vol. 1), edited by Philip M. Brown, Michael W. Corrigan and Ann Higgins-D'Alessandro. Lanham, MD: Rowman.

Corstange, Daniel and Erin A. York. 2018. "Sectarian Framing in the Syrian Civil War." *American Journal of Political Science* 62(2):441–55.

Cosculluela, Victor. 1995. *The Ethics of Suicide*. New York, NY: Garland.

Cosme, Danielle, and Elliot T. Berkman. 2018. "Autonomy Can Support Affect Regulation during Illness and in Health." *Journal of Health Psychology* 25(1):31–37.

Costa, Rosalina Pisco. 2013. "Family Rituals, Mapping the Postmodern Family through Time, Space and Emotion." *Journal of Comparative Family Studies* 44(3):269–289.

Costa-Requena, Gema, and Francisco Gil. 2009. "The Mental Adjustment to Cancer Scale: A Psychometric Analysis in Spanish Cancer Patients." *Psycho-Oncology* 18:984–991.

Costello, Barbara J., and Paul R. Vowell. 1999. "Testing Control Theory and Differential Association: A Reanalysis of the Richmond Youth Project Data." *Criminology* 37(4):815–842.

Costello, Barbara J., and Trina L. Hope. 2016. *Peer Pressure, Peer Prevention: The Role of Friends in Crime and Conformity*. New York: Routledge. (HM1246.C67) \d15–1.1, d14–2.7.

Costelloe, Laura. 2014. "Discourses of Sameness: Expressions of Nationalism in Newspaper Discourse on French Urban Violence in 2005." *Discourse & Society* 25(3):315–340.

Cote, James E. and Charles Levine. 1988. "The Relationship between Ego-Identity Status and Erikson's Notions of Institutionalized Moratoria, Value Orientation Stage, and Ego Dominance." *Journal of Youth & Adolescence* 17(1):81–99.

Cotterell, John. 2007. *Social Networks in Youth and Adolescence* (2nd ed.). London: Routledge.

Cotterill, Stewart. 2017. *Performance Psychology: Theory and Practice*. Abingdon, UK: Routledge.

Coulson, Neil S. 2019. "Online Support Communities." Pp. 241–260 n *The Oxford Handbook of Cyberpsychology*, edited by Alison Attrill-Smith, Chris Fullwood, Melanie Keep and Daria J. Kuss. Oxford, UK: Oxford University Press.

Coups, Elliot J., Bernard J. Park, Marc B. Feinstein, Richard M. Steingart, Brian L. Egleston, Donna J. Wilson, and Jamie S. Ostroff. 2009. "Correlates of Physical Activity and Lung Cancer Survivors." *Psycho-Oncology* 28:395–404.

Courtenay, Will H. 2000. "Constructions of Masculinity and Their Influence on Men's Well-being: A Theory of Gender and Health." *Social Science & Medicine* 50:1385–1401.

Cowden, Richard Gregory and Anna Meyer-Weitz. 2016. "Self-Reflection and Self-Insight Predict Resilience and Stress in Competitive Tennis." *Social Behavior & Personality* 44(7):1133–49.

Cox, Gary. 2012. The Existentialist's Guide to Death, the Universe and Nothingness. London: Continuum.

Cox, Martha J., and Blair Paley. 1997. "Families as Systems." *Annual Review of Psychology* 48:243–267.

Coyne, Sarah M., Laura M. Padilla-Walker, Hailey G. Holmgren, Emilie J. Davis, Kevin M. Collier, Madison K. Memmott-Elison, and Alan J. Hawkins. 2018. " A Meta-Analysis of Prosocial Media on Prosocial Behavior, Aggression, and Empathic Concern: A Multidimensional Approach." *Developmental Psychology* 54(2):331–347 \107–98.

Cradock, Angie L., Ichiro Kawachi, Graham A. Colditz, Steven L. Gortmaker, and Stephen L. Buka. 2009. "Neighborhood Social Cohesion and Youth Participation in Physical Activity in Chicago." *Social Science & Medicine* 68:427–435.

Crafter, Sarah, Rachel Maunder, and Laura Soulsby. 2019. *Developmental Transitions: Exploring Stability and Change through the Lifespan.*Abingdon, UK: Routledge.

Craig, Jessica M., Alex R. Piquero, and David P. Farrington. 2020. "Not All At-Risk Boys Have Bad Outcomes: Predictors of Later Life Success." *Crime & Delinquency* 66(3):392–419.

Craig, Lyn. 2007. Contemporary Motherhood: The Impact of Children on Adult Time. Aldershot, UK: Ashgate.

Cramm, J. M., V. Moller, and A. P. Nieboer. 2012. "Individual- and Neighbourhood-level Indicators of Subjective Well-Being in a Small and Poor Eastern Cape Township: The Effect of Health, Social Capital, Marital Status, and Income." *Social Indicators Research* 105(3):581–593.

Crandall, Christian S., and Ryan K. Beasley. 2001. "A Perceptual Theory of Legitimacy: Politics, Prejudice, Social Institutions, and Moral Value." Pp. 77–102 in *The Psychology of Legitimacy: Emerging Perspectives on Ideology, Justice, and Intergroup Relations*, edited by John T. Jost and Brenda Major. Cambridge, UK: Cambridge University Press.

Crane, M. F., B. J. Searle, M. Kangas, and Y. Nwiran. 2019. "How Resilience Is Strengthened by Exposure to Stressors: The Systematic Self-Reflection Model of Resilience Strengthening." *Anxiety, Stress, & Coping* 32(1):1–17.

Crawford, Emily, Margaret O'Dougherty Wright, Ann S. Masten. 2005. "Resilience and Spirituality in Youth." Pp. 355–370 in *The Handbook of Spiritual Development in Childhood and Adolescence*, edited by Eugene C. Roehlkepartain, Pamela Ebstyne King, Linda Wagener and Peter L. Benson. Thousand Oaks, CA: Sage.

Crawford, John R., and Julie D. Henry. 2003. "The Depression Anxiety Stress Scales (DASS): Normative Data and Latent Structure in a Large Non-clinical Sample." *British Journal of Clinical Psychology* 42:111–131.

Crede, Marcus, Michael Bushshur, and Sarah Niehorster. 2010. "Reference Group Effects or the Measurement of Personality and Attitudes." *Journal of Personality Assessment* 92(5):390–399.

Creed, Peter A. and Ruth-Eva Gagliardi. 2015. "Career Compromise, Career Distress, and Perceptions of Employability: The Moderating Roles of Social Capital and Core Self-Evaluations." *Journal of Career Assessment* 23(1):20–34.

Creed, Peter A., and Bronwyn M. Evans. 2002. "Personality, Well-being and Deprivation Theory." *Personality & Individual Differences* 33:1045–1054 \103–315.

Creed, Peter A., and Wendy Patton. 2003. "Predicting Two Components of Career Maturity in School-based Adolescents." *Journal of Career Development* 29(4):277–290.

Crespo, Carla, Isabel N. Davide, M. Emilia Costa, and Garth J. O. Fletcher. 2008. "Family Rituals in Married Couples: Links with Attachment, Relationship Quality, and Closeness." *Personal Relationships* 15(2):191–203.

Crisp, Richard J. and Rhiannon N. Turner. 2012. "The Imagined Contact Hypothesis." *Advances in Experimental Social Psychology* 46:125–82.

Criss, Michael M., Amy M. Smith, Amanda Sheffield Morris, Chao Liu, and Rebecca L. Hubbard. 2017. "Parents and Peers as Protective Factors among Adolescents Exposed to Neighborhood Risk." *Journal of Applied Developmental Psychology* 53:127–138.

Crocetti, Elisabetta, Seth J. Schwartz, Alessandra Fermani, and Wim Meeus. 2010. "The Utrecht-Management of Identity Commitments Scale (U-MICS) Italian Validation and Cross-National Comparisons." *European Journal of Psychological Assessment* 26(3):172–86.

Crocetti, Elisabetta, Silvia Moscatelli, Jolien Van der Graaff, Monica Rubini, Wim Meeus, and Susan Branje. 2016. "The Interplay of Self-Certainty and Prosocial Development in the Transition from Late Adolescence to Emerging Adulthood." *European Journal of Personality* 30(6):594–607.

Crocker, Jennifer, and Julie A. Garcia. 2010. "Internalized Devaluation and Structural Threat." Pp. 395–409 in *The SAGE Handbook of Prejudice, Stereotyping and Discrimination*, edited by John F. Dovidio, Miles Hewstone, Peter Glick and Victoria M. Esses. London, UK: SAGE.

Croll, Elisabeth J. 2006. "The Intergenerational Contract in the Changing Asian Family." *Oxford Development Studies* 34(4):473–491.

Crone, Eveline A. and Anna C. K. van Duijvenvoorde. 2021. "Multiple Pathways of Risk Taking in Adolescence." *Developmental Review* 62:100996.

Crosnoe, Robert, Rashmita S. Mistry, and Glen H. Elder, Jr. 2002. "Economic Disadvantage, Family Dynamics, and Adolescent Enrollment in Higher Education." *Journal of Marriage & Family* 64(3):690–702.

Cross, Jennifer L. Moren, and Nan Lin. 2008. "Access to Social Capital and Status Attainment in the United States: Racial/ethnic and Gender Differences." Pp. 364–379 in *Social Capital: An International Research Program*, edited by Nan Lin and Bonnie H. Erickson. Oxford, UK: Oxford University Press.

Crowe, Jessica. 2010. "Community Attachment and Satisfaction: The Role of a Community's Social Network Structure." *Journal of Community Psychology* 38(5):622–644.

Croy, Gerry, Paul Gerrans, and Craig Speelman. 2010. "The Role and Relevance of Domain Knowledge, Perceptions of Planning Importance, and Risk Tolerance in Predicting Savings Intentions." *Journal of Economic Psychology* 31(6):860–71.

Crume, Henry Joel, Paula S. Nurius, and Christopher M. Fleming. 2019. "Cumulative Adversity Profiles among Youth Experiencing Housing and Parental Care Instability." *Children & Youth Services Review* 100:129–135.

Crusius, Jan, Josephine Thierhoff, and Jens Lange. 2021. "Dispositional Greed Predicts Benign and Malicious Envy." *Personality & Individual Differences* 168:110361.

Crystal, David S., and Matthew DeBell. 2002. "Sources of Civic Orientation among American Youth: Trust, Religious Valuation, and Attributions of Responsibility." *Political Psychology* 23(1):113–132.

Csanyi, Gergely, Fanni Dés, and Anikó Gregor. 2023. "Pornification as Westernization on the Semi-Periphery: The History of the Hungarian "Porn Boom" in the 1990s." *Sexualities*.

Cuadrado, Esther, Carmen Tabernero, and Wolfgang Steinel. 2015. "Motivational Determinants of Prosocial Behavior: What Do Included, Hopeful Excluded, and Hopeless Excluded Individuals Need to Behave Prosocially?" *Motivation & Emotion* 39(3):344–58.

Cuesta, Jose. 2013. "Theory and Empirics of Democracy and Crime Revisited: How Much Further Can We Go with Existing Data and Methodologies?" *American Journal of Economics & Sociology* 72(3):645–74.

Cui, Lixian, Ganqi Tang, and Miner Huang. 2022. "Expressive Suppression, Confucian Zhong Yong Thinking, and Psychosocial Adjustment among Chinese Young Adults." *Asian Journal of Social Psychology* 25(4):715–30.

Cullen, Francis T., and Cheryl Lero Jonson. 2017. *Correctional Theory: Context and Consequences*. Thousand Oaks, CA: SAGE.

Cullen, Julie Berry, and Brian A. Jacob. 2009. "Is Gaining Access to Selective Elementary Schools Gaining Ground? Evidence from Randomized Lotteries." Pp. 43–84 in *The Problems of Disadvantaged Youth: An Economic Perspective*, edited by Jonathan Gruber. Chicago, IL: University of Chicago Press.

Cummings, C. Kim. 2000. "Regenerating Social Capital in Urban Neighborhoods: A Case Study." *Journal of Applied Sociology* 17(1):56–68.

Cummings, Janet R. 2014. "Contextual Socioeconomic Status and Mental Health Counseling Use among US Adolescents with Depression." *Journal of Youth & Adolescence* 43:1151–1162.

Cummings, Thomas G., and Cary L. Cooper. 1998. "A Cybernetic Theory of Organizational Stress." Pp. 101–121 in *Theories of Organizational Stress*, edited by Cary L. Cooper. Oxford, UK: Oxford University Press.

Cummins, Robert A., Richard Eckersley, Julie Pallant, Jackie van Vugt, and Roseanne Misajon. 2003. "Developing a National Index of Subjective Wellbeing: The Australian Unity." *Social Indicators Research* 64:159–190.

Cundiff, Jenny M., Timothy W. Smith, Jonathan Butner, Kenneth L. Critchfield, and Jill Nealey-Moore. 2015. "Affiliation and Control in Marital Interaction Interpersonal Complementarity Is Present but Is Not Associated with Affect or Relationship Quality." *Personality & Social Psychology Bulletin* 41(1):35–51.

Curl, Angela L., and Jerry G. Ingram. 2013 "Anticipatory Socialization for Retirement: A Multilevel Dyadic Model." *Clinical Gerontologist* 36(4):375–393.

Curley, Alexandra M. 2005. "Theories of Urban Poverty and Implications for Public Housing Policy." *Journal of Sociology & Social Welfare* 32(2):97–119.

Curley, Alexandra M. 2010. "Relocating the Poor: Social Capital and Neighborhood Resources." *Journal of Urban Affairs* 32(1):79–103

Currie, Janet, and Jeffrey Grozer. 2001. *Explaining Recent Declines in Food Stamp Program Participation*. Los Angeles, CA: University of California at Los Angeles \.

Curry, Oliver Scott, Lee A. Rowland, Caspar J. Van Lissa, Sally Zlotowitz, John McAlaney, and Harvey Whitehouse. 2018. "Happy to Help? A Systematic Review and Meta-Analysis of the Effects of Performing Acts of Kindness on the Well-Being of the Actor." *Journal of Experimental Social Psychology* 76:320–329.

Curtin, Nicola, Abigail J. Stewart, and Lauren E. Duncan. 2010. "What Makes the Political Personal? Openness, Personal Political Salience, and Activism." *Journal of Personality* 78(3):943–968.

Curtis, Guy J. and Serena Wee. 2021. "Are Individual Differences in Information-Processing Styles Related to Transformational Leadership? A Test of the Cognitive Experiential Leadership Model." *Frontiers in Psychology* 12:599008.

Curtis, Michael P., Anne E.B. Sales, Jean H. Sullivan, Shelly L. Gary, and Susan L. Hedrick. 2005 Satisfaction with Care among Community Residential Care Residents." *Journal of Aging & Health* 17(1):3–27.

Cutler, David M., Edward L. Glaeser, and Karen E. Norberg. 2001. "Explaining the Rise in Youth Suicide." Pp. 219–269 in *Risky Behavior among Youth: An Economic Analysis*, edited by Jonathan Gruber. Chicago, IL: University of Chicago Press.

Cutrona, Carolyn E., Daniel W. Russell, Robert M. Hessling, P. Adama, Brown, and Velma Murry. 2000. "Direct and Moderating Effects of Community Context on the Psychological Well-being of African American Women." *Journal of Personality & Social Psychology* 79(6):1088–1101.

Czajkowski, Susan M., Margaret A. Chesney, and Ashley W. Smith. 1998. "Adherence and the Placebo Effect." Pp. 515–534 in *The Handbook of Health Behavior Change*, 2nd ed., edited by Sally A Shumaker, Eleanor B. Schron, Judith K. Ockene and Wendy L. McBee. New York: Springer.

d'Astous, Alain and Dania Mouakhar-Klouz. 2022. "Self-Gift Giving and Satisfaction with Life: A Behavioural Tendency Perspective." *International Journal of Consumer Studies* 46(1):268–78.

D"Cruz, Heather, Philip Gillingham, and Sebastian Melendez. 2007. "Reflexivity, Its Meanings and Relevance for Social Work: A Critical Review of the Literature." *British Journal of Social Work* 37:73–90.

Da Costa Bizarro Morais, Diana Maria, Carla Maria Gomes Marques Faria, and Lia Paula Nogueira Sousa Fernandes. 2019. "Intergenerational Caregiving: The Role of Attachment and Mental Representation of Caregiving in Filial Anxiety of Middle-Aged Children," *Journal of Intergenerational Relationships* 17(4):468–487.

Dabbagh, Therese, Dorit Roer-Strier, and Jenny Kurman. 2017. "Perspectives on Filial Responsibility among Uprooted Families from South Lebanon." *Journal of Research on Adolescence* 27(3):506–520.

Dacey, John S., and Kathleen H. Lennon. 1998. Understanding Creativity: The Interplay of Biological, Psychological, and Social Factors. San Francisco, CA: Jossey-Bass.

Dageid, Wenche, and Anette Arnesen Gronlie. 2015. "Measuring Resilience and Its Association to Social Capital among HIV-positive South Africans Living in a Context of Adversity." *Journal of Community Psychology* 43(7):832–848.

Dahlback, Olof. 2003. "A Conflict Theory of Group Risk Taking." *Small Group Research* 34(3):251–289.

Dahlum, Sirianne and Tore Wig. 2019. "Educating Demonstrators: Education and Mass Protest in Africa." *Journal of Conflict Resolution* 63(1):3–30.

Dai, David Yun, Saiying Steenbergen-Hu, and Yehan Zhou. 2015. "Cope and Grow: A Grounded Theory Approach to Early College Entrants? Lived Experiences and Changes in a STEM Program." *Gifted Child Quarterly* 59(2):75–90.

Dalbert, Claudia. 2001. The Justice Motive as a Personal Resource: Dealing with Challenges and Critical Life Events. New York, NY: Kluwer.

Dalby, P. 2006. "Is There a Process of Spiritual Change in Development Associated with Ageing? A Critical Review of Research." *Ageing & Mental Health* 10(1):4–12.

Daley, Clare. 2009. "Exploring Community Connections: Community Cohesion and Refugee Integration at a Local Level." *Community Development Journal* 44(2):158–171.

Dallago, Lorenza, Douglas D. Perkins, Massimo Santinello, Will Boyce, Michal Molcho, and Antony Morgan. 2009. "Adolescent Place Attachment, Social Capital, and Perceived Safety: A Comparison of 13 Countries." *American Journal of Community Psychology* 44(1–2):148–160.

Damasio, Bruno Figueiredo, and Silvia Helena Koller. 2015. "Complex Experiences of Meaning in Life: Individual Differences among Sociodemographic Variables, Sources of Meaning and Psychological Functioning." *Social Indicators Research* 123(1):161–181.

Daniel, Ella, Anat Bardi, Ronald Fischer, Maya Benish-Weisman and Julie A. Lee. 2022. "Changes in Personal Values in Pandemic Times." *Social Psychological & Personality Science* 13(2):572–82.

Darnell, Simon C. 2012. "Olympism in Action, Olympic Hosting and the Politics of "Sport for Development and Peace": Investigating the Development Discourses of Rio 2016." *Sport in Society* 15(6):869–87.

Dash, Genevieve F. and Kristen G. Anderson. 2015. "Marijuana Use, Motives, and Change Intentions in Adolescents." *Journal of Psychoactive Drugs* 47(2):100–06.

Datler, Georg, Wolfgang Jagodzinski, and Peter Schmidt. 2013. "Two Theories on the Test Bench: Internal and External Validity of the Theories of Ronald Inglehart and Shalom Schwartz." *Social Science Research* 42:906–925.

Davelaar, Perine M., Fabiana S. Araujo. and David A. Kipper. 2008. "The Revised Spontaneity Assessment Inventory (Sai-R): Relationship to Goal Orientation, Motivation, Perceived Self-Efficacy, and Self-Esteem." *Arts in Psychotherapy* 35(2):117–28.

Davey, Gareth, Zhenghui Chen, and Anna Lau. 2009. "Peace in a Thatched Hut--That is Happiness: Subjective Wellbeing among Peasants in Rural China." *Journal of Happiness Studies* 10:239–252.

Davey, Gareth. 2012. "Happiness and Quality of Life in the People's Republic of China." Pp. 57–73 in *Happiness across Cultures*, edited by H. Selin and Gareth Davey. New York: Springer.

Davidson, Elsa. 2008. "Marketing the Self: The Politics of Aspiration among Middle-class Silicon Valley Youth." *Environment & Planning A* 40:2814–2830.

Davidson, Oranit B, David B. Feldman, and Malka Margalit. 2012. "A Focused Intervention for 1st-Year College Students: Promoting Hope, Sense of Coherence, and Self-Efficacy." *Journal of Psychology* 146(3):333–352.

Davies, Bleddyn, Andrew Bebbington, and Helen Charnley. 1990. Resources, Needs, and Outcomes in Community-based Care: A Comparative Study of the Production of Welfare for Elderly People in Ten Local Authorities in England and Wales. Aldershot, UK: Avebury.

Davies, Dilys, and Dinesh Bhugra. 2004. *Models of Psychopathology*. Maidenhead, UK: Open University Press.

Davis, Cindy, Catherine Tang, and Janet Ko. 1998. "Exploring Current Behaviors and Social Service Needs for Chinese Juvenile Delinquents in Hong Kong." *Children and Youth Services Review* 20(8):733–745.

Davis, Darren W., and Christian Davenport. 1999. "Assessing the Validity of the Postmaterialism Index." *American Political Science Review* 93(3):649–664.

Davis, Darren, and Kathleen M. Dooley. 1999. "Postmaterialism in World Societies: Is It Really a Value Dimension?" *American Journal of Political Science* 43(3):935–962.

Davis, Laurel, and Rebecca J. Shlafer. 2016. "Mental Health of Adolescents with Currently and Formerly Incarcerated Parents." *Journal of Adolescence* 54:120–134.

Davis, Mark S., Valerie J. Callanan, David D. Lester, and Janet Haines. 2009. "An Inquiry into Relationship Suicides and Reciprocity." *Suicide & Life-Threatening Behavior* 39(5):482–498.

Davis, Nancy J. and Robert V. Robinson. 1999. "Their Brothers" Keepers' Orthodox Religionists, Modernists, and Economic Justice in Europe." *American Journal of Sociology* 104(6):1631–65.

Davis, Tommy III, and Vera S. Paster. 2000. "Nurturing Resilience in Early Adolescence." *Journal of College Student Psychotherapy* 15(2):17–33.

Davis, William Eric. 2006. *Peace and Prosperity in an Age of Incivility*. Lanham, MD: University Press of America.

Davis-Lipman, Angelina, Tom R. Tyler, and Susan M. Andersen. 2007. "Building Community One Relationship at a Time: Consequences for the Seeking and Acceptance of Help." *Social Justice Research* 20(2):187–206.

Davydov, Dmitry M. Robert Stewart, Karen Ritchie, Isabelle Chaudieu. 2010. "Resilience and Mental Health." *Clinical Psychology Review* 30(5):479–495.

Dawson, Kevin M., Kimberly E. O'Brien. and Terry A. Beehr. 2016. "The Role of Hindrance Stressors in the Job Demand-Control-Support Model of Occupational Stress: A Proposed Theory Revision." *Journal of Organizational Behavior* 37(3):397–415.

Day, James. 2010. "Religion, Spirituality, and Positive Psychology in Adulthood: A Developmental View." *Journal of Adult Development* 17(4):215–229.

Day, Jennifer. 2013. Effects of Involuntary Residential Relocation on Household Satisfaction in Shanghai, China." *Urban Policy & Research* 31(1):93–117.

Dbaibo, Dania, Charles Harb, and Nathalie Van Meurs. 2010. "Values and Justice as Predictors of Perceived Stress in Lebanese Organisational Settings." *Applied Psychology* 59(4):701–20.

de Beer, Paul, and Ferry Kostere. 2009. Sticking Together or Falling Apart? Solidarity in an Era of Individualization and Globalization. Amsterdam, Netherlands: Amsterdam University Press.

De Bruyn, Eddy H., and Dymphna C. van den Boom. 2005. "Interpersonal Behavior, Peer Popularity, and Self-esteem in Early Adolescence." *Social Development* 1494).555–573.

de Bruyn, Eddy H., Maja Dekovic, and G. Wim Meijnen. 2003. "Parenting Goal Orientations, Classroom Behavior, and School Success in Early Adolescence." *Applied Developmental Psychology* 24:393–412.

De Carlo, Alessandro, Damiano Girardi, Alessandra Falco, Laura Dal Corso, and Annamaria Di Sipio. 2019. "When Does Work Interfere with Teachers' Private Life? An Application of the Job Demands-Resources Model." *Frontiers in Psychology* 10:1121.

de Castro Rodrigues, Andreia and Ana Sacau. 2015. "Judges" Perception on Causes of Criminality and Justifications for Crime." *European Journal of Probation* 7(2):124–42.

de Coster, Stacy. 2005. "Depression and Law Violation: Gendered Responses to Gendered Stresses." *Sociological Perspectives* 48(2):155–187.

de Courville Nicol, Valerie. 2011. Social Economies of Fear and Desire: Emotional Regulation, Emotion Management, and Embodied Autonomy. New York, NY: Palgrave. (BF575.F2C58)

De Graaf, Nan Dirk. 2013. "Secularization: Theoretical Controversies Generating Empirical Research." Pp. 322–354 in *The Handbook of Rational Choice Social Research*, edited by Rafael Wittek, Tom A. H. Snijders, and Victor Nee. Stanford, CA: Stanford University Press.

de Groot, Judith I.M., and Linda Steg. 2009. "Morality and Prosocial Behavior: The Role of Awareness, Responsibility, and Norms in the Norm Activation Model." *Journal of Social Psychology* 149(4):425–449.

De Haan, Laura G., and John Schulenberg. 1997. "The Covariation of Religion and Politics during the Transition to Young Adulthood: Challenging Global Identity Assumptions." *Journal of Adolescence* 20:537–552.

de Henestrosa, Martha Fernandez, Philipp E. Sischka, and Georges Steffgen. 2023. "Examining the Challenge-Hindrance-Threat Distinction of Job Demands Alongside Job Resources." *Frontiers in Psychology* 14:1011815.

de Jong, M. G., R. Pieters, and S. Stremersch. 2012. "Analysis of Sensitive Questions across Cultures: An Application of Multigroup Item Randomized Response Theory to Sexual Attitudes and Behavior." *Journal of Personality & Social Psychology* 103(3):543–64.

de la Haye, Kayla, Harold D. Green, Jr., Michael S. Pollard, David P. Kennedy, and Joan S. Tucker. 2015. "Befriending Risky Peers: Factors Driving Adolescents' Selection of Friends with Similar Marijuana Use." *Journal of Youth and Adolescence* 44(10):1914–1928.

de Lira, Aline Nogueira and Normanda Araujo de Morais. 2020. "Processes of Resilience Experienced by Families Composed of Same-Sex Couples." *Trends in Psychology* 28(2):249–69.

De Moortel, Deborah, Laia Palenciab, Lucia Artazcoz, Carme Borrell, and Christophe Vanroelen. 2015. "Neo-Marxian Social Class Inequalities in the Mental Well-Being of Employed Men and Women: The Role of European Welfare Regimes." *Social Science & Medicine* 128:188–200.

De Moulin, Donald F. 1993. "Re-conceptualizing the Self-efficacy Paradigm: Analysis of an Eight-year Study." *Education* 114(2):167–199.

De Silva, Mary J., Trudy Harpham, Tran Tuan, Rosario Bartolini, Mary E. Penny, and Sharon R. Hutty. 2006. "Psychometric and Cognitive Validation of a Social Capital Measurement Tool in Peru and Vietnam." *Social Science & Medicine* 22:941–953.

De Smedt, R. H., T. Jaarsma, A. V. Ranchor, K. van der Meer, K. H. Groenier, F. M. Haaijer-Ruskamp, and P. Denig. 2012. "Coping with Adverse Drug Events in Patients with Heart Failure: Exploring the Role of Medication Beliefs and Perceptions." *Psychology & Health* 27(5):570–87.

de Soysa, Indra. 2011. "The Hidden Hard Wrestles Rebellion: Theory and Evidence on How Economic Freedom Prevents Civil Violence." *Studies in Ethnicity & Nationalism* 11(2):285–297.

De Vos, Jan. 2010. "Christopher Lasch's *The Culture of Narcissism*: The Failure of a Critique of Psychological Politics." *Theory & Psychology* 20(4):528–548.

de Vries, Brian, and David Megathlin. 2009. "The Meaning of Friendship for Gay Men and Lesbians in the Second Half of Life." *Journal of GLBT Family Studies* 5(1–2):82–98.

DeBar, Lynn L., G. Terence Wilson, Bobbi Jo Yarborough, Beryl Burns, Barbara Oyler, Tom Hildebrandt, Gregory N. Clarke, John Dickerson, and Ruth H. Striegel. 2013. "Cognitive Behavioral Treatment for Recurrent Binge Eating in Adolescent Girls: A Pilot Trial." *Cognitive & Behavioral Practice* 20(2):147–161.

Debus, Maike E., Charlotte Fritz, and Michel Philipp. 2019. "A Story of Gains and Losses: Intra-Individual Shifts in Job Characteristics and Well-Being When Transitioning to a Managerial Role." *Journal of Business & Psychology* 34(5):637–655.

Deci, Edward L., Jennifer G. La Guardia, Arlen C. Moller, Marc J. Scheiner, and Richard M. Ryan. 2006. "On the Benefits of Giving as Well as Receiving Autonomy Support: Mutuality in Close Friendships." *Personality & Social Psychology Bulletin* 32(3):313–327.

Decuyper, Aron, Hanne Tack, Bénédicte Vanblaere, Mathea Simons, and Ruben Vanderlinde. 2023. "Collaboration and Shared Responsibility in Team Teaching: A Large-Scale Survey Study." *Education Sciences* 13(9):896.

Deeg, Richard. 2007. "Complementarity and Institutional Change in Capitalist Systems." *Journal of European Public Policy* 14(4):611–630.

Deemer, Eric D., Jessi L. Smith, and Dustin B. Thoman. 2014. "Precision in Career Motivation Assessment: Testing the Subjective Science Attitude Change Measures." *Journal of Career Assessment* 22(3):489–504.

Defoe, Ivy N., David P. Farrington, and Rolf Loeber. 2013. "Disentangling the Relationship Between Delinquency and Hyperactivity, Low Achievement, Depression, and Low Socioeconomic Status: Analysis of Repeated Longitudinal Data." *Journal of Criminal Justice* 41(2):100–107.

Defoe, Ivy N., Judith Semon Dubas, Bernd Figner, Marcel A. G.. van Aken. 2015. "A Meta-Analysis on Age Differences in Risky Decision Making: Adolescents versus Children and Adults." *Psychological Bulletin* 141(1):48–84.

Degenne, Alain, Marie-Odile Lebeaux, and Yannick Lemel. 2004. "Does Social Capital Offset Social and Economic Inequalities?" Social Capital in Everyday Life." Pp. 51–73 in *Creation and Returns of Social Capital: A New Research Program*, edited by Henk Flap and Beate Volker. London: Routledge.

DeGolyer, Michael E. 2001. "Conditional Citizenship: Hong Kong People's Attitudes toward the New Motherland." *Citizenship Studies* 5(2):165–183.

Dehejia, Rajeev Thomas DeLeire, Erzo F.P. Luttmer, and Josh Mitchell. 2009. "The Role of Religious and Social Organizations in the Lives of Disadvantaged Youth." Pp. 237–274 in *The Problems of Disadvantaged Youth: An Economic Perspective*, edited by Jonathan Gruber. Chicago, IL: University of Chicago Press.

Dekker, Henk, Darina Malova, Sander Heogendoorn. 2003. "Nationalism and Its Explanations." *Political Psychology* 24(2):345–376.

Dekkers, Gijs J.M. 2008. "Are You Unhappy? Then You Are Poor? Multi dimensional Poverty in Belgium." *International Journal of Sociology & Social Policy* 28(11/12):502–545.

Delang, Claudio O., and Ho Cheuk Lung. 2010. "Public Housing and Poverty Concentration in Urban Neighbourhoods: The Case of Hong Kong in the 1990s." *Urban Studies* 47(7):1391–1413.

Delanty, Gerard. 2008. "Fear of Others: Social Exclusion and the European Crisis of Solidarity." *Social Policy & Administration* 42(6):676–690.

Delanty, Gerard. 2009. *The Cosmopolitan Imagination: The Renewal of Critical Social Theory*. Cambridge, UK: Cambridge University Press.

Delgado, Melvin, and Lee Staples. 2008. *Youth-led Community Organizing: Theory and Action*. New York: Oxford University Press.

Delhey, Jan, and Kenneth Newton. 2005. "Predicting Cross-national Levels of Social Trust: Global Pattern or Nordic Exceptionalism?" *European Sociological Review* 21(4):311–327.

Delhey, Jan. 2010. "From Materialist to Post-materialist Happiness? National Affluence and Determinants of Life Satisfaction in Cross-national Perspective." *Social Indicators Research* 97:65–84.

DeLue, Steven M., and Timothy M. Dale. 2009. *Political Thinking, Political Theory, and Civil Society*. New York: Pearson.

DeMarree, Kenneth G. and Kimberly Rios. 2014. "Understanding the Relationship between Self-Esteem and Self-Clarity: The Role of Desired Self-Esteem." *Journal of Experimental Social Psychology* 50(1):202–09.

Demerath, Nicholas J., III. 2002. "A Sinner among the Saints. Confessions of a Sociologist of Culture and Religion." *Sociological Forum* 17(1):1–19.

Demerouti, Evangelia, Akihito Shimazu, Arnold B. Bakker, Kyoko Shimada, and Norito Kawakami. 2013. "Work-Self Balance: A Longitudinal Study on the Effects of Job Demands and Resources on Personal Functioning in Japanese Working Parents." *Work & Stress* 27(3).223–43.

Demertzis, Nicolas. 2020. *The Political Sociology of Emotions: Essays on Trauma and Ressentiment*. Abingdon, UK: Routledge.

DeNeve, Kristina M., and Harris Cooper. 1998. "The Happy Personality: A Meta-analysis of 137 Personality Traits and Subjective Well-being." *Psychological Bulletin* 124(2):197–229.

Denissen, Jaap J.A., Lars Penke, David P. Schmitt, and Marcel A.G. van Aken. 2008. "Self-esteem Reactions to Social Interactions: Evidence for Sociometer Mechanisms across Days, People, and Nations." *Journal of Personality & Social Psychology* 95(1):181–196.

Dennis, Jessica M., Jean S. Phinney, and Lizette Ivy Chuateco. 2005. "The Role of Motivation, Parental Support, and Peer Support in the Academic Success of Ethnic Minority First-generation College Students." *Journal of College Student Development* 46(3):223–236.

Denson, Nida and Nicholas Bowman. 2015. "The Development and Validation of an Instrument Assessing Student-Institution Fit." *Assessment & Evaluation in Higher Education* 40(8):1104–22.

Denver, David, and Gordon Hands. 1990. "Does Studying Politics Make a Difference? The Political Knowledge, Attitudes and Perceptions of School Students." *British Journal of Political Science* 20:263–288.

Deptula, Daneen P., and Robert Cohen. 2004. "Aggressive, Rejected, and Delinquent Children and Adolescents: A Comparison for Their Friendships." *Aggression & Violent Behavior* 9:75–104.

Derella, Olivia J., Jeffrey D Burke, Ari M Romano-Verthelyi, Emilie J Butler, and Oliver G Johnston. 2020. "Feasibility and acceptability of a brief cognitive-behavioral group intervention for chronic irritability in youth." *Clinical Child Psychology & Psychiatry.*

DeScioli, Peter and Robert Kurzban. 2009. "The Alliance Hypothesis for Human Friendship." *PLoS ONE* 4(6):e5802–e02.

Dess, Gregory g., and Steve Sauerwald. 2014. "Creating Values in Organizations: The Vital Role of Social Capital." *Organizational Dynamics* 43:1–8.

Detenber, Benjamin H., Shirley S. Ho, Rachel L. Neo, Shelly Malik, and Mark Cenite. 2013. "Influence of Value Predispositions, Interpersonal Contact, and Mediated Exposure on Public Attitudes toward Homosexuals in Singapore." *Asian Journal of Social Psychology* 16(3):181–96.

Devine, Joel A., Charles J. Brody, and James D. Wright. 1997. "Evaluating an Alcohol and Drug Treatment Program for the Homeless: An Econometric Approach." *Evaluation & Program Planning* 20(2):205–215.

Devos, Thierry, Dario Spini, and Shalom H. Schwartz. 2002. "Conflicts among Human Values and Trust in Institutions." *British Journal of Social Psychology* 41:481–494.

Dew, Jeffrey, Sonya Britt, and Sandra Huston. 2012. "Examining the Relationship between Financial Issues and Divorce." *Family Relations* 61(4):615–28.

Dhal, Espen, Tone Flotten, and Thomas Lorentzen. 2008. "Poverty Dynamics and Social Exclusion: An Analysis of Norwegian Panel Data." *Journal of Social Policy* 37(2):231–249.

Di Fabio, Annamaria, and Maureen E. Kenny. 2015. "The Contributions of Emotional Intelligence and Social Support for Adaptive Career Progress among Italian Youth." *Journal of Career Development* 42(1):48–59.

Diamond, Lisa M., and Karen L. Blair. 2018. "the Intimate Relationships of Sexual and Gender Minorities." Pp. 199–210 in *The Cambridge Handbook of Personal Relationships*, edited by Anita L. Vangelisti and Daniel Perlman. Cambridge, UK: Cambridge University Press.

Diekman, Amanda B., and Monica C. Schneider. 2010. "A Social Role Theory Perspective On Gender Gaps In Political Attitudes." *Psychology of Women Quarterly* 34:486–497.

Diener, Ed, and Frank Fujita. 1995. "Resources, Personal Strivings, and Subjective Well-being: A Nomothetic and Idiographic Approach." *Journal of Personality & Social Psychology* 68(5):926–935.

Diener, Ed, Richard E. Lucas, Ulrich Schimmack, and John F. Helliwell. 2009. *Well-being for Public Policy*. Oxford, UK: Oxford University Press.

Diener, Ed., and Richard E. Lucas. 1999. "Personality and Subjective Well-being." Pp. 213–229 in *Well-being: The Foundations of Hedonic Psychology*, edited by Daniel Kahneman, Ed Diener and Norbert Schwarz. New York: Russell Sage.

Dietrich, Julia, and Barbel Kracke. 2009. "Career-specific Parental Behaviors in Adolescents" Development." *Journal of Vocational Behavior* 75:109–119.

Difonzo, Nicholas. 2019. "Conspiracy Rumor Psychology." Pp. 257–268 in *Conspiracy Theories and the People Who Believe Them*, edited by Joseph E. Uscinski. New York, NY: Oxford University Press.

DiGiuseppe, Raymond, Russell Leaf, Bernard Gorman, and Mitchell W. Robin. 2017. "The Development of a Measure of Irrational/Rational Beliefs." *Journal of Rational-Emotive & Cognitive-Behavior Therapy* 36(1):47–79.

Dik, Bryan J., Ryan D. Duffy, and Michael F. Steger. 2012. "Enhancing Social Justice by Promoting Prosocial Values in Career Development Interventions." *Counseling & Values* 57(1):31–37.

Dillard, James Price. 2004. "The goals-plans-action Model of Interpersonal Influence." Pp. 185–206 in *Perspectives and Persuasion, Social Influence, and Compliance Gaining*, edited by John S. Seiter and Robert H. Gass. Boston, MA: Pearson.

Dillard, James, Price. 2015. "Goals-plan-action Theory of Message Production: Making Influence Messages." Pp. 63–74 in *Engaging Theories in Interpersonal Communication: Multiple Perspectives*, edited by Dawn O. Braithwaite and Paul Schrodt. Thousand Oaks, CA: SAGE.

Dilts, Andrew. 2017. "Justice as Failure." *Law, Culture & the Humanities* 13(2):184–92.

Dinerstein, Ana Cecilia. 2010. "Autonomy in Latin America: between Resistance and Integration. Echoes from the Piqueteros Experience." *Community Development Journal* 45(3):356–366.

Dinesen, Peter Thisted, and Kim Mannemar Sønderskov. 2015. "Ethnic Diversity and Social Trust Evidence from the Micro-Context." *American Sociological Review* 80(3):550–573.

Dinic, Bojana M. and Bojana Bodroza. 2021. "COVID-19 Protective Behaviors Are Forms of Prosocial and Unselfish Behaviors." *Frontiers in Psychology* 12:647710.

Dioale, William and Albert Seda. 2001. "Modernization as Changes in Cultural Complexity: New Cross-cultural Measurements." *Cross-Cultural Research* 35(2):129–153.

DiPrete, Thomas A., Dominique Goux, Eric Maurin, and Michael Tahlin. 2001. "Institutional Determinants of Employment Chances: The Structure of Unemployment in France and Sweden." *European Sociological Review* 17(3):233–254.

Dishon, Gideon. 2018. "Citizenship Education through the Pragmatist Lens of Habit." *Journal of Philosophy of Education* 52(3):483–97.

Distante, Roberta. 2013. "Subjective Well-being, Income and Relative Concerns in the UK." *Social Indicators Research* 113:81–105.

Dittman, Joerg, and Jan Goebel. 2010. "Your House Your Car, Your Education. The Socioeconomic Situation of the Neighborhood and Its Impact on Life Satisfaction in Germany." *Social Indicators Research* 96:497–513.

Doane, Leah D., Susan Mineka, Richard E. Zinbarg, Michelle Craske, and James W. Griffith. 2013. "Are Flatter Diurnal Cortisol Rhythms Associated with Major Depression and Anxiety Disorders in Late Adolescence? The Role of Life Stress and Daily Negative Emotion." *Development & Psychopathology* 25(3):629–642.

Doane, Woody. 2017. "Humanist Sociology." Pp. 322–329 in *The Cambridge Handbook of Sociology, Vol. 2: Specialty and Interdisciplinary Studies*, edited by Kathleen Odell Korgen. New York, NY: Cambridge University Press.

Dobson, Wendy L., and Paul T.P. Wong. 2008. "Women Living with HIV: The Role of Meaning and Spirituality." Pp. 173–207 in *Existential and Spiritual Issues in Death Attitudes*, edited by Adrian Tomer, Grafton T. Eliason and Paul T.P. Wong. New York: Lawrence Erlbaum.

Dodge, Tonya, and James Jaccard. 2002. "Participation in Athletics and Female Sexual Risk Behavior: The Evaluation of Four Causal Structures." *Journal of Adolescent Research* 17(1):42–67.

Dolinski, Dariusz. 2016. Techniques of Social Influence: The Psychology of Gaining Compliance. Hove, UK: Routledge.

Domeier, Markus et al. 2018. "Motivational Reasons for Biased Decisions: The Sunk-cost Effect's Instrumental Rationality." *Frontier in Psychology* 9:815.

Dominguez, Daniela G., Monte Bobele, Jacqueline Coppock, and Pea Ezequiel. 2015. "LGBTQ Relationally Based Positive Psychology: An Inclusive and Systemic Framework." *Psychological Services* 12(2):177–185.

Dominguez, Patricio, and Steven Raphael. 2015. "The Role of the Cost-of-Crime Literature in Bridging the Gap Between Social Science Research and Policy Making Potentials and Limitations." *Criminology & Public Policy* 14(4):589–632.

Donahue, Michael J., 1985. "Intrinsic and Extrinsic Religiousness: Review and Meta-analysis." *Journal of Personality & Social Psychology* 48(2):400–419.

Donald, William E., Yehuda Baruch, and Melanie Ashleigh. 2019. "The Undergraduate Self-Perception of Employability: Human Capital, Careers Advice, and Career Ownership." *Studies in Higher Education* 44(4):599–614.

Donaldson, Stewart I., John W. Graham, and William B. Hansen. 1994. "Testing the Generalizability of Intervening Mechanism Theories: Understanding the Effects of Adolescent Drug Use Prevention Intervention." *Journal of Behavioral Medicine* 17(2):195–216.

Donati, Pierpaolo, and Margaret S. Archer. 2015. *The Relational Subject*. Cambridge, UK: Cambridge University Press.

Dong, Zhiying. 1998. Development of Elderly Resources and Modern Civilized Society. Beijing, China: Economic Management.

Donnellan, M. Brent, Kali H. Trzesniewski, Richard W. Robins, Terrie E. Moffitt, and Avshalon Caspi. 2005. "Low Self-esteem Is Related to Aggression, Antisocial Behavior, and Delinquency." *Psychological Science* 16(4):328–335.

Donnellan, M. Brent, Monica J. Martin, Katherine J. Conger, and Rand D. Conger. 2013. "Economic Distress and Poverty in Families." Pp. 338–355 in *Handbook of Family Theories: A Content-based Approach*, edited by Mark A. Fine and Frank D. Fincham. New York: Routledge.

Donnelly, Gabrielle. 2013. "Reading the Signs of the Times: Centering Religion and Development." *Canadian Journal of Developmental Studies* 34(2):189–202.

Donohoe, Gill, and Tom Ricketts. 2012a. "Anxiety and Panic." Pp. 431–439 in *The SAGE Handbook of Counselling and Psychotherapy*, edited by Colin Feltham and Ian Horton. London: SAGE.

Dorahy, Martin J., Christopher Alan Lewis, Robert G. Millar, and Travis L. Gee. 2003. "Predictors of Nonpathological Dissociation in Northern Ireland: The Affects of Trauma and Exposure to Political Violence." *Journal of Traumatic Stress* 16(6):611–615.

Dorff, Cassy. 2017. "Violence, Kinship Networks, and Political Resilience: Evidence from Mexico." *Journal of Peace Research* 54(4):558–573.

Dorjee, Tenzin. 2013. "Intercultural and Intergroup Conflict Resolution: Nonviolence and Middle Way Approaches." Pp. 687–711 in *The SAGE Handbook of Conflict Communication,* edited by John G. Oetzel and Stelle Ting-Toomey. Thousand Oaks, CA: SAGE.

Dost-Gozkan, Ayfer. 2019. "Adolescents" Conflict Resolution with Their Parents and Best Friends: Links to Life Satisfaction." *Journal of Child & Family Studies* 28(10):2854–66.

Dou, Diya, Daniel T. L. Shek, Lindan Tan, and Li Zhao. 2023. "Family Functioning and Resilience in Children in Mainland China: Life Satisfaction as a Mediator." *Frontiers in Psychology* 14:1175934.

Doucete, Patrica A. 2004. "Walk and Talk: An Intervention for Behaviorally Challenged Youths." *Adolescence* 39(154):373–388.

Dougherty, Lea R. 2006. "Children's Emotionality and Social Status: A Meta-analysis Review." *Social Development* 15(3):394–417.

Douglas, Emily M. 2006. "Familial Violence Socialization in Childhood and Later Life Approval of Corporal Punishment: A Cross-cultural Perspective." *American Journal of Orthopsychiatry* 76(10:23–30.

Doumas, Michail, and Ralf Th. Krampe. 2015. "Ecological Relevance Determines Task Priority in Older Adults¡¯ Multitasking." *Journals of Gerontology, Series B: Psychological Sciences & Social Sciences* 70(3):377–385.

Dovidio, John F., Jane Allyn Piliavin, David Al Schroeder, and Louis A. Penner. 2006. *The Social Psychology of Prosocial Behavior*. Mahwah, NJ: Lawrence Erlbaum. (HM1140.S63)

Downey, Douglas B., and James W. Ainsworth-Darnell. 2002. "the Search for Oppositional Culture among Black Students." *American Sociological Review* 63:156–164.

Downie, Michelle, Genevieve A. Mageau, and Richard Koestner. 2008. "What Makes for Pleasant Social Interaction? Motivational Dynamics of Interpersonal Relations." *Journal of Social Psychology* 148(5):523–534.

Drake, David. 2018. "Narrative Coaching." Pp. 109–123 in *The Complete Handbook of Coaching*, edited by Elaine Cox, Tatiana Bachkirova, and David Clutterbuck. London, UK: SAGE.

Draper, Thomas W., and Thomas B. Holman. 2005. "Locating the Big Five Personality Factors in the Relate Relationship Evaluation Measures." *Psychological Reports* 97(3):877–886.

Dregan, Alex and David Armstrong. 2009. "Age, Cohort and Period Effects in the Prevalence of Sleep Disturbances among Older People: The Impact of Economic Downturn." *Social Science & Medicine* 69(10):1432–38.

Drezner, Noah D. 2013. "The Black Church and Millennial Philanthropy: Influences on College Student Prosocial Behaviors at a Church-Affiliated Black College." *Christian Higher Education* 12(5):363–382.

Drinkard, Allyson M., Nicolle Estevez, and Richard E. Adams. 2017. "Social Development Assets and Law-Abidingness among Urban Adolescents: Implications for Positive Youth Development." *Journal of Community Psychology* 45(3):363–79.

Droutman, Vita, Ilana Golub, Ani Oganesyan, and Stephen Read. 2018. "Development and Initial Validation of the Adolescent and Adult Mindfulness Scale (AAMS)." *Personality & Individual Differences* 123:34–43.

Drummond, Holli John M. Bolland, and Waverly Ann Harris. 2011. "Becoming Violent: Evaluating the Mediating Effect of Hopelessness on the Code of the Street Thesis." *Deviant Behavior* 32(3):191–223.

Dryden, Windy. 2003. Fundamentals of Rational Emotive Behavior Therapy: A Training Handbook. London: Whurr.

Duan, Wenjie and He Bu. 2019. "Randomized Trial Investigating of a Single-Session Character-Strength-Based Cognitive Intervention on Freshman's Adaptability." *Research on Social Work Practice* 29(1):82–92.

Dubar, Royette T., Nicole K. Watkins, and Grant C. Hill. 2021. "Examining the Direction of Effects between Covid-19 Experiences, General Well-Being, Social Media Engagement, and Insomnia Symptoms among University Students." *Emerging Adulthood* 9(6):655–69.

Duberstein, P. R., Y. Conwell, K. R. Conner, S. Eberly, J. S. Evinger, and E. D. Caine. 2004. "Poor Social Integration and Suicide: Fact or Artifact? A Case-control Study." *Psychological Medicine* 34:1331–1337.

Dubovska, Eva., Vladimír Chrz, Peter Tavel, Iva. Poláčková Šolcová, and Jiří Ruzicka. 2017. "Narrative Construction of Resilience: Stories of Older Czech Adults." *Ageing & Society* 37(9):1849–73.

Dufur, Mikaela J. Toby L. Parcel, and Benjamin A. McKune. 2013. "Does Capital at Home Matter More than Capital at School? The Case of Adolescent Alcohol and Marijuana Use." *Journal of Drug Issues* 43(1):85–102.

Duignan, Kieran. 2007. "Conversational Learning: Applying Personal Construct Psychology in Coaching." Pp. 229–252 in *Handbook of Coaching Psychology: A Guide for Practitioners*, edited by Stephen Palmer and Alison Whybrow. Hove, UK: Routledge.

Duncan, Greg J., Rachel E. Dunifon, Morgan B. Ward Doran, and W. Jean Yeung. 2001. "How Different Are Welfare and Working Families? And Do These Differences Matter for Children's Achievement?" Pp. 103–131 in *For Better and For Worse: Welfare Reform and the Well-being of Children and Families*, edited by Greg J. Duncan and P. Lindsay Chase-Lansdale. New York: Russell Sage.

Duncan, Susan C., Terry E. Duncan, and Lisa A. Strycker. 2006. "Alcohol Use from Age 9 to 16: A cohort-sequential Latent Growth Model." *Drug & Alcohol Dependence* 81:71–81.

Dunifon, Rachel, and Lori Kowaleski Jones. 2003. "The Influences of Participation in the National School Lunch Program and Food Insecurity on Child Well-being." *Social Service Review* 77:73–92.

Dunkel, Curtis S., Aaron W. Lukaszewski, and Kristine Chua. 2016. "The Relationships between Sex, Life History Strategy, and Adult Romantic Attachment Style." *Personality & Individual Differences* 98:176–178.

Dunkel-Schetter, Christine, and Tracy L. Bennett. 1990. "Differentiating the Cognitive and Behavioral Aspects of Social Support." Pp. 267–296 in *Social Support: An Interactional View*, edited by Barbara R. Sarason, Irwin G. Sarason and Gregory R. Pierce. New York: John Wiley & Sons.

Dunn, James R. 2013. "Security, Meaning, and the Home Conceptualizing Multiscalar Resilience in a Neoliberal Era." Pp. 183–205 in *Social Resilience in the Neoliberal Era*, edited by Peter A. Hall and Michele Lamont. Cambridge, UK: Cambridge University Press.

Durbin, Daniel T. 2020. "From Plato to St. Paul: Ancient Sport as Performative Public Discourse." *Journal of the Philosophy of Sport* 47(3):403–18.

Dust, Scott B., Peng Wang, and Lei Lai. 2020. "I'm Too Old for This: Time Demands and Older, Early-Career Employees" Receptivity to Supervisor Support." *Journal of Career Development* 47(2):220–236.

Dutton, Edward and J. O. A. Rayner-Hilles. 2022. *The Past Is a Future Country: The Coming Conservative Demographic Revolution*. Exeter, UK: Imprint Academic.

Dutton, Edward, Guy Madison, and Richard Lynn. 2016. "Demographic, Economic, and Genetic Factors Related to National Differences in Ethnocentric Attitudes." *Personality & Individual Differences* 101:137–143. \87–257

Duxbury, Linda, and Michael Halinski. 2018. "It's not all about Guns and Gangs: Role Overload as a Source of Stress for Male and Female Police Officers." *Policing & Society* 28(8):930–946.

Duxbury, Linda, Anne Bardoel, and Michael Halinski. 2021. "Bringing the Badge Home: Exploring the Relationship between Role Overload, Work-Family Conflict, and Stress in Police Officers." *Policing & Society* 31(8):997–1016.

Dwivedi, Chandra Bhal. 2017. "Spirituality, Culture and Resilience: A Virtue-informed Approach to Well-being." Pp. 334–345 in *The Routledge International Handbook of Psychosocial Resilience*, edited by Updesh Kumar. Abingdon, UK: Routledge.

Dworkin, Jodi B., Reed Larson, and David Hansen. 2003. "Adolescents" Accounts of Growth Experiences in Youth Activities." *Journal of Youth & Adolescence* 32(1):17–26.

Dwyer, Peter, and Irene Hardill. 2011. "Promoting Social Inclusion? The Impact of Village Services on the Lives of Older People Living in Rural England." *Ageing & Society* 31:243–264.

Dybicz, Phillip. 2011. "Interpreting the Strengths Perspective through Narrative Theory." *Families in Society* 92(3):247–53.

Dyck, Joshua J. 2012. "Racial Threat, Direct Legislation, and Social Trust." *Political Research Quarterly* 65(3):615–628.

Dy-Liacco, Gabriel S., Ralph L. Piedmont, Nichole A. Murray-Swank, Thomas E. Rodgerson, and Martin F. Sherman. 2009. "Spirituality and Religiosity as Cross-Cultural Aspects of Human Experience." *Psychology of Religion & Spirituality* 1(1):35–52.

Dynel, Marta and Fabio I. M. Poppi. 2018. "In Tragoedia Risus: Analysis of Dark Humour in Post-Terrorist Attack Discourse." *Discourse & Communication* 12(4):382–400.

Dzendolet, Ernest. 1999. "On the Theory of Behavioral Mechanics." *Psychological Reports* 85(3):707–42.

Dziengel, Lake. 2015. "A Be/Coming-Out Model: Assessing Factors of Resilience and Ambiguity." *Journal of Gay & Lesbian Social Services* 27(3):302–325.

Eagly, Alice H., Amanda B. Diekman, Mary C. Johannesen-Schmidt, and Anne M. Koenig. 2004. "Gender Gaps in Sociopolitical Attitudes: A Social Psychological Analysis." *Journal of Personality & Social Psychology* 87(6):796–816.

Eaton, William W., Carles Muntaner, Gregory Bovasso, and Corey Smith. 2001. "Socioeconomic Status and Depression Syndrome: The Role of Inter- and Intra-generational Mobility: Government Assistance and Work Environment." *Journal of Health & Social Behavior* 42:277–294.

Eatough, Virginia, Jonathan A. Smith, and Rachel Shaw. 2008. "Women, Anger, and Aggression: An Interpretative Phenomenological Analysis." *Journal of Interpersonal Violence* 23(12):1767–1799.

Eayrs, Caroline B., and Nick Ellis. 1990. "Charity Advertising: For or against People with a Mental Handicap?" *British Journal of Social Psychology* 29:349–360.

Eayrs, Caroline B., Nick Ellis, and Robert S.P. Jones. 1993. "Which Label? An Investigation into the Effect of Terminology on Public Perceptions of and Attitudes towards People with Learning Difficulties." *Disability, Handicap & Society* 8(2):111–127.

Eberl, Andreas. 2020. "The Effect of Informal Caregiving on Social Capital Investments." *Social Science Research* 85:102319.

Ebner, Katharina, Roman Soucek, and Simone Kauffeld. 2020. "Incongruities between Values, Motives, and Skills: Exploring Negative Effects of Self-Exploration in Career Coaching." *British Journal of Guidance & Counselling* 48(4):454–76.

Eccles, Jacquelynne S., and Bonnie L. Barber. 1999. "Student Council, Volunteering, Basketball, or Marching Band: What Kind of Extracurricular Involvement Matters?" *Journal of Adolescent Research* 14(1):10–43.

Eccles, Jacquelynne, and Jennifer Appleton Gootman. 2002. *Community Programs to Promote Youth Development*. Washington, DC: National Academy.

Ecclestone, Kathryn, and John Field. 2003. "Promoting Social Capital in a "Risk Society": A New Approach to Emancipatory Learning or a New Moral Authoritarianism?" *British Journal of Sociology of Education* 24(3):267–282.

Echezarraga, A., E. Calvete, A. M. González-Pinto, and C. Las Hayas. 2018. "Resilience Dimensions and Mental Health Outcomes in Bipolar Disorder in a Follow-up Study." *Stress & Health* 34(1):115–26.

Edara, Inna Reddy. 2021. "Role of Social, Civic, and Governance Aspects in Life Satisfaction and Psychological Distress: Insights from Taiwan." *Current Psychology*. 41(12):8668–77

Eddy, J. Mark, Jean Schumer, Joann Wu Shortt, Deborah M. Caldi, Stacey S. Tiberio, and Sabina Low. 2018. "A Life-course Model for the Development of Intimate Partner Violence." Pp. 52–64 *The Cambridge Handbook of Violent Behavior and Aggression*, edited by Alexander T. Vazsonyi, David J. Flannery and Matt DeLisi. Cambridge, UK: Cambridge University Press.

Edgerton, Jason, Tracey Peter, and Lance W. Roberts. 2008. "Back to the Basics: Socio-economic, Gender, and Regional Disparities in Canada." *Canadian Journal of Education* 31(4):861–888.

Edney, Kingsley. 2012. "Soft Power and the Chinese Propaganda System." *Journal of Contemporary China* 21(78):899–914.

Edwards, Jeffrey R., Robert D. Caplan, and R. Van Harrison. 1998. "Person-environment Fit Theory: Conceptual Foundations, Empirical Evidence, and Directions for Future Research." Pp. 28–67 in *Theories of Organizational Stress*, edited by Cary L. Cooper. Oxford, UK: Oxford University Press.

Edwards, Pearce and Daniel Arnon. 2021. "Violence on Many Sides: Framing Effects on Protest and Support for Repression." *British Journal of Political Science* 51(2):488–506.

Egan, Gerard. 2012. "The Skilled Helper Model." Pp. 372–376 in *The SAGE Handbook of Counselling and Psychotherapy*, edited by Colin Feltham and Ian Horton. London: SAGE.

Eggert, Janet, Alytia Levendosky, and Kelly Klump. 2007. "Relationships among Attachment Styles, Personality Characteristics, and Disordered Eating." *International Journal of Eating Disorders* 40(2):149–155.

Ehrensaft, Miriam K., Patricia Cohen, Jocelyn Brown, Elizabeth Smailes, Henian Chen, and Jeffrey G. Johnson. 2003. "Intergenerational Transmission of Partner Violence: A 20-year Prospective Study." *Journal of Consulting & Clinical Psychology* 71(4):741–753.

Eikemo, Terje Andreas, Arne Matekaasa, and Kristen Ringdal. 2008. "Health and Happiness." Pp. 48–64 in *Nordic Social Attitudes in a European Perspective*, edited by Heikki Ervasti, Torben Fridberg, Mikael Hjerm, and Kristen Ringdal. Cheltenham, UK: Edward Elgar.

Ein-Dor, Tsachi and Gilad Hirschberger. 2012. "Sexual Healing." *Journal of Social & Personal Relationships* 29(1):126–39.

Einhorn, Lois J. 1998. *Helen Keller: Public Speaker, Sightless but Seen, Deaf but Heard*. Westport, CT: Greenwood.

Eisenberg, Nancy, Richard A. Fabes, Ivanna K. Guthrie, and Mark Reiser. 2002. "The Role of Emotionality and Regulation in Children's Social Competence and Adjustment." Pp. 46–70 in *Paths to Successful Development: Personality in the Life Course*, edited by Lea Pulkkinen and Avshalom Caspi. Cambridge, UK: Cambridge University Press.

Eitle, Tamela McNutlty, and David J. Eitle. 2002. "Race, Cultural Capital, and the Educational Effects of Participation in Sports." *Sociology of Education* 75(2):123–146.

Ekholm, David, and Sofia Lindström Sol. 2019. "Mobilising Non-Participant Youth: Using Sport and Culture in Local Government Policy to Target Social Exclusion." *International Journal of Cultural Policy* 26(4):510–23

Elder, Todd E., and Elizabeth T. Powers. 2006. "The Incredible Shrinking Program: Trends in SSI Participation of the Aged." *Research on Aging* 28(3):341–358.

Elfenbein, Hillary Anger. 2013. "Individual Differences in Negotiation." Pp. 25–45 in *Handbook of Research on Negotiation*, edited by Mara Olekalns and Wendi L. Adair. Cheltenham, UK: Elgar.

Elfers, John, Patty Hlava, Farrah Sharpe, Sonia Arreguin, and Dawn Celeste McGregor. 2024. "Resilience and Loss: The Correlation of Grief and Gratitude." *International Journal of Applied Positive Psychology* 9(1):327–45. \110–310

Eliason, Grafton T., Jeff L. Samide, George Williams, and Mark F. Lepore. 2010. "Existential Theory and Our Search for Spirituality." *Journal of Spirituality in Mental Health* 12(2):86–111.

Elkan, Ruth, Denise Kendrick, Michael Dewey, Michael Hewitt, Jan Robinson, Mitch Blair, Deb Williams, and Kathy Brummell. 2001. Effectiveness of Home Based Support for Older People: Systematic Review and Meta Analysis." *British Medical Journal* 323(7315):719–727.

Ellemers, Naomi, and S. Alexander Haslam. 2012. "Social Identity Theory." Pp. 379–398 in *Handbook of Theories of Social Psychology* (vol. 2), edited by Paul A.M. Van Lange, Arie W. Kruglanski and E. Tory Higgins. London, CA: SAGE.

Ellingsen, Tore, and Magnus Johannesson. 2008. "Pride and Prejudice: The Human Side of Incentive Theory." *American Economic Review* 98(3):990–1008.

Elliott, Delbert S., and William Julius Wilson. 1996. "The Effects of Neighborhood Disadvantage on Adolescent Development." *Journal of Research in Crime & Delinquency* 33(4):389–416.

Elliott, Delbert S., Scott Menard, Bruce Rankin, Amanda Elliott, William Julius Wilson, and David Huizinga. 2006. *Good Kids from Bad Neighborhoods: Successful Development in Social Context*. New York: Cambridge University Press.

Elliott, Irina and Suzanne Coker. 2008. "Independent Self-Construal, Self-Reflection, and Self-Rumination: A Path Model for Predicting Happiness." *Australian Journal Of Psychology* 60(3):127–34.

Ellis, David A., and Kayleigh J. Renouf. 2018. "Predicting Fear of Crime: Personality Outperforms Prior Victimisation." *Journal of Forensic Psychiatry & Psychology* 29(3):403–418.

Ellis, Michael, and Jonathan Smith. 2012. "Gestalt Therapy." Pp. 315–319 in *The SAGE Handbook of Counselling and Psychotherapy*, edited by Colin Feltham and Ian Horton. London: SAGE.

Ellis, Robert M., 2022. *Absolutization: The Source of Dogma, Repression, and Conflict*. Sheffield, UK: Equinox.

Ellison, Christopher G., Jason D. Boardman, David R. Williams, and James S. Jackson. 2001. "Religious Involvement, Stress, and Mental Health: Findings from the 1995 Detroit Area Study." *Social Forces* 80(1):215–249.

Ellison, Nicole B., D. Yvette Wohn, and Christine M. Greenhow. 2014. "Adolescents" Visions of Their Future Careers, Educational Plans, and Life Pathways: The Role of Bridging and Bonding Social Capital Experiences." *Journal of Social & Personal Relationships* 31(4):516 –534.

Elsbach, Kimbergly D., and Greg Elofson. 2000. "How the Packaging of Decision Explanations Affects Perceptions of Trustworthiness." *Academy of Management Journal* 43(1):80–89.

Elvestad, Eiri and Arild Blekesaune. 2008. "Newspaper Readers in Europe: A Multilevel Study of Individual and National Differences." *European Journal of Communication* 23(4):425–47.

Emerson, Richard M. 1986. "Toward Theory of Value in Social Exchange." Pp. 11–46 in *Social Exchange Theory*, edited by Karen S. Cook. Newbury Park, CA: Sage.
Emery, Lydia F., Courtney Walsh, and Erica B. Slotter. 2015. "Knowing Who You Are and Adding to It." *Social Psychological & Personality Science* 6(3):259–66.
Emirbayer, Mustafa and Ann Mische. 1998. "What Is Agency?" *American Journal of Sociology* 103(4):962–1023.
Emjaian, Brian, Sarah Beth Bell, Zachary Whitt, and C. Nathan De Wall. 2018. "Social-cognitive Processes in the Development of Antisocial and Violent Behavior." Pp. 259–277 in *The Cambridge Handbook of Violent Behavior and Aggression*, edited by Alexander T. Vazsonyi, David J. Flannery and Matt DeLisi. Cambridge, UK: Cambridge University Press.
Emler, Nicholas, and Elizabeth Frazer. 1999. "Politics: The Education Effect." *Oxford Review of Education* 25(1/2):251–273.
Eneau, Jerome. 2008. "From Autonomy to Reciprocity, or Vice Versa? French Personalism's Contribution to a New Perspective on Self-Directed Learning." *Adult Education Quarterly* 58(3):229–248.
Engelstad, Fredrik. 2009. "Culture and Power." Pp. 210–238 in *The SAGE Handbook of Power*, edited by Stewart R. Clegg and Mark Haugaard. London, UK: SAGE.
Engle, Yuna, and tim Kasser. 2005. "Why Do Adolescent Girls Idolize Male Celebrities." *Journal of Adolescent Research* 20(2):263–283.
Ennett, Susan T., Vangie A. Foshee, Karl E. Bauman, Andrea Hussong, Li Cai, Heathe Reyes, Luz McNaughton, Robert Faris, John Hipp, and Robert DuRant. 2008. "The Social Ecology of Adolescent Alcohol Misuse." *Child Development* 79(6):1777–1791
Epstein, Ann S. and Christine Boisvert. 2006. "Let's Do Something Together: Identifying the Effective Components of Intergenerational Programs." *Journal of Intergenerational Relationships* 4(3):87–109.
Epstein, Seymour, Rosemary Pacini, Veronika Denes-Raj, and Harriet Heier. 1996. "Individual Differences in Intuitive-Experiential and Analytical-Rational Thinking Styles." *Journal of Personality & Social Psychology* 71(2):390–405.
Epstein, William M. 1997. *Welfare in America: How Social Service Fails the Poor*. Madison, WI: University of Wisconsin Press.
Erez, Ayelet, Mario Mikulincer, Mrinus H. van Ijzendoon, and Pieter M. Kroonenberg. 2008. "Attachment, Personality and Volunteering: Placing Volunteerism in an Attachment-theoretical Framework." *Personality & Individual Differences* 44:64–74.
Erford, Bradley T. Lauren E. Paul, Conor Oncken, Victoria E. Kress, and Matthew R. Erford. 2014. "Counseling Outcomes for Youth with Oppositional Behavior: A Meta-analysis." *Journal of Counseling & Development* 92:13–24.
Erford, Bradley T., Breann M. Erford, Gina Lattanzi Janet Weller, Hallie Schein, Emily Wolf, Meredith Hughes, Jenna Darrow, Janet Savin-Murphy, and Elizabeth Peacock. 2011. "Counseling Outcomes from 1990 to 2008 from School-age Youth with depression: A Meta-analysis." *Journal of Counseling & Development* 89:439–457.
Erickson, Rebecca J. 2008. "The Context of Care: Reconsidering Culture, Structure and the Performance of Emotional Labor among Registered Nurses." Pp. 259–286 in *Social Structure and Emotion*, edited by Jody Clay-Warner and Dawn T. Robinson. San Diego, CA: Academic.
Erickson, Rebecca J., and Christian Ritter. 2001. "Emotional Labor, Burnout, and Inauthenticity: Does Gender Matter?" *Social Psychology Quarterly* 64(2):146–163.
Erickson, Sarah J., and Sarah W. Feldstein. 2007. "Adolescent Humor and Its Relationship to Coping, Defense Strategies, Psychological Distress, and Well-being." *Child Psychology & Human Development* 37:255–371
Eriksson, Kimmo, Ali Kazemi, and Kjell Tornblom. 2015. "A New Look at Individual Differences in Perceptions of Unfairness: The Theory of Maximally Unfair Allocations in Multiparty Situations." *Social Justice Research* 28(4):401–414.

Eriksson, Malin and Maria Emmelin. 2013. "What Constitutes a Health-Enabling Neighborhood? A Grounded Theory Situational Analysis Addressing the Significance of Social Capital and Gender." *Social Science & Medicine* 97:112–23.

Erkkila, Tero. 2012. Government Transparency: Impacts and Unintended Consequences. Houndmills, UK: Palgrave.

Ertz, Myriam, Emine Sarigöllü, Fahri Karakas, and Omar Chehab. 2021. "Impact of TV Dramas on Consumers" Travel, Shopping and Purchase Intentions." *Journal of Consumer Behaviour* 20(3):655–69.

Eryilmaz, Ali. 2013. "A Model for Subjective Well-being in Adolescence: Need Satisfaction and Reasons for Living." *Social Indicators Research* 107:561–574.

Esbensen, Finn-Aage, and D. Wayne Osgood. 1999. "Gang Resistance Education and Training (GREAT) Results from the National Evaluation." *Journal of Research in Crime and Delinquency* 36(2):194–215.

Eshel, Yohanan, Shaul Kimhi, Mooli Lahad, and Dmitry Leykin. 2017. "Individual Attributes as Predictors of Protective and Risk Components of Resilience under Continuing Terror Attacks: A Longitudinal Study." *Personality & Individual Differences* 114:160–66.

Espelage, Dorothy L., Stanley Wasserman, and Mark Fleisher. 2007. "Social Networks and Violent Behavior." Pp. 450–464 in *The Cambridge Handbook of Violent Behavior and Aggression*, edited by Daniel J. Flannery, Alexander T. Vazsonyi and Irwin D. Waldman. Cambridge, UK: Cambridge University Press.

Esposito, John L. 2002. *What Everyone Needs to Know about Islam*. New York: Oxford University Press.

Espvall, Majen and Peter Dellgran. 2010. "Can We Count on Each Other? Reciprocity and Conflicts in Financial Support in Sweden." *International Journal of Social Welfare* 19(1):84–94.

Esteban, Esther J. 2006. "Parental Verbal Abuse: Culture-specific Coping Behavior of College Students in the Philippines." *Child Psychiatry & Human Development* 36(3):243–259.

Estes, Richard J. 2002. "Toward a Social Development Index of Hong Kong: The Process of Community Engagement." *Social Indicators Research* 58:313–341.

Estes, Thomas, and Susan L. Mintz. 2016. *Instruction: A Models Approach*. Upper Saddle River, NJ: Pearson.

Etezadi, Sarah, and Dolores Pushkar. 2013. "Why are Wise People Happier? An Explanatory Model of Wisdom and Emotional Well-Being in Older Adults." *Journal of Happiness Studies* 14(3):929–950.

Evans, F. Barton, III. 1996. Harry Stack Sullivan: Interpersonal Theory and Psychotherapy. London, UK: Routledge.

Evans, Geoffrey. 1996. "Putting Men and Women into Classes: An Assessment of the Cross-sex Validity of the Goldthorpe Class Schema." *Sociology* 30(2):209–234.

Evans, Jeremy. 2013. "The Moral Psychology of Determinism." *Philosophical Psychology* 26(5):639–61.

Evans, M.D.R., Jonathan Kelley, and Clayton D. Peoples. 2010. "Justifications of Inequality: The Normative Basis of Pay Differentials in 31 Nations." *Social Science Quarterly* 91(5):1405–1431.

Evans, Peter B., and William H. Sewell, Jr. 2013. "Neoliberalism: Policy, Regimes, International Regimes, and Social Effects." Pp. 35–68 in *Social Resilience in the Neoliberal Era*, edited by Peter A. Hall, and Michele Lamont. Cambridge, UK: Cambridge University Press.

Evers, Adalbert. 2009. "Civicness and Civility: Their Meanings for Social Services." *Voluntas* 20:239–259.

Ewart, Craig K., Randall S. Jorgensen, Sonia Suchday, Edith Chen, and Karen A. Matthews. 2002. "Measuring Stress Resilience and Coping in Vulnerable Youth: The Social Competence Interview." *Psychological Assessment* 14(3):339–352.

Ewick, Patricia, and Susan Silbey. 2003. "Narrating Social Structure: Stories of Resistance to Legal Authority." *American Journal of Sociology* 108(6):1328–1372.

Exline, Julie J. and Peter C. Hill. 2012. "Humility: A Consistent and Robust Predictor of Generosity." *Journal of Positive Psychology* 7(3):208–18.

Extremera, Natalio, Anxiliadora Duran, and Lourades Rey. 2007. "Perceived Emotional Intelligence and Dispositional Optimism-pessimism: Analyzing Their Roles in Predicting Psychological Adjustment among Adolescents." *Personality & Individual Differences* 42:1069–1079.

Fahmy, Eldin. 2006. "Social Capital and Civic Action: A Study of Youth in the United Kingdom." *Young* 14(2):101–118.

Fairbrother, Gregory P. 2003b. Toward Critical Patriotism: Student Resistance to Political Education in Hong Kong and China. Hong Kong, China: Hong Kong University Press.

Falci, Christina, and Clea McNeely. 2009. "Too Many Friends: Social Integration, Network Cohesion and Adolescent Depressive Symptoms." *Social Forces* 87(4):2031–2062.

Falk, John H. 2018. *Born to Choose: Evolution, Self, and Well-being*. New York, NJ: Routledge.

Falkenberg, Andrcas W. 1998. "Quality of Life: Efficacy, Equity and Freedom in the United States and Scandinavia." *Journal of Socio-Economics* 27(1):1–27.

Fall, Kevin A., Janice Miner Holden, and Andre Marquis. 2004. *Theoretical Models of Counseling and Psychotherapy*. New York: Brunner-Routledge.

Falon, Samantha L., Maria Kangas, and Monique F. Crane. 2021. "The Coping Insights Involved in Strengthening Resilience: The Self-Reflection and Coping Insight Framework." *Anxiety, Stress, & Coping* 34(6):734–50.

Fan, C. Simon, and Hon-Kwong Lui. 2004. "Extramarital Affairs, Marital Satisfaction, and Divorce: Evidence from Hong Kong." *Contemporary Economic Policy* 22(4):4442–452.

Fan, Juan, Wenhui Liang, and Hanyi Zheng. 2022b. "Government's Impression Management Strategies, Trust in Government and Social Cohesion: An Evidence from Songjiang University Town, China." *Frontiers in Psychology* 13:951579.

Fan, Lu, Swarn Chatterjee and Jinhee Kim. 2021. "An Integrated Framework of Young Adults" Subjective Well-Being: The Roles of Personality Traits, Financial Responsibility, Perceived Financial Capability, and Race." *Journal of Family & Economic Issues* 43(1):66–85.

Fan, Shenggen, Linxiu Zhang, and Xiaobo Zhang. 2004. "Reforms, Investment, and Poverty in Rural China." *Economic Development & Cultural Change* 52(2):395–421.

Fang, Lin, Deng-Min Chuang, and Maria Al-Raes. 2019. "Social Support, Mental Health Needs, and Hiv Risk Behaviors: A Gender-Specific, Correlation Study." BMC Public Health 19(1).

Fang, Litian. 2006. *Buddhist Philosophy*. Beijing, China: China People University.

Fang, Tongyi. 2003. Spirit of Chinese Wisdom: From the Realm of Heaven-Human to the Border between Dao-Tactics. Beijing, China: People.

Fang, Tony. 1999. *Chinese Business Negotiating Style*. Thousand Oaks, CA: Sage.

Fanning, Bryan, Trutz Haase, and Neil O'Boyle. 2011. "Well-being, Cultural Capital and Social Inclusion: Immigrants in the Republic of Ireland." *International Migration & Integration* 12(1):1–24.

Fararo, Thomas J., and Patrick Doreian. 1998. "The Theory of Solidarity: An Agenda of Problems." Pp. 1–31 in *The Problems of Solidarity: Theories and Models*, edited by Patrick Doreian and Thomas Fararo. Australia: Gordon & Breach.

Farber, Eugene W. 2010. "Humanistic-existential Psychotherapy Competencies and the Supervisory Process." *Psychotherapy Theory, Research, Practice, Training* 47(1):28–39.

Farr, James. 2004. "Social Capital: A Conceptual History." *Political Theory* 32(1):6–33.

Farrelly, Colin. 2007. *Justice, Democracy and Reasonable Agreement*. Houndmills, UK: Palgrave.

Farrington, David P. 2007. "Origins of Violent Behavior over the Life Span." Pp. 19–48 in *The Cambridge Handbook of Violent Behavior and Aggression*, edited by Daniel J. Flannery, Alexander T. Vazsonyi and Irwin D. Waldman. Cambridge, UK: Cambridge University Press.

Farrington, David P. 2018. "The Duration of Criminal Careers: How Many Offenders Do Not Desist up to Age 61?" *Journal of Developmental & Life Course Criminology* 5(1):4–21.

Farrington, David P., and Brandon C. Welsh. 2007. *Saving Children from a Life of Crime: Early Risk Factors and Effective Interventions*. New York: Oxford University Press.

Fasang, Anette Eva, William Mangino, and Hannah Bruckner. 2014. "Social Closure and Educational Attainment." *Sociological Forum* 29(1):137–164.

Fasoli, Allison DiBianca. 2017. "Moral Responsibility, Personal Regulation, and Helping Others: A Cultural Approach to Moral Reasoning in U.S. Evangelical Christian Cultures." *Culture & Psychology* 23(4):461–86.

Fauth, Rebecca C., Jodie L. Roth, and Jeanne Brooks-Gunn. 2007. "Does the Neighborhood Context Alter the Link between Youth after School Time Activities and Developmental Outcomes? A Multilevel Analysis." *Developmental Psychology* 43(3):760–777.

Fava, Giovanni A., and Chiara Ruini. 2014. "Well-being Therapy: Theoretical Background, Clinical Implications, and Future Directions." Pp. 1037–1049 in *The Oxford Handbook of Happiness*, edited by Susan A. David, Ilona Boniwell and Amanda Conley Ayers. Oxford, UK: Oxford University Press.

Fawcett, Barbara. 2012. "Mental Health." Pp. 515–530 in *The SAGE Handbook of Social Work*, edited by Mel Gray, James Midgley and Stephen A. Webb. London, UK: SAGE. (HV40.S24)

Fawzy, Fawzy I., Nancy W. Fawzy, and Andrea L. Canada. 2001. "Psychoeducational Intervention Programs for Patients with Cancer." Pp. 235–267 in *Psychosocial Interventions for Cancer*, edited by Andrew Baum and Barbara L. Andersen. Washington, DC: American Psychological Association.

Featherstone, Brid, and Kate Morris. 2012. "Feminist Ethics of Care." Pp. 341–354 in *The SAGE Handbook of Social Work*, edited by Mel Gray, James Midgley and Stephen A. Webb. London, UK: SAGE.

Feddes, Allard R., Liesbeth Mann, and Bertjan Doosje. 2015. "Increasing Self-Esteem and Empathy to Prevent Violent Radicalization: A Longitudinal Quantitative Evaluation of a Resilience Training Focused on Adolescents with a Dual Identity." *Journal of Applied Social Psychology* 45(7):400–411.

Federico, Christopher M., Agnieszka Golec De Zavala, and Wen Bu. 2023. "Collective Narcissism as a Basis for Nationalism." *Political Psychology* 44(1):177–96.

Feeney, Brooke C. and Nancy L. Collins. 2001. "Predictors of Caregiving in Adult Intimate Relationships: An Attachment Theoretical Perspective." *Journal of Personality & Social Psychology* 80(6):972–994.

Feeney, Brooke C., and Nancy L. Collins. 2018. "Social Support in Close Relationships." Pp. 281–296 in *The Cambridge Handbook of Personal Relationships*, edited by Anita L. Vangelisti and Daniel Perlman. Cambridge, UK: Cambridge University Press.

Fehr, Beverley, and Ross Broughton. 2001. "Gender and personality Differences in Conceptions of Love: An Interpersonal Theory Analysis." *Personal Relationships* 8(2):115–136.

Feinberg, Matthew and Robb Willer. 2019. "Moral Reframing: A Technique for Effective and Persuasive Communication across Political Divides." *Social & Personality Psychology Compass* 13(12):12501.

Feingold, Alan. 1994. "Gender Differences in Personality: A Meta-analysis." *Psychological Bulletin* 116(3):429–456.

Feinstein, Leon, and John Bynner. 2006. "Continuity and Discontinuity in Middle Childhood: Implications for Adult Outcomes in the UK 1970 Birth Cohort." Pp. 327–349 in *Developmental Contexts in Middle Childhood: Bridges to Adolescence and Adulthood*, edited by Aletha C. Huston and Marika N. Ripke. Cambridge, UK: Cambridge University Press.

Fekete, Anna, Eva Specker, Jan Mikuni, MacKenzie D. Trupp, and Helmut Leder. 2024. "When the Painting Meets Its Musical Inspiration: The Impact of Multimodal Art Experience on Aesthetic Enjoyment and Subjective Well-Being in the Museum." *Psychology of Aesthetics, Creativity, & the Arts*. \110–328

Feldman, Allan, Kory Bennett, and Vanessa Vernaza-Hernández. 2015. "Responsible Action Research for the Pursuit of Justice." *Educational Action Research* 23(1):85–103.

Feldman, Christina and Willem Kuyken. 2019. *Mindfulness: Ancient Wisdom Meets Modern Psychology*. New York, NY: Guilford.

Feldman, David B., and Diane E Dreher. 2012. "Can Hope be Changed in 90 Minutes? Testing the Efficacy of a Single-Session Goal-Pursuit Intervention for College Students." *Journal of Happiness Studies* 13(4):745–759.

Feldman, Stanley. 2003. "Enforcing Social Conformity: A Theory of Authoritarianism." *Political Psychology* 24(1):41–74.

Feldman, Yuval. 2018. *The Law of Good People: Challenging States" Ability to Regulate Human Behavior*. Cambridge, UK: Cambridge University Press.

Felker, Julie, and Martina Gianecchini. 2015. "Influence of Pre-Graduation International Experiences on Early Career Internationalization: The Mediation Effect of Career Capital." *European Management Journal* 33(1):60–70.

Felmlee, Diane H., and H. Colleen Sinclair. 2018. "Social Networks and Personal Relationships." Pp. 467–480 in *The Cambridge Handbook of Personal Relationships*, edited by Anita L. Vangelisti and Daniel Perlman. Cambridge, UK: Cambridge University Press.

Felson, Richard B. and Maureen C. Outlaw. 2007. "The Control Motive and Marital Violence." *Violence & Victims* 22(4):387–407.

Fenwick, Rudy, and Mark Tausig. 1994. "The Macroeconomic Context of Job Stress." *Journal of Health & Social Behavior* 35:266–282.

Fer, Seval. 2012. "Demographic Characteristics and Intellectual Styles." Pp. 109–130 in *Handbook of Intellectual Styles: Preferences in Cognition, Learning, and Thinking*. New York: Springer.

Ferguson, Amanda M., C. Daryl Cameron ,and Michael Inzlicht. 2020. "Motivational Effects on Empathic Choices." *Journal of Experimental Social Psychology* 90:104010.

Ferguson, Brian S. 2006. "Economic Modeling of the Rational Consumption of Addictive Substances." *Substance Use & Misuse* 41:573–603.

Ferguson, Christopher J., and Stephanie M. Rueda. 2010. "Violent Video Game Exposure Effects on Aggressive Behavior, Hostile Feelings, and Depression." *European Psychologist* 15(2):99–108.

Ferguson, Kitty. 2011. *Stephen Hawking: His Life and Work*. London, UK: Bantam.

Ferguson, Mark A., and Thomas E. Ford. 2008. "Disparagement Humor: A Theoretical and Empirical Review of Psychoanalytic, Superiority, and Social Identity Theories." Humor: *International Journal of Humor Research* 21(3):283–312.

Fernandes, April. 2018. "Red Lights and Handcuffs: The Effect of Arrests on the Fear of Crime." *Social Science Quarterly* 99(4):1390–1408.

Ferreira, Maria José, Rui Sofia, David F. Carreno, Nikolett Eisenbeck, Inês Jongenelen, and José Fernando A. Cruz. 2021. "Dealing with the Pandemic of Covid-19 in Portugal: On the Important Role of Positivity, Experiential Avoidance, and Coping Strategies." *Frontiers in Psychology* 12:647984.

Ferriss, Abbott L. 2002. "Studying and Measuring Civility: A Framework, Trends, and Scale." *Sociological Inquiry* 72(3):376–392.

Ferssizidis, Patty, Leah M. Adams, Todd B. Kashdan, Christine Plummer, Anjali Mishra and Joseph Ciarrochi. 2010. "Motivation for and Commitment to Social Values: The Roles of Age and Gender." *Motivation & Emotion* 34(4):354–62.

Festenstein, Matthew. 2010. "Pragmatism: Inquiry and Political Liberalism." *Contemporary Political Theory* 9(1):25–44.

Fett, Anne-Kathrin J., Sukhi S. Shergill, Paula M. Gromann, Iroise Dumontheil, Sarah-Jayne Blakemore, Farah Yakub, and Lydia Krabbendam. 2014. "Trust and Social Reciprocity in Adolescence: A Matter of Perspective-Taking." *Journal of Adolescence* 37(2):175–84.

Fevre, Ralph. 2006. Individualism and Inequality: The Future of Work and Politics. Cheltenham, UK: Elgar.

Fielding, R., J. Li, and Y.E. Tang. 1995. "Health Care Utilization as a Function of Subjective Health Status, Job Satisfaction, and Gender among Health Care Workers in Guangzhou, Southern China." *Social Science & Medicine* 41(8:1103–1110.

Fields, Scott A., and John R. McNamara. 2003. "The Prevention of Child and Adolescent Violence: A Review." *Aggression & Violent Behavior* 8:61–91.

Fierke, K. M. 2022. *Snapshots from Home: Mind, Action and Strategy in an Uncertain World*. Bristol, UK: Bristol University Press.

Fiese, Barbara H., and Amber Hammons. 2013. "Theories of Family Health: An Integrative Perspective and Look toward the Future." Pp. 398–416 in *Handbook of Family Theories: A Content-based Approach*, edited by Mark A. Fine and Frank D. Fincham. New York: Routledge.

Filip, Agneessens, Hans Waege, and John Lievens. 2006. "Diversity in Social Support by Role Relations: A Typology." *Social Networks* 28:427–441.

Fine, Gary Alan and Lori Holyfield. 1996. "Secrecy, Trust, and Dangerous Leisure: Generating Group Cohesion on Voluntary Organizations." *Social Psychology Quarterly* 59(1):22–38.

Fine, Michael D. 2007. A Caring Society? Care and the Dilemmas of Human Service in the Twenty-first Century. Houndmills, UK: Palgrave.

Finell, Eerika, and Karmela Liebkind. 2010. "National Symbols and Distinctiveness: Rhetorical Strategies in Creating Distinct National Identities." *British Journal of Social Psychology* 49(2):321–341.

Fingerman, Karen L., B. Bradford Brown, and Rosemary Blieszner. 2011. "Informal Ties across the Life Span: Peers, Consequential Strangers, and People We Encounter in Daily Life." Pp. 487–511 in *Handbook of Life-Development*, edited by Karen L. Fingerman, Cynthia A. Berg, Jacque Smith and Toni C. Antonucci. New York: Springer.

Finggerman, Karen L., Lindsay Pitzer, Eva S. Lefkowitz, Kira S. Birditt, and Daniel Mroczek. 2008. "Ambivalent Relationship Qualities between Adults and Their Parents: Implications for the Well-being of Both Parties." *Journal of Gerontology: Psychological Sciences* 63B(6):P362–P371.

Fink, Bruce. 1995. *The Lacanian Subject: Between Language and Jouissance.* Princeton, NJ: Princeton University Press.

Finkel, Eli J., Grainne M. Fitzsimons, and Michelle R. van Dellen. 2016. "Self-regulation as a Transactive Process: Reconceptualizing the Unit of Analysis for goal Setting, Pursuit, and Outcomes." Pp. 264–282 in *Handbook of Self-regulation: Research, Theory, and Application*, edited by Kathleen D. Vohs and Roy F. Baumeister. New York, NY: Guilford.

Finkel, Steven E., and James B. Rule. 1986. "Relative Deprivation and Related Psychological Theories of Civil Violence: A Critical Review." *Research in Social Movements, Conflicts & Change* 9:47–69.

Finne, Johannes. N., and Frode Svartdal. 2017. "Social Perception Training (SPT): Improving Social Competence by Reducing Cognitive Distortions." *International Journal of Emotional Education* 9(2):44–58.

Finnerty-Myers, Keli. 2011. "Understanding the Dynamics Behind the Relationship between Exposure to Negative Consequences of Risky Sex on Entertainment Television and Emerging Adults" Safe-Sex Attitudes and Intentions." *Mass Communication & Society* 14(6):743–64.

Finney, John W., Roger E. Mitchell, Ruth C. Cronkite, and Rudolph H. Moos. 1984. "Methodological Issues in Estimating Main and Interactive Effects: Examples from Coping/Social Support and Stress Field." *Journal of Health & Social Behavior* 25(Mar):85–98.

Firat, Rengin B. 2021. "A Neurosociological Theory of Culturally and Structurally Situated Cognition and Ethno-Racial Stress." *Frontiers in Sociology* 6:695042.

Firestone, Robert W., Lisa A. Firestone, and Joyce Catlett. 2006. *Sex and Love in Intimate Relationships*. Washington, DC: American Psychological Association.

First, Jennifer, Nathan L. First, and J. Brian Houston. 2018. "Resilience and Coping Intervention (RCI): A Group Intervention to Foster College Student Resilience." *Social Work with Groups* 41(3):198–210.

Fischer, Agneta, and Catharine Evers. 2013. "The Social Basis of Emotion in Men and Women." Pp. 183–215 in *The SAGE Handbook of Gender and Psychology*, edited by Michelle K. Ryan and Myla R. Branscombe. London, UK: SAGE.

Fischer, Claude S., Michael Hout, Martin Sanchez Jankowski, Samuel R. Lucas, Ann Swindler, and Kim Voss. 1996. *Inequality by Design: Cracking the Bell Curve Myth.* Princeton, NJ: Princeton University Press.

Fischer, Moritz, Mathias Twardawski, Peter Strelan, and Mario Gollwitzer. 2022. "Victims Need More Than Power: Empowerment and Moral Change Independently Predict Victims' Satisfaction and Willingness to Reconcile." *Journal of Personality & Social Psychology* 123(3):518–36.

Fischer, Peter, Tobias Greitemeyer, Suat Ilkay Omay, and Dieter Frey. 2007. "Mergers and Group Status: The Impact of High, Low and Equal Group Status on Identification and Satisfaction with a Company Merger, Experienced Controllability, Group Identity, and Group Cohesion." *Journal of Community & Applied Social Psychology* 17:203–217.

Fischer, Sophia, Claudia Dolitzsch, Klaus Schmeck, Jorg M. Fegert, and Marc Schmid. 2016. "Interpersonal Trauma and Associated Psychopathology in Girls and Boys Living in Residential Care." *Children & Youth Services Review* 67:203–211.

Fishbein, Joel N., Ruth A. Baer, Joshua Correll, and Joanna J. Arch. 2020. "The Questionnaire on Self-Transcendence (Quest): A Measure of Trait Self-Transcendence Informed by Contextual Cognitive Behavioral Therapies." *Assessment* 29(3):508–526.

Fisher, Ronald J., Herbert C. Kelman, and Susan Allen Nan. 2013. "Conflict Analysis and Resolution." Pp. 489–521 in *The Oxford Handbook of Political Psychology*, edited by Leone Huddy, David O. Sears and Jack S. Levy. New York: Oxford University Press. (JA74.5O355)

Fishkin, James 2018. *Democracy When the People Are Thinking: Revitalizing Our Politics through Public Deliberation*. Oxford, UK: Oxford University Press.

Fiske, Alan Page. 2000. "Complementarity Theory: Why Human Social Capacities Evolved to Require Cultural Complements." *Personality & Social Psychology Review* 4(1):76–94.

Fiske, Susan, Richard R. Lau, and Richard A. Smith. 1990. "On the Varieties and Utilities of Political Expertise." *Social Cognition* 8(1):31–48.

Fjellvang, Tormod. 2011. "Socialization Values, Cultural-religious Zones and Modernization Theory." *European Sociological Review* 27(2):196–211.

Flanagan, Constance A., and Michael Stout. 2010. "Developmental Patterns of Social Trust between Early and Late Adolescence: Age and School Climate Effects." *Journal of Research on Adolescence* 20(3):748–773.

Flanagan, Constance. 2003. "Trust, Identity, and Civic Hope." *Applied Developmental Science* 7(3):165–171.

Flanagan, Scott C., and Aie-Rie Lee. 2000. "Value Change and Democratic Reform in Japan and Korea." *Comparative Political Studies* 33(5):626–659.

Flanagan, Scott, and Aie-rie Lee. 2003. "The New Politics, Culture Wars, and the Authoritarian-libertarian Value Change in Advanced Industrial Democracies." *Comparative Political Studies* 36(3):235–270.

Flap, Henk, and Beate Volker. 2008. "Social, Cultural, and Economic Capital and Job Attainment: The Position Generator as a Measure of Cultural and Economic Resources." Pp. 65–80 in *Social Capital: An International Research Program*, edited by Nan Lin and Bonnie H. Erickson. Oxford, UK: Oxford University Press.

Flap, Henk, and Beate Volker. 2013. "Social Capital." Pp. 220–251 in *The Handbook of Rational Choice Social Research*, edited by Rafael Wittek, Tom A. H. Snijders, and Victor Nee. Stanford, CA: Stanford University Press.

Fleischmann, Fenella, and Karen Phalet. 2018. "Religion and National Identification in Europe: Comparing Muslim Youth in Belgium, England, Germany, the Netherlands, and Sweden." *Journal of Cross-Cultural Psychology* 49(1):44–61.

Fleischmann, Fenella, Lars Leszczensky, and Sebastian Pink. 2019. "Identity Threat and Identity Multiplicity among Minority Youth: Longitudinal Relations of Perceived Discrimination with Ethnic, Religious, and National Identification in Germany." *British Journal of Social Psychology* 58(4):971–90.

Flemming, Magne. 2013. "Putting Bourdieu to Work for Class Analysis. Reflections on Some Recent Contributions." *British Journal of Sociology* 64(2):325–343.

Flett, Gordon L. 2018. *The Psychology of Mattering: Understanding the Human Need to Be Significant*. London, UK: Academic.

Flintoff, Adam, Ewen Speed, and Susan McPherson. 2019. "Risk Assessment Practice within Primary Mental Health Care: A Logics Perspective." *Health* 23(6):656–74.

Flogie, Andrej, Andreja Barle Lakota, Boris Abersek. 2018. "The Psychosocial and Cognitive Influence of ICT on Competences of Stem Students." *Journal of Baltic Science Education* 17(2):267–276.

Flook, Lisa, and Andrew J. Fuligni. 2008. "Family and School Spillover in Adolescents¡¯ Daily Lives." *Child Development* 79(3):776–787.

Florida, Richard. 2005. *Cities and the Creative Class.* New York: Routledge.

Florsheim, Paul. 1997. "Chinese Adolescent Immigrants: Factors Related to Psychosocial Adjustment." *Journal of Youth & Adolescence* 26(2):143–163.

Flouri, Eirini, and Ann Buchanan. 2002. "The Protective Role of Parental Involvement in Adolescent Suicide." *Crisis* 23(1):17–22.

Floyd, Kory. 2019. *Affectionate Communication in Close Relationships.* Cambridge, UK: Cambridge University Press.

Flynn, Rachel M., Ashley A. Ricker, Curtis Dolezal, Mike Kunin, and Claude A. Mellins. 2019. "Residential Summer Camp for Youth with Special Needs: A Longitudinal Approach to Investigating Differences in Social Skills." *Children & Youth Services Review* 96:354–363.

Forestier, Katherine, and Michael Crossley. 2015. "International Education Policy Transfer-Borrowing Both Ways: The Hong Kong And England Experience." *Prometheus* 24(4):389–403.

Forgeard, Marie J. C., and Lizbeth Benson. 2019. "Extracurricular Involvement and Psychological Adjustment in the Transition from Adolescence to Emerging Adulthood: The Role of Mastery and Creative Self-Efficacy." *Applied Developmental Science* 23(1):41–58.

Forman, Tyrone A. 2001. "Social Determinants of White Youths" Racial Attitudes: Evidence from a National Survey." *Sociological Studies of Children and Youth* 8:173–207.

Forster, Daniel E., Eric J. Pedersen, Adam Smith, Michael E. McCullough and Debra Lieberman. 2017. "Benefit Valuation Predicts Gratitude." *Evolution & Human Behavior* 38(1):18–26.

Forsyth, James. 2003. *Psychological Theories of Religion.* Upper Saddle River, NJ: Prentice Hall.

Forsythe, Jeremy and Myriam Mongrain. 2023. "The Existential Nihilism Scale (Ens): Theory, Development, and Psychometric Evaluation." *Journal of Psychopathology & Behavioral Assessment* 45(3):865–83.

Forward, Catherine, Hafiz T. A. Khan, and Pauline Fox. 2023. "Older Women Living Alone in the UK: Does Their Health and Wellbeing Differ from Those Who Cohabit?" *Journal of Population Ageing* 16(1):103–19.

Foschi, Renato and Marco Lauriola. 2014. "Does Sociability Predict Civic Involvement and Political Participation?" *Journal of Personality & Social Psychology* 106(2):339–57.

Fosco, Gregory M, and Mark E Feinberg. 2015. "Cascading effects of Interparental Conflict in Adolescence: Linking Threat Appraisals, Self-Efficacy, and Adjustment." *Development & Psychopathology* 27(1):239–252.

Fosco, Gregory M. and David M. Lydon-Staley. 2020. "Implications of Family Cohesion and Conflict for Adolescent Mood and Well-Being: Examining within- and between-Family Processes on a Daily Timescale." *Family Process* 59(4):1672–89.

Foster, Vivien, Susana Mourato, David Pearce, and Ece Ozdemiroglu. 2001. *The Price of Virtue: The Economic Value of the Charitable Sector*. Cheltenham, UK: Edward Elgar.

Fouad, Nadya A., and John Bynner. 2008. "Work Transitions." *American Psychologist* 63(4):241–251.

Fournier, Marc A. 2009. "Adolescent Hierarchy Formation and the Social Competition Theory of Depression." *Journal of Social & Clinical Psychology* 28(9):1144–1172.

Fox, Claire L., and Ian Butler. 2009. "Evaluating the Effectiveness of a School-based Counseling Service in the UK." *British Journal of Guidance & Counselling* 37(2):95–106.

Fox, Greer Litton, Michael L. Benson, Alfred A. DeMaris, and Judy Van Wyk. 2002. "Economic Distress and Intimate Violence: Testing Family Stress and Resources Theories." *Journal of Marriage & Family* 64:793–807.

Fox, Jonathan. 1996. "How Does Civil Society Thicken? The Political Construction of Social Capital in Rural Mexico." *World Development* 24(6):1089–1103.
Foy, Steven, Robert Freeland, Andrew Miles, Kimberly B. Rogers, and Lynn Smith-Lovin. 2014. "Emotions and Affect as Source, Outcome and Resistance to Inequality." Pp. 295–324 in *Handbook of the Social Psychology of Inequality*, edited by Jane D. McLeod, Edward J. Lawler, and Michael Schwalbe. Dordrecht, Netherland: Springer.
Fraley, R. Chris, Marie E. Heffernan, Amanda M. Vicary, and Claudia Chloe Brumbaugh. 2011. "The Experiences in Close Relationships-Relationship Structures Questionnaire: A Method for Assessing Attachment Orientations across Relationships." *Psychological Assessment* 23(3):615–625.
Francis, Sophie, and Alison Zarecky. 2017. "Working with Strengths in Coaching." Pp. 361–380 in *The SAGE Handbook of Coaching*, edited by Tatiana Bachkirova, Gordon Spence, and David Drake. London, UK: SAGE.
Frank, Christine, Christopher G. Davis, and Frank J. Elgar. 2014. "Financial Strain, Social Capital, and Perceived Health During Economic Recession: A Longitudinal Survey in Rural Canada." *Anxiety, Stress, & Coping* 27(4):422–438.
Frankenmolen, Nikita L., Luciano Fasotti, Roy P. C. Kessels, and Joukje M. Oosterman. 2018. "The Influence of Cognitive Reserve and Age on the Use of Memory Strategies." *Experimental Aging Research* 44(2):117–134.
Franklin, Leanne. 2012. *Gender.* Houndmills, UK: Palgrave.
Franklin, Maureen. 1995. "The Effects of Differential College Environments on Academic Learning and Student Perceptions of Cognitive Development." *Research in Higher Education* 36(2):127–153.
Franks, Bradley, Adrian Bangerter, and Martin W. Bauer. 2013. "Conspiracy Theories as Quasi-Religious Mentality: An Integrated Account from Cognitive Science, Social Representations Theory, and Frame Theory." *Frontiers in Psychology* 4:424.
Fransella, Fay, and David Winter. 2012. "Personal Construct Counselling and Psychotherapy." Pp. 388–391 in *The SAGE Handbook of Counselling and Psychotherapy*, edited by Colin Feltham and Ian Horton. London: SAGE.
Franz, M., H. Lenshe, and N. Schmitz. 2003. "Psychological Distress and Socioeconomic Status in Single Mothers and Their Children in a German City." *Social Psychiatry & Psychiatric Epidemiology* 38:59–68.
Frazer, Elizabeth. 1999. *The Problems of Communitarian Politics: Unity and Conflict.* Oxford, UK: Oxford University Pres.
Frazier, Kathryn E. and Rachel Joffe Falmagro. 2014. "Empowered Victims? Women's Contradictory Positions on the Discourse of Violence Prevention." *Feminism & Psychology* 24(4):479–499.
Frazier, Leslie D., Frederick L. Newman, and James Jaccard. 2007. "Psychosocial Outcomes in Later Life: A Multivariate Model." *Psychological & Aging* 22(4):676–689.
Frederick, David A, Gaganjyot Sandhu, Patrick J. Morse, and Viren Swami. 2016. "Correlates of Appearance and Weight Satisfaction in a U.S. National Sample: Personality, Attachment Style, Television Viewing, Self-Esteem, and Life Satisfaction." *Body Image* 17:191–203.
Frederick-Recascino, Christina M., and Hana Schuster-Smith. 2003. "Competition and Intrinsic Motivation in Physical Activity: A Comparison of Two Groups." *Journal of Sport Behavior* 26(3):240–254.
Fredricks, Jennifer A., and Jacquelynne S. Eccles. 2005. "Developmental Benefits of Extracurricular Involvement: Do Peer Characteristics Mediate the Link between Activities and Youth Outcomes?" *Journal of Youth & Adolescence* 34(6):507–520.
Fredrickson, Barbara L., and Marcial F. Losada. 2005. "Positive Affect and the Complex Dynamics of Human Flourishing." *American Psychologist* 60(7):678–686.
Freeman, Daniel, Felicity Waite, Laina Rosebrock, Ariane Petit, Chiara Causier, Anna East, Lucy Jenner, Ashley-Louise Teale, Lydia Carr, Sophie Mulhall, Emily Bold, and Sinéad Lambe. 2022.

"Coronavirus Conspiracy Beliefs, Mistrust, and Compliance with Government Guidelines in England." *Psychological Medicine.* 52(2):251–63.
Frega, Roberto. 2012. Practice, Judgment, and the Challenge of Moral and Political Disagreement: A Pragmatist Account. Lanham, MD: Lexington.
Frei, Andreas, Kay W. Axhausen, and Timo Ohnmacht. 2009. "Mobilities and Social Network Geography: Size and Spatial Dispersion: The Zurich Case Study." Pp. 99–120 in *Mobilities and Inequality*, edited by Timo Ohnmacht, Hanja Maksim, and Marfred Max Bergman. Farnham, UK: Ashgate.
Freitag, Markus and Paul C. Bauer. 2016. "Personality Traits and the Propensity to Trust Friends and Strangers." *Social Science Journal* 53(4):467–476.
Freitag, Markus. 2003. "Social Capital in (Dis)similar Democracies: The Development of Generalized Trust in Japan and Switzerland." *Comparative Political Studies* 36(8):936–966.
Freitas, Daniela Fonseca, Susana Coimbra, Edna Maria Marturano, Susana C. Marques, Jos Egdio Oliveira, and Anne Marie Fontaine. 2017. "Resilience in the Face of Peer Victimisation and Discrimination: The Who, When and Why in Five Patterns of Adjustment." *Journal of Adolescence* 59:19–34.
Freund, Alexandra M. 2006. "Age-differential Motivational Consequences of Optimization versus Compensation Focus in Younger and Older Adults." *Psychology & Aging* 21(2):240–252.
Frey, Bruno S., Christine Benesch, and Alois Stutzer. 2007. "Does Watching TV Make Us Happy." *Journal of Economic Psychology* 28:283–313.
Frey, Lisa L., and Gangi Roysircar. 2006. "South Asian and East Asian International Students" Perceived Prejudice, Acculturation, and Frequency of Help Resource Utilization." *Journal of Multicultural Counseling & Development* 34:208–222.
Fridberg, Torben and Olli Kangas. 2008b. "Social Capital." Pp. 65–85 in *Nordic Social Attitudes in a European Perspective*, edited by Heikki Ervasti, Torben Fridberg, Mikael Hjerm, and Kristen Ringdal. Cheltenham, UK: Edward Elgar.
Friedman, Harris L., and Brent Dean Robbins. 2012. "The Negative Shadow Cast by Positive Psychology: Contrasting Views and Implications of Humanistic and Positive Psychology on Resiliency." *Humanistic Psychologist* 40(1):87–102.
Friedman, Harris L., and Douglas A. MacDonald. 2006. "Humanistic Testing and Assessment." *Journal of Humanistic Psychology* 46(4):510–529.
Friedman, Jed, Daniel Goodkind, Bui the Cuong, and Truong Si Anh. 2001. "Work and Retirement among the Elderly in Vietnam." *Research on Aging* 23(2):249–232.
Friedman, Maurice. 1992. *Religion and Psychology: A Dialogical Approach.* New York: Paragon House.
Frimpong-Manso, Kwabena. 2018. "Building and Utilising Resilience: The Challenges and Coping Mechanisms of Care Leavers in Ghana." *Children & Youth Services Review* 87:52–59.
Froh, Jeffrey J., Giacomo Bono, and Robert Emmons. 2010. "Being Grateful Is Beyond Good Manners: Gratitude and Motivation to Contribute to Society among Early Adolescents." *Motivation and Emotion* 34(2):144–157.
Froiland, John Mark, Paivi Mayor, and Marjaana Herlevi. 2015. "Motives Emanating from Personality Associated with Achievement in a Finnish Senior High School: Physical Activity, Curiosity, and Family Motives." *School Psychology International* 36(2):207–221.
Frost, Michelle Bellessa. 2007. "Texas Students" College Expectations: Does High School Racial Composition Matter?" *Sociology of Education* 80(1):43–66.
Fry, Prem S., and Dominique L. Debats. 2010. "Psychosocial Resources as Predictors of Resilience and Healthy Longevity of Older Widows." Pp. 185–212 in *New Frontiers in Resilient Aging: Life-strengths and Well-being in Late Life*, edited by Prom S. Fry and Corey L.M. Keyes. Cambridge, UK: Cambridge University Press.
Frydenberg, Erica. 2008. Adolescent Coping: Advances in Theory, Research and Practice. Hove, UK: Routledge.

Fu, Hongyu and Jinmei Tu. 2023. "Exploring the Influence of National Music Lessons on Subjective Well-Being, Self-Esteem, and National Identity among University Students: A Case Study from China." *Frontiers in Psychology* 14:1151007.

Fu, Jeanne Ho-ying, and Chi-yue Chiu. 2007. "Local Cultural Responses to Globalization: Exemplary Persons and Their Attendant Values." *Journal of Cross-Cultural Psychology* 38(5):636–653.

Fuchs, Christian. 2008. Internet and Society: Social Theory in the Information Age. New York: Routledge.

Fuchs, Christian. 2020. *Nationalism on the Internet: Critical Theory and Ideology in the Age of Social Media and Fake News.* New York, NY: Routledge.

Fuchs, Ester R., Robert Y. Shapiro, and Lorraine C. Minnite. 2001. "Social Capital, Political Participation, and the Urban Community." Pp. 290–324 in *Social Capital and Poor Communities,* edited by Susan Saegert, J. Phillip Thompson, and Mark R. Warren. New York: Russell Sage.

Fuertes, Jairo N., Arielle Toporovskya, Mariela Reyesa, and Jennifer Bennett Osborne. 2017. "The Physician-Patient Working Alliance: Theory, Research, and Future Possibilities." *Patient Education & Counseling* 100:610–615

Fujisawa, Yoshikazu, Tsuyashi Hamano, and Shogo Takegama. 2009. "Social Capital and Perceived Health in Japan: An Ecological and Multilevel Analysis." *Social Science & Medicine* 69:500–505.

Fujita, Frank. 2008. "The Frequency of Social Comparison and Its Relation to Subjective Wellobeing." Pp. 239–257 in *The Science of Subjective Well-being*, edited by Michael Eid and Randy J. Larsen. New York: Guilford.

Fujita, Masahiro. 2018. *Japanese Society and Lay Participation in Criminal Justice: Social Attitudes, Trust, and Mass Media.* Singapore: Springer.

Fukushima, Miyuki, Susan F. Sharp, and Emiko Kobayashi. 2009. "Bond to Society: Collectivism and Conformity: A Comparative Study of Japanese and American College Students." *Deviant Behavior* 30(5):434–460.

Fukuyama, Francis. 1999. The Great Disruption: Human Nature and the Constitution of Social Order. London: Profile.

Fukuyama, Francis. 2001. "Social Capital, Civil Society, and Development." *Third World Quarterly* 22(1):7–20.

Fukuyama, Francis. 2018. *Identity: The Demand for Dignity and the Politics of Resentment.* New York, NY: Farrar, Straus & Giroux.

Fukuyama, Francis. 2018b. "Why National Identity Matters." *Journal of Democracy* 29(4):5–15.

Fulle-Iglesias, Heather, Jacqui Smith, and Toni Antonucci. 2009. "Theories of Aging From a Life-Course and Life Span Perspective: An Overview." *Annual Review of Gerontology & Geriatrics* 29:3–25, R12–R13.

Fuller, Linda. 2000. "Socialism and the Transition in East and Central Europe: The Homogeneity Paradigm: Class and Economic Inefficiency." *Annual Revie of Sociology* 26:585–609.

Fung, Chi Keung Charles and Chi Shun Fong. 2019. "Going out under the Shadow of Red China: The Geopolitical Origin of Hong Kong's International Status." *Asian Education & Development Studies* 8(2):173–85.

Fung, Helene H., Derek M. Isaacowitz, Alice Y. Lu, Heather A. Wadlinger, Deborah Goren, and Hugh R. Wilson. 2008. "Age-related Positivity Enhancement Is Not Universal: Older Chinese Look away from Positive Stimuli." *Psychology & Aging* 23(2):440–446.

Fung, Kwok Kin. 2014. "Financial Crisis and the Developmental States: A Case Study of Hong Kong." *International Journal of Social Welfare* 23:321–332.

Furman, Wyndol, and Duane Buhrmester. 1992. "Age and Sex Differences in Perceptions of Networks of Personal Relationships." *Child Development* 63:603–115.

Furnham, Adrian, and Helen Cheng. 2000. "Lay Theories of Happiness." *Journal of Happiness Studies* 1:227–246.

Furnham, Adrian. 1990. "Commonsense Theories of Personality." Pp. 176–203 in *Everyday Understanding: Social and Scientific Implication*, edited by Gun R. Semin and Kenneth J. Gergen. London: Sage.

Furnham, Adrian. 1997. "Lay Theories of Work Stress." *Work Stress* 11(1):68–78.

Furnham, Adrian. 2003. "Belief in a Just World: Research Progress over the Past Decade." *Personality & Individual Differences* 34:795–817.

Furnham-Diggory, Syliva. 1992. *Cognitive Process in Education*. New York: HarperCollins.

Furstenberg, Frank F., Jr., and Mary Elizabeth Hughes. 1995. "Social Capital and Successful Development among At-risk Youth." *Journal of Marriage and the Family* 57(3):580–592. \76–205

Furstenberg, Frank F., Jr., Thomas D. Cook, Jacquelynne Eccles, Glen H. Elder, Jr., and Arnold Sameroff. 1999. *Managing to Make It: Urban Families and Adolescent Success*. Chicago, IL: University of Chicago Press.

Fyall, Rachel, and Beth Gazley. 2015. "Applying Social Role Theory to Gender and Volunteering in Professional Associations." *Voluntas* 26(1):288–314.

Fyhn, Tonje, Kristin Konglevoll Fjell, and Bjørn Helge Johnsen. 2016. "Resilience Factors among Police Investigators: Hardiness-Commitment a Unique Contributor." *Journal of Police & Criminal Psychology* 31(4):261–269.

Gabay-Egozi, Limor, Yossi Shavit, and Meir Yaish. 2010. "Curricular Choice: A Test of a Rational Choice Model of Education." *European Sociological Review* 26(4):447–463.

Gadsden, Vivian L. 2008. "The Arts and Education: Knowledge Generation, Pedagogy, and the Discourse of Learning." *Review of Research in Education* 32(1):29–61.

Gaertnel, Samuel L., John F. Dovidio, Mary C. Rust, Jason A. Nier, Brenda S. Banker, Christine M. Ward, Gary R. Mottola, and Missy Houlette. 1999. "Reducing Intergroup Bias: Elements of Intergroup Cooperation." *Journal of Personality & Social Psychology* 76(3):388–402.

Gaertner, Samuel L., and John F. Dovidio. 2012. "The Common Ingroup Identity Model." Pp. 439–457 in *Handbook of Theories of Social Psychology* (vol. 2), edited by Paul A.M. Van Lange, Arie W. Kruglanski and E. Tory Higgins. London, CA: SAGE.

Gagne, Marylene, and Edward L. Deci. 2005. "Self-determination Theory and Work Motivation." *Journal of Organizational Behavior* 26:331–362.

Gahlawat, Neha, Rina S. Phogat, and Subhash C. Kundu. 2019. "Evidence for Life Satisfaction among Dual-Career Couples: The Interplay of Job, Career, and Family Satisfaction in Relation to Workplace Support." *Journal of Family Issues* 40(18):2893–2921.

Gaitan-Rossi, Pablo, and Ce Shen. 2018. "Fear of Crime in Mexico: The Impacts of Municipality Characteristics." *Social Indicators Research* 135(1):373–399.

Galante, Julieta, Ignacio Galante, Marie-Jet Bekkers and John Gallacher. 2014. "Effect of Kindness-Based Meditation on Health and Well-Being: A Systematic Review and Meta-Analysis." *Journal of Consulting & Clinical Psychology* 82(6):1101–1114.

Galian, María D., Ester Ato, and María Angeles Fernández-Vilar. 2018. "Sociometric Status as Mediator in the Relation between Effortful Control and Achievement." *Merrill-Palmer Quarterly* 64(3):309–328.

Gall, Terry Lynn, Claire Charbonneau, Neil Henry Clarke, Karen Grant, Anjali Joseph, and Lisa Shouldice. 2005. "Understanding the Nature and Role of Spirituality in Relation to Coping and Heath: A Conceptual Framework." *Canadian Psychology* 46(2):88–104.

Galla, Brian M., Michael V. Esposito, and Hannah M. Fiore. 2020. "Mindfulness Predicts Academic Diligence in the Face of Boredom." *Learning & Individual Differences* 81:101864.

Gallie, Duncan, and Serge Paugam. 2004. "Unemployment, Poverty, and Social Isolation: An Assessment of the Current State of Social Exclusion Theory." Pp. 34–53 in *Resisting Marginalization: Unemployment Experience and Social Policy and the European Union*, edited by Duncan Gallie. Oxford, UK: Oxford University Press.

Gallie, Duncan, Michael White, Yuan Cheng, and Mark Tomlinson. 1998. *Restructuring the Employment Relationship*. Oxford, UK: Clarendon.

Gallie, Duncan. 2004. "Unemployment, Marginalization Risks and Welfare Policy." Pp. 1–33 in *Resisting Marginalization: Unemployment Experience and Social Policy and the European Union*, edited by Duncan Gallie. Oxford, UK: Oxford University Press.

Gallo, Linda C., Shiva G. Ghaed, and Wendy S. Bracken. 2004. "Emotions and Cognitions in Coronary Heart Disease: Risk, Resilience, and Social Context." *Cognitive Therapy & Research* 28(5):669–694.

Galperin, Andrew, and Martie Haselton. 2010. "Predictors of How Often and When People Fall in Love." *Evolutionary Psychology* 8(1):5–28.

Galston, William A. 2005. *The Practice of Liberal Pluralism*. Cambridge, UK: Cambridge University Press.

Gamson, William A. 1992. *Talking Politics*. Cambridge, UK: Cambridge University Press.

Gan, Yiqun and Fanny M. Cheung. 2010. "From Proactive Personality to Organizational Citizenship Behavior: Mediating Role of Harmony." *Psychological Reports* 106(3):755–65.

Gander, Fabian, Ines Gaitzsch, and Willibald Ruch. 2020. "The Relationships of Team Role- and Character Strengths-Balance with Individual and Team-Level Satisfaction and Performance." *Frontiers in Psychology* 11:566222.

Gangl, Markus. 2006. "Scar Effects of Unemployment: An Assessment of Institutional Complementarities." *American Sociological Review* 71(6):986–1013.

Ganster, Daniel and Bart Victor. 1988. The Impact of Social Support on Mental and Physical Health. *British Journal of Medical Psychology* 61:71–36.

Gant, Judy R., Robert J. Calsyn, and Joel Winter. 1999. "Predicting Agreement between Providers and Recipients of Social Support." *Journal of Social Behavior & Personality* 14(4):523–546.

Gao, Li and Weitao Jin. 2015. "Work-Family Conflict Mediates the Association between Job Demands and Life and Job Satisfaction in Chinese Middle Level Managers." *Current Psychology* 34(2):311–20.

Gao, Qin, Irwin Garfinkel, and Fuhua Zhai. 2009. "Anti-poverty Effectiveness of the Minimum Living Standard Assistance Policy in Urban China." *Review of Income & Wealth* 55(S1):630–655.

Gao, Shuqing, Hao Chen, Kaisheng Lai, and Weining Qian. 2021. "Predicting Regional Variations in Nationalism with Online Expression of Disgust in China." *Frontiers in Psychology* 12:564386.

Gao, Yunjiao, Dennis S.W. Wong, and Yanping Yu. 2015. "Maltreatment and Delinquency in China: Examining and Extending the Intervening Process of General Strain Theory." *International Journal of Offender Therapy & Comparative Criminology* 60(1):38–61.

Garcia, Enrique, and Juan Herrero. 2004. "Determinants of Social Integration in the Community: An Exploratory Analysis of Personal Interpersonal and Situational Variables." *Journal of Community & Applied Social Psychology* 14:1–15.

Garcia, Jeanette M., John R. Sirard, Nancy L. Deutsch, and Arthur Weltman. 2016. "The Influence of Friends and Psychosocial Factors on Physical Activity and Screen Time Behavior in Adolescents: A Mixed-Methods Analysis." *Journal of Behavioral Medicine* 39(4):610–623.

Garcia, Randi L., Hilary B. Bergsieker, and J. Nicole Shelton. 2017. "Racial Attitude (Dis)Similarity and Liking in Same-Race Minority Interactions." *Group Processes & Intergroup Relations* 20(4):501–18.

Garcia-Ruiz, Marta, Maria Jose Rodrigo, Juan Andres Hernandez-Cabrera, Maria Luisa Maiquez, and Maja Dekovic. 2013. "Resolution of Parent-Child Conflicts in the Adolescence." *European Journal of Psychology of Education* 28(2):173–88.

Gardner, Theodore W., Thomas J. Dishion, and Arin M Connell. 2008. "Adolescent Self-Regulation as Resilience: Resistance to Antisocial Behavior within the Deviant Peer Context." *Journal of Abnormal Child Psychology* 36(2):273–284.

Garfin, Dana Rose, E. Alison Holman, and Roxane Cohen Silver. 2015. "Cumulative Exposure to Prior Collective Trauma and Acute Stress Responses to the Boston Marathon Bombings." *Psychological Science* 26(6):675–83.

Garg, Naval and Ayatakshee Sarkar. 2020. "Vitality among University Students: Exploring the Role of Gratitude and Resilience." *Journal of Organizational Effectiveness* 7(3):321–37.

Garland, Ann F., and Edward F. Zigler. 1994. "Psychological Correlates of Help-seeking Attitudes among Children and Adolescents." *American Journal of Orthopsychiatry* 64(4):586–593.

Garner, Richard. 1994. *Beyond Morality*. Philadelphia, PA: Temple University Press.

Garnier, Helen E., and Judith A. Stein. 2002. "An 18-year Model of Family and Peer Effects on Adolescent Drug Use and Delinquency." *Journal of Youth & Adolescence* 31(1):45–56.

Garrett, Paul Michael. 2016. "Questioning Tales of 'Ordinary Magic': 'Resilience' and Neo-Liberal Reasoning." *British Journal of Social Work* 46(7):1909–1925.

Garriott, Patton O., Kristin M. Hultgren, and Julian Frazier. 2017b. "STEM Stereotypes and High School Student? Math/Science Career Goals." *Journal of Career Assessment* 25(4):585–600.

Garrod, Joan and Mursha Jones. 2009. *Religion and Belief.* Houndmills, UK: Palgrave.

Garst, Barry A., Ryan J. Gagnon, Thomas Clanton, and Jay Woodward. 2021. "Cultivating Youth Affinity for College within the Context of Campus-Based Summer Camps." *Journal of Youth Development* 16(5):64–85.

Gary, Tiffany L., Sarah A. Stark, and Thomas A. LaVeist. 2007. "Neighborhood Characteristics and Mental Health among African Americans and Whites Living in a Racially Integrated Urban Community." *Health & Place* 13:569–575.

Gasiorek, Jessica and R. Kelly Aune. 2021. *Creating Understanding: How Communicating Aligns Minds*. New York, NY: Lang.

Gass, Robert H., and John S. Seiter. 2004. "Theorizing about Persuasion: Cornerstones of Persuasion Research." Pp. 45–64 in *Perspectives and Persuasion, Social Influence, and Compliance Gaining*, edited by John S. Seiter and Robert H. Gass. Boston, MA: Pearson.

Gastil, John. 2000. "The Political Beliefs and Orientations of People with Disabilities." *Social Science Quarterly* 81(2):588–603.

Gatersleben, Birgitta, and Isabelle Griffin. 2017. "Environmental Stress." Pp. 469–485 in *Handbook of Environmental Psychology and Quality of Life Research*, edited by Ghozlane Fleury-Bahi, Graciela Tonon, Enric Pol, and Oscar Navarro. Cham, Switzerland: Springer.

Gattino, Silvia. Chiara Rollero, and Norma De Piccoli. 2015. "The Influence of Coping Strategies on Quality of Life from a Gender Perspective." *Applied Research in Quality of Life* 10(4):689–701.

Gault-Sherman, Martha. 2012. "It's a Two-Way Street: The Bidirectional Relationship between Parenting and Delinquency." *Journal of Youth & Adolescence* 41(2):121–145.

Gaunt, Ruth. 2011. "Effects of Intergroup Conflict and Social Contact on Prejudice: The Mediating Role of Stereotypes and Evaluations." *Journal of Applied Social Psychology* 41(6):1340–55.

Gay, David A. and John P. Lynxwiler. 2009. "The Impact of Race on Denominational Variations in Social Attitudes: The Issue and Its Dimensions." *Sociological Spectrum* 30(1):110–27.

Ge, Jingjing, Jingjing Yang, Jingjing Song, Guangyu Jiang, and Yong Zheng. 2020. "Dispositional Mindfulness and Past-Negative Time Perspective: The Differential Mediation Effects of Resilience and Inner Peace in Meditators and Non-Meditators." *Psychology Research & Behavior Management* 13:397–405.

Gearity, Brian T. and Melissa A. Murray. 2011. "Athletes' Experiences of the Psychological Effects of Poor Coaching." *Psychology of Sport & Exercise* 12(3):213–21.

Geboers, Ellen, Femke Geijsel, Wilfried Admiraal, Terrence Jorgensen, and Geert ten Dam. 2015. "Citizenship Development of Adolescents During the Lower Grades of Secondary Education." *Journal of Adolescence* 45:89–97.

Geeraert, Nicolas, and Stephanie Demoulin. 2013. "Acculturative Stress or Resilience? A Longitudinal Multilevel Analysis of Sojourners' Stress and Self-esteem." *Journal of Cross-Cultural Psychology* 44(8):1241–1262.

Gehring, Kai. 2013. "Who Benefits from Economic Freedom? Unraveling the Effect of Economic Freedom on Subjective Well-Being." *World Development* 50:74–90.

Gehrke, Sean J. 2008. "Leadership through Meaning-making: An Empirical Exploration of Spirituality and Leadership in College Students." *Journal of College Student Development* 49(4):351–359.

Geldard, Kathryn, and David Geldard. 2012a. "Counselling Children." Pp. 564–568 in *The SAGE Handbook of Counselling and Psychotherapy*, edited by Colin Feltham and Ian Horton. London: SAGE.

Geldard, Kathryn, and David Geldard. 2012b. "Counselling Young People." Pp. 669–675 in *The SAGE Handbook of Counselling and Psychotherapy*, edited by Colin Feltham and Ian Horton. London: SAGE.

Gelissen, John. 2002. Worlds of Welfare, Worlds of Consent? Public Opinion on the Welfare State. Leiden, Netherlands: Brill.

Geller, Daniel S., and J. David Singer. 1998. *Nations at War: A Scientific Study of International Conflict*. Cambridge, UK: Cambridge University Press.

Gelles, Richard J. 2007. "Family Violence." Pp. 403–417 in *The Cambridge Handbook of Violent Behavior and Aggression*, edited by Daniel J. Flannery, Alexander T. Vazsonyi and Irwin D. Waldman. Cambridge, UK: Cambridge University Press.

Georgas, Tames, Sophia Christakopoalou, Ype H. Poortinga, Alois Ahgleitner, Robin Goodwin, and Neophytos Charalambous. 1997. "The Relationship of Family Bonds to Family Structure and Function across Cultures." *Journal of Cross-Cultural Psychology* 28(3):303–320.

George, Login S., and Crystal L. Park. 2013. "Are Meaning and Purpose Distinct? An Examination of Correlates and Predictors." *Journal of Positive Psychology* 8(5):365–375.

Georgiades, Katholiki, and Michael H. Boyle, and Kelly A. Fife. 2013. "Emotional and Behavioral Problems among Adolescent Students: The Role of Immigrant, Racial/ethnic Congruence and Belongingness in Schools." *Journal of Youth & Adolescence* 42:1473–1492.

Gerard, Jean M., and Cheryl Buehler. 2004. "Cumulative Environmental Risk and Youth Problem Behavior." *Journal of Marriage & Family* 66(3):702–720.

Gerbasi, Alexandra, and Karen S. Cook. 2008. "The Effect of Perceived Trustworthiness on Affect in Negotiated and Reciprocal Exchange." Pp. 141–165 in *Social Structure and Emotion*, edited by Jody Clay-Warner and Dawn T. Robinson. San Diego, CA: Academic.

Gerber, Markus, Tim Hartmann, Serge Brand, Edith Holsboer-Trachsler, and Uwe Pühse. 2010. "The Relationship between Shift Work, Perceived Stress, Sleep and Health in Swiss Police Officers." *Journal of Criminal Justice* 38(6):1167–1175.

Gergen, Kenneth J., and Mary Gergen. 2010. "Positive Aging: Resilience and Reconstruction." Pp. 340–356 in *New Frontiers in Resilient Aging: Life-strengths and Well-being in Late Life*, edited by Prom S. Fry and Corey L.M. Keyes. Cambridge, UK: Cambridge University Press.

Gergen, Mary K., and Kenneth J. Gergen. 2006. "Narratives in Action." *Narrative Inquiry* 16(1):112–121.

German, Miguelina, Nancy A. Gonzales, and Larry Dumka. 2009. "Familism Values as a Protective Factor for Mexican-origin Adolescents Exposed to Deviant Peers." *Journal of Early Adolescence* 29(1):16–42.

Gerometta, Julia, Hartmut Haussermann, and Giulia Longo. 2005. "Social Innovation and Civil Society in Urban Governance: Strategies for an Inclusive City." *Urban Studies* 42(11):2007–2021.

Gershuny, Jonathan. 2000. *Changing Times: Work and Leisure in Postindustrial Society*. Oxford, UK: Oxford University Press.

Gersitel, Naomi, and Dan Clauson. 2014. "Class Advantage and the Gender Divide: Flexibility on the Job and at Home." *American Journal of Sociology* 120(2):394–431.

Gerstorf, Denis, Jacqui Smith, and Paul B. Baltes. 2006. "A Systemic-wholistic Approach to Differential Aging: Longitudinal Findings from the Berlin Aging Study." *Psychology & Aging* 21(4):645–663.

Geys, Benny, and Zuzana Murdoch. 2010. "Measuring the Bridging versus Bonding Nature of Social Networks: A Proposal for Integrating Existing Measures." *Sociology* 44(3):5230540.

Geys, Benny. 2012. "Association Membership and Generalized Trust: Are Connections between Associations Losing their Value?" *Journal of Civil Society* 8(1):1–15.

Gfellner, Barbara M. and Ana I. Cordoba. 2017. "Identity Problems, Ego Strengths, Perceived Stress, and Adjustment During Contextual Changes at University." *Identity* 17(1):25–39.

Gharaei, Nadya, Karen Phalet, and Fenella Fleischmann. 2018. "Contingent National Belonging: The Perceived Fit and Acceptance of Culturally Different Peers Predicts Minority Adolescents' Own Belonging." *Frontiers in Psychology* 9:1975.

Ghayas, Saba and Farah Malik. 2013. "Sociability and Academic Achievement as Predictors of Creativity Level among University Students." *Journal of the Indian Academy of Applied Psychology* 39(2):266–73.

Ghimire, Ramesh. 2021a. "Homeownership and Community Involvement: Results from the 2019 Metro Atlanta Speaks Survey." *Housing Policy Debate* 31(6):837–61.

Ghitterbuck, David Ashley, and Gordon Spence. 2017. "Working with goals in Coaching." Pp. 218–237 in *The SAGE Handbook of Coaching*, edited by Tatiana Bachkirova, Gordon Spence, and David Drake. London, UK: SAGE.

Ghoncheh, Shahyad and Jonathan C. Smith. 2004. "Progressive Muscle Relaxation, Yoga Stretching, and ABC Relaxation Theory." *Journal of Clinical Psychology* 60(1):131–36.

Ghorbani, Bima, Mark N. Bing, P.J. Watson, H. Knstl Davison, and Dan A. Mark. 2002. "Self-report Emotional Intelligence: Construct Similarity and Functional Dissimilarity of Higher-order Processing in Iran and the United States." *International Journal of Psychology* 37(5):297–308.

Giambra, Leonard. M. 2018. "Character Strengths: Stability and change from a military college education." *Military Psychology* 30(6):598–608.

Gibbs, Benjamin G., Lance D. Erickson, Mikael J. Dufur, and Aaron Miles. 2015. "Extracurricular Associations and College Enrollment." *Social Science Research* 50:367–381.

Gibbs, John C. 2014. Moral Development and Reality beyond the Theories of Kohlberg, Hoffman, and Haidt. New York: Oxford University Press.

Gibbs, John C., Karen S. Basinger, Rebecca L. Grime, and John R. Snarey. 2007. "Moral Judgment Development across Cultures: Revisiting Kohlberg's Universality Claims." *Developmental Review* 27(4):443–500.

Gibson, James L. 2001. "Social Networks, Civil Society, and the Prospects for Consolidating Russia's Democratic Transition." *American Journal of Political Science* 45(1):51–68.

Gibson, James L. 2008. "Group Identities and Theories of Justice: An Experimental Investigation into the Justice and Injustice of Land Squatting in South Africa." *Journal of Politics* 70(3):700–716.

Gibson, James L. 2013. "Measuring Political Tolerance and General Support for Pro-Civil Liberties Policies." *Public Opinion Quarterly* 77(S1):45–68.

Gibson-Davis, Christina M. 2009. "Money, Marriage, and Children: Testing the Financial Expectations and Family Formation Theory." *Journal of Marriage & Family* 71:146–160.

Gifford, Robert. 2011. "The Role of Nonverbal Communication in Interpersonal Relations." Pp. 171–190 in *Handbook of Interpersonal Psychology Theory, Research, Assessment, and Therapeutic Interventions*, edited by Leonard M. Horowitz and Stephen Strack. Hoboken, NJ: Wiley.

Giffords, Elissa D. 2009. "An Examination of Organizational Commitment and Professional Commitment and the Relationship to Work Environment, Demographic and Organizational Factors." *Journal of Social Work* 9(4):386–404.

Gil, Ana Isabel, and Jose Alberto Molina. 2007. "Human Development and Alcohol Abuse in Adolescence." *Applied Economics* 39:1315–1323.

Gilberbloom, John I., and John Po. Markham. 1995. "The Impact of Homeownership on Political Beliefs." *Social Forces* 73(4):1589–1607.

Giles, Howard, and Gordan Soliz. 2015. "Communication Accommodation Theory: A Situated Framework for Relational, Family, and Intergroup Dynamics." Pp. 161–173 in *Engaging Theories in Interpersonal Communication: Multiple Perspectives*, edited by Dawn O. Braithwaite and Paul Schrodt. Thousand Oaks, CA: SAGE.

Gill, Anthony. 2004. "Weber in Latin America: Is Protestant Growth Enabling the Consolidation of Democratic Capitalism?" *Democratization* 11(4):42–65.

Gillath, Omri, Phillip R. Shaver, Mario Mikulincer, Rachel E. Nitzberg, Ayelet Erez, Marinus H. Van Ijzendoorn. 2005. "Attachment, Caregiving, and Volunteering: Placing Volunteerism in an Attachment-theoretical Framework." *Personal Relationships* 12(4):425–446.

Gillespie, Alex. 2018. "Distinguishing Two Processes of Self-reflection." Pp. 245–259 in *The Cambridge Handbook of Sociocultural Psychology*, edited by Alberto Rosa and Jaan Valsiner. Cambridge, UK: Cambridge University Press.

Gilley, Bruce and Heike Holbig. 2009. "The Debate on Party Legitimacy in China: A Mixed Quantitative Qualitative Analysis." *Journal of Contemporary China* 18(59):339–358.

Gilligan, Robbie. 2009. "Positive Turning Points in the Dynamics of Change over the Life Course." Pp. 15–34 in *Pathways of Human Development: Explorations of Change*, edited by Jay A. Mancini and Karen A. Roberto. Lanham, MD: Lexington.

Gilman, Rich. 2000. "The Relationship between Life Satisfaction, Social Interest, and Frequency of Extracurricular Activities among Adolescent Students." *Journal of Youth & Adolescence* 30(6):749–767.

Gilman, Rich. 2001. "The Relationship between Life Satisfaction, Social Interest, and Frequency of Extracurricular Activities among Adolescent Students." *Journal of Youth & Adolescence* 30(6):749–767.

Gilmore, Linda, Marilyn Campbell, Ian Shochet, and Clare Roberts. 2013. "Resiliency Profiles of Children with Intellectual Disability and Their Typically Developing Peers." *Psychology in the Schools* 50(10):1032–43.

Gimpel, James G. and J. Celeste Lay. 2008. "Political Socialization and Reactions to Immigration-Related Diversity in Rural America." *Rural Sociology* 73(2):180–204.

Ginevra, Maria Cristina, Chiara Annovazzi, Sara Santilli, Ilaria Di Maggio, and Elisabetta Camussi. 2018. "Breadth of Vocational Interests: The Role of Career Adaptability and Future Orientation." *Career Development Quarterly* 66(3):233–245.

Ginevra, Maria Cristina, Susanna Pallini, Giovanni Maria Vecchio, Laura Nota, and Salvatore Soresi. 2016. "Future Orientation and Attitudes Mediate Career Adaptability and Decidedness." *Journal of Vocational Behavior* 95–96:102–110.

Gino, Francesca, and Adam D. Galinsky. 2012. "Vicarious Dishonesty: When Psychological Closeness Creates Distance from One's Moral Compass." *Organizational Behavior & Human Decision Processes* 119(1):15–26.

Giordano, Peggy C., Monica A. Longmore, Wendy D. Manning. 2006. "Gender and the Meanings of Adolescent Romantic Relationships: A Focus on Boys." *American Sociological Review* 71(2):260–287.

Giraldez-Garcia, Carolina, Maria Joas Forjaz, Maria-Eugenia Prieto-Flores, Fermina Rojo-Perez, Gloria Fernandez-Mayoralas, and Pablo Mortinez-Martin. 2013. "Individual's Perspective of Local Community Environment and Health Indicators in Older Adults." *Geriatrics & Gerontology International* 13:130–138.

Giri, Anaata Kumar. 2011. "Cultivating Transformative Reconciliation and Striving for Peace: Compassion, Confrontation and a New Art of Integration." *Current Sociology* 59(5):604–609.

Gitto, Lara, Yong-Hwan Noh, and Antonio Rodríguez Andrés. 2020. "Have Lifestyle Factors Led to Perceiving a Higher Level of Stress? Implications for Mental Health Policies from an Econometric Analysis for South Korea." *Journal of Asian Public Policy* 13(3):257–76.

Glaeser, Edward L., and Joshua D. Gottlieb. 2006. "Urban Resurgence and the Consumer City." *Urban Studies* 43(8):1275–1299.

Glaeser, Edward L., David L. Laibson, Jose A. Scheinkman, and Christine L. Soutter. 2000. "Measuring Trust." *Quarterly Journal of Economics* 115(5):811–846.

Glasberg, Davita Silfen, and Deric Shannon Contributors. 2018. "Resistance." Pp. 812–827 in *The SAGE Handbook of Political Sociology*, edited by William Outhwaite and Stephen Turner. London, UK: SAGE.

Glendinning, Anthony, Mark Nuttall, Leo Hendry, Marion Kleop, and Shila Wood. 2003. "Rural Communities and Well-being: A Good Place to Grow up?" *Sociological Review* 51(1):129–156.

Glendinning, Caroline. 2008. "Increasing Choice and Control for Older and Disabled People: A Critical Review of New Developments in England." *Social Policy & Administration* 42(5):451–469.

Glenn, Evelyn Nakano. 2000. "Creating a Caring Society." *Contemporary Sociology* 29(1):84–94.

Glover, Troy D., Diana C. Perry, and Kimberly J. Shinew. 2005. "Building Relationships Accessing Resources: Mobilizing Social Capital in Community Garden Contexts." *Journal of Leisure Research* 37(4):450–474.

Gluck, Judith, Susan Bluck, Jacqueline Baron, and Dan P. McAdams. 2005. "the Wisdom of Experience: Autobiographical Narratives across Adulthood." *International Journal of Behavioral Development* 29(3):197–208.

Godoy, Richardo, Victoria Reyes-Garcia, Tomas Huanca, William R. Leonard , Ramona G. Olvera, Jonathan Bauchet, Zhao Ma, Jonathan St. John, Marisa Miodowski, Oscar Zapata Rios, Vincent Vadez, and Craig Seyfried. 2007. "The Role of Community and Individuals in the Formation of Local Capital." *Human Ecology* 35:709–721.

Godwin, Emilie E., Herman R. Lukow, and Stephanie Lichiello. 2015. "Promoting Resilience Following Traumatic Brain Injury: Application of an Interdisciplinary, Evidence-Based Model for Intervention." *Family Relations* 64(3):347–362.

Goerres, Achim. 2007. "Why are Older People More Likely to Vote? The Impact of Ageing on Electoral Turnout in Europe." *British Journal of Politics & International Relations* 9(1):90–121.

Goertz-Dorten, Anja, Christina Benesch, Christopher Hautmann, Emel Berk-Pawlitzek, Martin Faber, Timo Lindenschmidt, Rahel Stadermann, Lioba Schuh, and Manfred Doepfner. 2017. "Efficacy of an Individualized Social Competence Training for Children with Oppositional Defiant Disorders/Conduct Disorders." *Psychotherapy Research* 27(3):326–337.

Goetz, Stephan J., Mark D. Partridge, Dan S. Rickman, and Shibalee Majumdar. 2011. "Sharing the Gains of Local Economic Growth: Race-to-the-Top versus Race-to-the Bottom Economic Development." *Environment & Planning C: Government & Policy* 29:428–456.

Golberstein, Ezra, Daniel Eisenberg, and Sarah E. Gollust. 2008. "Perceive Stigma and Mental Health Care Seeking." *Psychiatric Services* 59(4):392–399.

Gold, Alice Ross, Richard Christie, and Lucy Norman Friedman. 1976. *Fists and Flowers: A Social Psychological Interpretation of Student Dissent*. New York: Academic.

Goldberg, Abbie E., and Mauren Perry-Jenkins. 2004. "Division of Labor and Working-class Women's Well-being across the Transition to Parenthood." *Journal of Family Psychology* 18(1):225–236.

Goldberg, Steven. 1993. *Why Men Rule: A Theory of Male Dominance*. Chicago, IL: Open Court.

Goldenberg, Irina, Kimberly Matheson, and Janet Mantler. 2006. "The Assessment of Emotional Intelligence: A Comparison of Performance-based and Self-report Methodologies." *Journal of Personality Assessment* 86(1):33–45.

Goldman, Sharon, and Kobi Peleg. 2010. "Pupil Behaviour on School Buses and Potential Risk Factors for Injury: An Observational Study." *Bulletin of the World Health Organization* 88(8):570–575.

Goldner, Limor, Rachel Lev-Weisel, and Yael Schanan. 2019. "Caring About Tomorrow: The Role of Potency, Socio-Economic Status and Gender in Israeli Adolescents" Academic Future Orientation." *Child Indicators Research* 12(4):1333–1349.

Goldstein, Eda G. 1995. *Ego Psychology and Social Work Practices*. New York, NY: Free.

Goldstein, Eda G. 2001. *Object Relations Theory and Self Psychology in Social Work Practice*. New York, NY: Free.

Gomez-Baya, Diego, Ramon Mendoza, Margarida Gaspar de Matos, and Alvaro Tomico. 2019. "Sport Participation, Body Satisfaction and Depressive Symptoms in Adolescence: A Moderated-mediation Analysis of Gender Differences." *European Journal of Developmental Psychology* 16(2):183–197.

Gonzalez, Maru, Michael Kokozos, Christy M. Byrd, and Katherine E. McKee. 2020. "Critical Positive Youth Development: A Framework for Centering Critical Consciousness." *Journal of Youth Development* 15(6):24–43.

Gonzalez-Castro, José Luis, Silvia Ubillos-Landa, Alicia Puente-Martínez, and Marcela Gracia-Leiva. 2021. "Perceived Vulnerability and Severity Predict Adherence to Covid-19 Protection Measures: The Mediating Role of Instrumental Coping." *Frontiers in Psychology* 12:674032.
Gonzalez-Cutre, David, Álvaro Sicilia, Ana C Sierra, Roberto Ferriz, and Martin Hagger. 2016. "Understanding the Need for Novelty from the Perspective of Self-Determination Theory." *Personality & Individual Differences* 102:159–169.
Gonzalez-Jimenez, Hector. 2016. "Associations between Cosmopolitanism, Body Appreciation, Self-Esteem and Sought Functions of Clothing." *Personality & Individual Differences* 101:110–113.
Goodman, Fallon R., David J. Disabato, Todd B. Kashdan, and Kyla A. Machell. 2017. "Personality Strengths as Resilience: A One-Year Multiwave Study." *Journal of Personality* 85(3):423–434.
Goodwin, R. Kenneth, Jennifer W. Godwin, and Volerie Martinez-Ebers. 2004. "Civic Socialization in Public and Fundamentalist Schools." *Social Service Quarterly* 85(5):1097–1111.
Goodwin, Robin, George Nizharadze, Lan Anh Nguyen Luu, Eva Kosa, and Tatiana Emelyanava. 2001. "Social Support for a Changing Europe: An Analysis of Three Post-Communist Nations." *European Journal of Social Psychology* 31:379–393.
Gorbett, Kelly, and Theresa Kruczek. 2008. "Family Factors Predicting Social Self-esteem in Young Adults." *Family Journal of* 16(1):58–65.
Gordon, Kristin. 2008. "Tightening the Ship or Slowly Sinking? Reshaping Teachers" Work Conditions." *Research in Sociology of Education* 16:103–131.
Goren, Paul. 2005. "Party Identification and Core Political Values." *American Journal of Political Science* 49(4):881–896.
Gorman, Bridget K., Elaine Howard Ecklund, and Holly E. Heard. 2010. "Nativity Differences in Physical Health: The Roles of Emotional Support, Family, and Social Integration." *Sociological Spectrum* 30(6):671–94.
Gorsuch, Richard L., and William R. Miller. 1999. "Assessing Spirituality." Pp. 47–64 in *Integrating Spirituality into Treatment: Resources for Practitioners*, edited by William R. Miller. Washington, DC: American Psychological Association.
Gottfredson, Michael R. 2018. "Self-control Theory and Criminal Violence." Pp. 301–323 in *The Cambridge Handbook of Violent Behavior and Aggression*, edited by Alexander T. Vazsonyi, David J. Flannery and Matt DeLisi. Cambridge, UK: Cambridge University Press.
Gotzsche-Astrup, Oluf. 2020. "Pathways to Violence: Do Uncertainty and Dark World Perceptions Increase Intentions to Engage in Political Violence?" *Behavioral Sciences of Terrorism & Political Aggression* 13(2):142–59.
Gould-Williams, Julian, and Fiona Davies. 2005. "Using Social Exchange Theory to Predict the Effects of HRM Practice in Employee Outcomes: An Analysis of Public Sector Workers." *Public Management Review* 7(1):1–24.
Gountas, John, Sandra Gountas, Robert A. Reeves, and Lucy Moran. 2012. "Desire for Fame: Scale Development and Association with Personal Goals and Aspirations." *Psychology & Marketing* 29(9):680–689.
Gowans, Christopher W. 2003. *Philosophy of the Buddha*. London, Routledge.
Gowdy, Grace, Daniel P. Miller, and Renée Spencer. 2020. "Expanding and Deepening Our Understanding of Which Young People Are Most Likely to Have an Informal Mentor." *Children & Youth Services Review 108:104490*.
Graber, Rebecca, Rhiannon Turner, and Anna Madill. 2016. "Best Friends and Better Coping: Facilitating Psychological Resilience through Boys? and Girls? Closest Friendships." *British Journal of Psychology* 107(2):338–358.
Graeff, Peter and Gert Tinggaard Svendsen. 2013. "Trust and Corruption: The Influence of Positive and Negative Social Capital on the Economic Development in the European Union." *Quality & Quantity* 47(5):2829–46.
Graham, Carol, Soumya Chattopadhyay, and Mario Picon. 2010. "The Easterlin and Other Paradoxes: Why Both Sides of the Debate May be Correct." Pp. 247–288 in *International Differences*

*in Well-being*, edited by Ed Diener, John F. Helliwell and Daniel Kahneman. New York: Oxford University Press.

Graham, Steve, and Joe F. Donaldson. 1999. "Adult Students" Academic and Intellectual Development in College." *Adult Education Quarterly* 49(3):147–161.

Grandey, Alica A., and Russell Cropanzano. 1999. "The Conservation of Resources Model Applied to Work-family Conflict and Strain." *Journal of Vocational Behavior* 54:350–370.

Grant, Adam M. and Francesca Gino. 2010. "A Little Thanks Goes a Long Way: Explaining Why Gratitude Expressions Motivate Prosocial Behavior." *Journal of Personality & Social Psychology* 98(6):946–55.

Grant, Anthony M., and Michael J. Cavanagh. 2018. "The Solution-focused Approach to Coaching.} Pp. 35–51 in *The Complete Handbook of Coaching*, edited by Elaine Cox, Tatiana Bachkirova, and David Clutterbuck. London, UK: SAGE.

Grant, Nicholas J., Gabriel J. Merrin, Matthew T. King, and Dorothy L. Espelage. 2019. "Examining within-Person and between-Person Associations of Family Violence and Peer Deviance on Bullying Perpetration among Middle School Students." *Psychology of Violence* 9(1):18–27.

Granzin, Kent L., and Janeen E. Olsen. 1998. "Americans" Choice of Domestic over Foreign Products: A Matter of Helping Behavior?" *Journal of Business Research* 43:39–54.

Granzin, Kent L., and Lois M. Haggard. 2000. "An Integrative Explanation for Quality of Life: Development and Test of a Structural Model." Pp. 31–64 in *Advances in Quality of Life Theory and Research*, edited by Ed Diener and Don R. Rahtz. Dordrecht, Netherlands: Kluwer Academic.

Graser, Johannes, Volkmar Höfling, Charlotte Weβlau, Adriana Mendes, and Ulrich Stangier. 2016. "Effects of a 12-Week Mindfulness, Compassion, and Loving Kindness Program on Chronic Depression: A Pilot within-Subjects Wait-List Controlled Trial." *Journal of Cognitive Psychotherapy* 30(1):35–49.

Grasmick, Harold G., John Hagan, Brenda Sims Blackwell, and Bruce J. Arneklev. 1996. "Risk Preferences and Patriarchy: Extending Power-control Theory." *Social Forces* 75(1):177–199.

Grasner, Aviva Twersky. 2013. "Lonnie Athens Revisited: The Social Construction of Violence." *Aggression & Violent Behavior* 18:281–285.

Grasso, Maria T. 2014. "Age, Period and Cohort Analysis in A Comparative Context: Political Generations and Political Participation Repertoires in Western Europe." *Electoral Studies* 33:63–76.

Graupensperger, Scott, Jordan Sutcliffe, and Stewart A. Vella. 2021. "Prospective Associations between Sport Participation and Indices of Mental Health across Adolescence." *Journal of Youth & Adolescence* 50(7):1450–63.

Grawe, Klaus. 2004. *Psychological Therapy*. Cambridge, MA: Hogrefe.

Gray, Anne. 2009. "The Social Capital of Older People." *Ageing & Society* 29:5–31.

Gray, David E. 2017. "Towards a Systematic Model of Coaching Supervision." Pp. 662–679 in *The SAGE Handbook of Coaching*, edited by Tatiana Bachkirova, Gordon Spence, and David Drake. London, UK: SAGE.

Grayling, A. C. 2013. The God Argument: The Case against Religion and for Humanism. New York: Bloomsbury.

Graziano, William O., and Renee M. Tobin. 2009. "Agreeableness." Pp. 46–61 in *Handbook of Individual Differences in Social Behavior*, edited by Mark R. Leary and Rick H. Hoyle. New York, NY: Guilford.

Grealish, Annmarie, Sara Tai, Andrew Hunter, Richard Emsley, Trevor Murrells, and Anthony P. Morrison. 2017. "Does Empowerment Mediate the Effects of Psychological Factors on Mental Health, Well-Being, and Recovery in Young People?" *Psychology & Psychotherapy* 90(3):314–35.

Greeff, Abraham P., and Stephanus van der Merwe. 2004. "Variables Associated with Resilience in Divorced Families." *Social Indicators Research* 68:59–75.

Green, Andy, and Jan Germen Janmaat. 2011. *Regimes of Social Cohesion: Societies and the Crisis of Globalization*. Houndmills, UK: Palgrave.

Green, Judith, and Nicki Thorogood. 1998. *Analysing Health Policy: Sociological Approach.* London: Longman.

Green, Michael J., Colin A. Espie, Michael Benzeval. 2014. "Social Class and Gender Patterning of Insomnia Symptoms and Psychiatric Distress: A 20-year Prospective Cohort Study." *BMC Psychiatry* 14(1):263–280.

Greenberg Leslie S. and Juan Pascual-Leone. 2001. "A Dialectical Constructivist View of the Creation of Personal Meaning." *Journal of Constructivist Psychology* 14(3):165–86.

Greenberg, L.S. 2004. "Emotion-focused Therapy." *Clinical Psychology & Psychotherapy* 11:3–16.

Greenberg, Leslie S. and Catalina Woldarsky Meneses. 2019. *Forgiveness and Letting Go in Emotion-Focused Therapy.* Washington, DC: American Psychological Association.

Greene, Ida. 1991. *Soft Power Negotiation Skills.* San Diego, CA: PSI.

Greene, Kaylin M., Bora Lee, Nicole Constance, and Kathryn Hynes. 2013. "Examining Youth and Program Predictors of Engagement in out-of-School Time Programs." *Journal of Youth & Adolescence* 42(10):1557–72.

Greene, Roberta R., Shira Hantman, Adi Sharabi, and Harriet Cohen. 2012. "Holocaust Survivors: Three Waves of Resilience Research." *Journal of Evidence-Based Social Work* 9(5):481–497.

Greenfield, Patricia M. 2009. "Linking Social Change and Developmental Change: Shifting Pathways of Human Development." *Developmental Psychology* 45(2):401–18.

Greenman, Emily, and Yu Xie. 2008. "Is Assimilation Theory Dead? The Effect of Assimilation on Adolescent well-being." *Social Science Research* 37:109–137.

Greenstein, Theodore N. 1996. "Gender Ideology and Perceptions of the Fairness of the Division of Household Labor Effects on Marital Quality." *Social Forces* 74(3):1029–1042.

Greenwald, Howard P., Suzanne O'Keefe, and Mark Dicamill. 2004. "The Importance of Public Sector Health Care in an Underserved Population." *Journal of Health & Human Services Administration* 27(2):142–57.

Greenwood, Dara N., and Christopher R. Long. 2011. "Attachment, Belongingness Needs, and Relationship." *Communication Research* 38(2):278–297.

Greenwood, Verity Anne, and Larry Dwyer. 2017. "Reinventing Macau tourism: Gambling on Creativity?" *Current Issues in Tourism* 20(6):580–602.

Gregg, Benjamin. 2003. Coping in Politics with Indeterminate Norms: A Theory of Enlightened Localism. Albany, NY: State University of New York Press.

Greitemeyer, Tobias, Peter Fischer, Andreas Kastenmuller, and Dieter Frey. 2006. "Civil Courage and Helping Behavior: Differences and Similarities." *European Psychologists* 11(2):90–98.

Gremmen, Mariola Claudia, Jan KornelisDijkstra, Christian Steglich, and Ren? Veenstra. 2017. "First Selection, Then Influence: Developmental Differences in Friendship Dynamics Regarding Academic Achievement." *Developmental Psychology* 53(7):1356–1370.

Griciute, Ausra. 2015. "Optimal Level of Participation in Sport Activities According to Gender and Age Can Be Associated with Higher Resilience: Study of Lithuanian Adolescents." *School Mental Health* 8(2):257–67.

Griffin, Jennifer D., and Ivan Y. Sun. 2018. "Do Work-Family Conflict and Resiliency Mediate Police Stress and Burnout? A Study of State Police Officers." *American Journal of Criminal Justice* 43(2):354–370.

Griffiths, Mark D. 1999. "Counselling in the Treatment of Pathological Gambling: An Overview." *British Journal of Guidance & Counselling* 27(2):179–190.

Grimes, Marcia. 2006. "Organizing Consent: The Role of Procedural Fairness in Political Trust and Compliance." *European Journal of Political Research* 45(2):285–315.

Grimley, Bruce. 2007. "NLP Coaching." Pp. 193–210 in *Handbook of Coaching Psychology: A Guide for Practitioners*, edited by Stephen Palmer and Alison Whybrow. Hove, UK: Routledge.

Grimley, Bruce. 2018. "the NLP Approach to Coaching." Pp. 184–198 in *The Complete Handbook of Coaching*, edited by Elaine Cox, Tatiana Bachkirova, and David Clutterbuck. London, UK: SAGE.

Grodzicka, Elżbieta Drążkiewicz, and Jaron Harambam. 2021. "What Should Academics Do About Conspiracy Theories? Moving Beyond Debunking to Better Deal with Conspiratorial Movements, Misinformation and Post-Truth." *Journal for Cultural Research* 25(1):1–11.

Gronlund, Anne and Ida Oun. 2010. "Rethinking Work-Family Conflict: Dual-Earner Policies, Role Conflict and Role Expansion in Western Europe." *Journal of European Social Policy* 20(3):179–95.

Gronlund, Anne, and Ida Oun. 2012. "Rethinking Work-family Conflict: Dual-earner Policies, Role Conflict and Role Expansion in Western Europe." *Journal of European Social Policy* 20(3):170–195.

Grootaert, Christiaan, and Thierry van Bastelaer. 2002. *Understanding and Measuring Social Capital: A Multidisciplinary Tool for Practitioners*. Washington, DC: World Bank.

Gross, James J. 2015. "Emotion Regulation: Current Status and Future Prospects." *Psychological Inquiry* 26(1):1–26.

Gross, Michael L. 1995. "Moral Judgment, Organizational Incentives and Collective Action: Participation in Abortion Politics." *Political Research Quarterly* 48(3):507–534. \

Gross, Neil. 2009. "A Pragmatist Theory of Social Mechanisms." *American Sociological Review* 74(3):358–379.

Gross, Revital, Shuli Brammli-Greenberg. 2004. "Evaluating the Effect of Regulatory Prohibitions against Risk Selection by Health Status on Supplemental Insurance Ownership in Israel." *Social Science & Medicine* 58:1609–1622.

Gross, Stephen. 2001. "On Integrity.." *Psychodynamic Counselling* 7(2):207–216.

Grossman, Klaus E., Karin Grossmann, Monika Winter, and Pater Zimmermann. 2002. "Attachment Relationships and Appraisal of Partnership: From Early Experience of Sensitive Support to Later Relationship Representation." Pp. 73–105 in *Paths to Successful Development: Personality in the Life Course*, edited by Lea Pulkkinen and Avshalom Caspi. Cambridge, UK: Cambridge University Press.

Groves, Robert M., Eleanor Singer, and Amy Corning. 2000. "Leverage-saliency Theory of Survey Participation." *Public Opinion Quarterly* 64:299–308.

Growiec, Katarzyna, and Jakub Growiec. 2010. "Bridging Social Capital and Individual Earnings: Evidence for an Inverted U." *Social Indicators Research* 127(2):601–631.

Grundy, Emily, and Andy Sloggett. 2003. "Health Inequalities in the Older Population: The Role of Personal Capital, Social Resources and Socio-economic Circumstances." *Social Science & Medicine* 56:935–947.

Grunebaum, James O. 2003. *Friendship: Liberty, Equality, and Utility*. Albany, NY: State University of New York Press.

Grych, John H., and Kristen M. Kinsfogel. 2010. "Exploring the Role of Attachment Style in the Relation between Family Aggression and Abuse in Adolescent Dating Relationships." *Journal of Aggression, Maltreatment & Trauma* 19(6):624–640.

Grzegorek, Jennifer L., Robert B. Slaney, Sarah Franze, and Kenneth G. Rice. 2004. "Self-Criticism, Dependency, Self-Esteem, and Grade Point Average Satisfaction among Clusters of Perfectionists and Nonperfectionists." *Journal of Counseling Psychology* 51(2):192–200.

Grzywacz, Joseph G., and Brenda L. Bass. 2003. "Work, Family, and Mental Health: Testing Different Models of Work-family Fit." *Journal of Marriage & Family* 65:248–262.

Grzywacz, Joseph G., and David M. Almeida. 2008. "Stress and Binge Drinking: A Daily Process Examination of Stressor Pile-up and Socioeconomic Stress on Affect Regulation." *International Journal of Stress Management* 15(4):364–380.

Grzywacz, Joseph G., and Nadine F. Marks. 2001. "Social Inequalities and Exercise during Adulthood toward an Ecological Perspective." *Journal of Health & Social Behavior* 42(2):202–220.

Gu, Chuanhua, Bi Ying Hu, Flemmings Fishani Ngwira, Zhi Jing, and Zongkui Zhou. 2016. "The Effect of General Creative Personality and Freedom of Task Choice on Adolescents" Social Creativity." *Journal of Creative Behavior* 50(2):132–149.

Gu, Danan, Jessica Sautter, Robin Pipkin, and Yi Zeng. 2010. "Sociodemographic and Health Correlates of Sleep Quality and Duration among Very Old Chinese." *Sleep* 33(5):601–610.

Gu, Jibao, Yanbing Zhang, and Hefu Liu. 2014. "Importance of Social Capital to Student Creativity within Higher Education in China." *Thinking Skills & Creativity* 12:14–25.

Guan, Bin, Guoxian Bao, Qingchuan Liu and Raduziner Gary Raymond. 2021. "Two-Way Risk Communication, Public Value Consensus, and Citizens" Policy Compliance Willingness about Covid-19: Multilevel Analysis Based on a Nudge View." *Administration & Society* 53(7):1106–49.

Guan, Tianru and Yilu Yang. 2020. "Diversifying Conspiracy Beliefs and Populist Ideologies in the Chinese Context." *Social Science Quarterly* 101(2):459–72.

Guan, Yanjun, Hong Deng, and Michael Harris Bond. 2010. "Examining Stereotype Content Model in a Chinese Context: Inter-Group Structural Relations and Mainland Chineses Stereotypes Towards Hong Kong Chinese." *International Journal of Intercultural Relations* 34(4):393–99.

Guan, Yanjun, Michael Harris Bond, Zheng Huang, Zhiyong Zhang, Hong Deng, Tian Hu, and Haiyan Gao. 2009. "Role of Personal Endorsement of Outgroup Members" Distinctive Values and Need for Cognitive Closure in Attitude towards the Outgroup." *Asian Journal of Social Psychology* 12:54–62.

Guardiola, Jorge, and Teresa Garcia-Munoz. 2011. "Fulfilment of Basic Needs from a Subjective Point of View in Rural Guatemala." *International Journal of Social Welfare* 20(4):393–403.

Guay, Frederic, Catherine F. Ratelle, Caroline Senecal, Simon Larose, and Andree Deschenes. 2006. "Distinguishing Developmental From Chronic Career Indecision: Self-Efficacy, Autonomy, and Social Support." *Journal of Career Assessment* 14(2):235–251.

Gudmundsdottir, Dora Gudrun. 2013. "The Impact of Economic Crisis on Happiness." *Social Indicators Research* 110(3):1083–1101.

Guerra, Nancy G., and Catherine P. Bradshaw. 2008. "Linking the Prevention of Problem Behaviors and Positive Youth Development: Care Competencies for Positive Youth Development and Risk Prevention." *New Directions for Child & Adolescent Development* 122:1–17.

Guerrero, Laura K. 2013. "Emotion and Communication in Conflict Interaction." Pp. 105–131 in *The SAGE Handbook of Conflict Communication*, edited by John G. Oetzel and Stelle Ting-Toomey. Thousand Oaks, CA: SAGE.

Guerrero, Laura K. 2015. "Attachment Theory: A communication Perspective." Pp. 321–334 in *Engaging Theories in Interpersonal Communication: Multiple Perspectives*, edited by Dawn O. Braithwaite and Paul Schrodt. Thousand Oaks, CA: SAGE.

Gui, Yong, Ronggui Huang, and Yi Ding. 2020. "Three Faces of the Online Leftists: An Exploratory Study Based on Case Observations and Big-Data Analysis." *Chinese Journal of Sociology* 6(1):67–101.

Guilfoyle, Michael. 2005. "From Therapeutic Power to Resistance? Therapy and Cultural Hegemony." *Theory & Psychology* 15(1):101–24.

Guillen, Laura, Lluis Coromina and Willem E. Saris. 2011. "Measurement of Social Participation and Its Place in Social Capital Theory." *Social Indicators Research* 100(2):331–350.

Guillen-Royo, Monica. 2008. "Consumption and Subjective Wellbeing: Exploring Basic Needs, Social Comparison, Social Integration and Hedonism in Peru." *Social Indicators Research* 89(3):535–55.

Guisan, M.-C. 2009. "Government Effectiveness, Education, Economic Development and Well-Being: Analysis of European Countries in Comparison with the United States and Canada, 2000–2007." *Applied Econometrics & International Development* 9(1):39–55.

Guiso, Luigi, Paloa Sapienza, and Luigi Zingales. 2004. "The Role of Social Capital in Financial Development." *American Economic Review* 94(3):526–536.

Gullan, Rebecca L., Thomas J. Power, and Stephen S. Leff. 2013. "The Role of Empowerment in a School-Based Community Service Program with Inner City, Minority Youth." *Journal of Adolescent Research* 28(6):664–689.

Gullatz, Stefan. 2010. "Constructing the Collective Unconscious." *Journal of Analytical Psychology* 55(5):691–714.

Gulliford, Liz, Blaire Morgan, Emily Hemming, and Jenny Abbott. 2019. "Gratitude, Self-Monitoring and Social Intelligence: A Prosocial Relationship?" *Current Psychology* 38(4):1021–1032.

Gummerum, Michaela, and Monika Keller. 2008. "Affection, Virtue, Pleasure, and profit: Developing an Understanding of Friendship Closeness and Intimacy in Western and Asian Societies." *International Journal of Behavioral Development* 32(3):218–231.

Gundelach, Birte, and Anita Manatschal. 2017. "Ethnic Diversity, Social Trust and the Moderating Role of Subnational Integration Policy." *Political Studies* 65(2):413–431.

Gundersen, Craig, and James P. Ziliak. 2004. "Poverty and Macroeconomic Performance across Space, Race, and Family Structure." *Demography* 41(1):61–86.

Gundert, Stefanie and Christian Hohendanner. 2015. "Active Labour Market Policies and Social Integration in Germany: Do "One-Euro-Jobs" Improve Individuals" Sense of Social Integration?" *European Sociological Review* 31(6):780–97.

Guntzviller, Lisa M., Chelsea L. Ratcliff, Travis E. Dorsch, and Keith V. Osai. 2017. "How Do Emerging Adults Respond to Exercise Advice from Parents? A Test of Advice Response Theory." *Journal of Social & Personal Relationships* 34(6):936–960.

Guo, Qiyong. 2018. *Chinese People's Wisdom.* Beijing, China: China.

Guo, Xiaohui, Seth J. Schwartz, and Brian E. McCabe. 2008. "Aging, Gender, and Self: Dimensionality and Measurement Invariance Analysis in Self-Construal." *Self & Identity* 7(1):1–24.

Guo, Yu, Hongzhe Xiang, and Yuhan Wang. 2023. "Understanding Self-Protective Behaviors During COVID-19 Pandemic: Integrating the Theory of Planned Behavior and O-S-O-R Model." *Current Psychology.*

Guo, Zhen, Ying Yang, Wenqi Li, Xiaonan Yao, and Yu Kou. 2023. "Longitudinal Relations among Honesty-Humility, Moral Disengagement, and Unethical Behavior in Adolescents: A between- and within-person Analysis." *Journal of Research in Personality* 106:104401.

Guroglu, Berna. Cornelis F. M. van Lieshout, Gerbert J. T. Haselager, and Ron H. J. Scholte. 2007. "Similarity and Complementarity of Behavioral Profiles of Friendship Types and Types of Friends: Friendships and Psychosocial Adjustment." *Journal of Research on Adolescence* 17(2):357–386.

Gursimsek, Isik, and Melek Goregenli. 2005. "Humanistic Attitudes, Values, System Justification, and Control Beliefs in a Turkish Sample." *Social Behavior & Personality* 34(7):747–758.

Gurung, Regan A. R., Stephanie Byers, Jor Grapentine, and Arianna Stone. 2023. "I Believe I Can Try: Self-Efficacy, Pandemic Behaviors, Coping, and Learning." *Psychology Learning & Teaching* 22(2):124–36.

Gustavsson, Gina. 2012. "Freedom in Mass Values: Egocentric, Humanistic, or Both? Using Isaiah Berlin to Understand a Contemporary Debate." *European Political Science Review* 4(2):241–262.

Gutierrez, Ian A., Crystal L. Park, and Bradley R. E. Wright. 2017. "When the Divine Defaults: Religious Struggle Mediates the Impact of Financial Stressors on Psychological Distress." *Psychology of Religion & Spirituality* 9(4):387–98.

Gutman, Leslie Morrison, Vonnie C. McLoyd, and Teru Tokoyawa. 2005. "Financial Strain, Neighborhood, Stress, Parenting Behaviors, and Adolescent Adjustment in Urban African American Families." *Journal of Research on Adolescence* 15(4):425–449.

Haapanen-Niemi, Nina, Seppo Miilunpalo, Ilkka Nuori, Matti Pasanen, Pekka Oja. 1999. "The Impact of Smoking, Alcohol Consumption, and Physical Activity on Use of Hospital Services." *American Journal of Public Health* 989(5):691–698.

Haas, Anne, and Stanford W. Gregory, Jr. 2005. "The Impact of Physical Attractiveness on Women's Social Status and Interactional Power." *Sociological Forum* 20(3):449–469.

Haberkern, Klaus, and Mare Szydlik. 2010. "State Care Provision Societal Opinion and Children's Care of Older Parents in 11 European Countries." *Ageing & Society* 30:299–323.

Habibis, Daphne, Nicholas Hookway, and Anthea Vreugdenhil. 2016. "Kindness in Australia: An Empirical Critique of Moral Decline Sociology: Kindness in Australia." *British Journal of Sociology* 67(3):395–413.

Habigzang, Luísa Fernanda, Bruno Figueiredo Damásio, and Silvia Helena Koller. 2013. "Impact Evaluation of a Cognitive Behavioral Group Therapy Model in Brazilian Sexually Abused Girls." *Journal of Child Sexual Abuse* 22(2):173–190.

Hackman, Daniel A., Stephanie A. Robert, Jascha Grübel, Raphael P. Weibel, Eirini Anagnostou, Christoph Hölscher, and Victor R. Schinazi. 2019. "Neighborhood Environments Influence Emotion and Physiological Reactivity." *Scientific Report* 9(1):9498–11.

Hadden, Wilbur C., Gregory Pappas, and Abdul Qayyum Khan. 2003. "Social Stratification Development and Health in Pakistan: An Empirical Exploration of Relationships in Population-based National Health Examination Survey Data." *Social Science & Medicine* 57:1863–1874.

Haddorff, David W. 2000. "Religion and the Market Opposition, Absorption, or Ambiguity." *Review of Social Economy* 58(4):483–503.

Hadjar, Andreas, and Robin Samuel. 2015. "Does Upward Social Mobility Increase Life Satisfaction? A Longitudinal Analysis Using British and Swiss Panel Data." *Research in Social Stratification & Mobility* 39:48–58.

Haesevoets, Tessa, Chris Reinders Folmer, and Alain Van Hiel. 2015. "Cooperation in Mixed-Motive Games: The Role of Individual Differences in Selfish and Social Orientation." *European Journal of Personality* 29(4):445–458.

Hafer, Carolyn L., and Robbie Sutton. 2016. "Belief in a Just World." Pp 145–160 in *Handbook of Social Justice Theory and Research*, edited by Clara Sabbagh and Manfred Schmitt. New York, NY: Springer.

Hagan, John, and Bill McCarthy. 1997. *Mean Streets: Youth Crime and Homelessness*. Cambridge, UK: Cambridge University Press.

Hagan, John, and Holly Foster. 2001. "Youth Violence and the End of Adolescence." *American Sociological Review* 66:874–899.

Hagan, John, Joshua Kaiser, and Anna Hanson. 2016. "The Theory of Legal Cynicism and Sunni Insurgent Violence in Post-Invasion Iraq." *American Sociological Review* 81(2):316–46.

Hagan, John, Ross MacMillan, and Blair Wheaton. 1996. "New Kid in Town: Social Capital and the Life Course Effects of Family Migration on Children." *American Sociological Review* 67(3):368–385.

Hagger, Martin S. and Kyra Hamilton. 2018. "Motivational Predictors of Students" Participation in out-of-School Learning Activities and Academic Attainment in Science: An Application of the Trans-Contextual Model Using Bayesian Path Analysis." *Learning & Individual Differences* 67:232–44.

Hagger, Martin S., Mike W. L. Cheung, Icek Ajzen, and Kyra Hamilton. 2022. "Perceived Behavioral Control Moderating Effects in the Theory of Planned Behavior: A Meta-Analysis." *Health Psychology* 41(2):155–67.

Hahn, Elisabeth, Wendy Johnson, and Frank M. Spinath. 2013. "Beyond the Heritability of Life Satisfaction: The Roles of Personality and Twin-specific Influences." *Journal of Research in Personality* 47:757–767.

Hahn, Elizabeth A., David Cella, Rita K. Bode, and Rachel T. Hanrahan. 2010. "Measuring Social Well-Being in People with Chronic Illness." *Social Indicators Research* 96(3):381–401.

Haidt, Jonathan. 2012. The Righteous Mind: Why Good People Are Divided by Politics and Religion. New York: Pantheon.

Hair, M., K. V. Renaud and J. Ramsay. 2007. "The Influence of Self-Esteem and Locus of Control on Perceived Email-Related Stress." *Computers in Human Behavior* 23(6):2791–803.

Hakhverdian, Armen and Quinton Mayne. 2012. "Institutional Trust, Education, and Corruption: A Micro-Macro Interactive Approach." *Journal of Politics* 74(3):1739–1750.

Halas, Elzbieta. 2010. Towards the World Culture Society: Florian Znanieckis's Culturalism. Frankfurt, Germany: Peter Lang

Halbesleben, Jonathon R.B. 2006. "Sources of Social Support and Burnout: A Meta-analytic Test of the Conservation of Resources Model." *Journal of Applied Psychology* 91(5):1134–1145.

Hale, Carl S. 1999. "Eight Levels of Social Interest: Adult Development from an Adlerian Paradigm." *Adultspan Journal* 1(2):66–78.

Halevy, Nir, Eliran Halali, and Taya R. Cohen. 2019. "Brokering Orientations and Social Capital: Influencing Others' Relationships Shapes Status and Trust." *Journal of Personality & Social Psychology* 119(2):293–316.

Hall, M. Elizabeth Lewis, Jason McMartin, Crystal L. Park, Shane J. Sacco, Dahee Kim, Kelly Kapic, Eric Silverman, Laura Shannonhouse, Jamie Aten, Lindsay M. Snow, and Luis Lopez. 2022. "Suffering with Christ: Emic Christian Coping and Relation to Well-Being." *SSM: Mental Health* 2:100158.

Hall, Peter H., and Michele Lamont. 2013. "Social Resilience in the Neoliberal Era." Pp. 1–31 in *Social Resilience in the Neoliberal Era*, edited by Peter A. Hall, and Michele Lamont. Cambridge, UK: Cambridge University Press.

Hall, Todd W., and Keith J. Edwards. 2002. "The Spiritual Assessment Inventory: A Theistic Model and Measurement for Assessing Spiritual Development." *Journal of the Scientific Study of Religion* 41(2):341–357.

Haller, Max, and Markus Hadler. 2006. "How Social Relations and Structures Can Produce Happiness and Unhappiness: An International Comparative Analysis." *Social Indicators Research* 75:169–216.

Hallerod, Bjorn. 2006. "Sour Grapes: Relative Deprivation Adaptive Preferences and the Measurement of Poverty." *Journal of Social Policy* 35(3):371–390.

Hallsworth, Simon, and Tara Young. 2010. "Street Collectives and Group Delinquency: Social Disorganization, Subcultures and beyond." Pp. 72–95 in *The SAGE Handbook of Criminological Theory*, edited by Eugene McLaughlin and Tim Newburn. London, UK: SAGE.

Halnon, Karen Bettez. 2006. "Heavy Metal Carnival and Dis-Alienation: The Politics of Grotesque Realism." *Symbolic Interaction* 29(1):33–48.

Halvorsen, Knut. 2007. "Legitimacy of Welfare States in Transition from Homogeneity to Multiculturality: A Matter of Trust." Pp. 239–259 in *Social Justice, Legitimacy and the Welfare State*, edited by Steffen Mau and Benjamin Veghte. Aldershot, UK: Ashgate.

Hamermesh, David S. 2019. *Spending Time: The Most Valuable Resource*. New York, NY: Oxford University Press.

Hamilton, Vivian E. 2010. "Immature Citizens and the State." *Brigham Young University Law Review* 2010(4):1055–1147.

Hamm, Jeremy M., Carsten Wrosch, Meaghan A. Barlow, and Ute Kunzmann. 2021. "A Tale of Two Emotions: The Diverging Salience and Health Consequences of Calmness and Excitement in Old Age." *Psychology & Aging* 36(5):626–41.

Hammer, Torild. 2007. "Labour Market Integration of Unemployed Youth from a Life Course Perspective: The Case of Norway." *Internatinal Journal of Social Welfare* 16:249–257.

Hammond, John L. 2015. "The Anarchism of Occupy Wall Street." *Science & Society* 79(2):288–313.

Hampel, Petra, and Fran Petermann. 2005. "Age and Gender Effects on Coping in Children and Adolescents." *Journal of Youth & Adolescence* 34(2):73–83. \75–177

Hample, Dale. 2018. *Inrterpersonal Aruging*. New York, NY: Lang. Seabach, Swen. 2017. *Love and Society: Special Social Forms and the Master Emotion*. Abingdon, UK: Routledge.

Hampton, Keith N. 2007. "Neighborhoods in the Network Society the E-Neighbors Study." *Information, Communication & Society* 10(5):714–48.

Han, Yoonsun, and Andrew Grogan-Kaylor. 2012. "Parenting and Youth Psychosocial Well-being in South Korea Using Fixed-effects Models." *Journal of Family Issues* 34(5):689–715.

Han, Ziqiang, Ivan Y. Sun, and Rong Hu. 2017. "Social Trust, Neighborhood Cohesion, and Public Trust in the Police in China." *Policing* 40(2):380–394.

Hanaway, Monica, 2020. *An Existential Approach to Leadership Challenges* Abingdon, UK: Routledge.

Hand, Matthew M., Donna Thomas, Walter C. Buholtz, Eric D. Deemer, and Munkhsanaa Buyanjargal. 2013. "Facebook and Romantic Relationships: Intimacy and Couple Satisfaction Associated with Online Social Network Use." *Cyberpsychology, Behavior & Social Networking* 16(1):8–13.

Hanish, Laura D., Helene Barcelo, Carol Lynn Martin, Richard A. Fabes, Jennifer Holmwall, and Francisco Palermo. 2007. "Using the Q-connectivity Method to Study Frequency of Interaction with Multiple Peer Triads: Do Preschoolers Peer Group Interactions at School Relate to Academic Skills?" *New Directions for Child & Adolescent Development* 118:9–24.

Hanna, Jason. 2018. *In Our Best Interest: A Defense of Paternalism.* New York, NY: Oxford University Press.

Hannah, Sean T., Patrick J. Sweeney, and Paul B. Lester. 2007. "Toward a Courageous Mindset: The Subjective Act and Experience of Courage." *Journal of Positive Psychology* 2(2):129–135.

Hanna-Pladdy, Brenda and Alicia MacKay. 2011. "The Relation between Instrumental Musical Activity and Cognitive Aging." *Neuropsychology* 25(3):378–86.

Hansen, David M., Reed W. Larson, and Jodi B. Dworkin. 2003. "What Adolescents Learn in Organized Youth Activities: A Survey of Self-reported Developmental Experiences." *Journal of Research in Adolescence* 13(1):25–55.

Hansen-Nord, Nete, Sloth Mette Skar, Finn Kjaerulf, Juan Almendarez, Sergio Bohr, Oscar Sosa, Julio Castro, Anne-Marie Nybo Andersen, Jens Modvig. 2014. "Social Capital and Violence in Poor Urban Areas of Honduras." *Aggression & Violent Behavior* 19(6):643–648.

Hantula, Donald A. 2012. "Consumers Are Foragers, Not Rational Actors: Toward a Behavioral Ecology of Consumer Choice." Pp. 549–577 in *Handbook of Developments in Consumer Behavior*, edited by Victoria Wells and Gordon Foxall. Cheltenham, UK: Elgar.

Hao, Zhidong. 2015. "Social Stratification and Ethnic and Class Politics in Macao before and after the Handover in 1999." *China: An International Journal* 13(1):66–92.

Harambam, Jaron and Stef Aupers. 2015. "Contesting Epistemic Authority: Conspiracy Theories on the Boundaries of Science." *Public Understanding of Science* 24(4):466–80.

Harb, Charles, and Peter B. Smith. 2008. "Self-Construals across Cultures: Beyond Independence-Interdependence." *Journal of Cross-Cultural Psychology* 39(2):178–197.

Harber, Kent D., Joanne Kraenzle Schneider, Kelly M. Everard, and Edwin B. Fisher. 2005. "Directive support, Undirective support, and Morale." *Journal of Social & Clinical Psychology* 24(5):691–722.

Harding, David J. 2003. "Counterfactual Models of Neighborhood Effects: The Effect of Neighborhood Poverty or Dropping out and Teenage Pregnancy." *American Journal of Sociology* 109(3):676–719.

Hardy, Susan E., and Thomas M. Gill. 2004. "Resilience of Community-dwelling Older Persons." *Journal of American Geriatrics Society* 52(2):257–262.

Hareli, Shlomo, and Bernard Weiner. 2002. "Dislike and Envy as Antecedents of Pleasure at another's Misfortune." *Motivation & Emotion* 26(4):257–277.

Hariharan, Meena, and Suvashisa Rana. 2017. "Conceptual Complexity of Resilience: Synergy Approach to Measurement." Pp. 24–33 in *The Routledge International Handbook of Psychosocial Resilience*, edited by Updesh Kumar. Abingdon, UK: Routledge.

Harker, Kathryn. 2001. "Immigrant Generation, Assimilation, and Adolescent Psychological Well-being." *Social Forces* 79(3):969–1004.

Harper, Caroline, Rachel Marcus, and Karen Moore. 2003. "Enduring Poverty and the Conditions of Childhood; Lifecourse and Intergenerational Poverty Transmissions." *World Development* 31(3):535–554.

Harper, Charles L., and Kevin T. Leicht. 2011. *Exploring Social Change: America and the World.* Boston, MA: Prentice Hall.

Harpham, Trudy, Emma Grant, and Elizabeth Thomas. 2002. "Measuring Social Capital within Health Surveys: Key Issues." *Health Policy & Planning* 17(1):106–111.

Harre, Niki. 2007. "Community Service or Activism as an Identity Project for Youth." *Journal of Community Psychology* 35(6):711–724.

Harrington, Rick and Donald A. Loffredo. 2010. "Insight, Rumination, and Self-Reflection as Predictors of Well-Being." *Journal of Psychology* 145(1):39–57.

Harris, Angela, and Ken Laidlaw. 2012. "Counselling Older People." Pp. 631–640 in *The SAGE Handbook of Counselling and Psychotherapy*, edited by Colin Feltham and Ian Horton. London: SAGE.

Harris, David R. 2001. "Why Are Whites and Blacks Averse to Black Neighbors?" *Social Science Research* 30:100–116.

Harris, Kevin A., Desiree S. Howell, and Don W. Spurgeon. 2018. "Faith Concepts in Psychology: Three 30-Year Definitional Content Analyses." *Psychology of Religion & Spirituality* 10(1):1–29.

Harris, Phyllis Braudy. 2008. "Another Wrinkle in the Debate about Successful Aging: The Undervalued Concept of Resilience and the Lived Experience of Dementia." *International Journal of Aging & Human Development* 67(1):43–61.

Hart, Mechthild. 2005. "Class and Gender." *New Directions for Adult & Continuing Education* 106:63–71.

Harter, James K., and Raksha Arora. 2010. "The Impact of Time Spent Working and Job Fit onn Well-being around the World." Pp. 398–435 in *International Differences in Well-being*, edited by Ed Diener, John F. Helliwell and Daniel Kahneman. New York: Oxford University Press.

Hartley, Christie, and Lori Watson. 2012. "Political Liberalism, Marriage and the Family." *Law & Philosophy* 31(2):185–212.

Hartley, Michael T. 2013. "Investigating the Relationship of Resilience to Academic Persistence in College Students with Mental Health Issues." *Rehabilitation Counseling Bulletin* 56(4):240–250.

Harvey, Jacquelyn and Karen Boynton. 2021. "Self-Disclosure and Psychological Resilience: The Mediating Roles of Self-Esteem and Self-Compassion." *Interpersona* 15(1):90–104.

Hassan, Riaz. 1995. *Suicide Explained: The Australian Experience*. Victoria, Australia: Melbourne University Press.

Hassija, Christina M. and Matt J. Gray. 2012. "Negative Social Reactions to Assault Disclosure as a Mediator between Self-Blame and Posttraumatic Stress Symptoms among Survivors of Interpersonal Assault." *Journal of Interpersonal Violence* 27(17):3425–41.

Hassija, Christina M., and Marylane Cloitre. 2014. "the Skills Training in Affective and Interpersonal Regulation (STAIR) Narrative Model: A Treatment Approach to Promote Resilience." Pp. 285–298 in *The Resilience Handbook: Approaches to Stress and Trauman,* edited by Martha Kent, Mary C. Davis and John W. Reich. New York: NY: Routledge.

Hatch, Stephani L. 2007. "Economic Stressors, Social Integration, and Drug Use among Women in an Inner-city Community." *Journal of Drug Issues* 37:257–280.

Hatcher, Joe W., Samuel Cares, Rachel Detrie, Tessa Dillenbeck, Emma Goral, Katlyn Troisi, and Angela M. Whirry-Achten. 2018. "Conformity, Arousal, and the Effect of Arbitrary Information." *Group Processes & Intergroup Relations* 21(4):631–45.

Hati, Sri Rahayu Hijrah, Rahma Fitriasih, and Anya Safira. 2019. "E-Textbook Piracy Behavior." *Journal of Information, Communication & Ethics in Society* 18(1):105–23.

Hattery, Angela, and Earl Smith. 2012. *The Social Dynamics of Family Violence*. Boulder, CO: Westview.

Hatzidimitriadou, Eleni. 2002. "Political Ideology, Helping Mechanisms and Empowerment of Mental Health Self-help/Mutual Aid Groups." *Journal of Community & Applied Social Psychology* 12:271–285.

Haugaard, Mark. 2020. *The Four Dimensions of Power: Understanding Domination, Empowerment and Democracy*. Manchester, UK: Manchester University Press.

Hauser, Christoph, Urban Perkmann, Sibylle Puntscher, Janette Walde and Gottfried Tappeiner. 2016. "Trust Works! Sources and Effects of Social Capital in the Workplace." *Social Indicators Research* 128(2):589–608.

Haveman, Robert, Karen Holden, Kathryn Wilson, and Barbara Wolfe. 2003. "Social Security Age of Retirement and Economic Well-being: Intertemporal and Demographic Patterns among Retired Worker Beneficiaries." *Demography* 40(2):369–394.

Hawdon, James, Colin Bernatzky, and Matthew Costello. 2019. "Cyber-Routines, Political Attitudes, and Exposure to Violence-Advocating Online Extremism." *Social Forces* 98(1):329–54.

Hawking, Stephen. 2013. *My Brief History*. New York, NY: Bantam.

Hawkins, Robert L., and Katherine Mauer. 2012. "Unravelling Social Capital: Disentangling in Concept for Social Work." *British Journal of Social Work* 42:353–370.

Hawley, Patricia H. 2014. "Evolution, Prosocial Behavior, and Altruism: A Roadmap for Understanding Where the Proximate Meets the Ultimate." Pp. 3–69 in *Prosocial Development: A Multidimensional Approach*, edited by Laura M. Padilla-Walker and Gustavo Carlo. New York, NY: Oxford University Press.

Hawthorne, Graeme. 2006. "Measuring Social Isolation in Older Adults: Development and Initial Validation of the Friendship Scale." *Social Indicators Research* 77:521–548.

Hay, Carter, Edward N. Fortson, Dusten R. Hollist, Irshad Altheimer, and Lonnie M. Schaible. 2006. "The Impact of Community Disadvantage on the Relationship between the Family and Juvenile Crime." *Journal of Research in Crime & Delinquency* 43(4):326–356.

Hay, Carter. 2003. "Family Strain, Gender, and Delinquency." *Sociological Perspectives* 46(1):107–130.

Hayes, Louise. 2014. "Happiness in Valued Living: Acceptance and Commitment Therapy as a Model for Change." Pp. 994–1008 in *The Oxford Handbook of Happiness*, edited by Susan A. David, Ilona Boniwell and Amanda Conley Ayers. Oxford, UK: Oxford University Press.

Haynes, Jo and Raphaël Nowak. 2021. "We Were Never Cool: Investigating Knowledge Production and Discourses of Cool in the Sociology of Music." *British Journal of Sociology* 72(2):448–62.

Hays-Grudo, Jennifer, Amanda Sheffield Morris, Lana Beasley, Lucia Ciciolla, Karina Shreffler, and Julie Croff. 2021. "Integrating and Synthesizing Adversity and Resilience Knowledge and Action: The ICARE Model." *American Psychologist* 76(2):203–15. .

He, Alex Jingwei. 2019. "Long-Term Care Service Needs and Planning for the Future: A Study of Middle-Aged and Older Adults in Hong Kong." *Ageing & Society* 39(2):221–253. \102–306

He, Jia, and Jessica Fischer. 2020. "Differential Associations of School Practices with Achievement and Sense of Belonging of Immigrant and Non-Immigrant Students." *Journal of Applied Developmental Psychology* 66:101089.

He, Jia, Dave Bartram, Ilke Inceoglu, and Fons J. R. van de Vijver. 2014. "Response Styles and Personality Traits: A Multilevel Analysis." *Journal of Cross-Cultural Psychology* 45(7):1028–1045.

He, Shejing, and Fulong Wu. 2009. "China's Emerging Neoliberal Urbanism: Perspectives from Urban Redevelopment." *Antipode* 41(2):282–304.

He, Yaliu, Xiaohui Sophie Li, Jiaqi Zhao, and Yuanyuan An. 2022. "Family Resilience, Media Exposure, and Children's Mental Health in China During Covid-19." *Family Journal* 30(4):579–88.

He, Yinan. 2018. "Domestic Troubles, National Identity Discourse, and China's Attitude Towards the West, 2003–2012." *Nations & Nationalism* 24(3):741–66.

Headey, Bruce, and Derek Headey. 2003. "German Reunification: Welfare Gains and Losses East and West." *Social Indicators Research* 64:107–138.

Headey, Bruce, Fu Na, and Richard Zheng. 2001. "Pet Dogs" Benefit Owners" Health: A Natural Experiment in China." *Social Indicators Research* 87:481–493.

Heaphy, Brian. 2007. Late Modernity and Social Change: Reconstructing Social and Personal Life. Abingdon, UK: Routledge

Heath, Yuko, and Robert Gifford. 2006. "Free Market Ideology and Environmental Degradation: The Case of Belief in Global Climate Change." *Environment & Behavior* 38(1):48–71.

Heaven, Patrick C. L., and Joseph Ciarrochi. 2007. "Personality and Religious Values among Adolescents: A Three-Wave Longitudinal Analysis." *British Journal of Psychology* 98(4):681–694.

Hechanova, Regina, Terry A. Beehr, and Neil D. Christiansen. 2003. "Antecedents and Consequences of Employees" Adjustment to Overseas Assignment: A Meta-analytic Review." *Applied Psychology* 52(2):213–236.

Hechter, M., and D. Okamoto. 2001. "Political Consequences of Minority Group Formation." *Annual Review of Political Science* 4:189–215

Heckathorn, Douglas D., and Judith E. Rosenstein. 2002. "Group Solidarity as the Product of Collective Action: Creation of Solidarity in a Population of Injection Drug Uses." *Advances in Group Processes* 19:37–66.

Heckhausen, Jutta. 2002. "Developmental Regulation of Life-course Transitions: A Control Theory Approach." Pp. 257–280 in *Paths to Successful Development: Personality in the Life Course*, edited by Lea Pulkkinen and Avshalom Caspi. Cambridge, UK: Cambridge University Press.

Heckscher, Charles. 2015. *Trust in a Complex World: Enriching Community*. Oxford, UK: Oxford University Press.

Heenan, M. Colleen. 2012. "Feminist Psychotherapy." Pp. 607–611 in *The SAGE Handbook of Counselling and Psychotherapy*, edited by Colin Feltham and Ian Horton. London: SAGE.

Heffren, Cole D. J., and Peter A. Hausdorf. 2016. "Post-Traumatic Effects in Policing: Perceptions, Stigmas and Help Seeking Behaviours." *Police Practice & Research* 17(5):420–433.

Hegtvedt, Karen A., and Christie L. Parris. 2014. "Emotions in Justice Processes." Pp. 103–125 in *Handbook of the Sociology of Emotions*: Volume II, edited by Jan E. Stets and Jonathan H. Turner. Dordrecht, Netherlands: Springer.

Heidemeier, Heike, and Ursula M. Staudinger. 2012. "Self-evaluation Process in Life Satisfaction: Uncovering Measurement Non-equivalence and Age-related differences." *Social Indicators Research* 105:39–61.

Heiden Rootes, Katie M., Peter J. Jankowski, and Steven J. Sandage. 2010. "Bowen Family Systems Theory and Spirituality: Exploring the Relationship between Triangulation and Religious Questing." *Contemporary Family Therapy* 32(2):89–101.

Heilman, Renata M., and Petko Kusev. 2020. "Personal Values Associated with Prosocial Decisions." *Behavioral Sciences* 10(4):77.

Heiman, Tali, and Dafna Kariv. 2004. "Coping Experience among Students in Higher Education." *Educational Studies* 30(4):441–455.

Heinen, Eva. 2016. "Identity and Travel Behaviour: A Cross-Sectional Study on Commute Mode Choice and Intention to Change." *Transportation Research* 43:238–53.

Heinz, Walter R. 2009. "Youth Transitions in an Age of Uncertainty." Pp. 3–13 in *Handbook of Youth and Young Adulthood: New Perspectives and Agendas*, edited by Andy Furlong. Abingdon, UK: Routledge.

Heitmeyer, Wilhelm and Reimund Anhut. 2008. "Disintegration, Recognition, and Violence: A Theoretical Perspective." *New Directions for Youth Development* 119:25–37.

Held, David. 2010. *Cosmopolitanism: Ideals and Realities*. Cambridge, UK: Polity.

Helgeson, Vicki S. 2003. "Social Support and Quality of Life." *Quality of Life Research* 12(suppl.1):25–31.

Helgeson, Vicki, Kerry A. Reynolds, and Patricia L. Tomich. 2006. "A Meta-analytic Review of Benefit Finding and Growth." *Journal of Counseling & Clinical Psychology* 74(5):797–816.

Hellevik, Tale, and Richard A. Settersten, Jr. 2013. "Life Planning among Young Adults in 23 European Countries: The Effects of Individual and Country Security." *European Sociological Review* 29(5):923–938.

Helliwell, John F. 2006. "Well-being, Social Capital, and Public Policy." *Economic Journal* 116:C34–C45.

Helliwell, John F., and Robert D. Putnam. 2005. "The Social Context of Well-being." Pp. 435–459 in *The Science of Well-being*, edited by Felica A. Huppert, Nick Baylis and Barry Keverne. Oxford, UK: Oxford University Press.

Helliwell, John F., Chris Burrington-Leigh, Anthony Harris, and Haifang Huang. 2010. "International Evidence on the Social Context of Well-being." Pp. 291–327 in *International Differences in Well-being*, edited by Ed Diener, John F. Helliwell and Daniel Kahneman. New York: Oxford University Press.

Helliwell, John F., Haifang Huang, and Robert D. Putnam. 2009. "How's the Job? Are Trust and Social Capital Neglected Workplace Investment?" Pp. 87–144 in *Social Capital: Reaching out, Reaching in*, edited by Viva Ona Bartkus and James H. Davis. Cheltenham, UK: Edward Elgar.

Helmchen, Hanfrid, Margret M. Baltes, Bernhard Gewelmann, Siegfried Kanowski, Michael Linden, Friedel M. Reischies, Michael Wagner, Thomas Wernicke, and Hans-Ulrich Wilms. 1999. "Psychiatric Illnesses in Old Age." Pp. 167–196 in *The Berlin Aging Study: Aging from 70 to 100*, edited by Paul B. Baltes and Karl Ulrich Mayer. Cambridge, UK: Cambridge University Press.

Helson, Ravenna, and Sanjay Srivastava. 2001. "Three Paths of Adult Development: Conservers, Seekers, and Achievers." *Journal of Personality & Social Psychology* 80(6):995–1010.

Helwig, Andrew A. 2004. "A Ten-year Longitudinal Study of the Career Development of Students: Summary Findings." *Journal of Counseling & Development* 82:49–57.

Henderson, Craig E., Bert Hayslip, Jr., Leah M. Sanders, and Linda Louden. 2009. "Grandmother-grandchild Relationship Quality Predicts Psychological Adjustment among Youth from Divorced Families." *Journal of Family Issues* 30(9):1245–1264.

Henderson, Karla A., Leslie Scheuler Whitaker, M. Deborah Bialeschki, Margery M. Scanlin, and Christopher Thurber. 2007. "Summer Camp Experiences: Parental Perceptions of Youth Development Outcomes." *Journal of Family Issues* 28(8):987–1007.

Hendricks, Michael L. and Rylan J. Testa. 2012. "A Conceptual Framework for Clinical Work with Transgender and Gender Nonconforming Clients: An Adaptation of the Minority Stress Model." *Professional Psychology* 43(5):460–67.

Hendry, Leo B. and Marion Kloep. 2012. *Adolescence and Adulthood: Transitions And Transformations*. Houndmills, UK: Palgrave.

Hendry, Leo B., Janet Shucksmith, John G. Love, and Anthony Glendinning. 1993. *Young People's Leisure and Lifestyles*. London, UK: Routledge.

Henretta, John C. 1987. "Family Transitions, Housing Market Context and First Home Purchase by Young Married Households." *Social forces* 26:520–536.

Henry, Carolyn S., Andy L. Stephenson, Michelle Fryer Hanson, and William Harzett. 1993. "Adolescent Suicide and Families: An Ecological Approach." *Adolescence* 28(110):291–308.

Henry, Darla L. 2001. "Resilient Children: What They Tell Us about Coping with Maltreatment." *Social Work in Health Care* 34(3/4):283–298.

Henry, Mary Ellen, and John A. Capitman. 1995. "Finding Satisfaction in Adult Day Care: Analysis of a National Demonstration of Dementia Care and Respite Services." *Journal of Applied Gerontology* 14(3):302–320.

Hepper, Erica G., Tim Wildschut, Constantine Sedikides, Sara Robertson, and Clay D. Routledge. 2020. "Time Capsule: Nostalgia Shields Psychological Wellbeing from Limited Time Horizons." *Emotion* 21(3):644–64.

Herbert, James D., Brandon A. Gaudiano, Alyssa A. Rheingold, Valerie H. Myers, Kristy Dalrymple, and Elizabeth M. Nolan. 2005. "Social Skills Training Augments the Effectiveness of Cognitive Behavioral Group Therapy for Social Anxiety Disorder." *Behavior Therapy* 36(2):125–138.

Herd, Pamela, James S. House, and Robert F. Schoeni. 2008. "Income Support Policies and Health among the Elderly." Pp. 97–121 in *Making American Healthier: Social and Economic Policy as Health Policy*, edited by Robert F. Schoeni, James S. House, George A. Kaplan, and Harold Pollack. New York: Russell Sage.

Herek, Gregory M., Keith F. Widaman, and John P. Capitanto. 2005. "When Sex Equals AIDS: Symbolic Stigma and Heterosexual Adults" Inaccurate Beliefs about Sexual Transmission of AIDS." *Social Problems* 52(1):15–37.

Herian, Mitchel N., Louis Tay, Joseph A. Hamm, and Ed Diener. 2014. "Social Capital, Ideology, and Health in the United States." *Social Science & Medicine* 105:30–37.

Herman, Lise Esther. 2021. "Can Partisans Be Pluralist? A Comparative Study of Party Member Discourse in France and Hungary." *British Journal of Politics & International Relations* 23(1):22–42.

Herman-Kinney, Nancy J. 2003. "Deviance." Pp. 695–720 in *Handbook of Symbolic Interactionism*, edited by Larry T. Reynolds and Nancy J. Herman-Kinney. Lanham, MD: Rowman.

Hermanto, Nicola, David C. Zuroff, Allison C. Kelly, and Michelle J. Leybman. 2017. "Receiving Support, Giving Support, and Self-Reassurance: A Daily Diary Test of Social Mentality Theory." *Personality & Individual Differences* 107:37–42.

Hernandez, Ana, Fritz Drasgow, and Vicente Gonzalez-Roma. 2002. "Investigating the Functioning of a Middle Category by Means of a Mixed-measurement Model." *Journal of Applied Psychology* 89(4):687–699.

Herreros, Francisco. 2009. "The State." Pp. 179–196 in *Handbook of Social Capital: The Troika of Sociology, Political Science and Economics*, edited by Gert Tinggaard Svendsen and Gunnar Linad Haase Svendsen. Cheltenham, UK: Elgar.

Herrmann, Dorothy. 1998. *Helen Keller: A Life*. New York, NY: Knopf.

Hersberger-Langloh, Sophie E., Georg von Schnurbein1, Chulhee Kang, Michal Almog-Bar, Jacqueline Butcher, Garcia-Colin, and Marta Rey Garcia. 2022. "For the Love of Art? Episodic Volunteering at Cultural Events. *Voluntas* 33(3):428–442.

Hertzog, Christopher, and Daniela S. Jopp. 2010. "Resilience in the Face of Cognitive Aging: Experience, Adaptation, and Compensation." Pp. 130–161 in *New Frontiers in Resilient Aging: Life-strengths and Well-being in Late Life*, edited by Prom S. Fry and Corey L.M. Keyes. Cambridge, UK: Cambridge University Press.

Heshmati, Saeideh and Zita Oravecz. 2022. "I Feel Loved When Other People Feel Loved: Cultural Congruence in Beliefs on Love Is Related to Well-Being." *Journal of Social & Personal Relationships* 39(2):347–71.

Heward, Sue, Cheryl Hutchins and Helen Keleher. 2007. "Organizational Change—Key to Capacity Building and Effective Health Promotion." *Health Promotion International* 22(2):170–78.

Heyman, Richard E., and Amy M. Smith Slep. 2007. "Therapeutic Treatment Approaches to Violent Behavior." Pp. 602–617 in *The Cambridge Handbook of Violent Behavior and Aggression*, edited by Daniel J. Flannery, Alexander T. Vazsonyi and Irwin D. Waldman. Cambridge, UK: Cambridge University Press.

Heyman, Richard E., Heather M. Foran, and Jesse L. Wilkinson. 2013. "Theories of Intimate Partner Violence." Pp. 190–207 in *Handbook of Family Theories: A Content-based Approach*, edited by Mark A. Fine and Frank D. Fincham. New York: Routledge.

Heyns, Barbara. 1996. "Creating Capitalists: The Social Origins of Entrepreneurship in Post-communist Poland." Pp. 257–289 in *Generating Social Stratification: Toward a New Research Agenda*, edited by Alan C. Kerckhoff. Boulder, CO: Westview.

Hickman, Gregory P., Suanne Bartholomae, and Patrick C. McKenry. 2000. "Influence of Parenting Styles on the Adjustment and Academic Achievement of Traditional College Freshmen." *Journal of College Student Development* 41(1):41–54.

Hicks, Alexander, and Lane Kenworthy. 2003. "Varieties of Welfare Capitalism." *Socio-Economic Review* 1:27–61.

Hilbig, Benjamin E., Ingo Zettler, Felix Leist, and Timo Heydasch. 2013. "It Takes Two: Honesty-Humility and Agreeableness Differentially Predict Active versus Reactive Cooperation." *Personality & Individual Differences* 54(5):598–603.

Hildon, Zoe, Glenn Smith, Gopalakrishnan Netuveli, and David Blane. 2008. "Understanding Adversity and Resilience at Older Ages." *Sociology of Health & Illness* 30(5):726–740.

Hileman, Jacob, Marco T. A. Bastos, and Mark Lubell. 2018. "Robustness and the Paradox of Bridging Organizations: The Exit Problem in Regional Water Governance Networks in Central America," *Society & Natural Resources* 31(6):683–697.

Hill, Michael. 2000. "Asian Values as Reverse Orientalism: Singapore." *Asian Pacific Viewpoint* 41(2):177–190.

Hill, Patrick L., Leah H. Schultz, Joshua J. Jackson, and Judy A. Andrews. 2019. "Parent-Child Conflict During Elementary School as a Longitudinal Predictor of Sense of Purpose in Emerging Adulthood." *Journal of Youth & Adolescence* 48(1):145–53.

Hill-Briggs, Felicia, Tiffany L. Gary, Lee R. Bone, Martha N. Hill, David M. Levine, and Frederick L. Brancati. 2005. "Medication Adherence and Diabetes Control in Urban African Americans." *Health Psychology* 24(4):349–359.

Hillman, George Milton, Jr. 2008. "Leadership Practices of Non-traditional Seminary Students." *Journal of Research on Christian Education* 17:54–80.

Himes, Kenneth R. 2007. "Consumerism and Christian Ethics." *Theological Studies* 68:132–153.

Hines, Alice M., Paige Wigatt, and Joan Merdinger. 2005. "Former Foster Youth Attending College: Resilience and the Transition to Young Adulthood." *American Journal of Orthopsychiatry* 75(3):381–394.

Hintsanen, Mirka, Taina Hintsa, Anna Widell, Mika Kivimäki, Olli T. Raitakari, and Liisa Keltkangas-Järvinen. 2011. "Negative Emotionality, Activity, and Sociability Temperaments Predicting Long-Term Job Strain and Effort–Reward Imbalance: A 15-Year Prospective Follow-up Study." *Journal of Psychosomatic Research* 71(2):90–96.

Hipp, John R., George E. Tita, and Lyndsay N. Boggess. 2009. "Intergroup and Intragroup Violence: Is Violent Crime an Expression of Group Conflict or Social Disorganization?" *Criminology* 47(2):521–564.

Hirose, Iwao. 2015. *Egalitarianism.* Abington, UK: Routledge.

Hirschi, Andreas, and Fred W. Vondracek. 2009. "Adaptation of Career Goals to Self and Opportunities in Early Adolescence." *Journal of Vocational Behavior* 75:120–128.

Hitlin, Steven and Sarah K. Harkness. 2018. *Unequal Foundations: Inequality, Morality, and Emotions across Cultures.* New York, NY: Oxford University Press.

Hitlin, Steven. 2006. "Parental Influences on Children's Values and Aspirations: Bridging Two Theories of Social Class and Socialization." *Sociological Perspectives* 49(1):25–46.

Hjemdal, Odin, Antonio Roazzi, Maria da Graça, B. B. Dias, and Oddgeir Friborg. 2015. "The cross-cultural validity of the Resilience Scale for Adults: A comparison between Norway and Brazil." *BMC Psychology* 3(1):18.

Hlasny, Vladimir and Jieun Lee. 2020. "Investment in Social Capital by the Korean Elderly and Baby-Boomers." *Journal of the Economics of Ageing* 17:100256.

Ho, Chiew Siang Bryan. 2015. "Governance, Inclusion and Trust in Singapore, Hong Kong and Macao." *Asian Education & Development Studies* 4(3):250–264.

Ho, Chiew-Siang Bryan and Newman M. K. Lam. 2015. "Development Strategies of Small Economies: Singapore, Hong Kong and Macao." *Asian Education & Development Studies* 4(3):265–81.

Ho, Jeffrey C. F. and Ryan Ng. 2022. "Perspective-Taking of Non-Player Characters in Prosocial Virtual Reality Games: Effects on Closeness, Empathy, and Game Immersion." *Behaviour & Information Technology.*

Ho, Simon S.M., and Raymond S.Y. Chan. 2009. "Social Harmony in Hong Kong: Level, Determinants and Policy Implications." *Social Indicators Research* 91:37–58.

Ho, Wai-Yip. 2013. *Islam and China's Hong Kong: Ethnic Identity, Muslim Networks and the New Silk Road.* Abington, UK: Routledge.

Ho, Wing Chung and Lin Li. 2022. "The Time–Space Tactics of Chinese Buddhist and Taoist Believers under State–Religion Tension." *China Information* 36(2):241–61.

Hoang, Nam-Phuong T., Divna Haslam, and Matthew Sanders. 2020. "Coparenting Conflict and Cooperation between Parents and Grandparents in Vietnamese Families: The Role of Grandparent Psychological Control and Parent–Grandparent Communication." *Family Process* 59(3):1161–74.

Hoare, Carol Hren. 2002. Erikson on Development in Adulthood: New Insights from the Unpublished Papers. New York: Oxford University Press.

Hobfoll, Stevan E. 1998. Stress, Culture, and Community: The Psychology and Philosophy of Stress. New York: Plenum.

Hobson, Nicholas M., Francesca Gino, Michael I. Norton, and Michael Inzlicht. 2017. "When Novel Rituals Lead to Intergroup Bias: Evidence from Economic Games and Neurophysiology." *Psychological Science* 28(6):733–50.

Hocksmann, Hynn. 2004. *On Philosophy in China.* Toronto, Canada: Thomson. (B126.H57)

Hodge, Matthew. 2018. "Disney World: The Westernization of World Music in Epcot's Illuminations: Reflections of Earth." *Social Sciences* 7(8):136.

Hodson, Randy. 1996. "Dignity in the Workplace under Participative Management: Alienation and Freedom Revisited." *American Sociological Review* 61(5):719–738.

Hodson, Randy. 2001. *Dignity at Work.* Cambridge, UK: Campaign University Press.

Hoegh, Dana G., and Martin Bourgeois. 2002. "Prelude and Postlude to the Self: Correlates of Achieved Identity." *Youth & Society* 33(4):573–594.

Hoekstra, Erin. 2021. "Not a Free Version of a Broken System: Medical Humanitarianism and Immigrant Health Justice in the United States." *Social Science & Medicine* 285:114287.

Hofelich, Alicia J., and Stephanie D. Preston. 2014. "Different Strokes: Empathy, Individual Characteristics, and Helping." Pp. 247–255 in *The Resilience Handbook: Approaches to Stress and Trauman*, edited by Martha Kent, Mary C. Davis and John W. Reich. New York: NY: Routledge.

Hofferth, Sandra L., Johanne Boisjoly, and Greg J. Duncan. 1999. "The Development of Social Capital." *Rationality & Society* 11(1):79–110.

Hoffman, Kristi L., and John N. Edwards. 2004. "An Integrated Theoretical Model of Sibling Violence and Abuse." *Journal of Family Violence* 19(3):185–200.

Hoffman, Lily M. 2003. "The Marketing of Diversity in the Inner City: Tourism and Regulation in Harlem." *International Journal of Urban & Regional Research* 27(2):286–299.

Hoffman, Lisa. 2006. "Autonomous Choices and Patriotic Professionalism: On Governmentability in Late-socialist China." *Economy & Society* 35(4):550–570.

Hoffman, Louis, Nathaniel Granger, Lisa Vallejos, and Michael Moats. 2016. "An Existential–Humanistic Perspective on Black Lives Matter and Contemporary Protest Movements." *Journal of Humanistic Psychology* 56(6):595–611.

Hoffmann, John P. 2023. "Family Structure, Unstructured Socializing, and Delinquent Behavior." *Journal of Criminal Justice* 87:102086.

Hoffmann, John P., and Mikaela J. Dufur. 2008. "Family and School Capital Effects on Delinquency: Substitutes or Complements?" *Sociological Perspectives* 51(1):29–62.

Hoffmann, John P., and Mikaela J. Dufur. 2018. "Family Social Capital, Family Social Bonds, and Juvenile Delinquency." *American Behavioral Scientist* 62(11):1525–1544.

Hofstetter, C. Richard, David Barker, James T. Smith, Gina M. Zari, and Thomas A. Ingrassia. 1999. "Information, Misinformation, and Political Talk Radio." *Political Research Quarterly* 52(2):353–69.

Hogg, Michael A., Christie Meehan, and Jayne Farquharson. 2010. "The Solace of Radicalism: Self-Uncertainty and Group Identification in the Face of Threat." *Journal of Experimental Social Psychology* 46(6):1061–1066.

Holbrook, Allyson L., Melanie C. Green, and Jon A. Krosnick. 2003. "Telephone versus Face-to-face Interviewing of National Probability Samples with Long Questionnaires: Comparisons of Respondent Satisficing and Social Desirability Response Bias." *Public Opinion Quarterly* 67:79–125.

Holden, E. Wayne, Susan Rousseau O'Connell, Tim Connor, Ann Maria Brannan, E. Michael Foster, Gary Blau, and Heather Panciera. 2002. "Evaluation of the Connecticut Title IV-E Waiver Program: Assessing the Effectiveness, Implementation, Fidelity, and Cost Benefits of a Continuum of Care." *Children & Youth Services Review* 24(6/7):409–430.

Holl, Jane L., Kristen Shook Slack, and Amy Bush Stevens. 2005. "Welfare Reform and Health Insurance Consequences for Parents." *American Journal of Public Health* 95:279–285.

Hollander, Jocelyn A. 2018. "Women's Self-Defense and Sexual Assault Resistance: The State of the Field." *Sociology Compass* 12(8):e12597.

Hollenbaugh, Erin E. and Amber L. Ferris. 2015. "Predictors of Honesty, Intent, and Valence of Facebook Self-Disclosure." *Computers in Human Behavior* 50:456–64.

Holleran, Lori K., and Margaret A. Waller. 2003. "Sources of Resilience among Chicano/a Youth: Forging Identities in the Borderlands." *Child & Adolescent Social Work Journal* 20(5):335–350.

Holliday, Ian, and Waikeung Tam. 2001. "Social Capital in Hong Kong." *East Asia: An International Quarterly* 19(1/2):144–170.

Holliday, Ian, Ngok Ma, and Ray Yep. 2004. "After 1997: The Dialectics of Hong Kong Dependence." *Journal of Contemporary Asia* 34(2):254–270.

Holliman, Andrew, Daniel Waldeck, Bethany Jay, Summayah Murphy, Emily Atkinson, Rebecca J. Collie, and Andrew Martin. 2021. "Adaptability and Social Support: examining Links with Psychological Wellbeing among UK Students and Non-students." *Frontiers in Psychology* 12:636520.

Holloway, Katie, Navjot Bhullar, and Nicola S. Schutte. 2017. "A Latent Profile Analysis of Dispositional Hope and Defense Styles." *Personality & Individual Differences* 114(1):151–154.

Holman, E. Alison, Rachel G. Lucas-Thompson, and Tammy Lu. 2011. "Social Constraints, Genetic Vulnerability, and Mental Health Following Collective Stress." *Journal of Traumatic Stress* 24(5):497–505.

Holmstrom, Amanda J., Samantha J. Shebib, Josephine K. Boumis, Amanda Allard, Adam J. Mason, and Jong In Lim. 2021. "Support Gaps During the Covid-19 Pandemic: Sex Differences and Effects on Well-Being." *Journal of Social & Personal Relationships* 38(10):2985–3009.

Holowchak, M. Andrew. 2008. *The Stoics: A Guide for the Perplexed*. London, Continuum.

Holstein, James A., and Jaber F. Gubrium. 2000. Constructing the Life Course (2nd ed.). Dix Hills, NY: General Hall.

Holt-Lunstad, Julianne. 2022. "Social Connection as a Public Health Issue: The Evidence and a Systemic Framework for Prioritizing the "Social" in Social Determinants of Health." *Annual Review of Public Health* 43(1):193–213.

Holtom, Brooks C., Terence R. Mitchell, and Thomas W. Lee. 2006. "Increasing Human and Social Capital by Applying Job Embeddedness Theory." *Organizational Dynamics* 35(4):316–331.

Homant, Robert J. 2013. "Risky Altruism, Criminal Victimization, Fear of Crime, and Security Mindedness." *Journal of Applied Security Research* 8(2):203–221.

Homer, Melissa M., Patti A. Freeman, Raomn B. Zabriskie, and Dennis L. Eggett. 2007. "Rituals and Relationships: Examining the Relationship between Family of Origin Rituals and Young Adult Attachment." *Marriage & Family Review* 42(1):5–28.

Hong, Fang, Amanda R. Tarullo, Andrea E. Mercurio, Siyu Liu, Qiyue Cai, and Kathleen Malley-Morrison. 2018. "Childhood Maltreatment and Perceived Stress in Young Adults: The Role of Emotion Regulation Strategies, Self-Efficacy, and Resilience." *Child Abuse & Neglect* 86:36–146.

Hong, Ying-yi, Hsin-ha Lino, Gloria Chan, Rosanna Y.M. Wong, Chi-yue Chiu, Grace Wai-man Ip, Ho-ying Fu, and Ian G. Hansen. 2006. "Temporal Causal Links between Outgroup Attitudes and Social Categorization: The Case of Hong Kong 1997 Transition." *Group Processes & Intergroup Relations* 9^2):265–288.

Hoogervorst, Niek, Judith Metz, Lonneke Roza, and Eva van Baren. 2015. "How Perceptions of Altruism and Sincerity Affect Client Trust in Volunteers Versus Paid Workers." *Nonprofit & Voluntary Sector Quarterly* 45(3):593–611.

Hooghe, Marc. 2003. "Participation in Voluntary Associations and Value Indicators: The Effect of Current and Previous Participation Experiences." *Nonprofit & Voluntary Sector Quarterly* 32(1):47–69.

Hoover, Coty S., Jennifer M. Ragsdale, and Thomas B. Ayres. 2022. "An Experimental Test of Resource Recovery from Physical and Relaxation Work Break Activities." *Stress & Health* 38(3):477–89.

Hoover, Joe. 2016. Reconstructing Human Rights: A Pragmatist and Pluralist Inquiry on Global Ethics. Oxford, UK: Oxford University Press.

Hopcroft, Rosemary L. 2016. Evolution and Gender: Why It Matters for Contemporary Life. New York: Routledge.

Hopson, Laura M., Eunju Lee, and Ning Tang. 2014. "A Multi-Level Analysis of School Racial Composition and Ecological Correlates of Academic Success." *Children & Youth Services Review* 44:126–134.

Hordern, Joshua. 2013. *Political Affections: Civil Participation and Moral Theology*. Oxford, UK: Oxford University Press.

Horell, Harold D. 2014. "On Learning to See the World Religiously: Moral Awareness, Faith, and Public Moral Discourse." *Religious Education* 109(4):424–39.

Hornsey, Matthew J., Paul G. Bain, Emily A. Harris, Nadezhda Lebedeva, Emiko S. Kashima, Yanjun Guan, Roberto González, Sylvia Xiaohua Chen, and Sheyla Blumen. 2018. "How Much Is Enough in a Perfect World? Cultural Variation in Ideal Levels of Happiness, Pleasure, Freedom, Health, Self-Esteem, Longevity, and Intelligence." *Psychological Science* 29(9):1393–1404.

Horowitz, A., J.P. Reinhardt, and K. Boerner. 2005. "The Effect of Rehabilitation on Depression among Visually Disabled Older Adults." *Aging & Mental Health* 9(6):563–570.

Horowitz, Jonathan. 2018. "Relative Education and the Advantage of a College Degree." *American Sociological Review* 83(4):771–801.

Hoshino, Kazumi, Steven H. Zarit, and Makoto Nakayama. 2012. "Development of the Gerotranscendence Scale Type 2: Japanese Version." *International Journal of Aging & Human Development* 75(3):217–237.

Hospers, Harm J., and Anita Jansen. 2005. "Why Homosexuality Is a Risk Factor for Eating Disorders in Males." *Journal of Social & Clinical Psychology* 24(8):1188–1201.

Hou, Wai Kai, Brian J. Halld, Daphna Canettig, Kam Man Laua, Sin Man Nga, and Stevan E. Hobfoll. 2015. "Threat to Democracy: Physical and Mental Health Impact of Democracy Movement in Hong Kong." *Journal of Affective Disorders* 186(1):74–82.

Houldcroft, Laura, Emma Haycraft, and Claire Farrow. 2014. "Peer and Friend Influences on Children's Eating." *Social Development* 23(1):19–40.

Hounkpatin, Osafo, Hilda, Alex M. Wood, Christopher J. Boyce, and Graham Dunn. 2015. "An Existential-Humanistic View of Personality Change: Co-Occurring Changes with Psychological Well-Being in a 10 Year Cohort Study." *Social Indicators Research* 121(2):455–470.

House, Bailey, Joseph Henrich, Barbara Sarnecka, and Joan B. Silk. 2013. "The Development of Contingent Reciprocity in Children." *Evolution & Human Behavior* 34(2):86–93.

Houser, Daniel and Erte Xiao. 2015. "House Money Effects on Trust and Reciprocity." *Public Choice* 163(1/2):187–99.

Houts, Sandra, and Cathy Kassals. 1997. "Rotter's Social Learning Theory and Fear of Crime: Differences by Race and Ethnicity." *Social Science Quarterly* 78(1):122–136.

Hovden, Jorid. 2012. "Discourses and Strategies for the Inclusion of Women in Sport – the Case of Norway." *Sport in Society* 15(3):287–301.

Howard, Matt C. and Kent K. Alipour. 2014. "Does the Courage Measure Really Measure Courage? A Theoretical and Empirical Evaluation." *Journal of Positive Psychology* 9(5):449–59.

Howatt, William A. 2001. "The Evolution of Reality Therapy to Chronic Theory." *International Journal of Reality Therapy* 21(1):7–12.

Howe, Paul. 2010. Citizens Adrift: The Democratic Disengagement of Young Canadians. Vancouver, Canada: UBC Press.

Hoyer, Karlijn, Marcel Zeelenberg, and Seger Breugelmans. 2023. "Further Tests of the Scarcity and Luxury Hypotheses in Dispositional Greed: Evidence from Two Large-Scale Dutch and American Samples." *Current Psychology* 42(14):12045–54.

Hoyle, Rick H., and Erin K. Davison. 2016. "Varieties of Self-control and Their Personality Correlates." Pp. 396–413 in *Handbook of Self-regulation: Research, Theory, and Application*, edited by Kathleen D. Vohs and Roy F. Baumeister. New York, NY: Guilford.

Hraba, Joseph, Rehan Mullick, Frederick Lorenz, and Jiri Vecernik. 2001. "Age and Czechs" Attitudes toward the Postcommunist Economic Reforms." *Sociological Quarterly* 42(3):421–435.

Hrehorciuc-Caragea, Andreea and Lawrence T. White. 2017. "An Investigation of the Relationship between Psychological Flexibility and Bisexuality." *Journal of Bisexuality* 17(4):473–86.

Hrostowski, Susan, and Timothy Rehner. 2012. "Five Years Later: Resiliency among Older Adult Survivors of Hurricane Katrina." *Journal of Gerontological Social Work* 55:337–351.

Hu, Anning. 2013. "Generalized Trust among Christians in Urban China: Analysis Based on Propensity Score Matching." *Current Sociology* 61(7):1021–1039.

Huang, Han-Chung, T. C. E. Cheng, Wei-Fan Huang, and Ching-I Teng. 2018. "Who Are Likely to Build Strong Online Social Networks? The Perspectives of Relational Cohesion Theory and Personality Theory." *Computers in Human Behavior* 82:111–123.

Huang-Isherwood, Ke M. and Jorge Pena. 2021. "Testing Moral Disengagement and Proteus Effect Predictions on Feelings of Guilt and Self-Empowerment Attributed to Bearing Guns." *Frontiers in Psychology* 12:695086.

Huber, Alexandra, Cornelia Strecker, Timo Kachel, Thomas Höge, and Stefan Höfer. 2020. "Character Strengths Profiles in Medical Professionals and Their Impact on Well-Being." *Frontiers in Psychology* 11:566728.

Huber, Max A., Louis D. Brown, Rosalie N. Metze, Martin Stam, Tine Van Regenmortel, and Tineke N. Abma. 2022. "Exploring Empowerment of Participants and Peer Workers in a Self- Managed Homeless Shelter." *Journal of Social Work* 22(1):26–45.

Huddy, Leonie, and Nadia Khatib. 2007. "American Patriotism, National Identity, and Political Involvement." *American Journal of Political Science* 51(1):63–77.

Huddy, Leonie. 2004. "Contrasting Theoretical Approaches to Intergroup Relations." *Political Psychology* 25(6):947–967.

Huddy, Leonie. 2013. "From Group Identity to Political Cohesion and Commitment." Pp. 737–773 in *The Oxford Handbook of Political Psychology*, edited by Leone Huddy, David O. Sears and Jack S. Levy. New York: Oxford University Press.

Hudetz, Judith A., Anthony G. Hudetz, and Diane M. Reddy. 2004. "Effect of Relaxation on Working Memory and the Bispectral Index of the EEG." *Psychological Reports* 95(1):53–70.

Hudson, Christopher G. 2000. "From Social Darwinism to Self-organization: Implications for Social Change Theory." *Social Service Review* 74(4):533–559.

Hudson, Ray. 2019. *Co-produced Economics: Capital, Collaboration, Competition.* Abingdon, UK: Routledge.

Hudson, Tara D. and Jay Brandenberger. 2022. "College Students" Moral and Prosocial Responsibility: Associations with Community Engagement Experiences." *Journal of Experiential Education* 46(1):52–79.

Hue, Ming-Tak. 2011. "Developing Resiliency in Students with Behavioural Problems in Hong Kong Secondary Schools: Teachers' Narratives from a School Guidance Perspective." *Pastoral Care in Education* 29(4):261–72.

Huesmann, L. Rowell, and Lucyna Kirwil. 2007. "Why Observing Violence Increases the Risk of Violent Behavior by the Observer." Pp. 545–570 in *The Cambridge Handbook of Violent Behavior and Aggression*, edited by Daniel J. Flannery, Alexander T. Vazsonyi and Irwin D. Waldman. Cambridge, UK: Cambridge University Press.

Huesmann, L. Rowell. 2018. "The Contagion of Violence." Pp. 527–556 in *The Cambridge Handbook of Violent Behavior and Aggression*, edited by Alexander T. Vazsonyi, David J. Flannery and Matt DeLisi. Cambridge, UK: Cambridge University Press.

Huffman, Ann H., Satoris S. Culbertson, Heidi A. Wayment, and Louis H. Irving. 2015. "Resource Replacement and Psychological Well-Being during Unemployment: The Role of Family Support." *Journal of Vocational Behavior* 89:74–82.

Hughes, Honore M., Natalie N. Humphrey, and Terri L. Weaver. 2005. "Advances in Violence and Trauma: Toward Comprehensive Ecological Models." *Journal of Interpersonal Violence* 20(1):31–38.

Hughes, Jan N. 2011. "Longitudinal Effects of Teacher and Student Perceptions of Teacher-Student Relationship Qualities on Academic Adjustment." *Elementary School Journal* 112(1):38–60.

Huhe, Narisong. 2014. "Understanding the Multilevel Foundation of Social Trust in Rural China: Evidence from the China General Social Survey." *Social Science Quarterly* 95(2):581–597. \79–324

Hui, Bryant P. H., and Aleksandr Kogan. 2018a. "Daily Ups and Downs: An Event-Sampling Study of the Mediated Moderation of Prosocial Engagement on Well-Being." *Social Psychological & Personality Science* 9(6):675–688.

Hui, Bryant Pui Hung, and Aleksandr Kogan. 2018b. "Who Helping Helps: An Event-Sampling Study of How Basic Psychological Needs Moderate the Impact of Acting Prosocially." *Journal of Positive Psychology* 13(6):563–572.

Hui, Chin Ming, Daniel C. Molden, and Eli J. Finkel. 2013. "Loving Freedom: Concerns with Promotion or Prevention and the Role of Autonomy in Relationship Well-Being." *Journal of Personality & Social Psychology* 105(1):61–85.

Hui, Eddie Chi Man. 1999. "Willingness to Pay for Better Housing in Hong Kong: Theory and Evidence." *Urban Studies* 36(2):289–304.

Hui, Lai Hang Dennis, and Chi Yan Ryan Au. 2016. "Spatial Governance and the Rise of Post-Politics in Hong Kong." *Journal of Asian Public Policy* 9(3):227–242.

Hui, Victoria Ka-ying, Michael Harris Bond, and Timmy Sze Wing Ng. 2007. "General Beliefs about the World as Defensive Mechanisms against Death Anxiety." *Omega* 54(3):199–214.

Hull, Jay G., and Marilyn Mendolia. 1991. "Modeling the Relations of Attributional Style, Expectancies, and Depression." *Journal of Personality & Social Psychology* 61(1):85–97.

Hull, Pamela, Barbara Kilbourne, Michelle Reece, and Baqar Husaini. 2008. "Community Involvement and Adolescent Mental Health: Moderating Effects of Race/Ethnicity and Neighborhood Disadvantage." *Journal of Community Psychology* 36(4):534–551.

Hult, Carl, and Stefan Svallfors. 2002. "Production Regimes and Work Orientation: A Comparison of Sex Western Countries." *European Sociological Review* 18(3):315–331.

Hummelsheim, D., H. Hirtenlehner, J. Jackson and D. Oberwittler. 2011. "Social Insecurities and Fear of Crime: A Cross-National Study on the Impact of Welfare State Policies on Crime-Related Anxieties." *European Sociological Review* 27(3):327–345.

Hunter, Bronwyn A., Leonard A. Jason, and Christopher B. Keys. 2013. "Factors of Empowerment for Women in Recovery from Substance Use." *American Journal of Community Psychology* 51(1–2):91–102.

Hurd, Noelle M., Marc A. Zimmerman, and Thomas M. Reischl. 2011. "Role Model Behavior and Youth Violence: A Study of Positive and Negative Effects." *Journal of Early Adolescence* 31(2):323–354.

Hustinx, Lesley, and Femida Handy. 2009. "Where Do I Belong? Volunteer Attachment in a Complex Organization." *Administration in Social Work* 33(2):202–220.

Huta, Veronika. 2017. "An Overview of Hedonic and Eudaimonic Well-being Concepts." Pp. 14–33 in *The Routledge Handbook of Media Use and Well-being: International Perspectives on Theory and Research on Positive Media Effects*, edited by Leonard Reinecke and Mary Beth Oliver. New York, NY: Routledge.

Hutchings, Vincent L. 2003. Public Opinion and Democratic Accountability: How Citizens Learn about Politics. Princeton, NJ: Princeton University Press.

Huxhold, Oliver, Katherine L. Fiori, and Tim Windsor. 2022. "Rethinking Social Relationships in Adulthood: The Differential Investment of Resources Model." *Personality & Social Psychology Review* 26(1):57–82.

Huyck, Margaret Hellie, and David Leo Gutmann. 2006. "Men and Their Wives: Why Are Some Married Men Vulnerable at Midlife?" Pp. 27–50 in *Men in Relationships: A New Look from a Life Course Perspective*, edited by Victoria Hilkevitch Bedford and Barbara Formaniak Turner. New York: Springer.

Huynh, Jasmine-Yan, Jacques C. Metzer, and Anthony H. Winefield. 2012. "Engaged or Connected? A Perspective of the Motivational Pathway of the Job Demands-Resources Model in Volunteers Working for Nonprofit Organizations." *Voluntas* 23(4):870–898.

Hwang Hyesun, and Kee-Ok Kim. 2015. "Social Media as a Tool for Social Movements: The Effect of Social Media Use and Social Capital on Intention to Participate in Social Movements." *International Journal of Consumer Studies* 39(5):478–488.

Hwang, Sean-shong, Juan Xi, Yue Cao, Xiaotian Feng, and Xiaofei Qiao. 2007. "Anticipation of Migration and Psychological Stress and the Three Gorges Dam Project, China." *Social Science & Medicine* 65:1012–1024.

Hyggen, Christer. 2006. "Risks and Resources: Social Capital among Social Assistance Recipients in Norway." *Social Policy & Administration* 40(5):493–508.

Iceland, John, and Josh Kim. 2001. "Poverty among Working Families: New Insights from an Improved Poverty Measure." *Social Science Quarterly* 82(2):253–266. \72–331

Ickes, William, Anna Park, and Amanda, Johnson. 2012. "Linking Identity Status to Strength of Sense of Self: Theory and Validation." *Self & Identity* 11(4):531–544.

Imamoglu, E. Olcay. 2003. "Individuation and Relatedness: Not Opposing but Distinct and Complementary." *Genetic, Social & General Psychology Monographs* 129(4):367–402.

Immerzeel, Tim and Frank van Tubergen. 2013. "Religion as Reassurance? Testing the Insecurity Theory in 26 European Countries." *European Sociological Review* 29(2):359–372.

Ingleby, Ewan, and Jonathan Tummons. 2012. "Repositioning Professionalism: Teachers, Mentors, Policy and Praxis." *Research in Post-Compulsory Education* 17(2):163–178.

Ingledew, David K., David Markland, and Kate E. Sheppard. 2004. "Personality and Self-determination of Exercise Behavior." *Personality & Individual Differences* 36:1921–1932.

Inglehart, Ronald, and Christian Welzel. 2005. *Modernization, Cultural Change, and Democracy: The Human Development Sequence*. New York: Cambridge University Press.

Inglehart, Ronald, and Wayne E. Baker. 2000. "Modernization, Cultural Change, and the Persistence of Traditional Values." *American Sociological Review* 65:1–51.

Inglehart, Ronald. 1997. Modernization and Postmodernization: Cultural, Economic, and Political Change in 43 Societies. Princeton, NJ: Princeton University Press.

Inglehart, Ronald. 2003. "Modernization and Volunteering." Pp. 55–70 in *The Values of Volunteering: Cross-cultural Perspectives*, edited by Paul Dekker and Loek Halman. New York: Kluwer.

Inskipp, Francesca. 2012. "Generic Skills." Pp. 78–91 in *The SAGE Handbook of Counselling and Psychotherapy*, edited by Colin Feltham and Ian Horton. London: SAGE.

Inzlicht, Michael, and Brandon J. Schmeichel. 2016. "Beyond Limited Resources: Self-control Failure as the Product of Shifting Priorities." Pp. 165–181 in *Handbook of Self-regulation: Research*, Theory, and Application, edited by Kathleen D. Vohs and Roy F. Baumeister. New York, NY: Guilford.

Ip, Po-Keung. 2014. "Harmony as Happiness? Social Harmony in Two Chinese Societies." *Social Indicators Research* 117(3):719–41.

Irazabal, Clara, and Surajit Chakravarty. 2007. "Entertainment-retail Centres in Hong Kong and Los Angeles: Trends and Lessons." *International Planning Studies* 12(3):241–271.

Ireland, Leanna. 2021. "Predicting Online Target Hardening Behaviors: An Extension of Routine Activity Theory for Privacy-Enhancing Technologies and Techniques." *Deviant Behavior* 42(12):1532–48.

Irwin, Michael D. 2016. "The Concept of Community as Theoretical Ground: Contention and Compatibility across Levels of Analysis and Standpoints of Social Processes." Pp. 247–268 in *Handbook of Contemporary Sociological Theory*, edited by Seth Abrutyn. Cham, Switzerland: Springer.

Isaacowitz, Derek M., George E. Vaillant, and Martin E.P. Seligman. 2003. "Strengths and Satisfaction across the Adult Lifespan." *International Journal of Aging & Human Development* 57(2):181–201.

Isham, Jonathan, Jane Kolodinsky, and Garrett Kimberly. 2006. "The Effects of Volunteering for Nonprofit Organizations on Social Capital Formation: Evidence from a Statewide Survey." *Nonprofit & Voluntary Sector Quarterly* 35(3):367–83.

Ishii, Kenichi. 2009. "Nationalistic Sentiments of Chinese Consumers: The Effects and Determinants of Animosity and Consumer Ethnocentrism." *Journal of International Consumer Marketing* 21:299–308.

Ishii, Tatsunori and Katsumi Watanabe. 2023. "Do Empathetic People Have Strong Religious Beliefs? Survey Studies with Large Japanese Samples." *International Journal for the Psychology of Religion* 33(1):1–18.

Islam, Jonathan, Jane Kolodinsky, and Garrett Kimberly. 2006. "The Effects of Volunteering for Nonprofit Organizations on Social Capital Formation: Evidence from a Statewide Survey." *Nonprofit & Voluntary Sector Quarterly* 35(3):367–383.

Israelashvili, Moshe. 1999. "Adolescents" Help-seeking Behavior in Times of Community Crises." *International Journal for the Advancement of Counselling* 21:87–96.

Itzhaky, Haya, and Alan S. York. 2000. "Empowerment and Community Participation: Does Gender Make a Difference?" *Social Work Research* 24(4):225–234.

Iwai, Tatiana and João Vinícius de Franca Carvalho. 2022. "Would You Help Me Again? The Role of Moral Identity, Helping Motivation and Quality of Gratitude Expressions in Future Helping Intentions." *Personality & Individual Differences* 196:111719.

Iwanaga, Kanako, Emre Umucu, Jia-Rung Wu, Rana Yaghmaian, Hui-Ling Lee, Sandra Fitzgerald, and Fong Chan. 2017. "Assessing Vocational Outcome Expectancy in Individuals with Serious Mental Illness: A Factor-Analytic Approach." *Journal of Mental Health* 29(1):116–123.

Iyer, Aarti, Jolanda Jetten, Dimitrios Tsivrikos, Tom Postmes, and S. Alexander Haslam. 2009. "The More (and the More Compatible) the Merrier: Multiple Group Memberships and Identity Compatibility as Predictors of Adjustment after Life Transitions." *British Journal of Social Psychology* 48(4):707–733.

Izenstark, Dina and Aaron T. Ebata. 2016. "Theorizing Family-Based Nature Activities and Family Functioning: The Integration of Attention Restoration Theory with a Family Routines and Rituals Perspective: Theorizing Family-Based Nature Activities." *Journal of Family Theory & Review* 8:137–53.

Izzard, Susannah. 2000. "Psychoanalytic Psychotherapy." Pp. 106–121 in *Therapeutic Perspectives on Working with Lesbian, Gay and Bisexual Clients*, edited by Dominic Davies and Charles Neal. Buckingham, UK: Open University Press.

Izzo, Charles V., Roger P. Weissberg, Wesley J. Kasprow, and Michael Fendrich. 1999. "A Longitudinal Assessment of Teacher Perceptions of Parent Involvement in Children's Education and School Performance." *American Journal of Community Psychology* 27(6):817–839.

Jackman, Danielle M., and David MacPhee. 2017. "Self-Esteem and Future Orientation Predict Adolescents? Risk Engagement." *Journal of Early Adolescence* 37(3):339–366.

Jackson, Michelle. 2007. "You Have Full Text Access to This Content: How Far Merit Selection? Social Stratification and the Labour Market." *British Journal of Sociology* 58(3):367–390,

Jackson, Todd, Hong Chen, Cheng Guo, and Xiao Gao. 2006. "Stories We Love by: Conceptions of Love among Couples from the People's Republic of China and the United States." *Journal of Cross-Cultural Psychology* 37(4):446–464.

Jacobs, Lawrence R., Fay Lomax Cook, and Michael X. Delli Carpini. 2009. *Talking Together: Public Deliberative and Political Participation in America.* Chicago, IL: University of Chicago Press.

Jaeger, Mads Meier. 2008. "Does Left–Right Orientation Have a Causal Effect on Support for Redistribution? Causal Analysis with Cross-Sectional Data Using Instrumental Variables." *International Journal of Public Opinion Research* 20(3):363–74.

Jaeger, Mads, Meier. 2012. "The Extended Family and Children's Educational Success." *American Sociological Review* 77(6):903–922.

Jaeger, Wiliam K. 2004. "Status Seeking and Social Welfare: Is There Virtue in Vanity?" *Social Science Quarterly* 85(2):361–379.

Jaf, Darun, Metin Özdemir, and Therése Skoog. 2021. "Immigrant and Swedish Adolescents' Involvement in Organized Sports Activities: An Expectancy-Value Approach." *BMC Psychology* 9(1):12.

Jaffee, Sara R., and Robert Gallop. 2007. "Social, Emotional, and Academic Competence among Children Who Have Had Contact with Child Protective Services: Prevalence and Stability Estimates." *Journal of the American Academy of Child & Adolescent Psychiatry* 46(6):757–765.

Jakobsen, Tor Georg. 2010. "Public versus Private: The Conditional Effect of State Policy and Institutional Trust on Mass Opinion." *European Sociological Review* 26(3):307–318.

Jakoubek, Jane, and Robyn R. Swenson. 1993. "Differences in Use of Learning Strategies and Relation to Grades among Undergraduate Students." *Psychological Report* 73:787–793.

James, Rachel K., and Ye Luo. 1999. "The Culture of Poverty and African-American Culture: An Empirical Assessment." *Sociological Perspectives* 42(3):439–458.

James, Spencer L. and Paul R. Amato. 2013. "Self-Esteem and the Reproduction of Social Class." *Social Science Quarterly* 94(4):933–955.

James, Susan, and John Hunsley. 1995. "The Marital Adaptability and Cohesion Evaluation Scale III: Is the Relation with Marital Adjustment Linear or Curvilinear." *Journal of Family Psychology* 9(4):458–462.

Jamison, T. Rene; and Jessica Oeth Schuttler. 2017. "Overview and Preliminary Evidence for a Social Skills and Self-Care Curriculum for Adolescent Females with Autism: The Girls Night Out Model." *Journal of Autism & Developmental Disorders* 47(1):110–125.

Jang, Jongick, Tae-Hwan Kim, Hoon Hong, Chung Sik Yoo, and Jonghyun Park. 2018. "Statistical Estimation of the Causal Effect of Social Economy on Subjective Well-Being." *Voluntas* 29(3):511–525.

Jang, Sung Tae, Christine Halse, Daphnee Hui Lin Lee, and Queenie Chun Ki Hon. 2022. "Belongingness and National Belonging among Youth in Hong Kong." *Youth & Society* 54(8):1307–29.

Janion, Ludmila. 2020. "The Rise and Fall of the Progressive Drag Queen: Westernization of Cross-dressing in 1990s Poland." *Sexualities* 23(7):1179–1198.

Jankovic, Marija and Stefan Bogaerts. 2021. "Predicting Success in the Performing Arts: Ballet and Music." *Psychology of Music* 49(4):945–57.

Janoff-Bulman, Ronnie. 1992. Shattered Assumptions: Towards a New Psychology of Trauma. New York: Free Press.

Jans-Beken, Lilian. 2019. "The Dialectic Dynamics between Trait Gratitude, Subjective Well-Being, and Psychopathology across 30 Weeks." *Counselling Psychology Quarterly* 32(3–4):502–315.

Jarrett, Thomas A. 2013. "Warrior Resilience and Thriving (WRT): Rational Emotive Behavior Therapy (REBT) as a Resiliency and Thriving Foundation to Prepare Warriors and Their Families for Combat Deployment and Posttraumatic Growth in Operation Iraqi Freedom, 2005–2009." *Journal of Rational-Emotive & Cognitive-Behavior Therapy* 31(2):93–107.

Jarvis, Matt. 2004. Psychodynamic Psychology: Classical Theory and Contemporary Research. London, UK: Thomson.

Jasielska, Dorota. 2020. "The Moderating Role of Kindness on the Relation between Trust and Happiness." *Current Psychology* 39(6):2065–73.

Jasso, Guillermina. 2015. "Thinking, Saying, Doing in the World of Distributive Justice." *Social Justice Research* 28(4):435–478.

Jayawardana, Janaka, Renuka Priyantha, Michele Magni and Fausto Marincioni. 2019. "Disaster Resilience among War-Affected People Resettled in Northern Sri Lanka: Challenges Revisited." *International Journal of Disaster Risk Reduction* 34:356–62.

Jayawickreme, Eranda, Marie J. C. Forgeard, and Martin E. P. Seligman. 2012. "The Engine of Well-Being." *Review of General Psychology* 16(4):327–42.

Jeffries, Vincent. 2000. "Virtue and Marital Conflict: A Theoretical Formulation and Research Agenda." *Sociological Perspectives* 43(2):231–46.

Jen, Chun-Hui, Wei-Wen Chen, and Chih Wen Wu. 2019. "Flexible Mindset in the Family: Filial Piety, Cognitive Flexibility, and General Mental Health." Journal of Social & *Personal Relationships* 36(6):1715–1730.

Jenkins, Mikayla, and Marko Dragojevic. 2011. "Explaining the Process of Resistance to Persuasion: A Politeness Theory-based Approach." *Communication Research* 40(4):559–590.

Jennings, Freddie J. and Frank M. Russell. 2019. "Civility, Credibility, and Health Information: The Impact of Uncivil Comments and Source Credibility on Attitudes About Vaccines." *Public Understanding of Science* 28(4):417–32.

Jennings, Patricia K. 2004. "What Mothers Want: Welfare Reform and Maternal Desire." *Journal of Sociology & Social Welfare* 31(3):113–130.
Jensen, Gary F. 2007. "Social Learning and Violent Behavior." Pp. 636–646 in *The Cambridge Handbook of Violent Behavior and Aggression*, edited by Daniel J. Flannery, Alexander T. Vazsonyi and Irwin D. Waldman. Cambridge, UK: Cambridge University Press.
Jessop, Donna C., Ian P. Albery, Jean Rutter, Heather Garrod. 2008. "Understanding the Impact of Mortality-related Health-risk Information: A Terror Management Theory Perspective." *Personality & Social Psychology Bulletin* 34(7):951–964.
Ji, Qihao, Sophie H. Janicke-Bowles, Rebecca N. H. De Leeuw, and Mary Beth Oliver. 2021. "The Melody to Inspiration: The Effects of Awe-Eliciting Music on Approach Motivation and Positive Well-Being." *Media Psychology* 24(3):305–31.
Jiang, Da, Helene H. Fung, and Lynn Martire. 2022. "Daily Reciprocity and Well-Being: A Diary Study of Intergenerational Support between Mothers and Adult Children During the Covid-19 Pandemic." *Journals of Gerontology* 77(4):e46–e56.
Jiang, Yi, Mimi Bong, and Sung-il Kim. 2015. "Conformity of Korean Adolescents in Their Perceptions of Social Relationships and Academic Motivation." *Learning & Individual Differences* 40:41–54.
Jimenez-Anca, Juan J. 2013. "Beyond Power: Unbridging Foucault and Weber." *European Journal of Social Theory* 16(1):36–50.
Jinks, Gordon. 2012. "Specific Strategies and Techniques." Pp. 92–111 in *The SAGE Handbook of Counselling and Psychotherapy*, edited by Colin Feltham and Ian Horton. London: SAGE.
Jirsaraie, Robert Jesus, Krista Wilke Ranby, and David Scott Albeck. 2019. "Early Life Stress Moderates the Relationship between Age and Prosocial Behaviors." *Child Abuse & Neglect* 94:104029.
Jodl, Kathleen M., Alice Michael, Oksana Malanchuk, Jacquelynne S. Eccles, and Arnold Sameroff. 2001. "Parents' Roles in Shaping Early Adolescents' Occupational Aspirations." *Child Development* 72(4):1247–1265.
John, Karen. 2001. "Measuring Children's Social Functioning." *Child Psychology & Psychiatry Review* 6(4):181–88.
Johns, Amelia, Michele Grossman, and Kevin McDonald. 2014. "More than a Game: The Impact of Sport-Based Youth Mentoring Schemes on Developing Resilience toward Violent Extremism." *Social Inclusion* 2(2):57–70.
Johnson, Carolina. 2015. "Local Civic Participation and Democratic Legitimacy: Evidence from England and Wales." *Political Studies* 63(4):765–792.
Johnson, Daniel K.N., and Ayfer Ali. 2004. "a Tale of two Seasons: Participation and Medal Counts at the Summer and Winter Olympic Games." *Social Science Quarterly* 85(4):974–993.
Johnson, David W. and Roger T. Johnson. 2005. "New Developments in Social Interdependence Theory." *Genetic, Social, & General Psychology Monographs* 131(4):285–358.
Johnson, Elle P. and Jennifer A. Samp. 2022. "Stoicism and Verbal Aggression in Serial Arguments: The Roles of Perceived Power, Perceived Resolvability, and Frequency of Arguments." *Journal of Interpersonal Violence* 37(13–14):NP11836–NP56.
Johnson, Judith, Maria Panagioti, Jennifer Bass, Lauren Ramsey, and Reema Harrison. 2017. "Resilience to Emotional Distress in Response to Failure, Error or Mistakes: A Systematic Review." *Clinical Psychology Review* 52:19–42.
Johnson, Judy J. 2009. What's So Wrong with Being Absolutely Right: The Dangerous Nature of Dogmatic Beliefs. Amherst, NY: Prometheus.
Johnson, Lee Michael, Ronald L. Simons, and Rand D. Conger. 2004. "Criminal Justice System Involvement and Continuity of Youth Crime: A Longitudinal Analysis." *Youth & Society* 36(1):3–29.
Johnson, Malcolm. 2009. "Spirituality, Finitude, and Theories of the Life Span." Pp. 759–674 in *Handbook of Theories of Aging*, edited by Vern L. Bengtson, Merril Silverstein, Norella M. Putney and Daphna Gans. New York: Springer.

Johnson, Matthew D., Linh Nguyen, Jared R. Anderson, Wenli Liu, and Amber Vennum. 2015. "Pathways to Romantic Relationship Success among Chinese Young Adult Couples: Contributions of Family Dysfunction, Mental Health Problems, and Negative Couple Interaction." *Journal of Social & Personal Relationships* 32(1):5–23.

Johnson, Michael P., and Kathleen J. Ferraro. 2000. "Research on Domestic Violence in the 1990s." Making Distinctions." *Journal of Marriage & the Family* 62:948–963.

Johnson, Sara K., Mary H. Buckingham, Stacy L. Morris, Sara Suzuki, Michelle B. Weiner, Rachel M. Hershberg, Ettya R. Fremont, Milena Batanova, Caitlin C. Aymong, Cristina J. Hunter, Edmond Pya. Bowers, Jacqueline V. Lerner, and Richard M. Lerner. 2016. "Adolescents" Character Role Models: Exploring Who Young People Look up to as Examples of How to Be a Good Person." *Research in Human Development* 13(2):126–41.

Johnston, Britton W. 2010. "Breaching the Sacred Walls of Illness: A Girardian Model of Forgiveness as Healing." *Journal of Spirituality in Mental Health* 12(2):118–49. doi: 10.1080/19349631003730142.

Johnston, David W., Stefanie Sqhurer, Michael A. Shields. 2013. "Exploring the Intergenerational Persistence of Mental Health: Evidence from Three Generations." *Journal of Health Economics* 32:1077–1089.

Jokic, Biljana and Danka Puric. 2021. "Seeking Proxies for Internal States as a Possible Alternative for Rationality and Experientiality." *SAGE Open* 11(1):215824402098653.

Jones, Daniel N., and Delroy L. Paulhus. 2009. "Machiavellianism." Pp. 93–108 in *Handbook of Individual Differences in Social Behavior*, edited by Mark R. Leary and Rick H. Hoyle. New York, NY: Guilford.

Jones, Giavana and Kathryn Lafreniere. 2014. "Exploring the Role of School Engagement in Predicting Resilience among Bahamian Youth." *Journal of Black Psychology* 40(1):47–68.

Jones, Janelle M., and Jolanda Jetten. 2011. "Recovering from Strain and Enduring Pain." *Social Psychological & Personality Science* 2(3):239–244.

Jones, Lindsey, and Marco d'Errico. 2019. "Whose Resilience Matters? Like-for-Like Comparison of Objective and Subjective Evaluations of Resilience." *World Development* 124:104632.

Jones, Paul, Christopher Miller, David Pickernell, and Gary Packham. 2011. "The Role of Education, Training and Skills Development in Social Inclusion: The University of the Heads of the Valley Case Study." *Education + Training* 53(7):638–651.

Jones, Rebecca J., Stephen A. Woods, and Ying Zhou. 2021. "The Effects of Coachee Personality and Goal Orientation on Performance Improvement Following Coaching: A Controlled Field Experiment." *Applied Psychology* 70(2):420–58.

Jones, Russell, Derek Heim, Simon Hunter, and Anne Ellaway. 2014. "The Relative Influence of Neighbourhood Incivilities, Cognitive Social Capital, Club Membership and Individual Characteristics on Positive Mental Health." *Health & Place* 28:187–93.

Jones, Veronica Nyhan, and Michael Woolcock. 2010. "Measuring the Dimensions of Social Capital in Developing Countries." Pp. 537–559 in *The SAGE Handbook of Measurement*, edited by Geoffrey Walford, Eric Tucker, and Madhu Viswanathan. London, UK: SAGE.

Jones-Smith, Elsie. 2014. Strengths-based Therapy: Connecting Theory, Practice, and Skills. London, UK: SAGE.

Jonsson, Dagmar, Saga Johansson, Annika Rosengren, Georg Lappas, and Lars Wilhelmsen. 2003. "Self-Perceived Psychological Stress in Relation to Psychosocial Factors and Work in a Random Population Sample of Women." *Stress & Health* 19(6):149–62.

Jopp, Daniela, and Christoph Rott. 2006. "Adaptation in Very Old Age: Exploring the Role of Resource Beliefs and Attitudes for Centenarians" Happiness." *Psychology & Aging* 21(2):266–280.

Jorgensen, Bradley S., Robert D. Jamieson, and John F. Martin. 2010. "Income, Sense of Community and Subjective Well-being: Combining Economic and Psychological Variables." *Journal of Economic Psychology* 31:612–643.

Jorgensen, Nathan A., and Larry J. Nelson. 2018. "Moving toward and Away from Others: Social Orientations in Emerging Adulthood." *Journal of Applied Developmental Psychology* 58:66–76.

Joseph, Joanne M. 1994. The Resilient Child: Preparing Today's Youth for Tomorrow's World. New York: Plenum.

Joseph, Stephen, and Richard Bryant-Jefferies. 2007. "Person-centred Coaching Psychology." Pp. 211–228 in *Handbook of Coaching Psychology: A Guide for Practitioners*, edited by Stephen Palmer and Alison Whybrow. Hove, UK: Routledge.

Joseph, Stephen. 2018. "The Person-centered Approach to Coaching." Pp. 52–65 in *The Complete Handbook of Coaching*, edited by Elaine Cox, Tatiana Bachkirova, and David Clutterbuck. London, UK: SAGE.

Joshanloo, Mohsen and Aaron Jarden. 2016. "Individualism as the Moderator of the Relationship between Hedonism and Happiness: A Study in 19 Nations." *Personality & Individual Differences* 94:149–52.

Jost, John T. 2020. *A Theory of System Justification.* Cambridge, MA: Harvard University Press.

Jost, John T., and Jojanneke van der Toom. 2012. "System Justification Theory." Pp. 313–343 in *Handbook of Theories of Social Psychology* (vol. 2), edited by Paul A.M. Van Lange, Arie W. Kruglanski and E. Tory Higgins. London, CA: SAGE.

Jost, John t., and Orsolya Hunyady. 2005. "Antecedents and Consequences of System-justifying Ideologies:" *Current Directions in Psychological Science* 14(5):260–265.

Jost, John T., Brett W. Pelham, Oliver Sheldon, and Billian Ni Sullivan. 2003. "Social Inequality and the Reduction of Ideological Dissonance on Behalf of the System: Evidence of the Enhanced System Justification among the Disadvantaged." *European Journal of Social Psychology* 33:13–36.

Jowkar, Bahram, Oddgeir Friborg, And Odin Hjemdal. 2010. "Cross-cultural validation of the Resilience Scale for Adults (RSA) in Iran." *Scandinavian Journal of Psychology* 51(5):418–25.

Juanchich, Marie, Lukasz Walasek, and Miroslav Sirota. 2018. "Decision-Makers Are Resilient in the Face of Social Exclusion." *British Journal of Psychology* 109(3):604–630.

Juanchich, Marie, Miroslav Sirota, Daniel Jolles, and Lilith A. Whiley. 2021. "Are COVID-19 Conspiracies a Threat to Public Health? Psychological Characteristics and Health Protective Behaviours of Believers." *European Journal of Social Psychology* 51(6):969–89.

Judge, Timothy A., Amir Erez, Joyce E. Bono, and Carl J. Thoresen. 2002. "Are Measures of Self-esteem, Neuroticism, Locus of Control, and Generalized Self-efficacy Indicators of a Common Core Construct?" *Journal of Personality & Social Psychology* 83(3):693–710.

Juhl, Jacob, Tim Wildschut, Constantine Sedikides, Tara Diebel, Wing-Yee Cheung, and Ad J. J. M. Vingerhoets. 2020a. "Nostalgia Proneness and Empathy: Generality, Underlying Mechanism, and Implications for Prosocial Behavior." *Journal of Personality* 88(3):485–500.

Jung, Jinkyung J., and Eunsun E. Kwon. 2011. "Trust Development in Volunteering: An Exploratory Study of Social Trust and Volunteer Activities in Korea." *International Review of Public Administration* 16(1):157–179.

Juni, Samuel. 2009. "Conceptualization of Hostile Psychopathology and Sadism: Drive Theory and Object Relations Perspectives." *International Forum of Psychoanalysis* 18:11–22.

Junttila, Niina, Marinus Voeten, Ari Kaukiainen, and Marja Vauras. 2006. "Multisource Assessment of Children's Social Competence." *Educational & Psychological Measurement* 66(5):874–895.

Jurik, Verena, Alexander Gröschner, and Tina Seidel. 2014. "Predicting Students" Cognitive Learning Activity and Intrinsic Learning Motivation: How Powerful Are Teacher Statements, Student Profiles, and Gender?" *Learning & Individual Differences* 32:132–39.

Jutengren, Göran, and Eva Medin. 2019. "Cross-Ethnic Friendship and Prosocial Behavior's Potential Significance to Elementary Children's Academic Competence." *Journal of Educational Research* 112(1):38–45.

Juvonen, Yaana. 1991. "Deviance, Perceived Responsibility, and Negative Peer Reactions." *Developmental Psychology* 27(4):672–681.

Kabiri, Saeed, Seyyedeh Masoomeh Shadmanfaat, Hayden Smith, and John Cochran. 2020. "A Social Learning Model of Antisocial Coaching Behavior." *International Journal of Offender Therapy & Comparative Criminology* 64(8):860–879.

Kachadonrian, Lirig K. et al. 2013. "Maladaptive Dependency Schemas, Posttraumatic Stress Hyperarousal Symptoms, and Intimate Partner Aggressive Perpetration." *Journal of Traumatic Stress* 26:580–587.

Kachanoff, Frank J., Donald M. Taylor, Julie Caouette, Thomas H. Khullar, and Michael J. A. Wohl. 2019. "The Chains on All My People Are the Chains on Me: Restrictions to Collective Autonomy Undermine the Personal Autonomy and Psychological Well-Being of Group Members." *Journal of Personality & Social Psychology* 116(1):141–165.

Kachiga, Jean. 2021. *The Rise of China and International Relations Theory*. New York, NY: Lang.

Kaczmarek, Lukasz D. and Dariusz Drążkowski. 2014. "MMORPG Escapism Predicts Decreased Well-Being: Examination of Gaming Time, Game Realism Beliefs, and Online Social Support for Offline Problems." *Cyberpsychology, Behavior & Social Networking* 17(5):298–302.

Kadushin, Charles, and Delmos J. Jones. 1992. "Social Networks and Urban Neighborhoods in New York City." *City & Society* 58–75.

Kadushin, Charles. 2004. "Too Much Investment in Social Capital?" *Social Networks* 26(1):75–90.

Kafashun, Sara, Adam Spork, Amanda Rotella, and Pat Barclay. 2017. "What Heroism Exists: Evolutionary Perspectives on Extreme Helping." Pp. 36–57 in *Handbook of Heroism and Heroic Leadership*, edited by Scott T. Allison, George R. Goethals and Roderick M. Kramer. New York: Routledge.

Kafetsio, Konstantinos, and Georgios D. Sideridis. 2006. "Attachment, Social Support and Well-being in Young and Older Adults." *Journal of Health Psychology* 11(6):863–876.

Kahneman, Daniel, David A. Schkade, Calude Fishler, Alan B. Krueger, and Amy Krilla. 2010. "The Structure of Well-being in Two Cities: Life Satisfaction and Experience and Happiness in Columbus, Ohio and Rennes, France." Pp. 16–33 in *International Differences in Well-being*, edited by Ed Diener, John F. Helliwell and Daniel Kahneman. New York: Oxford University Press.

Kalish, Yuval. 2008. "Bridging in Social Networks: Who Are the People on Structural Holes and Why Are They There?" *Asian Journal of Social Psychology* 11:53–66.

Kalkstein, Solomon, and Roni Beth Tower. 2009. "The Daily Spiritual Experiences Scale and Well-being: Demographic Comparisons and Scale Validation with Older Jewish Adults and a Diverse Internet Sample." *Journal of Religion & Health* 48:402–417.

Kanan, James W., and Matthew V. Pruitt. 2002. "Modeling Fear of Crime and Perceived Victimization Risk: The (In)significance of Neighborhood Integration." *Sociological Inquiry* 72(4):527–548.

Kane, Emily W. 2019. "Beliefs About Family Policy among Us Mothers in Publicly-Subsidised Housing: Collective Responsibility or Individual Self-Sufficiency." *Journal of Poverty & Social Justice* 27(3):333–49.

Kane Frieder, Rachel E., Wayne A. Hochwarter, and Gerald R. Ferris. 2013. "Terms of Engagement: Political Boundaries of Work Engagement-Work Outcomes Relationships." *Human Relations* 67(3):357–382.

Kang, Ziyoung, and Gary D. Gottfredson. 2015. "Environments Diversity in Theoretical Foundations of Career Intervention." Pp. 159–181 in *APA Handbook of Career Intervention, Vol: Foundations,* edited by Paul J. Hartung, Mark L. Savickas, and W. Bruce Walsh. Washington, DC: American Psychological Association.

Kangas, Olli. 2003. "The Grasshopper and the Ants: Popular Opinions of Just Distribution in Australia and Finland." *Journal of Socio-Economics* 31:721–743.

Kanji, Mebs, and Neil Nevitte. 1997. "Environmental Support, Concern and Action: An Exploratory Crossnational Analysis." *International Journal of Public Opinion Research* 9(1):66–76.

Kanmeyer-Mueller, John D., and Timothy A. Judge. 2007. "A Quantitative Review of Mentoring Research: Test of a Model." *Journal of Vocational Behavior* 72:269–283.

Kanno, Hanae, and Gary F. Koeske. 2010. "MSW Students Satisfaction with Their Placements: The Role of Preparedness and Supervision Quality." *Journal of Social Work Education* 46(1):23–38.

Kaplan, Celia P. Pamela I. Erickson, and Maria Juarez-Reyes. 2002. "Acculturation, Gender Role Orientation, and Reproductive Risk-taking Behavior among Latina Adolescent Family Planning Clients." *Journal of Adolescent Research* 17(2):103–121.

Kaplan, Howard B. 2012. "Reconceptualizing Resilience." Pp. 39–55 in *Handbook of Resilience in Children*, edited by Sam Goldstein and Robert B. Brooks. New York, NY: Springer.

Kaplan, Howard B., Feodor A. Gostjev, and Robert J. Johnson. 2013. "Social Psychological Perspectives on Deviance." Pp. 563–594 in *Handbook of Social Psychology*, edited by John Delamater and Amanda Ward. Dordrecht, Netherlands: Springer.

Kapoutsis, Ilias, Roger Volkema, and Antonia Lampaki. 2017. "Mind the First Step: The Intrapersonal Effects of Affect on the Decision to Initiate Negotiations under Bargaining Power Asymmetry." *Frontiers in Psychology* 8:1313.

Karasawa, Minoru. 2003. "Projecting Group Liking and Ethnocentrism on In-group Members: False consensus Effect of Attitude Strength." *Asia Journal of Social Psychology* 6:103–116.

Karoly, Paul, and Linda S. Ruehlman. 2006. "Psychological Resilience and Its Correlates in Chronic Pain: Findings from a National Community Sample." *Pain* 123:90–97.

Karpinski, Jakub. 1990. *Causality in Sociological Research*. Dordrecht, Netherlands: Kluwer.

Karpov, Yuriy V. 2014. *Vygotsky for Educators*. New York, NY: Cambridge University Press.

Karremans, Johan C., Melanie P. J. Schellekens, and Gesa Kappen. 2017. "Bridging the Sciences of Mindfulness and Romantic Relationships: A Theoretical Model and Research Agenda." *Personality & Social Psychology Review* 21(1):29–49.

Karuza, Jurgis, Michael A. Zevon, Timothy A. Gleason, Colleen M. Karuza, and Linda Nash. 1990. "Models of Helping and Coping Responsibility Attributions and Well-being in Community Elderly and Their Helpers." *Psychology & Aging* 5(2):194–208.

Karwowski, Maciej, and Izabela Lebuda. 2017. "Creative Self-concept: A Surface Characteristic of Creative Personality." Pp. 84–101 in *The Cambridge Handbook of Creativity and Personality Research*, edited by Gregory J. Feist, Roni Reiter-Palmon, and James C. Kaufman. New York, NY: Cambridge University Press.

Karwowski, Maciej, Marta Czerwonka, Izabela Lebuda, Dorota Maria Jankowska, and Aleksandra Gajda. 2020. "Does Thinking About Einstein Make People Entity Theorists? Examining the Malleability of Creative Mindsets." *Psychology of Aesthetics, Creativity, & the Arts* 14(3):361–66.

Kas, Judith, Joyce Delnoij, Rense Corten, and Paolo Parigi. 2022. "Trust Spillovers in the Sharing Economy: Does International Airbnb Experience Foster Cross-National Trust?". *Journal of Consumer Behaviour* 21(3):509–22.

Kasen, Stephanie; Henian Chen, Joel Sneed, Thomas Crawford, and Patricia Cohen. 2006. "Social Role and Birth Cohort Influences on Gender-Linked Personality Traits in Women: A 20-Year Longitudinal Analysis." *Journal of Personality & Social Psychology: Personality Processes and Individual Differences* 91(5):944–958.

Kasser, Tim. 2016. "Materialistic Values and Goals." *Annual Review Psychology* 67:489–514.

Kast, Verena. 2006. "Anima/animus." Pp. 113–119 in *The Handbook of Jungian Psychology: Theory, Practice and Applications*, edited by Ronosk Papadopoulos. Hove, UK: Routledge.

Katartzi, Eugenia. 2018. "Unpacking Young People's National Identities: The Role of Ethno-Cultural and Religious Allegiances, History and "Others"." *Young* 26(3):215–231.

Kato, Tsukasa. 2015. "Effects of Flexibility in Coping with Chronic Headaches on Depressive Symptoms." *International Journal of Behavioral Medicine* 22(4):506–11.

Katz-Gerro, Tally, and Yossi Shavit. 1998. "The Stratification of Leisure and Taste: Classes and Lifestyles in Israel." *European Sociological Review* 14(4):369–386.

Kaukinen, Catherine. 2004. "Status Compatibility, Physical Violence, and Emotional Abuse in Intimate Relationships." *Journal of Marriage & Family* 66:452–471.

Kaurin, Pauline Shanks. 2020. *On Obedience: Contrasting Philosophies for the Military, Citizenry and Community*. Annapolis, MD: Naval.

Kavussanu, Maria, and Glyn C. Roberts. 2001. "Moral Functioning in Sport: An Achievement Goal Perspective." *Journal of Sport & Exercise Psychology* 23:37–54.

Kawachi, Ichiro, Bruce P. Kennedy, Kimberly Lochner, and Deborah Prothrow-Stith. 1997. "Social Capital, Income Inequality, and Mortality." *American Journal of Public Health* 87(9):1491–1498.

Kawakami, K., D. M. Amodio, and K. Hugenberg. 2017. "Intergroup Perception and Cognition: An Integrative Framework for Understanding the Causes and Consequences of Social Categorization." *Advances in Experimental Social Psychology* 55:1–80.

Kay, Aaron C., Danielle Gaucher, Jamie L. Napier, Mitchell J. Callan and Kristin Laurin. 2008. "God and the Government: Testing a Compensatory Control Mechanism for the Support of External Systems." *Journal of Personality & Social Psychology* 95(1):18–35.

Kayabol, Nazlı Büşra Akçabozan, and Zeynep Hatipoğlu Sümer. 2022. "How to Maintain a Marriage: Maintenance Behaviors, Equity, and Appreciation in Understanding Marital Satisfaction." *Current Psychology* 41(9):5781–94.

Kaye-Tzadok, Avital, and Bilha Davidson-Arad. 2017. "The Contribution of Cognitive Strategies to the Resilience of Women Survivors of Childhood Sexual Abuse and Non-Abused Women." *Violence against Women* 23(8):993–1015.

Keeting, Caroline F. 2016. "The Life and Times of Nonverbal Communication Theory and Research: Past, Present, Future." Pp. 17–42 in *APA Handbook of Nonverbal Communication*, edited by David Matsumoto, Hyisung C. Hwang and Mark G. Frank. Washington, DC: American Psychological Association.

Kegler, Michelle C., and Vicki Harris Wyatt. 2003. "A Multiple Case Study of Neighborhood Partnerships for Positive Youth Development." *American Journal of Health Behavior* 27(2):156–169.

Kegler, Michelle Crozier, Roy F. Oman, Sara K. Veskly, Kenneth R. McLeroy, Cheryl B. Aspy, Sharon Rodine, and La Donna Marshall. 2005. "Relationships among Youth Assets and Neighborhood and Community Resources." *Health Education & Behavior* 32(3):380–397.

Keightley, Michelle L., Gordon Winocur, Hana Burianova, Donaya Hongwanishkul, and Cheryl L. Grady. 2006. "Age Effects on Social Cognition: Faces Tell a Different Story." *Psychology & Aging* 21(3):558–572

Keijsers, Loes, Rolf Loeber, Susan Branje, and Wim Meeus. 2011. "Bidirectional Links and Concurrent Development of Parent-child Relationships and Boys" Offending Behavior." *Journal of Abnormal Psychology* 120(4):878–889.

Keillor, Bruce, Deborah Owens, and Charles Pettijohn. 2001. "A Cross-cultural Cross-national Study of Influencing Factors and Socially Desirable Response Biases." *International Journal of Market Research* 43(1):63–84.

Kekes, John. 1998. *A Case of Conservatism*. Ithaca, NY: Cornell University Press.

Kekes, John. 2003. *The Illusions of Egalitarianism*. Ithaca, NY: Cornell University Press.

Kelley, Douglas L., Vincent R. Waldron, and Dayna N. Kloeber. 2019. *A Communicative Approach to Conflict, Forgiveness, and Reconciliation: Reimagining Our Relationships*. New York, NY: Routledge.

Kelley, Susan J., Deborah M. Whitley, and Peter E. Campos. 2011. "Behavior Problems in Children Raised by Grandmothers: The Role of Caregiver Distress Family Resources, and the Home Environment." *Children & Youth Services Review* 33:2138–2145.

Kellner, Douglas. 1989. *Critical Theory, Marxism and Modernity*. Cambridge: Polity Press.

Kelly, Brendan D. 2012. "Contemplative Traditions and Meditation." Pp. 307–325 in *The Oxford Handbook of Psychology and Spirituality*, edited by Lisa J. Miller. New York, NY: Oxford University Press.

Kelly, Gail J., and Lyndall S. Steed. 2004. "Communities Coping with Change: A Conceptual Model." *Journal of Community Psychology* 32(2):209–216.

Kelly, Kevin R., and Wei-chien Lee. 2002. "Mapping the Domain of Career Decision Problems." *Journal of Vocational Behavior* 61:302–326.

Keltener, Dacher, Gerben A. Van Kleef, Serena Chen, and Michael W. Kraus. 2008. "A Reciprocal Influence Model of Social Power: Emerging Principles and Lines of Inquiry." *Advances in Experimental Social Psychology* 40:151–192.

Kemp, Candace L. 2007. "Grandparent-grandchild Ties: Reflections on Continuity and Change across Three Generations." *Journal of Family Issues* 28(7):855–881.

Kemshall, Hazel. 2002. *Risk, Social Policy and Welfare.* Buckingham, UK: Open University Press.

Kende, Judit, Charis Psaltis, Julia Reiter, Kyriaki Fousiani, Huseyin Cakal, and Eva Green. 2022. "Past and Present Intergroup Contact and Conflict among Inhabitants of Former Mixed Villages of Cyprus: The Role of Individual and Collective Experiences in Predicting Attitudes and Trust." *Political Psychology* 43(4):751–68.

Kendler, K. S., H. Ohlsson, B. Mezuk, K. Sundquist, and J. Sundquist. 2015. "Exposure to Peer Deviance During Childhood and Risk for Drug Abuse: A Swedish National Co-Relative Control Study." *Psychological Medicine* 45(4):855–64.

Kendler, Kenneth S., Charles O. Gardner, and Carol A. Prescott. 2006. "Toward a Comprehensive Developmental Model for Major Depression in Men." *American Journal of Psychiatry* 163(1):115–124.

Kennedy, Bruce D. Ichiro Kawachi, and Elizabeth Brainerd. 1998. "The Role of Social Capital in the Russia Mortality Crisis." *World Development* 26(11):2029–2043.

Kennedy, Gary J., and Bruce W. Tuckman. 2013. "An Exploration into The Influence of Academic and Social Values, Procrastination, and Perceived School Belongingness on Academic Performance." *Social Psychology of Education* 16(3):435–470.

Kenny, Sue, Ismet Fanany, and Sutria Rahayu. 2013. "Community Development in Indonesia: Westernization or Doing It Their Way?" *Community Development Journal* 48(2):280–97.

Kent, Martha and Mary C. Davis. 2010. "The Emergence of Capacity-building Programs and Models of Resilience." Pp. 427–449 in *Handbook of Adult Resilience*, edited by John W. Reich, Alex J. Zautra and John Stuart Hall. New York, NY: Guilford.

Keown, Damien. 2001. *The Nature of Buddhist Ethics.* Houndmills, UK: Palgrave.

Kern, Margaret L., Lea E. Waters, Alejandro Adler & Mathew A. White. 2015. "A multidimensional approach to measuring well-being in students: Application of the PERMA framework." *Journal of Positive Psychology* 10(3):262–271.

Kernis, Michael H., and Brian M. Goldman. 2006. "A Multicomponent Conceptualization of Authenticity: Theory and Research." *Advances in Experimental Social Psychology* 38:283–357.

Kerns, Kathryn A. Amanda J. Koehn, Manfred H. M. van Dulmen, Kaela L. Stuart-Parrigon, and Karin G. Coifman. 2016. "Preadolescents' Relationships with Pet Dogs: Relationship Continuity and Associations with Adjustment." *Applied Developmental Science* 21(1):67–80.

Kerr, Margaret, and Hakan Stattin. 2000. "What Parents Know, How They Know It, and Several Forms of Adolescent Adjustment: Further Support for a Reinterpretation of Monitoring." *Developmental Psychology* 36(3):366–380.

Kerrissey, Jasmine, and Evan Schofer. 2013. "Civic and Political Participation: Union Membership and Political Participation in the United States." *Social Forces* 91(3):895–928.

Kershaw, Tace, Laurel Northouse, Charuwan Kritpracha, Ann Schafenacker, and Darlene Mood. 2004. "Coping Strategies and Quality of Life in Women with Advanced Breast Cancer and Their Family Caregivers." *Psychology & Health* 19(2):139–155.

Kerstein, Samuel J. 2002. *Kant's Search for the Supreme Principle of Morality.* Cambridge, UK: Cambridge University Press.

Kertzer, Joshua D., Kathleen E. Powers, Brian C. Rathbun, and Ravi Iyer. 2014. "Moral Support: How Moral Values Shape Foreign Policy Attitudes." *Journal Of Politics* 76(3):825–840.

Kessler, Ronald C., Kristin D. Michelson, and David R. Williams. 1999. "The Prevalence, Distribution, and Mental Health Correlates of Perceived Discrimination in the United States." *Journal of Health & Social Behavior* 40(3):208–230.

Ketelaars, Pauline, Stefaan Walgrave and Ruud Wouters. 2017. "Protesters on Message? Explaining Demonstrators" Differential Degrees of Frame Alignment." *Social Movement Studies* 16(3):340–54.

Keyes, Corey L.M. 2002. "Social Civility in the United States." *Sociological Inquiry* 72(3):393–408.

Khalaila, Rabia. 2016. "Depression Statuses and Related Predictors in Later Life: A 10-Year Follow-up Study in Israel." *European Journal of Ageing* 13(4):311–321.

Khamis, Vivian. 2006. "Family Environment and Parenting as Predictors of Attention-deficient and Hyperactivity among Palestinian Children." *Journal of Social Service Research* 32(4):99–116.

Khattab, Nabil, and Steve Fenton. 2009. "What Makes Young Adults Happy? Employment and Non-work as Determinants of Life Satisfaction." *Sociology* 43(1):11–26.

Khodabakhsh, Sonia and Chia Sin Ooi. 2022. "Gratitude and Well-Being During COVID-19 Pandemic in Malaysia: Mediating Role of Resilience." *Psychological Thought* 15(1):189–214.

Khoo, Shuna Shiann, Wei Xing Toh, and Hwajin Yang. 2021. "Seeking Control during Uncontrollable Times: Control Abilities and Religiosity Predict Stress during Covid-19." *Personality & Individual Differences* 175:110675.

Khoshneviss, Hadi, and Robert D. Benford. 2018. "Social Movements." Pp. 828–842 in *The SAGE Handbook of Political Sociology*, edited by William Outhwaite and Stephen Turner. London, UK: SAGE.

Kiecolt, K. Jill. 2003. "Satisfaction with Work and Family Life: No Evidence of a Cultural Reversal." *Journal of Marriage & Family* 65(1):23–35.

Kilian, Britta, Manfred Hofer, and Claudia Kuhnle. 2013. "Conflicts between on-Task and Off-Task Behaviors in the Classroom: The Influences of Parental Monitoring, Peer Value Orientations, Students" Goals, and Their Value Orientations." *Social Psychology of Education* 16(1):77–94.

Killian, Timothy, and Lawrence H. Ganong. 2002. "Ideology, Context, and Obligations to Assist Older Persons." *Journal of Marriage & Family* 64(4).

Kilminster, Richard. 2008. "Narcissism or Informalization? Christopher Lasch, Norbert Elias and Social Diagnosis." *Theory, Culture & Society* 25(3):131–151.

Kim, Changsoo, Sang-Gun Lee, and Minchoel Kang. 2012. "I Became an Attractive Person in The Virtual World: Users? Identification with Virtual Communities and Avatars." *Computers in Human Behavior* 28(5):1663–1669.

Kim, Daniel, and Ichiro Kawachi. 2007. "U.S. State-Level Social Capital and Health-Related Quality of Life: Multilevel Evidence of Main, Mediating, and Modifying Effects." *Annals of Epidemiology* 17(4):258–269.

Kim, Emily, and Dov Cohen. 2017. "Roads More and Less Traveled: Different Emotional Routes to Creativity among Protestants and Catholics." *Journal of Personality and Social Psychology* 112(6):901–925.

Kim, Harris Hyun-Boo. 2017. "Strength of Weak Ties, Neighborhood Ethnic Heterogeneity, and Depressive Symptoms among Adults: A Multilevel Analysis of Korean General Social Survey (Kgss) 2012." *Social Sciences* 6(2):65.

Kim, Heejung S., David K. Sherman, and John A. Updegraff. 2016. "Fear of Ebola." *Psychological Science* 27(7):935–944.

Kim, Hyungsook. 2015. "Community and Art: Creative Education Fostering Resilience through Art." *Asia Pacific Education Review* 16(2):193–201.

Kim, Jeong Han, Carolyn E. Hawley, Rene Gonzalez, Abigail K. Vo, Lara A. Barbir, Brian T. Mcmahon, Dong-Hun Lee, Jung Hee Lee, and Yun Woo Lee. 2018. "Resilience from a Virtue Perspective." *Rehabilitation Counseling Bulletin* 61(4):195–204.

Kim, Jeong Han, Carolyn E. Hawley, Rene Gonzalez, Lara A. Barbir, Dong-Hun Lee, Abigail K. Vo, Brian T. McMahon, Jung Hee Lee, and Yun Woo Lee. 2018. "Resilience from a Virtue Perspective." *Rehabilitation Counseling Bulletin* 61(4).195–204.

Kim, Jun Won, Hye-Kyung Lee, and Kounseok Lee. 2013. "Influence of Temperament and Character on Resilience." *Comprehensive Psychiatry* 54(7):1105–10.

Kim, Seoyong and Sunhee Kim. 2021. "Searching for General Model of Conspiracy Theories and Its Implication for Public Health Policy: Analysis of the Impacts of Political, Psychological, Structural Factors on Conspiracy Beliefs about the Covid-19 Pandemic." *International Journal of Environmental Research & Public Health* 18(1):266–28.

Kim, Sungmoon. 2018. *Democracy after Virtue: Toward Pragmatic Confucian Democracy*. New York, NY: Oxford University Press.

Kim, Tae Kuen, and Karen A. Zurlo. 2007. "Factors that Influence Workfare Program Participants: Focusing on South Korea's Self-sufficiency Program." *International Social Work* 50(6):796–808.

Kim, Yeung Yun. 2013. "The Identity Factor in Intercultural Conflict." Pp. 639–660 in *The SAGE Handbook of Conflict Communication*, edited by John G. Oetzel and Stelle Ting-Toomey. Thousand Oaks, CA: SAGE.

Kim, Young K., Christopher S. Collins, Liz A. Rennick, and David Edens, 2017. "College Experiences and Outcomes among International Undergraduate Students at Research Universities in the United States: A Comparison to Their Domestic Peers." *Journal of International Students* 7(2):395–420.

Kim-Cohen, Julia, Terrie E. Moffitt, Avshnlom Caspi, and Alan Taylor. 2004. "Genetic and Environmental Processes in Young Children's Resilience and Vulnerability to Socioeconomic Deprivation." *Child Development* 75(3):651–668.

Kimhi, Shaul,Yohanan Eshel, Hadas Marciano, and Bruria Adini. 2021. "Prediction of Hope and Morale during COVID-19." *Frontiers in Psychology* 12:739645.

Kincade, Jean, Donna J. Rabiner, Shulamit L. Bernard, Alison Wwoomert, Thomas R. Konrad, Gordon H. DeFriese, and Marcia G. Ory. 1998. "Older Adults as a Community Resource: Results from the National Survey of Self-care and Aging." *Gerontologist* 36(4):474–482.

King, Eden B., Jennifer L. Knight, and Michelle R. Hebl. 2010. "The Influence of Economic Conditions on Aspects of Stigmatization." *Journal of Social Issues* 66(3):446–60.

King, Gillian A. 2003. "Tying It All Together: Frames of Reference and Meaning in Life." Pp. 153–194 in *Resilience: Learning from People with Disabilities and the Turning Point in Their Lives*, edited by Gillian A. King, Elizabeth G. Brown and Linda K. Smith. Westport, CT: Praeger.

King, Gillian A., Tamzin Cathers, Elizabeth G. Brown, and Elizabeth MacKinnon. 2003. "Turning Points: Emotionally Compelling Life Experiences." Pp. 31–88 in *Resilience: Learning from People with Disabilities and the Turning Point in Their Lives*, edited by Gillian A. King, Elizabeth G. Brown and Linda K. Smith. Westport, CT: Praeger.

King, Ian T. 2008. The Political Theory of Darwinism: Zoon Politikon and the Evolutionary Case for Social Democracy. Lewiston, NY: Edwin Mellen.

King, Pamela Ebstyne, and James L. Furrow. 2004. "Religion as a Resource for Positive Youth Development: Religion, Social Capital, and Moral Outcomes." *Developmental Psychology* 40(5):703–713.

King, Pamela Ebstyne, and Robert W. Roeser. 2009. "Religion and Spirituality in Adolescent Development." Pp. 435–478 in *Handbook of Adolescent Psychology* (3rd ed., Vol. 1), edited by Richard M. Lerner and Laurence Steinberg. Hoboken, NJ: Wiley.

King, Pamela Ebstyne. 2007. "Adolescent Spirituality and Positive Youth Development: A Look at Religion, Social Capital, and Moral Functioning." Pp. 227–242 in *Approaches to Positive Youth Development*, edited by Rainer K. Sibereisen and Richard M. Lerner. London: Sage.

Kirk, David S. 2009. "Unraveling the Contextual Effects on Student Suspension and Juvenile Arrest: The Independent and Interdependent Influences of School, Neighborhood, and Family Social Controls." *Criminology* 47(2):479–520.

Kirk, David S., and Andrew V. Papachristos. 2011. "Cultural Mechanisms and the Persistence of Neighborhood Violence." *American Journal of Sociology* 116(4):1190–1233.

Kirkpatrick, Lee A., Christian E. Waugh, Alelhie Valencia, and Gregory D. Webster. 2002. "The Functional Domain Specificity of Self-esteem and the Differential Prediction of Aggression." *Journal of Personality & Social Psychology* 82(5):756–767.

Kirmanoglu, Hasan, and Cem Baslevent. 2014. "Life Satisfaction of Ethnic Minority Members: An Examination of Interactions with Immigration, Discrimination, and Citizenship." *Social Indicators Research* 116:173–184.

Kitayama, Shinobu. 1997. "Affective Influence in Perception: Some Implications of the Amplification Model." Pp. 193–258 in *Cognitive Science Perspectives on Personality and Emotion*, edited by Gerald Matthews. Amsterdam, Netherlands: Elsevier. (BF698.9E45C64)

Kitayama, Shinsbu, and Anzel Rose Markus. 2000. "The Pursuit of Happiness and the Realization of Sympathy: Cultural Patterns of Self, Social Relations, and Well-being." Pp. 113–161 in *Culture and Subjective Well-being*, edited by Ed Diener and Eunkook M. Suh. Cambridge, MA: MIT.

Kitts, James. 2003. "Egocentric Bias on Information Management? Selective Disclosure and the Social Roots of Norm Misperception." *Social Psychology Quarterly* 66(3):222–237.

Kivimaki, Timo A. 2012. "What Generates, Constitutes and Causes Opportunity-driven Violence? The Case of West Kalimantan." *Asian Journal of Political Science* 20(3):284–303.

Kjell, O. N. E., D. Daukantaitė, K. Hefferon, and S. Sikström. 2016. "The Harmony in Life Scale Complements the Satisfaction with Life Scale: Expanding the Conceptualization of the Cognitive Component of Subjective Well-Being." *Social Indicators Research* 126(2):893–919.

Kleiman, Evan M. and John H. Riskind. 2014. "Negative Cognitive Style and Looming Cognitive Style Synergistically Predict Stress Generation." *Anxiety, Stress, & Coping* 27(3):347–59.

Kleiman, Evan M., Leah M. Adams, Todd B. Kashdan, and John H. Riskind. 2013. "Gratitude and Grit Indirectly Reduce Risk of Suicidal Ideations by Enhancing Meaning in Life: Evidence for a Mediated Moderation Model." *Journal of Research in Personality* 47:539–546.

Klein, Jill Gabrielle, Richard Ettenson, and Marlene D. Morris. 1998. "The Animosity Model of Foreign Product Purchases: An Empirical Test in the People's Republic of China." *Journal of Marketing* 62(1):89–100.

Klein, Markus. 2015. "The Increasing Unemployment Gap between the Low and High Educated in West Germany. Structural or Cyclical Crowding-Out?" *Social Science Research* 50:110–125.

Klein, Renate C.A., and Robert M. Milardo. 2000. "The Social Context of Couple Conflict: Support and Criticism from Informal Third Parties." *Journal of Social & Personal Relationships* 17(4/5):618–637.

Kleine, Robert, III, Susan Schultz Kleine, and Gray J. Brunswick. 2009. "Transformational Consumption Choices Building on Understanding by Integrating Social Identity and Multi-attribute Attitude Theories." *Journal of Consumer Behavior* 8:54–70.

Kleinhans, Reinout, Hugo Priemus, and Godfried Engbersen. 2007. "Understanding Social Capital in Recently Restructured Urban Neighborhoods: Two Case Studies in Rotterdam." *Urban Studies* 44(5/6):1069–1091.

Kleinke, Chris L. 2007. "What Does It Mean to Cope?" Pp. 289–308 in *The Praeger Handbook in Stress and Coping* (vol. 2), edited by Alan Monat, Richard S. Lazarus and Gretchen Reevy. Westport, CT: Praeger.

Kleinman, Arthur, Joan Kleinman, and Sing Lee. 1999. "Introduction to the Transformation of Social Experience in Chinese Society: Anthropological, Psychiatric and Social Medicine Perspectives." *Culture, Medicine & Psychiatry* 23:1–6.

Klingle, Renee Storm. 2004. "Compliance Gaining in Medical Contexts." Pp. 289–315 in *Perspectives and Persuasion, Social Influence, and Compliance Gaining*, edited by John S. Seiter and Robert H. Gass. Boston, MA: Pearson.

Kloep, M., N. Guney, F. Cok, O.F. Simsek. 2009. "Motives for Risk-taking in Adolescence: A Cross-cultural Study." *Journal of Adolescence* 32:135–151.

Kloep, Marion. 1999. "Love is All You Need? Focusing on Adolescents" Life Concerns from an Ecological Point of View." *Journal of Adolescence* 22:49–63.

Klucarova, Sona and Xie He. 2021. "Status Consumption and Charitable Donations: The Power of Empowerment." *Psychology & Marketing* 39:1116–1128.

Kluegal, James R., and Lawrence D. Bobo. 2001. "Perceived Group Discrimination and Policy Attitudes: The Sources and Consequences of the Race and Gender Gaps." Pp. 163–213 in *Urban Inequality: Evidence from Four Cities*, edited by Alice O'Connor, Chris Tilly and Lawrence D. Bobo. New York: Russell Sage.

Kluegel, James, and Eliot R. Smith. 1986. Beliefs about Inequality: Americans" Views of What is and What Ought to Be. New York: Aldine de Gruyter.

Kluemper, Donald H. 2008. "Trait Emotional Intelligence: The Impact of Core-self Evaluation and Social Desirability." *Personality & Individual Differences* 44:1402–1412.

Klussman, Kristine, Austin Lee Nichols, and Julia Langer. 2020. "The Role of Self-Connection in the Relationship between Mindfulness and Meaning: A Longitudinal Examination." *Applied Psychology: Health & Well-being* 12(3):636–59.

Klyukanov, Igor E. 2021. *Principles of Intercultural Communication*. New York, NY: Routledge.

Knab, Jean, Irv Garfinkel, and Sara McLanahan. 2008. "The Effects of Welfare and Child Support Policies on Maternal Health and Well-being." Pp. 281–303 in *Making American Healthier: Social and Economic Policy as Health Policy*, edited by Robert F. Schoeni, James S. House, George A. Kaplan, and Harold Pollack. New York: Russell Sage.

Knack, Stephen. 2002. "Social Capital, Growth, and Poverty: A Survey of Cross-country Evidence." Pp. 42–84 in *The Role of Social Capital in Development: An Empirical Assessment*, edited by Christiaan Grootaert and Thierry van Bastelaer. Cambridge, UK: Cambridge University Press.

Kneeland, Elizabeth T. and John F. Dovidio. 2020. "Emotion Malleability Beliefs and Coping with the College Transition." *Emotion* 20(3):452–61.

Kneezel, Teresa T., and Robert A. Emmons. 2005. "Personality and Spiritual Development." Pp. 266–278 in *The Handbook of Spiritual Development in Childhood and Adolescence*, edited by Eugene C. Roehlkepartain, Pamela Ebstyne King, Linda Wagener and Peter L. Benson. Thousand Oaks, CA: Sage.

Kneipp, Lee B., Kathryn E. Kelly, and Benita Cyphers. 2009. "Feeling at Peace with College: Religiosity, Spiritual Well-Being, and College Adjustment." *Individual Differences Research* 7(3):188–96.

Knies, Gundi. 2012. "Income Comparisons among Neighbors and Satisfaction in East and West Germany." *Social Indicators Research* 106:471–489.

Knight, Jack, and James Johnson. 2011. *The Priority of Democracy: Political Consequences of Pragmatism*. New York: Russell Sage.

Knight, Sarah, and Victoria Edwards. 2008. "In the Company of Wolves: The Physical, Social, and Psychological Benefits of Dog Ownership." *Journal of Aging & Health* 20(4):437–455.

Knoarska, Joanna. 2005. "Sources of Social Activity of People with Visual and Motor Impairments." *Social Behavior & Personality* 33(8):751–766.

Kochenderfer-Ladd, Becky. 2004. "Peer Victimization: The Role of Emotions in Adaptive and Maladaptive Coping." *Social Development* 13(3):329–349.

Koegl, Christopher J., and David M. Day. 2019. "The Monetary Costs of Crime for a Sample of Offenders in Ontario." *Canadian Journal of Criminology & Criminal Justice* 61(3):21–44.

Koehler, Daniel and Verena Fiebig. 2019. "Knowing What to Do: Academic and Practitioner Understanding of How to Counter Violent Radicalization." *Perspectives on Terrorism* 13(3):44–62.

Koerner, Ascan. 2018. "Relationship Typologies." Pp. 65–76 in *The Cambridge Handbook of Personal Relationships*, edited by Anita L. Vangelisti and Daniel Perlman. Cambridge, UK: Cambridge University Press.

Koerner, Kelly. 2012. Doing Dialectical Behavior Therapy: A Practical Guide. New York, NY: Guilford.

Kohlhammer, Y., M. Schnoor, M. Schwartz, H. Raspe, and T. Schafer. 2007. "Determinants of Influenza and Pneumococcal Vaccination in Elderly People: A Systematic Review." *Public Health* 121:742–751.

Kohn, Melvin L., and Kazimierz M. Slomczynski. 1990. Social Structure and Self-direction: A Comparative Analysis of the United States and Poland. Cambridge, MA: Basil Blackwell.

Kohn, Melvin L., Carmi Schooler, Joanne Miller, Karen A. Miller, Carrie Schoenbach, and Ronald Schoenberg. 1983. *Work and Personality: An Inquiry into the Impact of Social Stratification*. Norwood, NJ: Ablex.

Kohn, Melvin L., Kazimicrz M. Slomczynski, Krystyna Janicka, Valeri Khmelko, Bogdan W. Mach, Vladrmir Paniotto, Wojciech Zoborowski, Roberto Gutrerez, and Cary Heyman. 1997. "Social Structure and Personality under Conditions of Radical Social Change: A Comparative Analysis of Poland and Ukraine." *American Sociological Review* 62(4):614–638.

Kokkinos, Constantinos M., and Stamatia Hatzinikolaou. 2011. "Individual and Contextual Parameters Associated with Adolescents¡¯ Domain Specific Self-Perceptions." *Journal of Adolescence* 34(2):349–360.

Koltko-Rivera, Mark E. 2004. "The Psychology of Worldviews." *Review of General Psychology* 8(1):3–58.

Konarska, Joanna. 2005. "Sources of Social Activity of People with Visual and Motor Impairments." *Social Behavior & Personality* 33(8):751–766.

Kondili, Elvita, Dana Isawi, Claudia Interiano-Shiverdecker, and Olivia Maleckas. 2022. "Predictors of Cultural Humility in Counselors-in-Training." *Counselor Education & Supervision* 61(2):129–40.

Kondo, Ayumi, and Kiyoshi Wada. 2009. "The Effectiveness of a Mutual-help Group Activity for Drug Users and Family Members in Japan." *Substance Use & Misuse* 44:472–489.

Konig, Susanne, and Judith Gluck. 2013. "Individual Differences in Wisdom Conceptions: Relationships to Gratitude and Wisdom." *International Journal of Aging & Human Development* 77(2):127–147.

Koning, Lukas, and Eric van Dijk. 2013. "Motivational Cognition in Negotiation." Pp. 46–74 in *Handbook of Research on Negotiation*, edited by Mara Olekalns and Wendi L. Adair. Cheltenham, UK: Elgar.

Kono, Shintaro and Eiji Ito. 2021. "Effects of Leisure Constraints and Negotiation on Activity Enjoyment: A Forgotten Part of the Leisure Constraints Theory." *Annals of Leisure Research* 26(5):647–666.

Koole, S. L., M. E. McCullough, J. Kuhl, and P. H. M. P. Roelofsma. 2010. "Why Religion's Burdens Are Light: From Religiosity to Implicit Self-Regulation." *Personality & Social Psychology Review* 14(1):95–107.

Koole, Sander L., and Amolia Aldas. 2016. "The Self-regulation of Emotion: Theoretical and Empirical Advances." Pp. 24–41 in *Handbook of Self-regulation: Research, Theory, and Application*, edited by Kathleen D. Vohs and Roy F. Baumeister. New York, NY: Guilford.

Koomen, Wilem, and Joop van der Pligt. 2016. *The Psychology of Radicalization and Terrorism*. Abingdon, UK: Routledge.

Koramaz, Elif Kisar. 2014. "The Spatial Context of Social Integration." *Social Indicators Research* 119(1):49–71.

Korkeila, Katariina, Sirkka-Liisa Kivela, Sakari Suominen, Jussi Vahtera, Mika Kivimaki, Jari Sundell, Hans Helenius, and Markku Koskenvuo. 2004. "Childhood Adversities, Parent-child Relationships and Dispositional Optimism in Adulthood." *Social Psychiatry & Psychiatric Epidemiology* 39:286–292.

Kornienko, Olga, Thomas J. Dishion, and Thao Ha. 2018. "Peer Network Dynamics and the Amplification of Antisocial to Violent Behavior among Young Adolescents in Public Middle Schools." *Journal of Emotional & Behavioral Disorders* 26(1):21–30.

Koromeckyj-Cox, Tanya, Amy Mehraban Pienta, and Tyson H. Brown. 2007. "Women of the 1950s and the Normative Life Course: The Implications of Childlessness, Fertility Timing, and Marital Status for Psychological Well-being in Late Midlife." *International Journal of Aging & Human Development* 64(4):299–330.

Kotler, Philip, Ned Roberto, and Tory Leisner. 2006. "Alleviating Poverty: A Macro/micro Marketing Perspective." *Journal of Macromarketing* 26(2):233–239.

Kou, Xiaonan, Sara Konrath, and Thalia R. Goldstein. 2019. "The Relationship among Different Types of Arts Engagement, Empathy, and Prosocial Behavior." *Psychology of Aesthetics, Creativity, & the Arts* 14(4):481–92.

Kouzis, Anthony C., and William W. Eaton. 1998. "Absence of Social Networks, Social Support and Health Services Utilization." *Psychological Medicine* 28(6):1301–1310

Kowal, John, and Michele S. Fortier. 1999. "Motivational Determinants of Flow: Contributions from Self-determination Theory." *Journal of Social Psychology* 139(3):355–368.

Kozbelt, Aaron, Ronald A. Beghetto, and Mark A. Runco. 2010. "Theories of Creativity." Pp. 20–47 in *The Cambridge Handbook of Creativity*, edited by James C. Kaufman and Robert J. Sternberg. New York, NY: Cambridge University Press.

Kozlowski, Christine, Joseph R. Ferrari, Charlynn Odahl. 2014. "Social Justice and Faith Maturity: Exploring Whether Religious Beliefs Impact Civic Engagement." *Education* 134(4):427–432.

Krahe, Barbara. 2001. *The Social Psychology of Aggression*. Hove, UK: Psychology.

Krahe, Barbara. 2013. *The Social Psychology of Aggression*. Hove, UK: Psychology.

Kraimer, Maria L., Margaret A. Shaffer, Mark C. Bolino, Steven D. Charlier, and Olivier Wurtz. 2022. "A Transactional Stress Theory of Global Work Demands: A Challenge, Hindrance, or Both?" *Journal of Applied Psychology* 107(12):2197–219.

Kral, Michael J. 2019. *The Idea of Suicide: Contagion, Imitation, and Cultural Diffusion*. New York, NY: Routledge.

Kramer, Patricia and Linda Frazer. 1990. *The Dynamics of Relationships: A Guide for Developing Self-esteem and Social Skills for Preteens and Young People*. Silver Spring, MY: Equal Partners.

Kramer, Roderick M. 1999. "Trust and Distrust in Organizations: Emerging Perspectives, Enduring Questions." *Annual Review of Psychology* 50:569–598.

Krause, Neal. 2010. "Close Companion Friends, Self-Expression, and Psychological Well-Being in Late Life." *Social Indicators Research* 95:199–213.

Krause-Parello, Cheryl A., and Elsie E. Gulick. 2013. "Situational Factors Related to Loneliness and Loss Over Time Among Older Pet Owners." *Western Journal of Nursing Research* 35(7):905–919.

Krauss, Steven Eric, Jessica Collura, Shepherd Zeldin, Adriana Ortega, Haslinda Abdullah, and Abdul Hadi Sulaiman. 2014. "Youth–Adult Partnership: Exploring Contributions to Empowerment, Agency and Community Connections in Malaysian Youth Programs." *Journal of Youth & Adolescence* 43(9):1550–62.

Krebs, Simone, Anke Baaken, Ramona Wurst, Wiebke Goehner. and Reinhard Fuchs. 2019. "Effects of a Worksite Group Intervention to Promote Physical Activity and Health: The Role of Psychological Coaching." *Applied Psychology: Health & Well-Being* 11(3):584–605.

Kreitler, Shulamith, and Hernan Casakin. 2009. "Motivation for Creativity in Design Students." *Creativity Research Journal* 21(2-3):282–293.

Krippner, Greta R., and Anthony S. Alvarez. 2007. "Embeddedness and the Intellectual Projects of Economic Sociology." *Annual Review of Sociology* 33:219–240.

Krishna, Anirudh, and Norman Uphoff. 2002. "Mapping and Measuring Social Capital through Assessment of Collective Action to Conserve and Develop Watersheds in Rajasthan, India." Pp. 85–124 in *The Role of Social Capital in Development: An Empirical Assessment*, edited by Christiaan Grootaert and Thierry van Bastelaer. Cambridge, UK: Cambridge University Press.

Krishnakumar, Ambika, and Maureen M. Black. 2003. "Family Processes within Three-generation Households and Adolescent Mothers" Satisfaction with Father Involvement." *Journal of Family Psychology* 17(4):488–498.

Kristjansson, Kristjan. 2013. *Virtues and Vices in Positive Psychology: A Philosophical Critique*. New York: Cambridge University Press.

Kroll, Christian. 2011. "Different Things Make Different People Happy: Examining Social Capital and Subjective well-being by Gender and Parental Status." *Social Indicators Research* 104:157–177.

Krossa, Anne Sophie. 2013. *Theorizing Society in a Global Context*. Hondmills, UK: Palgrave.

Kruesi, Markus J.P. 2007. "Psychopharmacology of Violence." Pp. 618–635 in *The Cambridge Handbook of Violent Behavior and Aggression*, edited by Daniel J. Flannery, Alexander T. Vazsonyi and Irwin D. Waldman. Cambridge, UK: Cambridge University Press.

Krug, Gerhard and Sebastian Prechsl. 2020. "The Role of Social Integration in the Adverse Effect of Unemployment on Mental Health – Testing the Causal Pathway and Buffering Hypotheses Using Panel Data." *Social Science Research* 86:102379.

Krulichova, Eva. 2019. "The Relationship between Fear of Crime and Risk Perception across Europe." *Criminology & Criminal Justice* 19(2):197–214.

Krumrei-Mancuso, Elizabeth J. 2017. "Intellectual Humility and Prosocial Values: Direct and Mediated Effects." *Journal of Positive Psychology* 12(1):13–28.

Krumrei-Mancuso, Elizabeth J., and Brian Newman. 2021. "Sociopolitical Intellectual Humility as a Predictor of Political Attitudes and Behavioral intentions." *Journal of Social & Political Psychology* 9(1):52–68.

Krys, Kuba, Yukiko Uchida, Shigehiro Oishi, and Ed Diener. 2019. "Open Society Fosters Satisfaction: Explanation to Why Individualism Associates with Country Level Measures of Satisfaction." *Journal of Positive Psychology* 14(6):768–78.

Kryshko, Olena, Jens Fleischer, Carola Grunschel, and Detlev Leutner. 2023. "University Students' Self-Efficacy for Motivational Regulation, Use of Motivational Regulation Strategies, and Satisfaction with Academic Studies: Exploring between-Person and within-Person Associations." *Journal of Educational Psychology* 115(4):571–88. \94–236

Ku, Agnes Shuk-mei. 2009. "Contradictions in the Development of Citizenship in Hong Kong: Governance without Democracy." *Asian Survey* 49(3):505–527.

Ku, Agnes Shuk-mei. 2012. "Remaking Places and Fashioning an Opposition Discourse: Struggle over the Star Ferry Pier and the Queen's Pier in Hong Kong." *Environment & Planning D: Society & Place* 30:5–22.

Kuah-Pearce, Kuhn Eng, and Yiu Chak Fong. 2010. "Identity and Sense of Belonging in Post-Colonial Education in Hong Kong." *Asia Pacific Journal of Education* 30(4):433–448.

Kuentzel, Walter F. 2000. "Self-identity, Modernity, and the Rational Actor in Leisure Research." *Journal of Leisure Research* 32(1):87–92.

Kuiper, Nicholas A., and Melanie Borowicz-Sibenik. 2005. "A Good Sense of Humor Doesn't Always Help: Agency and Communion as Moderators of Psychological Well-being." *Personality & Individual Differences* 38:365–377.

Kulik, Liat. 2006. "The Impact of Spousal Variables on Life Satisfaction of Individuals in Life Adulthood." *International Journal of Comparative Sociology* 67(1):54–72.

Kulik, Liat. 2007. "Explaining Responses to Volunteering: An Ecological Model." *Nonprofit & Voluntary Sector Quarterly* 36(2):239–255.

Kulin, Joakim and Alexander Seymer. 2014. "What's Driving the Public? A Cross-Country Analysis of Political Attitudes, Human Values and Political Articulation." *Sociological Research Online* 19(1):145–58.

Kullgen, John. 1995. *Autonomy and Intervention: Parentalism in the Caring Life.* New York: Oxford University Press.

Kumkale, G. Tarcan, Dolores Albarracín, and Paul J. Seignourel. 2010. "The Effects of Source Credibility in the Presence or Absence of Prior Attitudes: Implications for the Design of Persuasive Communication Campaigns." *Journal of Applied Social Psychology* 40(6):1325–56.

Kung, Winnie W. 2003. "Chinese Americans' Help Seeking for Emotional Distress." *Social Service Review* 77:110–134.

Kunovich, Robert M. 2009. "The Sources and Consequences of National Identification." *American Sociological Review* 74:573–593.

Kunovich, Robert M., and Randy Hudson. 1999. "Civil War, Social Integration and Mental Health in Croatia." *Journal of Health & Social Behavior* 40:323–343.

Kunovich, Robert M., and Randy Hodson. 1999. "Conflict, Religious Identity, and Ethnic Intolerance in Croatia." *Social Forces* 78(2):643–669.

Kuntla, Shrikant, Srinivas Goli, T. V. Sekherm and Riddhi Doshi. 2013. "Consanguineous Marriages and Their Effects on Pregnancy Outcomes in India." *International Journal of Sociology & Social Policy* 33(7/8):437–452.

Kuppens, Toon, Russell Spears, Antony S. R. Manstead, Bram Spruyt, and Matthew J. Easterbrook. 2018. "Educationism and the Irony of Meritocracy: Negative Attitudes of Higher Educated People Towards the Less Educated." *Journal of Experimental Social Psychology* 76:429–47.

Kurata, Toru. 2015. "Support for and Opposition to Democratization in Hong Kong." *Asia-Pacific Review* 22(1):16–33. \105–163

Kurtz, Steven P. 2008. "Arrest Histories of High-risk Gay and Bisexual Men in Miami: Unexpected Additional Evidence for Syndemic Theory." *Journal of Psychoactive Drugs* 40(4):513–521.

Kurz, Karin, Nikolei, Steinhage, and Katrin Golsch. 2005. "Case Study Germany: Global Competition, Uncertainty and the Training to Adulthood." Pp. 58–81 in *Globalization, Uncertainty and Youth in Society*, edited by Hans-Peter Blossfeld, Erik Klijzing, Melinda Mills and Karin Kurz. London: Routledge.

Kutnick, Peter, and Alison Kington. 2005. "Children's Friendships and Learning in School: Cognitive Enhancement through Social Interaction?" *British Journal of Educational Psychology* 75(4):521–538.

Kutsyuruba, Benjamin. 2012. "Teacher Induction and Mentorship Policies: The Pan-Canadian Overview." *International Journal of Mentoring and Coaching in Education* 1(3):235–256.

Kuwabara, Ko. 2015. "Do Reputation Systems Undermine Trust? Divergent Effects of Enforcement Type on Generalized Trust and Trustworthiness." *American Journal of Sociology* 120(5):1390–1428.

Kwak, Dae-Hoon, Chaudia E. San Miguel, and Diana L. Carreon. 2010. "Political Legitimacy and Public Confidence in Police: An Analysis of Attitudes toward Mexican Police." *Policing* 35(1):124–146.

Kwan, Simon Shui-man. 2007. "Clinical Efficacy of Ritual Healing and Pastoral Ministry." *Pastoral Psychology* 55(6):741–49.

Kwan, Y.K. 2010. "Life Satisfaction and Self-assessed Health among Adolescents in Hong Kong." *Journal of Happiness Studies* 11:383–393.

Kwarikunda, Diana, Nakalema Gladys, Charles Magoba Muwonge, Joseph Ssenyonga, and Ulrich Schiefele. 2023. "Adjusting to and Thriving in a New School: Role of Students' Expectations, Educational Attitudes, and Resilience During Secondary School Transition." *International Journal of School & Educational Psychology* 11(3):259–73.

Kwok, Sylvia Y. C. L., Leveda Cheng, Bonnie W. Y. Chow, and Chloe C. Y. Ling. 2015. "The Spillover Effect of Parenting on Marital Satisfaction Among Chinese Mothers." *Journal of Child and Family Studies* 24(3):772–783.

Kwon, Ik-Whan G. and Daniel W. Baack. 2005. "The Effectiveness of Legislation Controlling Gun Usage. A Holistic Measure of Gun Control Legislation." *American Journal of Economics & Sociology* 64(2):533–47.

Kwong, Man-Kit, Rainbow Tin-Hung Ho, and Yu-Te Huang. 2019. "A Creative Pathway to a Meaningful Life: An Existential Expressive Arts Group Therapy for People Living with Hiv in Hong Kong." *Arts in Psychotherapy* 63:9–17.

Kwong, Ying-ho and Mathew W. H. Wong. 2017. "State Size and Democratization in Hybrid Regimes: The Chinese Island Cities of Macau and Hong Kong." *Island Studies Journal* 12(2):113–26.

Kyle, Gerard, and Garry Chick. 2004. "Enduring Leisure Involvement: The Importance of Personal Relationships." *Leisure Studies* 23(3):243–266.

Kyriacou, Andreas P. 2020. *Inequality and Governance.* Abingdon, UK: Routledge.

La Grange, Adrienne, and Frederik Pretorius. 2000. "Ontology, Policy and the Market: Trends to Home-ownership in Hong Kong." *Urban Studies* 37(9):1561–1582.

Labrecque, Lauren I. 2014. "Fostering Consumer-Brand Relationships in Social Media Environments: The Role of Parasocial Interaction." *Journal of Interactive Marketing* 28(2):134–148.

Lacourse, Eric, Michel Claes, and Martine Villeneuve. 2001. "Heavy Metal Music and Adolescent Suicidal Risk." *Journal of Youth & Adolescence* 30(3):321–332.

Ladany, Nicholas, and Tiffany O'Shaughnessy. 2014. "Training and Supervision in Career Counseling." Pp. 375–387 in *APA Handbook of Career Intervention, Vol: Foundations*, edited by Paul J. Hartung, Mark L. Savickas, and W. Bruce Walsh. Washington, DC: American Psychological Association.

Ladouceur, Robert, Normand Boudreault, Christian Jacques, and Frank Vitaro. 1999. "Pathological Gambling and Related Problems among Adolescents." *Journal of Child & Adolescent Substance Abuse* 8(4):55–68.

Lagergren, Marten. 1996. "Transferring to an Institution: An Analysis of Factors behind the Transfer to Institutional Long-Term Care." *Canadian Journal on Aging* 15(3):427–441.

Laguna, Mariola, Zofia Mazur, Michał Kędra, and Karol Ostrowski. 2020. "Interventions Stimulating Prosocial Helping Behavior: A Systematic Review." *Journal of Applied Social Psychology* 50(11):676–696.

Lai, Chun, Mark S.K. Shum, and Bennan Zhang. 2014. International Mindedness In An Asian Context: The Case of the International Baccalaureate in Hong Kong." *Educational Research* 56(1):77–96.

Lai, Daniel W.L. 2011. "Perceived Impact of Economic Downturn on Worry Experienced by Elderly Chinese Immigrants in Canada." *Journal of Family & Economic Issues* 32:521–531.

Lai, Dicky W. L. 2017. "A Comparative Study of Social Assistance Systems in Macao and Hong Kong." *Asia Pacific Journal of Social Work & Development* 27(1):39–52.

Lai, Yan-ho. 2023. "Securitisation or Autocratisation? Hong Kong's Rule of Law under the Shadow of China's Authoritarian Governance." *Journal of Asian & African Studies* 58(1):8–25.

Lakey, Brian, and Edward Orehek. 2011. "Relational Regulation Theory: A New Approach to Explain the Link between Perceived Social Support and Mental Health." *Psychological Review* 118(3):482–495.

Lakin, Rebecca, and Annette Mahoney. 2006. "Empowering Youth to Change Their World: Identifying Key Components of a Community Service Program to Promote Positive Development." *Journal of School Psychology* 44:513–531.

Lalot, Fanny, Gaëlle Marinthe, Alice Kasper, and Dominic Abrams. 2023. "Mobilising Ideas in the Covid-19 Pandemic: Anti-Lockdown Actions and the Identity-Deprivation-Efficacy-Action-Subjective Well-Being Model." *Journal of Social & Political Psychology* 11(1):145–66.

Lalot, Fanny, Maria S. Heering, Marika Rullo, Giovanni A. Travaglino, and Dominic Abrams. 2022. "The Dangers of Distrustful Complacency: Low Concern and Low Political Trust Combine to Undermine Compliance with Governmental Restrictions in the Emerging Covid-19 Pandemic." *Group Processes & Intergroup Relations* 25(1):106–121

Lalwani, Ashok K., L. J. Shrum, and Chi-yue Chiu. 2009. "Motivated Response Styles: The Role of Cultural Values, Regulatory Focus, and Self-Consciousness in Socially Desirable Responding." *Journal of Personality & Social Psychology* 96(4):870–882.

Lam, Carlos Siu and Malcolm Greenlees. 2017. "Casino Money Laundering Regulations – Macao and USA." *Journal of Money Laundering Control* 20(1):52–69.

Lam, Cindy L.K., I.J. Lauder, T.P. Lam, and B. Gandek. 1999. "Population Based Norming of the Chinese (HK) Version of the SF-36 Health Survey." *Hong Kong Practitioner* 21:460–470.

Lam, Stacy, Angus Kuok, and Tat Ming Sze. 2023. "Self-Efficacy, Stress and Job Satisfaction among Pre-Service, Novice and Experienced English Teachers: A Study of Their Occupational Health." *Health Psychology Report* 11(2):108–23.

Lambie, John A. 2008. "On the Irrationality of Emotion and the Rationality of Awareness." *Consciousness & Cognition* 17(3):946–71.

Lamont, Michele, Jessica S. Welburn, and Crystal M. Fleming. 2013. "Responses to Discrimination and Social Resilience under Neoliberalism: The United States Compared." Pp. 129–157 in *Social Resilience in the Neoliberal Era*, edited by Peter A. Hall and Michele Lamont. Cambridge, UK: Cambridge University Press.

LaMothe, Ryan. 2012. "State-Corporate Capitalism, Political Polarization, and a Culture of Unquiet Desperation: A Pastoral Analysis and Responses." *Pastoral Psychology* 61(1):15–29.

Lan, Xiaoyu and Wenchao Wang. 2019. "Direct and Interactive Effects of Peer Support and Resilience on Psychosocial Adjustment in Emerging Adults with Early Left-Behind Experiences." *Psychology Research & Behavior Management* 12:277–88.

Lancee, Bram, and Jaap Dronkers. 2011. "Ethnic, Religious and Economic Diversity in Dutch Neighbourhoods: Explaining Quality of Contact with Neighbours, Trust in the Neighbourhood and Inter-Ethnic Trust." *Journal of Ethnic & Migration Studies* 37(4):597–618.

Landmann, Helen and Anette Rohmann. 2020. "Being Moved by Protest: Collective Efficacy Beliefs and Injustice Appraisals Enhance Collective Action Intentions for Forest Protection via Positive and Negative Emotions." *Journal of Environmental Psychology* 71:101491.

Landolfi, Alfonso, Massimiliano Barattucci, Assunta De Rosa, and Alessandro Lo Presti. 2021. "The Association of Job and Family Resources and Demands with Life Satisfaction through Work-Family Balance: A Longitudinal Study among Italian Schoolteachers during the COVID-19 Pandemic." *Behavioral Sciences* 11(10):136.

Lane, Robert E. 2000. *The Loss of Happiness in Market Democracies*. New Haven, CT: Yale University Press.

Lang, Frieder R., and Laura L. Carstensen. 2002. "Time Counts: Future Time Perspective, Goals, and Social Relationships." *Psychology & Aging* 17(1):125–139.

Langenderfer, Jeff, and Terence A. Shimp. 2001. "Consumer Vulnerability to Scams, Swindles, and Fraud: A New Theory of Visceral Influences on Persuasion." Psychology & Marketing 18(7):763–783.

Langer, Nieli. 2004. "Resiliency and Spirituality: Foundations of Strengths Perspective Counseling with the Elderly." *Educational Gerontology* 30:611–617.

Langner, Carrie A., Elissa S. Epel, Karen A. Matthews, Judith T. Moskowitz, and Nancy E. Adler. 2012. "Social Hierarchy and Depression: The Role of Emotion Suppression." *Journal of Psychology* 146(4):417–436.

Lansford, Jennifer E., Michael M. Criss, Gregory S. Pettit, Kenneth A. Dodge, and John E. Bates. 2003. "Friendship Quality, Peer Group Affiliation, and Peer Antisocial Behavior as Moderators of the Link between Negative Parenting and Adolescent Externalizing Behavior." *Journal of Research on Adolescence* 13(2):161–184.

Lantz, Paula M., James S. House. Richard P. Mero, and David R. Williams. 2005. "Stress, Life Events, and Socioeconomic Disparities in Health: Results from the Americans" Changing Lives Study." *Journal of Health & Social Behavior* 46(3):274–288.

Lapan, Richard T., Norman C. Gysbers, and Gregory F. Petroski. 2001. "Helping Seventh Graders Be Safe and Successful: A Statewide Study of the Impact of Comprehensive Guidance and Counseling Programs." *Journal of Counseling & Development* 79:320–330.

Laroche, Hervé, Véronique Steyer, and Christelle Théron. 2019. "How Could You Be So Gullible? Scams and over-Trust in Organizations." *Journal of Business Ethics* 160(3):641–56.

Larose, Simon, Donald U. Robertson, Roland Roy, and Frederic Legautt. 1998. "Nonintellectual Learning Factors as Determinants for Success in College." *Research in Higher Education* 39(3):275–297

Larrick, Richard P., Richard E. Nisbett, and James N. Morgan. 1993. "Who Uses the Cost-benefit Rules of Choice? Implications for the Normative Status of Microeconomic Theory." *Organizational Behavior & Human Decision Processes* 56:331–349.

Larsen, Christian Albrekt. 2006. The Institutional Logic of Welfare Attitudes: How Welfare Regimes Influence Public Support. Aldershot, UK: Ashgate.

Larsen, Knud S. 2018. *Adaptation and Well-Being: Meeting the Challenges of Life*. Abingdon, UK: Routledge.

Larson, Justine J., Sarah W. Whitton, Stuart T. Hauser, and Joseph P. Allen. 2007. "Being Close and Being Social: Peer Ratings of Distinct Aspects of Young Adult Social Competence." *Journal of Personality Assessment* 89(2):136–148.

Larson, Lisa M., Wayne C. Piersel, Rosalie A.K. Imao, and Sarah J. Allen. 1990. "Significant Predictions of Problem-Solving Appraisal." *Journal of Counseling Psychology* 37(4):482–490.

Larson, Reed. 2006. "Positive Youth Development, Willful Adolescents, and Mentoring." *Journal of Community Psychology* 34(6):677–689.

Lasch, Christopher. 1984. *The Minimal Self: Psychic Survival in Troubled Times*. New York, NY: Norton.

Laser, Julie Anne, and George Stuart Leibowitz. 2009. "Promoting Positive Outcomes for Healthy Youth Development: Utilizing Social Capital Theory." *Journal of Sociology & Welfare* 36(1):87–102.

Lashley, Conrad. 2001. *Empowerment: HR Strategies for Service Excellence.* Oxford, UK: Butterworth-Heinemann.

Lassri, Dana, Noa Bregman-Hai, Nirit Soffer-Dudek, and Golan Shahar. 2023. "The Interplay between Childhood Sexual Abuse, Self-Concept Clarity, and Dissociation: A Resilience-Based Perspective." *Journal of Interpersonal Violence* 38(3–4):2313–36.

Latham, Mark. 2000. "The Search for Social Capital." *Social Capital* 2000:7–47. \75–197

Latimer, Melissa. 1999. "A Longitudinal Analysis of Unemployment Insurance Receipt: 1987–1991." *Sociological Focus* 32(4):383–400.

Lau, Anna L.D., Iris Chi, Robert A. Cummins, Tatia M.C. Lee, Kee-L. Chou, and Lawrence W.M. Chung. 2008. "The SARS (Severe Acute Respiratory Syndrome) Pandemic in Hong Kong: Effects on the Subjective Wellbeing of Elderly and Younger People." *Ageing & Mental Health* 12(6):746–760.

Lau, Bobo H. P., Cecilia L. W. Chan, and Siu-Man Ng. 2021. "Resilience of Hong Kong People in the Covid-19 Pandemic: Lessons Learned from a Survey at the Peak of the Pandemic in Spring 2020." *Asia Pacific Journal of Social Work & Development* 31(1–2):105–14.

Lau, Joseph T. F., Yoona Kim, Anise M. S. Wu, Zixin Wang, Bishan Huang, and Phoenix K. H. Mo. 2017. "The Occupy Central (Umbrella) Movement and Mental Health Distress in the Hong Kong General Public: Political Movements and Concerns as Potential Structural Risk Factors of Population Mental Health." *Social Psychiatry & Psychiatric Epidemiology* 52(5):525–536.

Lau, Patrick S.Y., Man Tak Yuen, and Raymond M.C. Chan. 2005. "Do Demographic Characteristics Make a Difference to Burnout among Hong Kong Secondary School Teachers." *Social Indicators Research* 71:491–516.

Lau, Siu-kai, and Hsin-chi Kuan. 1988. *The Ethos of the Hong Kong Chinese.* Hong Kong: Chinese University Press.

Lau, Yuk King, Joyce Lai Chong Ma, Ying Keung Chan, and Liping He. 2012. "Risk and Protective Factors of Marital Adjustment to Cross-Border Work Arrangement of Hong Kong Residents: The Perspective of Stationary Spouses." *Journal of Comparative Family Studies* 43(5):715–730.

Lauder, Hugh, Philip Brown, and Sin-Yi Cheung. 2018. "Fractures in the Education-Economy Relationship: The End of the Skill Bias Technological Change Research Programme?" *Oxford Review of Economic Policy* 34(3):495–515.

Lauder, William, Kerry Mummery, Siobhan Sharkey. 2006. "Social Capital, Age and Religiosity In People Who Are Lonely." *Journal of Clinical Nursing* 15(3):334–340.

Lauermann, Fani and Johannes Konig. 2016. "Teachers" Professional Competence and Wellbeing: Understanding the Links between General Pedagogical Knowledge, Self-Efficacy and Burnout." *Learning & Instruction* 45:9–19.

Laurence, James. 2011. "The Effect of Ethnic Diversity and Community Disadvantage on Social Cohesion: A Multi-level Analysis of Social Capital and Interethnic Relations in UK Communities." *European Sociological Review* 27(1):70–89.

Laverie, Debra A., and Dennis B. Arnett. 2000. "Factors Affecting Fan Attendance: The Influence of Identity Salience and Satisfaction." *Journal of Leisure Research* 32(2):225–246.

Lavigne, Katie M., Samantha Hofman, Angela J. Ring, Andrew G. Ryder, and Todd S. Woodward. 2013. "The Personality of Meaning in Life: Associations between Dimensions of Life Meaning and the Big Five." *Journal of Positive Psychology* 8(1):34–43.

Lavretsky, Helen, and Michael R. Irwin. 2007. "Resilience and Aging." *Aging Health* 3(3):309–323.

Lavy, Shiri, Mario Mikulincer, and Phillip R. Shaver. 2010. "Autonomy's Proximity Imbalance: An Attachment Theory Perspective on Intrusiveness in Romantic Relationships." *Personality & Individual Differences* 48:552–556.

Law, Ho. 2007. "Narrative Coaching and Psychological Learning from Multicultural Perspectives." Pp. 174–192 in *Handbook of Coaching Psychology: A Guide for Practitioners*, edited by Stephen Palmer and Alison Whybrow. Hove, UK: Routledge.

Law, Kam-yee. 2014. "The Red Line over European Colonialism: Comparison of the Macao Museum and Hong Kong Museum of History after Their Return to China." *International Journal of Heritage Studies* 20(5):534–555.

Lawler, Edward J. 2002. "Micro Social Order." *Social Psychology Quarterly* 65(1):4–17.
Lawler, Edward J. Shane R. Thye, and Jeongkoo Yoon. 2009. *Social Commitments in a Depersonalized World*. New York: Russell Sage.
Lawler, Edward J., Shane R. Thye, and Jeongkoo Yoon. 2014. "Emotions and Group Ties in Social Exchange." Pp. 77–101 in *Handbook of the Sociology of Emotions*: Volume II, edited by Jan E. Stets and Jonathan H. Turner. Dordrecht, Netherlands: Springer.
Lawler, Margaret, Caroline Heary, and Elizabeth Nixon. 2020. "Peer Support and Role Modelling Predict Physical Activity Change among Adolescents over Twelve Months." *Journal of Youth & Adolescence* 49(7):1503–16.
Lawrence, Rich L., and Steven E. Daniels. 1997. "Procedural Justice and Public Involvement in Natural Resource Decision Making." *Society & Natural Resources* 10(6):577–589.
Lawton Smith, Carmelina. 2017. "Coaching for Resilience and Well-being." Pp. 346–362 in *The SAGE Handbook of Coaching*, edited by Tatiana Bachkirova, Gordon Spence, and David Drake. London, UK: SAGE.
Lawton, M. Powell, Miriam S. Moss, Laraine Winter, and Christine Hoffman. 2002. "Motivation in Later Life: Personal Projects and Well-being." *Psychology & Aging* 17(4):539–547.
Lawy, Robert. 2002. "Risky Stories: Youth Identities, Learning and Everyday Risk." *Journal of Youth Studies* 5(4):407–423.
Layous, Kristin, S. Katherine Nelson, Eva Oberle, Kimberly A. Schonert-Reichl, Sonja Lyubomirsky, and Frank Krueger. 2012. "Kindness Counts: Prompting Prosocial Behavior in Preadolescents Boosts Peer Acceptance and Well-Being." *PloS One* 7(12):e51380.
Layte, Richard, Henrik Levin, John Hendrickx, and Ivano Bison. 2000. "Unemployment and Cumulative Disadvantage in the Labour Market." pp. 153–174 in *Welfare Regimes and the Experience of Unemployment in Europe*, edited by Duncan Gallie and Serge Paugam. Oxford, UK: Oxford University Press.
Lazar, Lee and Naomi I. Eisenberger. 2022. "The Benefits of Giving: Effects of Prosocial Behavior on Recovery from Stress." *Psychophysiology* 59(2):13954.
Le Bosse, Yann, Marguerite, Lavallee, Denis Lacerte, Mathalie Dube, Josee Nadeau, Eric Porcher, and Line Vandette. 1998. "Is Community Participation Empirical Evidence for Psychological Empowerment? A Distinction between Passive and Active Participation." *Social Work & Social Sciences Review* 8(1):59–82.
Leander, N. Pontus, and Tanya L. Chartrand. 2017. "On Thwarted Goals and Displaced Aggression: A Compensatory Competence Model." *Journal of Experimental Social Psychology* 72:88–100.
Leary, Mark R., and Catherine A. Cottrell. 2013. "Evolutionary Perspectives on Interpersonal Acceptance and Rejection." Pp. 9–19 in *The Oxford Handbook of Social Exclusion*, edited by C. Nathan DeWall. New York: Oxford University Press.
Ledbetter, Andrew M. 2015. "Media Multiplexity Theory: Technology Use and Interpersonal Tie Strength." Pp. 363–375 in *Engaging Theories in Interpersonal Communication: Multiple Perspectives*, edited by Dawn O. Braithwaite and Paul Schrodt. Thousand Oaks, CA: SAGE.
Ledbetter, Andrew M., Heather M. Stassen-Ferrara, and Megan M. Dowd. 2013. "Comparing Equity and Self-Expansion Theory Approaches to Relational Maintenance." *Personal Relationships* 20(1):38–51.
Ledoux, Tracey, Carrie Winterowd, Tamara Richardson, and Julie Dorton Clark. 2010. "Relationship of Negative Self-Schemas and Attachment Styles with Appearance Schemas." *Body Image* 7(3):213–217.
Lee, Barrett A., Karen E. Campbell, and Oscar Miller. 1991. "Racial Differences in Urban Neighboring." *Sociological Forum* 6(3):525–550.
Lee, Bora and Yoonhee Lee. 2020. "A Study Examining the Effects of a Training Program Focused on Problem-Solving Skills for Young Adults." *Thinking Skills And Creativity* 37:100692.
Lee, Chien-Ti, Laura M. Padilla-Walker, and Madison K. Memmott-Elison. 2017. "The Role of Parents and Peers on Adolescents" Prosocial Behavior and Substance Use." *Journal of Social & Personal Relationships* 34(7):1053–69.

Lee, Chien-Ti. 2011. "The Impact of Marital Discord of Parents on Taiwanese Adolescents' Academic Achievement: The Mediating and Moderating Effect of Maternal Parenting Practice." *Journal of Comparative Family Studies* 42(6):827–850.
Lee, Francis L. F. and Chi-kit Chan. 2023. "Legalization of Press Control under Democratic Backsliding: The Case of Post-National Security Law Hong Kong." *Media, Culture, & Society* 45(5):916–31.
Lee, Francis L. F., and Joseph Man Chan. 2009. "The Political Consequences of Ambivalence: The Case of Democratic Reform in Hong Kong." *International Journal of Public Opinion Research* 21(1):47–64.
Lee, Francis L. F., and Joseph Man Chan. 2016. "Digital Media Activities and Mode of Participation in a Protest Campaign: A Study of the Umbrella Movement, Information," *Communication & Society* 19(1):4–22.
Lee, Francis L.F. 2009. "The Impact of Political Discussion in a Democratizing Society: The Moderating Role of Disagreement and Support for Democracy." *Communication Research* 36(3):379–391.
Lee, Francis L.F. 2010. "The Perceptual Bases of Collective Efficacy and Protest Participation: The Case of Pro-democracy Protests in Hong Kong." *International Journal of Public Opinion Research* 22(3):392–411.
Lee, Graham. 2018. "The Psychodynamic Approach to Coaching." Pp. 3–16 in *The Complete Handbook of Coaching*, edited by Elaine Cox, Tatiana Bachkirova, and David Clutterbuck. London, UK: SAGE.
Lee, Heeuk D., Francis D. Boateng, David Kim, and Cooper Maher. 2022. "Residential Stability and Fear of Crime: Examining the Impact of Homeownership and Length of Residence on Citizens' Fear of Crime." *Social Science Quarterly* 103(1):141–54.
Lee, Juyeon. 2018. "Prosocial Parent-to-Peer Path Model for South Korean School-Aged Children." *Child Indicators Research* 11(6):1867–88.
Lee, Kibeom and Michael C. Ashton. 2012. "Getting Mad and Getting Even: Agreeableness and Honesty-Humility as Predictors of Revenge Intentions." *Personality & Individual Differences* 52(5):596–600.
Lee, Kibeom, Michael C. Ashton, Jocelyn Wiltshire, Joshua S. Bourdage, Beth A. Visser, and Alissa Gallucci. 2013. "Sex, Power, and Money: Prediction from the Dark Triad and Honesty-Humility." *European Journal of Personality* 27:169–184.
Lee, Kim Ming, Benny Ho-Pong, and Ka Ming Yu. 2014. "The New Paradox of Thrift." *China Perspectives* 2014(1):15–24.
Lee, Kyunghee. 2009. "Impact of the 1996 Welfare Reform on Child and Family Well-being." *Journal of Community Psychology* 37(5):602–617.
Lee, Richard M., and Steven B. Robbins. 1998. "The Relationship between Social Connectedness and Anxiety, Self-esteem and Social Identity." *Journal of Counseling Psychology* 45(3):338–345.
Lee, Seung Pil. 2020. "Sustainable Reciprocity Mechanism of Social Initiatives in Sport: The Mediating Effect of Gratitude." *Sustainability* 12(21):9279.
Lee, Sunwoo and Sangwoo Lee. 2019. "Relationships among Financial Satisfaction, Life Satisfaction, and Political Action: A Comparative Study of the United States and South Korea." *Asian Social Work & Policy Review* 13(3):252–62.
Lee, Tak-yan, Wai-man Kwong, Chau-kiu Cheung, Michael Ungar, and Maria Y.L. Cheung. 2010. "Children's Resilience-related Beliefs as a Predictor of Positive Child Development in Face of Adversities: Implications for Intervention to Enhance Children's Quality of Life." *Social Indicators Research* 95(3):437–453.
Lee, Yeen-ju, and Zhenyu Xiao. 1998. "Children's Support for Elderly Parents in Urban and Rural China: Results from a National Surveys." *Journal of Cross-Cultural Gerontology* 13:39–82.
Lee, Yejin, Juliette L. Ratchford, Mason S. Ming, Rosemary L. Al-Kire, Perry L. Glanzer, Kevin D. Dougherty, and Sarah A. Schnitker. 2023. "A Person-Centered Approach to the Dark Triad

Traits and Religiousness: Examining Differences in Intellectual Humility, Prosociality, and Mental Health in U.S. College Students." *Psychology of Religion & Spirituality.*

Lee, Yueh-Ting. 2003. "Daoistic Humanism in Ancient China: Broadening Personality and Counseling Theories in the 21st Century." *Journal of Humanistic Psychology* 43(1):64–85.

Lee-Baggley, Dayna, Anita DeLongis, Paul Voorhoeave, and Esther Greenglass. 2004. "Coping with the Threat of Severe Acute Respiratory Syndrome: Role of Threat Appraisals and Coping Responses in Health Behaviors." *Asian Journal of Social Psychology* 7:9–12.

Lefcourt, Herbert M., Karina Davidson, Kenneth M. Prkachin, and David E. Mills. 1997. "Humor as a Stress Moderation in the Prediction of Blood Pressure Obtained During Five Stressful Tasks." *Journal of Research in Personality* 31:523–542.

Lefrancois, Mélanie, Karen Messing, and Johanne Saint-Charles. 2017. "Time Control, Job Execution and Information Access: Work/Family Strategies in the Context of Low-Wage Work and 24/7 Schedules." *Community, Work & Family* 20(5):600–22.

Lehmann, Curtis S. and Richard L. Gorsuch. 2017. "The Relevance of Religiousness and Reasoned Action for Adolescent Moral and Immoral Behavioral Intentions." *Psychology of Religion & Spirituality* 9(S1):S49–S59.

Lehmann, Michal, Sarit Pery, Avraham N. Kluger, David R. Hekman, Bradley P. Owens, and Thomas E. Malloy. 2023. "Relationship-Specific (Dyadic) Humility: How Your Humility Predicts My Psychological Safety and Performance." *Journal of Applied Psychology* 108(5):809–25.

Lei, Chang. 2004. "The Role of Classroom Norms in Contextualizing the Relations of Children's Social Behaviors to Peer Acceptance." *Developmental Psychology* 40(5):691–702.

Leibovitz, Talia, Amanda L. Shamblaw, Rachel Rumas, and Michael W. Best. 2021. "Covid-19 Conspiracy Beliefs: Relations with Anxiety, Quality of Life, and Schemas." *Personality & Individual Differences* 175:110704.

Leigert, Beverly D., and Lind Reutter. 2005. "Developing Resilience: How Women Maintain Their Health in Northern Geographically Isolated Settings." *Qualitative Health Research* 15(1):49–65.

Leighton, D. C., M. J. Brandt, and L. A. Kennedy. 2020. "Political Extremity, Social Media Use, Social Support, and Well-Being for Emerging Adults During the 2016 Presidential Election Campaign." *Emerging Adulthood* 8(4):285–96.

Leimberg, Anna and Peter S. Lehmann. 2022. "Unstructured Socializing with Peers, Low Self-Control, and Substance Use." *International Journal of Offender Therapy & Comparative Criminology* 66(1):3–27.

Leiser, David, Sacha Bourgeois-Gironde, and Rinat Benita. 2010. "Human Foibles or Systemic Failure: Lay Perceptions of the 2008-2009 Financial Crisis." *Journal of Socio-Economics* 39:132–141.

Leitner, Larry M., and Franz R. Epting. 2015. "Constructivist Approaches to Therapy." Pp. 523–533 in *The Handbook of Humanistic Psychology: Theory, Research, and Practice*, edited by Kirk J. Schneider, J. Fraser Pierson and James F. Bugental. Thousand Oaks, CA: SAGE.

Lelli, Sara. 2008. "Operationalizing Sen's Capability Approach: The Influence of the Selected Technique." Pp. 310–361 in *The Capability Approach: Concepts, Measures and Applications*, edited by Flavio Comim, Mozaffar Qizilbash and Sabina Alinre. Cambridge, UK: Cambridge University Press.

Lemaire, Gail Schoen, and Kali Mallik. 2002. "Expanding Horizons: A Model Academic and Vocational Training Program for Out-of-school Youth with Disabilities." *Journal of Rehabilitation* 68(2):39–45.

Lemay, Edward P., Arie W. Kruglanski, Erica Molinario, Maximilian Agostini, Jocelyn J. Bélanger, Ben Gützkow, Jannis Kreienkamp, Anne Margit Reitsema, Michelle R vanDellen, PsyCorona Collaboration, and N. Pontus Leander. 2023. "The Role of Values in Coping with Health and Economic Threats of COVID-19." Journal of Social Psychology 163(6): 755–72.

Lemay, Edward P., Jr., Margaret S. Clark, and Brooke C. Feeney. 2007. "Proportion of Responsiveness to Needs and the Construction of Satisfying Communal Relationships." *Journal of Personality & Social Psychology* 92(5):834–853.

Lemyre, Louise, Jennifer E.C. Lee, Pierre Mercier, Louise Bouchard, and Daniel Krewski. 2006. "The Structure of Canadians" Health Risk Perceptions, Environmental Therapeutic and Social Health Risks." *Health, Risk & Society* 8(2):185–195.

Lennartsson, Carin. 2010. "Need and Support: Determinants of Intra-familial Financial Transfers in Sweden." *International Journal of Social Welfare* 20:66–74.

Lent, Robert W. 2013. "Career-life Preparedness: Revisiting Career Planning and Adjustment in the New Workplace." *Career Development Quarterly* 61:2–14.

Lenz, A. Stephen, Rachel Holman, and Denise Dominguez. 2010. "Encouraging Connections: Integrating Expressive Art and Drama into Therapeutic Social Skills Training with Adolescents." *Journal of Creativity in Mental Health* 5(2):142–157.

Lepkowski, James M., and Mick P. Couper. 2002. "Nonresponse in the Second Wave of Longitudinal Household Surveys." Pp. 259–272 in *Survey Nonresponse*, edited by Robert M. Groves, Don A. Dillman, John L. Eltinge and Roderick J.A. Little. New York: John Wiley.

Lerner, Richard M, Michelle B. Weiner, Miriam R. Arbeit, Paul A. Chase, Jennifer P. Agans et al. 2012. "Resilience Across the Life Span." *Annual Review of Gerontology & Geriatrics* 32:275–299.

Lessard, Jared, Ellen Greenberger, Chuansheng Chen, and Susan Farruggia. 2011. "Are Youths" Feelings of Entitlement Always Bad? Evidence for a Distraction between Exploitive and Non-exploitive Dimensions of Entitlement." *Journal of Adolescence* 34:521–529.

Leu, Chao-Hsien. Ke-Mei Chen, and Hsiu-Hui Chen. 2016. "A Multidimensional Approach to Child Poverty in Taiwan." *Children & Youth Services Review* 66:35–44.

Leung, Angel Nga-man, and Catherine McBride-Chang. 2013. "Game On? Online Friendship, Cyberbullying, and Psychosocial Adjustment in Hong Kong Chinese Children." *Journal of Social & Clinical Psychology* 32(2):159–185.

Leung, Beeto Wai-chung, Giovanni B. Maneta, and Catherine McBride-Chang. 2005. "Think Positively and Feel Positively: Optimism and Life Satisfaction in Late Life." *International Journal of Aging & Human Development* 61(4):335–365.

Leung, Kwok, Pamela Tremain Koch, and Lin Lu. 2002. "A Dualistic Model of Harmony and Its Implications for Conflict Management in Asia." *Asia Pacific Journal of Management* 19(2,3):201–220.

Lever, Joaquina Palomar, Nuria Lanzagorta Pinol, and Jorge Hernandez Uralde. 2005. "Poverty, Psychological Resources and Subjective Well-being." *Social Indicators Research* 73:375–408. \84–9

Levesque, Ariane, Julianne Béliveau, David Ogez, Valérie Marcil, Daniel Curnier, Caroline Laverdière, Daniel Sinnett, Katherine Péloquin, and Serge Sultan. 2023. "Do Problem-Solving Skills Help Mitigate Emotional Distress through Perceived Control and Self-Efficacy in Parents of Children with Cancer?" *Psycho-Oncology* 32(2):247–55.

Levesque-Bristol, Chantal, Timothy D. Knapp, and Bradley J. Fisher. 2011. "The Effectiveness of Service-Learning: It's Not Always What You Think." *Journal of Experiential Education* 33(3):208–24.

Levi, Margaret, and Laura Strker. 2000. "Political Trust and Trustworthiness." *Annual Review of Political Science* 3:475–507.

Levi, Margaret. 2003. "A State of Trust." Pp. 27–101 in *Trust and Governance*, edited by Valerie A. Braithwaite and Margaret Levi. New York, NY: Russell Sage.

Levidi, Myrto Dafni Chatzimike, Andrew McGrath, Peter Kyriakoulis, and Danielle Sulikowski. 2024. "Understanding Criminal Decision-Making: Links between Honesty-Humility, Perceived Risk and Negative Affect." *Psychology, Crime & Law*. \110–259

Levin, Jeffrey S., and Linda M. Chatters. 1998. "Research on Religion and Mental Health: An Overview on Empirical Findings and Theoretical Issues." Pp. 33–50 in *Handbook of Religion and Mental Health*, edited by Harold G. Koenig. San Diego, CA: Academic.

Levine, Mark, Amy Prosser David Evans, and Stephen Recher. 2005. "Identity and Emergency Intervention: How Our Group Membership and Inclusiveness of Group Boundaries Shape Helping Behavior." *Personality & Social Psychology Bulletin* 31(4):443–453.

Levitt, Heidi M., Caroline M. Stanley, Zeev Frankel, and Karina Raina. 2005. "An Evaluation of Outcome Measures Used in Humanistic Psychotherapy Research: Using Thermometers to Weigh Oranges." *Humanist Psychologist* 33(2):113–130.

Levitt, Mary J., and Ayse Cici-Gokaltun. 2011. "Close Relationships across the Life Span." Pp. 457–486 in *Handbook of Life-Development*, edited by Karen L. Fingerman, Cynthia A. Berg, Jacque Smith and Toni C. Antonucci. New York: Springer.

Levitt, Mary J., Sherrilyn Coffman, Nathalie Guacci-Franco, and Stephen C. Loveless. 1994. "Attachment Relationships and Life Transitions: An Expectancy Model." Pp. 232–255 in *Attachment in Adults: Clinical and Developmental Perspectives*, edited by Michael B. Sperling and William H. Berman. New York: Guilford.

Lewicki, Roy J., and Beth Polin. 2013. "Trust and Negotiation." Pp. 161–190 in *Handbook of Research on Negotiation*, edited by Mara Olekalns and Wendi L. Adair. Cheltenham, UK: Elgar.

Lewin, Epstein Noah, Smit Kaplan, and Asaf Levanon. 2003. "Distributive Justice and Attitudes toward the Welfare State." *Social Justice Research* 16(1):1–27.

Lewin-Epstein, Noah, Amit Kaplan, and Asaf Levanon. 2003. "Distributive Justice and Attitudes toward the Welfare State." *Social Justice Research* 16(1):1–27.

Lewinsohn, Peter M., Paul Rohde, and John R. Seeley. 1994. "Psychosocial Risk Factors for Future Adolescent Suicide Attempts." *Journal of Consulting & Clinical Psychology* 62(2):297–305.

Lewis, Megan A., Colleen M. McBride, Kathryn I. Pollak, Elaine Puleo, Rita M. Butterfield, and Karen M. Emmons. 2006a. "Health-related Social Control and Relationship Interdependence among Gay Couples." *Health Education Research* 21(4):488–500.

Lewis, Megan A., Colleen M. McBride, Kathryn I. Pollak, Elaine Puleo, Rita M. Butterfield, and Karen M. Emmons. 2006b. "Understanding Health Behavior Change among Couples: An Interdependence and Communal Coping Approach." *Social Science & Medicine* 62(6):1369–80.

Leybman, Michelle J., David C. Zuroff, Marc A. Fournier, Allison C. Kelly, and Martin Alia. 2011. "Social Exchange Styles: Measurement, Validation, and Application." *European Journal of Personality* 25(3):198–210.

Li, Babai, and Andrew G. Walder. 2001. "Career-advancement as Party Patronage: Sponsored Mobility into the Chinese Administrative Elite, 1949–1996." *Americal Journal of Sociology* 106(5):1371–1408.

Li, Chunkai, Qiunv Zhang, and Na Li. 2018. "Does Social Capital Benefit Resilience for Left-Behind Children? An Evidence from Mainland China." *Children & Youth Services Review* 93:255–262.

Li, Euli, and Kwok Leung. 2012. "Effects of Evaluation of Societal Conditions and Work-family Conflict on Social Cynicism and Distress: A Longitudinal Analysis." *Journal of Applied Social Psychology* 42(3):717–734.

Li, Haibin, Dorothy Bottrell, and Derrick Armstrong. 2018. "Understanding the Pathways to Resilience: Voices from Chinese Adolescents." *Young* 26(2):126–144.

Li, Ji. 2006. "The Interactions between Person-organization Fit and Leadership Styles in Asian Firms, an Empirical Study." *International Journal of Human Resource Management* 17(10):1689–1706.

Li, Jia, Ling Xu, and Chi, Iris. 2018. "Challenges and Resilience Related to Aging in the United States among Older Chinese Immigrants." *Aging & Mental Health* 22(12):1548–55.

Li, Jin, Kaina Zhou, Xiaomei Li, Miao Liu, Shaonong Dang, Duolao Wang, and Xia Xin. 2016. "Mediator Effect of Sleep Hygiene Practices on Relationships Between Sleep Quality and Other Sleep-Related Factors in Chinese Mainland University Students." *Behavioral Sleep Medicine* 14(1):85–99.

Li, Kui-Wai. 2012. *Economic Freedom: Lessons of Hong Kong*. Singapore: World Scientific.

Li, Liman Man Wai. 2018. "Dialectical Beliefs and Savings Tendency: Opposite Patterns in Good Versus Bad Current Status." *Journal of Applied Social Psychology* 48(3):128–135.

Li, Shuxian, Xinyuan Fu, Mengyuan Zhang, Ruoran Fu, Mei Zhang, and Yu Kou. 2024. "*Effect of Economic Inequality on Generosity: A Social Norm Perspective.*" *International Journal of Psychology.*

Li, Tianyuan, Chun Bun Lam, and Kevin Ka-shing Chan. 2018. "Grandparental Involved and Young Adults" Cognitive and Social Adjustment: The Moderating Role of Filial Piety in Hong Kong." *Journal of Social & Personal Relationships* 35(7):999–1018.

Li, Yunqing, and Kenneth F. Ferraro. 2006. "Volunteering in Middle and Later Life: Is Health a Benefit, Barrier or Both?" *Social Forces* 85(1):497–518.

Li, Yu-sheng, and Ying-chih Chung. 2008. "Neighborhood Effects on an Individual's Health Using Neighborhood Measurements Developed by Factor Analysis and Cluster Analysis." *Journal of Urban Health* 86(1):5–18.

Li, Zhengmin. 2022. "How Organizations Create Employee Based Brand Equity: Mediating Effects of Employee Empowerment." *Frontiers in Psychology* 13:862678.

Li, Zhigang and Fulong Wu. 2013. "Residential Satisfaction in China's Informal Settlements: A Case Study of Beijing, Shanghai, and Guangzhou." *Urban Geography* 34(7):923–49.

Liang, Belle, Renée Spencer, Deirdre Brogan, and Macarena Corral. 2008. "Mentoring Relationships from Early Adolescence through Emerging Adulthood: A Qualitative Analysis." *Journal of Vocational Behavior* 72(2):168–182.

Liang, Hai and Francis L. F. Lee. 2022. "Opinion Leadership in a Leaderless Movement: Discussion of the Anti-Extradition Bill Movement in the "Lihkg" Web Forum." *Social Movement Studies.*

Liao, Pei-Shan, Yang-Chih Fu, and Chin-Chun Yi. 2005. "Perceived Quality of Life in Taiwan and Hong Kong: An Intra-culture Comparison." *Journal of Happiness Studies* 6:43–67.

Lichbach, Mark Irving. 1988. "An Evaluation of "Does Economic Inequality Breed Political Conflict's Studies." *World Politics* 41(4):431–470.

Lichter, David T., and Diane K. McLaughlin, and David C. Ribar. 2002. "Economic Restructuring and the Retreat from Marriage." *Social Science Research* 31:230–256.

Lichterman, Paul. 2012. "Religion in Public Action." *Sociological Theory* 30(1):15–36.

Lie, Mabel, Susan Baines, and Jane Wheelock. 2009. "Citizenship, Volunteering and Active Ageing." *Social Policy & Administration* 43(7):702–718.

Liebenberg, Linda and Jeff Christopher Moore. 2018. "A Social Ecological Measure of Resilience for Adults: The RRC-ARM." *Social Indicators Research* 136(1):1–19.

Liebig, Stefan, and Steffen Mau. 2007. "When Is a Taxation System Just? Attitudes towards General Taxation Principles Are towards the Justice of One's Own Tax Burden." Pp. 97–122 in *Social Justice, Legitimacy and the Welfare State*, edited by Steffen Mau and Benjamin Veghte. Aldershot, UK: Ashgate.

Lieneman, Corey C., Laurel A. Brabson, April Highlander, Nancy M. Wallace, and Cheryl B. McNeil. 2017. "Parent-Child Interaction Therapy: Current Perspectives." *Psychological Research & Behavioral Management* 10:239–256.

Light, John M., Joel W. Grube, Patricia A. Madden, and Jill Gover. 2003, "Adolescent Alcohol Use and Suicidal Ideation: A Nonrecursive Model." *Addictive Behaviors* 28:705–724.

Light, M. John, and Thomas J. Dishion. 2007. "Early Adolescent Antisocial Behavior and Peer Rejection: A Dynamic Test of a Developmental Process." *New Directions for Child & Adolescent Development* 118:77–89.

Like, Taya Z. 2011. "Urban Inequality and Racial Differences in Risk for Violent Victimization." *Crime & Delinquency* 57(3):432–457.

Lilly, J. Robert, Francis T. Cullen, and Richard A. Ball. 2011. *Criminological Theory: Context and Consequences.* Los Angeles, CA: SAGE.

Lim, Chaeyoon, and Robert D. Putnam. 2010. "Religion, Social Networks, and Life Satisfaction." *American Sociological Review* 75(6):914–933.

Lim, Lena L. 2009. "The Influences of Harmony Motives and Implicit Beliefs on Conflict Styles of the Collectivist." *International Journal of Psychology* 44(6):401–09.

Lin, Delia. 2017. Civilising Citizens in Post-Mao China: Understanding the Rhetoric of Suzhi. Abington, UK: Routledge.

Lin, Ka, Yun Xu, Tianhai Huang, and Jiahua Zhang. 2013. "Social Exclusion and Its Cause in East Asian Societies: Evidence from SQSQ Survey Data." *Social Indicators Research* 112(3):641–660.

Lin, Shen. 2018. "We Work Like Ants…We Avoid Being Troublemaker: An Exploratory Inquiry on Resilience of Chinese Street Vendors in the Urban Village." *International Journal of Sociology & Social Policy* 38(11/12):1024–40.
Lin, Thunghong, and Xiaogang Wu. 2009. "The Transformation of the Chinese Class Structure, 1978–2005." *Social Transformations in Chinese Societies* 5:81–112.
Lin, Yi-Ying, Dena Phillips Swanson, and Ronald David Rogge. 2021. "The Three Teachings of East Asia (TTEA) Inventory: Developing and Validating a Measure of the Interrelated Ideologies of Confucianism, Buddhism, and Taoism." *Frontiers in Psychology* 12:626122.
Lin, Y-J., C-S. Chen, T-C. Liu, and H-C. Lin. 2008. "Taiwan's National Health Insurance System and the Application of Preventive Care: The Case of Pal Smear Testing." *Public Health* 122:857–861.
Linares, Leticia, Paula Jauregui, David Herrero-Fernández, and Ana Estévez. 2016. "Mediating Role of Mindfulness as a Trait between Attachment Styles and Depressive Symptoms." *Journal of Psychology* 150(7):881–896.
Lincoln, Karen, Linda M. Chatters, and Robert Joseph Taylor. 2003. "Psychological Distress among Black and White Americans: Differential Effects of Social Support, Negative Interaction, and Personal Control." *Journal of Health & Social Behavior* 44:390–407.
Linden-Andersen, Stine, Dorothy Markiewicz, and Anna-Beth Doyle. 2009. "Perceived Similarity among Adolescent Friends: The Role of Reciprocity, Friendship Quality, and Gender." *Journal of Early Adolescence* 29(5):617–637.
Lindstrom, Martin, and Maria Rosvall. 2012. "Marital Status, Social Capital, Economic Stress, and Mental Health: A Population-Based Study." *Social Science Journal* 49(3):339–342.
Lindstrom, Martin, and Maria Rosvall. 2015. "Life Course Perspectives on Economic Stress and Generalized Trust in Other People." *Social Science Journal* 53(1):7–13.
Lindstrom, Martin. 2006. "Psychosocial Work Conditions, Social Participation and Social Capital: A Causal Pathway Investigated in Longitudinal Study." *Social Science & Medicine* 62:280–291.
Lindwall, Magnus. 2004. "Factorial Structure and Invariance across Gender of the Swedish Self-consciousness Scale." *Journal of Personality Assessment* 82(2):233–240.
Lineres, L. Oriann. 2004. "Social Connection to Neighbors, Multiple Victimization, and Current Health among Women Residing in High Crime Neighborhoods." *Journal of Family Violence* 19(6):355–366.
Lintz, Mario J., Christian Thurstone, Madelyne Hull, and Kristie Ladegard. 2019. "Development of a School-Based Substance Treatment Model." *Journal of Child & Adolescent Substance Abuse* 28(2):127–131.
Lipford, Jody W., and Bruce Yandle. 2009. "The Determinants of Purposeful Voluntarism." *Journal of Socio-Economics* 38(1):72–79.
Lipkus, Isaac M., and Victor Bissonette. 1998. "The Belief in a Just World and Willingness to Accommodate among Married and Dating Couples." Pp. 127–140 in *Responses to Victimizations and Belief in a Just World*, edited by Leo Montada and Melvin J. Lerner. New York: Plenum.
Lipschitz-Elhawi, Racheli. 2009. "Ways of Enhancing Hope among Social Workers Working with Adolescents in Residential Treatment Centres." *British Journal of Social Work* 39(3):451–466.
Lipshits-Braziler, Yuliya, and Moshe Tatar. 2012. "Perceived Career Barriers and Coping among Youth in Israel: Ethnic and Gender Differences." *Journal of Vocational Behavior* 80:545–554.
Lipsitt, Lewis P. and Jack Demick. 2012. "Theory and Measurement of Resilience: Views from Development." Pp. 43–52 in *The Social Ecology of Resilience: Handbook of Theory and Practice*, edited by Michael Ungar. New York, NY: Springer.
Little, Todd D., Takahiro Miyashita, Mayumi Karasawa, Mari Mashima, Gabriele Dettingen, Hiroshi Azuma, and Paul B. Baltes. 2003. "The Links among Action-control Beliefs, Intellective Skill, and School Performance in Japanese, US, and German School Children." *International Journal of Behavioral Development* 27(1):41–48.
Littlejohn, Stephen W., Karen A. Foss, and John G. Oetzel. 2017. *Theories of Human Communication*. Long Grove, IL: Waveland.

Littleton, Heather, Samantha Horsley, Siji John, and David V. Nelson. 2007. "Trauma Coping Strategies and Psychological Distress: A Meta-analysis." *Journal of Traumatic Stress* 20(6):977–988.
Littman-Ovadia, Hadassah, Vered Lazar-Butbul, and Benny A. Benjamin. 2014. "Strengths-Based Career Counseling: Overview and Initial Evaluation." *Journal of Career Assessment* 22(3):403–19.
Liu, Airan, and Xie, Yu. 2016. "Why Do Asian Americans Academically Outperform Whites? The Cultural Explanation Revisited." *Social Science Research* 58:210–226.
Liu, Chang-Jiang and Fang Hao. 2017. "Reciprocity Belief and Gratitude as Moderators of the Association between Social Status and Charitable Giving." *Personality & Individual Differences* 111:46–50.
Liu, Cong, Ling Li, Hai Li, Valentina Bruk-Lee, Jie Ma, and Ying Liu. 2023. "Supervisor–Employee Task Conflict and Supervisor Ostracism: The Moderating Effect of Interpersonal Harmony Values." *Applied Psychology* 72(3):971–97.
Liu, Cong, Margaret M. Nauta, Liu-Qin Yang, and Paul E. Spector. 2018. "How Do Coworkers "Make the Place"? Examining Coworker Conflict and the Value of Harmony in China and the United States." *Applied Psychology* 67(1):30–60.
Liu, Eric Y. 2010. "Fatalistic Voluntarism and Life Happiness in Post-socialist China." *Sociological Spectrum* 30:270–288.
Liu, Haidong, Baojuan Ye and Yong Hu. 2022. "Stressful Life Events and Depression During the Recurrent Outbreak of COVID-19 in China: The Mediating Role of Grit and the Moderating Role of Gratitude." *Psychology Research & Behavior Management* 15:1359–70.
Liu, James H., Mei-chih Li, and Xiaodong Yue. 2010. "Chinese Social Identity and Intergroup Relations: The Influence of Benevolent Authority." Pp. 579–597 in *The Oxford Handbook of Chinese Psychology*, edited by Michael Harris Bond. Oxford, UK: Oxford University Press.
Liu, Jianhong and Siyu Liu. 2016. "Are Children of Rural Migrants More Delinquent Than Their Peers? A Comparative Analysis of Delinquent Behaviors in the City of Guangzhou, China." *Crime, Law, & Social Change* 66(5):465–89.
Liu, Jianhong, Steven F. Messner, Lening Zhang, and Yue Zhuo. 2009. "Socio-Demographic Correlates of Fear of Crime and the Social Context of Contemporary Urban China." *American Journal of Community Psychology* 44(1–2):93–108.
Liu, Leiph Ann, and Wei Cai. 2013. "Shared Cognition and Identity in Negotiation." Pp. 75–102 in *Handbook of Research on Negotiation*, edited by Mara Olekalns and Wendi L. Adair. Cheltenham, UK: Elgar.
Liu, Weidong. 2019. *The Belt and Road Initiative: A Pathway towards Inclusive Globalization.* Abington, UK: Routledge.
Liu, Ying, and Sek-yum Ngai. 2019. "The Impact of Social Capital, Self-Efficacy, and Resilience on the Prosocial Involvement of Adolescents from Families with and without Economic Disadvantages." *Child Indicators Research* 12(5):1735–1757.
Liu, Yuli. 2004. The Unity of Rule and Virtue: A Critique of a Supposed Parallel between Confucian Ethics and Virtue Ethics. Singapore: Eastern Universities Press.
Liu, Zhangming. 2008. *Pondering Harmonious Development*. Beijing, China: People.
Livingstone, Sonia, Nick Couldry, and Tim Markham. 2007. "Youthful Steps towards Civic Participation: Does the Internet Help?" Pp. 21–34 in *Young Citizens in the Digital Age: Political Engagement, Young People and New Media*, edited by Brian D. Loader. London: Routledge.
Lizardo, Omar. 2006. "How Cultural Tastes Shape Personal Networks." *American Sociological Review* 71(5):778–807.
Lloyd, Christopher E. M., Brittney S. Mengistu, and Graham Reid. 2022. "His Main Problem Was Not Being in a Relationship with God": Perceptions of Depression, Help-Seeking, and Treatment in Evangelical Christianity." *Frontiers in Psychology* 13:831534.
Lloyd, Helen, and Rudi Dallos. 2008. "First Session Solution-focused Brief Therapy with Families Who Have a Child with Severe Intellectual Disabilities: Mothers" Experiences and Views." *Journal of Family Therapy* 30:5–28.

Lo, Alex Y.H., and C.Y. Jim. 2012. "Citizen Attitude and Expectation towards Greenspace Provision in Compact." *Land Use Policy* 29:577–586.

Lo, Sonny Shiu-Hing. 2018b. "The New Democracy Movement, Interest Group Politics and Implications for China." Pp. 243–256 in *Interest Groups and New Democracy Movement in Hong Kong*, edited by Sonny Shiu-Hing Lo. Abingdon, UK: Routledge.

Lo, Sonny Shiu-Hing. 2021. *The Dynamics of Peaceful and Violent Protests in Hong Kong: The Anti-Extradition Movement*, Singapore: Palgrave.

Lo, T. Wing. 2012. "Triadization of Youth Gangs in Hong Kong." *British Journal of Criminology* 52:556–576.

Lochner, Kimberly, Ichiro Kawachi, and Bruce L. Kennedy. 1999. "Social Capital: A Guide to Its Measurement." *Health & Place* 5:259–270.

Lochner, Kimberly, Ichiro Kawachi, Robert T. Brennan, and Stephen L. Burka. 2003. "Social Capital and Neighborhood Mortality Rates in Chicago." *Social Science & Medicine* 36:1797–1805.

Lock, Samantha, Clare S. Rees, and Brody Heritage. 2020. "Development and Validation of a Brief Measure of Psychological Resilience: The State-Trait Assessment of Resilience Scale." *Australian Psychologist* 55(1):10–25.

Locke, Kenneth D. 2003. "Status and Solidarity in Social Comparison: Agentic and Communal Values and Vertical and Horizontal Directions." *Journal of Personality & Social Psychology* 84(3):619–631.

Lodewijkx, Hein F. M., Gaby L. E. Kersten, and Martijn van Zomeren. 2008. "Dual Pathways to Engage in "Silent Marches" against Violence: Moral Outrage, Moral Cleansing and Modes of Identification." *Journal of Community & Applied Social Psychology* 18(3):153–67.

Loewy, Erich H. 1993. *Freedom and Community: The Ethics of Interdependence*. Albany, NY: State University of New York Press.

Lofors, Jonas, and Kristina Sundquist. 2007. "Law-linking Social Capital as a Predictor of Mental Disorders: A Cohort Study of 4.5 Million Swedes." *Social Science & Medicine* 64:21–34.

Logan, Jill M., and Rebecca J. Cobb. 2013. "Trajectories of Relationship Satisfaction: Independent Contributions of Capitalization and Support Perceptions." *Personal Relationships* 20(2):277–293.

Logan, John R., and Glenna D. Spitze. 1994. "Family Neighbors." *American Journal of Sociology* 100(2):453–476.

Logan, John R., Yanjie Bian, and Fuqin Bian. 1999. "Housing Inequality in Urban China in the 1990s." *International Journal of Urban and Regional Research* 23:7–25.

London, Rebecca A. 2003. "Which TANF Applicants Are Diverted and What Are Their Outcomes?" *Social Service Review* 77(3):373–398.

Long, D. Adam, and Douglas D. Perkins. 2007. "Community Social and Place Predictors of Sense of Community: A Multilevel and Longitudinal Analysis." *Journal of Community Psychology* 35(5):563–581.

Long, Jonathan, and Peter Bramham. 2006. "Joining up Policy Discourages and Fragmented Practices: the Precarious Contribution of Cultural Projects to Social Inclusion?" *Policy & Practices* 34(1):133–151

Lopez, J. Humberto, K. Schmidt-Hebbel, and Luis Servén. 2000. "How Effective Is Fiscal Policy in Raising National Saving?" *Review of Economics & Statistics* 82(2):226–38.

Loptson, Peter. 2001. *Theories of Human Nature* (2nd ed.). Peterborough, Canada: Broadview.

Lorant, Vincent, and Pablo Nicaise. 2015. "Binge Drinking at University: A Social Network Study in Belgium." *Health Promotion International* 30(3):675–683.

Lord, Sarah, Julie Brevard, and Simon Budman. 2011. "Connecting to Young Adults: An Online Social Network Survey of Beliefs and Attitudes Associated with Prescriptive Opioid Misuse among College Students." *Substance Use & Misuse* 66:66–76.

Loriol, Marc. 2016. "Collective Forms of Coping and the Social Construction of Work Stress among Industrial Workers and Police Officers in France." *Theory & Psychology* 26(1):112–29. doi: 10.1177/0959354315616877.

Loscocco, Karyn A., and Glenna Spitze. 1990. "Working Conditions, Social Support, and the Well-Being of Female and Male Factory Workers." *Journal of Health and Social Behavior* 31:313–327.

Lou, Vivian W. Q. and Jimmy W. Ng. 2012. "Chinese Older Adults' Resilience to the Loneliness of Living Alone: A Qualitative Study." *Aging & Mental Health* 16(8):1039–46.

Lou, Vivian Wei-qun, and Iris Chi. 2008. "Measuring Grandparenthood Stress and Reward: Developing a Scale Based on Perceptions by Grandparents with Adolescent Grandchildren in Hong Kong." *Geriatric Gerontology International* 8:291–299.

Lou, Yunfei, Emily P. Taylor, and Simona Di Folco. 2018. "Resilience and Resilience Factors in Children in Residential Care: A Systematic Review." *Children & Youth Services Review* 89:83–92.

Louis, Vincent V., and Shanyang Zhao. 2002. "Effects of Family Structure, Family SES, and Adulthood Experience on Life Satisfaction." *Journal of Family Issues* 23(8):986–1005.

Louis, Winnifred, Emma Thomas, Craig McGarty, Morgana Lizzio-Wilson, Catherine Amiot, and Fathali Moghaddam. 2020. "The Volatility of Collective Action: Theoretical Analysis and Empirical Data." *Political Psychology* 41(S1):35–74.

Loukakis, Angelos and Martín Portos. 2020. "Another Brick in the Wall? Young People, Protest and Nonprotest Claims Making in Nine European Countries." *American Behavioral Scientist* 64(5):669–85.

Loukopoulos, Peter, Cecilia Jakobsson, Tommy Garling, Cldudia M. Schneider, and Satoshi Fujii. 2005. "Public Attitudes towards Policy Measures for Reducing Private Car Use: Evidence from a Study in Sweden." *Environmental Science & Policy* 8:57–66.

Low, Sabina, and Joann Wu Shortt. 2017. "Family, Peer, and Pubertal Determinants of Dating Involvement among Adolescents." *Journal of Research on Adolescence* 27(1):78–87.

Low, Xiao Qing and Shue Ling Chong. 2024. "Helicopter Parenting and Resilience among Malaysian Chinese University Students: The Mediating Role of Fear of Negative Evaluation." *Journal of Adult Development.*

Lowe, Sarah R., Jean E. Rhodes, Liza Zwiebach, and Christian S. Chan. 2009. "The Impact of Pet Loss on the Perceived Social Support and Psychological Distress of Hurricane Survivors." *Journal of Traumatic Stress* 22(3):244–247.

Lowis, Michael J., Anthony C. Edwards, and Mary Burton. 2009. "Coping with Retirement: Wellbeing, Health, and Religion." *Journal of Psychology* 143(4):427–448.

Lowndes, Vivien, and Mark Roberts. 2013. *Why Institutions Matter: The New Institutionalism in Political Science.* Houndmills, UK: Palgrave.

Loxbo, Karl. 2018. "Ethnic Diversity, out-Group Contacts and Social Trust in a High-Trust Society." *Acta Sociologica* 61(2):182–201.

Lu, Aitao, Simin Cai, Shuang Zheng, Huiqing Hu, and Pingfang Song. 2018. "Stereotype and National Attachment in Hong Kong Chinese Context: A Moderated Mediation Model of Perceived Inter-group Relationship and Age." *Social Indicators Research* 135(1):357–371.

Lu, Luo, and Shu-fang Kao. 2002. "Traditional and Modern Characteristics across the Generations: Similarities and Discrepancies." *Journal of Social Psychology* 142(1):45–59.

Lu, Mai, and Mingliang Feng. 2008. "Reforming the Welfare System in the People's Republic of China." *Asian Development Review* 25(1):58–80.

Lubbers, Mareel, Marcel Coenders, and Peer Scheepers. 2006. "Objections to Asylum Seeker Centres: Individual and Contextual Determinants of Resistance to Small and Large Centres in the Netherlands." *European Sociological Review* 32(3):243–257.

Lubell, Mark. 2003. "Collaborative Institutions, Belief-systems, and Perceived Policy Effectiveness." *Political Research Quarterly* 56(3):309–323.

Lubis, Syahid Izharuddin and Agnes Sianipar. 2022. "How Religious Tolerance Can Emerge among Religious People: An Investigation on the Roles of Intellectual Humility, Cognitive Flexibility, and Trait Aggressiveness." *Asian Journal of Social Psychology* 25(2):276–87.

Lucas, Brian J. and Nour S. Kteily. 2018. "(Anti-)Egalitarianism Differentially Predicts Empathy for Members of Advantaged Versus Disadvantaged Groups." *Journal of Personality & Social Psychology* 114(5):665–92.

Lucas, Margaretha S. 2012. "Counseling on Campus: Client Persistence and Progress." *Journal of College Student Psychotherapy* 26(3):227–240.

Lucas, Todd, Ludmila Zhdanova, Craig A. Wendorf, and Sheldon Alexander. 2013. "Procedural and Distributive Justice Beliefs for Self and Others: Multilevel Associations with Life Satisfaction and Self-Rated Health." *Journal of Happiness Studies* 14(4):1325–1341.

Ludigdo, Unti and Ali Mashuric. 2021. "Negative Evaluations of National Ethics and Its Impact on Islamic Radicalism." *SAGE Open* 11(3).

Luk, Pattie Fong Yuk Yee. 2001. "Competing Contents for Developing Personal and Social Education in Hong Kong." *Comparative Education Review* 37(1):65–87.

Luk-Fong, Pattie Yuk Yee. 2006. "Hybridity in a Guidance Curriculum in Hong Kong." *International Journal of Advancement in Counselling* 28:331–342.

Luk-Fong, Pattie Yuk Yee. 2007. "Primary School Teachers" Perceptions of School Children Coping with Changing Family Situations – a Hybrid Hong Kong Experience." *Social Psychology of Education* 9(4):425–41.

Lundasen, Susanne Wallman, and Dag Wollebaek. 2013. "Diversity and Community Trust in Swedish Local Communities." *Journal of Elections, Public Opinion & Parties* 23(3):299–321.

Lupien, Sonia J., Bruce S. McEwen, Megan R. Gunnar, and Christine Heim. 2009. "Effects of Stress throughout the Lifespan on the Brain, Behavior and Cognition." *Nature Reviews: Neuroscience* 10:434–445.

Lupton, Deborah. 2013. *Risk*. Milton Park, UK: Routledge.

Luria, Gil, Ram A. Cnaan, and Amnon Boehm. 2019. "National Culture of Indulgence as Predictor of Prosocial Behavior: Governmental Effectiveness as Boundary Condition." *Voluntas* 30(5):1164–75.

Luschen, Gunther, William Cockerham, and Gerhard Kunz. 1996. "The Sociocultural Context of Sport and Health Problems of Causal Relations and Structural Interdependence." Sociology of Sport Journal 13:197–213.

Luskin, Robert C. 1990. "Explaining Political Sophistication." *Political Behavior* 12(4):331–361.

Luszczynska, Aleksandra, and Benicio Gutierrez-Dona. 2005. "General Self-efficacy in Various Domains of Human Functioning: Evidence from Five Countries." *International Journal of Psychology* 40(2):80–89.

Lutgen-Sandvik, Pamela, and Courtney Vail Fletcher. 2013. "Conflict Motivations and Tactics of Targets, Bystanders, and Bullies." Pp. 349–376 in *The SAGE Handbook of Conflict Communication*, edited by John G. Oetzel and Stelle Ting-Toomey. Thousand Oaks, CA: SAGE.

Luthans, Fred, Carolyn M. Youssef-Morgan, and Bruce J. Avolio. 2015. *Psychological Capital and Beyond. Oxford*, UK: Oxford University Press.

Luthar, Suniya S., Dante Cicchetti, and Bronwyn Becker. 2000. "The Construct of Resilience: A Critical Evaluation and Guidelines for Future Work." *Child Development* 21(3):543–562.

Luttmer, Erzo F.P. 2005. "Neighbors is Negatives: Relative Earnings and Well-being." *Quarterly Journal of Economics* 963–1002.

Lyness, Karen S., Janet C. Gornick, Pamela Stone, and Angela R. Grotto. 2012. "It's All About Control." *American Sociological Review* 77(6):1023–1049.

Lyng, Stephen, Rick Matthews, and William J. Miller. 2009. "Existentialism Edgework and the Contingent Body: Exploring the Criminalized Implications of Ultimate Fighting." Pp. 94–126 in *Existentialist Criminology*, edited by Ronnie Lippens and Don Crewe. Abingdon, UK: Routledge-Cavendish.

Lyng, Stephen. 2012. "Existential Transcendence in Late Modernity: Edgework and Hermeneutic Reflexivity." *Human Studies* 35(3):401–14.

Lyubomirsky, Sonja, Chris Tkach, and M. Robin DiMatteo. 2005. "What Are the Differences between Happiness and Self-esteem?" *Social Indicators Research* 78:363–404.

Ma, Guizhen. 2019. "Similar or Different? A Comparison of Environmental Behaviors of US-Born Whites and Chinese Immigrants." *Journal of International Migration & Integration* 20(4):1203–23.

Ma, Hing Keung, Ping Chung Cheung, and Daniel T.L. Shek. 2007. "The Relation of Prosocial Orientation to Peer Interactions, Family Social Environment and Personality of Chinese Adolescents." *International Journal of Behavioral Development* 31(1):12–18.

Ma, Hing Keung, Sandy C. Li, and Jacky W.C. Pow. 2011. "The Relation of Internet Use to Prosocial and Antisocial Behavior in Chinese Adolescents." *Cyberpsychology, Behavior, & Social Networking* 14(3):123–130.

Ma, Joyce L.C., Timothy K.Y. Wong, Yuk King Lau, and Shuk Han Pun. 2009. "Perceived Family Functioning and Family Resources of Hong Kong Families: Implications for Social Work Practice." *Journal of Family Social Work* 12:244–263.

Ma, Minjie et al. 2022. "Family Adaptability and Cohesion and The Subjective Well-being of Parents of Children with Disabilities: The Mediating Role of Coping Style and Resilience." *Current Psychology* 42:19065–75.

Ma, Ngok. 2009. "Reinventing the Hong Kong Sate or Rediscovering It? From Low Interventionism to Eclectic Corporatism." *Economy & Society* 38(3):492–519.

Ma, Ngok. 2011b. "Value Changes and Legitimacy Crisis in Post-industrial Hong Kong." *Asian Survey* 51(4):683–712.

Maatta, Sami, and Jari-Erik Nurmi. 2007. "Achievement Orientations, School Adjustment, and Well-being: A Longitudinal Study." *Journal of Research on Adolescence* 17(4):789–812.

Macdonald, Alexandra, and Tibor Palfai. 2008. "Predictors of Exercise Behavior among University Student Women: Utility of a Goal-Systems/Self-Regulation Theory Framework." *Personality & Individual Differences* 44(4):921–931.

MacDonald, Douglas A. 2000. "Spirituality: Description, Measurement, and Relation to the Five-factor Model of Personality." *Journal of Personality* 68(1):153–197.

MacDonald, Douglas A., and Harris L. Friedman. 2002. "Assessment of Humanistic, Transpersonal, and Spiritual Constructs: States of the Science." *Journal of Humanistic Psychology* 42(4):102–125.

MacDonald, Geoff, and Mark R. Leary. 2005. "Why Does Social Exclusion Hurt? The Relationship between Social and Physical Pain." *Psychological Bulletin* 131(2):202–223.

MacDonald, Robert, Tracy Shildrick, Colin Webster, and Donald Simpson. 2005. "Growing up in Poor Neighborhoods: The Significance of Class and Place in the Extended Transitions of Socially Excluded Young Adults." *Sociology* 39(5):873–891.

MacDonell, Elliott T. and Teena Willoughby. 2020. "Investigating Honesty-Humility and Impulsivity as Predictors of Aggression in Children and Youth." *Aggressive Behavior* 46(1):97–106

Macias, Thomas. 2015. "Risks, Trust, and Sacrifice: Social Structural Motivators for Environmental Change." *Social Science Quarterly* 96(5):1264–1276.

MacKay, Kevin. 2017. Radical Transformation: Oligarchy, Collapse, and the Crisis of Civilization. Toronto, Canada: Between the Lines.

Mackinnon, Sean P. 2012. "Perceived Social Support and Academic Achievement: Cross-Lagged Panel and Bivariate Growth Curve Analyses." *Journal of Youth and Adolescence* 41(4):474–485.

MacLeod, Andrew K. 2015. "Well-Being: Objectivism, Subjectivism or Subjectivism?" *Journal of Happiness Studies* 16(4):1073–1089

MacLeod, Andrew. 2017. *Prospection, Well-being, and Mental Health*. Oxford, UK: Oxford.

MacPherson, Heather A., Jennifer S. Cheavens, and Mary A. Fristad. 2013. "Dialectical Behavior Therapy for Adolescents: Theory, Treatment Adaptations, and Empirical Outcomes." *Clinical Child & Family Psychology Review* 16:59–80.

Maes, Jurgen. 1998. "Immanent Justice and Ultimate Justice: Two Ways of Believing in Justice." Pp. 9–40 in *Responses to Victimizations and Belief in a Just World*, edited by Leo Montada and Melvin J. Lerner. New York: Plenum.

Magi, Katrin, Eve Kikas, and Piret Soodla. 2018. "Effortful Control, Task Persistence, and Reading Skills." *Journal of Applied Developmental Psychology* 54:42–52.

Magliano, Lorenza, Andrea Fiorillo, Claudio Malangone, Corrado De Rosa, and Mario Maj. 2006. "Social Network in Long-term Diseases: A Comparative Study in Relatives of Persons with Schizophrenia and Physical Illnesses versus a Sample from the General Population." *Social Science & Medicine* 62:1392–1402.

Magnani, Elisabetta, and Rong Zhu. 2018. "Does Kindness Lead to Happiness? Voluntary Activities and Subjective Well-Being." *Journal of Behavioral & Experimental Economics* 77:20–28.

Magnuson, Katherine, Greg J. Duncan, and Ariel Kalil. 2006. "The Contribution of Middle Childhood Contexts to Adolescent Achievement and Behavior." Pp. 150–172 in *Developmental Contexts in Middle Childhood: Bridges to Adolescence and Adulthood*, edited by Aletha C. Huston and Marika N. Ripke. Cambridge, UK: Cambridge University Press.

Mahajna, Sami. 2017b. "The Effect of Proximal and Psychological Factors on Future Orientation and Developmental Outcomes: The Case of Palestinian Adolescents in Israel." *Psychological Studies* 62(4):345–356.

Mahler, Elizabeth Bussman. 2011. "Midlife Work Role Transitions: Generativity and Learning in 21st-century Careers." Pp. 186–214 in *The Oxford Handbook of Reciprocal Adult Development Learning*, edited by Carol Hoare, New York: Oxford University Press.

Mahoney, Dennis J. 2004. Politics and Progress: The Emergence of American Political Science. Lanham, MD: Lexington.

Mahoney, Joseph L., Deborah Lowe Vandell, Sandra Simpkins, and Nicole Zarrett. 2009. "Adolescent Out-of-school Activities." Pp. 228–269 in *Handbook of Adolescent Psychology, Vol. 2: Contextual Influences and Adolescent Development*, edited by Richard M. Lerner and Laurence Steinberg. Hoboken, NJ: Wiley.

Mahoney, Joseph L., Heather Lord, and Erica Carry. 2005. "An Ecological Analysis of After-school Program Participation and the Development of Academic Performance and Motivational Attributes for Disadvantaged Children." *Child Development* 76(4):811–825.

Major, Brenda, and Sarah S. M. Townsend. 2010. "Coping with Bias." Pp. 410–425 in *The SAGE Handbook of Prejudice, Stereotyping and Discrimination*, edited by John F. Dovidio, Miles Hewstone, Peter Glick and Victoria M. Esses. London, UK: SAGE. (HM1091.S24) \d12–1.20

Major, Wayne F. 2001. "The Benefits and Costs of Serious Running." *World Leisure Journal* 43(2):12–25.

Mak, S., and Jason Mueller. 2000. "Job Insecurity, Coping Resources and Personality Dispositions in Occupational Strain." *Work & Stress* 14(4):312–328.

Mak, Winnie W. S., Ivy S. W. Ng, Celia C. Y. Wong, and Rita W. Law. 2019. "Resilience Style Questionnaire: Development and Validation among College Students and Cardiac Patients in Hong Kong." *Assessment* 26(4):706–25.

Makarios, Matthew D., and Tara L. Sams. 2013. "Social Support and Crime." Pp. 160–185 in *The Oxford Handbook of Criminological Theory*, edited by Francis T. Cullen and Pamela Wilcox. New York: Oxford University Press.

Malat, Jennifer. 2001. "Social Distance and Patients" Rating of Healthcare Providers." *Journal of Health and Social Behavior* 42:360–372.

Males, Mike A. 2010. "Is Jumping Off the Roof Always a Bad Idea? A Rejoinder on Risk Taking and the Adolescent Brain." *Journal of Adolescent Research* 25(1):48–63.

Maliepaard, Mieke and Karen Phalet. 2012. "Social Integration and Religious Identity Expression among Dutch Muslims." *Social Psychology Quarterly* 75(2):131–48.

Malka, Ariel and Christopher J. Soto. 2011. "The Conflicting Influences of Religiosity on Attitude toward Torture." *Personality & Social Psychology Bulletin* 37(8):1091–103.

Mallard, Graham. 2020. *Bounded Rationality*. Newcastle, UK: Agenda.

Mallick, Jane, and Mike Watts. 2008. "Drugsbridge: A Humanistic Approach to Drug Education." *Research in Education* 78:110–128.

Mallick, Jane. 2007. "Parent Drug Education: A Participatory Action Research Study into Effective Communication about Drugs between Parents and Unrelated Young People." *Drugs: Education, Prevention & Policy* 14(3):247–260.

Malloy, Thomas E. 2018. *Social Relations Modeling of Behavior in Dyads and Groups*. London, UK: Academic.

Maltby, John, Liz Day, Magdalena Zemojtel-Piotrowska, Jaroslaw Piotrowski, Hidefumi Hitokoto, Tomasz Baran, Ceri Jones, Anjalee Chakravarty-Agbo and Heather D. Flowe. 2016. "An Ecological Systems Model of Trait Resilience: Cross-Cultural and Clinical Relevance." *Personality & Individual Differences* 98:96–101.

Maltby, John, Liz Day, Sophie S. Hall, and Sally Chivers. 2019. "The Measurement and Role of Ecological Resilience Systems Theory across Domain-Specific Outcomes: The Domain-Specific Resilient Systems Scales." *Assessment* 26(8):1444–61.

Maltseva, Kateryna. 2016. "Prosocial Morality in Individual and Collective Cognition." *Journal of Cognition & Culture* 16(1–2):1–36.

Manassis, Katharina. 2017. *Developing Empathy: A Biopsychosocial Approach to Understanding Compassion for Therapists and Parents*. New York, NY: Routledge.

Mancini, Anthony D., Gabriele Prati, and George A. Bonanno. 2011. "Do Shattered Worldviews Lead to Complicated Grief? Prospective and Longitudinal Analyses." *Journal of Social & Clinical Psychology* 30(2):184–215.

Mandel, Tobey, David M. Dunkley, and Claire J. Starrs. 2018. "Self-Critical Perfectionism, Daily Interpersonal Sensitivity, and Stress Generation: A Four-Year Longitudinal Study." *Journal of Psychopathological Behavioral Assessment* 40(4):701–13.

Mangion, Claude. 2011. *Philosophical Approaches to Communication*. Bristol, UK: Intellect.

Manglos-Weber, Nicolette D. and Jade Avelis. 2019. "Expanding the Reflexive Space: Resilient Young Adults, Institutional Cultures, and Cognitive Schemas." *Sociological Forum* 34(3):664–84.

Manners, John, and Kevin Durkin. 2000. "Processes Involved in Adult Ego Development: A Conceptual Framework." *Developmental Review* 20(4):475–513.

Manning, Lydia K. 2014. "Enduring as Lived Experience: Exploring the Essence of Spiritual Resilience for Women in Late Life." *Journal of Religious Health* 53:352–362.

Manning, Matthew, Christopher M. Fleming, and Christopher L. Ambrey. 2016. "Life Satisfaction and Individual Willingness to Pay for Crime Reduction." *Regional Studies* 50(12):2024–39.

Manroveli, Stella, K.V. Petrides, Carolien Rieffe, and Femke Bakker. 2007. "Trait Emotional Intelligence, Psychological Well-being and Peer-reported Social Competence in Adolescence." *British Journal of Developmental Psychology* 25:263–275.

Mansfield, Nick. 2000. *Subjectivity: Theories of the Self from Freud to Haraway*. New York, NY: New York University Press.

Manturuk, Kim, Mark Lindblad, and Roberto Quercia. 2010. "Friends and Neighbors: Homeownership and Social Capital among Low- to Moderate-Income Families." *Journal of Urban Affairs* 32(4):471–488.

Maoz, Ifat. 2018. "Intergroup Contact in Settings of Protracted Ethnopolitical Conflict." Pp. 353–355 in *The Oxford Handbook of Social Psychology*, edited by Philip L. Hammack. New York, NY: Oxford University Press.

Mapelli, Vittorio. 1993. "Health Needs, Demand for Health Services and Expenditure across Social Groups in Italy: An Empirical Investigation." *Social Science & Medicine* 36(8):999–1009.

Marchetti, Igor, Jason Shumake, Ivan Grahek, and Ernst H. W. Koster. 2018. "Temperamental Factors in Remitted Depression: The Role of Effortful Control and Attentional Mechanisms." *Journal of Affective Disorders* 235:499–505.

Marcia, James E. 1980. "Identity in Adolescence." *Pp. 159–187 in (Ed.), Handbook of Adolescent Psychology,* edited by Joseph Adelson. New York, NY: Wiley.

Marcks, Brook A. and Douglas W. Woods. 2007. "Role of Thought-Related Beliefs and Coping Strategies in the Escalation of Intrusive Thoughts: An Analog to Obsessive-Compulsive Disorder." *Behaviour Research & Therapy* 45(11):2640–51.

Marcum, Christopher Steven. 2013. "Age Differences in Daily Social Activities." *Research on Aging* 35(5):612–640.

Marcus, George E., W. Russell Neuman, and Michael MacKuen. 2000. *Affective Intelligence and Political Judgment*. Chicago, IL: University of Chicago Press.

Marcus, Paul 2014. *They Shall Beat Their Swords into Plowshares: Military Strategy, Psychoanalysis and the Art of Living*. Milwaukee, WI: Marquette University Press.

Marien, Sofie, and Marc Hooghe. 2011. "Does Political Trust Matter? An Empirical Investigation into The Relation Between Political Trust and Support for Law Compliance." *European Journal of Political Research* 50(2):267–291.

Mark, Noah P. 2018. "Status Organizes Cooperation: An Evolutionary Theory of Status and Social Order." *American Journal of Sociology* 123(6):1601–34.

Markey, Patrick M., David C. Funder, and Daniel J. Ozer. 2003. "Complementarity of Interpersonal Behaviors in Dyadic Interactions." *Personality & Social Psychology Bulletin* 29(9):1082–1090.

Markiewicz, Dorothy, Anna Beth Doyle, and Mara Brendgen. 2001. "The Quality of Adolescents" Friendships: Associations with Mothers" Interpersonal Relationships, Attachments to Parents and Friends, and Prosocial Behaviors." *Journal of Adolescence* 24(4):429–445.

Markowitz, Fred E. 2001. "Modeling Processes in Recovery from Mental Illness: Relationships between Symptoms, Life Satisfaction, and Self-concept." *Journal of Health & Social Behavior* 42(1):64–79.

Marks, Nadine F., Larry L. Bumpass, and Heyjung Jun. 2004. "Family Roles and Well-being during the Middle Life Course." Pp. 514–549 in *How Healthy Are We: A National Study of Well-being at Midlife*, edited by Orville Gilbert Brim, Carol D. Ryff and Ronald C. Kessler. Chicago, IL: University of Chicago Press.

Marks, Ronald, Douglas W. Vorhies, and Gordon J. Badovick. 1996. "A Psychometric Evaluation of the ADAPTS Scale: A Critique and Recommendations." *Journal of Personal Selling & Sales Management* 16(4):53–65.

Markstrom, Carol A., Sheila K. Marshall, and Robin J. Tryon. 2000. "Resiliency, Social Support, and Coping in Rural Low-Income Appalachian Adolescents from Two Racial Groups." *Journal of Adolescence* 23(6):693–703.

Marmot, Michael G., and Rebecca Fuhrer. 2004. "Socioeconomic Position and Health across Midlife." Pp. 64–89 in *How Healthy Are We: A National Study of Well-being at Midlife*, edited by Orville Gilbert Brim, Carol D. Ryff and Ronald C. Kessler. Chicago, IL: University of Chicago Press.

Marquis, Andre, Kathryn Z. Douthit, and Ari J. Elliot. 2011. "Best Practices: A Critical yet Inclusive Vision for the Counseling Profession." *Journal of Counseling & Development* 89:397–405.

Marschall, Melissa J., and Dietlind Stolle. 2004. "Race and the City: Neighborhood Context and Development of Generalized Trust." *Political Behavior* 26(2):125–153.

Marsh, Berbert W., K.T. Hau, R.Y.T. Sung, and C.W. Yu. 2007. "Childhood Obesity, Gender, Actual-ideal Body Image, Discrepancies, and Physical Self-concept in Hong Kong Children: Cultural Differences in the Value of Moderation." *Developmental Psychology* 43(3):647–662.

Marsh, Dylan R. and Bryan J. Dik. 2021. "Beyond-the-Self Callings: The Role of a Transcendent Summons for Undergraduates and Working Adults." *Journal of Career Assessment* 29(4):570–88.

Marsh, Herbert W. 1993. "The Effects of Participation in Sport during the Last Two Years of High School." *Sociology of Sport Journal* 10:18–43.

Marshall, Douglas A. 2002. "Behavior, Belonging, and Belief: A Theory of Ritual Practice." *Sociological Theory* 20(3):360–380.

Marshall, Nancy L. 2001. "Health and Illness Issues Facing an Aging Workforce in the New Millennium." *Sociological Spectrum* 21(3):431–439.

Martela, Frank and Richard M. Ryan. 2016. "The Benefits of Benevolence: Basic Psychological Needs, Beneficence, and the Enhancement of Well-Being." *Journal of Personality* 84(6):750–64.

Martela, Frank, and Tapani J. J. Riekki. 2018. "Autonomy, Competence, Relatedness, and Beneficence: A Multicultural Comparison of the Four Pathways to Meaningful Work." *Frontiers in Psychology* 9:01157.

Marti, Joel, Mireia Bolíbar, and Carlos Lozares. 2017. "Network Cohesion and Social Support." *Social Networks* 48:192–201.

Martin, John Levi, James P. Murphy, and Rick Moore. 2018. "Protest Movements and Citizen Discontent: Occupy Wall Street and the Tea Party." *Sociological Forum* 33(3):575–95.

Martin, Meredith J., Melissa L. Sturge-Apple, Patrick T. Davies, Christine V. Romero and Abigail Buckholz. 2017. "A Process Model of the Implications of Spillover from Coparenting Conflicts into the Parent-child Attachment Relationship in Adolescence." *Development & Psychopathology* 29(2):417–431

Martin, Michelle E. 2012. "Philosophical and Religious Influences on Social Welfare Policy in the United States: The Ongoing Effect of Reformed Theology and Social Darwinism on Attitudes toward the Poor and Social Welfare Policy and Practice." *Journal of Social Work* 12(1):51–64.

Martin, Rod A. 2007. The Psychology of Humor: An Integrative Approach. Burlington, MA: Elsevier.

Martin, Rod A., Patricia Puhlik-Doris, Gwen Larsen, Jeanette Gray, and Kelly Weir. 2003. "Individual Differences in Uses of Humor and Their Reaction to Psychological Well-being: Development of the Humor Styles Questionnaire." *Journal of Research in Personality* 37:48–75.

Martin, Sam. 2016. "How Can You Be Strong All the Time? Discourses of Stoicism in the First Counselling Session of Young Male Clients." *Counselling & Psychotherapy Research* 16(2):100–08.

Martin, Teresa J., Susan Holtzman, and Anita DeLongis. 2007. "Coping and the Response of Others." *Journal of Social & Personal Relationships* 24(6):951–969.

Martin, Virginia. 2000. "The Effect of Neighborhood Racial Heterogeneity and Income Inequality on the Level of Home Ownership." *Research in Community Sociology* 10:345–362.

Martin, William E., Jr., Jody L. Swartz-Kulstad, and Michael Madson. 1999. "Psychosocial Factors that Predict the College Adjustment of First-year Undergraduate Students: Implications for College Counselors." *Journal of College Counseling* 2(2):121–133.

Martinez-Marti, María Luisa, and Willibald Ruch. 2017. "Character Strengths Predict Resilience over and above Positive Affect, Self-Efficacy, Optimism, Social Support, Self-Esteem, and Life Satisfaction." *Journal of Positive Psychology* 12(2):110–19.

Marx, Paul. 2014. "Labour Market Risks and Political Preferences: The Case of Temporary Employment." *European Journal of Political Research* 53(1):136–159.

Marzana, Daniela, Elena Marta, and Maura Pozzi. 2012. "Social Action in Young Adults: Voluntary and Political Engagement." *Journal of Adolescence* 35(3):497–507.

Mascaro, Nathan, and David H. Rosen. 2005. "Existential Meaning's Role in the Enhancement of Hope and Prevention of Depressive Symptoms." *Journal of Personality* 73(4):985–1014.

Maslach, Christina, Wilmar B. Schaufeli, and Michael P. Leiter. 2001. "Job Burnout," *Annual Review of Psychology* 52.397–422.

Massengale, Kelley E. C., Alice Ma, Kelly L. Rulison, Jeffrey J. Milroy, David L. Wyrick. 2017. "Perceived Norms and Alcohol Use Among First-Year College Student-Athletes" Different Types of Friends." *Journal of American College Health* 65(1):32–40.

Massey, Garth, Randy Hodson, and Dusko Sekulic. 2003. "Nationalism, Liberalism and Liberal Nationalism In Post-War Croatia." *Nations & Nationalism* 9(1):55–82.

Mastain, Lisa. 2007. "A Phenomenological Investigation of Altruism as Experienced by Moral Exemplars." *Journal of Phenomenological Psychology* 38:62–99.

Masten, Ann S. 2014. *Ordinary Magic: Resilience in Development*. New York, NY: Guilford.

Masten, Ann S., Glenn I. Roisman, Jeffrey D. Long, Keith B. Burt, Jelena Obradovic, Jennifer R. Riley, Kristen Boelcke-Stesnes, and Auke Tellgen. 2005. "Developmental Cascade: Linking Academic Achievement and Externalizing and Internalizing Symptoms over 20 Years." *Developmental Psychology* 41(5):733–746.

Masten, Ann S., J. J. Cutuli, Janette E. Herbers, and Marie Gabrielle J. Read. 2009. "Resilience in Development." Pp. 117–131 in *Oxford Handbook of Positive Psychology*, edited by C. R. Synder and Shane J. Lopez. New York, NY: Oxford University Press.

Masters, Stephanie Laura, and Amy Roberson Hayes. 2020. "Pathways among Masculinity, Femininity, and Health Behaviors in Emerging Adulthood." *Current Psychology* 41(5):2848–59.

Mata, Fernando, and Ravi Pendakur. 2014. "Social Capital, Diversity and Giving or Receiving Help Among Neighbours." *Social Indicators Research* 118(1):329–347.

Mathis, Arlesia, Ronica Rooks, and Daniel Kruger. 2016. "Improving the Neighborhood Environment for Urban Older Adults: Social Context and Self-Rated Health." *International Journal of Environmental Research and Public Health* 13(3):1–13.

Matsueda, Ross L., and Maria S. Grigoryeva. 2014. "Social Inequality, Crime, and Deviance." Pp. 683–714 in *Handbook of the Social Psychology of Inequality*, edited by Jane D. McLeod, Edward J. Lawler, and Michael Schwalbe. Dordrecht, Netherlands: Springer.

Matsuo, Makoto. 2020. "The Role of Work Authenticity in Linking Strengths Use to Career Satisfaction and Proactive Behavior: A Two-Wave Study." *Career Development International* 25(6):617–30.

Matthewman, Steve. 2011. *Technology and Social Theory*. Houndmills, Palgrave.

Matthews, Gerald, Amanda K. Emo, Gregory Funke, Moshe Zeidner, Richard D. Roberts, Paul T. Costa, and Ralf Schulze. 2006. "Emotional Intelligence, Personality, and Task-Induced Stress." *Journal of Experimental Psychology: Applied* 12(2):96–107.

Matthews, Gerald, Moshe Zeidner, and Richard D. Roberts. 2012. *Emotional Intelligence*. New York: Springer.

Matthews, Gerald. 1997. "An Introduction to the Cognitive Science of Personality and Emotion." Pp. 3–30 in *Cognitive Science Perspectives on Personality and Emotion*, edited by Gerald Matthews. Amsterdam, Netherlands: Elsevier.

Matts, Jacqueline S., Wizdom Powell Hammond, Nyusha Grayman, Meredith Bonacci-William Brennan, Sheri-Ann Cowie, and Lina Ladyzhenskaya, and Sara So. 2009. "The Social Production of Altruism: Motivations for Caring Action in a Low-income Urban Community." *American Journal of Community Psychology* 43:71–84.

Matusitz, Jonathan. 2017. "Martyrdom as a Result of Psychosocial Resilience: The Case of Palestinian Suicide Terrorists." Pp. 285–295 in *The Routledge International Handbook of Psychosocial Resilience*, edited by Updesh Kumar. Abingdon, UK: Routledge.

Mau, Steffen. 2005a. "Democratic Demand for a Social Europe? Preferences of the European Citizenry." *International Journal of Social Welfare* 14:76–85.

Maule, Linda S., and Robert K. Goidel. 2003. "Adultery, Drugs, and Sex: An Experimental Investigation of Individual Reactions to Unethical Behavior by Public Officials." *Social Science Journal* 40:65–78.

Maume, David J. 2006. "Gender Differences in Taking Vacation Time." *Work & Occupations* 33(2):161–190.

Maxwell, Jessica A., Stephanie S. Spielmann, Samantha Joel, and Geoff Macdonald. 2013. "Attachment Theory as a Framework for Understanding Responses to Social Exclusion." *Social & Personality Psychology Compass* 7(7):444–456.

Maybery, D.J., Jenny Jones-. Jason Neale, and Alexandra Arentz. 2006. "The Positive Event Scale: Measuring Uplift Frequency and Intensity in an Adult Sample." *Social Indicators Research* 78:61–83.

Mayer, John D., Peter Salovey, and David R. Caruso. 2004. "Emotional Intelligence: Theory, Findings, and Implications." *Psychological Inquiry* 15(3):197–215.

Mayer, John D., Peter Salovey, and David R. Caruso. 2008. "Emotional Intelligence: New Ability or Eclectic Traits?" *American Psychologist* 63(6):503–517.

Mayer, Margit. 2003. "The Onward Sweep of Social Capital: Causes and Consequences for Understanding Cities, Communities and Urban Movements." *International Journal of Urban & Regional Research* 27(1):110–132.

Maypole, Joanne, and Timothy Gray Davies. 2001. "Students" Perceptions of Constructivist Learning in a Community College." American History II." *Community College Review* 29(2):54–79.

Mayrl, Damon, and Jeremy E. Uecker. 2011. “Higher Education and Religious Liberalization among Young Adults.” *Social Forces* 90(1):181–208.

Mazumdar, Shampa, and Sanjoy Mazumdar. 2004. “Religion and Place Attachment: A Study of Sacred Places.” *Journal of Environmental Psychology* 24(3):385–397.

Mazziotta, Agostino, Amélie Mummendey, and Stephen C. Wright. 2011. “Vicarious Intergroup Contact Effects.” *Group Processes & Intergroup Relations* 14(2):255–74.

Mbiba, Monicah, Mark Collinson, Lori Hunter and Wayne Twine. 2019. “Social Capital Is Subordinate to Natural Capital in Buffering Rural Livelihoods from Negative Shocks: Insights from Rural South Africa.” *Journal of Rural Studies* 65:12–21.

McBride, Duane C., Holly Van Buren, Yvonne M. Terry, and Burton J. Goldstein. 2000. “Depression, Drug Use, and Health Service Need, Utilization, and Cost.” *Advances in Medical Sociology* 7:67–99.

McCabe, Brian J. 2012. “Homeownership and Social Trust in Neighbors.” *City & Community* 11(4):389–408.

McCabe, Brian J. 2014. “Are Homeowners Better Citizens? Homeownership and Community Participation in the United States.” *Social Forces* 91(3):929–954.

McCarthy, Lauren P., Jennifer L. Siegel, and Orrin D. Ware. 2022. “Supporting Social Work Field Instructors: Empowerment as a Strategy for Preventing Burnout.” *Journal of Social Work* 22(5):1153–69.

McCarthy, Mary B., Alan M. Collins, Sarah Jane Flaherty, and Sinead N. McCarthy. 2017. “Healthy Eating Habit: A Role for Goals, Identity, and Self-Control?” *Psychology & Marketing* 34(8):772–85.

McCarthy, Wanda C., and Irene Hanson Frieze. 1999. “Negative Aspects of Therapy: Client Perceptions of Therapists” Social Influence, Burnout, and Quality of Care.” *Journal of Social Issues* 55(1):33–50.

McCay, Elizabeth, Celina Carter, Andria Aiello, Susan Quesnel, John Langley, Steven Hwang, Heather Beanlands, Linda Cooper, Carol Howes, Bjorn Johansson, Bruce MacLaurin, Jean Hughes, and Jeff Karabanow. 2015. “Dialectical Behavior Therapy as a Catalyst For Change in Street-Involved Youth: A Mixed Methods Study.” *Children & Youth Services Review* 58:187–199.

McClaran, Nikki, Nancy Rhodes, and Shay Xucjing Yao. 2022. “Trust and Coping Beliefs Contribute to Racial Disparities in Covid-19 Vaccination Intention.” *Health Communication* 37(12):1457–64.

McClemon, James 2013. “Cognitive Resource Depletion and the Ritual Healing Theory.” *Religion, Brain & Behavior* 3(1):71–73.

McClendon, McKee J. 1991. “Acquiescence and Recency Response-order Effects in Interview Surveys.” *Sociological Methods & Research* 20(1):60–103.

McClurg, Scott D. 2006. “The Electoral Resources of Political Talk: Examining Disagreement and Expertise Effects in Social Networks on Political Participation.” *American Journal of Political Science* 50(3):737–754.

McCormack, Teresa, and Aidan Feeney. 2015. “The Development of the Experience and Anticipation of Regret.” *Cognition & Emotion* 29(2):266–280.

McCormick, Meghan P., Erin E. O¡¯Connor, and Sophie P. Barnes. 2016. “Mother-child Attachment Styles and Math and Reading Skills in Middle Childhood. The Mediating Role of Children’s Exploration and Engagement.” *Early Childhood Research Quarterly* 36:295–306.

McCray, Janet, Adam Palmer, and Nik Chmiel. 2016. “Building Resilience in Health and Social Care Teams.” *Personnel Review* 45(6):1132–1155.

McCullars, Adrianne, Fallon J. Richie, Jeffrey J. Klibert, and Jennifer Langhinrichsen-Rohling. 2021. “What’s So Funny? Adaptive Versus Maladaptive Humor Styles as Mediators between Early Maladaptive Schemas and Resilience.” *Humor* 34(1):93–111.

McDonald, Matthew and Stephen Wearing. 2013. *Soc8ial Ps6ychology and Theories of Consumer Culture: A Political Economy Perspective.* Hove, UL: Routledge.

McDougall, Janette, David J. DeWit, Gillian King, Linda T. Miller, and Steve Killip. 2004. "High School-aged Youths" Attitudes toward Their Peers with Disabilities: The Role of School and Student Interpersonal Factors." *International Journal of Disability, Development & Education* 51(3):288–313.

McDowell, Michael and Nathan Robert Brown. 2009. *World Religions: At Your Fingertips*. New York, NY: Alpha.

McEachan, Rosemary, Natalie Taylor, Reema Harrison, Rebecca Lawton, Peter Gardner, and Mark Conner. 2016. "Meta-Analysis of the Reasoned Action Approach (Raa) to Understanding Health Behaviors." *Annals of Behavioral Medicine* 50(4):592–612.

McFarland, Cathy, Roger Buehler, Rebecca von Ruti, Lewis Nguyen, and Celeste Alvaro. 2007. "The Impact Of Negative Moods On Self-Enhancing Cognitions: The Role Of Reflective Versus Ruminative Mood Orientations." *Journal of Personality & Social Psychology* 93(5):728–750.

McFarland, Daniel A., Dan Turafsky, and Craig Rawlings. 2013. "Making the Connection: Social Bonding in Courtship Situations." *American Journal of Sociology* 118(6):1596–1649.

McFee, Graham. 2004. *Sport, Rules and Values: Philosophical Investigations into the Nature of Sport*. Abingdon, UK: Routledge.

McGhee, Derek. 2003. "Moving to Our Common Ground: A Critical Examination of Community Cohesion Discourse in Twenty-First Century Britain." *Sociological Review* 51(3):376–404.

McGinley, Meredith and Alexandria M. Evans. 2020. "Parent and/or Peer Attachment? Predicting Emerging Adults" Prosocial Behaviors and Internalizing Symptomatology." *Journal of Child & Family Studies* 29(7):1833–44.

McGurk, Dennis, and Carl Andrew Castro. 2010. "Courage in Combat." Pp. 167–185 in the *Psychology of Courage: Modern Research on an Ancient Virtue*, edited by Cynthia L.S. Pury and Bhane J. Lopez. Washington, DC: American Psychological Association.

McIlveen, Peter. 2015. "Psychotherapy, Counseling, and Career Counseling." Pp. 403–417 in *APA Handbook of Career Intervention, Vol: Foundations*, edited by Paul J. Hartung, Mark L. Savickas, and W. Bruce Walsh. Washington, DC: American Psychological Association.

McIntosh, John L., John F. Santos, Richard W. Hubbard., and James C. Overholser. 1994. *Elder Suicide: Research, Theory, and Treatment*. Washington, DC: American Psychological Association.

McIntyre, Kevin P., Brent A. Mattingly, Sarah C. E. Stanton, Xiaomeng Xu, Timothy J. Loving, and Gary W. Lewandowski. 2023. "Romantic Relationships and Mental Health: Investigating the Role of Self-Expansion on Depression Symptoms." *Journal of Social & Personal Relationships* 40(1):3–28.

McKay, Samuel, Jason L. Skues, and Ben J. Williams. 2018. "With Risk May Come Reward: Sensation Seeking Supports Resilience through Effective Coping." *Personality & Individual Differences* 121:100–105.

McKie, John, Jeff Richardson, Peter Singer, and Helga Kuhse. 1998. The Allocation of Health Care Resources: An Ethical Evaluation of the "QALY" Approach. Aldershot, UK: Ashgate.

McKnight, D. Harrison, and Norman L. Chervany. 2006. "Reflection on an Initial Trust-building Model." Pp. 29–51 in *Handbook of Trust Research*, edited by Reinhard Bachmann and Akbar Zaheer. Cheltenham, UK: Elgar.

McLaren, Lauren M. 2003. "Anti-immigrant Prejudice in Europe: Contact, Threat Perception, and Preferences for the Exclusion of Migrants." *Social Forces* 81(3):909–930.

McLaren, Rachel M., and Denise Haunami Solomon. 2015. "Relational Framing Theory: Drawing Inferences about Relationships from Interpersonal Interactions." Pp. 115–127 in *Engaging Theories in Interpersonal Communication: Multiple Perspectives*, edited by Dawn O. Braithwaite and Paul Schrodt. Thousand Oaks, CA: SAGE.

McLeod, John. 2012. "Narrative Therapy." Pp. 379–382 in *The SAGE Handbook of Counselling and Psychotherapy*, edited by Colin Feltham and Ian Horton. London: SAGE.

McMahon, Sarah, N. Andrew Peterson, Samantha C. Winter, Jane E. Palmer, Judy L. Postmus, and Ruth Anne Koenick. 2015. "Predicting Bystander Behavior to Prevent Sexual Assault on

College Campuses: The Role of Self-Efficacy and Intent." *American Journal of Community Psychology* 56(1–2):46–56.
McManus, Ruth. 2017. "The Sociology of Death and Dying." Pp. 256–262 in *The Cambridge Handbook of Sociology, Vol. 2: Specialty and Interdisciplinary Studies*, edited by Kathleen Odell Korgen. New York, NY: Cambridge University Press.
McMullin, Julie Ann, and John Cairney. 2004. "Self-esteem and the Intersection of Age, Class, and Gender." *Journal of Aging Studies* 18(1):75–90.
McMunn, Anne M., James Y. Nazroo, Michael G. Marmot, Richard Boreham, and Robert Goodman. 2001. "Children's Emotion and Behavioral Well-being and the Family Environment: Findings from the Health Survey for England." *Social Science & Medicine* 53:423–440.
McNeal, Ralph B., Jr. 1997. "High School Dropouts: A Closer Examination of School Effects." *Social Science Quarterly* 78(1):209–222.
McNeal, Ralph B., Jr. 1999. "Participation in High School Extracurricular Activities: Investigating School Effects." *Social Science Quarterly* 80(2):291–309.
McNeeley, Susan and Yue Yuan. 2017. "A Multilevel Examination of the Code of the Street's Relationship with Fear of Crime." *Crime & Delinquency* 63(9):1146–1167.
McNeill, Donald. 2014. "Airports and Territorial Restructuring: The Case of Hong Kong." *Urban Studies* 51(14):2996–3010.
McNicholas, J., and G. M. Collis. 2001. "Children's Representations of Pets in Their Social Networks." *Child: Care, Health & Development* 27(3):279–294.
McPherson, Miller, Lynn Smith-Lovin, and Matthew E. Brashears. 2006. "Social Isolation in America: Changes in Core Discussion Networks over Two Decades." *American Sociological Review* 71(3):353–375.
McVicar, Duncan, and Arnold Polanski. 2014. "Peer Effects in UK Adolescent Substance Use: Never Mind the Classmates?" *Oxford Bulletin of Economics & Statistics* 26(4):589–604.
McWhirter, Ellen Hawley. 1994. *Counseling for Empowerment*. Alexandra, VA: American Counseling Association.
McWilliams, Nancy. 2011. Psychoanalytic Diagnosis: Understanding Personality Structure in the Clinical Process. New York: Guilford.
Meadows, Chris M. 2014. A Psychological Perspective on Joy and Emotional Fulfillment. New York: NY: Routledge.
Medai, Evelyn and Charles N. Noussair. 2021. "Positive Emotion and Honesty." *Frontiers in Psychology* 12:694841.
Medvedovski, Dmitri, and Kirk Allison. 2017. "Paternal Religious Affiliation and Practice in Lithuania: Spiritual Goods or Secular Utilities?". *International Journal of Social Economics* 44(12):1758–1777.
Meeus, Wim Jurjen Iedema, Gerard Maassena, and Rutger Engels. 2005. "Separation-individuation Revisited: on the Interplay of Parent-Adolescent Relations, Identity and Emotional Adjustment in Adolescence." *Journal of Adolescence* 28(1):89–106.
Meeus, Wim, Annereke, Oosterwegel, and Wilma Vollebergh. 2002. "Parental and Peer Attachment and Identity Development in Adolescence." *Journal of Adolescence* 25:93–106.
Meeus, Wim. 2019. *Adolescent Development: Longitudinal Research into the Self, Personal Relationships, and Psychopathology*. Abingdon, UK: Routledge.
Meeusen, Cecil, Thomas de Vroome, and Marc Hooghe. 2013. "How Does Education Have an Impact on Ethnocentrism? A Structural Equation Analysis of Cognitive, Occupational Status and Network Mechanisms." *International Journal of Intercultural Relations* 37(5):507–522.
Mehlsen, Mimi, Merete Platz, and Pia Fromholt. 2003. "Life Justification across the Life Course: Evaluations of the Most and Least Satisfying Decades of Life." *International Journal of Aging & Human Development* 57(3):217–236.
Mehmood, Anam, Rubina Hanif, and Irum Noureen. 2020. "Influence of Trait-Patience in Goal Pursuit and Subjective Well-Being among University Students." *Pakistan Journal of Psychological Research* 35(4):707–23.

Mehrabian, Albert. 2000. "Beyond IQ: Broad-based Measurement of Individual Success Potential or Empirical Intelligence." *Genetic, Social, & General Psychology Monographs* 126(2):123–239.

Mei, Mei, Fu Yang, and Mingfeng Tang. 2021. "Does Practice Enhance Adaptability? The Role of Personality Trait, Supervisor Behavior, and Career Development Training" *Frontiers in Psychology* 11:594791.

Mele, Domenec. 2010. "The Practice of Networking: An Ethical Approach." *Journal of Business Ethics* 90:487–503.

Melrose, Margaret. 2002. "Labour Pains: Some Considerations on the Difficulties of Researching Juvenile Prostitution." *International Journal of Social Research Methodology* 5(4):333–351.

Melton, Laura M. 2016. "If I Don't Laugh, I'll Cry: Exploring Humor Coping in Breast Cancer." *Journal of Psychosocial Oncology* 34(6):530–541

Melzer, Silvia Maja. 2011. "Does Migration Make You Happy? The Influence of Migration on Subjective Well-being." *Journal of Social Research & Policy* 2(2):73–92.

Menard, A. Dana, and Alia Offman. 2009. "The Interrelationships between Sexual Self-Esteem, Sexual Assertiveness and Sexual Satisfaction." *Canadian Journal of Human Sexuality* 18(1–2):35–45.

Menard, Scott, and Barbara J. Mose. 1984. "A Structuralist Critique of the IQ-Delinquency Hypotheses: Theory and Evidence." *American Journal of Sociology* 89:1347–1378.

Menard, Scott. 1995. "A Developmental Test of Mertonian Anomie Theory." *Journal of Research in Crime and Delinquency* 32(2):136–174.

Menec, Verena H., and Judith G. Chipperfield. 1997. "Remaining Active in Later Life: The Role of Locus of Control in Seniors Leisure Activity Participation, Health, and Life Satisfaction." *Journal of Aging & Health* 9(1):105–125.

Menesini, Ersilia, Elena Codecasa, Beatrice Benelli, and Helen Cowie. 2003. "Enhancing Children's Responsibility to Take Action against Bullying: Evaluation of a Befriending Intervention in Italian Middle Schools." *Aggressive Behavior* 29(1):1–14.

Meng, Tianguang, and He Chen. 2014. "A Multilevel Analysis of Social Capital and Self-Rated Health: Evidence From China." *Health & Place* 27:38–44.

Merolla, Andy J. 2014. "Forgive Like You Mean It: Sincerity of Forgiveness and the Experience of Negative Affect." *Communication Quarterly* 62(1):36–56.

Merrell, Kenneth W. 2009. "Linking Prevention Science and Social and Emotional Learning: The Oregon Resiliency Project." *Psychology in the Schools* 47(1):55–70.

Mesch, Gustavo S. 2009. "Social Bonds and Internet Pornographic Exposure among Adolescents." *Journal of Adolescence* 32:601–618.

Mesch, Gustavo S., and Orit Manor. 1998. "Social Ties, Environmental Perception, and Local Attachment." *Environment & Behavior* 30(4):504–519.

Mesirow, Jack. 2003. "Transformative Learning as Discourse." *Journal of Transformative Education* 1(1):58–63.

Messner, Steven F., Helmut Thome, and Richard Rosenfeld. 2008. "Institutions, Anomie, and Violent Crime: Clarifying and Elaborating Institutional-anomie Theory." *International Journal of Conflict & Violence* 2(2):163–181.

Messner, Steven F., Richard Rosenfeld, and Susanna Karstedt. 2013. "Social Institutions and Crime." Pp. 405–423 in *The Oxford Handbook of Criminological Theory*, edited by Francis T. Cullen and Pamela Wilcox. New York: Oxford University Press.

Mestre, Maria Vicenta, Gustavo Carlo, Paula Samper, Elizabeth Malonda, and Ana Llorca Mestre. 2019. "Bidirectional Relations among Empathy-Related Traits, Prosocial Moral Reasoning, and Prosocial Behaviors." *Social Development* 28(3):514–528.

Mesurado, Belén, María José Distefano, Gabriela Robiolo, and María Cristina Richaud. 2018. "The Hero Program: Development and Initial Validation of an Intervention Program to Promote Prosocial Behavior in Adolescents." *Journal of Social & Personal Relationships* 36(8):2566–2584.

Metzl, Einat S., and Malissa A. Morrell. 2008. "The Role of Creativity in Models of Resilience: Theoretical Exploration and Practical Applications." *Journal of Creativity in Mental Health* 3(3):303–318.

Meulemann, Heiner. 2010. "Self-concern, Self-transcendence, and Well-being." *European Sociological Review* 26(4):385–399.

Mevarech, Zemira R. and Ditza Maskit. 2015. "The Teaching Experience and the Emotions It Evokes." *Social Psychology of Education* 18(2):241–53.

Mewes, Jan, Malcolm Fairbrother, Giuseppe Nicola Giordano, Cary Wu, and Rima Wilkes. 2021. "Experiences Matter: A Longitudinal Study of Individual-Level Sources of Declining Social Trust in the United States." *Social Science Research* 95:102537.

Meyer, Ilan H., and David M. Frost. 2013. "Minority Stress and the Health of Sexual Minorities." Pp. 252–266 in *Handbook of Psychology and Sexual Orientation*, edited by Charlotte J. Patterson and Anthony R. D'Augelli. New York: Oxford University Press.

Meyerson, Denise. 1991. *False Consciousness*. Oxford: Clarendon Press.

Mgbeoji, Ikechi. 2006. "The Civilised Self and the Barbaric Other: Imperial Delusions of Order and the Challenges of Human Security." *Third World Quarterly* 27(5):855–869.

Mialet, Helene. 2012. *Hawking Incorporated: Stephen Hawking and the Anthropology of the Knowing Subject*. Chicago, IL: University of Chicago Press.

Miao, Shanshan, Wim Heijman, Xueqin Zhu, Dan Qiao, and Qian Lu. 2018. "Income Groups, Social Capital, and Collective Action on Small-Scale Irrigation Facilities: A Multigroup Analysis Based on a Structural Equation Model." *Rural Sociology* 83(4):882–911.

Michael, John, Luke McEllin and Annalena Felber. 2020. "Prosocial Effects of Coordination – What, How and Why?" *Acta Psychologica* 207:103083.

Michael, Scott T., Julia D. Taylor, and Jen Cheavens. 2000. "Hope Theory as Applied to Brief Treatments: Problem-solving and Soution-focused Therapies." Pp. 151–166 in *Handbook of Hope: Theory, Measures, Applications*, edited by C.R. Snyder. San Diego, CA: Academic.

Michaeli, Yossi, Daniel J. Dickson, Maor Kalfon Hakhmigari, Miri Scharf, and Shmuel Shulman. 2022. "Change in Self-Criticism across Emerging Adulthood and Psychological Well-Being at Age 35: The Mediating Role of Reflectivity." *Emerging Adulthood* 10(2):323–34.

Michalos, Alex C., Bruno D. Zumbo, and Anita Hubley. 2000. "Health and the Quality of Life." *Social Indicators Research* 51:245–286.

Michalski, Joseph H. 2005. "Explaining Intimate Partner Violence: The Sociological Limitation of Victimization Studies." *Sociological Forum* 20(4):623–640.

Mickler, Charlotte, and Ursula M. Staudinger. 2008. "Personal Wisdom: Validation and Age-related Differences of a Performance Measure." *Psychology & Aging* 23(4):787–799.

Midlarsky, Elizabeth, and Eva Kahana. 1994. *Altruism in Late Life*. Thousand Oaks, CA: Sage.

Midtgaard, Julie, Reinhard Stelter, Mikael Rorth, and Lis Admsen. 2007. "Regaining a Sense of Agency and Shared Self-reliance: The Experience of Advanced Disease Cancer Patients Participating in a Multidimensional Exercise Intervention While Undergoing Chemotherapy: Analysis of Patient Diaries." *Scandinavian Journal of Psychology* 48:181–190.

Migerode, Femke, Bea Maes, Ann Buysse, and Ruben Brondeel. 2012. "Quality of Life in Adolescents with a Disability and Their Parents: The Mediating Role of Social Support and Resilience." *Journal of Developmental & Physical Disabilities* 24(5):487–503.

Miglietta, Anna, Stefano Tartaglia, and Barbara Loera. 2018. "Personal Values and the Acceptance of Immigrants: Why National Identification Matters." *International Journal of Social Psychology* 33(3):682–714.

Miguel, Maria L. Mondolfi and Margarita Pino-Juste. 2021. "Therapeutic Achievements of a Program Based on Drama Therapy, the Theater of the Oppressed, and Psychodrama with Women Victims of Intimate Partner Violence." *Violence Against Women* 27(9):1273–96.

Mikula, Gerold, Bernhard Riederer, and Otto Bodi. 2012. "Perceived Justice in The Division of Domestic Labor: Actor and Partner Effects." *Personal Relationships* 19(4):680–695.

Mikula, Gerold, Dominik Schoebi, Sonja Jagoditsch, and Silvia Macher. 2009. "Roots and Correlates of Perceived Injustice in the Division of Family Work." *Personal Relationships* 16(4):553–574.

Mikulincer, Mario, and Michal Selinger. 2001. "The Interplay between Attachment and Affiliation Systems in Adolescents" Same-Sex Friendships: The Role of Attachment Style." *Journal of Social & Personal Relationships* 18(1):81–106.

Mikulincer, Mario, and Phillip R. Shaver. 2014. "An Attachment Perspective on Resilience to Stress and Trauma." Pp. 156–168 in *The Resilience Handbook: Approaches to Stress and Trauman*, edited by Martha Kent, Mary C. Davis and John W. Reich. New York: NY: Routledge.

Mikulincer, Mario, Victor Florian, and Gilad Hirschberger. 2003. "The Existential Function of Close Relationships: Introducing Death into the Science of Love." *Personality & Social Psychology Review* 7(1):20–40.

Miles, Andrew. 2015. "The (Re)Genesis of Values." *American Sociological Review* 80(4):680–704.

Milioni, Michela, Guido Alessandri, Nancy Eisenberg, Valeria Castellani, Antonio Zuffian¨°, Michele Vecchione, and Gian Vittorio Caprara. 2015. "Reciprocal Relations Between Emotional Self-Efficacy Beliefs and Ego-Resiliency Across Time." *Journal of Personality* 83(5):552–563.

Millar, Anthen, and Jenny Warner. 2012. "Alderian Therapy." Pp. 249–253 in *The SAGE Handbook of Counselling and Psychotherapy*, edited by Colin Feltham and Ian Horton. London: SAGE.

Miller, Alan S. 1995. "A Rational Choice Model of Religious Behavior in Japan." *Journal for the Scientific Study of Religion* 34(2):234–244.

Miller, Alan S., and Tomoko Mitamura. 2003. "Are Surveys on Trust Trustworthy?" *Social Psychology Quarterly* 66(1):62–70.

Miller, Delbert C. 1983. Handbook of Research Design and Social Measurement. New York: Longman.

Miller, Jacob T. and Paul Verhaeghen. 2022. "Mind Full of Kindness: Self-Awareness, Self-Regulation, and Self-Transcendence as Vehicles for Compassion." *BMC Psychology* 10(1).

Miller, Marianne McInnes and Nicole Van Ness Sheppard. 2014. "What Does Spirituality Mean to You? Mapping the Spiritual Discourses of Psychotherapy Graduate Students." *Journal of Spirituality in Mental Health* 16(4):286–310.

Miller-Day, Michelle A. 2004. Communication among Grandmothers, Mothers, and Adult Daughters: A Qualitative Study of Maternal Relationships. Mahwah, NJ: Lawrence Erlbaum.

Milner, Henry. 2002. *Civic Literacy: How Informed Citizens Make Democracy Work*. Hanover, NH: University Press of New England.

Milner, Judith, and Steve Myers. 2007. Working with Violence: Policies and Practices in Risk Assessment and Management. Houndmills, UK: Palgrave.

Milton, Martin. 2000. "Existential-phenomenological Therapy." Pp. 39–53 in *Therapeutic Perspectives on Working with Lesbian, Gay and Bisexual Clients*, edited by Dominic Davies and Charles Neal. Buckingham, UK: Open University Press.

Miner, Sonia. 1995. "Racial Differences in Family Support and Formal Service Utilization among Older Persons: A Nonrecursive Model." *Journal of Gerontology* 50B:S143–153.

Miner-Rubino, Kathi and Whitney D. Reed. 2010. "Testing a Moderated Mediational Model of Workgroup Incivility: The Roles of Organizational Trust and Group Regard." *Journal of Applied Social Psychology* 40(12):3148–3168.

Mingo, Isabella and Maria Paola Faggiano. 2020. "Trust in Institutions between Objective and Subjective Determinants: A Multilevel Analysis in European Countries." *Social Indicators Research* 151(3):815–39.

Minnaert, Alexander, and Piet J. Janssen. 1992. "Success and Progress in Higher Education: A Structural Model of Studying." *British Journal of Educational Psycholog*y 62:184–192.

Minnebo, Jurgen. 2006. "The Relation between Psychological Distress, Television Exposure, and Television-Viewing Motives in Crime Victims." *Media Psychology* 8(2):65–93.

Minogue, Kenneth. 2010. The Servile Mind: How Democracy Erodes the Moral Life. New York: Encounter.

Mintz, Alex, Nicholas A. Valentino, and Carly Wayne. 2022. *Beyond Political Science in the 21$^{st}$ Century*. Cambridge, UK: Cambridge University Press.
Miranti, Riyana, and Mark Evans. 2019. "Trust, Sense of Community, and Civic Engagement: Lessons from Australia." *Journal of Community Psychology* 47(2):254–271.
Mirivel, Julien C. 2014. The Art of Positive Communication: Theory and Practice. New York, NY: Lang.
Mirowsky, John, and Catherine E. Ross. 1989. *Social Causes of Psychological Distress*. New York: Aldine de Gruyter.
Mirowsky, John, and Catherine E. Ross. 1990. "The Consolation-Prize Theory of Alienation." *American Journal of Sociology* 95(6):1505–1535.
Mirowsky, John, and Catherine E. Ross. 1999. "Economic Hardship across the Life Course." *American Sociological Review* 64(4):548–569.
Mirowsky, John, and Catherine E. Ross. 2001. "Age and Effect of Economic Hardship on Depression." *Journal of Health & Social Behavior* 42:132–150.
Mishna, Faye. 2012. *Bullying: A Guide to Research, Intervention, and Prevention*. New York< NY: Oxford University Press.
Misra, Joya. 1997. "Teaching Stratification: Stimulating Interest and Critical Thinking through Research Projects." *Teaching Sociology* 25:278–291.
Misra, Ranjita, and Linda G. Castillo. 2004. "Academic Stress among College Students: Comparison of American and International Students." *International Journal of Stress Management* 11(2):132–148.
Mitchell, Katharyne. 2017. "Factivism: A New Configuration of Humanitarian Reason." *Geopolitics* 22(1):110–28.
Mitchell, Neil J. 2005. "Calculating and Believing: Ideological Norms in the Cradle of Utility Maximization." *Social Justice Research* 18(3):243–256.
Mitchell, Wendy A., Paul Crawshaw, Robin Bunton, and Eileen E. Green. 2001. "Situating Young People's Experiences of Risk and Identity." *Health, Risk & Society* 3(2):217–233.
Mithaug, Dennis E. 2000. *Learning to Theorize: A Four-step Strategy*. Thousand Oaks, CA: Sage.
Mitoma, Glenn and Kerry Bystrom. 2013. "Humanitarianism and Responsibility." *Journal of Human Rights* 12(1):1–20.
Mitrut, Andreea and Francois-Charles Wolff. 2011. "Do Private and Public Transfers Received Affect Life Satisfaction: Evidence from Romania." *Journal of Economic Psychology* 32:969–979.
Mitsis, Phillip. 2003. "Stoicism." Pp. 253–267 in *The Blackwell Guide to Ancient Philosophy*, edited by Christopher Shields. Malden, MA: Blackwell.
Miyata, Kakuto, and Tetsuro Kubayashi. 2008. "Causal Relationship between Internet Use and Social Capital in Japan." *Asian Journal of Social Psychology* 11:42–52.
Miyazaki, Anthony D., Jeff Langenderfer, and David E. Sprott. 1999. "Government-sponsored Lotteries: Exploring Purchase and Nonpurchase Motivation." *Psychology & Marketing* 16(1):1–20.
Moeller, Hans-Georg. 2004. Daoism Explained: From the Dream of the Butterfly to the Fishnet Allegory. Chicago, IL: Open Court.
Moeller, Hans-Georg. 2006. *The Philosophy of the Daodejing*. New York: Columbia Univesity Press.
Moeller, Scott J., Jennifer Crocker, and Brad J. Bushman. 2009. "Creating Hostility and Conflict: Effects of Entitlement and Self-Image Goals." *Journal of Experimental Social Psychology* 45(2):448–52.
Moen, Phyllis, Erin L. Kelly, and Jack Lam. 2013. "Healthy Work Revisited: Do Changes in Time Strain Predict Well-Being?" *Journal of Occupational Health Psychology* 18(2):157–172.
Moen, Phyllis, Mary Ann Erickson, and Donna Dempster McClain. 2000. "Social Role Identities among Older Adults in a Continuing Care Retirement Community." *Research on Aging* 22(5):559–579.

Moen, Phyllis, Stephen Sweet, and Rachelle Hill. 2010. "Risk, Resilience, and Life-course Fit: Older Couples' Encores Following Job Loss." Pp. 283–309 in *New Frontiers in Resilient Aging: Life-strengths and Well-being in Late Life*, edited by Prom S. Fry and Corey L.M. Keyes. Cambridge, UK: Cambridge University Press.

Moffitt, Leonard Caum. 2018. *Challenge of Change: Perspective for Our Twenty-First Century.* Washington, DC: Academica.

Molana, Hanieh H. and Richard E. Adams. 2019. "Evaluating Sense of Community in the Residential Environment from the Perspectives of Symbolic Interactionism and Architectural Design." *Journal of Community Psychology* 47(7):1591–602.

Molitor, Fred, Melissa Rossi, Lisa Branton, and Julie Field. 2011. "Increasing Social Capital and Personal Efficacy through Small-Scale Community Events." *Journal of Community Psychology* 39(6):749–754.

Moller, Arlen C., Edward L. Deci, and Richard M. Ryan. 2006. "Choice and Ego-Depletion: The Moderating Role of Autonomy." *Personality & Social Psychology Bulletin* 32(8):1024–1036.

Moller, Jorgen, and Svend-Erik Skaaning. 2014. "Respect for Civil Liberties During the Third Wave of Democratization: Presenting a New Dataset." *Social Indicators Research* 117(3):1069–1087.

Moller, Stephanie, David Bradley, Everlyne Huber, Francois Nielsen, and John D. Stephens. 2003. "Determinants of Relative Poverty in Advanced Capitalist Democracies." *American Sociological Review* 68(1):22–51.

Molm, Linda D. 1997. *Coercive Power in Social Exchange.* Cambridge, UK: Cambridge University Press.

Molm, Linda D. 2008. "The Structure of Reciprocity and Integrative Bonds: The Role Emotions." Pp. 167–192 in *Social Structure and Emotion*, edited by Jody Clay-Warner and Dawn T. Robinson. San Diego, CA: Academic.

Molz, Ashleigh R., Chelsea L. Black, Benjamin G. Shapero, Rachel E. Bender, Lauren B. Alloy, and Lyn Y. Abramson. 2013. "Aggression and Impulsivity as Predictors of Stress Generation in Bipolar Spectrum Disorders." *Journal of Affective Disorders* 146(2):272–80.

Momonoki, Yoshie S. and Hidetoki Ishii. 2023. "Modeling the Direct and Indirect Relationships between Cognitive Style, Daily Life Stress and Mental Distress." *Journal of Affective Disorders Reports* 13:100594.

Monahan, Kathryn C., Lawrence Steinberg, Elizabeth Cauffman, and Edward P. Mulvey. 2013. "Psychosocial (Im)maturity from Adolescence to Early Adulthood: Distinguishing between Adolescence-limited and Persisting Antisocial Behavior." *Development & Psychopathology* 25(4):1093–1105.

Mondak, Jeffery J., and Jon Hurwitz. 2012. "Examining the Terror Exception: Terrorism and Commitments to Civil Liberties." *Public Opinion Quarterly* 76(2):193–213.

Moneta, Giovanni B., Barbara Schneider, and Mihaly Csikszentmihalyi. 2001. "A Longitudinal Study of the Self-concept and Experiential Components of Self-worth and Affect across Adolescence." *Applied Developmental Science* 5(2):125–142.

Monroe, Andrew E., James B. Wyngaarden, and E. Ashby Plant. 2021. "They Should Have Followed the Rules: Trade-Offs between Fairness and Authority Values Predict Judgments of Social Justice Protests." Social Psychological & Personality Science.

Monroe, Pamela, and Vicky V. Tiller. 2001. "Commitment to Work among Welfare Reliant Women." *Journal of Marriage & the Family* 63(3):816–828.

Montazer, Shirin. 2022. "Immigration, Homeownership, and Mental Health." *Socius* 8:237802312211393.

Montgomery, Diane, Pamela A. Hodges, and Judith S. Kaufman. 2004. "An Exploratory Study of the Relationship between Mood States and Creativity Self-perceptions." *Creativity Research Journal* 16(2&3):341–344.

Mookerjee, Rajer, and Krista Beron. 2004. "Gender, Religion, and Happiness." *Journal of Socio-Economics* 34:674–685.

Moore, Dahlia, and Salem Aweiss. 2003. "Outcome Expectations in Prolonged Conflicts: Perceptions of Sense of Control and Relative Deprivation." *Sociological Inquiry* 73(2):190–211.

Moore, Margaret. 2010. "Defending Community: Nationalism, Patriotism, and Culture." Pp. 130–145 in *Ethics and World Politics*, edited by Duncan Bell. Oxford, UK: Oxford University Press.
Moore, Simon, and Jonathan P. Shepherd. 2006. "The Cost of Fear: Shadow Pricing the Intangible Costs of Crime." *Applied Economics* 38(3):293–300.
Moos, Rudolf H., and Sonne Lemke. 1996. Evaluating Residential Functions: The Multiphasic Environmental Assessment Procedure. Thousand Oaks, CA: Sage.
Moote, Gerald T., Jr., Nancy J. Smyth, and Jah S. Wodarski. 1999. "Social Skills Training with Youth in Social Setting: A Review." *Research on Social Work Practice* 9(4):427–465.
Mordeno, Imelu G., Jelli Grace C. Luzano, I. Marie Joy S. Gallemit, and Edmarie Zoe J. Gonzaga. 2023. "Prevalence and Predictors of Psychological Distress and Common Mental Health Concerns among Filipino University Teachers Amid the Covid-19 Pandemic." *Psychology in the Schools* 60(9):3542–74.
Morenoff, Jeffrey D., Ana V. Diez Roux, Ben B. Hansen, and Theresa L. Osypuk. 2008. "Residential Environments and Obesity: What Can We Learn about Policy Interventions from Observational Studies?" Pp. 309–343 in *Making American Healthier: Social and Economic Policy as Health Policy*, edited by Robert F. Schoeni, James S. House, George A. Kaplan, and Harold Pollack. New York: Russell Sage.
Moreno-Jimenez, M. Pilar, and M. Carmin Hidalgo Villodres. 2010. "Prediction of Burnout in Volunteers." *Journal of Applied Social Psychology* 40(7):1798–1818.
Morgan, Jessica; and Oliver Robinson. 2013. "Intrinsic Aspirations and Personal Meaning across Adulthood: Conceptual Interrelations and Age/Sex Differences." *Developmental Psychology* 49(5):999–1010.
Morgan, Seiriol. 2021. "Entitlement, Domination and Violence: A Philosophical Model of a Deviant Sense of Justification, and Its Implications for Understanding Human Rights Abuses." *International Journal of Human Rights* 25(9):1543–73.
Morgan, Stephen L., and Christopher Winship. 2007. *Counterfactuals and Causal Inference: Methods and Principles for Social Research.* Cambridge, UK: Cambridge University Press.
Morgan, William, and Matthew Streb. 2001. "Building Citizenship: How Student Voice in Service-learning Develops Civic Values." *Social Science Quarterly* 82(1):154–169.
Morimoto, Hiroshi, Hironori Shimada, and Kenichi Ozaki. 2014. "Sociocultural Beliefs, as Well as Goodness of Fit, Influence the Effectiveness of Coping in Japanese Workers." *International Journal of Behavioral Medicine* 21(3):447–55.
Morin, Alain. 2011. "Self-Awareness Part 1: Definition, Measures, Effects, Functions, and Antecedents." *Social & Personality Psychology Compass* 5(10):807–823.
Morizot, Julien, and Marc Le Blanc. 2007. "Behavioral, Self, and Social Control Predictors of Desistance from Crime: A Test of Launch and Contemporaneous Effect Models." *Journal of Contemporary Criminal Justice* 23(1):50–71.
Morody, Mioslawa and Anna Giza-Poleszczuk. 2018. *Transformation of Social Bonds: The Outline of the Theory of Social Change.* Berlin, Germany: Lang.
Morokoff, Patricia J., Colleen A. Redding, Lisa L. Harlow, Sookhyun Cho, Joseph S. Rossi, Kathryn S. Meier, Kenneth H. Mayer, Beryl Koblin, and Pamela Brown-Peterside. 2009. "Associations of Sexual Victimization, Depression, and Sexual Assertiveness with Unprotected Sex: A Test of the Multifaceted Model of HIV Risk across Gender." *Journal of Applied Biobehavioral Research* 14(1):30–54,
Morris, Anjana Madan, Sylvie Mrug and Michael Windle. 2015. "From Family Violence to Dating Violence: Testing a Dual Pathway Model." *Journal of Youth & Adolescence* 44(9):1819–1835.
Morris, Matthew C., Chrystyna D. Kouros, Kim Janecek, Rachel Freeman, Alyssa Mielock, and Judy Garber. 2017. "Community-level Moderators of a School-Based Childhood Sexual Assault Prevention Program." *Child Abuse & Neglect* 63:295–306.
Morris, Nina Jane and Kate Orton-Johnson. 2024. "Camping at Home: Escapism, Self-Care, and Social Bonding During the Covid-19 Pandemic." *Annals of Leisure Research* 27(1):14–35.

Morris, Pamela, and Ariel Kaljl. 2006. "Out-of-school time Use During Middle Childhood in a Low-income Sample: Do Combinations of Activities Affect Achievement and Behavior?" Pp. 237–259 in *Developmental Contexts in Middle Childhood: Bridges to Adolescence and Adulthood*, edited by Aletha C. Huston and Marika N. Ripke. Cambridge, UK: Cambridge University Press.

Morris, Stephen D., and Joseph L. Klesner. 2010. "Corruption and Trust: Theoretical Considerations and Evidence from Mexico." *Comparative Political Studies* 43(10):1258–1285

Morriss, Peter. 2009. "Power and Liberalism." Pp. 54–69 in *The SAGE Handbook of Power*, edited by Stewart R. Clegg and Mark Haugaard. London, UK: SAGE.

Morrissey, Mary Beth Quaranta. 2015. *Suffering Narratives of Older Adults: A Phenomenological Approach to Serious Illness, Chronic Pain, Recovery and Maternal Care*. Abingdon, UK: Routledge.

Morrissey, Sean Afnan. 2008. "Performing Risks: Catharsis Carnival, and Capital in the Risk Society." *Journal of Youth Studies* 11(4):413–427.

Morrow, Virginia. 1999. "Conceptualising Social Capital in Relation to the Well-being of Children and Young People: A Critical Review." *Sociological Review* 47(4):744–765.

Morselli, Davide and Stefano Passini. 2018. "Exclusive and Inclusive Protest in Europe: Investigating Values, Support for Democracy, and Life Conditions." *Journal of Community & Applied Social Psychology* 28(3):123–41.

Morton, Thomas A., and Julie M. Duck. 2001. "Communication and Health Beliefs: Mass and Interpersonal Influences on Perceptions of Risk to Self and Others." *Communication Research* 28(5):602–626.

Moschis, George P., and Fon Sim Ong. 2011. "Religiosity and Consumer Behavior of Older Adults: A Study of Subcultural Influences in Malaysia." *Journal of Consumer Behavior* 10:8–17.

Moscoso-Sanchez, David, Álvaro Rodríguez-Díaz, and Jesús Fernández-Gavira. 2015. "Elitist Rhetoric and the Sports Gap. Examining the Discourse and Reality of Sport in Spain." *European Journal for Sport & Society* 12(1):31–51.

Moshman, David. 2003. ¡°Developmental Change in Adulthood.? Pp. 43–61 in *Handbook of Adult Development*, edited by Jack Demick and Carrie Andreoletti. New York: Kluwer Academic.

Moss, Jeremy. 2014. *Reassessing Egalitarianism*. Houndmills, UK: Palgrave. (JC575.M677)

Mota, Catarina Pinheiro, and Paula Mena Matos. 2015. "Does Sibling Relationship Matter to Self-Concept and Resilience in Adolescents under Residential Care?" *Children & Youth Services Review* 56:97–106.

Motschenbacher, Heiko. 2010. Language, Gender and Sexual Identity: Poststructuralist Perspectives. Amsterdam, Netherlands: John Benjamin.

Mouatsou, Chrysi and Katerina Koutra. 2023. "Emotion Regulation in Relation with Resilience in Emerging Adults: The Mediating Role of Self-Esteem." *Current Psychology* 42(1):734–47.

Mouw, Ted, and Barbara Entwisle. 2006. "Residential Segregation and Interracial Friendship in Schools." *American Journal of Sociology* 112(2):394–441.

Mrazek, Alissa J., Elliott D. Ihm, Daniel C. Molden, Michael D. Mrazek, Claire M. Zedelius and Jonathan W. Schooler. 2018. "Expanding Minds: Growth Mindsets of Self-Regulation and the Influences on Effort and Perseverance." *Journal of Experimental Social Psychology* 79:164–180.

Mroczek, Daneil K., and David M. Almeida. 2004. "The Effect of Daily Stress, Personality, and Age on Daily Negative Affect." *Journal of Personality* 72(2):355–378. person-centered

Mruk, Christopher J. 2006. Self-esteem, Research, Theory and Practice: Toward a Positive Psychology of Self-esteem. New York: Springer.

Mruk, Christopher J. 2019. Feeling Good by Doing Good: A Guide to Authentic Self-esteem and Well-being. New York, NY: Oxford University Press.

Muenks, Katherine, Veronica X. Yan, and Nina K. Telang. 2021. "Who Is Part of the Mindset Context? The Unique Roles of Perceived Professor and Peer Mindsets in Undergraduate Engineering Students" Motivation and Belonging." *Frontiers in Education* 6:633570.

Muennig, Peter, Alison K. Cohen, Aileen Palmer, and Wenyi Zhu. 2013. "The Relationship between Five Different Measures of Structural Social Capital, Medical Examination Outcomes, and Mortality." *Social Science & Medicine* 85:18–26.

Muffels, Ruud, and Didier Fouarge. 2004. "The Role of European Welfare Status in Explaining Resources Deprivation." *Social Indicators Research* 68:299–330.

Mukherjee, Swaiti, and Updesh Kumar. 2017. "Psychological Resilience: A Conceptual Review of Theory and Research." Pp. 3–12 in *The Routledge International Handbook of Psychosocial Resilience*, edited by Updesh Kumar. Abingdon, UK: Routledge.

Mulford, Matthew, John Orbell, Catherine Shatto, and Jean Stockard. 1998. "Physical Attractiveness, Opportunity, and Success in Everyday Exchange." *American Journal of Sociology* 103(6):1565–1592.

Muller, Chandra. 1998. "Gender Differences in Parental Involvement and Adolescents" Mathematics Achievement." *Sociology of Education* 71(4):336–356.

Mullet, Etienne, Felix Neto, and Sheila Riviere. 2005. "Personality and Its Effects on Resentment, Revenge, Forgiveness, and Self-forgiveness." Pp. 159–181 in *Handbook of Forgiveness*, edited by Everett L. Worthington, Jr. New York, NY: Routledge.

Mullin, Walter J., and Miguel Arce. 2008. "Resilience of Families Living in Poverty." *Journal of Family Social Work* 11(4):424–446.

Mullins, Larry C., and Elizabeth Dugan. 1991. "Elderly Social Relationships with Adult Children and Close Friends and Depression." *Journal of Social Behavior and Personality* 6(2):315–328.

Muluk, Hamdi, Nathanael G. Sumaktoyo, and Dhyah Madya Ruth. 2013. "Jihad as Justification: National Survey Evidence of Belief in Violent Jihad as a Mediating Factor for Sacred Violence among Muslims in Indonesia." *Asian Journal of Social Psychology* 16(2):101–11.

Munch, Richard. 1987. *Theory of Action: Towards a New Synthesis Going beyond Parsons*. London: Routledge & Kegan Paul.

Munch, Richard. 1988. Understanding Modernity: Toward a New Perspective Going beyond Durkheim and Weber. London: Routledge.

Munch, Richard. 1989. "Structures, Cultures, and Knowledge: A Historical and Comparative Exploration." Pp. 39–66 in *Social Structure and Culture*, edited by Hans Haferkamp. Berlin, Germany: Walter de Gruyter.

Munch, Richard. 2012. *Inclusion and Exclusion in the Liberal Competition State: The Cult of the Individual*. Abington, UK: Routledge.

Mundia, Lawrence. 2011. "Social Desirability, Non-Response Bias and Reliability in a Long Self-Report Measure: Illustrations from the MMPI-2 Administered to Brunei Student Teachers." *Educational Psychology* 31(2):207–24.

Munro, Rolland. 2009. "Actor-Network Theory." Pp. 125–139 in *The SAGE Handbook of Power*, edited by Stewart R. Clegg and Mark Haugaard. London, UK: SAGE.

Munroe, Melanie, Mohamed Al-Refae, Helen W. Chan, and Michel Ferrari. 2022. "Using Self-Compassion to Grow in the Face of Trauma: The Role of Positive Reframing and Problem-Focused Coping Strategies." *Psychological Trauma* 14(S1):S157–S64.

Muradwij, Nawal and Maureen Allwood. 2022. "Making Meaning of Community Violence among Adolescents: Associations between Exposure, Pro-Violence Attitudes and Psychological Symptoms." *Journal of Community Psychology* 50(3):1315–30.

Murayama, Yoh, Hiroshi Murayama, Masami Hasebe, Jan Yamaguichi, and Yosninori fujiwara. 2019. "The Impact of Intergenerational Programs on Social Capital in Japan: A Randomized Population-based Cross-sectional Study." *BMC Public Health* 19:156.

Murer, Jeffrey Stevenson and Tilman Schwarze. 2022. "Social Rituals of Pain. The Socio-Symbolic Meaning of Violence in Gang Initiations." *International Journal of Politics, Culture, & Society* 35(1):95–110.

Muris, Peter Cor Meesters, and Frank van den Berg. 2003. "The Strengths and Difficulties Questionnaire (SDQ): Further Evidence of Its Reliability and Validity in a Community Sample of Dutch Children and Adolescents." *European Child & Adolescent Psychiatry* 12:1–8.

Muris, Peter, Anne Jeurissen, Morgan Rooswinkel, and Cor Meesters. 2022. "Good Traits, Bad Traits, and "Ugly" Behavior: Relations between the Dark Triad, Honesty-Humility, Other Hexaco Personality Traits, and Externalizing Problems in Adolescents." *Journal of Child & Family Studies* 31(12):3247–57.

Muris, Peter, Birgit Mayer, and Tinke-Schubert. 2010. "Your Might Belong in Gryffindor: Children's Courage and Its Relationships to Anxiety Symptoms, Big Five Personality Traits and Sex Roles." *Child Psychiatry & Human Development* 41:204–213.

Murphy, P. Karen, Jeffrey A. Greene, Carla M. Firetto, Mengyi Li, Nikki G. Lobczowski, Rebekah F. Duke, Liwei Wei, and Rachel M. V. Croninger. 2017. "Exploring the Influence of Homogeneous versus Heterogeneous Grouping on Students" Text-Based Discussions and Comprehension." *Contemporary Educational Psychology* 51:336–55.

Murray, Joy. 2009. "The wider social benefits of higher education: What do we know about them?" *Australian Journal of Education* 53(3):230–244.

Music, Graham, 2014. *The Good Life: Wellbeing and the New Science of Altruism, Selfishness and Immorality*. Hove, UK: Routledge.

Musick, Marc A., and John Wilson. 2008. *Volunteers: A Social Profile*. Bloomington, IN: Indiana University Press.

Muskett, Judith A. 2012. "From Vicarious Religion to Vicarious Social Capital? Information and Passive Participation in Voluntary Associations." *Research in the Social Scientific Study of Religion* 23:29–52.

Mussel, Patrick, and Johannes Hewig. 2016. "The Life and Times of Individuals Scoring High and Low on Dispositional Greed." *Journal of Research in Personality* 64:52–60.

Mussen, Paul. 1982. "Personality Development and Liberal Sociopolitical Attitudes." Pp. 363–370 in *The Development of Prosocial Behavior*, edited by Nancy Eisenberg. New York: Academic Press.

Mussweiler, Thomas, Katja Ruter, and Kai Epstude. 2006. "The Why, Who, and How of Social Comparison: A Social-cognitive Perspective." Pp. 33–54 in *Social Comparison and Social Psychology: Understanding Cognitive, Intergroup Relations, and Culture*, edited by Berge Guimond. Cambridge, UK: Cambridge University Press.

Muthuswamy, Moorthy S. 2022. "Does Sharia Act as Both a Mediator and Moderator in Salafi Radicalism?" *Cogent Social Sciences* 8(1).2030452.

Mutz, Diana C., and Byron Reeves. 2005. "The New Videomalaise: Effects of Televised Incivility on Political Trust." *American Political Science Review* 99(1):1–15.

Mutz, Diana C., and Jeffery J. Mondak. 2006. "The Workplace as a Context for Cross-cutting Political Discourse." *Journal of Politics* 68(1):140–155.

Muuss, Rolf E. 1996. *Theories of Adolescence*. New York: McGraw-Hill.

Myer, Landon, Dan J. Stein, Anna Grimsrud, Soraya Seedat, and David R. Williams. 2008. "Social Determinants of Psychological Distress in a Nationally Representative Sample of South African Adults." *Social Science & Medicine* 60:1828–1840.

Myers, David G. 1999. "Close Relationships and Quality of Life." Pp. 374–391 in *Well-being: The Foundations of Hedonic Psychology*, edited by Daniel Kahneman, Ed Diener and Norbert Schwarz. New York: Russell Sage.

Myers, David G. 2008. "Religion and Human Flourishing." Pp. 323–343 in *The Science of Subjective Well-being*, edited by Michael Eid and Randy J. Larsen. New York: Guilford.

Myers, David G. 2014. "Religious Engagement and Well-being." Pp. 88–100 in *theOxfordHandbook of Happiness*, edited by Susan A. David, Ilona Boniwell and Amanda Conley Ayers. Oxford, UK: Oxford University Press.

Myers, Jane E., and Melanie C. Harper. 2004. "Evidence-based Effective Practices with Older Adults." *Journal of Counseling & Development* 82:207–218.

Myers, Scott A., Barbara Lorene Ropog, R. Pierre Rodgers. 1997. "Sex Differences in Humor." *Psychological Reports* 81(1):221–222.

Mytton, Jill. 2012. "Cognitive Therapy." Pp. 286–297 in *The SAGE Handbook of Counselling and Psychotherapy*, edited by Colin Feltham and Ian Horton. London: SAGE.

Na, Chongmin, and Ray Paternoster. 2019. "Prosocial Identities and Youth Violence." *Journal of Research in Crime & Delinquency* 56(1):84–128.

Nagayoshi, Kikuko, and Yoshimichi Sato. 2014. "Who Supports Redistributive Policies in Contemporary Japan? An Integrative Approach To Self-Interest And Trust Models." *International Sociology* 29(4):302–323.
Nagurney, Alexander J. 2007. "The Effects of Relationship Stress and Unmitigated Communion on Physical and Mental Health Outcomes." *Stress & Health* 23:267–273. \73–374
Nahapiet, Janine. 2009. "Capitalizing on Connections: Social Capital and Strategic Management." Pp. 205–236 in *Social Capital: Reaching out, Reaching in*, edited by Viva Ona Bartkus and James H. Davis. Cheltenham, UK: Edward Elgar.
Nahum-Shani, Inbal, Melanie M. Henderson, Sandy Lim, and Amiram D. Vinokur. 2014. "Does Supervisor Support Buffer or Exacerbate the Adverse Effects of Supervisor Undermining?" *Journal of Applied Psychology* 99(3):484–503.
Nai, Jared, Jayanth Narayanan, Ivan Hernandez, and Krishna Savani. 2018. "People in More Racially Diverse Neighborhoods Are More Prosocial." *Journal of Personality & Social Psychology* 114(4):497–515.
Nail, Paul R., Julia I. Misak, and Randi M. Davis. 2004. "Self-affirmation versus Self-consistency: A Comparison of Two Competing Self-theories of Dissonance Phenomena." *Personality & Individual Differences* 36:1893–1905.
Nakashima, Ken"ichiro, Kuniaki Yanagisawa, and Mitsuhiro Ura. 2013. "Dissimilar Effects of Task-relevant and Interpersonal Threat on Independent-interdependent Self-construal in Individuals with High Self-esteem." *Asian Journal of Social Psychology* 16(1):50–59.
Nakashima, Mitsuko, and Edward R. Canda. 2005. "Positive Dying and Resiliency in Later Life: A Qualitative Study." *Journal of Aging Studies* 19:109–125.
Nalis, Irina, Bettina Kubicek, and Christian Korunka. 2022. "Resources to Respond: A Career Construction Theory Perspective on Demands, Adaptability, and Career Crafting." *Career Development Quarterly* 70(2):138–52.
Namini, Sussan, Claudia Appel, Ralph Jurgensen, and Sebastian Murken. 2010. "How is Well-Being Related to Membership in New Religious Movements? An Application of Person-Environment Fit Theory." *Applied Psychology: An International Review* 59(2):181–201.
Napier, Jaime L., and John T. Jost. 2008. "Why Are Conservatives Happier Than Liberals?" *Psychological Science* 19(6):565–572.
Napper, Rosemary, and Tradi Newton. 2018. "Transactional Analysis and Coaching." Pp. 167–183 in *The Complete Handbook of Coaching*, edited by Elaine Cox, Tatiana Bachkirova, and David Clutterbuck. London, UK: SAGE.
Narayan, Despa, and Michael F. Cassidy. 2001. "A Dimensional Approach to Measuring Social Capital: Development and Validation of a Social Capital Inventory." *Current Sociology* 49(2):59–102.
Naruse, Sayuri M., Piers L. Cornelissen, and Mark Moss. 2020. "To Give Is Better Than to Receive? Couples Massage Significantly Benefits Both Partners" Wellbeing." *Journal of Health Psychology* 25(10–11):1576–86.
Narvaez, Darcia. 2008. "Human Flourishing and Moral Development: Cognitive and Neurobiological Perspectives of Virtue Development." Pp. 310–327 in *Handbook of Moral and Character Education*, edited by Larry P. Nucci and Darcia Narvaez. New York: Routledge.
Narvaez, Darcia. 2014. Neurobiology and the Development of Human Morality: Evolution, Culture, and Wisdom. New York, NY: Norton.
Nash, James K., Lawrence L. Kupper, and Mark W. Fraser. 2004. "Using Multilevel Statistical Models Social Work Intervention Research." *Journal of Social Service Research* 30(3):35–54.
Nassauer, Anne. 2019. *Situational Breakdowns: Understanding Protest Violence and Other Supporting Outcomes*. New York, NY: Oxford University Press.
Navarra, Melissa Quetulio, Anke Niehof, Wander Van Der Vaart, Hilje Van Der Horst and Hester Moerbeek. 2018. "History and Institutions in the Rebuilding of Social Capital after Forced Resettlement in the Philippines and Indonesia." *Journal of Development Studies* 54(8):1392–405.

Naveed, Amjad and Cong Wang. 2021. "Can Attitudes toward Immigrant Explain Social Integration in Europe? EU Versus Non-EU Migrant." *Social Indicators Research* 153(1):345–383.

Nee, Victor, and Jimy Sanders. 2001. "Trust in Ethnic Ties: Social Capital and Immigrants." Pp. 374–392 in *Trust in Society*, edited by Karen S. Cook. New York: Russell Sage Foundation.

Nelis, Sharon M., Gordon Rae, and Christine Liddell. 2006. "Factor Analyses and Score Validity of the Family Emotional Involvement and Criticism Sale in an Adolescent Sample." *Educational & Psychological Measurement* 66(4):676–686.

Nelson, Julie A. 2015. "Fearing Fear: Gender and Economic Discourse." *Mind & Society* 14(1):129–39.

Nelson, L.J., and L.M.Padilla-Walker. 2013. "Flourishing and Floundering in Emerging Adult College Students." *Emerging Adulthood* 1(1):67–78.

Nelson, Larry J., Laura M. Padilla-Walker, and Matthew G. Nielson. 2015. "Is Hovering Smothering or Loving? An Examination of Parental Warmth as a Moderator of Relations between Helicopter Parenting and Emerging Adults" Indices of Adjustment." *Emerging Adulthood* 3(4):282–285.

Nelson, Larry J., Sarah Badger, and Bo Wu. 2004. "The Influence of Culture in Emerging Adulthood: Perspectives of Chinese College Students." *International Journal of Behavioral Development*. 28(1):26–36.

Nelson-Becker, Holly B. 2006. "Voices of Resistance: Older Adults in Hospice Care." *Journal of Social Work in En-of-Life & Palliative Care* 2(3):87–106.

Nelson-Becker, Holly. 2005. "Religion and Coping in Older Adults: A Social Work Perspective." *Journal of Gerontological Social Work* 45(1/2):51–67.

Nelson-Coffey, S. Katherine, Kristin Layous, John K. Coffey, and Linda C. Mayes. 2023. "The Effects of Social Belonging and Kindness on Stress and Well-Being during the COVID-19 Pandemic: A Longitudinal Experiment." *Social & Personality Psychology Compass* 2023:e12798.

Nemeth, Darlyne G., and Trace W. Olivier. 2017. *Innovative Approaches to Individual and Community Resilience: From Theory to Practice*. London, UK: Academic.

Nemeth, Lilla, and László Bernath. 2022. "The Mediating Role of Global and Contingent Self-Esteem in the Association Between Emerging Adults" Perceptions of Family Cohesion and Test Anxiety," *Journal of Adult Development* 29(3):192–204.

Nes, Lise Soblerg, and Suzanne C. Segerstrom. 2006. "Dispositional Optimism and Coping: A Meta-analytic Review." *Personality & Social Psychology Review* 10(3):235–251.

Neto, Felix and Jose Barros. 2003. "Predictors of Loneliness among Students and Nuns in Angola and Portugal." *Journal of Psychology* 137(4):351–362.

Nettle, Daniel. 2000. "Linguistic Fragmentation and the Wealth of Nations: The Fishman-Post Hypothesis Reexamined." *Economic Development & Cultural Change* 48(2):335–48.

Nevarez, Leonard. 2011. Pursuing Quality of Life: From the Affluent Society to the Consumer Society. New York: Routledge.

Newby, Wendy Levin, Ronald T. Brown, Teresa M. Pawletko, Stuart H. Gold, and J. Kenneth Whitt. 2000. "Social Skills and Psychological Adjustment of Child and Adolescent Cancer Survivors." *Psycho-Oncology* 9:113–120.

Newman, David B. and John B. Nezlek. 2019. "Private Self-Consciousness in Daily Life: Relationships between Rumination and Reflection and Well-Being, and Meaning in Daily Life." *Personality & Individual Differences* 136:184–89.

Newton, Kenneth. 1999. "Social and Political Trust in Established Democracies." Pp. 169–203 in *Critical Citizens: Global Support for Democratic Government*, edited by Pippa Norris. Oxford, UK: Oxford University Press.

Nezlek, John B., Kristof Vansteelandt, Iven Van Mechelen, and Peter Kuppens. 2008. "Appraisal-Emotion Relationships in Daily Life." *Emotion* 8(1):145–50.

Nezu, Arthur M., Christine Maguth Nezu, and Thomas J. D"Zurilla. 2013. *Problem-Solving Therapy: A Treatment Manual*. New York, NY: Springer.

Ng, Chung-hung, and Thomas W.P. Wong. 1999. "The Ethos of the Hong Kong People: Taking Stock in 1997." Pp. 233–253 in *Indicators of Social Development: Hong Kong 1997*, edited by

Siu-kai Lau, Ming-kwan Lee, Po-san Wan and Siu-lun Wong. Hong Kong: Hong Kong Institute of Asia-Pacific Studies, Chinese University of Hong Kong.

Ng, Eddie Chi Wai, and Adrian T. Fisher. 2016. "Protestant Spirituality and Well-Being of People in Hong Kong: The Mediating Role of Sense of Community." *Applied Research in Quality of Life* 11(4):1253–1267.

Ng, Mark. 2016. "Factors Influencing the Consumer Adoption of Facebook: A Two-Country Study of Youth Markets." *Computers in Human Behavior* 54:491–500.

Ng, Sik Hung, and Michael W. Allen. 2005. "Perception of Economic Distributive Justice: Exploring Leading Theories." *Social Behavior & Personality: An international journal*. 33(5):435–453.

Ng, Sik Hung, Anping He, and Cynthia Loong. 2004. "Tri-generational Family Conversation: Communication Accommodation and Brokering." *British Journal of Social Psychology* 43:449–464.

Ng, Siu-man, Cecilia L. W. Chan, David Y. F. Ho, Yu-yeuk Wong, and Rainbow T. H. Ho. 2006. "Stagnation as a Distinct Clinical Syndrome: Comparing Yu (Stagnation) in Traditional Chinese Medicine with Depression." *British Journal of Social Work* 36:467–484.

Ni, Hong, Chieh Li, and Cixin Wang. 2016. "Students' Perceptions of Resilience Promoting Factors in Chinese and American Middle Schools." *School Psychology International* 37(5):435–455.

Ni, Hong, Chieh Li, and Cixin Wang. 2016. "Students" Perceptions of Resilience Promoting Factors in Chinese and American Middle Schools." *School Psychology International* 37(5):435–455.

Nicholas, Angela, Thomas Niederkrotenthaler, Nicola Reavley, Jane Pirkis, Anthony Jorm and Matthew J. Spittal. 2020. "Belief in Suicide Prevention Myths and Its Effect on Helping: A Nationally Representative Survey of Australian Adults." *BMC Psychiatry* 20:303.

Nickerson, Carol, Norbert Schwarz, and Ed Diener. 2007. "Financial Aspirations, Financial Success, and Overall Life Satisfaction: Who? And How?" *Journal of Happiness Studies* 8:467–515.

Nicolai, Susanne, Philipp Franikowski, and Susanne Stoll-Kleemann. 2022. "Predicting Pro-Environmental Intention and Behavior Based on Justice Sensitivity, Moral Disengagement, and Moral Emotions – Results of Two Quota-Sampling Surveys." *Frontiers in Psychology* 13:914366.

Niditch, Laura A., and R. Enrique Varela. 2011. "Mother-child Disagreement in Reports of Child Anxiety: Effects of Child Age and Maternal Anxiety." *Journal of Anxiety Disorders* 25(3):450–455.

Niemi, Richard G., and Jonathan D. Klingler. 2012. "The Development of Political Attitudes and Behaviour Among Young Adults." *Australian Journal of Political Science* 47(1):31–54.

Nieminen, Tarja, Tuija Martelin, Seppo Koshinen, Jussi Simpura, Erkki ALanen, Tommi Harkanen, and Arpo Aromaa. 2008. "Measurement and Socio-demographic Variation of Social Capital in a Large Population-based Survey." *Social Indicators Research* 85:405–423.

Nieuwenhuis, Jaap, Maarten van Ham, Rongqin Yu, Susan Branje, Wim Meeus, and Pieter Hooimeijer. 2017. "Being Poorer Than the Rest of the Neighborhood: Relative Deprivation and Problem Behavior of Youth." *Journal of Youth & Adolescence* 46(9):1891–1904.

Nifadkar, Sushil S. and Talya N. Bauer. 2016. "Breach of Belongingness: Newcomer Relationship Conflict, Information, and Task-Related Outcomes During Organizational Socialization." *Journal of Applied Psychology* 101(1):1–13.

Nikolayenko, Olena. 2014. "Trust in Government and Goal Pursuit in a Transition Society." *Comparative Sociology* 13(5):618–38.

Nilsen, Wendy, Evalill Karevold, Espen Røysamb, Kristin Gustavson, and Kristin S. Mathiesen. 2013. "Social Skills and Depressive Symptoms across Adolescence: Social Support as a Mediator in Girls Versus Boys." *Journal of Adolescence* 36(1):11–20.

Nilson, Linda Burzotta. 1981. "Reconsidering Ideological Lines: Beliefs about Poverty in America." *Sociological Quarterly* 22:531–548.

Nip, Patrick T.K. 2010. "Social Welfare Development in Hong Kong: Changes and Challenges in Building a Caring and Harmonious Society." *Asian Pacific Journal of Social Work & Development* 20(1):65–81.

Nivette, Amy, Denis Ribeaud, Aja Murray, Annekatrin Steinhoff, Laura Bechtiger, Urs Hepp, Lilly Shanahan, and Manuel Eisner. 2021. "Non-Compliance with Covid-19-Related Public Health Measures among Young Adults in Switzerland: Insights from a Longitudinal Cohort Study." *Social Science & Medicine* 268:113370.

Njoh, Ambe J. 2009. "Ideology and Public Health Elements of Human Settlement Policies in Sub-Saharan Africa." *Cities* 26(1):9–18.

Noack, Peter, Christine Krettek, and Sabine Walper. 2001. "Peer Relations of Adolescents from Nuclear and Separated Families." *Journal of Adolescence* 24:535–548.

Noack, Peter. [1999] 2000. "Adolescent Peer Relations in Times of Social Change." Pp. 137–156 in *Negotiating Adolescence in Times of Social Change*, edited by Lisa J. Crockett and Rainer K. Silbereisen. Cambridge, UK: Cambridge University Press.

Noller, Patricia, Judith A. Feeney, and Candida Petersca. 2001. *Personal Relationships across the Lifespan*. Hove, UK: Psychology.

Nollmann, Gerd, and Hermann Strasser. 2007. "The Twofold Class Concept: Traditional Limitations and New Perspectives of Class Research." *Canadian Journal of Sociology* 32(3):371–397.

Nordin, Andreas. 2011. "Making the Lisbon Strategy Happen: A New Phase of Lifelong Learning Discourse in European Policy?" *European Educational Research Journal* 10(1):11–20.

Norris, Fran H., Susan P. Stevens, Betty Pfefferbaum, Karen F. Wyche, and Rose L. Pfefferbaum. 2008. "Community Resilience as a Metaphor Theory, Set of Capacities and Strategy for Disaster Readiness." *American Journal of Community Psychology* 41:127–150.

Norris, Pippa, and Ronald Inglehart. 2002. "Islamic Culture and Democracy: Testing the Clash of Civilizations Thesis." *Comparative Sociology* 1(3–4):235–263.

Norris, Pippa, and Ronald Inglehart. 2009. *Cosmopolitan Communications: Cultural Diversity in a Globalized World*. Cambridge, UK: Cambridge University Press.

Norris, Pippa. 2002. *Democratic Phoenix: Reinventing Political Activism*. Cambridge, UK: Cambridge University Press.

Norris, Pippa. 2011. *Democratic Deficit: Critical Citizens Revisited*. New York: Cambridge University Press.

North, Adrian C., Mark Tarrant, and David J. Hargreaves. 2004. "The Effects of Music on Helping Behavior: A Field Study." *Environment & Behavior* 36(2):266–275.

North, Michael S., and Susan T. Fiske. 2013. "Driven to Exclude: How Core Social Motives Explain Social Exclusion." Pp. 32–42 in *The Oxford Handbook of Social Exclusion*, edited by C. Nathan DeWall. New York: Oxford University Press.

Norvilitis, Jill M., P. Bernard Szablicki, and Sandy D. Wilson. 2003. "Factors Influencing Levels of Credit-card Debt in College Students." *Journal of Applied Social Psychology* 33(5):935–947.

Nosko, Amanda, Thanh-Thanh Tieu, and Heather Lawford, and Michael W. Pratt. 2011. "How Do I Love Thee? Let Me Count The Ways: Parenting during Adolescence, Attachment Styles, and Romantic Narratives in Emerging Adulthood." *Developmental Psychology* 47(3):645–657.

Notter, Megan L., Katherine A. MacTavish, and Devora Shamah. 2008. "Pathways toward Resilience among Women in Rural Trailer Parks." *Family Relations* 57:613–624.

Novak, Michael. 1993. *The Catholic Ethic and the Spirit of Capitalism*. New York: Free Press.

Novak, William J. 2001. "The American Law of Association: The Legal-Political Construction of Civil Society." *Studies in American Political Development* 15(2):163–88.

Ntontis, Evangelos, Angélique M. Blackburn, Hyemin Han, Sabrina Stöckli, Taciano L. Milfont, Jarno Tuominen, Siobhán M. Griffin, Gözde Ikizer, Alma Jeftic, Stavroula Chrona, Aishath Nasheedha, Liudmila Liutsko, and Sara Vestergren. 2023. "The Effects of Secondary Stressors, Social Identity, and Social Support on Perceived Stress and Resilience: Findings from the Covid-19 Pandemic." *Journal of Environmental Psychology* 88:102007.

Nucci, Larry. 2006. "Education for Moral Development." Pp. 657–681 in *Handbook of Moral Development*, edited by Melanie Killen and Judith S. Smetana. Mahwah, NJ: Lawrence Erlbaum.

Nudelman, Gabriel, Shira Peleg, and Shoshana Shiloh. 2021. "The Association between Healthy Lifestyle Behaviours and Coronavirus Protective Behaviours." *International Journal of Behavioral Medicine* 28(6):779–87.

Nudelman, Gabriel. 2013. "The Belief in a Just World and Personality: A Meta-Analysis." *Social Justice Research* 26(2):105–19.
Nunkoo, Robin. 2015. "Tourism Development and Trust in Local Government." *Tourism Management* 46:623–634.
Nussio, Enzo. 2019. "Can Crime Foster Social Participation as Conflict Can?" *Social Science Quarterly* 100(3):653–665.
O'Brien, Daniel Tumminelli. 2014. "An Evolutionary Model of the Environmental Conditions That Shape the Development of Prosociality." *Evolutionary Psychology* 12(S2):386–402.
O'Brien, John. 2015. "Individualism as a Discursive Strategy of Action." *Sociological Theory* 33(2):173–99.
O'Callaghan, Paul, John McMullen, Harry Rafferty, Ciaran Shannon, and Alastair Black. 2013. "A Randomized Controlled Trial of Trauma-Focused Cognitive Behavioral Therapy for Sexually Exploited, War-Affected Congolese Girls." *Journal of the American Academy of Child & Adolescent Psychiatry* 52(4):359–369.
O'Connell, Bill, and Stephen Palmer. 2007. "Solution-focused Coaching." Pp. 278–292 in *Handbook of Coaching Psychology: A Guide for Practitioners*, edited by Stephen Palmer and Alison Whybrow. Hove, UK: Routledge.
O'Connell, Bill. 2012. "Solution-focused Therapy." Pp. 392–395 in *The SAGE Handbook of Counselling and Psychotherapy*, edited by Colin Feltham and Ian Horton. London: SAGE.
O'Connor, Alison M., Rebecca A. Judges, Kang Lee, and Angela D. Evans. 2022. "Examining Honesty–Humility and Cheating Behaviors across Younger and Older Adults." *International Journal of Behavioral Development* 46(2):112–17.
O'Mahony, Patrick. 2013. *The Contemporary Theory of the Public Sphere*. Bern, Switzerland: Lang.
O'Neill, H. Katherine, and Blake A. Evans. 1999. "Psychological Distress during the Red River Flood: Predictive Utility of the Conservation of Resources Model." *Applied Behavioral Science Review* 7(2):159–161.
O'Neill, John. 2012. "Rationality and Rationalisation in Teacher Education Policy Discourse in New Zealand." *Education Research* 54(2):225–37.
O'Neill, Shane. 2000. "The Politics of Inclusive Agreements towards a Critical Discourse Theory of Democracy." *Political Studies* 48:503–521.
Oades, Lindsay G., Trevor P. Crowe, and Frank P. Deane. 2014. "The Collaborative Recovery Model: Developing Positive Institutions to Facilitate Recovery in Enduring Mental Illness." Pp. 1050–1066 in *The Oxford Handbook of Happiness*, edited by Susan A. David, Ilona Boniwell and Amanda Conley Ayers. Oxford, UK: Oxford University Press.
Oberle, Eva, Xuejun Ryan Ji, Martin Guhn, Kimberly A. Schonert-Reichl, and Anne M. Gadermann. 2019. "Benefits of Extracurricular Participation in Early Adolescence: Associations with Peer Belonging and Mental Health." *Journal of Youth & Adolescence* 48(11):2255.
Obucina, Ognjen. 2013. "The Patterns of Satisfaction among Immigrants." *Social Indicators Research* 113:1105–1127.
Oei, Tian Po, James Lin, and Namrata Raylu. 2008. "The Relationship between Gambling Cognitions, Psychological States, and Gambling: A Cross-cultural Study of Chinese and Caucasians in Australia." *Journal of Cross-Cultural Psychology* 39(2):147–161.
Oettingen, Gabriele, and Malin Patricia Chromick. 2018. "How Hope Influences Goal-directed Behavior." Pp. 69–79 in *The Oxford Handbook of Hope*, edited by Matthew W. Gallagher and Shane J. Lopez. New York, NY: Oxford University Press.
Offe, Claus, and Susanne Fuchs. 2002. "A Decline of Social Capital? The German Case." Pp. 188–243 in *Democracies in Flux: The Evolution of Social Capital in Contemporary Society*, edited by Robert Putnam. New York: Oxford University Press.
Ogbuanya, Theresa Chinyere and Samson Onyeluka Chukwuedo. 2017. "Career-Training Mentorship Intervention Via the Dreyfus Model: Implication for Career Behaviors and Practical Skills Acquisition in Vocational Electronic Technology." *Journal of Vocational Behavior* 103:88–105.
Oglensky, Bonnie D. 2008. "The Ambivalent Dynamics of Loyalty in Mentorship." *Human Relations* 61(3):419–448.

Ogolsky, Brian G., and J. Kale Monk. 2018. "Maintaining Relationships." Pp. 523–537 in *The Cambridge Handbook of Personal Relationships*, edited by Anita L. Vangelisti and Daniel Perlman. Cambridge, UK: Cambridge University Press.

Oh, In-Sue, Kibeom Lee, Michael C. Ashton, and Reinout E. de Vries. 2011. "Are Dishonest Extraverts More Harmful Than Dishonest Introverts? The Interaction Effects of Honesty-Humility and Extraversion in Predicting Workplace Deviance." *Applied Psychology* 60(3):496–516.

Oh, Jiyoung and Heykyung Park. 2023. "Effects of Covid-19 Stress on Healing Behavior in Residential Spaces." *Behavioral Sciences* 13(7):524.

Oh, Joong-hwan. 2003. "Assessing the Social Bonds of Elderly Neighbors: the Roles of Length of Residence, Crime Victimization, and Parental Disorder." *Sociological Inquiry* 73(4):490–510.

Ohbuchi, Ken-ichi, Osamu Fukushima, and James T. Tedeschi. 1999. "Cultural Values in Conflict Management: Goal Orientation, Goal Attainment and Tactical Decision." *Journal of Cross-Cultural Psychology* 30(1):51–71.

Ohmer, Mary L. 2007. "Citizen Participation in Neighborhood Organizations and Its Relationship to Volunteers" Self- and Collective Efficacy and Sense of Community." *Social Work Research* 31(2):109–120.

Oinas, Tomi, Petri Ruuskanen, Mari Hakala, and Timo Anttila. 2020. "The Effect of Early Career Social Capital on Long-Term Income Development in Finland." *International Journal of Sociology & Social Policy* 40(11–12):1373–90.

Oishi, Shigehiro, Jaime L. Kurtz, Felicity F. Miao, Jina Park, and Erin Whitchurch. 2011. "The Role of Familiarity in Daily Well-Being: Developmental and Cultural Variation." *Developmental Psychology* 47(6):1750–56.

Oishi, Shigehiro, Janetta Lun, and Gary D. Sherman. 2007. "Residential Mobility, Self-concept and Positive Affect in Social Interactions." *Journal of Personality & Social Psychology* 93(1):131–141.

Oksanen, Kaisa. 2011. "Framing the Democracy Debate in Hong Kong." *Journal of Contemporary China* 20(7):479–497.

Oleksy, Tomasz, Anna Wnuk, Małgorzata Gambin, and Agnieszka Łyś. 2021. "Dynamic Relationships between Different Types of Conspiracy Theories About Covid-19 and Protective Behaviour: A Four-Wave Panel Study in Poland." *Social Science & Medicine* 280:114028.

Oliver, J. Eric. 2003. "Mental Life and the Metropolis in Suburban America: The Psychological Correlates of Metropolitan Place Characteristics." *Urban Affairs Review* 39(2):228–253.

Oliver, Steve. 2006. "Moral Dilemmas of Participation in Dangerous Leisure Activities." *Leisure Studies* 25(1):95–109.

Olson, Amanda, and Stephanie Reiland, Susan Davies, and Amy Reitmaier Koehler. 2016. "Learning about the Experience of Living With Chronic Conditions: A Framework Analysis of Nursing Students' Reflections on Their Conversations with Older Adults." *Gerontology & Geriatrics Education* 17:1–21.

Olson, James M., and Crolyn L. Hafer. 2001. "Tolerance of Personal Deprivation." Pp. 157–175 in *The Psychology of Legitimacy: Emerging Perspectives on Ideology, Justice, and Intergroup Relations*, edited by John T. Jost and Brenda Major. Cambridge, UK: Cambridge University Press.

Olsson, Craig A., Lyndal Bond, Jane M. Burns, Dianne A. Vella-Brodick, and Susan M. Sawyer. 2003. "Adolescent Resilience: A Concept Analysis." *Journal of Adolescence* 26:1–11.

Oltean, Lia-Ecaterina, Andrei C. Miu, Radu Şoflău, and Aurora Szentágotai-Tătar. 2022. "Tailoring Gratitude Interventions. How and for Whom Do They Work? The Potential Mediating Role of Reward Processing and the Moderating Role of Childhood Adversity and Trait Gratitude." *Journal of Happiness Studies* 23(6):3007–30.

Oman, Doug, Carl E. Thoresen, and Kay McMahon. 1999. "Volunteerism and Mortality among the Community-dwelling Elderly." *Journal of Health Psychology* 4(3):301–316.

Ongen, Demet Erol. 2007. "The Relationships between Sensation Seeking and Gender Role Orientations among Turkish University Students." *Sex Roles* 57(1–2):111–18.

Onu, Diana, Thomas Kessler, Daniela Andonovska Trajkovska, Immo Fritsche, Georgia R. Midson, and Joanne R. Smith. 2016. "Inspired by the Outgroup: A Social Identity Analysis of Intergroup Admiration." *Group Processes & Intergroup Relations* 19(6):713–731.

Onwuegbuzie, Anthony, Philip Bailey, and Christine E. Daily. 2001. "Cognitive, Affective, Personality, and Demographic Predictors of Foreign-language Achievement." *Journal of Educational Research* 94(1):3–15.

Onyx, Jenny, and Paul Bullen. 2000. "Measuring Social Capital in Five Communities." *Journal of Applied Behavioral Science* 36(1):23–42.

Opp, Karl-Dieter. 1989. The Rationality of Political Protest: A Comparative Analysis of Rational Choice Theory. Boulder, CO: Westview.

Opp, Karl-Dieter. 2001. "Social Networks and the Emergence of Protest Norms." Pp. 234–273 in *Social Norms*, edited by Michael Hechter and Karl-Dieter Opp. New York: Russell Sage.

Opp, Karl-Dieter. 2005. "Decline of the Nation State? How the European Union Creates National and Sub-national Identifications." *Social Forces* 84(2):653–680.

Orjuela, Camilla. 2020. "Countering Buddhist Radicalisation: Emerging Peace Movements in Myanmar and Sri Lanka." *Third World Quarterly* 41(1):133–50.

Orlowski, Johannes and Pamela Wicker. 2015. "The Monetary Value of Social Capital." *Journal of Behavioral & Experimental Economics* 57:26–36.

Ormel, Johan, Judith Rosmalen, and Ann Farmer. 2004. "Neuroticism: A Non-Informative Marker of Vulnerability to Psychopathology." *Social Psychiatry & Psychiatric Epidemiology* 39(11):906–912.

Orthner, Dennis K., Hinckley Jones-Sanpei, and Sabrina Williamson. 2004. "The Resilience and Strengths of Low-income Families." *Family Relations* 53(2):159–167.

Ortner, Catherine N. M. and Pia Pennekamp. 2020. "Emotion Malleability Beliefs and Event Intensity and Importance Predict Emotion Regulation in Daily Life." *Personality & Individual Differences* 159:109887.

Osborne, Danny, Petar Milojev, and Chris G Sibley. 2017. "Authoritarianism and National Identity: Examining the Longitudinal Effects of SDO and RWA on Nationalism and Patriotism." *Personality & Social Psychology Bulletin* 43(8):1086–1099.

Oshio, Takashi and Mari Kan. 2019. "Which Is Riskier for Mental Health, Living Alone or Not Participating in Any Social Activity? Evidence from a Population-Based Eleven-Year Survey in Japan." *Social Science & Medicine* 233:57–63.

Oshio, Takashi, and Miki Kobayashi. 2010. "Income Inequality, Perceived Happiness, and Self-rated Health: Evidence from Nationwide Surveys in Japan." *Social Science & Medicine* 70:1358–1366.

Oshri, Assaf; Erinn B. Duprey, Steven M. Kogan, Matthew W. Carlson, and Sihong Liu. 2018. "Growth Patterns of Future Orientation among Maltreated Youth: A Prospective Examination of the Emergence of Resilience." *Developmental Psychology* 54(8):1456–1471.

Ossewaarde, Marinus. 2007. "Cosmopolitanism and the Society of Strangers." *Current Sociology* 55(3):367–388.

Osswald, Silvia, Tobias Greitemeyer, Peter F. Scher, and Dieter Frey. 2010. "What Is Moral Courage? Definition, Explication, and Classification of a Complex Construct." Pp. 149–164 in the *Psychology of Courage: Modern Research on an Ancient Virtue*, edited by Cynthia L.S. Pury and Shane J. Lopez. Washington, DC: American Psychological Association.

Osterling, Kathy Lemon, and Alice M. Hines. 2006. "Mentoring Adolescent Foster Youth: Promoting Resilience during Developmental Transitions." *Child & Family Social Work* 11(3):242–253.

Ostrom, Elinor. 2009. "What Is Social Capital." Pp. 17–38 in *Social Capital. Reaching out, Reaching in*, edited by Viva Ona Bartkus and James H. Davis. Cheltenham, UK: Edward Elgar.

Ou, Suh-Ruu, Irma Arteaga, and Arthur J. Reynolds. 2019. "Dosage Effects in the Child-Parent Center Prek-to-3rd Grade Program: A Re-Analysis in the Chicago Longitudinal Study." *Children & Youth Services Review* 101:285–98.

Ouweneel, Piet and Ruut Veenhoven. 2016. "Happy Protest Voters: The Case of Rotterdam 1997–2009." *Social Indicators Research* 126(2):739–56.

Overall, Nickda C. et al. 2020. "Effects of the COVID-19 Pandemic and Nationwide Lockdown on Trust, Attitudes toward Government, and Well-being." *American Psychologist* 75(5):618–630.

Overholt, William H. 2004. *Hong Kong at the Crossroads*. Santa Monica, CA: RAND.

Owen, Joel. 2023. "Psychological Resilience: Connecting Contemporary Psychology to Ancient Practical Philosophy." *Theory & Psychology* 33(3):366–85.

Owens, Laurence, Anthony Daly, and Phillip Slee. 2005. "Sex and Age Differences in Victimisation and Conflict Resolution among Adolescents in a South Australian School." *Aggressive Behavior* 31:1–12.

Owens, Timothy. 1992. "Where Do We Go from Here? Post-high School Choices of American Men." *Youth & Society* 23(4):452–477.

Owusu-Agyeman Yaw and Pertrude Amoakoheme. 2021. "Student Engagement and Perceived Gains in Transnational Education in Ghana." *International Journal of Comparative Education & Development* 23(4):297–311.

Oyserman, Daphna, Heather M. Coon, and Markus Kemmelmeier. 2002. "Rethinking Individualism and Collectivism: Evaluation of Theoretical Assumptions and Meta-analyses." *Psychological Bulletin* 128(1):3–72.

Ozbay, Ozben. 2008. "Does Social Capital Deter Youth from Cheating, Alcohol Use and Violence in Turkey? Bringing Torpil in." *Journal of Criminal Justice* 36:403–415.

Ozkirimli, Umut. 2005. Contemporary Debates on Nationalism: A Critical Engagement. Houndsmills, UK: Palgrave.

Paakkanen, Miia A., Frank Martela, and Anne B. Pessi. 2021. "Responding to Positive Emotions at Work – the Four Steps and Potential Benefits of a Validating Response to Coworkers" Positive Experiences." *Frontiers in Psychology* 12:668160.

Pabilonic, Sabrina Wulff. 2001. "Evidence on Youth Employment, Earnings, and Parental Transfers in the National Longitudinal Survey of Youth 1997." *Journal of Human Resources* 36(4):795–822.

Pachankis, John E., Kirsty A. Clark, Charles L. Burton, Jaclyn M. White Hughto, Richard Bränström, and Danya E. Keene. 2020. "Sex, Status, Competition, and Exclusion: Intraminority Stress from within the Gay Community and Gay and Bisexual Men's Mental Health." *Journal of Personality & Social Psychology,* 119(3):713–740.

Pacini, Rosemary and Seymour Epstein. 1999. "The Relation of Rational and Experiential Information Processing Styles to Personality, Basic Beliefs, and the Ratio-Bias Phenomenon." *Journal of Personality & Social Psychology* 76(6):972–87.

Padilla-Walker, Laura M., Larry J. Nelson, Xinyuan Fu, and Carolyn McNamara Barry. 2018. "Bidirectional Relations between Parenting and Prosocial Behavior for Asian and European-American Emerging Adults." *Journal of Adult Development* 25(2):107–120.

Paez, Dario, Bernard Rimé, Nekane Basabe, Anna Wlodarczyk, and Larraitz Zumeta. 2015. "Psychosocial Effects of Perceived Emotional Synchrony in Collective Gatherings." *Journal of Personality & Social Psychology* 108(5):711–29.

Paez, Dario, Nekane Basabe, Silvia Ubillos, and Jose Luis Gonzalez-Castro. 2007. "Social Sharing, Participation in Demonstrations, Emotional Climate, and Coping with Collective Violence after the March 11th Madrid Bombings." *Journal of Social Issues* 63(2):323–337.

Pai, Manacy, and Joongbaeck Kim. 2017. "Neighborhood Physical Disorder and Psychological Distress: Does the Risk Increase With Age?" *International Journal of Aging & Human Development* 84(4):378–402.

Paige, Katie J., Nolan E. Ramer, and Craig R. Colder. 2022. "Developmental Cascade Effects of Maternal Depression on Offspring Substance Use across Adolescence: Pathway through Mother-Child Relationship Quality and Peer Deviancy." *Research on Child & Adolescent Psychopathology* 50(7):933–44.

Paine, David R., Peter J. Jankowski, and Steven J. Sandage. 2016. "Humility as a Predictor of Intercultural Competence." *Family Journal* 24(1):15–22.

Pakulshi, Jan, and Bruce Tranter. 2000. "Civic, National and Denizen Identity in Australia." *Journal of Sociology* 36(2):205–222.

Palacios, Diego, Christian Berger, Bernadette Paula Luengo Kanacri, René Veenstra, and Jan Kornelis Dijkstra. 2019. "The Interplay of Adolescents" Aggression and Victimization with Friendship and Antipathy Networks within an Educational Prosocial Intervention." *Journal of Youth & Adolescence* 48(10):2005–2022.

Palacios, Margarita. 2013. Radical Sociality: On Disobedience, Violence and Belonging. Houndmills, UK: Palgrave.

Pallas, Aaron M. 2002. "Educational Participation across the Life Course: Do the Rich Get Richer?" *Advances in Life Course Research* 7:327–354.

Palmer, Neal A., Douglas D. Perkins, and Qingwen Xu. 2011. "Social Capital and Community Participation among Migrant Workers in China." *Journal of Community Psychology* 39(1):89–105.

Palmer, Stephen E. and William S. Griscom. 2013. "Accounting for Taste: Individual Differences in Preference for Harmony." *Psychonomic Bulletin & Review* 20(3):453–61.

Palmer-Rubin, Brian, Candelaria Garay, and Mathias Poertner. 2021. "Incentives for Organizational Participation: A Recruitment Experiment in Mexico." *Comparative Political Studies* 54(1):110–43.

Pan, Jia-Yan, Daniel Fu Keung Wong, Kin Sun Chan, and Cecilia Lai Wan Chan. 2008. "Development and Validation of the Chinese Making Sense of Adversity Scale: Acculturative Stressors as an Example." *Research on Social Work Practice* 18(5):479–486.

Pang, Zhenjing, Ce Zhao, and Lan Xue. 2022. "What Drives People's Protective Behaviors During the Early Stage of the COVID-19 Pandemic in China." *Frontiers in Psychology* 13:781279.

Pangallo, Antonio, Lara Zibarras, Rachel Lewis, and Paul Flaxman. 2015. "Resilience through the Lens of Interactionism: A Systematic Review." *Psychological Assessment* 27(1):1–20.

Panitch, Leo. 2008. Renewing Socialism: Transforming Democracy, Strategy and Imagination. Pontypool, UK: Merlin.

Panter-Brick, Catherine. 2015. "Culture and Resilience: Next Steps for Theory and Practice." Pp. 233–244 in *Youth Resilience and Culture: Commonalities and Complexities*, edited by Linda C. Theron, Michael Ungar, and Liebenberg Linda. Dordrecht, Netherlands: Springer.

Paoline, Eugene A. and Eric G. Lambert. 2012. "The Issue of Control in Jail: The Effects of Professionalism, Detainee Control, and Administrative Support on Job Stress, Job Satisfaction, and Organizational Commitment among Jail Staff." *American Journal of Criminal Justice* 37(2):179–99.

Papadakis, Elim. 1993. "Public Opinion, Sexual Difference and the Welfare State." *Australian and New Zealand Journal of Sociology* 29(3):343–366.

Papastephanou, Marianna. 2015. "The Lifeblood of Science and Its Politics: Interrogating Epistemic Curiosity as an Educational Aim." *Education Sciences* 6(4):1.

Parade, Stephnie H., Esther M. Leekes, and A. Nayena Blankson. 2010. "Attachment to Parents, Social Anxiety, and Close Relationships of Female Students over the Transition to College." *Journal of Youth & Adolescence* 39:127–137.

Paraskevopoulos, Christos J. 2010. "Social Capital: Summing up the Debate on a Conceptual Tool of Comparative Politics and Public Policy." *Comparative Politics* 42(4):475–94.

Pargament, Kenneth I. 1997. The Psychology of Religion and Coping: Theory, Research, Practice. New York: Guilford.

Pargament, Kenneth I., and Annette Mahoney. 2009. "Spirituality: The Search for the Sacred." Pp. 611–619 in *Oxford Handbook of Positive Psychology*, edited by C. R. Synder and Shane J. Lopez. New York, NY: Oxford University Press.

Pargament, Kenneth, Margaret Feuille, and Donna Burdzy. 2011. "The Brief Rcope: Current Psychometric Status of a Short Measure of Religious Coping." *Religions* 2(1):51–76.

Park, Crystal L., and Jeanne M. Slattery. 2014. "Resilience Interventions with a Focus on Meaning and Values." Pp. 270–282 in *The Resilience Handbook: Approaches to Stress and Trauma*, edited by Martha Kent, Mary C. Davis and John W. Reich. New York: NY: Routledge.

Park, Crystal L., Dalnim Cho, and Philip J. Moore. 2018. "How Does Education Lead to Healthier Behaviours? Testing the Mediational Roles of Perceived Control, Health Literacy and Social Support." *Psychology & Health* 33(11):1416–29

Park, Crystal. 2017. "Meaning Making and Resilience." Pp. 162–172 in *The Routledge International Handbook of Psychosocial Resilience*, edited by Updesh Kumar. Abingdon, UK: Routledge.

Park, Gum-Ryeong, HyunJee Park, and Jinho Kim. 2022. "Homeownership and Psychological Resources among Older Adults: Do Gender and Mortgage Status Moderate Homeownership Effects?" *Journal of Aging & Health* 34(1):88–99.

Park, Hong-Jae. 2015. "Legislating for Filial Piety: An Indirect Approach to Promoting Family Support and Responsibility for Older People in Korea." *Journal of Aging & Social Policy* 27(3):280–93.

Park, Hwanjin, Byung Seong Suh, Won Sool Kim, Hye-Kyung Lee, Seon-Cheol Park, and Kounseok Lee. 2015. "Character Profiles and Life Satisfaction." *Comprehensive Psychiatry* 58:172–177.

Park, Julie J. 2012. "When Race and Religion Collide: The Effect of Religion on Interracial Friendship During College." *Journal of Diversity in Higher Education* 5(1):8–21.

Park, Sung Hee, Choong-Ki Lee, and Joseph C. Miller. 2015. "A Comparative Study of the Motivations, Activities, Overall Satisfaction, and Post-Trip Behaviors of International Tourists in Macau: Mainland Chinese, Hongkongese, Taiwanese, and Westerners." *Asia Pacific Journal of Tourism Research* 20(10):1174–93

Parker, Ian. 2002. *Critical Discursive Psychology*. Houndsmills, UK: Palgrave. (BF455.P345)

Parker, Ian. 2011. *Lacanian Psychoanalysis: Revolutions in Subjectivity*. Hove, UK: Routledge.

Parker, Jennifer S., and Mark J. Benson. 2004. "Parent-adolescent Relations and Adolescent Functioning: Self-esteem, Substance Abuse, and Delinquency." *Adolescence* 39(155):519–530.

Parker, John, and Hilary Stanworth. 2005. "Go for It: Towards a Critical Realist Approach to Voluntary Risk Taking." *Health, Risk & Society* 7(4):319–336.

Parkes, Alison, Ade Kearns, and Rowland Atkinson. 2002. "What Makes People Dissatisfied with Their Neighbourhoods?" *Urban Studies* 39(13):2413–2438.

Parrott, Dominic J., Kevin M. Swartout, Andra Teten Tharp, Danielle M. Purvis, and Volkan Topalli. 2020. "Speak Up! Prosocial Intervention Verbalizations Predict Successful Bystander Intervention for a Laboratory Analogue of Sexual Aggression." *Sexual Abuse* 32(2):220–243.

Parslow, Ruth A., Anthony F. Jorm, Helen Christensen, Bryan Rodgers, and Patricia Jacomb, 2005. "Pet Ownership and Health in Older Adults: Findings from a Survey of 2,551 Community-Based Australians Aged 60-64." *Gerontology* 51(1):40–47.

Parsons, Talcott. 1968. *The Structure of Social Action*. New York: Free.

Parviniannasab, Ali Mohammad, Mahnaz Rakhshan, Marzieh Momennasab, Mitra Soltanian, Masoume Rambod, and Mahdi Akbarzadeh. 2022. "The Mediating Role of Courageous Coping in the Relations between Spirituality and Social Support with Resilience among Adolescents with Hemophilia." *Clinical Child Psychology & Psychiatry* 27(4):1141–54.

Pascarella, Ernest T., and Patrick T. Terenzini. 2005. *How College Affects Students, Vol. 2: A Third Decade of Research*. San Francisco, CA: Jossey-Bass.

Pascarella, Ernest T., Louise Bohr, Amaury Nora, and Patrick T. Terenzini. 1995. "Intercollegiate Athletic Participation and Freshman-year Cognitive Outcomes." *Journal of Higher Education* 66(4):369–387.

Passini, Stefano and Davide Morselli. 2011. "In the Name of Democracy: Disobedience and Value-Oriented Citizenship." *Journal of Community & Applied Social Psychology* 21(3):255–67.

Passini, Stefano and Davide Morselli. 2015. "Supporting Protest Movements: The Effect of the Legitimacy of the Claims." *International Journal of Psychological Research* 8(2):10–22.

Patall, Erika A., Harris Cooper, and Jorgianne Civey Robinson. 2008. "The Effects of Choice of Intrinsic Motivation and Related Outcomes: A Meta-analysis of Research Findings." *Psychological Bulletin* 134(2):270–300.

Patch, Kartikeya C. 2012. "Eastern Traditions, Consciousness, and Spirituality." Pp. 343–357 in *The Oxford Handbook of Psychology and Spirituality*, edited by Lisa J. Miller. New York, NY: Oxford University Press.

Paterson, Ian. 2018. "Any Room at the Inn? The Impact of Religious Elite Discourse on Immigration Attitudes in the United Kingdom." *British Journal of Politics & International Relations* 20(3):594–612.

Patrick, Heather, C. Raymond Knee, Amy Canevello, and Cynthia Lonsbary. 2007. "The Role of Need Fulfillment in Relationship Functioning and Well-being: A Self-determination Theory Perspective." *Journal of Personality & Social Psychology* 92(3):434–457.

Pattie, Charles, Patrick Seyd, and Paul Whiteley. 2004. *Citizenship in Britain: Values, Participation and Democracy*. Cambridge, UK: Cambridge University Press.

Patton, Wendy and Mary McMahon. 2021. *Career Development and Systems Theory: Connecting Theory and Practice*. Leiden, Netherlands:: Brill.

Patulny, Roger Vincent, and Alan Morris. 2012. "Questioning the Need for Social Mix: The Implications of Friendship Diversity amongst Australian Social Housing Tenants." *Urban Studies* 49(15):3365–3384.

Patwardhan, Vidya, Manuel Alector Ribeiro, Valsaraj Payini, and Kyle M. Woosnam, Jyothi Mallya, and Parvadhavardhini Gopalakrishnan. 2019. "Visitors? Place Attachment and Destination Loyalty: Examining the Roles of Emotional Solidarity and Perceived Safety." *Journal of Travel Research* 59(1):3–21.

Paul, Iman, Smaraki Mohanty, and Rumela Sengupta. 2022. "The Role of Social Virtual World in Increasing Psychological Resilience during the On-Going COVID-19 Pandemic." *Computers in Human Behavior* 127:107036.

Paul, Stephen. 2012. "Group Counselling and Therapy." Pp. 617–625 in *The SAGE Handbook of Counselling and Psychotherapy*, edited by Colin Feltham and Ian Horton. London: SAGE.

Paulhus, Delroy L. 1991. "Measurement and Control of Response Bias." Pp. 17–60 in *Measures of Personality and Social Psychological Attitudes, Vol. 1 of Measures of Social Psychological Attitudes*, edited by John P. Robinson, Phillip R. Shaver and Lawrence S. Wrightsman. San Diego, CA: Academic Press.

Pauwels, Lieven and Maarten De Waele. 2014. "Youth Involvement in Politically Motivated Violence: Why Do Social Integration, Perceived Legitimacy, and Perceived Discrimination Matter?" *International Journal of Conflict & Violence* 8(1):134–53.

Pavlova, Maria K., Astrid Körner, and Rainer K. Silbereisen. 2015. "Perceived Social Support, Perceived Community Functioning, and Civic Participation across the Life Span: Evidence from the Former East Germany." *Research in Human Development* 12(1–2):100–117.

Pawson, Hal, and Keith Kintrea. 2002. "Part of the Problem or Part of the Solution? Social Housing Allocation Policies and Social Exclusion in Britain." *Journal of Social Policy* 31(4):643–667.

Payne, Yasser, Arafat. 2011. "Site of Resilience: A Reconceptualization of Resiliency and Resilience in Street Life-oriented Black Men." *Journal of Black Psychology* 37(4):P426–451.

Paz-Fuchs, Amir. 2008. "Welfare to Work: Myth and Fact, Social Inclusion and Labour Exclusion." *Oxford Journal of Legal Studies* 28(4):797–817.

Pe, Madeline L. Ian H. Gotlib, Wim Van Den Noortgate, and Peter Kuppens. 2016. "Revisiting Depression Contagion as a Mediator of the Relation Between Depression and Rejection: A Speed-Dating Study." *Clinical Psychological Science* 4(4):675–682.

Peacock, Robert B., Priscilla A. Day, and Thomas D. Peacock. 1999. "Adolescent Gambling on a Great Lakes Indian Preservation." *Journal of Human Behavior in the Social Environment* 2(1/2):8–17.

Pearrow, Melissa M. 2011. "Opportunity for Unity Collaborative: Building Healthy Communities by Empowering Young Adults." *Community Development*. 42(2):167–180.

Peciuliauskiene, Palmira, Lina Kaminskienė, and Erno Lehtinen. 2023. "Science Teachers" Collaborative Innovative Activities: The Role of Professional Development and Professional Experience." *Humanities & Social Sciences Communications* 10:324.

Pedahzur, Ami, and Daphna Canetti-Nisim. 2004. "Support for Right-wing Extremist Ideology: Socio-economic Indicators and Socio-psychological Mechanisms of Social Identification." *Comparative Sociology* 3(1):1–36.

Pedersen, Daphne E., Jenelle Swenberger, and Katlyn E. Moes. 2017. "School Spillover and College Student Health," *Sociological Inquiry* 87(3):524–546.

Pedersen, Morten Axel. 2018. "Becoming What You Are: Faith and Freedom in a Danish Lutheran Movement." *Social Anthropology* 26(2):182–96.

Peet, Richard and Elaine Hatwick. 2009. *Theories of Development: Contentions, Arguments, Alternatives*. New York: Guilford.

Peeters, Miranda A. G., and Christel G. Rutte. 2005. "Time Management Behavior as in Moderation for the Job Demand-Control Interaction." *Journal of Occupational Health Psychology* 10(1):64–75.

Peifer, J. L. 2010. "The Economics and Sociology of Religious Giving: Instrumental Rationality or Communal Bonding?" *Social Forces* 88(4):1569–94.

Pelham, Brett W., and William B. Swann, Jr. 1989. "From Self-conceptions to Self-worth: On the Source and Structure of Global Self-esteem." *Journal of Personality & Social Psychology* 57(4):672–680.

Pellegrini, Anthony D., and Peter Blatchford. 2000. *The Child at School: Interactions with Peers and Teachers*. London: Arnold.

Pena, Pablo A. 2020. "Relative Age and Investment in Human Capital." *Economics of Education Review* 78:102039.

Pena-Lopez, José Atilano and José Manuel Sanchez-Santos. 2016. "Individual Social Capital: Accessibility and Mobilization of Resources Embedded in Social Networks." *Social Networks* 49:1–11.

Penarroja, Vicente, Miguel A. Serrano, Esther Gracia, Adrian Alacreu-Crespo, Patricia Gonzalez, and Vicente Martinez-Tur. 2017. "Rational-Experiential Thinking Style and Rational Intergroup Cooperation: The Moderating Role of Intergroup Conflict." *International Journal of Social Psychology* 32(1):23–51.

Peng, He. 2022. "Similar or Different Effects? Quantifying the Effects of Humility and Modesty on Job Performance." *Frontiers in Psychology* 13:809841.

Peng, Ito. 2012. "Social and Political Economy of Care in Japan and South Korea." *International Journal of Sociology & Social Policy* 32(11/12):636–49.

Peng, Zongchao, Ben Ma, and Taoxiong Liu. 2017. *Chinese Cooperative-Harmonious Democracy*. Abington, UK: Routledge.

Penner, Louis A. 2002. "Dispositional and Organizational Influences on Sustained Volunteerism: An Interactionist Perspective." *Journal of Social Issues* 58(3):447–467.

Penningroth, Suzanna L. and Walter D. Scott. 2012. "Age-Related Differences in Goals: Testing Predictions from Selection, Optimization, and Compensation Theory and Socioemotional Selectivity Theory." *International Journal of Aging & Human Development* 74(2):87–111.

Pentz, Marty. 2005. "Resilience among Older Adults with Cancer and the Importance of Social Support and Spirituality-faith: I Don"t Have Time to Die." *Journal of Gerontological Social Work* 44(3/4):3–22.

Peplak, Joanna and Tina Malti. 2022. "Toward Generalized Concern: The Development of Compassion and Links to Kind Orientations." *Journal of Adolescent Research* 37(6):776–804. \112–245

Percival, Garrick L. 2009. "Testing the Impact of Racial Attitudes and Racial Diversity on Prisoner Reentry Policies in the U.S. States." *State Politics & Policy Quarterly* 9(2):176–203.

Perdrix, Sphie, Sarah Stauffer, Jonas Masdonati, Koorosh Massoudi, and Jerome Rossier. 2012. "Effectiveness of Career Counseling: A One Year Follow-up." *Journal of Vocational Behavior* 80:265–278.

Pereyra-Rojas, Milagros, Enrique Mu, James Gaskin, and Tony Lingham. 2017. "The Higher-Ed Organizational-Scholar Tension: How Scholarship Compatibility and the Alignment of Organizational and Faculty Skills, Values and Support Affects Scholar's Performance and Well-Being." *Frontiers in Psychology* 8:450.

Perez, Tony, Jennifer G. Cromley, and Avi Kaplan. 2014. "The Role of Identity Development, Values, and Costs in College Stem Retention." *Journal of Educational Psychology* 106(1):315–29.

Perkins, Douglas D., and D. Adam Long. 2002. "Neighborhood Sense of Community and Social Capital: A Multi-level Analysis." Pp. 291–318 in *Psychological Sense of Community: Research, Applications and Implications*, edited by Adrian T. Fisher, Christopher C. Sonn and Brian J. Bishop. New York: Kluwer Academic.

Perks, Thomas and Michael Haan. 2011. "Youth Religious Involvement and Adult Community Participation: Do Levels of Youth Religious Involvement Matter?" *Nonprofit and Voluntary Sector Quarterly* 40(1):107–129.

Perlin, Jonah. 2011. "Religion as a Conversation Starter: What Liberal Religious Political Advocates Add to the Debate about Religion's Place in Legal and Political Discourse." *Georgetown Law Journal* 100(1):331–65.

Perner, Josef and Frank Esken. 2015. "Evolution of Human Cooperation in Homo Heidelbergensis: Teleology Versus Mentalism." *Developmental Review* 38:69–88.

Perrig, Chiello P., W.j. Perrig, and H.B. Stahelin. 1999. "Health Control Beliefs in Old Age: Relationship with Subjective and Objective Health, and Health Behavior." *Psychology, Health & Medicine* 4(1):83–94.

Perry, John L., Peter J. Clough, Lee Crust, Keith Earle, and Adam N. Nicholls. 2013. "Factorial Validity of the Mental toughness Questionnaire-48." *Personality & Individual Differences* 54:587–592.

Persell, Caroline Hodges. 1997. "The Interdependence of Social Justice and Civil Society." *Sociological Forum* 12(3):149–171.

Peruzzi, Agnese. 2014. "Understanding Social Exclusion from a Longitudinal Perspective: A Capability-Based Approach." *Journal of Human Development & Capabilities* 15(4):335–354.

Pervez, Adam, and Jonathan Halbesleben. 2017. "Burnout and Well-being." Pp. 101–122 in *Research Handbook on Work and Well-being*, edited by Ronald J. Burke and Kathryn M. Page. Cheltenham, UK: Elgar.

Petersen, Alan R. 1996. "Risk and the Regulated Self: The Discourse of Health Promotion as Politics of Uncertainty." *Australian and New Zealand Journal of Sociology* 32(1):44–57.

Petersen, Michael, Rune Slothuus, Rune Stubager, and Lise Togeby. 2011. "Freedom for All? The Strength and Limits of Political Tolerance." *British Journal of Political Science* 41(3):581–597.

Peterson, Bill E., and Eva C. Klohnen. 1995. "Realization of Generativity in Two Samples of Women at Midlife." *Psychology & Aging* 10(1):20–29.

Peterson, Christopher, and Martin E.P. Seligman. 2004. *Character Strengths and Virtues: A Handbook and Classification*. Washington, DC: American Psychological Association.

Peterson, Christopher, and Nansook Park. 2009. "Classifying and Measuring Strength of Character." Pp. 25–33 in *Oxford Handbook of Positive Psychology*, edited by C. R. Synder and Shane J. Lopez. New York, NY: Oxford University Press.

Peterson, Christopher, Nansook Park, and Patrick J. Sweeney. 2008. "Group Well-being: Morale from a Positive Psychology Perspective." *Applied Psychology* 57:19–36.

Peterson, Christopher. 1999. "Personal Control and Well-being." Pp. 288–301 in *Well-being: The Foundations of Hedonic Psychology*, edited by Daniel Kahneman, Ed Diener and Norbert Schwarz. New York: Russell Sage.

Peterson, Dana, and Finn-Aage Esbensen. 2004. "The Outlook Is G.R.E.A.T.: What Educators Say about School-based Education and Training (G.R.E.A.T.) Program." *Evaluation Review* 28(3):218–245.

Peterson, Gary W., Jose A. Cobas, Kevin R. Bush, Andrew Supple, and Stephan M. Wilson. 2006. "Parent-youth Relationships and the Self esteem of Chinese Adolescents: Collectivism versus Individualism." *Marriage & Family Review* 36(3–4):173–200.

Peterson, N. Andrew, and Joseph Huphey. 2004. "Social Cohesion and Intrapersonal Empowerment: Gender as Moderator." *Health Education Research* 19(5):533–542.

Peterson, Steven A., and Robert Maiden. 1993. "Personality and Politics among Older Americans: A Rural Case Study." *International Journal of Aging and Human Development* 36(2):157–169.

Petress, Kenneth C. 1995. "Coping with a New Educational Environment: Chinese Students" Imagined Interactions before Commencing Studies in the U.S." *Journal of Instructional Psychology* 22(1):50–63.

Petro, Nicolai N. 2001. "Creating Social Capital in Russia: The Novgorod Model." *World Development* 29(2):229–244.

Petrou, Michalis, and George Kandylis. 2016. "Violence and Extreme Right Activism: The Neo-Nazi Golden Dawn in a Greek Rural Community." *Journal of Intercultural Studies* 37(6):589–604.

Petrovic, Katja, Arthur A. Stukas, and Mathew D. Marques. 2020. "Religiosity, Motivations, and Volunteering: A Test of Two Theories of Religious Prosociality." *Journal of Theoretical Social Psychology* 4(4):157–68.

Pett, James. 2000. "Gay Lesbian and Bisexual Therapy and Its Supervision." Pp. 54–72 in *Therapeutic Perspectives on Working with Lesbian, Gay and Bisexual Clients*, edited by Dominic Davies and Charles Neal. Buckingham, UK: Open University Press.

Pettit, Gregory S., John E. Bates, Amy Holtzworth-Munroe, Amy D. Marshall, Lori D. Harach, David J. Cleary, and Kenneth A. Dodge. 2006. "Aggression and Insecurity in Late Adolescent Romantic Relationships: Antecedents and Developmental Pathways." Pp. 41–61 in *Developmental Contexts in Middle Childhood: Bridges to Adolescence and Adulthood*, edited by Aletha C. Huston and Marika N. Ripke. Cambridge, UK: Cambridge University Press.

Pfattheicher, Stefan, Mattis Geiger, Johanna Hartung, Selina Weiss, and Simon Schindler. 2017. "Old Wine in New Bottles? The Case of Self-compassion and Neuroticism." *European Journal of Personality* 31(2):160–169.

Pfeifer, Hanna. 2019. "The Normative Power of Secularism. Tunisian Ennahda's Discourse on Religion, Politics, and the State (2011–2016)." *Politics & Religion* 12(3):478–500.

Pfister, Isabel Barbara, Nicola Jacobshagen, Wolfgang Kälin, and Norbert Karl Semmer. 2020. "How Does Appreciation Lead to Higher Job Satisfaction?". *Journal of Managerial Psychology* 35(6):465–79.

Pfundmair, Michaela and Luisa A. M. Mahr. 2022. "Regaining Power: How Feelings of Exclusion During Covid-19 Are Associated with Radicalism among Critics of Containment Policies." *Frontiers in Psychology* 13:952760.

Phan, Mai B., Nadine Blumer, and Erin I. Demaiter. 2009. "Helping Hands: Neighborhood Diversity, Deprivation, and Reciprocity of Support in Non-kin Networks." *Journal of Social & Personal Relationships* 26(6–7):899–918.

Phelan, Elizabeth A., Lynda A. Anderson, Andrea Z. LaCroix, and Eric B. Larson. 2004. "Older Adults" Views of Successful Aging: How Do They Compare with Researchers" Definitions?" *Journal of American Geriatrics Society* 52:211–216.

Phillips, David. 2006. Quality of Life: Concept, Policy and Practice. London: Routledge.

Phinney, Jean S., Anthony Ong, and Tanya Madden. 2000. "Cultural Values and Intergenerational Value Discrepancies in Immigrant and Non-immigrant Famiies." *Child Development* 71(2):528–539.

Phipps, Shelley. 2003. "Social Cohesion and the Well-being of Canadian Children." Pp. 79–120 in *Economic Implications of Social Cohesion*, edited by Lars Osberg. Toronto, Canada: University of Toronto Press.

Phipps, Warwick D., and Charl Vorster. 2011 "Narrative Therapy: A Return to the Intrapsychic Perspective?" *Journal of Family Psychotherapy* 22(2):128–147.

Phongsavan, Philayrath, Tien Chey, Adrian Bauman, Robert Brooks, and Derrick Silove. 2006. "Social Capital, Socio-Economic Status and Psychological Distress among Australian Adults." *Social Science & Medicine* 63(10):2546–2561.

Phye, Gary D. 1997. "Inductive Reasoning and Problem Solving: The Early Grades." Pp. 451–471 *Handbook of Academic Learning: Construction of Knowledge*, edited by Gary D. Phye. San Diego, CA: Academic.

Pianta, Robert, Bridget Hamre, Jason Downer, Margaret Burchinal, Amanda Williford, Jennifer LoCasale-Crouch, Carollee Howes, Karen La Paro. and Catherine Scott-Little. 2017. "Early

Childhood Professional Development: Coaching and Coursework Effects on Indicators of Children's School Readiness." *Early Education & Development* 28(8):956–75.
Piatak, Jaclyn Sched. 2016. "Public Service Motivation, Prosocial Behaviours, and Career Ambitions." *International Journal of Manpower* 37(5):804–821.
Pickover, Clifford A. 2018. *Archimedes to Hawking: Laws of Science and the Great Minds Behind*. Oxford, UK: Oxford University Press.
Piedmont, Ralph L. 2012. "Overview and Development of a Trait-based Measure of Numinous Constructs: The Assessment of Spirituality and Religious Sentiments (ASPIRES) Scale." Pp. 104–122 in *The Oxford Handbook of Psychology and Spirituality*, edited by Lisa J. Miller. New York, NY: Oxford University Press.
Pierce, Barbara Decker, and Roderick E. White. 2006. "Resource Context and Emergent Social Structure: An Empirical Investigation of an Evolutionary Theory." *Journal of Organizational Behavior* 27:221–239.
Pierce, Kayla D. R., and Christopher S. Quiroz. 2018. "Who Matters Most? Social Support, Social Strain, and Emotions." *Journal of Social & Personal Relationships* 36(10):3273–3292.
Piercy, Kathleen W. 2000. "When It is More than a Job: Close Relationships between Home Health Aides and Older Clients." *Journal of Aging & Health* 13(3):362–387.
Piko, Bettina F., Noemi Keresztes, and Zsuzsanna F. Pluhar. 2006. "Aggressive Behavior and Psychosocial Health among Children." *Personality & Individual Differences* 40:885–895.
Piliavin, Jane Allyn, and Peter L. Callero. 1991. *Giving Blood: The Development of an Altruistic Identity*. Baltimore, MY: Johns Hopkins University Press.
Pincione, Guido, and Fernando R. Teson. 2006. *Rational Choice and Democratic Deliberation: A Theory of Discourse Failure*. New York: Cambridge University Press.
Pinker, Steven. 2011. The Better Angels of Our Nature: Why Violence Has Declined. New York. Viking.
Pinkerton, John, and Pat Dolan. 2007. "Family Support, Social Capital, Resilience and Adolescent Coping." *Child & Family Social Work* 12:219–228.
Pinto, Isabel R., Catarina L. Carvalho, Carina Dias, Paula Lopes, Sara Alves, Cátia de Carvalho, and José M. Marques. 2020. "A Path toward Inclusive Social Cohesion: The Role of European and National Identity on Contesting vs. Accepting European Migration Policies in Portugal." *Frontiers in Psychology* 11:1875.
Pintrich, Paul R., Akane Zusho, Ulrich Schiefele, and Reinhard Pekrun. 2001. "Goal Orientation and Self-regulated Learning in the College Classroom: A Cross-cultural Comparison." Pp. 149–169 in *Student Motivation: The Culture and Context of Learning*, edited by Farideh Salili, Chi Yue Chiu and Ying Yi Hong. New York: Kluwer.
Pires, Carla. 2022. "Global Predictors of COVID-19 Vaccine Hesitancy: A Systematic Review." *Vaccines* 10(8):1349.
Pitonak, Michal, Jiří Kožený, and Martin Čihák. 2023. "Disparities in Psychological Distress between Czech General Population and LGB + Community Sample." *Journal of Bisexuality*,
Pitzer, Jennifer and Ellen Skinner. 2017. "Predictors of Changes in Students' Motivational Resilience over the School Year." *International Journal of Behavioral Development* 41(1):15–29.
Plagnol, Anke, and Richard A. Easterlin. 2008. "Aspirations, Attainments, and Satisfaction: Life Cycle Differences between American Women and Men." *Journal of Happiness Studies* 9:601–619.
Pleiss, Mary K., and John F. Feldhusen. 1995. "Mentors, Role Models, and Heroes in the Lives of Gifted Children." *Educational Psychologists* 30(3):159–169.
Plohl, Nejc and Bojan Musil. 2023. "Assessing the Incremental Value of Intellectual Humility and Cognitive Reflection in Predicting Trust in Science." *Personality & Individual Differences* 214:112340.
Plouffe, Rachel A., Hiten P. Dave, Claire A. Wilson, Gabriela Topa, Alex Riggin, Chloe Lau, Vanessa M. Sinclair, Donald H. Saklofske, and Sandra Prince-Embury. 2020. "Validity and

Cross-Cultural Invariance of the Resiliency Scale for Young Adults - Spanish Version." *European Journal of Psychological Assessment* 36(5):918–922.

Plutzer, Eric, Adith Maney, and Robert E. O'Connor. 1998. "Ideology and Elite's Perceptions of the Safety of New Technologies." *American Journal of Political Science* 42:190–209.

Plutzer, Eric. 1987. "Determinants of Leftist Radical Belief in the United States: A Test of Competing Theories." *Social Forces* 65:1002–1019.

Pohling, Rico, Rhett Diessner, and Anja Strobel. 2018. "The Role of Gratitude and Moral Elevation in Moral Identity Development." *International Journal of Behavioral Development* 42(4):405–415.

Poku, Nana K., and Jim Whitman. 2011. "The Millennium Development Goals and Development after 2005." *Third World Quarterly* 32(1):181–198.

Policarpo, Verónica. 2015. "What Is a Friend? An Exploratory Typology of the Meanings of Friendship." *Social Sciences* 4(1):171–91.

Pollack, Detlef, and Gert Pickel. 2007. "Religious Individualization or Secularization? Testing Hypotheses of Religious Change: The Case of Eastern and Western Germany." *British Journal of Sociology* 58(4):623–632.

Pollio, Howard R., Tracy B. Henley, and Craig J. Thompson. 1997. *The Phenomenology of Everyday Life.* Cambridge, UK: Cambridge University Press. (BF204.5P65) \102–178

Pomerleau, Julie M., Kenneth I. Pargament, Neal Krause, Gail Ironson, and Peter Hill. 2020. "Religious and Spiritual Struggles as a Mediator of the Link between Stressful Life Events and Psychological Adjustment in a Nationwide Sample." *Psychology of Religion & Spirituality* 12(4):451–59.

Pompili, Maurizio, Marco Innamorati, David Lester, Srena Brunetti, Roberto Tatarelli, and Paolo Girardi. 2007. "Gender Effects among Undergraduates Relating to Suicide Risk, Impulsivity, Aggression and Self-efficacy." *Personality & Individual Differences* 43:2047–2056.

Pong, Suet-ling, and Vivien W. Chen. 2010. "Co-resident Grandparents and Grandchildren's Academic Performance in Taiwan." *Journal of Comparative Family Studies* 41(1):111–129.

Poortinga, Wouter. 2012. "Community Resilience and Health: The Role of Bonding, Bridging, and Linking Aspects of Social Capital." *Health & Place* 18(2):286–95.

Portes, Alejandro and Erik Vickstrom. 2011. "Diversity, Social Capital, and Cohesion." *Annual Review of Sociology* 37:467–479.

Portes, Alejandro. 2000. "The Two Meanings of Social Capital." *Sociological Forum* 15(1):1–12.

Portnoy, Galina A., Mark R. Relyea, Suzanne Decker, Andrea Shamaskin-Garroway, Mary Driscoll, Cynthia A. Brandt, and Sally G. Haskell. 2018. "Understanding Gender Differences in Resilience among Veterans: Trauma History and Social Ecology." *Journal of Traumatic Stress* 31(6):845–55.

Posel, Dorrit Ruth, and Daniela Maria Casale. 2011. "Relative Standing and Subjective Well-being in South Africa: The Role Perceptions, Expectations and Income Mobility." *Social Indicators Research* 104:195–223.

Posthumus, Hanneke, Gideon Bolt, and Ronald van Kempen. 2013. "Why Do Displaced Residents Move to Socioeconomically Disadvantaged Neighborhoods?" *Housing Studies* 28(2):272–293.

Potash, Jordan S. 2019. "Actually, Hong Kong Is a Small Town: Art Therapy and Multiple Relationships within a Community." Pp. 191–197 in *Exploring Ethical Dilemmas in Art Therapy: 50 Clinicians from 20 Countries Share Their Stories*, edited by Audrey Di Maria.

Poveda, Alexander Cotte. 2011. "Economic Development, Inequality, and Poverty: An Analysis of Urban Violence in Columbia." *Oxford Development Studies* 39(4):453–468.

Powdthavee, Nattavudh. 2009. "I Can't Smile without You: Spousal Correlation in Life Satisfaction." *Journal of Economic Psychology* 30(4):675–89.

Powell, Fred. 2007. The Politics of Civil Society: Big Society, Small Government? Bristol, UK: Policy Press.

Powell, William E. 1994. "The Relationship between Feelings of Alienation and Burnout in Social Work." *Families in Society* 75(4):229–234.

Power, Ann Marie R., and Vladimir T. Khmelkov. 1999. "The Effects of Service Participation on High School Students" Social Responsibility." *Research in Sociology of Education & Socialization* 12:185–210.

Power, Mick, and Tim Dalgleish. 2008. *Cognition and Emotion: From Order to Disorder*. Hove, UK: Psychology.

Powley, Edward H. 2009. "Reclaiming Resilience and Safety: Resilience Activation in the Critical Period of Crisis." *Human Relations* 62(9):1289–1326.

Poynton, Timothy A., Richard T. Lapan, and Amanda M. Marcotte. 2015. "Financial Planning Strategies of High School Seniors: Removing Barriers to Career Success." *Career Development Quarterly* 63(1):57–73. \101–248

Praszkier, Ryszard. 2018. *Empowering Leadership of Tomorrow*. Cambridge, UK: Cambridge University Press.

Pratt, Michael W., and M. Kyle Matsuba. 2018. The Life Story, Domains of Identity, and Personality Development in Emerging Adulthood: Integrating Narrative and Traditional Approaches. New York, NY: Oxford University Press.

Pratt, Michael W., Rhett Diessner, Adelle Pratt, Bruce Hunsberger, and S. Mark Pancer. 1996. "Moral and Social Reasoning and Perceptive Testing in Later Life: A Longitudinal Study." *Psychology & Aging* 11(1):66–73.

Pratt, Travis C., Kristy Holtfreter, and Michael D. Reisig. 2010. "Routine Online Activity and Internet Fraud Targeting: Extending the Generality of Routine Activity Theory." *Journal of Research in Crime & Delinquency* 47(3):267–296.

Preda, Adina. 2013. "Group Rights and Shared Interests." *Political Studies* 61(2):250–66.

Prelow, Hazel M., Scott R. Weaver, and Rebecca R. Swenson. 2006. "Competence, Self-esteem, and Coping Efficacy as Mediators of Ecological Risk and Depressive Symptoms in Urban African American and European American Youth." *Journal of Youth & Adolescence* 35:507–517.

Premo, Joshua, Richard Lamb, and Andy Cavagnetto. 2018. "Conditional Cooperators: Student Prosocial Dispositions and Their Perceptions of the Classroom Social Environment." *Learning Environment Research* 21(2):229–244.

Prenda, Kimberly M., and Margie E. Lachman. 2001. "Planning for the Future: A Life Management Strategy for Increasing Control and Life Satisfaction in Adulthood." *Psychology & Aging* 16(2):206–216.

Pressgrove, Geah, Cristobal Barra, and Melissa Janoske. 2020. "Using STOPS to Predict Prosocial Behavioral Intentions: Disentangling the Effects of Passive and Active Communicative Action." *Public Relations Review* 46(4):101956.

Preston, Jesse L. and Abdullah Khan. 2024. "Comparing the Influence of Intellectual Humility, Religiosity, and Political Conservatism on Vaccine Attitudes in the United States, Canada, and the United Kingdom." *Public Understanding of Science* . 33(3):343–52. \110–256

Preston, Mark S. 2018. "Does Job Control Moderate Work Demands" Nonlinear Association with Job Strain? A Two-Sample Study Using Human Service Case Managers." *Human Service Organizations, Management, Leadership & Governance* 42(3):300 17.

Pretsch, Johanna and Natalie Ehrhardt-Madapathi. 2018. "Experiences of Justice in School and Attitudes Towards Democracy: A Matter of Social Exchange?" *Social Psychology of Education* 21(3):655–75.

Pretty, Jules, and Hugh ward. 2001. "Social Capital and the Environment." *World Development* 29(2):209–227.

Prezza, Miretta, Matilde Amici, Tiziana Roberti, and Gloria Tedeschi. 2001. "Sense of Community Referred to the Whole Town: Its Relations with Neighboring, Homelessness, Life Satisfaction and Area of Residence." *Journal of Community Psychology* 29(1):29–52.

Price, Vincent, Clarissa David, Brian Goldthorpe, Marci Mccoy Roth, and Joseph N. Cappella. 2006. "Locating the Issue Public: The Multi dimensional Nature of Engagement with Health Care Reform." *Public Behavior* 28(1):33–63.

Prilleltensky, Isaac. 2012. "Wellness as Fairness." *American Journal of Community Psychology* 49:1–21.

Primoratz, Igor. 1999. *Ethics and Sex*. London, UK: Routledge.

Prince-Embury, Sandra, Donald H. Saklofshe, and Kateryna V. Keefer. 2017. "Three-factor Model of Personal Resilience." Pp. 34–45 in *The Routledge International Handbook of Psychosocial Resilience*, edited by Updesh Kumar. Abingdon, UK: Routledge.

Prince-Embury, Sandra. 2013b "Community-level Resiliency Intervention in a Post-disaster Environment: The Three Mile Island Health and Environmental Information Series—Theoretical Assumptions, Implementation, and Participant Response." Pp. 227–242 in *Resilience in Children, Adolescents, and Adults: Translating Research into Practice*, edited by Sandra Prince-Embury and Donald H. Saklofske. New York, NY: Springer.

Prince-Embury, Sandra. 2013c. "Bowen Systems Theory Aplied to Systemic Resilience versus Vulnerability." Pp. 315–333 in *Resilience in Children, Adolescents, and Adults: Translating Research into Practice*, edited by Sandra Prince-Embury and Donald H. Saklofske. New York, NY: Springer.

Prince-Embury, Sandra. 2014a. "Three-factor Model of Individual resiliency and Related Interventions." Pp. 13–23 in *Resilience Interventions for Youth in Diverse Populations*, edited by Sandra Prince-Embury and Donald H. Saklofske. New York, NY: Springer.

Principi, Andrea, Henrike Galenkamp, Roberta Papa, Marco Socci, Bianca Suanet, Andrea Schmidt, Katharine Schulmann, Stella Golinowska, Agnieszka Sowa, Amilcar Moreira, and Dorly J. H. Deeg. 2016. "Do Predictors of Volunteering in Older Age Differ by Health Status?" *European Journal of Ageing* 13(2):91–102.

Prins, Karin, Bram P. Buunk, and Nico W. VanYperen. 1993. "Equity, Normative Disapproval and Extramarital Relationships." *Journal of Social & Personal Relationships* 10:39–53.

Prins, R.G.., M.A. Beenackers, M.C. Boog, F.J. Van Lenthe, J. Brug, and A. Oenema. 2014. "Neighbourhood Social Capital as a Moderator Between Individual Cognitions and Sports Behaviour among Dutch Adolescents." *Social Science & Medicine* 105:9–15.

Prinstein, Mitchell J., and Shirley S. Wang. 2005. "False Consensus and Adolescent Peer Contagion: Examining Discrepancies between Perceptions and Actual Reported Levels of Friends" Deviant and Health Risk Behaviors." *Journal of Abnormal Child Psychology* 33(3):293–306.

Printz, Brian L., Mark D. Shermis, and Patrick M. Webb. 1999. "Stress-buffering Factors Related to Adolescent Coping: A Path Analysis." *Adolescence* 34(136):715–734.

Proulx, Travis and Steven J. Heine. 2006. "Death and Black Diamonds: Meaning, Mortality, and the Meaning Maintenance Model." *Psychological Inquiry* 17(4):309–18.

Prouteau, Liopel, and Francois-Charles Wolff. 2008. "On the Relational Motive for Volunteer Work." *Journal of Economic Psychology* 29:314–335.

Proyer, Rene T., Willibald Ruth, and Claudia Bnschor. 2013. "Testing Strengths-based Interventions: A Preliminary Study on the Effectiveness of a Program Targeting Curiosity, Gratitude, Hope, Humor, and Zest for Enhancing Life Satisfaction." *Journal of Happiness Studies* 14:275–292.

Pryor, Robert G.L., & Jim E.H. Bright. 2007. "Applying Chaos Theory to Careers: Attraction and Attractors." *Journal of Vocational Behavior* 71:375–400.

Puig, Marieva, Michael Canute Lambert, George T. Rowan, Tyrone Winfrey, Miilchail Lyubansky, Stanley D. Hannan, and Martin F. Hill. 1999. "Behavioral and Emotional Problems among Jamaican and African American Children, Ages 6 to 11: Teacher Reports versus Direct Observations." *Journal of Emotional & Behavioral Disorders* 7(4):240–250.

Pulkkinen, Lea, Anna-Liisa Lyyra, and Katja Kokko. 2009. "Life Success of Males on Nonoffender, Adolescence-Limited, Persistent, and Adult-Onset Antisocial Pathways: Follow-up from Age 8 to 42." *Aggressive Behavior* 35(2):117–135.

Pulkkinen, Lea. 2018. "Longitudinal Study of Personality and Social Development: Insights about Aggression after Five Decades." Pp. 31–51 *The Cambridge Handbook of Violent Behavior and Aggression*, edited by Alexander T. Vazsonyi, David J. Flannery and Matt DeLisi. Cambridge, UK: Cambridge University Press.

Puntscher, Sibylle, Christoph Hauser, Janette Walde, and Gottfried Tappeiner. 2016. "Measuring Social Capital with Aggregated Indicators: A Case of Ecological Fallacy?" *Social Indicators Research* 125(2):431–449.

Putman, Daniel. 2010. "Philosophical Roots of the Concept of Courage." Pp. 9–22 in the *Psychology of Courage: Modern Research on an Ancient Virtue*, edited by Cynthia L.S. Pury and Bhane J. Lopez. Washington, DC: American Psychological Association.

Putnam, Robert D. 2007. "E Pluribus Unum: Diversity and Community in the Twenty-first Century." *Scandinavian Political Studies* 30(2):137–174.

Putnam, Robert. 2002. Democracies in Flux: The Evolution of Social Capital in Contemporary Society. New York: Oxford University Press.

Pyszkowska, Anna and Michael Ronnlund. 2021. "Psychological Flexibility and Self-Compassion as Predictors of Well-Being: Mediating Role of a Balanced Time Perspective." *Frontiers in Psychology* 12:671746.

Pyszkowska, Anna. 2020. "Personality Predictors of Self-Compassion, Ego-Resiliency and Psychological Flexibility in the Context of Quality of Life." *Personality & Individual Differences* 161:109932.

Qin, Chu. 2013. *Daoist Living, Scholarist Pracice*, Buddhist Cultivation. Beijing, China: Foreing Languages.

Qiu, Lin and Jinyan Fan. 2015. "Family Boundary Characteristics, Work-Family Conflict and Life Satisfaction: A Moderated Mediation Model." *International Journal of Psychology* 50(5):336–44.

Qu, Diyang, Jiasheng Huang, Chrystyna D. Kouros, and Nancy Xiaonan Yu. 2021. "Dyadic Effects of Fluid Mindset on Psychological Growth in Immigrant Mothers and Their Children: Indirect Effect of Resilience." *Family Process* 60:1507–22.

Quackenbush, Steven W., Alanah K. Lockwood, and Travis G. Cyr. 2016. "And yet Your Duty Is to Hope: The Positive Psychology of Jean-Paul Sartre." *Theory & Psychology* 26(3):360–376.

Quick, James Campbell, Debra L. Nelson, Jonathan D. Quick, and Dusty K. Orman. 2001. "An Isomorphic Theory of Stress: The Dynamics of Person-environment Fit." *Stress & Health* 17:147–157.

Quilty, Lena C., Jonathan M. Oakman, and Evan Risoo. 2006. "Correlates of the Rosenberg Self-esteem Scale Method Effects." *Structural Equation Modeling* 13(1):99–117.

Quinn, Jane. 1995. "Positive Effects of Participation in Youth Organizations." Pp. 274–304 in *Psychosocial Disturbances in Young People*: Challenges for Prevention, edited by Michael Rutter. Cambridge, UK: Cambridge University Press.

Raab, Jurgen. 2019. *Erving Goffman: From the Perspective of the New Sociology of Knowledge.* Abington, UK: Routledge.

Rabin, Carolyn. 2011. "Review of Health Behaviors and Their Correlates among Young Adult Cancer Survivors." *Journal of Behavioral Medicine* 34:41–52.

Radley, Keith C., William R. Jenson, Elaine Clark, Julia A. Hood, and Peter Nicholas. 2014. "Using a Multimedia Social Skills Intervention to Increase Social Engagement of Young Children with Autism Spectrum Disorder." *Intervention in School & Clinic* 50(1):22–28.

Raffo, Carlo, and Helen Gunter. 2008. "Leading Schools to Promote Social Inclusion: Developing a Conceptual Framework for Analysing Research, Policy and Practice." *Journal of Educational Policy* 23(4):397–414.

Ragheb, Mounir G., and Charles A. Griffith. 1982. "The Contribution of Leisure Participation and Leisure Satisfaction to Life Satisfaction of Older Persons." *Journal of Leisure Research* 14:295–306.

Rahn, Wendy. 2008. "Cooperation with and without Trust: Evidence from Local Settings." Pp. 259–274 in *Cooperation: The Political Psychology of Effective Human Interaction*, edited by Brandon A. Sullivan, Mark Snyder and John L. Sullivan. Malden, MA: Blackwell.

Raijman, Rebeca, Eldad Davidov, Peter Schmidt, and Oshrat Hochman. 2008. "What Does a Nation Owe Non-Citizens?" *International Journal of Comparative Sociology* 49(2–3):195–220.

Raijman, Rebeca, Moshe Semyonov, and Peter Schmidt. 2003. "Do Foreigners Deserve Rights? Determinants of Public Views towards Foreigners in Germany and Israel." *European Sociological Review* 19(4):379–392.

Raitakari, Suvi, Riikka Haahtela, and Kirsi Juhila. 2016. "Tackling Community Integration in Mental Health Home Visit Integration In Finland." *Health & Social Care in the Community* 24(5):e53–e62,

Rajan-Rankin, Sweta. 2014. "Self-Identity, Embodiment and the Development of Emotional Resilience." *British Journal of Social Work* 44(8):242624–42.

Rakap, Salih and Serife Balikci. 2023. "Training Preservice Teachers to Use Evidence-Based Practices: Effects of Coaching with Performance Feedback on Teacher and Child Outcomes." *Learning & Instruction* 86:101755.

Ralph, Jason. 2018. "What Should Be Done? Pragmatic Constructivist Ethics and the Responsibility to Protect." *International Organization* 72(1):173–203.

Ram, Rati. 2009. "Government Spending and Happiness of the Population: Additional Evidence from Large Cross-country Samples." *Public Choice* 138:483–490.

Ramadier, Thierry. 2017. "Adjustment to Geographical Space and Psychological Well-Being." Pp. 291–307 in *Handbook of Environmental Psychology and Quality of Life Research*, edited by Ghozlane Fleury-Bahi, Graciela Tonon, Enric Pol, and Oscar Navarro. Cham, Switzerland: Springer.

Ramasubramanian, Srividya. 2017. "Mindfulness, Stress Coping and Everyday Resilience among Emerging Youth in a University Setting: A Mixed Methods Approach." *International Journal of Adolescence & Youth* 22(3):308–321.

Rampichini, Carla, and Silvana Schifini D"Andrea. 1998. "A Hierarchical Ordinal Probit Model for the Analysis of Life Satisfaction in Italy." *Social Indicators Research* 44(1):41–69.

Ramsay, Maureen. 1997. *What's Wrong with Liberalism? A Radical Critque of Liberal Political Philosophy.* London, UK: Leicester University Press.

Ramsey, Janet L., and Rosemary Blieszner. 1999. *Spiritual Resiliency in Older Women: Models of Strength for Challenges through the Life Span.* Thousand Oaks, CA: Sage.

Ramsey, Meagan A., and Amy L. Gentzler. 2015. "An upward Spiral: Bidirectional Associations between Positive Affect and Positive Aspects of Close Relationships across the Life Span." *Developmental Review* 36:58–104.

Ran, Jingliang, Huiyue Liu, Yue Yuan, Xuan Yu, and Tiantian Dong. 2023. "Linking Career Exploration, Self-Reflection, Career Calling, Career Adaptability and Subjective Well-Being: A Self-Regulation Theory Perspective." *Psychology Research & Behavior Management* 16:2805–17.

Rand, David G. 2016. "Cooperation, Fast and Slow." *Psychological Science* 27(9):1192–1206.

Randall, William L., and A. Elizabeth McKim. 2008. *Reading Our Lives: The Poetics of Growing Old.* New York: Oxford University Press.

Rantanen, Johanna, Pessi Lyyra, Taru Feldt, Mikko Villi, and Tiina Parviainen. 2021. "Intensified Job Demands and Cognitive Stress Symptoms: The Moderator Role of Individual Characteristics." *Frontiers in Psychology* 12:607172.

Raper, Mitchell J., Paula Brough, and Amanda Biggs. 2019. "Evidence for the Impact of Organisational Resources versus Job Characteristics in Assessments of Occupational Stress over Time." *Applied Psychology* 69(3):715–740.

Raphals, Lisa. 1992. Knowing Words: Wisdom and Cunning in the Classical Traditions of China and Greece. Ithaca, NY: Cornell University Press.

Raposa, Elizabeth B., Holly B. Laws, and Emily B. Ansell. 2016. "Prosocial Behavior Mitigates the Negative Effects of Stress in Everyday Life." *Clinical Psychological Science* 4(4):691–698.

Rashid, Tayyab. 2014. "Positive Psychology in Practice: Positive Psychotherapy." Pp. 978–993 in *The Oxford Handbook of Happiness*, edited by Susan A. David, Ilona Boniwell and Amanda Conley Ayers. Oxford, UK: Oxford University Press.

Rasmussen, Stig Hebbelstrup Rye, and AsbjØRn Sonne NØRgaard. 2018. "When and Why Does Education Matter? Motivation and Resource Effects in Political Efficacy." *European Journal of Political Research* 57(1):24–46.

Ratelle, Jean-François, and Emil Aslan Souleimanov. 2017. "Retaliation in Rebellion: The Missing Link to Explaining Insurgent Violence in Dagestan." *Terrorism & Political* 29(4):573–592.

Raty, Hannu, Ulla Hytti, Kati Kasanen, Katri Komulainen, Päivi Siivonen, and Inna Kozlinska. 2020. "Perceived Employability and Ability Self among Finnish University Students." *European Journal of Psychology of Education* 35(4):975–93.

Ravanera, Zenaida R., Fernando Rajalton, and Pierre Turcotta. 2003. "Youth Integration and Social Capital: An Analysis of the Canadian Social Surveys in Time Use." *Youth & Society* 35(2):158–182.

Rawlings, Mary A. 2012. "Assessing BSW Student Direct Practice Skill Using Standardized Clients and Self-efficacy Theory." *Journal of Social Work Education* 48(2):553–576.

Rawwas, Mohammed Y. A., Jamal A. Al-Khatib, and Scott J. Vitell. 2004. "Academic Dishonesty: A Cross-cultural Comparison of U.S. and Chinese Marketing Students." *Journal of Marketing Education* 26(1):89–100.

Ray, Larry. 2014. "Shame and the City: Looting, Emotions and Social Structure." *Sociological Review* 62:117–136.

Raymo, James M. 2015. "Living Alone in Japan: Relationships with Happiness and Health." *Demographic Research* 32(1):1267–98.

Reardon, Sean F., and Kendra Bischoff. 2011. "Income Inequality and Income Segregation." *American Journal of Sociology* 116(4):1092–1153.

Reavy, Matthew. 2023. *Professional Communication Ethics*. Long Grove, IL: Waveland.

Reay, Diane. 2004. "Gendering Bourdieu's Concepts of Capitals? Emotional Capital, Women and Social Class."*Sociological Review* 52:S57–S74.

Recchia, Holly E., and Nina Howe. 2010. "When Do Siblings Compromise? Associations with Children's Descriptions of Conflict Issues, Culpability, and Emotions." *Social Development* 18(4):838–857.

Redmond, Mark V. 2018. *Social Decentering: A Theory of Other orientation Encompassing Empathy and Perspective-taking*. Berlin, Germany: Walter de Gruyter.

Reed, Isaac Ariail. 2013. "Power: Relational, Discursive, and Performative Dimensions." *Sociological Theory* 31(3):193–218.

Rees, C. Roger, and Frank M. Howell. 1990. "Do High School Sports Build Character? A Quasi-experiment on a National Sample." *Social Science Journal* 27(3):76–92.

Rees, Peter. 2023. "Rhetoric and Rights: Citizenship and the Politics of Persuasion." *Political Studies*,

Reese, Gerhard, Amir Rosenmarnn, and James E. Cameron. 2019. *The Psychology of Globalization: Identity, Ideology, and Action*. London, UK: Academic.

Reeskens, Tim and Leen Vandecasteele. 2017. "Economic Hardship and Well-Being: Examining the Relative Role of Individual Resources and Welfare State Effort in Resilience against Economic Hardship." *Journal of Happiness Studies* 18(1):41–62.

Reeskens, Tim, and Wim van Oorschot. 2013. "Equity, Equality, or Need? A Study of Popular Preferences for Welfare Redistribution: Principles across 24 European Countries." *Journal of European Public Policy* 20(8):1174–1195.

Regev, Rotem, and Marion F. Ehrenberg. 2012. "A Pilot Study of a Support Group for Children in Divorcing Families: Aiding Community Program Development and Marking Pathways to Resilience." *Journal of Divorce & Remarriage* 53(3):220–230.

Regnerus, Mark D. 2003. "Religion and Positive Adolescent Outcomes: A Review of Research and Theory." *Review of Religious Research* 44(4):394–413.

Rego, Armenio, Fernanda Machado, Susana Leal, and Miguel Pima E. Cunha. 2009. "Are Hopeful Employees More Creative? An Empirical Study." *Creativity Research Journal* 21(2–3):223–231.

Reich, Sabine, Frank M. Schneider, and Leonie Heling. 2018. "Zero Likes: Symbolic Interactions and Need Satisfaction Online." *Computers in Human Behavior* 80.97–102.

Reicher, Stephen, Russell Spears, and S. Alexander Haslam. 2010. "The Social Identity Approach in Social Psychology." Pp. 45–62 in *The SAGE Handbook of Identities*, edited by Margaret Wetherell and Chandra Talpade Mohanty. London, UK: SAGE,

Reichert, Frank and Murray Print. 2017. "Mediated and Moderated Effects of Political Communication on Civic Participation." *Information, Communication & Society* 20(8):1162–84. \92–359

Reid, John B., J. Mark Eddy, Rebecca Ann Fetrow, and Mike Stoolmiller. 1999. "Description and Immediate Impacts of a Preventive Intervention for Conduct Problems." *American Journal of Community Psychology* 27(4):483–517.

Reilly, Jacqueline, Orla T. Muldoon, and Clare Byrne. 2004. "Young Men as Victims and Perpetrators of Violence in Northern Ireland: A Qualitative Analysis." *Journal of Social Issues* 60(3):469–484.

Reis, Olaf, and Heike M. Buhl. 2008. "Individuation during Adolescence and Emerging Adulthood: 5 German Studies." *International Journal of Behavioral Development* 32(5):369–371.

Reitzes, Donald C., and Elizabeth J. Mutran. 2004. "The Transition to Retirement: Stages and Factors that Influence Retirement Adjustment." *Internal Journal of Aging & Human Development* 59(1):63–84.

Reitzle, Matthias, Fred W. Vondracek, and Rainer K. Silbereisen. 1998. "Timing of School-to-work Transitions: Developmental-contextual Perspective." *International Journal of Behavioral Development* 22(1):7–28.

Renfrow, Daniel G., and Judith A. Howard. 2013. "Social Psychology of Gender and Race." Pp. 491–531 in *Handbook of Social Psychology*, edited by John Delamater and Amanda Ward. Dordrecht, Netherlands: Springer.

Renger, Daniela, and Gerhard Reese. 2017. "From Equality-Based Respect to Environmental Activism: Antecedents and Consequences of Global Identity." *Political Psychology* 38(5):867–879.

Renger, Daniela, Silke Eschert, Mimke L. Teichgräber, and Sophus Renger. 2020. "Internalized Equality and Protest against Injustice: The Role of Disadvantaged Group Members" Self-Respect in Collective Action Tendencies." *European Journal of Social Psychology* 50(3):547–60.

Rentziou, Aikaterini, Christina Milioti, Konstantina Gkritza, and Matthew G. Karlaftis. 2011. "Urban Road Pricing: Modeling Public Acceptance." *Journal of Urban Planning & Development* 137(1):56–64.

Requena, Felix. 2003. "Social Capital, Satisfaction and Quality of Life in the Workplace." *Social Indicators Research* 61:331–360.

Requena, Miguel and Mikolaj Stanek. 2014. "Religiosity and Politics in Spain and Poland: A Period Effect Analysis." *Sociological Compass* 61(3):348–67.

Reyna, Valerie F., and Frank Farley. 2006. "Risk and Rationality in Adolescent Decision Making: Implications for Theory, Practice, and Public Policy." *Psychological Science in the Public Interest* 7(1):1–44.

Reynolds, Jill, Margaret Wetherell, and Stephanie Taylor. 2007. "Choice and Chance: Negotiating Agency in Narratives of Singleness." *Sociological Review* 55(2):331–351. \a00–1–2

Reynolds, Nicola. 2015. "Discourses of Love, Compassion, and Belonging: Reframing Christianity for a Secular Audience." *Journal Contemporary Religion* 30(1):39–54.

Riad, Jasmin K., and Fran H. Norris. 1992. "The Influence of Relocation on the Environmental, Social, and Psychological Stress Experienced by disaster Victims." *Environment & Behavior* 28(2):163–182.

Richards, Lindsay. 2016. "For Whom Money Matters Less: Social Connectedness as a Resilience Resource in the UK." *Social Indicators Research* 125(2):509–535.

Richards, P. Scott. 2012. "Honoring Religious Diversity and Universal Spirituality in psychotherapy." Pp. 237–254 in *The Oxford Handbook of Psychology and Spirituality*, edited by Lisa J. Miller. New York, NY: Oxford University Press.

Richardson, Glenn E. 2002. "The Metatheory of Resilience and Resiliency." *Journal of Clinical Psychology* 58(3):307–321.

Richardson, Glenn E. 2017. “The Applied Metatheory of Resilience and Resiliency.” Pp. 124–135 in *The Routledge International Handbook of Psychosocial Resilience*, edited by Updesh Kumar. Abingdon, UK: Routledge.

Richardson, Michael Joseph. 2018. “Occupy Hong Kong? Gweilo Citizenship and Social Justice.” *Annals of the American Association of Geographers* 108(2):486–498.

Richert, Alphons J. 2002. “The Self Narrative Therapy: Thoughts from a Humanistic/Existential Perspective.” *Journal of Psychotherapy Integration* 12(1):77–104.

Richey, Sean, and Ken’ichi Ikeda. 2009. “Institutional Incentives and Trust: Marginalized Groups and the Creation of Trust in Local Government.” *Social Science Quarterly* 90(4):911–926.

Richey, Sean. 2010. “The Impact of Corruption on Social Trust.” *American Politics Research* 38(4):676–690.

Richter, Jörg, Beate Krecklow, and Matrin Eisemann. 2002. “Interrelations between Temperament, Character, and Parental Rearing among Delinquent Adolescents: A Cross-Validation.” *Comprehensive Psychiatry* 43(3):210–14.

Rick, Blake M., Eric W. Mania, and Samuel L. Guertner. 2006. “Intergroup Threat and Outgroup Attitudes: A Meta-analytic Review.” *Personality & Social Psychology Review* 10(4):336–353.

Ridenour, Ty A., Mark T. Greenberg, Elizabeth T. Cook. 2006. “Structure and Validity of People in My Life: A Self-report Measure of Attachment in Late Childhood.” *Journal of Youth & Adolescence* 35:1037–1053.

Ridgeway, Cecilia L. 2001. “Gender Status, and Leadership.” *Journal of Social Issues* 57(4):637–655.

Ridley-Duff, Rory. 2007. “Communitarian Perspective on Social Enterprise.” *Corporate Governance* 15(2):382–392.

Rijken, Mieke, and Peter P. Groenewegen. 2008. “Money Does Not Bring Well being, But It Does Help? The Relationship between Financial Resources and Life Satisfaction of the Chronically Ill Meidated by Social Deprivation and Loneliness.” *Journal of Community & Applied Social Psychology* 18:3–33.

Riley, Michael A., Michael J. Richardson, Kevin Shockley, and Veronica C. Ramenzoni. 2011. “Interpersonal Synergies.” *Frontiers in Psychology* 2(38).

Rindermann, Heiner. 2008. “Relevance of Education and Intelligence for the Political Development of Nations: Democracy, Rule of Law and Political Liberty.” *Intelligence* 36(4):306–322.

Ringen, Stein. 2007. *What Democracy Is for: On Freedom and Moral Goernment*. Princeton, NJ: Princeton University Press.

Rip, Blanka, Robert J. Vallerand, and Mare-Andre K. Lafreniere. 2012. “Passion for a Cause, Passion for a Creed: On Ideological Passion, Identity Threat, and Extremism.” *Journal of Personality* 80(3):573–602.

Rippl, Suzanne, Nicola Bücker, Anke Petrat, and Klaus Boehnke. 2010. “Crossing the Frontier: Transnational Social Integration in the EU’s Border Regions.” *International Journal of Comparative Sociology* 51(1–2):5–31.

Ritchie, Liesel Ashley. 2012. “Individual Stress, Collective Trauma, and Social Capital in the Wake of the Exxon Valdez Oil Spill: Individual Stress, Collective Trauma, and Social Capital.” *Sociological Inquiry* 82(2):187–211.

Ritschel, Lorie A., and Christopher S. Sheppard. 2018. “Hope and Depression.” Pp. 209–219 in The Oxford Handbook of Hope, edited by Matthew W. Gallagher and Shane J. Lopez. New York, NY: Oxford University Press.

Rivera, Jason D. 2018. “Reliance on Faith-Based Organizations for Tangible Assistance in Times of Disaster: Exploring the Influence of Bonding Social Capital.” *Sociological Spectrum* 38(1):39–50.

Robert, Peter and Erzsebet Bukodi. 2005. “The Effects of the Globalization Process in the Transition to Adulthood in Hungary.” Pp. 177–213 in *Globalization, Uncertainty and Youth in Society*, edited by Hans-Peter Blossfeld, Erik Klijzing, Melinda Mills and Karin Kurz. London: Routledge.

Roberto, Karen A. 2009. "Placing Developmental Paradigms in Context: Health and Adaptation in Later Life." Pp. 127–147 in *Pathways of Human Development: Explorations of Change*, edited by Jay A. Mancini and Karen A. Roberto. Lanham, MD: Lexington.

Roberto, Karen A., and Erica K. Husser. 2007. "Social Relationships: Resources and Obstacles to Older Women's Health Adaptation and Well-being." *Advances in Life Course Research* 12:383–410.

Roberts, Alden E., Jerome R. Koch, and D. Paul Johnson. 2001. "Religious Reference Groups and the Persistence of Normative Behavior: An Empirical Test." *Sociological Spectrum* 21:81–98.

Roberts, Brent W., and Wendy F. DelVecchio. 2000. "The Rank-order Consistency of Personality Traits from Childhood to Old Age: A Quantitative Review of Longitudinal Studies." *Psychological Bulletin* 126(1):3–25.

Roberts, Donald F., Lisa Henriksen, and Ulla G. Foehr. 2009. "Adolescence, Adolescents, and Media." Pp. 314–344 in *Handbook of Adolescent Psychology, Vol. 2: Contextual Influences and Adolescent Development*, edited by Richard M. Lerner and Laurence Steinberg. Hoboken, NJ: Wiley.

Roberts, James A., and Aimee Clement. 2007. "Materialism and Satisfaction with over all Quality of Life and Eight Life Domains." *Social Indicators Research* 82:79–92.

Roberts, Ken.. 2004. "Leisure Inequalities, Class Divisions and Social Exclusion in Present-day Britain." *Cultural Trends* 13(2):57–71.

Roberts, Richard D., Moshe Zeidner, and Gerald Matthews. 2001. "Does Emotional Intelligence Meet Traditional Standards for Intelligence? Some New Data and Conclusions." *Emotion* 1(3):196–231.

Roberts, Vega Zagier, and Halina Brunning. 2007. "Psychodynamic and Systems: Psychodynamic Coaching." Pp. 253–277 in *Handbook of Coaching Psychology: A Guide for Practitioners*, edited by Stephen Palmer and Alison Whybrow. Hove, UK: Routledge.

Robinson, Elizabeth, and Graham Dyson. 2012. "Interpersonal Psychotherapy." Pp. 356–360 in *The SAGE Handbook of Counselling and Psychotherapy*, edited by Colin Feltham and Ian Horton. London: SAGE.

Robison, Lindon J., A. Allan Schmid, and Marcelo E. Siles. 2002. "Is Social Capital Really Capital?" *Review of Social Economy* 60(1):1–21.

Robison, Lindon J., and Bryan K. Ritchie. 2010. Relationship Economics: The Social Capital Paradigm and Its Application to Business, Politics and Other Transactions. Furnham, UK: Gower.

Roch, Christine H. and Na Sai. 2015. "Nonprofit, for-Profit, or Stand-Alone? How Management Organizations Influence the Working Conditions in Charter Schools." *Social Science Quarterly* 96(5):1380–95.

Roche, Maurice. 2002. "Social Citizenship: Grounds of Social Change." Pp. 69–86 in *Handbook of Citizenship Studies*, edited by Engin F. Isin and Bryan S. Turner. London: Sage.

Rochelle, Tina L. 2015. "Diversity and Trust in Hong Kong: An Examination of Tin Shui Wai, Hong Kong's City of Sadness." *Social Indicators Research* 120:437–454.

Rocke, Christina and Margie E. Lachman. 2008. "Perceived Trajectories of Life Satisfaction across Past, Present, and Future: Profiles and Correlates of Subjective Change in Young, Middle-aged, and Older Adults." *Psychology & Aging* 23(4):833–847.

Rodebaugh, Thomas L. and Richard G. Heimberg. 2008. "Measurement of Ambivalent and Purposeful Engagement after Aversive Social Experiences." *Journal of Anxiety Disorders* 22(4):693–706.

Rodrigo-Gonzalez, Amalia, María Caballer-Tarazona, and Aurora García-Gallego. 2019. "Active Learning on Trust and Reciprocity for Undergraduates." *Sustainability* 11(16):4399.

Rodrigo-Gonzalez, Amalia, María Caballer-Tarazona, and Aurora García-Gallego. 2021. "Effects of Inequality on Trust and Reciprocity: An Experiment with Real Effort." *Frontiers in Psychology* 12:745948–48.

Rogers, Mary E., and Peter A. Creed. 2011. "A Longitudinal Examination of Adolescent Career Planning and Exploration Using a Social Cognitive Career Theory Framework." *Journal of Adolescence* 34(1):163–172.

Rogers, Meghan L., and William Alex Pridemore. 2018. "Research on Social Structure and Cross-national Homicide Rates." Pp. 418–437 in *The Cambridge Handbook of Violent Behavior and Aggression*, edited by Alexander T. Vazsonyi, David J. Flannery and Matt DeLisi. Cambridge, UK: Cambridge University Press.

Rojas, Joanne P., and Kenneth M. Tyler. 2018. "Measuring the Creative Process: A Psychometric Examination of Creative Ideation and Grit." *Creativity Research Journal* 30(1):29–40.

Rojek, Chris. 2005. "Leisure and Tourism." Pp. 302–313 in *The SAGE Handbook of Sociology*, edited by Craig Calhoun, Chris Rojek, and Bryan Turner. London, UK: SAGE.

Rojewski, Jay W., and Heejn Kim. 2003. "Career Choice Patterns and Behavior of Work-bound Youth During Early Adolescence." *Journal of Employment Counseling* 30(2):89–108.

Roller, Bill and Philip Zimbardo. 2017. "The Berkeley Civic Courage and Heroism Experiment: The Group Dynamics of Individuals Acting in Concert to Advance Ethical Goals in the Public Interest." *International Journal of Group Psychotherapy* 67(3):433–47.

Roloff, Michael E., and Courtney N. Wright. 2013. "Social Cognition and Conflict." Pp. 133–160 in *The SAGE Handbook of Conflict Communication*, edited by John G. Oetzel and Stelle Ting-Toomey. Thousand Oaks, CA: SAGE.

Romaioli, Diego, Alessio Nencini, and Anna Maria Meneghini. 2016. "How to Foster Commitment among Volunteers: A Social Constructionist Study in Italian Nonprofit Organizations." *Journal of Social Service Research* 42(5):718–728.

Romanowicz, Magdalena, Stephen S. O'Connor, Kathryn M. Schak, Cosima C. Swintak, and Timothy W. Lineberry. 2013. "Use of the Suicide Status Form-II to Investigate Correlates of Suicide Risk Factors in Psychiatrically Hospitalized Children and Adolescents." *Journal of Affective Disorders* 151(2):467–473.

Romer, Daniel and Kathleen Hall Jamieson. 2020. "Conspiracy Theories as Barriers to Controlling the Spread of COVID-19 in the U.S." *Social Science & Medicine* 263:113356.

Romero-Simpson, J.E. 1995. "The Importance of Learning Styles in Total Quality Management-oriented College and University Courses." Pp. 99–115 in *The Importance of Learning Styles: Understanding the Implications for Learning, Course Design, and Education*, edited by Ronald R. Sims and Serbrenia J. Sims. Westport, CT: Greenwood.

Ronel, Natti and Dana Segev. 2014. "Positive Criminology in Practice." *International Journal of Offender Therapy & Comparative Criminology* 58(11):1389–407.

Rook, Karen S., and Philip H.G. Ituarte. 1999. "Social Control, Social Support, and Companionship in Older Adults" Family Relationships and Friendships." *Personal Relationships* 6:199–211

Rose, Christopher D. 2003. "Making the Grade in the Prison Yard: Who Takes Advantage of Educational Programming While Incarcerated?" *Journal of Crime & Justice* 26(2):101–24.

Rose, Debra J. 2002. "Promoting Functional Independence among at Risk and Physically Frail Older Adults through Community-based Fall-risk-reduction Programs." *Journal of Aging & Physical Activity* 10(2):207–225.

Rose, Stephen M. 2000. "Reflections on Empowerment-based Practice." *Social Work* 45(5):403–412.

Rose-Krasnor, Linda, Michael A. Busseri, Teena Willoughby, and Heather Chalmers. 2005. "Breadth and Intensity of Youth Activity Involvement as Contexts of Positive Development." *Journal of Youth & Adolescence* 35(3):385–399.

Rosenbaum, Emily, and Jessie Anne Rochford. 2008. "Generational Patterns in Academic Performance: The Variable Effects of Attitudes and Social Capital." *Social Science Research* 37:350–372.

Rosenfeld, Lawrence B., and Jack M. Richman. 1997. "Developing Effective Social Support: Team Building and the Social Support Process." *Journal of Applied Sport Psychology* 9:133–153.

Rosler, Nimrod, Keren Sharvit, and Daniel Bar-Tal. 2018. "Perceptions of Prolonged Occupation as Barriers to Conflict Resolution." *Political Psychology* 39(3):519–38.

Ross, Catherine E., and John Mirowsky. 1989. "Explaining the Social Patterns of Depression: Control and Problem Solving--or Support and Talking?" *Journal of Health and Social Behavior* 30(2):206–219.

Ross, Catherine E., and John Mirowsky. 1995. "Does Employment Affect Health?" *Journal of Health & Social Behavior* 36(3):230–243.

Ross, Catherine E., and John Mirowsky. 2009. "Neighborhood Disorder, Subjective Alienation, and Distress." *Journal of Health & Social Behavior* 50:49–64.

Ross, Catherine E., and Patricia Drentea. 1998. "Consequences of Retirement Activities for Distress and the Sense of Personal Control." *Journal of Health & Social Behavior* 39:317–334.

Ross, Catherine E., and Sung Joon Jang. 2000. "Neighborhood Disorder, Fear, and Mistrust: The Buffering Role of Social Ties with Neighbors." *American Journal of Community Psychology* 28(4):401–420.

Ross, Catherine E., John R. Reynolds, Karlyn J. Geis. 2000. "The Contingent Meaning of Neighborhood Stability for Residents" Psychological Well-being." *American Sociological Review* 65:581–597.

Ross, William, and Jessica LaCroix. 1996. "Multiple Meaning of Trust in Negotiation Theory and Research: A Literature Review and Integrative Model." *International Journal of Conflict Management* 7(4):314–320.

Rossi, Alice S. 2001. "Contemporary Dialogue on Civil Society and Social Responsibility." Pp. 3–74 in *Caring and Doing for Others: Social Responsibility in the Domain of Family, Work, and Community*, edited by Alice S. Rossi. Chicago, IL: University of Chicago Press.

Rossi, Alice S. 2004a. "The Menopausal Transition and Aging Processes." Pp. 153–201 in *How Healthy Are We: A National Study of Well-being at Midlife*, edited by Orville Gilbert Brim, Carol D. Ryff and Ronald C. Kessler. Chicago, IL: University of Chicago Press.

Rossner, Meredith, and Mythily Meher. 2014. "Emotions in Ritual Theories." Pp. 199–219 in *Handbook of the Sociology of Emotions*: Volume II, edited by Jan E. Stets and Jonathan H. Turner. Dordrecht, Netherlands: Springer.

Rostan, Susan M. 1997. "A Study of Young Artists: The Development of Artistic Talent and Creativity." *Creativity Research Journal* 10(2/3):175–192.

Rostosky, Sharon Scales, Olga Dekhtyar, Pamela K. Cupp, and Eric M. Anderman. 2008. "Sexual Self-concept and Sexual Self-efficacy in Adolescents: A Possible Clue to Promoting Sexual Health." *Journal of Sex Research* 45(3):277–286.

Roth, Guy, and Avi Assor. 2012. "The Costs of Parental Pressure to Express Emotions: Conditional Regard and Autonomy Support as Predictors of Emotion Regulation and Intimacy." *Journal of Adolescence* 35(4):799–808.

Roth, Marcus and Philipp Yorck Herzberg. 2017. "The Resilient Personality Prototype: Resilience as a Self-Deception Artifact?" *Journal of Individual Differences* 38(1):1–11.

Rothmund, Tobias, Anna Baumert, and Axel Zinkernagel. 2014. "The German "Wutbürger": How Justice Sensitivity Accounts for Individual Differences in Political Engagement." *Social Justice Research* 27(1):24–44.

Rothschild, Zachary K. and Lucas A. Keefer. 2022. "Meaningful Outrage: Anger at Injustice Bolsters Meaning for Justice Sensitive Individuals." *European Journal of Social Psychology* 52(1):124–46.

Rothstein, Bo, and Eric M Uslaner. 2005. "All for All: Equality, Corruption, and Social Trust." *World Politics* 58(1):41–72.

Rothwell, David W., Mohammad N. Khan, and Katrina Cherney. 2016. "Building Financial Knowledge Is Not Enough: Financial Self-Efficacy as a Mediator in the Financial Capability of Low-Income Families." *Journal of Community Practice* 24(4):368–388,

Rotkirch, A. 2014. "Gratitude for Help Among Adult Friends and Siblings." *Evolutionary Psychology* 12(4):673–686.

Rovio, Esa, Jari Eskola, Stephen A. Kozub, Joan L. Duda, and Taru Lintunen. 2009. "Can High Group Cohesion Be Harmful? A Case Study of a Junior Ice-hockey Team." *Small Group Research* 40(4):421–435.

Rowan, John. 1998. The Reality Game: A Guide to Humanistic Counselling and Psychotherapy. London: Routledge.

Rowan, John. 2001. Ordinary Ecstasy: The Dialectics of Humanistic Psychology. Hove, UK: Brunner-Routledge.

Rowatt, Wade C., Jordan LaBouff, Megan Johnson, Paul Froese and Jo-Ann Tsang. 2009. "Associations among Religiousness, Social Attitudes, and Prejudice in a National Random Sample of American Adults." *Psychology of Religion & Spirituality* 1(1):14–24.

Roy, Kakoli, and Anoshua Chaudhuri. 2008. "Influence of Socioeconomic Status, Wealth and Financial Empowerment on Gender Differences in Health and Healthcare Utilization in Later Life: Evidence from India." *Social Science & Medicine* 66:1951–1962.

Roy, Sanjit Kumar. 2009. "Internet Uses and Gratifications: A Survey in the Indian Context." *Computers in Human Behavior* 25:878–886.

Rubin, Kenneth, Bridget Fredstrom, and Gulie Bowker. 2008. "Future Directions in... Friendship in Childhood and Early Adolescence." *Social Development* 17(4):1085–1096.

Rudd, Jill E. and D. Timothy Hughes. 2020. *Negotiation Preparation in a Global World: Symptoms of Success and Failure*. New York, NY: Routledge.

Rudkin, Laura, Glen H. Elder, Jr., and Rand Conger. 1994. "Influences on the Migration: Intentions of Rural Adolescents." *Sociological Studies of Children* 6:87–106.

Rudolph, Thomas, and Elizabeth Popp. 2009. "Bridging the Ideological Divide: Trust and Support for Social Security Privatization." *Political Behavior* 31:331–351.

Rudowicz, Elisabeth, and Xiao-dong Yue. 2002. "Concepts of Creativity: Similarities and Differences among Mainland, Hong Kong, and Taiwanese Children." *Journal of Creative Behavior* 34(3):175–192.

Ruffman, Ted, Marc Wilson, Julie D. Henry, Abigail Dawson, Yan Chen, Natalie Kladnitski, Ella Myttari, Janice Murray, Jamin Halberstadt, and John A. Hunter. 2016. "Age Differences in Right-Wing Authoritarianism and Their Relation to Emotion Recognition." *Emotion* 16(2):226–36.

Ruggiero, Vincenzo. 2020. *Visions of Political Violence*. Abingdon, UK: Routledge.

Ruiter, Robert A. C., Bas Verplanken, Gerjo Kok, and Marieke Q. Werri. 2003. "The Role of Coping Appraisal in Reactions to Fear Appeals: Do We Need Threat Information?" *Journal of Health Psychology* 8(4):465–474.

Ruiter, Robert C. C., Bas Verplanken, and David De Cremer, and Gerjo Kok. 2004. "Danger and Fear Control in Response to Fear Appeals: The Role of Need for Cognition." *Basic & Applied Social Psychology* 26(1):13–24.

Ruiz, Ignacio Elpidio Domínguez, Alèxia Rué, and Olga Jubany. 2023. "Police Resilience as a Multilevel Balance: Needs and Resources for Victim Support Officers." *Police Quarterly* 26(2):213–44.

Rullo, Marika, Emilio Paolo Visintin, Stella Milani, Alessandra Romano, and Loretta Fabbri. 2022. "Stay Humble and Enjoy Diversity: The Interplay between Intergroup Contact and Cultural Humility on Prejudice." *International Journal of Intercultural Relations* 87:169–82.

Rumbaut, Ruben G. 1997. "Ties That Bind: Immigration and Immigrant Families in the United States." Pp. 3–46 in *Immigration and the Family: Research and Policy on U.S. Immigrants*, edited by Alan Booth, Ann C. Crouter, and Nancy Landale. Mahwah, NJ: Lawrence Erlbaum.

Rundman, Laurie A., and Peter Glick. 2008. The Social Psychology of Gender: How Power and Intimacy Shape Gender Relations. New York, NY: Guilford.

Ruppanner, Leah. 2010. "Conflict and Housework: Does Country Context Matter?" *European Sociological Review* 26(5):557–570.

Rusbutt, Caryl E., Michael K. Coolsen, Jeffrey L. Kirchner, and Jennifer A. Clarke. 2006. "Commitment." Pp. 615–635 in *The Cambridge Handbook of Personal Relationships*, edited by Anita L. Vangelisti and Daniel Perlman. New York: Cambridge University Press.

Russell, Mary N. 1990. "Consumer Satisfaction: An Investigation of Contributing Factors." *Journal of Social Service Research* 13(4):43–56.

Rutter, Michael. 2012. "Resilience: Causal Pathways and Social Ecology." Pp. 33–42 in *The Social Ecology of Resilience: Handbook of Theory and Practice*, edited by Michael Ungar. New York, NY: Springer.

Ryan, Richard M., and Edward L. Deci. 2017. *Self-determination Theory: Basic Psychological Needs in Motivation, Development, and Wellness*. New York, NY: Guilford.

Ryb, Gabriel E., Patricia C. Dischinger, Joseph A. Kufera, and Kathy M. Read. 2006. "Risk Perception and Impulsivity: Association with Risky Behaviors and Substance Abuse Disorders." *Accident Analysis & Prevention* 38:567–573.

Rydin, Yvonne, and Nancy Holman. 2004. "Re-evaluating the Contributing of Social Capital in Achieving Sustainable Development." *Local Environment* 9(2):117–133.

Ryff, Carol D., Corey L.M. Keyes, and Diane L. Hughes. 2004. "Psychological Well-being in MIDUS: Profiles of Ethnic/racial Diversity and Life-course Uniformity." Pp. 398–422 in *How Healthy Are We: A National Study of Well-being at Midlife*, edited by Orville Gilbert Brim, Carol D. Ryff and Ronald C. Kessler. Chicago, IL: University of Chicago Press.

Ryu, Young-Ju, Irmak Olcaysoy Okten, Anton Gollwitzer, and Gabriele Oettingen. 2023. "Intellectual Humility Predicts Covid-19 Preventive Practices through Greater Adoption of Data-Driven Information and Feelings of Responsibility." *Social & Personality Psychology Compass* 17(8):12766.

Sabatier, Colette, and Lyda Lannegrand-Willems. 2005. "Transmission of Family Values and Attachment: A French Three-Generation Study." *Applied Psychology* 54(3):378–395.

Sabatini, Fabio, and Francesco Sarracino. 2019. "Online Social Networks and Trust." *Social Indicators Research* 142(1):229–260.

Sabbagh, Clara. 2002. "A Taxonomy of Normative and Empirically Oriented Theories of Distributive Justice." *Social Justice Research* 14(3):277–263.

Sabet, Naser Shafiei and Sogand Khaksar. 2022. "The Performance of Local Government, Social Capital and Participation of Villagers in Sustainable Rural Development." *Social Science Journal*.

Sabia, Joseph J. and Brittany Bass. 2017. "Do Anti-Bullying Laws Work? New Evidence on School Safety and Youth Violence." *Journal of Population Economics* 30(2):473–502.

Sadler, Pamela, Nicole Etheir, and Erik Woody. 2011. "Interpersonal Complementarity." Pp. 123–142 in *Handbook of Interpersonal Psychology Theory, Research, Assessment, and Therapeutic Interventions*, edited by Leonard M. Horowitz and Stephen Strack. Hoboken, NJ: Wiley.

Saegert, Susan, and Gary Winkel. 2004. "Crime, Social Capital, and Community Participation." *American Journal of Community Psychology* 34(3/4):219–233.

Sagy, Shifra, Emda Orr, and Dan Bar-On. 1999. "Individualism and Collectivism in Israeli Society: Comparing Religious and Secular High-school Students." *Human Relations* 52(3):327–348.

Sahi, Shalini Kalra. 2017. "Psychological Biases of Individual Investors and Financial Satisfaction." *Journal of Consumer Behaviour* 16(6):511–35.

Sahin, Nail, Nesrin H. Sahin, and Sibel Turner. 1994. "Stereotypes of Suicide Causes for Three Age/Gender Cohorts." *International Journal of Psychology* 29(2):213–233.

Salazar, Laura F., Charlene K. Baker, Ann W. Price, and Kathleen Carlin. 2003. "Moving Beyond the Individual: Examining the Effects of Domestic Violence Policies on Social Norms." *American Journal of Community Psychology* 32(3/4):253–264.

Saldana, Christopher M., Kevin G. Welner, Susan Malcolm, and Eleanore Tisch. 2021. "Teachers as Market Influencers: Towards a Policy Framework for Teacher Brand Ambassador Programs in K-12 Schools." *Education Policy Analysis Archives* 29(109). \83–355

Samios, Christina and Shayne Baran. 2018. "Couple Adjustment to a Stressful Life Event: A Dyadic Investigation of the Roles of Positive Reframing and Perceived Benefits." *Anxiety, Stress, & Coping* 31(2):188–205.

Sampson, Robert J. 1991. "Linking the Micro- and Macrolevel Dimensions of Community Social Organization." *Social Forces* 70(1):43–64.

Sampson, Robert J., and Stephen W. Raudenbush. 2004. "Social Disorder: Neighborhood Stigma and the Social Construction of Broken Windows." *Social Psychology Quarterly* 67(4):319–342.

Samuels, Andrew. 1985. *Jung and the Post-Jungians*. London, UK: Routledge.
Samuels, Andrew. 2006. "Transference/countertransference." Pp. 178–195 in *The Handbook of Jungian Psychology: Theory, Practice and Applications*, edited by Ronosk Papadopoulos. Hove, UK: Routledge.
Samuels, Gina Miranda, and Julia M. Pryce. 2008. "What Doesn't Kill You Makes You Stronger: Survivalist Self-reliance as Resilience and Risk among Young Adults Aging out of Former Care." *Children & Youth Services Review* 30:1198–1210.
Sanchez-Perez, Noelia, Luis J. Fuentes, Nancy Eisenberg, and Carmen González-Salinas. 2018. "Effortful Control Is Associated with Children's School Functioning Via Learning-Related Behaviors." *Learning and Individual Differences* 63:78–88.
Sandage, Steven J., and Ian Williamson. 2005. "Forgiveness in Cultural Context." Pp. 41–55 in *Handbook of Forgiveness*, edited by Everett L. Worthington, Jr. New York, NY: Routledge.
Sandage, Steven J., Peter J. Jankowski, Cheryl D. Bissonette, and David R. Paine. 2017. "Vulnerable Narcissism, Forgiveness, Humility, and Depression: Mediator Effects for Differentiation of Self." *Psychoanalytic Psychology* 34(3):300–10.
Sandel, Michael J. 2020. *The Tyranny of Merit: What's Become of the Common Good?* New York, NY: Farrar, Straus & Giroux.
Sanders, Jackie, Robyn Munford, Tewaporn Thimasarn-Anwar, Linda Liebenberg, and Michael Ungar. 2015. "The Role of Positive Youth Development Practices in Building Resilience and Enhancing Wellbeing for At-Risk Youth." *Child Abuse & Neglect* 42:40–53.
Sanders, Jimy M. 1990. "Public Transfers: Safety Net or Inducement into Poverty?" *Social Forces* 68(3):813–834.
Sanderson, Alex, Anne McKeough, Jennifer Malcolm, Darlene Omstead, Lynn Davis, and Keoma Thorne. 2016. "The Life Stories of Troubled and Non-Troubled Youth: Content and Meaning Making Analyses." *North American Journal of Psychology* 18(3):499–524.
Sanderson, Cynthia, and Marsha M. Linehan. 1999. "Acceptance and Forgiveness." Pp. 199–216 in *Integrating Spirituality into Treatment: Resources for Practitioners*, edited by William R. Miller. Washington, DC: American Psychological Association.
Sanderson, Stephen K. 2001. The Evolution of Human Sociality: A Darwinian Conflict Perspective. Lanham, MY: Rowman & Littlefield.
Sandler, Irwin. 2001. "Quality and Ecology of Adversity as Common Mechanisms of Risk and Resilience." *American Journal of Community Psychology* 29(1):19–61.
Sandoval, Jennifer M. 2017. *A Psychological Inquiry into the Meaning and Concept of Forgiveness*. New York, NY: Routledge.
Sandstrom, Kent L., Kathryn J. Lively, Daniel D. Martin, and Gary Alan Fine. 2014. *Symbols, Selves, and Social Reality: A Symbolic Interactionist Approach to Social Psychology and Sociology*. New York, NY: Oxford University Press.
Sani, Fabio, Mhairi Bowe, and Marina Herrera. 2008. "Perceived Collective Continuity and Social Well-being: Exploring the Connections." *European Journal of Social Psychology* 38:365–374.
Sant, Edda, and Chris Hanley. 2018. "Political Assumptions Underlying Pedagogies of National Education: The Case of Student Teachers Teaching British Values in England." *British Educational Research Journal* 44(2):319–337.
Santoro, Wayne A., and Lisa Broidy. 2014. "Gendered Rioting: A General Strain Theoretical Approach." *Social Forces* 93(1):329–354.
Saraglou, Vassilis. 2004. "Being Religious Implies Being Different in Humor: Evidence from Self- and Peer ratings." *Mental Health, Religion & Culture* 7(3):255–267.
Sarasa, Sebastian. 2008. "Do Welfare Benefits Affect Women's Choices of Adult Care Giving?" *European Sociological Review* 24(1):37–51
Sargent-Cox, Kerry A., Peter Butterworth, and Kaarin J. Anstey. 2015. "Role of Physical Activity in the Relationship between Mastery and Functional Health." *Gerontologist* 55(1):120–131.
Saroglou, Vassilis, and Lydwine Anciaux. 2004. "Liking Sick Humor: Coping Styles and Religion as Predictors." *Humor: International Journal of Humor Research* 17(3):257–277.

Sarpila, Outi. 2014. "Attitudes Towards Performing, and Developing Erotic Capital in Consumer Culture." *European Sociological Review* 30(3):302–14.

Sasaki, M.S. 1979. "Status Inconsistency and Religious Commitment." Pp. 135–156 in *The Religious Dimension: New Directions in Quantitative Research*, edited by Robert Wuthnow. New York: Academic.

Sassler, Sharon L. 2006. "School Participation among Immigrant Youths: The Care of Segmented Assimilation in the Early 20th Century." *Sociology of Education* 79:1–24.

Satariano, William A. Thaddeus J. Haight, and Ira B. Tager. 2002. "Living Arrangements and Participation in Leisure-time Physical Activities in an Older Population." *Journal of Aging & Health* 14(4):427–451.

Sato, Yoshimichi. 2002. "Trust Assurance and Inequality: A Rational Choice Model of Natural Trust." *Journal of Mathematical Sociology* 26:1–16.

Sattler, Kierra M. P., and Sarah A. Font. 2018. "Resilience in Young Children Involved with Child Protective Services." *Child Abuse & Neglect* 75:104–114.

Saucier, Gerard, and Katarzyna Skrzypinska. 2006. "Spiritual but Not Religious? Evidence for Two Independent Dispositions." *Journal of Personality* 74(5):1257–1292.

Saunders, Peter, and Melissa Wong. 2012. "Examining Australian Attitudes to Inequality and Redistribution." *Journal of Australian Political Economy* 71:51–75.

Savage, Joanne, and Satoshi Kanazawa. 2004. "Social Capital and the Human Psyche: Why Is Social Life Capital." *Sociological Theory* 22(3):504–522.

Savage, Joanne. 2014. "The Association between Attachment, Parental Bonds and Physically Aggressive and Violent Behavior: A Comprehensive Review." *Aggression & Violent Behavior* 19(2):164–78.

Savelkoul, Michael, Maurice Gesthuizen, and Peer Scheepers. 2011. "Explaining Relationships between Ethnic Diversity and Informal Social Capital across European Countries and Regions: Tests of Constrict, Conflict and Contact Theory." *Social Science Research* 40(4):1091–1107.

Savelkoul, Michael, Maurice Gesthuizen, and Peer Scheepers. 2014. "The Impact of Ethnic Diversity on Participation in European Voluntary Organizations." *Nonprofit & Voluntary Sector Quarterly* 43(6):1070–1094.

Savelkoul, Michael, Miles Hewstone, Peer Scheepers, and Dietlind Stolle. 2015. "Does Relative Out-Group Size in Neighborhoods Drive down Associational Life of Whites in the U.S.? Testing Constrict, Conflict and Contact Theories." *Social Science Research* 52:236–252.

Savickas, Mark L. 2015. "Career Counseling Paradigms: Guiding, Developing, and Designing." Pp. 129–143 in APA *Handbook of Career Intervention, Vol: Foundations*, edited by Paul J. Hartung, Mark L. Savickas, and W. Bruce Walsh. Washington, DC: American Psychological Association.

Sawyer, Patricia, and Richard M. Allman. 2010. "Resilience in Mobility in the Context of Chronic Disease and Aging: Cross-sectional and Prospective Findings from the University of Alabama at Birmingham (UAB) Study of Aging." Pp. 310–339 in *New Frontiers in Resilient Aging: Life-strengths and Well-being in Late Life*, edited by Prom S. Fry and Corey L.M. Keyes. Cambridge, UK: Cambridge University Press.

Sawyers, Chelsea, Erin D. Kurtz, Christina Sheerin, Hermine H. Maes, Kenneth S. Kendler, and Ananda B. Amstadter. 2020. "A Behavioral Genetic Investigation of Conceptualizations of Resilience in a Female Twin Sample." *Depression & Anxiety* 37(6):532–39.

Saxton, Gregory D. and Michelle A. Benson. 2006. "Structure, Politics, and Action: An Integrated Model of Nationalist Protest and Rebellion." *Nationalism & Ethnic Politics* 12(2):137–75.

Scabini, Eugenia, and Vittorio Cigoli. 1997. "Young Adult Families: An Evlutionary Slowdown or a Breakdown in the Generational Transition?" *Journal of Family Issues* 18(6):608–626.

Scaff, Lawrence. 2014. *Weber and the Weberians*. Houndmills, UK: Palgrave.

Scafuto, Francesca, and Francesco La Barbera. 2016. "Protest Against Waste Contamination in the Land of Fires: Psychological Antecedents for Activists and Non-activists." *Journal of Community & Applied Social Psychology* 26(6):481–495.

Scales, Peter, Dale A. Blyth, Thomas H. Berkas, and James C. Kielsmeier. 2000. "The Effects of Service-learning on Middle School Students" Social Responsibility and Academic Success." *Journal of Early Adolescence* 20(3):332–358.

Scannell, Leila, and Robert Gifford. 2017. "The Experienced Psychological Benefits Of Place Attachment." *Journal of Environmental Psychology* 51:256–269.

Schaafsma, Juliette and Kipling D. Williams. 2012. "Exclusion, Intergroup Hostility, and Religious Fundamentalism." *Journal of Experimental Social Psychology* 48(4):829–37.

Schafer, Karl. 2015. "Realism and Constructivism in Kantian Metaethics (2): The Kantian Conception of Rationality and Rationalist Constructivism." *Philosophy Compass* 10(10):702–713.

Schaie, K. Warner. 2013. Developmental Influences on Adult Intelligence: The Seattle Longitudinal Study. New York: Oxford University Press.

Schaller, Mark, and Justin H. Park. 2011. "The Behavioral Immune System (and Why It Matters)." *Current Directions in Psychological Science* 20(2):99–103.

Scharf, Miri, and Miri Levy. 2015. "The Contribution of Familial Characteristics and Idolization to Children's Body and Eating Attitudes." *Journal of Child & Family Studies* 24(7):1943–1954.

Scharrer, Erica. 2008. "Media Exposure and Sensitivity to Violence in News Reports: Evidence of Desensitization?" *Journalism & Mass Communication Quarterly* 85(2):291–310.

Schaufeli, Wilmar B. 2016. "Heavy Work Investment, Personality and Organizational Climate." *Journal of Managerial Psychology* 31(6):1057–73.

Schbley, Ayla, and Clark McCauley. 2005. "Political, Religious, and Psychological Characteristics of Muslim Protest Marchers in Eight European Cities: Jerusalem Day 2002." *Terrorism & Political Violence* 17(4):551–572.

Schenke, Katerina, Arena C. Lam, Anne Marie M. Conley, and Stuart A. Karabenick. 2015. "Adolescents" Help Seeking In Mathematics Classrooms: Relations Between Achievement And Perceived Classroom Environmental Influences over One School Year." *Contemporary Educational Psychology* 41:133–146.

Scherger, Simone. 2009. "Cultural Practices, Age and the Life Course." *Cultural Trends* 18(1):23–45.

Schiefer, David and Jolanda van der Noll. 2017. "The Essentials of Social Cohesion: A Literature Review." *Social Indicators Research* 132(2):579–603.

Schieman, Scott, and Atsushi Narisada. 2014. "In Control or Fatalistically Ruled? The Sense of Mastery among Working Canadians." *Canadian Review of Sociology* 51(4):343–374.

Schieman, Scott, and Gabriele Plickert. 2008. "How Knowledge is Power: Education and the Sense of Control." *Social Forces* 87:153–183.

Schieman, Scott, and Janice E. Campbell. 2001. "Age Variations in Personal Agency and Self-esteem: The Context of Physical Disability." *Journal of Aging & Health* 13(2):155–185.

Schieman, Scott, and Marisa Young. 2010. "Is There a Downside to Schedule Control for the Work-Family Interface?" *Journal of Family Issues* 31(10):1391–1414.

Schieman, Scott. 2001. "Age, Education, and the Sense of Contrl: A Test of the Cumulative Advantage Hypothesis." *Research on Aging* 23(2):153–178.

Schieman, Scott. 2002. "Socioeconomic Status, Job Conditions, and Well-being: Self-concept Explanations for Gender-contingent Effects." *Sociological Quarterly* 43(4):627–646.

Schieman, Scott. 2006. "Gender, Dimension of Work and Supportive Coworker Relations." *Sociological Quarterly* 47:195–214

Schieman, Scott. 2013. "Job-Related Resources and the Pressures of Working Life." *Social Science Research* 42(2):271–282.

Schiff, Miriam, and David Bargal. 2000. "Helping Characteristics of Self-Help and Support Groups: Their Contribution to Participants~{!/~} Subjective Well-Being." *Small Group Research* 31(3):275–304.

Schilbach, Miriam, Anja Baethge, and Thomas Rigotti. 2021. "Do Challenge and Hindrance Job Demands Prepare Employees to Demonstrate Resilience?" *Journal of Occupational Health Psychology* 26(3):155–74.

Schimmack, Ulrich, Phanikiran Radhakrishnan, Shigehiro Oishi, and Vivian Dzokoto. 2002. "Cultural, Personality, and Subjective Well-being: Integrating Process Models of Life Satisfaction." *Journal of Personality & Social Psychology* 82(4):582–593.

Schindler, Ines, Christopher P. Fagundes, and Kyle W. Murdock. 2010. "Predictors of Romantic Relationship Formation: Attachment Style, Prior Relationships, and Dating Goals." *Personal Relationships* 17(1):97–105.

Schindler, Ines, Juliane Paech, and Fabian Löwenbrück. 2015. "Linking Admiration and Adoration to Self-Expansion: Different Ways to Enhance One's Potential." *Cognition & Emotion* 29(2):292–310.

Schinkel, Willem. 2010. *Aspects of Violence: A Critical Theory*. Houndmills, UK: Palgrave.

Schjoedt, Uffe, Jesper Sørensen, Kristoffer L. Nielbo, Dimitris Xygalatas, Panagiotis Mitkidis, and Joseph Bulbulia. 2013b. "The Resource Model and the Principle of Predictive Coding: A Framework for Analyzing Proximate Effects of Ritual." *Religion, Brain & Behavior* 3(1):79–86.

Schjoedt, Uffe, Jesper Sørensen, Kristoffer L. Nielbo, Dimitris Xygalatas, Panagiotis Mitkidis, and Joseph Bulbulia. 2013. "Cognitive Resource Depletion in Religious Interactions." *Religion, Brain & Behavior* 3(1):39–54.

Schludermann, Eduard H., Shirin M. Schludermann., and Cam-loi Huynh. 2000. "Religiosity, Prosocial Value, and Adjustment among Students in Catholic High Schools in Canada." *Journal of Beliefs & Values* 21(1):99–115.

Schmid, Christine. 2012. "The Value "Social Responsibility" as a Motivating Factor for Adolescents" Readiness to Participate in Different Types of Political Actions, and Its Socialization in Parent and Peer Contexts." *Journal of Adolescence* 35(3):533–547.

Schmid, Katharina and Orla T. Muldoon. 2015. "Perceived Threat, Social Identification, and Psychological Well-Being: The Effects of Political Conflict Exposure." *Political Psychology* 36(1):75–92.

Schmid, Petra C. 2022. "The Effort Investment Theory of Power." *Journal of Applied Social Psychology* 52(3):145–57.

Schmidt, Christopher, and Donna E. Little. 2007. "Qualitative Insights into Leisure as a Spiritual Experience." *Journal of Leisure Research* 39(2):222–247.

Schmidt, Steffen. 2010. "A Challenge-response Model in Research on Social Change." Pp. 31–49 in *Social Change and Human Development: Concept and Results*, edited by Rainer K. Silbereisen. Los Angeles, CA: SAGE.

Schmidtz, David. 2006. *Elements of Justice*. New York: Cambridge University Press.

Schmitt, Manfred, Jürgen Maes, and Keith Widaman. 2010. "Longitudinal Effects of Egoistic and Fraternal Relative Deprivation on Well-Being and Protest." *International Journal of Psychology* 45(2):122–30.

Schmitt, Randee M. and Ho Phi Huynh. 2024. "Stay (Close to) Humble: Intellectual Humility Negatively Predicts Stigma toward and Social Distance from Individuals with Posttraumatic Stress Disorder." *Psychological Reports* 13:332941231157233.

Schmitt-Redermund, Eva, and Fred W. Vondracek. 2002. "Occupational Dreams, Choices, and Aspirations: Adolescents" Entrepreneurial Prospect and Orientations." *Journal of Adolescence* 25:65–78.

Schmitt-Rodermund, Eva. 2004. "Pathways to Successful Entrepreneurship: Parenting, Personality, Early Entrepreneurial Competence, and Interests." Journal of Vocational Behavior 65:498–518.

Schmuck, Desirée, Nayla Fawzi, Carsten Reinemann, and Claudia Riesmeyer. 2022. "Social Media Use and Political Cynicism among German Youth: The Role of Information-Orientation, Exposure to Extremist Content, and Online Media Literacy." *Journal of Children & Media* 16(3):313–31.

Schneck, Stefan. 2014. "Why the Self-employed Are Happier: Evidence from 25 European Countries." *Journal of Business Research* 67:1043–1048.

Schneider, Barbara, Karoline Lukaschek, Jens Baumert, Christa Meisinger, Natalia Erazo, and Karl-Heinz Ladwig. 2014. "Living Alone, Obesity, and Smoking Increase Risk for Suicide

Independently of Depressive Mood Findings from the Population Based Monica/Kora Augsburg Cohort Study." *Journal of Affective Disorders* 152–154(1):416–21.

Schneider, Barry H. 1993. Children's Social Competence in Context: The Contributions of Family, School and Culture. Oxford, UK: Pergamon.

Schneider, Claudia R. and Elke U. Weber. 2020. "Reducing Discrimination and Fostering Prosociality Towards Ex-Prisoners in Nigeria and the United States." *Journal of Social Issues* 76(1):172–99.

Schneider, Jennifer P. 2000. "Effects of Cybersex Addiction on the Family: Results of a Survey Sexual." *Addiction & Compulsivity* 7:31–58.

Schneider, Silke L. 2007. "Anti-immigrant Attitudes in Europe: Outgroup Size and Perceived Ethnic Threat." *European Sociological Review* 24(1):53–67.

Schnell, Tatjana, and Peter Becker. 2006. "Personality and Meaning in Lie." *Personality & Individual Differences* 41:117–129.

Schnittker, Jason, and Jere R. Behrman. 2012. "Learning to Do Well or Learning to Do Good? Estimating the Effects of Schooling on Civic Engagement, Social Cohesion, and Labour Market Outcomes in the Presence of Endowments." *Social Science Research* 41:306–320.

Schnittker, Jason. 2020. "Religion, Social Integration, and Depression in Europe: Evidence from the European Social Survey." *Social Science & Medicine* 267:112376.

Schoeni, Robert F., and Karen E. Ross. 2005. "Material Assistance from Families During the Transition to Adulthood." Pp. 396–416 in *On the Frontier of Adulthood: Theory, Research, and Public Policy*, edited by Richard A. Settersten Jr., Frank F. Furstenberg Jr., and Ruben G. Rumbaut. Chicago, IL: University of Chicago Press

Scholz, Urte and Alexandra M. Freund. 2021. "Determinants of Protective Behaviours During a Nationwide Lockdown in the Wake of the COVID-19 Pandemic." *British Journal of Health Psychology* 26(3):935–57.

Schoon, Ingrid. 2006. *Risk and Resilience: Adaptations in Changing Times*. Cambridge, UK: Cambridge University Press.

Schram, Danford. 2015. The Return of Ordinary Capitalism: Neoliberalism, Precarity, Occupy. New York: Oxford University Press.

Schreck, Christopher J., Melissa W. Burek, Eric A. Stewart, and J. Mitchell Miller. 2007. "Distress and Violent Victimization among Young Adolescents: Early Puberty and the Social Interactionist Explanation." *Journal of Research in Crime and Delinquency* 44(4):381–405.

Schroeder, Ralph. 2013. *An Age of Limits: Social Theory for the 21st Century*. Houndmills, UK: Palgrave.

Schulte, Aileen. 2002. "Consensus Versus Disagreement in Disease-Related Stigma: A Comparison of Reactions to AIDS and Cancer Patients." *Sociological Perspectives* 45(1):81–104

Schulz, Sonja. 2014. "Individual Differences in the Deterrence Process: Which Individuals Learn (Most) from Their Offending Experiences?" *Journal of Quantitative Criminology* 30(2):215–36.

Schulz, Wolfgang. 1995. "Multiple-discrepancies Theory versus Resource Theory." *Social Indicators Research* 34:153–169.

Schumann, Frank, Michael B. Steinborn, Jens Kürten, Liyu Cao, Barbara Friederike Händel, and Lynn Huestegge. 2022. "Restoration of Attention by Rest in a Multitasking World: Theory, Methodology, and Empirical Evidence." *Frontiers in Psychology* 13:867978.

Schunk, Dale H., and Ellen L. Usher. 2019. "Social Cognitive Theory and Motivation." Pp. 11–26 in *The Oxford Handbook of Human Motivation*, edited Y. Richard M. Ryan. New York, NY: Oxford University Press.

Schunk, Dale. 2020. *Learning Theories: An Educational Perspective*. Hoboken, NJ: Pearson.

Schunk, Fabian, Natalie Wong, Gen Nakao, and Gisela Trommsdorff. 2023. "Different functions of emotion regulation in linking harmony seeking and rejection avoidance to life satisfaction and social support in Germany, Hong Kong, and Japan." *Asian Journal of Social Psychology* 26(2):254–69.

Schuster, Carolin, Gregg Sparkman, Gregory M. Walton, Anna Alles, and David D. Loschelder. 2023. "Egalitarian Norm Messaging Increases Human Resources Professionals" Salary Offers to Women." *Journal of Applied Psychology* 108(4):541–52.

Schutte, Nicola S., and John M. Malouff. 2020. "Connections between Curiosity, Flow and Creativity." *Personality & Individual Differences* 152:109555.

Schutte, Nicola, John M. Malouff, Maureen Simunek, Jamie McKenley, and Sharon Hollander. 2002. "Characteristics Emotional Intelligence and Emotional Well-being." *Cognition & Emotion* 16(6):769–785.

Schutte, Sebastian. 2015. "Geography, Outcome, and Casualties." *Journal of Conflict Resolution* 59(6):1101–28.

Schwager, Susanne, and Klaus Rothermund. 2014. "The Automatic Basis of Resilience: Adaptive Regulation of Affect and Cognition." Pp. 55–72 in *The Resilience Handbook: Approaches to Stress and Trauman*, edited by Martha Kent, Mary C. Davis and John W. Reich. New York: NY: Routledge.

Schwartz, Lisa B. 2012. "Mixed-Orientation Marriages: Coming out, Staying Together." *Journal of GLBT Family Studies* 8(1):121–36.

Schwartz, Robert H., Mojisola F. Tiamiyu, and Dale J. Dwyer. 2007. "Social Worker Hope and Perceived Burnout: The Effects of Age, Years in Practice, and Setting." *Administration in Social Work* 31(4):103–119.

Schwartz, Shalom H. and Gila Melech. 2000. "National Differences in Mirco and Macro Worry: Social, Economic, and Cultural Explanations." Pp. 219–256 in *Culture and Subjective Well-being*, edited by Ed Diener and Eunkook M. Suh. Cambridge, MA: MIT.

Schwartz, Shalom H., Gian Vittorio Caprara, Michele Vecchione, Paul Bain, Gabriel Bianchi, Maria Giovanna Caprara, Jan Cieciuch, Hasan Kirmanoglu, Cem Baslevent, Jan-Erik Lonnqvist, Catalin Mamali, Jorge Manzi, Vassilis Pavlopoulos, Tetyana Posnova, Harald Schoen, Jo Silvester, Carmen Tabernero, Claudio Torres, Markku Verkasalo, and Eva Vondrokov. 2014. "Basic Personal Values Underlie and Give Coherence to Political Values: A Cross National Study in 15 Countries." *Political Behavior* 36(4):899–930.

Schwarz, Silke. 2018. "Resilience in Psychology: A Critical Analysis of the Concept." *Theory & Psychology* 28(4):528–541.

Schwarzer, Ralf, and Nina Knoll. 2007. "Functional Roles of Social Support within the Stress and Coping Process: A Theoretical and Empirical Overview." *International Journal of Psychology* 42(4):243–252.

Schwendinger, Herman, and Julia Siegel Schwendinger. 1985. *Adolescent Subcultures and Delinquency*. New York: Praeger.

Schyns, Peggy. 2000. "The Relationship between Income Changes in Income and Life Satisfaction in West Germany and the Russian Federation: Relative, Absolute, or a Combination of Both?" Pp. 83–109 in *Advances in Quality of Life Theory and Research*, edited by Ed Diener and Don R. Rahtz. Dordrecht, Netherlands: Kluwer Academic.

Schyns, Peggy. 2001. "Income and Satisfaction in Russia." *Journal of Happiness Studies* 2:173–204.

Scott, Susie. 2015. *Negotiating Identity: Symbolic Interactionist Approaches to Social Identity*. Cambridge, UK: Polity.

Scott, W. Richard. 2008. *Institutions and Organizations: Ideas and Interests* (3rd ed.). Los Angeles, CA: Sage.

Scruton, Roger. 2014. *How to Be a Conservative*. London, UK: Bloomsbury.

Searle, Mark S., Michael J. Mahon, Seppo E. Iso-Ahola, Heather Adam Sdrolias, and Joanne van Dyck. 1998. "Examining the Long-term Effects of Leisure Education on a Sense of Independence and Psychological Well-being among the Elderly." *Journal of Leisure Research* 30(3):331–340.

Seaton, Cherisse L., and Sherry L Beaumont. 2015. "Pursuing the Good Life: A Short-Term Follow-Up Study of the Role of Positive/Negative Emotions and Ego-Resilience in Personal Goal Striving and Eudaimonic Well-Being." *Motivation & Emotion* 39(5):813–826.

Seaton, Cherisse L., and Sherry L. Beaumont. 2008. "Individual Differences in Identity Styles Predict Proactive Forms of Positive Adjustment." *Identity* 8(3):249–268.

Secker, Jenny, Sue Hacking, Lyn Kent, Jo Shenton, and Helen Spandler. 2009. "Development of a Measure of Social Inclusion for Arts and Mental Health Project Participants." *Journal of Mental Health* 18(1):65–72.

Seder, J. Patrick, and Shigehiro Oishi. 2009. "Ethnic/racial Homogeneity in College Students" Facebook Friendship Networks and Subjective Well-being." *Journal of Research in Personality* 43:438–443.

Sedikides, Constantine, and Jochen E. Gebauer. 2010. "Religiosity as Self-enhancement: A Meta-analysis of the Relation between Socially Desirable Responding and Religiosity." *Personality & Social Psychology Review* 14(1):17–36.

Sedikides, Constantine, Eric A. Rudich, Aiden P. Gregg, Madoka Kumashiro, and Caryl Rusbult. 2004. "Are Normal Narcissists Psychologically Healthy? Self-esteem Matters." *Journal of Personality & Social Psychology* 87(3):400–416.

Seeman, Don. 2004. "Otherwise Than Meaning: On the Generosity of Ritual." *Social Analysis* 48(2):55–71.

Seeman, Melvin, and Alice Z. Seeman. 1992. "Life Strains, Alienation, and Drinking Behavior." *Alcoholism* 16(2):199–205.

Segal, Julia. 2012. "Psychodynamic Therapy." Pp. 273–277 in *The SAGE Handbook of Counselling and Psychotherapy*, edited by Colin Feltham and Ian Horton. London: SAGE.

Segal, Robert A. 1989. "Religionist and Social Scientific Strategies." *Religion* 19(4):310–16.

Segrin, Chris and Jeanne Flora. 2019. *Family communication*, New York, NY: Routledge.

Seibert, Ashley C., and Kathryn A. Kerns. 2009. "Attachment Figures in Middle Childhood." *International Journal of Behavioral Development* 33(4):347–355.

Seidlitz, Larry, Alexis D. Abernethy, Paul R. Duberstein, James S. Evinger, Theresa H. Chang, and Barbara L. Lewis. 2002. "Development of the Spiritual Transcendence Index." *Journal of the Scientific Study of Religion* 41(3):439–453.

Selim, Sibel. 2008. "Life Satisfaction and Happiness in Turkey." *Social Indicators Research* 88:531–562.

Sellers, Sherrill L., and Harold W. Neighbors. 2008. "Effects of Goal-striving Stress on the Mental Health of Black Americans." *Journal of Health & Social Behavior* 49(1):92–103.

Selvanathan, Hema Preya. and Brian Lickel. 2019. "A Field Study around a Racial Justice Protest on a College Campus: The Proximal Impact of Collective Action on the Social Change Attitudes of Uninvolved Bystanders." *Journal of Social & Political Psychology* 7(1):598–619.

Selznick, Philip. 2008. *A Humanistic Science: Values and Ideals in Social Inquiry*. Stanford, CA: Stanford University Press.

Semenova, Galina N., Elena I. Larionova, Oleg G. Karpovich, Sergei V. Shkodinsky, and Fatima M. Ouroumova. 2020. "Social Integration as a Factor of Economic Growth: Experience and Perspectives of Developing Countries." *International Journal of Sociology & Social Policy* 41(1/2):37–49.

Semple, Randye J. and Sean P. Hott. 2012. "Translation of Eastern Meditation Disciplines into Western Psychotherapy." Pp. 326–342 in *The Oxford Handbook of Psychology and Spirituality*, edited by Lisa J. Miller. New York, NY: Oxford University Press.

Sengupta, Nikhil K. and Chris G. Sibley. 2019. "The Political Attitudes and Subjective Wellbeing of the One Percent." *Journal of Happiness Studies* 20(7):2125–40.

Seo, Dong-Chul, Mohammad R. Torabi, Ming Kai Chin, Sen Fang Huang, Chee Keong Chen, Magdalena Mo Ching Mok, Patricia Wong, Michael Chia, Chung Gun Lee, and Chunyun Wang. 2012. "A Comparison of Factors Associated with Physical Inactivity among East Asian College Students." *International Journal of Behavioral Medicine* 19(3):316–23.

Sereny, Melanie D., and Danan Gu. 2011. "Living Arrangement Concordance and Its Association with Self-rated Health among Institutionalized and Community-residing Older Adults in China." *Journal of Cross-Cultural Gerontology* 26:239–259.

Sereny, Melanie. 2011. "Living of Older Adults in China: The Interplay among Preferences, Realities, and Health." *Research on Aging* 33(2):172–204.

Serna, Loretta, Elizabeth Nielsen, Katina Lambros, and Steven Forness. 2000. "Primary Prevention with Children at Risk for Emotional or Behavioral Disorders: Data on a Universal Intervention for Head Start Classrooms." *Behavioral Disorders* 26(1):70–84.

Seyd, Patrick, and Paul Whiteley. 1992. *Labor's Grass Roots: The Politics of Party Membership.* Oxford: Clarendon Press. (

Sgambati, Tyrone J. and Ozlem N. Ayduk. 2023. "Intellectual Humility and Political Polarization: An Exploration of Social Networks, Attitudes, and Affect." *Political Psychology* 44(4):807–28.

Shah, Dhavan V. and Dietram A. Scheufele. 2006. "Explicating Opinion Leadership: Nonpolitical Dispositions, Information Consumption, and Civic Participation." *Political Communication* 23(1):1–22.

Shahzalal, Md and Hamedi Mohd Adnan. 2022. "Attitude, Self-control, and Prosocial Norm to Predict Intention to Use Social Media Responsibly: From Scale to Model Fit towards a Modified Theory of Planned Behavior." *Sustainability* 14:9822.

Shakib, Shalila, and Michele D. Dunbar. 2002. "The Social Construction of Female and Male High School Basketball Participation: Reproducing the Gender Order through a Two-Tiered Sporting Institution." *Sociological Perspectives* 45(4):353–378.

Shamir, Ronen. 2008. "The Age of Responsibilization: On Market-embedded Morality." *Economy & Society* 37(1):1–19.

Shanahan, Mackenzie L., Ian C. Fischer, and Kevin L. Rand. 2020. "Hope, Optimism, and Affect as Predictors and Consequences of Expectancies: The Potential Moderating Roles of Perceived Control and Success." *Journal of Research in Personality* 84:103903.

Shandra, John M., Bruce London, and John B. Williamson. 2003. "Environmental Degradation, Environmental Sustainability, and Overurbanization in the Developing World: A Quantitative Cross-national Analysis." *Sociological Perspectives* 46(3):309–329.

Shane, Jon M. 2013. "Daily Work Experiences and Police Performance." *Police Practice & Research* 14(1):17–34.

Shane, Matthew S., and Jordan B. Peterson. 2004. "Defensive Copers Show a Deficit in Passive Avoidance Learning on Newman's Go/No-go Task: Implications for Self-deception and Socialization." *Journal of Personality* 72(5):939–965.

Shank, Daniel B. 2012. "Perceived Justice and Reactions to Coercive Computers1." *Sociological Forum* 27(2):372–91.

Shao, Lei, Yan Dong and Denghao Zhang. 2021. "Effects of Security on Social Trust among Chinese Adults: Roles of Life Satisfaction and Ostracism." *Journal of Social Psychology* 161(5):560–69.

Shapiro, Jerrold Lee. 2016. *Pragmatic Existential Counseling and Psychotherapy: Intimacy, Intuition, and the Search for Meaning.* Thousand Oaks, CA: SAGE.

Sharabany, Ruth. 1994. "Intimate Friendship Scale: Conceptual Underpinnings, Psychometric Properties and Construct Validity." *Journal of Social & Personal Relationships* 11(3):449–469.

Sharma, Neeru. 2003. "The Role of Pure and Quasi-moderators in Services: An Empirical Investigation of Ongoing Customer-service-provider Relationships." *Journal of Retailing & Consumer Services* 10:253–262.

Sharp, Elizabeth A., and Lawrence Ganong. 2011. "I'm a Loser, I'm not Married, Let's Just All Look at Me: Ever-single Women's Perceptions of Their Environment." *Journal of Family Issues* 32(7):956–980.

Shaver, Phillip R., and Mario Mikulincer. 2012. "Attachment Theory." Pp. 160–179 in *Handbook of Theories of Social Psychology* (vol. 2), edited by Paul A.M. Van Lange, Arie W. Kruglanski and E. Tory Higgins. London, CA: SAGE.

Shaw, Benjamin A. 2005. "Anticipated Support from Neighbors and Physical Functioning during Later Life." *Research on Aging* 27(5):503–525.

Shaw, Rachael, Katie J. Paige, Jennifer A. Livingston, Craig R. Colder, and Jennifer P. Read. 2023. "Effectiveness of Sexual Assault Protective Behaviors on the Daily Level: The Roles of Intoxication and Executive Control." *Journal of Interpersonal Violence* 38(15–16):9015–38.

Shaw, William H. 1999. Contemporary Ethics: Taking Account of Utilitarianism. Malden, MA: Blackwell.

Shechtman, Zipora, Yaffa Friedman, Ytzhak Kashti, and Ruth Sharabany. 2002. "Group Counseling to Enhance Adolescents' Close Friendships." *International Journal of Group Psychotherapy* 52(4):537–553.

Shek, Daniel T. L. 2010. "The Spirituality of the Chinese People: A Critical Review." Pp. 343–366 *in The Oxford Handbook of Chinese Psychology*, edited by Michael Harris Bond. Oxford, UK: Oxford University Press.

Shek, Daniel T. L. and Xiaoqin Zhu. 2018. "Self-Reported Risk and Delinquent Behavior and Problem Behavioral Intention in Hong Kong Adolescents: The Role of Moral Competence and Spirituality." *Frontiers in Psychology* 9:430.

Shek, Daniel T. L., Diya Dou, Xiaoqin Zhu, and Xiang Li. 2022a. "Law Abidance Leadership Education for University Students in Hong Kong: Post-Lecture Evaluation." *Frontiers in Psychology* 13: 994448.

Shek, Daniel T.L. 2002. "Parenting Characteristics and Parent-adolescent Conflict: A Longitudinal Study in the Chinese Culture." *Journal of Family Issues* 23(2):189–208.

Shek, Daniel T.L. 2005. "Perceived Parental Control Processes, Parent-child Relational Qualities, and Psychological well-being in Chinese Adolescents with and without Economic Disadvantage." *Journal of Genetic Psychology* 166(2):171–188.

Sheldon, Kennon M. and B. Ann Bettencourt. 2002. "Psychological Need-satisfaction and Subjective Well-being within Social Groups." *British Journal of Social Psychology* 41:25–38.

Sheldon, Kennon M., and Lawrence S. Krieger. 2007. "Understanding the Negative Effects of Legal Education on Law Students: A Longitudinal Test of Self-determination Theory." *Personality & Social Psychology Bulletin* 33(6):883–897.

Sheldon, Kennon M., and Linda Hower-Marko. 2001. "Self-concordance, Goal Attainment, and the Pursuit of Happiness: Can There Be an Upward Spiral?" *Journal of Personality & Social Psychology* 80(1):152–165.

Sheldon, Kennon M., and Tim Kasser. 2001. "Getting Older, Getting Better? Personal Strivings and Psychological Maturity across the Life Span." *Developmental Psychology* 37(4):491–501.

Shell, Duane F., and Jenefer Husman. 2008. "Control Motivation, Affect, and Strategic Self-regulation in the College Classroom: A Multidimensional Phenomenon." *Journal of Educational Psychology* 100(2):443–459.

Shemmings, David. 2006. "Quantifying Qualitative Data: an Illustrative Example of the Use of Q Methodology in Psychosocial Research." *Qualitative Research of Psychology* 3:147–165.

Shen, April Chiang-Too. 2009. "Self-esteem of Young Adults Experiencing Interparental Violence and Child Physical Maltreatment: Parental and Peer Relationships as Mediators." *Journal of Interpersonal Violence* 24(5):770–794.

Sheridan, Zachariah, Peter Boman, Amanda Mergler, Michael J. Furlong, and Stefan Elmer. 2015. "Examining Well-Being, Anxiety, and Self-Deception in University Students." *Cogent Psychology* 2(1):993850.

Sherkat, Darren E., and Christopher G. Ellison. 2007. "Structuring the Religion-environment Connection: Identifying Religious Influences on Environmental Concern and Activism." *Journal of the Scientific Study of Religion* 46(1):71–85.

Sherman, David K., and Geoffrey L. Cohen. 2006. "The Psychology of Self-defense: Self-affirmation Theory." *Advances in Experimental Social Psychology* 38:183–242.

Shewark, Elizabeth A., Miranda Matern, Kelly L. Klump, Alytia A. Levendosky and S. Alexandra Burt. 2022. "Interpersonal Complementarity as a Predictor of Parent-Child Relationship Quality." *Journal of Family Psychology* 6(6):885–895.

Shi, Kan, Hongxin Fan, Jianming Jia, Wendong Li, Zhaoli Song, Jing Gao, Xuefeng Chen, Jiafang Lu, and Weipeng Hu. 2003. "The Risk Perception of SARS and Socio-psychological Behaviors for Urban People in China." *Acta Psychologica Sinica* 35(4):546–554.

Shibue, Yuko, and Makiko Kasai. 2014. "Relations between Attachment, Resilience, and Earned Security in Japanese University Students." *Psychological Reports* 115(1):279–295.

Shields, David Light, and Brenda Light Bredemeier. 2005. "Can Sports Build Character?" Pp. 121–139 in *Character Psychology and Character Education*, edited by Daniel K. Lapsley and F. Clark Power. Notre Dame, IN: University of Notre Dame Press.

Shields, David Light, and Brenda Light Bredemeier. 2008. "Sport and the Development of Character." Pp. 500–519 in *Handbook of Moral and Character Education*, edited by Larry P. Nucci and Darcia Narvaez. New York, NY: Routledge.

Shimai, Satoshi, Keiko Otake, Nansook Park, Christopher Peterson, and Martin E.P. Seligman. 2006. "Convergence of Character Strengths in American Young Adults." *Journal of Happiness Studies* 7:311–322.

Shin, Hyon-Uk. 2012. Vulnerability and Courage: A Pastoral Theology of Poverty and the Alienated Self. New York: Peter Lang.

Shippee, Nathan D. 2012. "Victimization, Fear of Crime, and Perceived Risk: Testing a Vulnerability Model of Personal Control." *Sociological Perspectives* 55(1):117–140.

Shirzadifard, Maysam, Ehsan Shahghasemi, Elaheh Hejazi, Zahra Naghsh, and Ghafar Ranjbar. 2018. "Psychometric Properties of Rational-Experiential Inventory for Adolescents." *SAGE Open* 8(1):215824401876721.

Shmueli, Amir. 1999. "Survival vs. Quality of Life: A Study of the Israeli Public Priorities in Medical Care." *Social Science & Medicine* 49:497–302.

Shor, Eran and Yuval Yonay. 2010. "Sport, National Identity, and Media Discourse over Foreign Athletes in Israel." *Nationalism & Ethnic Politics* 16(3–4):483–503.

Shorey, Hal S., Steve Bisgaier, and Scott R. Thien. 2018. "Attachment Process and the Social Developmental Bases of Hope." Pp. 313–325 in *The Oxford Handbook of Hope*, edited by Matthew W. Gallagher and Shane J. Lopez. New York, NY: Oxford University Press.

Short, Tim, 2018. *The Psychology of Successful Trading: Behavioral Strategies for Profitability*. New York, NY: Routledge.

Shortall, Sally, and Mildred E. Warner. 2010. "Social Inclusion or Market Competitiveness? A Comparison of Rural Development Policies in the European Union and the United States." *Social Policy & Administration* 44(5):575–597.

Shorthose, Jim, and Neil Maycroft. 2017. *Where in Creativity? A Multi-disciplinary Approach*. Abington, UK: Routledge.

Shoss, Mindy K. and Clair Reynolds Kueny. 2022. "From Speculation to Substantiation: Empirically-Testing Societal Changes in Impact of Fit on Job Satisfaction from 1989, 1998, 2006, and 2016." *Group & Organization Management* 47(6):1181–217.

Shoukry, Hany. 2017. "Coaching for Social Change." Pp. 176–191 in *The SAGE Handbook of Coaching*, edited by Tatiana Bachkirova, Gordon Spence, and David Drake. London, UK: SAGE.

Shrira, Amit. 2012. "The Effect of Life Time Cumulative Adversity on Change and Chronicity in Depressive Symptoms and Quality of Life in Older Adults." *International Psychogeriatrics* 24(12):1988–1997.

Shtudiner, Ze¡¯ev, Galit Klein, and Jeffrey Kanto. 2017. "Who is Responsible for Economic Failures? Self-Serving Bias and Fundamental Attribution Error in Political Context." *Quality & Quantity* 51(1):335–350.

Shumow, Lee, Deborah Lowe Vandell, and Jill K. Posner. 1998. "Harsh, Firm, and Permissive Parenting in Low-income Families: Relations to Children's Academic Achievement and Behavioral Adjustment." *Journal of Family Issues* 19(5):483–507.

Shure, Myrna B., and Bonnie Aberson. 2012. "Enhancing the Process of Resilience through Effective Thinking." Pp. 481–503 in *Handbook of Resilience in Children*, edited by Sam Goldstein and Robert B. Brooks. New York, NY: Springer.

Sibley, Chris G., and John Duckitt. 2009. "Big-Five Personality, Social Worldviews, and Ideological Attitudes: Further Tests of a Dual Process Cognitive-motivational Model." *Journal of Social Psychology* 149(5):545–561.

Sidanius, Jim and Felicia Pratto. 1999. *Social Dominance: An Intergroup Theory of Social Hierarchy and Oppression*. Cambridge, UK: Cambridge University Press.

Sidanius, Jim, and Robert Kurzban. 2013. "Toward an Evolutionarily Informed Political Psychology." Pp. 205–236 in *The Oxford Handbook of Political Psychology*, edited by Leone Huddy, David O. Sears and Jack S. Levy. New York: Oxford University Press. (JA74.5O355)

Sidanius, Jim, Yesilernis Pena, and Mark Sawyer. 2001. "Inclusionary Discrimination: Pigmentocracy and Patriotism in the Dominican Republic." *Political Psychology* 22(4):827–851.

Sieber, Vanda, Lavinia Flückiger, Jutta Mata, Katharina Bernecker, and Veronika Job. 2019. "Autonomous Goal Striving Promotes a Nonlimited Theory about Willpower." *Personality & Social Psychology Bulletin* 45(8):1295–307.

Siegling, Alexander B., Donald H. Sakofske, Azshley K. Vesely, and David W. Nordstokke. 2012. "Relations of Emotional Intelligence with Gender-linked Personality: Implications for a Refinement of EI Constructs." *Personality & Individual Differences* 52:776–781.

Sieler, Alan. 2018. "Ontological Coaching." Pp. 95–123 in *The Complete Handbook of Coaching*, edited by Elaine Cox, Tatiana Bachkirova, and David Clutterbuck. London, UK: SAGE.

Sieroda, Helen. 2012. "Psychosynthesis Therapy." Pp. 330–334 in *The SAGE Handbook of Counselling and Psychotherapy*, edited by Colin Feltham and Ian Horton. London: SAGE.

Siisiainen, Lauri. 2019. *Foucault, Biopolitics and Resistance*. Abington, UK: Routledge.

Siisiainen, Martti. 2003. "One Concept, Two Approaches: Bourdieu and Putnam on Social Capital." *International Journal of Contemporary Sociology* 40(2):83–203.

Sikka, Pilleriin, Antti Revonsuo, and James J. Gross. 2023. "Individual Differences in Peace of Mind Reflect Adaptive Emotion Regulation." *Personality & Individual Differences* 215:112378.

Sikora, Joanna. 2005. "Public Attitudes to Economic Policy in East and West: Efficiency, Subsidies and Public Ownership." *Research in Social Stratification & Mobility* 23:229–274.

Silbereisen, Rainer K., and Margit Wiesner. 2002. "Lessons from Research on the Consequences of German Unification: Continuity and Discontinuity of Self-Efficacy and the Timing of Psychosocial Transitions." *Applied Psychology* 5(2):291–317.

Silbereisen, Rainer K., Martin Pinquart, and Martin J. Tomasik. 2010. "Demands of Social Change and Psychosocial Adjustment: Results from the Jena Study." Pp. 125–147 in *Social Change and Human Development: Concept and Results*, edited by Rainer K. Silbereisen. Los Angeles, CA: SAGE.

Silk, Jennifer S., Ella Vanderbilt-Adriance, Daniel S. Shaw, Erika E. Forbes, Diana J. Whalen, Neal D. Ryan, and Ronald E. Dahl. 2007. "Resilience among Children and Adolescents at Risk for Depression: Mediation and Moderation across Social and Neurobiological Contexts." *Development & Psychopathology* 19:841–865.

Silver, Daniel. 2011. "The Moodiness of Action." *Sociological Theory* 29(3):199–222.

Silvester, Keith. 2000. "Psychosynthesis." Pp. 122–143 in *Therapeutic Perspectives on Working with Lesbian, Gay and Bisexual Clients*, edited by Dominic Davies and Charles Neal. Buckingham, UK: Open University Press.

Simmons, Solon. 2020. *Root Narrative Theory and Conflict Resolution: Power, Justice and Values*. Abington, UK: Routledge.

Simon, Dan, and Stephen J. Read. 2018. "Neither Cognitive nor Consistency: A Comment on Cognitive Consistency Theory in Social Psychology: A Paradigm Reconsidered." *Psychological Inquiry* 29(2):97–108.

Simon, Gaiul, and Gwyn Whitfield. 2000. "Social Constructionist and Systemic Therapy." Pp. 144–162 in *Therapeutic Perspectives on Working with Lesbian, Gay and Bisexual Clients*, edited by Dominic Davies and Charles Neal. Buckingham, UK: Open University Press.

Simon, Joan B., John J. Murphy, and Shelia M. Smith. 2005. "Understanding and Fostering Family Resilience." *Family Journal* 13(4):427–436.

Simon, Robin W., and Kathryn Lively. 2010. "Sex, Anger and Depression." *Social Forces* 88(4):1543–1568.

Simons, Leslie Gordon, Tara E. Sutton, Ronald L. Simons, Frederick X. Gibbons, and Velma McBride Murry. 2016. "Mechanisms that Link Parenting Practices to Adolescents' Risky Sexual Behavior: A Test of Six Competing Theories." Journal of Youth & Adolescence 45(2):255–270.

Simons, Raluca M., Kyle J. Walters, Jessica A. Keith and Jeffrey S. Simons. 2021. "Posttraumatic Stress Disorder and Conduct Problems: The Role of Self-Control Demands." *Journal of Traumatic Stress* 34(2):298–308.

Simons, Ronald L., Les B. Whitbeck, Rand D. Conger, and Katherine J. Conger. 1991. "Parenting Factors, Social Skills, and Value Commitments as Precursors to School Failure, Involvement with Deviant Peers, and Delinquent Behavior." *Journal of Youth and Adolescence* 20(6):645–664.

Simonton, Kelly L. and Alex C. Garn. 2020. "Control–Value Theory of Achievement Emotions: A Closer Look at Student Value Appraisals and Enjoyment." *Learning & Individual Differences* 81:101910.

Simpkins, Sandra D., Jennifer A. Fredricks, Pamela E. Davis-Kean, and Jacquelynne S. Eccles. 2006. "Healthy Mind, Healthy Habits: The Influence of Activity Involvement and Middle Childhood." Pp. 283–302 in *Developmental Contexts in Middle Childhood: Bridges to Adolescence and Adulthood*, edited by Aletha C. Huston and Marika N. Ripke. Cambridge, UK: Cambridge University Press.

Simpson, David B., Jody L. Newman, and Dale R. Euqua. 2008. "Understanding the Role of Relational Factors in Christian Spirituality." *Journal of Psychology & Theology* 36(2):124–134.

Simpson, Jeffry A., Vladas Griskevicius, and John S. Kim. 2011. "Evolution, Life History Theory, and Personality." Pp. 75–89 in *Handbook of Interpersonal Psychology Theory, Research, Assessment, and Therapeutic Interventions*, edited by Leonard M. Horowitz and Stephen Strack. Hoboken, NJ: Wiley.

Simsek, Omer Faruk. 2013. "Self-Absorption Paradox Is Not a Paradox: Illuminating the Dark Side of Self-Reflection." *International Journal of Psychology* 48(6):1109–21.

Sin, Wai Man, and Yiu Wai Chu. 2000. "Postcolonial Law in the Global Economy: The Case of Hong Kong." *International Journal of the Sociology of Law* 28:291–309.

Sing, Ming. 2004. "Origins of Anti-partyism in Hong Kong." *East Asia* 21(3):37–57.

Singelis, Theodore M., and Harry C. Triandis. 1995. "Horizontal and Vertical Dimensions of Individualism and Collectivism: A Theoretical and Measurement Refinement." *Cross-Cultural Research* 29(3):240–275.

Singer, Alexa J., Cecilia Chouhy, Peter S. Lehmann, Jessica N. Walzak, Marc Gertz, and Sophia Biglin. 2019. "Victimization, Fear of Crime, and Trust in Criminal Justice Institutions: A Cross-National Analysis." *Crime & Delinquency* 65(6):822–44.

Sinha, Shilpi. 2013. "Derrida, Friendship and Responsible Teaching in Contrast to Effective Teaching." *Educational Philosophy & Theory* 45(3):259–71.

Sinn, Jeffrey S. and Matthew W. Hayes. 2018. "Is Political Conservatism Adaptive? Reinterpreting Right-Wing Authoritarianism and Social Dominance Orientation as Evolved, Sociofunctional Strategies." *Political Psychology* 39(5):1123–39.

Sirgy, M. Joseph. 2012. The Psychology of Quality of Life: Hedonic Well-Being, Life Satisfaction, and Eudaimonia. Dordrecht, Netherlands: Springer.

Sirois, Fuschia M., Danielle S. Molnar, and Jameson K. Hirsch. 2015. "Self-Compassion, Stress, and Coping in the Context of Chronic Illness." *Self and Identity* 14(3):334–347.

Sitzer, David L., and Ann B Stockwell. 2015. "The Art of Wellness: A 14-Week Art Therapy Program for At-Risk Youth." *Arts in Psychotherapy* 45:69–81.

Siu, Andrew M. H., and Daniel T. L. Shek. 2005. "Validation of the Interpersonal Reactivity Index in a Chinese Context." *Research on Social Work Practice* 15(2):118–126.

Siu, Andrew M.H., and Daniel T.L. Shek. 2005. "The Chinese Version of the Social Problem-solving Inventory: Some Initial Results on Reliability and Validity." *Journal of Chinese Psychology* 61(3):347–360.

Siu, Kin Wai Michael, and Jia Xin Xiao. 2015. "Quality of Life and Recycling Behaviour in High-Rise Buildings: A Case in Hong Kong." *Applied Research in Quality* of Life 1–18.

Sivami, Viren. 2016. Attraction Explained: The Science of How We Form Relationships. Abington, UK: Routledge.

Six, Benjamin. 2014. "A Pragmatic Contribution for a More Reflexive Institution-Based Trust." *Journal of Trust Research* 4(2):132–46.

Sjoberg, Lennart. 2003. "Distal Factors in Risk Perception." *Journal of Risk Research* 6(3):187–211.

Skerkat, Darren E. 1998. "Counterculture or Continuity? Competing Influence on Baby Boomers" Religious Orientation and Participation." *Social Force* 76(3):1087–1104.

Skerkat, Darren E., and Christopher G. Ellison. 1999. "Recent Developments and Current Controversies in the Sociology of Religion." *Annual Review of Sociology* 25:363–394.

Skinner, Ellen A., Thomas A. Kindermann, and Andrew J. Mashburn. 2019. *Lifespan Developmental Systems: Meta-Theory, Methodology and the Study of Applied Problems*, New York, NY: Routledge.

Skomoravsky, Alla, Kimberly Matheson, and Hymie Anisman. 2006. "The Buffering Role of Social Support Perceptions of Relation to Eating Disturbances among Women and Abuse Dating Relationships." *Sex Roles* 54:627–638.

Skopek, Jan, Florian Schulz, and Hans-Peter Blossfeld. 2011. "Who Contacts Whom? Educated Homophily in Online Mate Selection." *European Sociological Review* 27(2):180–195.

Skyttner, Lars. 2005. General Systems Theory: Problems, Perspectives, Practices. Singapore: World Scientific.

Slaby, Jan, and Achim Stephan. 2008. "Affective Intentionality and Self-Consciousness." *Consciousness & Cognition* 17(2):506–513.

Slagsvold, Britt, and Annemette Sorensen. 2008. "Age, Education, and the Gender Gap in the Sense of Control." *International Journal of Aging & Human Development* 67(1):25–42.

Small, Brent J., Christopher Hertzog, Daivd F. Hultsch, and Roger A. Dixon. 2003. "Stability and Change in Adult Personality over 6 Years: Findings from the Victoria Longitudinal Study." *Journal of Gerontology: Psychological Sciences* 58B(3):P166–P176.

Smart, Alan, and Josephine Smart. 2008. "Time-space Punctuation: Hong Kong's Border Regime and Limits on Mobility." *Pacific Affairs* 81(2):175–193.

Smart, Barry. 2003. *Economy, Culture and Society: A Sociological Critique of Neo-liberalism*. Buckingham, UK: Open University Press.

Smidt, Hannah. 2020. "Mitigating Election Violence Locally: UN Peacekeepers" Election-Education Campaigns in Côte D"Ivoire." *Journal of Peace Research* 57(1):199–216.

Smith, Anthony D. 2010. *Nationalism: Theory, Ideology, History*. Cambridge, UK: Polity.

Smith, Brian N., and Mark F. Stasson. 2000. "A Comparison of Health Behavior Constructs: Social Psychological Predictors of AIDS preventive Behavioral Intentions." *Journal of Applied Social Psychology* 30(3):443–462.

Smith, Elizabeth, Fiona Ross, Sheila Donovan, Jill Manthorpe, Sally Brearley, John Sitzia, and Peter Beresford. 2006. "Service User Involvement in Nursing, Midwifery and Health Visiting Research: A Review of Evidence and Practice." *International Journal of Nursing Studies* 45(2):298–315.

Smith, Eric N., Carissa Romero, Brian Donovan, Rachel Herter, David Paunesku, Geoffrey L. Cohen, Carol S. Dweck, and James J. Gross. 2018. "Emotion Theories and Adolescent Well-Being: Results of an Online Intervention." *Emotion* 18(6):781–788.

Smith, Glen. 2024. "You Know You're Right: How Intellectual Humility Decreases Political Hostility." *Political Psychology*.

Smith, Huston. 1991. The World's Religions: Our Great Wisdom Traditions. New York: Harper-Collins.

Smith, Jonathan C. and Aaron D. Karmin. 2002. "Idiosyncratic Reality Claims, Relaxation Dispositions, and ABC Relaxation Theory: Happiness, Literal Christianity, Miraculous Powers, Metaphysics, and the Paranormal." *Perceptual & Motor Skills* 95(3_suppl):1119–28.

Smith, Mario Luis, and Katherine Newman. 2001. "Urban Poverty after the Family Disadvantaged: The Rediscovery of the Family, the Neighborhood, and Culture." Annual Review of Sociology 27:23–45.

Smith, Nick, and Peter Hawkins. 2018. "Transformational Coaching." Pp. 231–246 in *The Complete Handbook of Coaching*, edited by Elaine Cox, Tatiana Bachkirova, and David Clutterbuck. London, UK: SAGE.

Smith, Peter B., Matthew J. Easterbrook, Goksu Cagil Celikkol, Sylvia Xiaohua Chen, Hu Ping, and Muhammad Rizwan. 2016. "Cultural Variations in the Relationship between Anger Coping Styles, Depression, and Life Satisfaction." *Journal of Cross-Cultural Psychology* 47(3):441–456.

Smith, Suzanne R., and Raeann R. Hamon. 2012. *Exploring Family Theories*. New York: Oxford University Press.

Smith, Tom W. 1997. "The Impact of the Presence of Others in a Respondent's Answers to Questions." *International Journal of Public Opinion Research* 9(1):31–47.

Smoktunowicz, Ewelina, Roman Cieslak, and Evangelia Demerouti. 2017. "Interrole Conflict and Self-Efficacy to Manage Work and Family Demands Mediate the Relationships of Job and Family Demands with Stress in the Job and Family Domains." *Anxiety, Stress, & Coping* 30(5):485–497.

Sneed, Joel R., Susan Krauss Whitbourne, and Michelle E. Culang. 2006. "Trust, Identity, and Ego Integrity: Modeling Erikson's Core Stages over 34 Years." *Journal of Adult Development* 13:148–157.

Snijders, Chris, and Gideon Keren. 1999. "Determinants of Trust." Pp. 355–385 in *Games and Human Behavior: Essays in Honor of Annon Rapoport*, edited by David V. Budescu, Ido Ercv, and Rani Jwick. Mahwah, NJ: Lawrence Erlbaum.

Snir, Raphael, and Itzhak Harpaz. 2002. "Work Leisure Relations: Leisure Orientation and the Meaning of Work." *Journal of Leisure Research* 34(2):178–203.

Snyder, Eldon E., and Elmer Spreitzer. 1992. "Social Psychological Concomitants of Adolescents' Role Identities as Scholars and Athletes: A Longitudinal Analysis." *Youth & Society* 23(4):507–522.

Snyder, Jordan D., David Boan, Jamie D. Aten, Edward B. Davis, Leif Van Grinsven, Tao Liu, and Everett L. Worthington. 2020. "Resource Loss and Stress Outcomes in a Setting of Chronic Conflict: The Conservation of Resources Theory in the Eastern Congo." *Journal of Traumatic Stress* 33(3):227–37.

Snyder, Karrie Ann, Alexandra Tate, and Ethan Roubenoff. 2018. "Younger Women with Breast Cancer and Treatment Decision-Making: Rethinking Patient Involvement and Empowerment." *Research in the Sociology of Health Care* 36:37–58.

Sobeck, Joanne, Joanne Smith-Darden, Megan Hicks, Poco Kernsmith, Paul E. Kilgore, Lara Treemore-Spears, and Shawn McElmurry. 2020. "Stress, Coping, Resilience and Trust During the Flint Water Crisis." *Behavioral Medicine* 46(3–4):202–16.

Sobek, David. 2009. *The Causes of War.* Cambridge, UK: Polity.

Soccio, Douglas. 2004. *Archetypes of Wisdom: An Introduction to Philosophy*. Belmont, CA: Wadsworth Thomson.

Soenens, Bart, and Wim Beyers. 2012. "The Cross-cultural Significance of Control and Autonomy in Parent-adolescent Relationships." *Journal of Adolescence* 35:243–248.

Sokolowski, S. Wojciech. 1996. "Show Me the Way to the Next Worthy Seed: Towards a Microstructural Theory of Volunteering and Giving." *Voluntas* 7(3):259–278.

Soller, Brian, Aubrey L Jackson, and Erin R. Coleman. 2017. "Violent Peers and Street Efficacy in Legally Cynical Neighborhoods." *Social Currents* 4(2):156–174.

Solomon, Brittany C. and Joshua J. Jackson. 2014. "Why Do Personality Traits Predict Divorce? Multiple Pathways through Satisfaction." *Journal Personality of Social Psychology* 106(6):978–96.

Solomon, Denise Hannani, and Michael E. Roloff. 2018. "Relationship Initiation and Growth." Pp. 79–89 *The Cambridge Handbook of Personal Relationships*, edited by Anita L. Vangelisti and Daniel Perlman. Cambridge, UK: Cambridge University Press.

Solomon, Lewis D. 2006. From Athens to America: Virtues and the Formulation of Public Policy. Lanham, MD: Lexington.

Solomon, Robert C. 2003. *Living with Nietzsche: What the Great Immoralist Has to Teach Us*. Oxford, UK: Oxford University Press.

Somma, Nicolás M. and Rodrigo M. Medel. 2019. "What Makes a Big Demonstration? Exploring the Impact of Mobilization Strategies on the Size of Demonstrations." *Social Movement Studies* 18(2):233–51.

Sommer, Kristin L., Kipling D. Williams, Natalie J. Ciarocco, and Roy F. Baumeister. 2001. "When Silence Speaks Louder Than Words: Explorations into the Intrapsychic and Interpersonal Consequences of Social Ostracism." *Basic & Applied Social Psychology* 23(4):225–243.

Son Hag, Leanne S. 2013. "Stigmatization, Neoliberalism, and Resilience." Pp. 158–182 in *Social Resilience in the Neoliberal Era*, edited by Peter A. Hall and Michele Lamont. Cambridge, UK: Cambridge University Press.

Son, Joonmo, and John Wilson. 2012. "Using Normative Theory to Explain the Effect of Religion and Education on Volunteering." *Sociological Perspectives* 55(3):473–499.

Son, Joonmo. 2013. Social Capital and Institutional Constraints: A Comparative Analysis of China, Taiwan and the US. Abingdon, UK: Routledge.

Song, Ahyoung, Suzanne L. Wenzel, Jae Yop Kim, and Boyoung Nam. 2017. "Experience of Domestic Violence During Childhood, Intimate Partner Violence, and the Deterrent Effect of Awareness of Legal Consequences." *Journal of Interpersonal Violence* 32(3):357–72.

Song, Geng, and Tracy K. Lee. 2010. "Consumption, Class Formation and Sexuality: Reading Men's Lifestyle Magazines in China." *China* 64:159–177.

Song, Jaeki, and Fatemeh Mariam Zahedi. 2005. "A Theoretical Approach to Web Design in E-commerce: A Belief Reinforcement Model." *Management Science* 51(8):1219–1235.

Soodak, Leslie C., and David M. Podell. 1994. "Teachers" Thinking about Difficult-to-teach Students." *Journal of Educational Research* 88(1):44–51.

Sorens, Jason. 2011. "Mineral Production, Territory, and Ethnic Rebellion: The Role of Rebel Constituencies." *Journal of Peace Research* 48(5):571–85.

Sorensen, Silvia, Jameson K. Hirsch, and Jeffrey M. Lyness. 2014. "Optimism and Planning for Future Care Needs among Older Adults." *GeroPsych: Journal of Gerontopsychology & Geriatric Psychiatry* 27(1):5–22.

Sorge, Antonio. 2008. "Divergent Visions: Localist And Cosmopolitan Identities in Highland Sardinia." *Journal of the Royal Anthropological Institute* 14(4):808–824.

Sosa, Teresa, and Kimberley Gomez. 2012. "Connecting Teacher Efficacy Beliefs in Promoting Resilience to Support of Latino Students." *Urban Education* 47(5):876–909.

Sotirovic, Mira. 2000. "Effects of Media Use on Audience Framing and Support for Welfare." *Mass Communication & Society* 3(2&3):269–296.

Soto, Christopher J., Oliver P. John, and Samuel D. Gosling. 2008. "The Development Psychometrics of Big Five Self-reports: Acquiescence, Factor Structure, Coherence, and Differentiation from Ages 10 to 20." *Journal of Personality & Social Psychology* 94(4):718–737.

South, Scott J., Amy Lutz, and Eric P. Baumer. 2005. "Adolescent Residential Mobility and Premature Life-course Transitions: The Role of Peer Networks." *Sociological Studies of Children & Youth* 11:23–52.

Sovereign, Genevieve and Benjamin R. Walker. 2021. "Mind, Body and Wellbeing: Reinforcement Sensitivity Theory and Self-Cultivation Systems as Wellbeing Influencers." *Journal of Happiness Studies* 22(1):1–20.

Speed, David, Thomas J. Coleman, and Joseph Langston. 2018. "What Do You Mean, "What Does It All Mean?" Atheism, Nonreligion, and Life Meaning." *SAGE Open* 8(1):2158244017754238.

Speer, Paul W., and Joseph Hughey. 1995. "Community Organizing: An Ecological Route to Empowerment and Power." *American Journal of Community Psychology* 23(5):729–748.

Spelman, William. 2004. "Optimal Targeting of Incivility-reduction Strategies." *Journal of Quantitative Criminology* 20(1):63–88.

Spence, Gordon B., and Anthony M. Grant. 2014. "Coaching and Well-being: A Brief Review of Existing Evidence, Relevant Theory, and Implications for Practitioners." Pp. 1008–1025 in *The Oxford Handbook of Happiness*, edited by Susan A. David, Ilona Boniwell and Amanda Conley Ayers. Oxford, UK: Oxford University Press.

Spencer-Rodgers, Julie, Helen C. Boucher, Kaiping Peng, and Lei Wang. 2009. "Cultural Differences in Self-verification: The Role of Naive Dialecticism." *Journal of Experimental Social Psychology* 45:860–866.

Spengler, Marion, Rodica Ioana Damian, and Brent W. Roberts. 2018. "How You Behave in School Predicts Life Success Above and Beyond Family Background, Broad Traits, and Cognitive Ability." *Journal of Personality & Social Psychology* 114(4):620–636.

Sperry, Len. 2012. "Spiritually Sensitive Psychotherapy: An Impending Paradigm Shift in Theory and Practice." Pp. 223–236 in *The Oxford Handbook of Psychology and Spirituality*, edited by Lisa J. Miller. New York, NY: Oxford University Press.

Spinelli, Ernesto, Peter. 2018. "Existential Coaching." Pp. 66–80 in *The Complete Handbook of Coaching*, edited by Elaine Cox, Tatiana Bachkirova, and David Clutterbuck. London, UK: SAGE.

Spitzberg, Brian H. 2013. "Intimate Partner Violence." Pp. 187–210 in The SAGE *Handbook of Conflict Communication*, edited by John G. Oetzel and Stelle Ting-Toomey. Thousand Oaks, CA: SAGE.

Spreitzer, Elmer. 1994. "Does Participation in Interscholastic Athletics Affect Development? A Longitudinal Analysis of an 18–24 Age Cohort." *Youth & Society* 25(3):368–387.

Ssewamala, Fred M., Margaret Lombe, and Jami C. Curley. 2006. "Using Individual Development Accounts for Microenterprise Development." *Journal of Developmental Entrepreneurship* 11(2):117–131.

Stacki, Sandra L., and Karen Monkman. 2003. "Change through Empowerment Processes: Women's Stories from South Asia and Latin America." *Compare* 33(2):173–189.

Stadtfeld, Christoph and Alex Pentland. 2015. "Partnership Ties Shape Friendship Networks: A Dynamic Social Network Study." *Social Forces* 94(1):453–77.

Stafford, Ian. 2000. "Children with Movement Difficulties, Primary Education and the Development of Performance Indicators." *British Journal of Special Education* 27(2):81–86.

Stafford, Laura. 2015. "Social Exchange Theories: Calculating the Rewards and Costs of Personal Relationships." Pp. 403–415 in *Engaging Theories in Interpersonal Communication: Multiple Perspectives*, edited by Dawn O. Braithwaite and Paul Schrodt. Thousand Oaks, CA: SAGE.

Stafford, M., S. Cummins, S. Macintyre, A. Ellaway, and M. Marmot. 2005. "Gender Differences in the Associations between Health and Neighborhood Environment." *Social Science & Medicine* 60:1681–1692.

Stagnaro, Michael N., Antonio A. Arechar, and David G. Rand. 2017. "From Good Institutions to Generous Citizens: Top-Down Incentives to Cooperate Promote Subsequent Prosociality but Not Norm Enforcement." *Cognition* 167:212–254.

Stake, Jayne E. 2006. "The Critical Mediating Role of Social Encouragement for Science Motivation and Confidence among Higher School Girls and Boys." *Journal of Applied Social Psychology* 36(4):1017–1045.

Stalker, Glenn John. 2008. "Measuring Diversity in Daily Social Contact: The Contribution of Social Context, Work and Leisure on the Opportunity for Engagement." *Social Indicators Research* 86(2):275–295.

Stankov, Lazar, Goran Knežević, Gerard Saucier, Borislav Radović, and Biljana Milovanović. 2018. "Militant Extremist Mindset and the Assessment of Radicalization in the General Population." *Journal of Individual Differences* 39(2):88–98.

Stanley, Jennifer Tehan, Monika Lohani, and Derek M. Isaacowitz. 2014. "Age-related Differences in Judgments of Inappropriate Behavior Are Related to Humor Style Preferences." *Psychology & Aging* 29(3):528–541.

Stanley, John K., David A. Heasher, Janet R. Stanley, and Dianne Vella-Brodrick. 2011. "Mobility, Social Exclusion, and Well-being: Exploring the Links." *Transportation Research* Part A 45:789–801.

Stanton, Sarah C. E., Katie Spence, Jenni E. Kähkönen, and Kiersten Dobson. 2020. "Individual and Dyadic Associations among Relational Self-expansion Potential, Affect, and Perceived Health." *Personal Relationships* 27(3):550–70.

Stanton-Salazar, Ricardo D. 2011. "A Social Capital Framework for the Study of Institutional Agents and Their Role in the Empowerment of Low-Status Students and Youth." *Youth & Society* 43(3):1066–1109.

Staples, Susan L., Randolph R. Cornelius, and Margaret S. Gibbs. 1999. "Noise Disturbance from a Developing Airport: Perceived Risk or General Annoyance?" *Environment & Behavior* 31(5):692–710.

Starrin, Bengt, Cecilia Aslund, and Kent W. Nilsson. 2009. "Financial Stress, Shaming Experiences and Psychosocial Ill-health: Studies into the Finances-shame Model. " *Social Indicators Research* 91:283–298.

Stater, Keely Jones and Mark Stater. 2019. "Is It "Just Work"? The Impact of Work Rewards on Job Satisfaction and Turnover Intent in the Nonprofit, For-Profit, and Public Sectors." *American Review of Public Administration* 49(4):495–511.

Staton-Tindall, Michele, Ginny Sprang, and James Clark. 2012. "Caregiver Drug Use and Arrest as Correlates of Child Trauma Exposure," *Journal of Evidence-Based Social Work* 9(3):265–282.

Staub, Ervin. 2003. "Notes on Cultures of Violence, Cultures of Caring and Peace, and the Fulfillment of Basic Human Needs." *Political Psychology* 24(1):1–21.

Staudinger, Ursula M., William Fleeson, and Paul B. Baltes. 1999. "Predictors of Subjective Physical Health and Global Well-being: Similarities and Differences between the United States and Germany." *Journal of Personality & Social Psychology* 76(2):305–329.

Stavrova, Olga and Daniel Ehlebracht. 2018. "Education as an Antidote to Cynicism." *Social Psychological & Personality Science* 9(1):59–69.

Stavrova, Olga and Pascal Siegers. 2014. "Religious Prosociality and Morality across Cultures." *Personality & Social Psychology Bulletin* 40(3):315–33.

Stavrova, Olga. 2014. Fitting in and Getting Happy: How Conformity to Societal Norms Affect Subjective Well-being. Frankfurt, Germany: Campus.

Stebleton, Michael J. Krista M. Soria, Ronald L. Huesman, Jr., and Vasti Torres. 2014. "Recent Immigrant Students at Research Universities: The Relationship between Campus Climate and Sense of Belonging." *Journal of College Student Development* 55(2):196–202.

Steca, P., Greco Baretta, and Monzani D"Addario. 2017. "Associations between Personality, Sports Participation and Athletic Success. A Comparison of Big Five in Sporting and Non-Sporting Adults." *Personality & Individual Differences* 121:176–183.

Steel, Liz, Warren Kidd, and Anne Brown. 2012. *The Family*. Houndmills, UK: Palgrave.

Stefaniak, Anna, Michał Bilewicz, and Maria Lewicka. 2017. "The Merits of Teaching Local History: Increased Place Attachment Enhances Civic Engagement and Social Trust." *Journal of Environmental Psychology* 51:217–225.

Steffen, Jordan and Jiuqing Cheng. 2022. "The Influence of Gain-Loss Framing and Its Interaction with Political Ideology on Social Distancing and Mask Wearing Compliance During the Covid-19 Pandemic." *Current Psychology* 42(10):8028–38.

Steg, Linda, and Judith de Groot. 2010. "Explaining Prosocial Intentions: Testing Causal Relationships in the Norm Activation Model." *British Journal of Social Psychology* 49(4):725–743.

Steger, Michael F., Shigehiro Oishi, and Todd B. Kashdan. 2009. "Meaning in Life Across the Life Span: Levels and Correlates of Meaning in Life from Emerging Adulthood to Older Adulthood." *Journal of Positive Psychology* 4(1):43–52.

Steger, Michael F., Yeshito Karsabata, Satoshi Shimai, and Keiko Otake. 2008. "The Meaningful Life in Japan and the United States: Levels and Correlates of Meaning in Life." *Journal of Research in Personality* 42:660–678.

Stehr, Nico. 2008. Moral Markets: How Knowledge and Affluence Change Consumers and Products. Boulder, CO: Paradigm.

Steijn, Bram. 2001. "Work Systems, Quality of Working Life and Attitudes of Workers; An Empirical Study toward the Effects of Team and Non-teamwork." *New Technology, Work & Employment* 16(3):191–203.

Stein, Catherine H., Erica Hoffmann, Erin E. Bonar, Jaclyn E. Leith, Kristen M. Abraham, Alexis C. Hamill, Shane W. Kraus, Shinakee Gumber, and Wendy R Fogo. 2013. "The United States

Economic Crisis: Young Adults" Reports of Economic Pressures, Financial and Religious Coping and Psychological Well-Being." *Journal of Family & Economic Issues* 34(2):200–210.

Stein, Janice Gross. 2013. "Threat Perception in International Relations." Pp. 364–394 in *The Oxford Handbook of Political Psychology*, edited by Leone Huddy, David O. Sears and Jack S. Levy. New York: Oxford University Press.

Steiner, Jurg. 2012. The Foundations of Deliberative Democracy: Empirical Research and Normative Implications. New York: Cambridge University Press.

Steinhardt, H. Christoph 2012. "How is High Trust in China Possible? Comparing the Origins of Generalized Trust in Three Chinese Societies." *Political Studies* 60(2):434–454.

Steinhardt, H. Christoph, Linda Chelan Li. and Yihong Jiang. 2018. "The Identity Shift in Hong Kong since 1997: Measurement and Explanation." *Journal of Contemporary China* 27(110):261–276.

Steinhausen, Hans-Christoph, Cinzia Bearth-Carrari, and Christa Winkler Metzke. 2009. "Psychosocial Adaptation of Adolescent Migrants in a Swiss Community Survey." *Social Psychiatry & Psychiatric Epidemiology* 44:308–316.

Steinkamp, Marjorie W., and John B. Kelly. 1987. "Social Integration, Leisure Activity, and Life Satisfaction in Older Adults: Activity Theory Revisited." *International Journal of Aging and Human Development* 25(4):293–307.

Stelter, Reinhard. 2017. "Working with Values in Coaching." Pp. 331–345 in *The SAGE Handbook of Coaching*, edited by Tatiana Bachkirova, Gordon Spence, and David Drake. London, UK: SAGE.

Stephens, Nicole M., Jessica S. Cameron, and Sarah S.M. Townsend. 2014. "Lower Social Class Does Not (Always) Mean Greater Interdependence: Women in Poverty Have Fewer Social Resources than Working-class Women." *Journal of Cross-Cultural Psychology* 45(7):1061–1073.

Stern, Jessica A. and Jude Cassidy. 2018. "Empathy from Infancy to Adolescence: An Attachment Perspective on the Development of Individual Differences." *Developmental Review* 47:1–22.

Sternberg, Robert J. 2004. "What Is Wisdom and How Can We Develop It?" *Annals of the American Academy of Political & Social Science* 591:164–174.

Sternberg, Robert J., Linda Jarvin, and Elena J. Grigorenko. 2011. *Explorations in Giftedness*. New York: Cambridge University Press.

Stets, Jan E., Michael J. Carter, Michael M. Harrod, Christine Cerven, and Seth Abrutyn. 2008. "The Moral Identity, Status, Moral Emotions, and the Normative Order." Pp. 227–251 in *Social Structure and Emotion*, edited by Jody Clay-Warner and Dawn T. Robinson. San Diego, CA: Academic.

Stevens, Elizabeth S., Alexander A. Jendrusina, Alison C. Legrand, Erica R. Nahin, Michelle Goldwin Kaufman, Thomas D. Borkovec, and Evelyn Behar. 2018. "The Effects of Worry and Relaxation on Flexibility During Cognitive Restructuring." *Behavior Modification* 42(6):838–63.

Stevens, Fred C. J., Charles D. Kaplan, Rudolf W. H. M. Ponds, and Jellemer Jolles. 2001. "The Importance of Active Lifestyles for Memory Performance and Memory Self-knowledge." *Basic & Applied Social Psychology* 23(2):137–145.

Stevens, Irene, and Peter Hassett. 2007. "Applying Complexity Theory to Risk in Child Protection Practice." *Children* 14(1):128–144. \99–171

Stevens-Long, Judith, and Greg Michaud. 2003. "Theory in Adult Development: The New Paradigm and the Problem of Direction." Pp. 3–22 in *Handbook of Adult Development,* edited by Jack Demick and Carrie Andreoletti. New York: Kluwer Academic. (BF724.5H36)

Stevenson, Clifford and Rachel Manning. 2010. "National Identity and International Giving: Irish Adults" Accounts of Charitable Behaviour." *Journal of Community & Applied Social Psychology* 20(4):249–61.

Stevenson, Fiona A., Miranda Leontowitsch, and Catherine Duggan. 2008. "Over-the-Counter Medicines: Professional Expertise and Consumer Discourses." *Sociology of Health & Illness* 30(6):913–28.

Stevenson, Nick. 2011. *Education and Cultural Citizenship*. Los Angeles, CA: SAGE.
Steverink, Nardi, and Siegwurt Lindenberg. 2006. "Which Social Needs Are Important for Subjective Well-being? What Happiness to Them with Aging?" *Psychology & Aging* 21(2):281–290.
Stewart, Donna E., and Tracy Yuen. 2011. "A Systematic Review of Resilience in the Physically Ill." *Psychosomatics* 52:199–209.
Stewart, Miriam J. 1989. "Social Support: Diverse Theoretical Perspectives." *Social Science & Medicine* 28(12):1275–1282.
Stichter, Matt. 2018. *The Skillfulness of Virtue: Improving Our Moral and Epistemic Lives*. Cambridge, UK: Cambridge University Press.
Stiles, William B. 2012. "The Client-therapist Relationship." Pp. 67–76 in *The SAGE Handbook of Counselling and Psychotherapy*, edited by Colin Feltham and Ian Horton. London: SAGE.
Stober, Joachim. 2001. "The Social Desirability Scale-17 (SDS-17): Convergent Validity, Discriminant Validity and Relationship with Age." *European Journal of Psychological Assessment* 17(3):222–232.
Stoddard, Sarah A., and Jennifer Pierce. 2018. "Alcohol and Marijuana Use and Intentions among Adolescents: The Role of the Reasoned Action Approach and Positive Future Orientation." *Youth & Society* 50(6):758–779.
Stoeger, Heidrun, Tobias Debatin, Michael Heilemann, and Albert Ziegler. 2019. "Online Mentoring for Talented Girls in Stem: The Role of Relationship Quality and Changes in Learning Environments in Explaining Mentoring Success." *New Directions for Child & Adolescent Development*. 2019(168):75–99.
Stogner, John, Chris L. Gibson, and J. Mitchell Miller. 2014. "Examining the Reciprocal Nature of the Health-Violence Relationship: Results from a Nationally Representative Sample." *Justice Quarterly* 31(3):473–99.
Stojanov, Ana and Jamin Halberstadt. 2019. "The Conspiracy Mentality Scale: Distinguishing between Irrational and Rational Suspicion." *Social Psychology* 50(4):215–32.
Stokes, Charles E., and Mark D. Regnerus. 2008. "When Faith Divides Family: Religious Discord and Adolescent Reports of Parent-child Relations." *Social Science Research* 38:155–167.
Stoll, Michael A. 2001. "Race, Neighborhood Poverty, and Participation in Voluntary Associations." *Sociological Forum* 16(3):529–557.
Stolle, Dietlind and Allison Harell. 2013. "Social Capital and Ethno-Racial Diversity: Learning to Trust in an Immigrant Society." *Political Studies* 61(1):42–66.
Stolle, Dietlind, and Michele Micheletti. 2013. *Political Consumerism: Global Responsibility in Action*. New York, NY: Cambridge University Press.
Stolz, Jorg.2011. "The "social integration" of religious groups in society: A social mechanisms approach." *Annual Review of the Sociology of Religion* 2:85–116.
Stone, Walter J., and Matthew K. Buttice. 2010. "Voters in Context: The Politics of Citizen Behavior." Pp. 555–576 in *The Oxford Handbook of American Elections and Political Behavior*, edited by Jan E., Leighley. Oxford, UK: Oxford University Press. (JK1976.O935)
Stotsky, Miriam T., Julie C. Bowker, and Rebecca G. Etkin. 2019. "Receiving Prosocial Behavior: Examining the Reciprocal Associations between Positive Peer Treatment and Psychosocial and Behavioral Outcomes." *Journal of Research on Adolescence* 30(2):458–470.
Stott, Clifford, John Drury, and Steve Reicher. 2017. "On the Role of a Social Identity Analysis in Articulating Structure and Collective Action: The 2011 Riots in Tottenham and Hackney." *British Journal of Criminology* 57(4):964–981.
Stoynoff, Steve. 1997. "Factors Associated with International Students" Academic Achievement." *Journal of Instructional Psychology* 24(1):56–68.
Straughn, Jeremy Brooke, and Angie L. Andriot. 2011. "Education, Civic Patriotism and Democratic Citizenship: Unpacking the Education Effect on Political Involvement." *Sociological Forum* 26(3):556–580.
Straume, Sivert, and Magnus Odeen. 2010. "International and Domestic Altruism: A Study among the Adult Population in Norway." *Journal of Applied Social Psychology* 40(3):618–635.

Strauser, David R., Daniel C. Lustig, Pamela A. Cogdal, and Ayse Ciftci Uruk. 2006. "Trauma Symptoms: Relationship with Career Thoughts Vocational Identity and Developmental Work Personality." *Career Development Quarterly* 54:346–360.

Strelan, Peter, Jan-Willem Van Prooijen, and Mario Gollwitzer. 2020. "When Transgressors Intend to Cause Harm: The Empowering Effects of Revenge and Forgiveness on Victim Well-Being." *British Journal of Social Psychology* 59(2):447–69.

Strenger, Carlo. 2011. *The Fear of Insignificance: Searching for Meaning in the Twenty-first Century*. Houndmills, UK: Palgrave.

Strepparava, Maria Grazia et al. 2016. "Cognitive Counselling Intervention: Treatment Effectiveness in an Italian University Centre." *British Journal of Guidance in Counselling* 44(4):423–433.

Strong, Tom. 2002. "Collaborative Expertise after the Discursive Turn." *Journal of Psychotherapy Integration* 12(2):218–232.

Strydom, Piet. 2002. *Risk, Environment and Society: Ongoing Debates, Current Issues and Future Prospects*. Buckingham, UK: Open University Press.

Stuart, Scott, and Michael Robertson. 2003. *Interpersonal Psychotherapy: A Clinician's Guide*. London, UK: Arnold.

Stuhr, John J. 2003. Pragmatism, Postmodernism and the Future of Philosophy. New York: Routledge.

Sturgis, Patrick, Caroline Roberts, and Nick Allum. 2005. "A Different Take on the Deliberative Poll: Information, Deliberation, and Attitude Constraint." *Public Opinion Quarterly* 69(1):30–65.

Sturm, Douglas. 1998. *Solidarity and Suffering: Toward a Politics of Relationality*. Albany, NY: State University of New York Press.

Sturmer, Stefan, Bernd Simon, and Michael I. Loewy. 2008. "Intraorganizational Respect and Organizational Participation: The Mediating Role of Collective Identity." *Group Processes & Intergroup Relations* 11(1):5–20.

Stutchbury, Kristina. 2022. "Critical Realism: An Explanatory Framework for Small-Scale Qualitative Studies or an Unhelpful Edifice?" *International Journal of Research & Method in Education* 45(2):113–28.

Stutzer, Alois. 2004. "The Role of Income Aspirations in Individual Happiness." *Journal of Economic Behavior & Organization* 54:89–109.

Su, Lujun, Binli Tang and Jeroen Nawijn. 2021. "How Tourism Activity Shapes Travel Experience Sharing: Tourist Well-Being and Social Context." *Annals of Tourism Research* 91:103316.

Su, Yan, Danielle Ka Lai Lee, and Porismita Borah. 2021. "The Conditional Indirect Effects of Political Social Media Information Seeking and Expression on Government Evaluation in Hong Kong: Revisiting the Communication Mediation Model." *International Journal of Communication* 15:277–99.

Su, Yang and Shizheng Feng. 2013. "Adapt or Voice: Class, Guanxi, and Protest Propensity in China." *Journal of Asian Studies* 72(1):45–67.

Su, Zhenhua, Yanyu Ye, and Pu Wang. 2019. "Social Change and Generalized Anomie: Why Economic Development Has Reduced Social Trust in China." *International Sociology* 34(1):58–82.

Suchweh, Patrick. 2012. "The Moral Economy of Inequality: Popular Views on Income Differentiation, Poverty and Wealth." *Socio-Economic Review* 10:419–445.

Suhay, Elizabeth. 2015. "Explaining Group Influence: The Role of Identity and Emotion in Political Conformity and Polarization." *Political Behavior* 37(1):221–51.

Sui, Xiaoming. 2011. *Daoist Wisdom*. Beijing, China: Golden City.

Sukabdi, Zora A. 2019. "Psychological Rehabilitation for Ideology-based Terrorism Offenders." Pp. 95–116 in *Deradicalisation and Terrorist Rehabilitation: A Framework for Police Making and Implementation*, edited by Rohan Gunaratina and Subariah Hussin. Abingdon, UK: Routledge.

Sukys, Saulius, Ausra Lisinskiene, and Ilona Tilindiene. 2015. "Adolescents' Participation in Sport Activities and Attachment to Parents and Peers." *Social Behavior & Personality* 43(9):1507–17.

Sulemana, Iddisah. 2015. "The Effect of Fear of Crime and Crime Victimization on Subjective Well-Being in Africa." *Social Indicators Research* 121(3):849–872.
Sullivan, Alice. 2001. "Cultural Capital and Education Attainment." *Sociology* 35(4):893–912.
Sullivan, Daniel, Sheridan A. Stewart, and Joseph Diefendorf. 2015. "Simmel's Time-Space Theory: Implications for Experience of Modernization and Place." *Journal of Environmental Psychology* 41:45–57.
Sumter, Sindy R., Patti M. Valkenburg, and Jochen Peter. 2013. "Perceptions of Love Across the Lifespan Differences in Passion, Intimacy, and Commitment." *International Journal of Behavioral Development* 37(5):417–427.
Sun, Jessie, Scott Barry Kaufman, and Luke D. Smillie. 2018. "Unique Associations between Big Five Personality Aspects and Multiple Dimensions of Well-Being." *Journal of Personality* 86(2):158–72.
Sun, Jiaming, and Xun Wang. 2010. "Value Differences between Generations in China: A Study in Shanghai." *Journal of Youth Studies* 13(1):65–81.
Sun, Jing, and Donald Stewart. 2007. "Development of Population-based Resilience Measures in the Primary School Setting." *Health Education* 107(6):575–599.
Sun, Rachel C.F., and Daniel T.L. Shek. 2013. "Longitudinal Influences of Positive Youth Development and Life Satisfaction Problem Behaviour among Adolescents in Hong Kong." *Social Indicators Research* 14:1171–1197.
Sun, Shaojing, Alan M. Rubin, and Paul M. Haridakis. 2008. "The Role of Motivation and Media Involvement in Explaining Internet Dependency." *Journal of Broadcasting & Electronic Media* 52(3):408–431.
Sun, Shufang, and James Robert Bitter. 2012. "From China to South Korea: Two Perspectives on Individual Psychology in Asia." *Journal of Individual Psychology* 68(3):233–248.
Sun, Wenkai, and Xianghong Wang. 2012. "Do Government Actions Affect Trust? Cross-city Evidence in China." *Social Science Journal* 49:447–457.
Sun, Yu, Shangpeng Li, and Zheng Li 2024. "Student-perceived Social Interactions in University Musical Ensembles Predicted Group Identification." *Psychology of Music.*
Sundquist, Kristina, and Min Yang. 2007. "Linking Social Capital and Self-rated Health: A Multilevel Analysis of 11,775 Men and Women in Sweden." *Health & Place* 13:324–334.
Sunstein, Caso R., and Adrian Vermeule. 2009. "Conspiracy Theories: Causes and Cures." *Journal of Political Philosophy* 17(2):202–227.
Suntikul, Wantanee, and Timothy Jachna. 2016. "Profiling the Heritage Experience in Macao's Historic Center." *International Journal of Tourism Research* 18(4):308–318.
SunWolf. 2008. Peer Groups: Expanding Our Study of Small Group Communication. Los Angeles, CA: Sage.
Supkoff, Laura, Jennifer Puig, and L. Alan Sroufe. 2012. "Situating Resilience in Developmental Context." Pp. 127–156 in *The Social Ecology of Resilience: Handbook of Theory and Practice*, edited by Michael Ungar. New York, NY: Springer.
Sussman, Steve, and Susan L. Ames. 2001. *The Social Psychology of Drug Abuse*. Buckingham, UK: Open University Press.
Sutherland, Claire. 2012. Nationalism in the Twenty-first Century: Challenges and Responses. Houndmills, UK: Palgrave.
Sutherland, Lynette F., and Gerard J. Fogarty. 1995. "Congruence as a Predictor of Occupational Stress." *Journal of Vocational Behavior* 46:292—309.
Sutherland, Siobhan and Uzma S. Rehman. 2018. "Viewing Sexual Desire as Stable Versus Fluid: The Impact of Implicit Beliefs on Women's Coping with Sexual Desire Problems." *Journal of Sex & Marital Therapy* 44(4):410–20.
Svara, J.H. 2001. "The Myth of the Dichotomy: Complementarity of Politics and Administration in the Past and Future of Public Administration." *Public Administration Review* 61(2):176–183.
Svebak, Sven, K. Gunnar Gotestam, and Eva Naper Jensen. 2004. "The Significance of Sense of Humor, Life Regard, and Stressors for Bodily Complaints among High School Students." *Humor* 17(1/2):67–83.

Svendsen, Gunner Lin Haase, and Gert Tinggaard Svendsen. 2003. “On the Wealth of Nations: Bourdieuconomics and Social Capital.” *Theory & Society* 32:607–631.

Svetina, Matija. 2014. “Resilience in the Context of Erikson’s Theory of Human Development.” *Current Psychology* 33(3):393–404.

Swales, Michaela, and Christine Dunkley. 2012. “Dialectical Behavior Therapy.” Pp. 293–297 in *The SAGE Handbook of Counselling and Psychotherapy*, edited by Colin Feltham and Ian Horton. London: SAGE.

Swami, Viren, Jakob Pietschnig, Ulrich S. Tran, Ingo W. Nader, Stefan Stieger, and Martin Voracek. 2013. “Lunar Lies: The Impact of Informational Framing and Individual Differences in Shaping Conspiracist Beliefs About the Moon Landings.” *Applied Cognitive Psychology* 27(1):71–80.

Swann, William B., Jr. 2012. “Self-verification Theory.” Pp. 23–42 in *Handbook of Theories of Social Psychology* (vol. 2), edited by Paul A.M. Van Lange, Arie W. Kruglanski and E. Tory Higgins. London, CA: SAGE.

Swanson, Jeffrey W., Arthur O. Linskey, Ruben Quintero-Salinas, Andres J. Pumariega, and Charles E. Holzer, III. 1992. “A Binational School Survey of Depressive Symptoms, Drug Use, and Suicidal Ideation.” *Journal of the American Academy of Child & Adolescent Psychiatry* 31(4):669–678.

Swanson, Vivien, and Kevin Power. 2001. “Employee’s Perceptions of Organizational Restructuring: The Roles of Social Support.” *Work & Stress* 1592):161–178.

Swarbrick, Dana and Jonna Katariina Vuoskoski. 2023. “Collectively Classical: Connectedness, Awe, Feeling Moved, and Motion at a Live and Livestreamed Concert.” *Music & Science* 6:1–24.

Swart, Lu-Anne, Sarah Day, Rajen Govender, and Mohamed Seedat. 2020. “Participation in (Non)Violent Protests and Associated Psychosocial Factors: Sociodemographic Status, Civic Engagement, and Perceptions of Government’s Performance.” *South African Journal of Psychology* 50(4):480–92.

Swartz, David L. 2013. Symbolic Power, Politics, and Intellectuals: The Political Sociology of Pierre Bourdieu. Chicago, IL: University of Chicago Press.

Sweeting, Helen, and Patrick West. 2003. “Young People’s Leisure and Risk Taking Behaviors: Changes in Gender Patterning in the West of Scotland during the 1990s.” *Journal of Youth Studies* 6(4):391–412.

Sy, Thomas, And Stephane Cote. 2005. “The Contagious Leader: In Part of the Leader’s Mood on the Mood of Group Members, Group Affective Tone, and Group Processes.” *Journal of Applied Psychology* 90(2):295–305.

Syme, Gabrielle. 2012. “Beavement.” Pp. 450–455 in *The SAGE Handbook of Counselling and Psychotherapy*, edited by Colin Feltham and Ian Horton. London: SAGE

Sympson, Susie C., and Myra Qualls Elder. 2000. “Feminist Therapy in Empowering Hope.” Pp. 167–182 in *Handbook of Hope: Theory, Measures, Applications*, edited by C.R. Snyder. San Diego, CA: Academic.

Szabo, Attila, Szilvia Boros, Sándor Mezei, Viktoria Németh, István Soós, Ricardo de la Vega, Roberto Ruíz-Barquín, and Júlia Patakiné Bősze. 2019. “Subjective Psychological Experiences in Leisure and Competitive Swimming.” *Annals of Leisure Research* 22(5):629–41.

Szinovacy, Maximiliane. 1997. “Adult Children Taking Parents into Their Homes: Effects of Childhood Living Arrangements.” *Journal of Marriage & Family* 59(3):700–717.

Tacher, Elisa Levy, and Christine Anderson Readdick. 2006. “The Relation between Aggression and Creativity among Second Graders.” *Creativity Research Journal* 18(3):261–267.

Tak, Sangdong. 2017. “Cooperative Membership and Community Engagement: Findings from a Latin American Survey.” *Sociological Forum* 32(3):566–586.

Takahashi, Lois M., and Sharon Lord Gaber. 1998. “Controversial Facility Siting in the Urban Environment: Resident and Planner Perceptions in the United States.” *Environment & Behavior* 30(2):184–215.

Takahashi, Masami, and Willis F. Overton. 2002. “Wisdom: A Culturally Inclusive Developmental Perspective.” *International Journal of Behavioral Development* 26(3):269–277.

Takahashi, Miho, Shinichiro, Morita, and Kazuko Ishidu. 2015. "Stigma and Mental Health in Japanese Unemployed Individuals." *Journal of Employment Counseling* 52(1):18–28.
Takano, Yohtaro, and Shunya Sogon. 2008. "Are Japanese More Collectivistic Than Americans? Examining Conformity in In-Groups and the Reference-Group Effect." *Journal of Cross-Cultural Psychology* 39(3):237–250.
Talisse, Robert B. 2009. *Democracy and Moral Conflict*. Cambridge, UK: Cambridge University Press.
Tam, Frank Wai-ming, and Mitsuru Taki. 2007 "Bullying among Girls in Japan and Hong Kong: An Examination of the Frustration-aggression Model," *Educational Research & Evaluation* 13(4):373–399.
Tam, Kim-Pong. 2014. "Anthropomorphism of Nature and Efficacy in Coping with the Environmental Crisis." *Social Cognition* 32(3):276–296.
Tam, May Yeuk-mui, and Stephen Chiu. 2010. "Job Training Prevision by Employers: An Institutional Analysis of Employees in Hong Kong." *International Journal of Human Resource Management* 21(12):2194–2217.
Tam, May, and Chung Yan Ip. 2017. "Experience and Coping of Employment Risks in Hong Kong." *International Journal of Sociology & Social Policy* 37(3–4):166–185.
Tam, Vicky Chiu-man, and Rebecca Siu-yuk Lam. 2005. "Stress and Coping among Migrant and Local-born Adolescents in Hong Kong." *Youth & Society* 36(3):312–332.
Tan, Mingran. 2008. "Emptiness, Being and Non-being: Sengzhao's Reinterpretation of the Laozi and Zhuangzi in a Buddhist Context." *Dao* 7:195–209.
Tan, Siu-Lan, Peter Pfordresher, and Rom Harré. 2010. *Psychology of Music: From Sound to Significance*. Hove, UK: Psychology.
Tan, Tony Xing and Linda A. Camras. 2011. "Social Skills of Adopted Chinese Girls at Home and in School: Parent and Teacher Ratings." *Children & Youth Services Review* 33(10):1813–1821.
Tan, Vnna E., and David A. Snow. 2015. "Cultural Conflicts and Social Movements." Pp. 513–533 in *Oxford Handbook of Social Movements*, edited by Donatella della Porta and Mario Diani. Oxford, UK: Oxford University Press.
Taneja, Shilpa and Liaqat Ali. 2021. "Determinants of Customers" Intentions towards Environmentally Sustainable Banking: Testing the Structural Model." *Journal of Retailing & Consumer Services* 59:102418.
Tang, Fengyan, and Nancy Morrow-Howell. 2008. "Involvement in Voluntary Organizations: How Older Adults Access Volunteer Roles?" *Journal of Gerontological Social Work* 51(3-4):210–227.
Tang, Fengyan. 2006. "What Resources Are Needed for Volunteerism? A Life Course Perspective." *Journal of Applied Gerontology* 25(5):375–390.
Tang, Gary, Eva Hung, Ho-Kong Au- Yeung, and Samson Yuen. 2020. "Politically Motivated Internet Addiction: Relationships among Online Information Exposure, Internet Addiction, FOMO, Psychological Well-Being, and Radicalism in Massive Political Turbulence." *International Journal of Environmental Research & Public Health* 17(2):633.
Tang, Min. 2011. "The Political Behavior of the Chinese Middle Class." *Journal of Chinese Political Sciences* 16:373–387.
Tang, Shih-che. 2009. "The Club and the Carrot of China's Globalization." *Inter-Asia Cultural Studies* 10(2):326–329.
Tang, Wenfang. 2001. "Religion and Society in China and Taiwan." Pp. 298–319 in *Chinese Political Culture, 1989–2000*, edited by Shiping Hua. Armonk, NY: Sharpe.
Tang, Wenfang. 2014. "The Worshipping Atheist: Institutional and Diffused Religiosities in China." *China* 12(3):1–26.
Tani, Franca, and Barry Schneider. 1997. "Self-reported Symptomatology of Socially Rejected and Neglected Italian Elementary School Children." *Child Study Journal* 27(4).
Tanner, Denise. 2007. "Starting with Lives: Supporting Older People's Strategies and ways of Coping." *Journal of Social Work* 7(1):7–30.

Tanner, Jennifer Lynn, and Jeffrey Jensen Arnett. 2009. "The Emergence of Emerging Adulthood: The New Life Stage between Adolescence and Young Adolthood." Pp. 39–45 in *Handbook of Youth and Young Adulthood: New Perspectives and Agendas*, edited by Andy Furlong. Abingdon, UK: Routledge.

Tanner-Smith, Emily E., Sandra J. Wilson, and Mark W. Kipsey. 2013. "Risk Factors and Crime." Pp. 89–111 in *The Oxford Handbook of Criminological Theory*, edited by Francis T. Cullen and Pamela Wilcox. New York: Oxford University Press.

Tao, Yu. 2015. "Unlikely Friends of the Authoritarian and Atheist Rules: Religious Groups and Collective Contention in rural China." *Politics & Religion* 8:86–110.

Tapia, Mike. 2011. "U.S. Juvenile Arrests: Gang Membership, Social Class, and Labeling Effects." *Youth & Society* 43(4):1407–1432.

Taplin, Ross H., Rosemary Kerr, and Alistair M. Brown. 2013. "Who Pays for Blended Learning? A Cost-Benefit Analysis." *Internet & Higher Education* 18:61–68.

Tartakovsky, Eugene. 2011. "National Identity of High-School Adolescents in an Era of Socio-Economic Change: Russia and Ukraine in the Post-Perestroika Period." *Journal of Youth & Adolescence* 40(2):231–244.

Taubman-Ben-Ari, Orit, and Liora Findler. 2003. "Reckless Driving and Gender: An Examination of a Terror Management Theory Explanation." *Death Studies* 27:603–618.

Tausch, Nicole, Julia C. Becker, Russell Spears, Oliver Christ, Rim Saab, Purnima Singh and Roomana N. Siddiqui. 2011. "Explaining Radical Group Behavior: Developing Emotion and Efficacy Routes to Normative and Nonnormative Collective Action." *Journal of Personality & Social Psychology* 101(1):129–48.

Tavares, Susana M., Daan van Knippenberg, and Rolf van Dick, 2016. "Organizational Identification and Currencies of Exchange: Integrating Social Identity and Social Exchange Perspectives." *Journal of Applied Social Psychology* 46:34–45.

Taylor, Alan C., Mihaela Robila, and Hae Seung Leo. 2005. "Distance, Contact, and Intergenerational Relationships: Grandparents and Adult Grandchildren from an International Perspective." Journal of Adult Development 12(1):33–41.

Taylor, Eileen Z. and Mary B. Curtis. 2018. "Mentoring: A Path to Prosocial Behavior." *Journal of Business Ethics* 152:1133–1148.

Taylor, Morgan M. and Hannah R. Snyder. 2022. "Dependent Stress Generation Mediates the Relation between Poor Cognitive Control and Repetitive Negative Thinking in Emerging Adults." *Emerging Adulthood* 11(2):216769682110549.

Taylor, Ralph B., Brian R. Wyant, and Brian Lockwood. 2015. "Variable Links within Perceived Police Legitimacy? Fairness and Effectiveness across Races and Places." *Social Science Research* 49:234–248.

Taylor, Richard. 2002. *Virtue Ethics: an Introduction. Amherst*, NY: Prometheus.

Taylor, Sherria D. and Brian Distelberg. 2016. "Predicting Behavioral Health Outcomes among Low-Income Families: Testing a Socioecological Model of Family Resilience Determinants." *Journal of Child & Family Studies* 25(9):2797–807.

Taylor, Verta, Katrina Kimport, Nella Van Dyke, and Ellen Ann Andersen. 2009. "Culture and Mobilization: Tactical Repertoires, Same-sex Weddings, and the Impact on Gay Activism." *American Sociological Review* 74:865–890.

Taylor-Gooby, Peter. 2005. *New Approaches to Expert and Institutional Trust: Issues*. Kent, UK: University of Kent.

Teachman, Jay D. 1996. "Intellectual Skill and Academic Performance: Do Families Bias the Relationship?" *Sociology of Education* 69(1):35–48.

Tebes, Jacob Kraemer, Julie T. Irish, Mary Jo Puglisi Vosquez, and David V. Perkins. 2004. "Cognitive Transformation as a Marker of Resilience." *Substance Use & Misuse* 39(5):769–788.

Teets, Jessica C. 2014. *Civil Society under Authoritarianism: The China Model*. New York: Cambridge University Press.

Temple, Matthew and Terry Lynn Gall. 2018. "Working through Existential Anxiety toward Authenticity: A Spiritual Journey of Meaning Making." *Journal of Humanistic Psychology* 58(2):168–93.

ten Brinke, Leanne and Dacher Keltner. 2020. "Theories of power: Perceived strategies for gaining and maintaining power." *Journal of Personality & Social Psychology.*

TenHouten, Warren D. 2017. *Alienation and Affect.* Abingdon, UK: Routledge.

Tenorio, Kimberly A., and Celia C. Lo. 2011. "Social Location, Social Integration, and the Co-Occurrence of Substance Abuse and Psychological Distress." *American Journal of Drug & Alcohol Abuse* 37(4):218–223.

Teovanovic, Predrag, Petar Lukić, Zorana Zupan, Aleksandra Lazić, Milica Ninković, and Iris Žeželj. 2021. "Irrational Beliefs Differentially Predict Adherence to Guidelines and Pseudoscientific Practices During the COVID-19 Pandemic." *Applied Cognitive Psychology* 35(2):486–96.

Tepper, Robin L. 2001. "Parental Regulation and Adolescent Discretionary Time-use Decisions: Findings from the NLSY97." Pp. 79–105 in *Social Awakening: Adolescent Behavior as Adulthood Approaches*, edited by Robert T. Michael. New York: Russell Sage.

Terhune, Victoria and Jonathan Matusitz. 2016. "The Uighurs Versus the Chinese Government: An Application of Realistic Conflict Theory." *Journal of Applied Security Research* 11(2):139–48.

Tett, Kevin E. Fox, and Alvin Wang. 2005. "Development and Validation of a Self-report Measure of Emotional Intelligence as a Multidimensional Trait Domain." *Personality & Social Psychology Bulletin* 31(7):859–888.

Teunisse, Alessandra K., Trevor I. Case, Julie Fitness and Naomi Sweller. 2020. "I Should Have Known Better: Development of a Self-Report Measure of Gullibility." *Personality & Social Psychology Bulletin* 46(3):408–23.

Tew, Jerry. 2002. *Social Theory, Power and Practice.* Houndmills, UK: Palgrave.

Teymoori, Ali, Jolanda Jetten, Brock Bastian, Amarina Ariyanto, Frederique Autin, Nadia Ayub, Constantina Badea, Tomasz Besta, Fabrizio Butera, Rui Costa-Lopes, Lijuan Cui, Carole Fantini, Gillian Finchilescu, Lowell Gaertner, Mario Gollwitzer, Angel Gomez, Roberto Gonzalez, Ying Yi Hong, Dorthe Hoj Jensen, and Minoru Karasawa. 2016. "Revisiting the Measurement of Anomie." *PLoS ONE* 11(7):1–27.

Thapa, Shreena, Shelley L. Brown, and Tracey A. Skilling. 2021. "The Relationship between Self-Esteem, Gender, Criminal Attitudes, and Recidivism in a Youth Justice Sample." *Criminal Justice & Behavior* 48(4):539–55.

Tharp, Derek T., Martin Seay, Cherie Stueve and Somer Anderson. 2020. "Financial Satisfaction and Homeownership." *Journal of Family & Economic Issues* 41(2):255–80.

The Freedom to Pursue Happiness: Belief in Free Will Predicts Life Satisfaction and Positive Affect among Chinese Adolescents." *Frontiers in Psychology* 7:02027.

Theeboom, Tim, Bianca Beersma, and Annelies E. M. van Vianen. 2014. "Does Coaching Work? A Meta-Analysis on the Effects of Coaching on Individual Level Outcomes in an Organizational Context." *Journal of Positive Psychology* 9(1):1–18.

Theiss, Jennifer A. 2018. *The Experience and Expression of Uncertainty in Close Relationships.* Cambridge, UK: Cambridge University Press.

Thelen, Kathleen. 2012. "Varieties of Capitalism: Trajectories of Liberalization and the New Politics of Social Solidarity." *Annual Review of Political Science* 15:135–159. \116–220

Theobald, Maryanne. 2016. "Achieving Competence: The Interactional Features of Children's Storytelling." *Childhood* 23(1):87–104.

Theron, L., Ann Cameron, Lau Didkowsky, and Ungar Liebenberg. 2011. "A Day in the Lives of Four Resilient Youths." *Youth & Society* 43(3):799 818.

Theron, Linda C. and Linda Liebenberg. 2015. "Understanding Cultural Contexts and Their Relationship to Resilience Processes." Pp. 23 36 in *Youth Resilience and Culture: Commonalities and Complexities*, edited by Linda C. Theron, Michael Ungar, and Liebenberg Linda. Dordrecht, Netherlands: Springer.

Thielmann, Isabel, and Benjamin E. Hilbig. 2019. "No Gain without Pain: The Psychological Costs of Dishonesty." *Journal of Economic Psychology* 71:126–317.

Thielmann, Isabel, Giuliana Spadaro, and Daniel Balliet. 2020. "Personality and Prosocial Behavior: A Theoretical Framework and Meta-Analysis." *Psychological Bulletin* 146(1):30–90.

Thin, Neil. 2012. Social Happiness: Theory into Policy and Practice. Bristol, UK: Polity.

Thoits, Peggy A., and Lyndi N. Hewitt. 2001. "Volunteer Work and Well-being." *Journal of Health & Social Behavior* 42:115–131.

Thoits, Peggy. 2011. "Mechanisms Linking Social Ties and Support to Physical and Mental Health." *Journal of Health & Social Behavior* 52(2):145–161.

Thomas, David C. 1999. "Cultural Diversity and Work Group Effectiveness: An Experimental Study." *Journal of Cross-Cultural Psychology* 30(2):242–263.

Thomas, David C., and Kevin Au. 2002. "The Effect of Cultural Differences and Behavioral Responses to Low Job Satisfaction." *Journal of International Business Studies* 33(2):309–326.

Thomas, Elaine R. 2002. "Who Belongs?" *European Journal of Social Theory* 5(3):323–349.

Thomas, Kyle J. and Jean Marie McGloin. 2013. "A Dual-Systems Approach for Understanding Differential Susceptibility to Processes of Peer Influence." *Criminology* 51(2):435–74.

Thomas, R. Murray. 1997. Moral Development Theories: Secular and Religius: A Comparative Study. Westport, CT: Greenwood.

Thompson, Cynthia A., Laura L. Beauvais, and Karen S. Lyness. 1999. "When Work-family Benefits and Not Enough: The Influence of Work-family Culture on Benefit Utilization, Organization Attachment, and Work-family Conflict." *Journal of Vocational Behavior* 54:392–415.

Thompson, Leigh, Margaret Neale, and Marwan Sinaceur. 2004. "The Evolution of Cognition and Biases in Negotiation and Emotion." Pp. 7–44 in *The Handbook of Negotiation and Culture*, edited by Michele J. Gelfand and Jeanne M. Brett. Stanford, CA: Standord University Press.

Thompson, Martie P., and Fran H. Norris. 1992. "Crime, Social Status, and Alienation." *American Journal of Community Psychology* 20(1):97–119.

Thompson, Mindi, and Jason Dahling. 2010. "Image Theory and Career Aspirations: Indirect and Interactive Effects of Status-related Variables." *Journal of Vocational Behavior* 77:21–29.

Thompson, Neil, and Sue Thompson. 2001. "Empowering Older People beyond the Care Model." *Journal of Social Work* 1(1):61–76.

Thompson, Rosemary A. 2006. *Nurturing Future Generations: Promoting Resilience in Children and Adolecents through Social, Emotional and Cognitive Skills.* New York, NY: Routledge.

Thorisdottir, Hulda, John T. Jost, Ido Liviatan, and Patrick E. Shrout. 2007. "Psychological Needs and Values Underlying Left-right Political Orientation: Cross-national Evidence from Eastern and Western Europe." *Public Opinion Quarterly* 71(2):175–203.

Thorlindsson, Thorolfur, and Jon Gunnar Bernburg. 2006. "Peer Groups and Substance Use: Examining the Direct and Interactive Effect of Leisure Activity." *Adolescence* 41(162):321–339.

Thornton, Arland, William G. Axinn, and Yu Xie. 2007. *Marriage and Cohabitation.* Chicago, IL: University of Chicago Press.

Thorson, James A. 1998. "Religion and Anxiety: Which Anxiety? Which Religion?" Pp. 147–160 in *Handbook of Religion and Mental Health*, edited by Harold G. Konenig. San Diego, CA: Academic.

Thrash, Todd M., Andrew J. Elliot, Laura A. Maruskin, and Scott E. Cassidy. 2010. "Inspiration and the Promotion of Well-Being: Tests of Causality and Mediation." *Journal of Personality & Social Psychology* 98(3):488–506.

Thrasher, James F., Marci Kramish Campbell, and Veronica Oates. 2004. "Behavior-specific Social Support for Healthy Behaviors among African American Church Members: Applying Optimal Matching Theory." *Health Education & Behavior* 31(2):193–205.

Thulin, Elyse J., Dan B. Lee, Andria B. Eisman, Tom M. Reischl, Pete Hutchison, Susan Franzen, and Marc A. Zimmerman. 2022. "Longitudinal Effects of Youth Empowerment Solutions: Preventing Youth Aggression and Increasing Prosocial Behavior." *American Journal of Community Psychology* 70:75–88.

Thunberg, Sara and Åsa Kallstrom. 2018. "Does Professional or Social Network Support Meet the Needs of Victimized and Polyvictimized Youths in Sweden?". *Victims Offenders* 13(3):390–408.
Thye, Shane R., David Willer, and Barry Markovsky. 2006. "From Status to Power: New Models at the Intersection of Two Theories." *Social Forces* 84(3):1471–1495.
Thye, Shane R., Edward J. Lawler, and Jeongkoo Yoon. 2008. "Social Exchange and the Maintenance of Order in Status-Stratified Systems." Pp. 37–63 in *Social Structure and Emotion*, edited by Jody Clay-Warner and Dawn T. Robinson. San Diego, CA: Academic.
Thye, Shane, and Will Kalkhoff. 2014. "Theoretical Perspectives on Power and Resource Inequality." Pp. 27–47 in *Handbook of the Social Psychology of Inequality*, edited by, Jane D. McLeod, Edward J. Lawler, and Michael Schwalbe. Dordrecht, Netherland: Springer.
Tian, Allen Ding, Juliana Schroeder, Gerald Haubl, Jane L. Risen, Michael I. Norton, and Francesca Gino. 2018. "Enacting Rituals to Improve Self-Control." *Journal of Personality & Social Psychology* 114(6):851–876.
Tiedens, Larissa Z., and Alison R. Fragale. 2003. "Power Moves: Complementarity in Dominant and Submissive Nonverbal Behavior." *Journal of Personality & Social Psychology* 84(3):558–568.
Tierney, Kathleen. 2015. "Resilience and the Neoliberal Project." *American Behavioral Scientist* 59(10):1327–1342.
Tiliouine, Habib, Robert A. Cummins, and Melanie Davern. 2006. "Measuring Wellbeing in Developing Countries: The Case of Algeria." *Social Indicators Research* 75:1–30.
Till, Benedikt, Peter Vitouch, Arno Herberth, Gernot Sonneck, and Thomas Niederkrotenthaler. 2013. "Personal Suicidality in Reception and Identification with Suicidal Film Characters." *Death Studies* 37(4):383–392.
Tillmar, Malin, and Lars Lindkvist. 2007. "Cooperation against All Odds: Finding Reasons for Trust Where Formal Institutions Fail." *International Sociology* 22(3):343–366.
Timmer, Erika, and Marja Aartsen. 2003. "Mastery Beliefs and Productive Leisure Activities in the Third Age." *Social Behavior & Personality* 31(7):643–656.
Timulak, Ladislav. 2015. *Transforming Emotional Pain in Psychotherapy: An Emotion Focused Approach*. Hove, UK: Routledge.
Tindall, D.B., and Barry Wellman. 2001. "Canada as Social Structure: Social Network Analysis and Canadian Sociology." *Canadian Journal of Sociology* 26(3):265–307.
Ting-Toomey, Stella. 2004. "Translating Conflict Face-negotiating Theory into Practice." Pp. 217–248 in *Handbook of Intercultural Training*, edited by Dan Landis, Janet M. Bennett and Milton J. Bennett. Thousand Oaks, CA: Sage.
Tink, Lisa N., Danielle Peers, Candace I. J. Nykiforuk, and Bethan C. Kingsley. 2020. "Moving beyond ideology: contemporary recreation and the neoliberal discourses of new public health." *Leisure Studies* 39(6):767–781.
Tiwari, Dharmendra Nath and Girishwar Misra. 2021. "Personality and Value Preference as Predictors of Social Well-Being." *Journal of Human Values* 27(2):161–74.
Todorova, Zdravka. 2013. "Conspicuous Consumption as Routine Expenditure and Its Place in the Social Provisioning Process." *American Journal of Economics & Sociology* 72(5):1183–1204.
Tokunaga, Robert S. 2016. "Interpersonal Surveillance over Social Network Sites." *Journal of Social & Personal Relationships* 33(2):171–90.
Tolentino, Laramie R., Patrick Raymund James M. Garcia, Vinh Nhat Lu, Simon Lloyd D. Restubog, Prashant Bordia, and Carolin Plewa. 2014. "Career Adaptation: The Relation of Adaptability to Goal Orientation, Proactive Personality, and Career Optimism." *Journal of Vocational Behavior* 84(1):39–48.
Tolmatcheff, Chloé, Benoit Galand, Isabelle Roskam, and René Veenstra. 2022. "The Effectiveness of Moral Disengagement and Social Norms as Anti-Bullying Components: A Randomized Controlled Trial." *Child Development* 93(6):1873–88.
Tolonen, Tarja. 2008. "Success, Coping and Social Exclusion in Transitions of Young Finns." *Journal of Youth Studies* 11(2):233–249.
Toma, Catalina L. 2017. "Taking the Good with the Bad: Effects of Facebook Self-presentation on Emotional Well-being." Pp. 170–182 in *The Routledge Handbook of Media Use and Well-being:*

*International Perspectives on Theory and Research on Positive Media Effects*, edited by Leonard Reinecke and Mary Beth Oliver. New York, NY: Routledge.

Tomas, Joso M., Amparo Oliver, Laura Galiana, Patricia Sancho, and Marisol Lila. 2013. "Explaining Method Effects Associated with Negatively Worded Items in Trait and State Global and Domain-Specific Self-Esteem Scales." *Structural Equation Modeling* 20(2):299–313,

Tomasello, Michael. 2019. "The Moral Psychology of Obligation." *Behaviour & Brain Science* 43:e56–e56.

Tomich, Patricia L., and Vicki S. Helgeson. 2002. "Five Years Later: A Cross-sectional Comparison of Breast Cancer Survivors with Healthy Women." *Psycho-Oncology* 11:154–169.

Tomlinson, Jennifer M., Arthur Aron, and Elaine Hatfield. 2018. "Romantic Love." Pp. 407–421 in *The Cambridge Handbook of Personal Relationships*, edited by Anita L. Vangelisti and Daniel Perlman. Cambridge, UK: Cambridge University Press.

Tompson, George H., and Parshotam Dass. 2000. "Improving Students" Self-efficacy in Strategic Management: The Relative Impact of Cases and Simulations." *Simulation & Gaming* 31(1):22–41.

Toporek, Rebecca L. and Rachel Fuld Cohen. 2017. "Strength-Based Narrative Résumé Counseling: Constructing Positive Career Identities from Difficult Employment Histories." *Career Development Quarterly* 65(3):222–36.

Torlo, Vanina Jasmine, and Alessandro Lomi. 2017. "The Network Dynamics of Status: Assimilation and Selection." *Social Forces* 96(1):389–422.

Torsvik, Gaute. 2000. "Social Capital and Economic Development." *Rationality & Society* 12(4):451–476. \76–205

Toth-Kiraly, István, Beáta Bőthe, Éva Gál, Gábor Orosz, and Adrien Rigó. 2021. "Perceived Parenting Practices as Predictors of Harmonious and Obsessive Passion among High Schoolers and Adults." *Journal of Happiness Studies* 22(7):2981–99.

Totton, Nick. 2012. "Body Psychotherapy." Pp. 305–310 in *The SAGE Handbook of Counselling and Psychotherapy*, edited by Colin Feltham and Ian Horton. London: SAGE.

Toussaint, Loren L., Grant S. Shields, and George M. Slavich. 2016. "Forgiveness, Stress, and Health: A 5-Week Dynamic Parallel Process Study." *Annals of Behavioral Medicine* 50(5):727–35.

Towsley, Gail L., Susan L. Beck, and John F. Watkins. 2007. "Learning to Live with It: Coping with the Transition to Cancer Survivorship in Older Adults." *Journal of Aging Studies* 21:93–106. \v11–16

Tracey, Terence J. G., Jessica E. Rohlfing. 2010. "Variations in the Understanding of Interpersonal Behavior: Adherence to the Interpersonal Circle as a Moderator of the Rigidity? Psychological Well-Being Relation." *Journal of Personality* 78(2):711–746.

Tracey, Terence J., Patrick Sherry, and Merle Keitel. 1986. "Distress and Help-Seeking as a Function of Person-Environment Fit and Self-Efficacy: A Causal Model." *American Journal of Community Psychology* 14(6):657–676.

Tracy, Jessica A., Joey T. Cheng, Richard W. Robins, and Kali H. Trzesniewski. 2009. "Authentic and Hubristic Pride: The Affective Core of Self-esteem and Narcissism." *Self & Identity* 8:196–213.

Trang, Duyen T. and Tuppett M. Yates. 2020. "(in)Congruent Parent–Child Reports of Parental Behaviors and Later Child Outcomes." *Journal of Child & Family Studies* 29(7):1845–60.

Trapman, Sabrina, Benedikt Hell, Jan-Oliver W. Hirn, and Heinz Schuler. 2007. "Meta-analysis of the Relationship between the Big Five and Academic Success at University." *Journal of Psychology* 215(2):132–151.

Trauernicht, Mareike, Elisa Oppermann, Uta Klusmann, and Yvonne Anders. 2021. "Burnout Undermines Empathising: Do Induced Burnout Symptoms Impair Cognitive and Affective Empathy?" *Cognition & Emotion* 35(1):185–192.

Traunmuller, Richard. 2011. "Moral Communities? Religion as a Source of Social Trust in a Multilevel Analysis of 97 German Regions." *European Sociological Review* 27(3):346–363.

Traut-Mattausch, Eva, Stephanie Guter, Mark P. Zanna, Eva Jonas, and Dieter Frey. 2011. "When Citizens Fight Back: Justice Sensitivity and Resistance to Political Reform." *Social Justice Research* 24(1):25–42.

Treas, Judith. 2011. "Revisiting the Bott Thesis on Kin Networks and Marriage." *Social Science Research* 40(3):716–26.

Trebilcock, Michael J. 2014. Dealing with Losers: *The Political Economy of Policy Transitions*. New York, NY: Oxford University Press.

Treno, Andrew J., and Harold D. Holder. 1997. "Community Mobilization, Organizing, and Media Advocacy." *Evaluation Review* 21(2):166–190.

Triandis, Harry C. 1995. *Individualism and Collectivism*. Boulder, CO: Westview.

Triandis, Harry C., and Eunkook M. Suh. 2002. "Cultural Influences on Personality." *Annual Review Psychology* 53:133–160.

Troyer, Daniela, and Tobias Greitemeyer. 2018. "The Impact of Attachment Orientations on Empathy in Adults: Considering the Mediating Role of Emotion Regulation Strategies and Negative Affectivity." *Personality and Individual Differences* 122:198–205.

Truebridge, Sara. 2016. "Resilience: It Begins with Beliefs." *Kappa Delta Pi Record* 52(1):22–27.

Trumbo, Craig W., Katherine A. McComas, and John C. Besley. 2008. "Individual-and-community-level Effects on Risk Perception in Cancer Cluster Investigations." *Risk Analysis* 28(1):161–178.

Tsai, Jack, and Robert A. Rosenheck. 2012. "Conceptualizing Social Integration among Formerly Homeless Adults with Severe Mental Illness." *Journal of Community Psychology* 40(4):456–467.

Tsai, Jack, Laurie Harkness, Katelyn Kang, and Mary Sperrazza. 2018. "Measuring Citizenship among U.S. Veterans with Chronic Mental Illness: A Psychometric Evaluation." *Journal of Community Psychology* 46(1):107–16.

Tsai, Jenny Hsin-chun. 2006. "Xenophobia, Ethnic Community, and Immigrant Youths" Friendship Network Formation." *Adolescence* 41(162):285–298.

Tsaur, Sheng-Hshiung, Ying-Wen Liang, and Szu-Chun Weng. 2014. "Recreationist-environment fit and place attachment." *Journal of Environmental Psychology* 40:421–429.

Tse, Thomas Kwan Choi. 2007. "Remaking Chinese Identity: Hegemonic Struggles over National Education in Post-colonial Hong Kong." *International Studies in Sociology of Education* 17(3):231–248.

Tsfati, Yario, Riva Turkachinsky, and Yorom Peri. 2009. "Exposure to News, Political Comedy, and Entertainment Talk Shows: Concern about Security and Political Mistrust." *International Journal of Public Opinion Research* 21(4):399–423.

Tsou, Meng-Wen, and Jin-Tan Liu. 2001. "Happiness and Domain Satisfaction in Taiwan." *Journal of Happiness Studies* 2(3):269–288.

Tsutsumi, Akizumi, and Norito Kawakami. 2004. "A Review of Empirical Studies on the Model of Effort-reward Imbalance at Work: Reducing Occupational Stress by Implementing a New Theory." *Social Science & Medicine* 59:2335–2359.

Tudor, Keith, and Charlotte Sills. 2012. "Transactional Analysis." Pp. 335–340 in *The SAGE Handbook of Counselling and Psychotherapy*, edited by Colin Feltham and Ian Horton. London: SAGE.

Tugade, Michele M., and Barbara L. Fredrickson. 2004. "Resilient Individuals Use Positive Emotions to Bounce Back from Negative Emotional Experiences." *Journal of Personality & Social Psychology* 86(2):320–333.

Tulin, Marina, Bram Lancee, and Beate Volker. 2018. "Personality and Social Capital." *Social Psychology Quarterly* 81(4):295–318.

Tumkaya, Songul. 2007. "Burnout and Humor Relationship among University Lecturers." *Humor* 20(1):73–92.

Turner, Bryan S. 2009. "Talcott Parsons's Sociology of Religion and the Expressive Revolution." *Journal of Classical Sociology* 5(3):303–318.

Turner, Bryan. 2005a. "The Sociology of the Family." Pp. 135–153 in *The SAGE Handbook of Sociology*, edited by Craig Calhoun, Chris Rojek, and Bryan Turner. London, UK: SAGE.

Turner, Heather A., David Finkelhor, and Richard Ormrod. 2007. "Predictors of Receiving Counseling in a National Sample of Youth: The Relative Influence of Symptoms, Victimization Exposure, Parent-Child Conflict, and Delinquency." *Journal of Youth & Adolescence* 36(7):861–76.

Turner, Jonathan H. 1988. *A Theory of Social Interaction*. Stanford, CA: Stanford University Press.

Turner, Jonathan H. 2003. *Human Institutions: A Theory of Societal Evolution*. Lanham, MD: Rowman & Littlefield.

Turner, Jonathan H. 2006. "Psychoanalytic Sociological Theories and Emotions." Pp. 276–294 in *Handbook of the Sociology of Emotions*, edited by Jan E. Stets and Jonathan H. Turner. Boston, MA: Springer.

Turner, Jonathan H. 2013. *Contemporary Sociological Theory*. Thousand Oaks, CA: SAGE.

Turner, Jonathan H. 2013. Theoretical Principles of Sociology Vol. 3: Mesodynamics. New York: Springer.

Turner, Jonathan H. and Alexandra Maryanski. 2005. *Incest: Origins of the Taboo*. Boulder, CO: Paradigm.

Turner, Jonathan, H.. 2007. "Self, Emotions, and Extreme Violence: Extending Symbolic Interactionist Theorizing." *Symbolic Interaction* 30(4):501–30.

Turner, Jonathan. 2021. *On Human Nature: The Biology and Sociology of What Made Us Human*. New York, NY: Routledge.

Turner, Rhiannon N., Miles Hewstone, and Alberto Voci. 2007. "Reducing Explicit and Implicit Outgroup Prejudice via Direct and Extended Contact: The Mediating Role of Self-disclosure and Intergroup Anxiety." *Journal of Personality & Social Psychology* 93(3):369–388.

Turner, Sherri L. and Julia L. Conkel. 2010. "Evaluation of a Career Development Skills Intervention with Adolescents Living in an Inner City." *Journal of Counseling & Development* 88(4):457–65.

Tusicisny, Andrej. 2017. "Reciprocity and Discrimination: An Experiment of Hindu-Muslim Cooperation in Indian Slums." *Political Psychology* 38(3):409–26.

Twardawski, Mathias, Lena Steindorf, and Isabel Thielmann. 2021. "Three Pillars of Physical Distancing: Anxiety, Prosociality, and Rule Compliance during the COVID-19 Pandemic." *Collabra Psychology* 7(1).

Twenge, Jean M., Roy F. Baumeister, C. Nathan DeWall, Natalie J. Ciarocco, and J. Michael Bartels. 2007. "Social Exclusion Decreases Prosocial Behavior." *Journal of Personality & Social Psychology* 92(1):56–66.

Tybur, Joshua M., Willem E. Frankenhuis, and Thomas V. Pollet. 2014. "Behavioral Immune System Methods: Surveying the Present to Shape the Future." *Evolutionary Behavioral Sciences* 8(4):274–283.

Tyler, Tom R., Robert J. Boerkmann, Heather J. Smith, and Yuen J. Huo. 1997. Social Justice in a Diverse Society. Boulder, CO: Westview.

Tyson, Mandy, Judith Covey, and Harriet E. S. Rosenthal. 2014. "theory of Planned Behavior Interventions for Reducing Heterosexual Risk Behaviors: A Meta-analysis." *Health Psychology* 33(12);1454–1467.

Ullman, Chana, and Moshe Tatar. 2001. "Psychological Adjustment among Israeli Adolescent Immigrants: A Report on Life Satisfaction, Self-concept, and Self-esteem." *Journal of Youth & Adolescence* 30(4):449–463.

Ullrich, Simone, David P. Farrington, and Jeremy W. Cold. 2007. "Dimensions of DSM-IV Personality Disorders and Life-success." *Journal of Personality Disorders* 21(6):657–663.

Umana-Taylor, Adriana J., Olga Kornienko, Elana R. McDermott, and Frosso Motti-Stefanidi. 2020. "National Identity Development and Friendship Network Dynamics among Immigrant and Non-Immigrant Youth." *Journal of Youth & Adolescence* 49 (3), p.706–723.

Umeh, Kanayo. 2003. "Social Cognitions and Past Behavior as Predictors of Behavioral Intentions Related to Cardiovascular Health." *Journal of Applied Social Psychology* 33(7):1417–1436.

Umeh, Kanayo. 2004. "Cognitive Appraisals, Maladaptive Coping, and Past Behavior in Protective Motivation." *Psychology & Health* 19(6):719–735.

Umezawa, Yoshiko, Qian Lu, Jin You, Marjorie Kagawa-Singer, Barbara Leake, and Rose C. Maly. 2012. "Belief in Divine Control, Coping, and Race/Ethnicity among Older Women with Breast Cancer." *Annals of Behavioral Medicine* 44(1):21–32.

Umino, Ayumi and Jesper Dammeyer. 2016. "Effects of a Non-Instructional Prosocial Intervention Program on Children's Metacognition Skills and Quality of Life." *International Journal of Educational Research* 78:24–31.

Umino, Ayumi and Jesper Dammeyer. 2018. "Effects of a Danish Student-Centered Prosocial Intervention Program among Japanese Children." *Japanese Psychological Research* 60(2):77–86.

Unantenne, Nalika, Narelle Warren, Rachel Canaway, and Lenore Manderson. 2013. "The Strength to Cope: Spirituality and Faith in Chronic Disease." *Journal of Religious Health* 52:1147–1161.

Ungar, Michael, Camille Dumond, and Wanda Mcdonald. 2005. "Risk, Resilience and Outdoor Programmes for At-risk Children." *Journal of Social Work* 5(3):319–338.

Ungar, Michael, Marion Brown, Linda Liebenberg, Rasha Otman, Wai Man Kwong, Mary Armstrong, and Jane Gilgun. 2007. "Unique Pathways to Resilience across Cultures." *Adolescence* 42(166):287–310.

Ungar, Michael. 2004. "A Constructionist Discourse of Resilience: Multiple Contexts, Multiple Realities among At-risk Children and Youth." *Youth & Society* 35(3):341–365.

Ungar, Michael. 2010. "Cultural Dimensions of Resilience among Adults." Pp. 404–423 in *Handbook of Adult Resilience*, edited by John W. Reich, Alex J. Zautra and John Stuart Hall. New York, NY: Guilford.

Ungar, Michael. 2011. "Community Resilience for Youth and Families: Facilitative Physical and Social Capital in Contexts of Adversity." *Children & Youth Services Review* 33:1742–1748.

Ungar, Michael. 2012. "Social Ecologies and Their Contribution to Resistance." Pp. 13–31 in The Social Ecology of Resilience." Pp. 13–31 in *The Social Ecology of Resilience: Handbook of Theory and Practice*, edited by Michael Ungar. New York, NY: Springer.

Ungar, Michael. 2015. "Resilience and Culture: The Diversity of Protective Processes and Positive Adaptation." Pp. 37–48 in *Youth Resilience and Culture: Commonalities and Complexities*, edited by Linda C. Theron, Michael Ungar, and Liebenberg Linda. Dordrecht, Netherlands: Springer.

Ungar, Michael. 2018. "The Differential Impact of Social Services on Young People's Resilience." *Child Abuse & Neglect* 78:4–12.

Urbanaviciute, Ieva, Birute Pociute, Antanas Kairys, and Audrone Liniauskaite. 2016. "Perceived Career Barriers and Vocational Outcomes among University Undergraduates: Exploring Mediation and Moderation Effects." *Journal of Vocational Behavior* 92:12–21.

Urbatsch, R. 2014. Families" Values: How Parents, Siblings, and Children Affect Political Attitudes New York. Oxford University Press.

Ursache, Alexandra, Kimberly G. Noble, and Clancy Blair. 2015. "Socioeconomic Status, Subjective Social Status, and Perceived Stress: Associations with Stress Physiology and Executive Functioning." *Behavioral Medicine* 41(3):145–54.

Uscinski, Joseph E. 2019. "Down the Rabit Hole We Go!" Pp. 1–32 in *Conspiracy Theories and the People Who Believe Them*, edited by Joseph E. Uscinski. New York, NY: Oxford University Press.

Usher, Ellen L., and Frank Pajares. 2006. "Sources of Academic and Self-regulatory Efficacy Beliefs of Entering Middle School Students." *Contemporary Educational Psychology* 3:125–141.

Uskul, Ayse K., Michaela Hynie, and Richard N. LaLonde. 2004. "Interdependence as a Mediator between Culture and Interpersonal Closeness for Euro-Canadians and Turks." *Journal of Cross-Cultural Psychology* 31(2):174–191.

Uslaner, Eric M. 2002. *The Moral Foundations of Trust*. Cambridge, UK: Cambridge University Press.

Uslaner, Eric M. 2008. Corruption, Inequality, and the Rule of Law: The Bulging Pocket Makes the Easy Life. Cambridge, UK: Cambridge University Press.

Uslaner, Eric M., and Mitchell Brown. 2005. "Inequality, Trust, and Civic Engagement." *American Politics Research* 33(6):868–894.

Utz, Sonja and Johannes Breuer. 2017. "The Relationship between Use of Social Network Sites, Online Social Support, and Well-Being: Results from a Six-Wave Longitudinal Study." *Journal of Media Psychology* 29(3):115–25.

Vaccaro, Christian, Melissa Swauger, Shayna Morrison and Alex Heckert. 2021. "Sociological Conceptualizations of Compassion Fatigue: Expanding Our Understanding." *Sociology Compass* 15(2):e12844.

Vadher, Kiren, and Martyn Barrett. 2009. "Boundaries of Britishness in British Indian and Pakistani Young Adults." *Journal of Community & Applied Social Psychology* 19:442–458.

Vahhab, Marzie, Zohreh Latifi, Mehdi Marvi, Mohammad Soltanizadeh, and Alexander Loyd. 2024. "Effects of Self-Healing Training on Perfectionism and Frustration Tolerance in Mothers of Single-Parent Students." *Journal of General Psychology*. doi: 10.1080/00221309.2023.2275305.

Vaillant, George E. 1977. *Adaptation to Life*. Boston, MA: Little, Brown.

Valarino, Isabel, Gerardo Meil, and Jesús Rogero-García. 2018. "Family or State Responsibility? Elderly- and Childcare Policy Preferences in Spain." *International Journal of Sociology & Social Policy* 38(11–12):1101–15.

Valdivia, Ibis Alvarez, Barry H. Schneider, Kenia Lorenzo Chavez, and Xinyin Chen. 2005. "social Withdrawal and Maladjustment in a Very Group-oriented Society." *International Journal of Behavioral Development* 29(3):219–228.

Valiente, Celia. 2018. "Gender and Political Sociology." Pp. 143–154 in *The SAGE Handbook of Political Sociology*, edited by William Outhwaite and Stephen Turner. London, UK: SAGE.

Valle, Ron. 2019. "Toward a Psychology of Silence." *Humanistic Psychologist* 47(3):219–61.

Vallejos, Elvira Perez, Mark John Ball, Poppy Brown, David Crepaz-Keay, Emily Haslam-Jones et al. 2016. "Kundalini Yoga as Mutual Recovery: A Feasibility Study Including Children in Care and Their Carers." *Journal of Children's Services* 11(4):261–282.

Vallerand, Robert J., and Robert Bissonnette. 1992. "Intrinsic, Extrinsic, and Amotivational Styles vs Predictors of Behavior: A Prospective Study." *Journal of Personality* 60(3):599–620.

Vallerand, Robert J., Paul Deshaies, Jean-Pierre Cuerrier, Luc G. Pelletier, and Claude Mongeau. 1992. "Ajzen and Fishbein's Theory of Reasoned Action as Applied to Moral Behavior: A Confirmatory Analysis." *Journal of Personality & Social Psychology* 62:98–109.

van Aken, Marcel A.G. 1994. "The Transactional Relation between Social Support and Children's Competence." Pp. 131–141 in *Social Networks and Social Support in Childhood and Adolescence*, edited by Frank Nestmann and Klaus Hurrelmann. Berlin, Germany: Walter de Gryter.

Van Damme, Anjuli. 2017. "The Impact of Police Contact on Trust and Police Legitimacy in Belgium." *Policing & Society* 27(2):205–28.

van de Rakt, Marieke, Joseph Murray, and Paul Nieuwbeerta. 2012. "The Long-Term Effects of Paternal Imprisonment on Criminal Trajectories of Children." *Journal of Research in Crime and Delinquency* 49(1):81–108.

van de Ven, Niels, Marce Zeelenberg, and Rik Pieters. 2011. "Why Envy Outperforms Admiration." *Personality & Social Psychology Bulletin* 37(6):784–795.

Van de Vyver, Julie and Dominic Abrams. 2018. "The Arts as a Catalyst for Human Prosociality and Cooperation." *Social Psychological & Personality Science* 9(6):664–74.

Van den Broeck, Evert, Karolien Poels, and Michel Walrave. 2015. "Older and Wiser? Facebook Use, Privacy Concern, and Privacy Protection in the Life Stages of Emerging, Young, and Middle Adulthood." *Social Media + Society* 1(2):205630511561614.

Van Der Gaag, Martin, and Tom A.B. Snijders. 2005. "The Resource Generator: Social Capital Quantification with Concrete Items." *Social Networks* 27:1–29.

Van der Stede, Wim A. 2014. "A Manipulationist View of Causality in Cross-Sectional Survey Research." *Accounting, Organizations & Society* 39(7):567–574.

van der Toorn, Jojanneke, Miholy Berkics, and John T. Jost. 2010. "System Justification, Satisfaction, and Perceptions of Fairness and Typicality at Work: A Cross-System Comparison Involving the U.S. and Hungary." *Social Justice Research* 23(2):189–210.

van Deth, Jan W. 2003. "Measuring Social Capital: Orthodox and Continuing Controversies." *International Journal of Social Research Methodology* 6(1):79–92. \

Van Deurzen, Emmy. 1997. *Everyday Mysteries: Existential Dimensions of Psychotherapy*. London, UK: Routledge.

van Deurzen, Emmy. 2012. "Existential Counseling and Therapy." Pp. 311–314 in *The SAGE Handbook of Counselling and Psychotherapy*, edited by Colin Feltham and Ian Horton. London: SAGE.

van Deurzen, Emmy. 2021. *Rising from Existential Crisis: Life beyond Calamity*. Monmouth, UK: PCCS.

Van Dierendonck, Dirk, and Wilmar B. Schaufeli. 2001. "Burnout and Inequity among Human Service Professionals: A Longitudinal Study." *Journal of Occupational Health Psychology* 6(1):43–52.

van Dijk, E.M., E. van Dulmen-den Broeder, G.J.L. Kaspers, W.C.M. van Dam, K.I. Braam, and J. Huisman. 2008. "Psychosexual Functioning of Childhood Cancer Survivors." *Psycho-Ontology* 17:506–511.

Van Dyke, Nella, and Sarah A. Soule. 2002. "Structural-social Change and the Mobilizing Effect of Threat: Explaining Levels of Patriot and Militia Organizing in the United States." *Social Problems* 49(4):497–520.

Van Eijck, Koen. 2001. "Social Differentiation in Musical Taste Patterns." *Social Forces* 79(3):1163–1185.

Van Haaften, E. Heleen, Zhenrong Yu, and Fons J.R. Van de Vijver. 2004. "Human Resilience in a Degrading Environment: A Case Study in China." *Asian Journal of Social Psychology* 7:205–219.

Van Heel, Martijn, Patricia Bijttebier, Hilde Colpin, Luc Goossens, Wim Van Den Noortgate, Karine Verschueren, and Karla Van Leeuwen. 2019. "Investigating the Interplay between Adolescent Personality, Parental Control, and Externalizing Problem Behavior across Adolescence." *Journal of Research in Personality* 81:176–86.

van Hemert, Dianne A., Fons J.R. van de Viver, Ype H. Poortinger, and James Georgas. 2002. "Structural and Functional Equivalence of the Eysenck Personality Questionnaire within and between Countries." *Personality & Individual Differences* 33:1229–1249.

van Hiel, Alain, and Maarten Vansteenkiste. 2009. "Ambitions Fulfilled? The Effects of Intrinsic and Extrinsic Goal Attachment on Older Adults" Ego-integrity and Death Attitudes." *International Journal of Aging & Human Development* 68(1):27–51.

Van Hook, Jennifer. 2002. "Immigration and African American Educational Opportunity: The Transformation of Minority Schools." *Sociology of Education* 75:169–189.

van Ingen, Erik, and Rene Bekkers. 2015. "Generalized Trust through Civic Engagement? Evidence from Five National Panel Studies." *Political Psychology* 36(3):277–294.

Van Kenhove, Patrick, Kristof De Wulf, and Sarah Steenhaut. 2003. "The Relationship between Consumers Unethical Behavior and Customer Loyalty in a Retail Environment." *Journal of Business Ethics* 44:261–278.

Van Lange, Paul A. M., René Bekkers, Antonio Chirumbolo, and Luigi Leone. 2012. "Are Conservatives Less Likely to Be Prosocial Than Liberals? From Games to Ideology, Political Preferences and Voting. Are Conservatives Less Prosocial?" *European Journal of Personality* 26(5):461–73.

Van Lange, Paul A.M., and Caryl E. Rusbutt. 2012. "Interdependence Theory." Pp. 251–272 in *Handbook of Theories of Social Psychology* (vol. 2), edited by Paul A.M. Van Lange, Arie W. Kruglanski and E. Tory Higgins. London, CA: SAGE.

Van Lange, Paul A.M., Daniel Balliet, Craig D. Parks, and Mark Van Vugt. 2014. *Social Dilemmas: The Psychology of Human Cooperation*. New York: NY: Oxford University Press.

Van Oorschot, Wim. 2000. "Why Pay for Welfare? A Sociological Analysis of Reasons for Welfare Solidarity." Netherlands" *Journal of Social Sciences* 36(1):15–36.

van Praag, B.M.S., P. Frijters, and A. Ferrer-i-Carbonell. 2003. "The Anatomy of Subjective Well-being." *Journal of Economic Behavior & Organization* 51:29–49.

van Praag, Bernard M.S., and Paul Frijters. 1999. "The Measurement of Welfare and Well-being: The Layden Approach." Pp. 413–433 in *Well-being: The Foundations of Hedonic Psychology*, edited by Daniel Kahneman, Ed Diener and Norbert Schwarz. New York: Russell Sage.

Van Praag, Bernard M.S., Dmitri Romanov, and Ada Ferrer-i-Carbonell. 2010. "Happiness and Financial Satisfaction in Israel: Effects of Religiosity, Ethnicity, and War." *Journal of Economic Psychology* 31:1008–1020.

van Praag, Bernard, and Ada Ferrer-I-Carbonell. 2004. *Happiness Quantified: A Satisfaction Calculus Approach*. Oxford, UK: Oxford University Press.

van Prooijen, J. W., Gallucci, M., and G. Toeset. 2008. "Procedural Justice in Punishment Systems: Inconsistent Punishment Procedures Have Detrimental Effects on Cooperation." *British Journal of Social Psychology* 47(2):311–324.

van Prookjen, Jan-Willem, Kees van den Bos, and Henk A.M. Wilke. 2004. "Group Belongingness and Procedural Justice: Social Inclusion and Exclusion by Peers Affects the Psychology of Voice." *Journal of Personality & Social Psychology* 87(1):66–79.

van Rensburg, Angelique, Linda Theron, and Sebastiaan Rothmann. 2019. "A Social Ecological Modeled Explanation of the Resilience Processes of a Sample of Black Sesotho-Speaking Adolescents." *Psychological Reports* 122(4):1211–34.

van Rijsewijk, Loes, Jan Kornelis Dijkstra, Kim Pattiselanno, Christian Steglich, and Ren? Veenstra. 2016. "Who Helps Whom? Investigating the Development of Adolescent Prosocial Relationships." *Developmental Psychology* 52(6):894–908.

Van Rooy, David L., and Chockalingam Viswesvaran. 2004. "Emotional Intelligence: A Meta-analytic Investigation of Prediction Validity and Nomological Net." *Journal of Vocational Behavior* 65:71–95.

van Schalkwyk, G.J., and, H.H.Y. Sit. 2013. "Evaluating School-Based Psychological and Counselling Services in Macao Using a Qualitative Approach." *School Psychology International* 34(2):154–165.

van Scheppingen, Manon A., Joshua J. Jackson, Jule Specht, Roos Hutteman, Jaap J. A. Denissen, and Wiebke Bleidorn. 2016. "Personality Trait Development During the Transition to Parenthood." *Social Psychological & Personality Science* 7(5):452–62.

van Seggelen-Damen, Inge and Karen van Dam. 2016. "Self-Reflection as a Mediator between Self-Efficacy and Well-Being." *Journal of Managerial Psychology* 31(1):18–33.

van Swol, Lyn M. 2003. "The Effects of Regulation on Trust." *Basic & Applied Social Psychology* 25(3):221–233.

van Tilburg, Wijnand A. P., and Eric R. Igou. 2011. "On Boredom and Social Identity." *Personality & Social Psychology Bulletin* 37(12):1679–1691.

Van Tongeren, Daryl R., C. Nathan DeWall, Don E. Davis, and Joshua N. Hook. 2023. "Intellectual Humility and Existentially Relevant Moral Decisions." *Journal of Positive Psychology* 18(3):363–69.

Van Vianen, Annelies E.M., Bernard A. Nijstad, and Olga F. Voskuijl. 2008. "A Person-environment Fit Approach to Volunteerism: Volunteer Personality Fit and Culture Fit as Predictors of Affective Outcomes." *Basic & Applied Social Psychology* 38:153–166.

Van Vliet, K. Jessica. 2008. "Shame and Resilience in Adulthood: A Grounded- Theory Study." *Journal of Counseling Psychology* 55(2):233–245.

Van Voorhis, Rebecca Morrison, and Carol Hostetter. 2006. "The Impact of Msw Education on Social Worker Empowerment and Commitment to Client Empowerment through Social Justice Advocacy." *Journal of Social Work Education* 42(1):105–21.

van Zalk, Maarten Herman Walter, Margaret Kerr, Susan J. T. Branje, Hakan Stattin, and Wim H. J. Meeus. 2010. "Peer Contagion and Adolescent Depression: The Role of Failure Anticipation." *Journal of Clinical Child & Adolescent Psychology* 39(6):837–848.

Van Zandt, Shannon, and William M. Rohe. 2006. "Do First-time Home Buyers Improve Their Neighborhood Quality?" *Journal of Urban Affairs* 28(5):491–510.

Van, Hung Tran. 2017. "Liberal Reforms & Economic Growth: Current Issues and Interrelations." *Journal of International Studies* 10(4):109–118.

Vandell, Deborah L., Kenneth T. H. Lee, Anamarie A. Whitaker, and Kim M. Pierce. 2020. "Cumulative and Differential Effects of Early Child Care and Middle Childhood Out-of-School Time on Adolescent Functioning." *Child Development* 91(1):129–144.

Vander Elst, Tinne, Anja Van den Broeck, Nele De Cuyper, and Hans De Witte. 2014. "On the Reciprocal Relationship between Job Insecurity and Employee Well-Being: Mediation by Perceived Control?" *Journal of Occupational & Organizational Psychology* 87(4):671–693.

Vander Ven, Thomas M., Francis T. Cullen, Mark A. Carrozza, and John Paul Wright. 2001. "Home Alone: The Impact of Maternal Employment on Delinquency." *Social Problems* 48(2):236–257.

Vandermeer, James, Christine Hosey, Nicholas Epley, and Boaz Keysar. 2019. "Escalation of Negative Social Exchange: Reflexive Punishment or Deliberative Deterrence?". *Journal of Experimental Social Psychology* 84:103823.

Vanderplaat, Madine. 2016. "Activating the Sociological Imagination to Explore the Boundaries of Resilience Research and Practice." *School Psychology International* 37(2):189–203.

Vandervoort, Debra J. 2006. "Hostility and Health: Mediating Effects of Belief Systems and Coping Styles." *Current Psychology* 25(1):50–66.

Vandoninck, Sofie, and Leen d'Haenens. 2015. "Children's Online Coping Strategies: Rethinking Coping Typologies in a Risk-Specific Approach." *Journal of Adolescence* 45:225–236. \109–100

Vandsburger, Etty, Victoria S. Curtis, and Bethany A. Imbody. 2012. "Professional Preparedness to Address Abuse and Neglect among Elders Living in the Rural South: Identifying Resiliency where Stress Prevails." *Ageing International* 37:356–372

VanFleet, Rise, Andrea E. Sywulak, and Cynthia Caparosa Sniscak. 2010. *Child-centered Play Therapy*. New York, NY: Guilford.

Vanhee, Gaëlle, Gilbert M. D. Lemmens, Lara Stas, Tom Loeys, and Lesley L. Verhofstadt. 2018. "Why Are Couples Fighting? A Need Frustration Perspective on Relationship Conflict and Dissatisfaction." *Journal of Family Therapy* 40(S1):S4–S23.

vanOyen Witvliet, Charlotte, Nathaniel J. DeYoung, Alicia J. Hofelich, and Paul A. DeYoung. 2011. "Compassionate Reappraisal and Emotion Suppression as Alternatives to Offense-Focused Rumination: Implications for Forgiveness and Psychophysiological Well-Being." *Journal of Positive Psychology* 6(4):286–99.

Vansteenkiste, Maarten, Willy Lens, Hans De Witte, and N.T. Feather. 2005. "Understanding Unemployed People's Job Search Behaviour, Unemployment Experience and Well-being: A Comparison of Expectancy-value Theory and Self-determination Theory." *British Journal of Social Psychology* 44:269–287.

Varda, Danielle M. 2011. "A Network Perspective on State-Society Synergy to Increase Community-Level Social Capital." *Nonprofit & Voluntary Sector Quarterly* 40(5):896–923.

Vargas-Salfate, Salvador, Dario Paez, Xavier Oriol, Silvia da Costa, Sonia Gondim, and Elza Techio. 2020. "Nationalistic Collective Rituals, Intergroup Relations, and Legitimation of National Social Systems." *Revue Internationale de Psychologie Sociale* 33(1).

Vargova, Lenka, Lubica Zibrinova, and Gabriel Banik. 2020. "The Way of Making Choices: Maximizing and Satisficing and Its Relationship to Well-Being, Personality, and Self-Rumination." *Judgment & Decision Making* 15(5):798–806.

Vartanian, Thomas P. 1999. "Adolescent Neighborhood Effects on Labor Market and Economic Outcomes." *Social Service Review* 73(2):142–167.

Vaughan, Tyler J., Jeffrey T. Ward, Jeff Bouffard, and Alex R. Piquero. 2019. "The General Factor of Self-Control and Cost Consideration: A Critical Test of the General Theory of Crime." *Crime & Delinquency* 65(6):731–771.

Veenhoven, Ruut. 1998. "Quality-of-life in Individualistic Society: A Comparison of 43 Nations in the Early 1990s." Social Indicators Research 48:157–186.

Veenhoven, Ruut. 2005. "Return of Inequality in Modern Society? Test by Dispersion of Life Satisfaction across Time and Nations." *Journal of Happiness Studies* 6:457–487.

Veenstra, Gerry, Isaac Luginnah, Sarah Wakefield, Stephen Birth, John Eyles, and Susan Elliott. 2005. "Why You Know, Where You Live: Social Capital, Neighbourhood and Health." *Social Science & Medicine* 60:2799–2818.

Veg, Sebastian. 2017. "The Rise of "Localism" and Civic Identity in Post-Handover Hong Kong: Questioning the Chinese Nation-State." *China Quarterly* 230:323–347.

Vega, William A., Andres G. Gil, George J. Warheit, Rick S. Zimmerman, and Eleni Apospori. 1993. "Acculturation and Delinquent Behavior among Cuban American Adolescents: Toward an Empirical Model." *American Journal of Community Psychology* 21(1):113–125.

Velladics, Katalin, Kene Henkens, and Hendrik P. Van Dolen. 2006. "Do Different Welfare States Engender Different Policy Preferences? Options on Pension Reforms in Eastern and Western Europe." *Ageing & Society* 26:475–495.

Vera-Toscano, Esperanza, Fernando E. Garrido-Fernandez, Jose A. Gomez-Limon, and Jose L Canadas-Reche. 2013. "Are Theories about Social Capital Empirically Supported? Evidence from the Farming Sector." *Social Indicators Research* 114(3):1331–1359.

Verba, Sidney, Kay Lehman Schlozman, and Henry E. Brady. 1995. *Voice and Equality: Civic Voluntarism in American Politics*. Cambridge, MA: Harvard.

Verba, Sidney, Kay Lehman Schlozman, and Henry E. Brady. 2004. "Political Equality: What Do We Know about It?" Pp. 635–666 in *Social Inequality*, edited by Kathryn M. Neckerman. New York: Russell Sage.

Vermeer, Paul and Peer Scheepers. 2019. "Bonding or Bridging? Volunteering among the Members of Six Thriving Evangelical Congregations in the Netherlands." *Voluntas* 30(5):962–75.

Vermeersch, Hans, Guy T'Sjoen, Jean-Marc Kaufman, and Mieke Van Houtle. 2011. "Social Science Theories on Adolescent Risk-taking: The Relevance of Behavioral Inhibition and Activation." *Youth & Society* 45(1):27–53.

Vermunt, Rië, and Herman Steensma. 2016. "Procedural Justice." Pp. 219–236 in *Handbook of Social Justice Theory and Research*, edited by Clara Sabbagh and Manfred Schmitt. New York, NY: Springer.

Vernon, Philip A., Rod A. Martin, Julie Aitken Schermer, and Ashley Mackie. 2008. "A Behavioral Genetic Investigation of Humor Styles and Their Correlations with the Big-5 Personality Dimensions." *Personality & Individual Differences* 44:1116–1125.

Verona, Suman, and Madelene Sta. Maria. 2006. "The Changing Global Context of Adolescent Spirituality." Pp. 124–136 in *The Handbook of Spiritual Development in Childhood and Adolescence*, edited by Eugene C. Roehlkepartain, Pamela Ebstyne King, Linda Wagener and Peter L. Benson. Thousand Oaks, CA: Sage.

Veronese, Guido, and Gianpiero Barola. 2018. "Healing Stories: An Expressive-Narrative Intervention for Strengthening Resilience and Survival Skills in School-Aged Child Victims of War and Political Violence in the Gaza Strip." *Clinical Child Psychology & Psychiatry* 23(2):311–332.

Verschuur, Margot J. , Marija Maric, and Philip Spinhoven. 2010. "Differences in Changes in Health-Related Anxiety Between Western and Non-Western Participants in a Trauma-Focused Study." *Journal of Traumatic Stress* 23(2):300–303.

Vertsberger, Dana, and Itamar Gati. 2016. "Career Decision-making Difficulties and Help-seeking among Israeli Young Adults." *Journal of Career Development* 43(2):145–159.

Vess, Matthew, Jamie Arndt, Cathy R. Cox, Clay Routledge, and Jamie L. Goldenberg. 2009. "Exploring the Existential Function of Religion: The Effect of Religious Fundamentalism and Mortality Salience on Faith-based Medical Refusals." *Journal of Personality & Social Psychology* 97(2):334–350.

Vestergaard, Anne. 2013. "Humanitarian Appeal and the Paradox of Power." *Critical discourse studies* 10(4):444–67.

Vestergren, Sara, John Drury, and Eva Hammar Chiriac. 2017. "The Biographical Consequences of Protest and Activism: A Systematic Review and a New Typology." *Social Movement Studies* 16(2):203–221,

Vezzali, Loris, Miles Hewstone, Dora Capozza, Dino Giovannini, and Ralf Wölfer. 2014. "Improving Intergroup Relations with Extended and Vicarious Forms of Indirect Contact." *European Review of Social Psychology* 25(1):314–389.

Vieira, Edward T. 2015. "Family Communication Patterns, Sympathy, Perspective-Taking, and Girls¡¯ Thoughts about Interpersonal Violence." *Journal of family Violence* 30(5):607–619.

Viewiebe, Roland, and Bernd Wegener. 2000. "Social Inequality and the Perceived Income Justice Gap." *Social Justice Research* 13(2):123–149.

Vignansky, Efrat and Uri Timor. 2017. "Domestic Violence against Partners According to Wife-Beaters: Construction of Lifestyle and Life Meaning." *International Journal of Offender Therapy & Comparative Criminology* 61(10):1125–50.

Viklund, Mattias and Lennart Sjoberg. 2008. "An Expectancy-Value Approach to Determinants of Trust." *Journal of Applied Social Psychology* 38(2):294–313.

Vilhjalmsson, Runar, and Thorolfur Thorlindsson. 1998. "Factors Related to Physical Activity: A Study of Adolescents." *Social Science & Medicine* 47(5):665–675.

Village, Andrew, and Leslie J. Francis. 2010. "All in the Mind? Psychological, Social, and Religious Predictors of Civic Volunteerism among Churchgoers in England." *Research on the Social Scientific Study of Religion* 21:1–26.

Villasana, Mercedes, Jesús Alonso-Tapia, and Miguel A. Ruiz. 2017. "Personal Factors Underlying Resilience in Adolescence: Cross-Cultural Validity of the Prince-Embury Model." *Spanish Journal of Psychology* 20:E42–E42.

Vincens, Natalia, Maria Emmelin, and Martin Stafström. 2018. "Social Capital, Income Inequality and the Social Gradient in Self-Rated Health in Latin America: A Fixed Effects Analysis." *Social Science & Medicine* 196:115–122.

Viola, Thiago Wendt Giovanni Abrahio Salum, Bruno Kluwe Schiavon, Breno Sanvicente-Vieira, Mateus Luz Levandowski, and Rodrigo Grassi-Oliveir. 2016. "The Influence of Geographical and Economic Factors in Estimates of Childhood Abuse and Neglect Using the Childhood Trauma Questionnaire: A Worldwide Meta-Regression Analysis." Child Abuse & Neglect 51:1–11.

Viry, Gil, Vincent Kaufmann, and Eric D. Widmer. 2009. "Social Integration Faced with Commuting: More Widespread and Less Dense Support Networks." Pp. 121–143 in *Mobilities and Inequality*, edited by Timo Ohnmacht, Hanja Maksim, and Marfred Max Bergman. Farnham, UK: Ashgate.

Visaria, Abhijit, Rahul Malhotra, June May-Ling Lee, and Angelique Chan. 2023. "Enhancing Psychological Resilience at the Cusp of Older Ages: The Role of Social Networks." *Ageing & Society*.

Visher, Glenn S. 1997. Human Values: From the Greeks to Modern Times. Commack, NY: Nova.

Vitaro, Frank, Mara Brendgen, and Brigitte Wanner. 2005. "Patterns of Affiliation with Delinquent Friends during Late Childhood and Early Adolescence: Correlates and Consequences." *Social Development* 14(1):82–108.

Vittengl, J.R., C.N. White, R.J. McGovern, and B.J. Morton. 2006. "Comparative Validity of Seven Scoring Systems for the Instrumental Activities of Daily Living Scale in Rural Elders." *Aging & Mental Health* 10(1):40–47.

Vogel, David L., Nathaniel G. Wade, and Shawn Haake. 2006. "Measuring the Self-stigma Associated with Seeking Psychological Health." *Journal of Counseling Psychology* 53(3):325–337.

Volker, Beate, and Henk Flap. 1997. "The Comrade's Belief: Intended and Unintended Consequences of Communism for Neighborhood Relations in the Former GDR." *European Sociological Review* 13(3):241–265.

Volker, Beate, and Henk Flap. 2001. "Work Ties as a Liability. The Case of East Germany." *Rationality & Society* 13(4):397–428 \63–265.

Volker, Beate, and Henk Flap. 2007. "Sixteen Million Neighbors: A Multilevel Study of the Role of Neighbors in the Personal Networks of the Dutch." *Urban Affairs Review* 43(2):256–284.

Volker, Beate, Henk Flap, and Siegwart Lindenberg. 2007. "When Are Neighborhoods Communities? Community in Dutch Neighborhoods." *European Sociological Review* 23(1):99–114.

Vollhardt, Johanna R., and Ervin Staub. 2011. "Inclusive Altruism Born of Suffering: The Relationship Between Adversity and Prosocial Attitudes and Behavior toward Disadvantaged Outgroups." *American Journal of Orthopsychiatry* 81(3):307–315.

Von Culin, Katherine R., Eli Tsukayama, and Angela L. Duckworth. 2014. "Unpacking Grit: Motivational Correlates of Perseverance and Passion for Long-Term Goals." *Journal of Positive Psychology* 9(4):306–12.

von Dras, Dean D., and Herman T. Blumenthal. 2000. "Biological, Social-environmental and Psychological Dialecticism: An Integrated Model of Aging." *Basic & Applied Social Psychology* 22(3):199–212.

Von Krogh, Georg, and Martin W. Wallin. 2011. "The Firm, Human Capital and Knowledge Creation." Pp. 261–286 in *The Oxford Handbook of Human Capital*, edited by Alan Burton-Jones and J. C. Spender. Oxford, UK: Oxford University Press.

von Soest, Tilmann, Svein Mossige, Kari Stefansen, and Odin Hjemdal. 2010. "A Validation Study of the Resilience Scale for Adolescents (READ)." *Journal of Psychopathology & Behavioral Assessment* 32(2):215–225.

von Stuckrad, Kocku. 2013. "Secular Religion: A Discourse-Historical Approach to Religion in Contemporary Western Europe." *Journal of Contemporary Religion* 28(1):1–14.

Vorhaus, John. 2014. "Function and Functional Explanation in Social Capital Theory: A Philosophical Appraisal." *Studies in Philosophy & Education* 33(2):185–99.

Votruba-Drzal, Elizabeth. 2006. "Economic Disparities in Middle Childhood Development: Does Income Matter?" *Developmental Psychology* 42(6):1154–1167.

Vrangalova, Zhana, and Ritch C. Savin-Williams. 2011. "Adolescent Sexuality and Positive Well-being: A Group Norms Approach." *Journal of Youth & Adolescence* 40:931–944.

Vuori, Miika. 2015. "Revisiting Local Responses to Mass Violence." *Journal of Risk Research* 19(4):515–532.

Waanders, Christine Julia L. Mendez, Jason T. Downer. 2007. "Parent Characteristics, Economic Stress and Neighborhood Context as Predictors of Parent Involvement in Preschool Children's Education." *Journal of School Psychology* 45:619–636.

Wacquant, Loic. 2008. Urban Outcasts: A Comparative Sociology of Advanced Marginality. Cambridge, UK: Polity.

Wadds, Phillip, Bianca Fileborn, and Stephen Tomsen. 2022. "Carnival, Sexual Violence and Harm at Australian Music Festivals." *British Journal of Criminology* 62(1):1–17.

Wade-Benzoni, Kimberly A., and Leigh Plunkett Tost. 2009. "The Egoism and Altruism of Intergenerational Behavior." *Personality & Social Psychology Review* 13(3):165–193.

Wagenaar, Alexander C., and Cheryl L. Perry. 1994. "Community Strategies for the Reduction of Youth Drinking: Theory and Application." *Journal of Research on Adolescence* 4(2):319–345.

Wagener, Linda M., and H. Newton Malony. 2006. "Spiritual and Religious Pathology in Childhood and Adolescence." Pp. 137–149 *The Handbook of Spiritual Development in Childhood and Adolescence*, edited by Eugene C. Roehlkepartain, Pamela Ebstyne King, Linda Wagener and Peter L. Benson. Thousand Oaks, CA: Sage.

Wager, Nadia M. 2012. "Respondents" Experiences of Completing a Retrospective Web-Based, Sexual Trauma Survey: Does a History of Sexual Victimization Equate with Risk for Harm?" *Violence & Victims* 27(6):991–1004.

Waines, Alison. 2012. "Low Self-esteem." Pp. 482–486 in *The SAGE Handbook of Counselling and Psychotherapy*, edited by Colin Feltham and Ian Horton. London: SAGE.

Wakefield, Sarah E.L., and Blake Poland. 2005. "Family, Friend or Foe? Critical Reflections on the Reliance and Role of Social Capital in Health Promotion and Community Development." *Social Science & Medicine* 60:2819–2832.

Wakimoto, Shinobu, and Takehiro Fujihara. 2004. "The Correlation between Intimacy and Objective Similarity in Interpersonal Relationships." *Social Behavior & Personality* 32(1):95–102.

Walder, Andrew G. 1995. "Career Mobility and the Communist Political Order." *American Sociological Review* 60(3):309–328.

Waldstrom, Christian, Gunnar Lind, and Haase Svendsen. 2008. "On the Capitalization And Cultivation of Social Capital: Towards A Neo-Capital General Science?" *Journal of Socio-Economics* 37(4):1495–1514.

Walen, Heather R., and Margie E. Lachman. 2016. "Social Support and Strain from Partner, Family, and Friends: Costs and Benefits for Men and Women in Adulthood." *Journal of Social & Personal Relationships* 17(1):5–30.

Walker, Gordan, R. Bruce Hall, IV, and Joseph W. Roggenbuck. 1998. "On-site Optimal Experiences and Their Relationship to Off-site Benefits." *Journal of Leisure Research* 30(4):453–471.

Walker, Ja'Nina J., Buffie Longmire-Avital. 2013. "The Impact of Religious Faith and Internalized Homonegativity on Resiliency for Black Lesbian, Gay, and Bisexual Emerging Adults." *Developmental Psychology* 49(9):1723–1731.

Walker, Karen. 1995. "Always There for Me: Friendship Patterns and Expectations among Middle- and Working-class Men and Women." *Sociological Forum* 10(2):273–296.

Walker, Lawrence J., and Karl H. Hennig. 1999. "Parenting Style and the Development of Moral Reasoning." *Journal of Moral Education* 28(3):357–374.

Walker, Moira. 2012. "Sexual Abuse in Childhood." Pp. 533–538 in *The SAGE Handbook of Counselling and Psychotherapy*, edited by Colin Feltham and Ian Horton. London: SAGE.

Walker, Robert, David Greenberg, Karl Ashworth, and Andreas Cebulla. 2003. "Successful Welfare-to-work Programs: Were Riverside and Portland Really That Good?" *Focus* 22(3):10–18.

Walker, Robert, Mark Tomlinson, and Glenn Williams. 2010. "The Problem with Poverty: Definition, Measurement and Interpretation." Pp. 353–376 in *The SAGE Handbook of Measurement*, edited by Geoffrey Walford, Eric Tucker, and Madhu Viswanathan. London, UK: SAGE.

Walkner, Paul, and Nicholas Finney. 1999. "Skill Development and Critical Thinking in Higher Education." *Teaching in Higher Education* 4(4):531–547.

Walkowitz, Gari. 2021. "Dictator Game Variants with Probabilistic (and Cost-Saving) Payoffs: A Systematic Test." *Journal of Economic Psychology* 85:102387.

Wallace, Claire, and Florian Pichler. 2009. "More Participation, Happier Society? A Comparative Study of Civil Society and the Quality of Life." *Social Indicators Research* 93:255–274.

Wallace, Sandi D. and Jake Harwood. 2018. "Associations between Shared Musical Engagement and Parent-Child Relational Quality: The Mediating Roles of Interpersonal Coordination and Empathy." *Journal of Family Communication* 18(3).202–16.

Wallenius, Mariut A. 2006. "Personal Project Content and Stress: Relations to Subjective Health and Depressive Mood." *Social Indicators Research* 81:35–50.

Waller, Margaret A. 2001. "Resilience in Ecosystemic Context: Evolution of the Concept." *American Journal of Orthopsychiatry* 71(3):290–297.

Walls, Theodore A., and Todd D. Little. 2005. "Relations among Personal Agency, Motivation, and School Adjustment in Early Adolescence." *Journal of Educational Psychology* 97(1):23–31.

Walsh, Anthony. 2014. Criminological Theory: Assessing Philosophical Assumptions. Waltham, MA: Anderson.

Walsh, Forma. 2009. "Human-animal Bond II: The Role of Pets in Family Systems and Family Therapy." *Family Process* 48(4):481–499.

Walsh, Froma. 2002. "A Family Resilience Framework: Innovative Practice Applications." *Family Relations* 51(2):130–137.

Walters, Glenn D. 2016. "The Parent-Peer Interface." *Youth Violence & Juvenile Justice* 14(4):411–425.

Walters, Glenn D. 2019. "Prosocial Peers as Risk, Protective, and Promotive Factors for the Prevention of Delinquency and Drug Use." *Journal of Youth & Adolescence* 49(3):618–30.

Walters, Glenn D. 2020. "Perceived Peer Delinquency, Proactive Criminal Thinking, Neighborhood Disorder, and Serious Offending: Moderated Mediation and Theoretical Integration." *Journal of Crime & Justice* 43(4):467–85

Walton, David. 2012. *Doing Cultural Theory*. London, UK: SAGE.

Walton, Douglas. 2007. *Dialog Theory for Critical Argumentation*. Amsterdam, Netherland: Benjamins.

Wampold, Bruce E. 2007. "Psychotherapy: The Humanistic (and Effective) Treatment." *American Psychology* 62:857–873.

Wan, Min, Thomas K. Kelemen, Yejun Zhang, and Samuel H. Matthews. 2023. "An Island of Sanity During COVID-19 Pandemic: Does Pet Attachment Support Buffer Employees" Stress Due to Job Insecurity?". Psychological Reports.

Wang, C.-W., C.L.W. Chan, S.-M. Ng, and A.H.Y. Ho. 2008. "The Impact of Spirituality on Health-related Quality of Life among Chinese Older Adults with Vision Impairment." *Aging & Mental Health* 12(2):267–275.

Wang, Dongdong, Zhichao Qian, and Linyi Ouyang. 2022. "'One Glories, All Glory': Role of Inclusiveness Behaviour in Creativity." *Current Psychology* 41(12):8449–60.

Wang, Faming, Ronnel B. King and Shing On Leung. 2022. "Beating the Odds: Identifying the Top Predictors of Resilience among Hong Kong Students." *Child Indicators Research* 15(5):1921–44.

Wang, Fang, and Yaoru Sun. 2008. "Self-organizing Peer-to-peer Social Networks." *Computational Intelligence* 24(3):213–233.

Wang, Guishui. 2012. *Confucian Ways to Conduct in Society*. Beijing, China: Sea Tide.

Wang, Jian. 2006. "The Politics of Goods: A Case Study of Consumer Nationalism and Media Discourse in Contemporary China." *Asian Journal of Communication* 16(2):187–206.

Wang, Jin-Liang, Da-Jun Zhang, and Marc A. Zimmerman. 2015. "Resilience Theory and Its Implications for Chinese Adolescents." *Psychological Reports* 117(2):354–375.

Wang, Kate Yeong-Tsyr, Chack-kie Wong, and Kwong-leung Tang. 2013. "Citizens" Attitudes towards Economic Insecurity and Government after the 2007 Financial Tsunami: A Hong Kong and Taiwan Comparison." *International Journal of Social Welfare* 22:152–163.

Wang, Lili, and Elizabeth Graddy. 2008. "Social Capital, Volunteering, and Charitable Giving." *Voluntas* 19:23–42.

Wang, Ming-Te, Feifei Ye, and Jessica Lauren Degol. 2017. "Who Chooses Stem Careers? Using a Relative Cognitive Strength and Interest Model to Predict Careers in Science, Technology, Engineering, and Mathematics." *Journal of Youth & Adolescence*. 46(8):1805–20.

Wang, Ning. 2012. *The Rise of the Consumer in Modern China*. Reading, UK: Paths International.

Wang, Peigang and Tyler J. VanderWeele. 2011. "Empirical Research on Factors Related to the Subjective Well-being of Chinese Urban Residents." *Social Indicators Research* 101:447–459.

Wang, Quanquan, Hui Wang, and Xia Liu. 2020. "Loneliness, Non-Suicidal Self-Injury, and Friendship Quality among Chinese Left-Behind Adolescents: The Role of Parent-Child Cohesion." *Journal of Affective Disorders* 271:193–200.

Wang, Songhua, Naiquan Shen, Fengchen Li, Zhaoshuang Wu, Jinhua Zhang, and Xiaolan Xu. 1998. *Philosophy and Art* (vol. 1). Tianjin, China: Tianjin Social Science Academy \68–267.

Wang, Wei, Xixi Li, and Jj Po-An Hsieh. 2013. "The Contingent Effect of Personal It Innovativeness and It Self-Efficacy on Innovative Use of Complex It." *Behaviour & Information Technology* 32(11):1105–1124.

Wang, Weiquan, Lingyun Qiu, Dongmin Kim, and Izak Benbasat. 2016. "Effects of Rational and Social Appeals of Online Recommendation Agents on Cognition- and Affect-Based Trust." *Decision Support Systems* 86:48–60.

Wang, Wenhua, Shuaiqi Li, Jianbiao Li, and Yujun Wang. 2021. "The Covid-19 Pandemic Changes the Nudging Effect of Social Information on Individuals" Blood Donation Intention." *Frontiers in Psychology* 12:736002.

Wang, Yongsheng. 1997. *On the Strategy of Leadership*. Beijing, China: People.

Wang, Zeying. 1999. *Nature and Morality: Daoist Ethics Selection*. Changsha, China: Hunan University.

Wang. Zheng, and Jerome Busemeyer. 2015. "Reintroducing the Concept of Complementarity into Psychology." *Frontier in Psychology* 6:1822.

Wansink, Brian, and Robert van Itterum. 2012. "Fast Food Restaurant Lighting and Music Can Reduce Calorie Intake and Increase Satisfaction." *Psychology Reports* 111(1):228–232.

Wapner, Seymour, and Jack Demick. 2003. "Adult Development: The Holistic Developmental, and Systems-oriented Perspective." Pp. 63–83 in *Handbook of Adult Development*, edited by Jack Demick and Carrie Andreoletti. New York: Kluwer Academic.
Ward, Jeffrey T. and Megan Forney. 2020. "Unpacking within- and between-Person Effects of Unstructured Socializing and Differential Association on Solo- and Co-Offending." *Journal of Criminal Justice* 70:101720.
Ward, Jeffrey T., John H. Boman, IV, and Shayne Jones. 2015. "Hirschi's Redefined Self-Control: Assessing the Implications of the Merger between Social- and Self-Control Theories." *Crime & Delinquency* 61(9):1206–1233.
Ward, Jeffrey T., Marvin D. Krohn, and Chris L. Gibson. 2014. "The Effects of Police Contact on Trajectories of Violence: A Group-Based, Propensity Score Matching Analysis." *Journal of Interpersonal Violence* 29(3):440–475.
Ward, Russell E., Jr. 2002. "Fan Violence: Social Problem or Moral Panic?" *Aggression & Violent Behavior* 7(5):453–475.
Warner, Barbara D., and Shannon K Fowler. 2003. "Strain and Violence: Testing a General Strain Theory Model of Community Violence." *Journal of Criminal Justice* 31(6):511–521.
Warner, Tara D., Tara Leigh Tober, Tristan Bridges, and David F. Warner. 2022. "To Provide or Protect? Masculinity, Economic Precarity, and Protective Gun Ownership in the United States." *Sociological Perspectives* 65(1):97–118.
Warr, Mark. 2005. "Making Delinquent Friends: Adult Supervision and Children's Affiliations." *Criminology* 43(1):77–105.
Warren, Mark E. 2011. "Democracy." Pp. 517–529 in *The Oxford Handbook of the History of Political Philosophy*, edited by George Klosko. Oxford, UK: Oxford University Press.
Waterman, Alan S. 2008. "Reconsidering Happiness: A Eudaimonist's Perspective." *Journal of Positive Psychology* 3(4):234–252.
Waterman, Alan S. 2013. "The Humanistic Psychology Positive Psychology Divide: Contrasts in Philosophical Foundations." *American Psychologist* 68(3):124–133.
Waterman, Emily A., Victoria L. Banyard, Katie M. Edwards, and Victoria A. Mauer. 2022. "Youth Perceptions of Prevention Norms and Peer Violence Perpetration and Victimization: A Prospective Analysis." *Aggressive Behavior* 48(4):402–17.
Watkins, David, Shahrenaz Mortazavi, and Irina Trofimova. 2000. "Independent and Interdependent Conceptions of Self: An Investigation of Age, Gender, and Culture Differences in Importance and Satisfaction Ratings." *Cross-Cultural Research* 34(2):113–134.
Watkins, Leo, Marcia Wilson, and Richard Buscombe. 2022. "Examining the Diversity of Ultra-Running Motivations and Experiences: A Reversal Theory Perspective." *Psychology of Sport & Exercise* 63:102271.
Watkins, Philip C. 2016. *Positive Psychology*. New York, NY: Springer.
Watson, Jeanne C., and Arthur C. Bohart. 2015. "The Roots and Genealogy of Humanistic Psychology." Pp. 585–600 in *The Handbook of Humanistic Psychology: Theory, Research, and Practice*, edited by Kirk J. Schneider, J. Fraser Pierson and James F. Bugental. Thousand Oaks, CA: SAGE.
Watson, Marlene F., and Howard O. Protinsky. 1988. "Black Adolescent Identity Development Effects of Perceived Family Structure." *Family Relations* 37:288–292.
Watt, Margo C., and Sherry H. Stewart. 2003. "Dyscontrol Experiences Questionnaire: Development, Reliability and Validity." *Journal of Psychopathology & Behavioral Assessment* 25(3):155–165.
Watts, Meredith W., and Ofer Feldman. 2001. "Are Nativists a Different Kind of Democrat? Democratic Values and "Outsiders" in Japan." *Political Psychology* 22(4):639–663.
Watts, Randolph H., Craigs Cashwell, and Wendo K. Schweiger. 2004. "Fostering Intrinsic Motivation in Children: A Humanistic Counseling Process." *Journal of Humanistic Counseling Education & Development* 43:16–24.
Watts, Rob. 2020. *Criminalizing Dissent: The Liberal State and the Problem of Legitimacy*. Abingdon, UK: Routledge.

Wawrytko, Sandra A. 2005. "The Viability (Dao) and Virtuosity (De) of Daoist Ecology: Reversion (Fu) as Renewal." *Journal of Chinese Philosophy* 32(1):89–103.
Wayment, Heidi A., Steven D. Barger, Lauren Woodward Tolle, and Erin M. O'Mara. 2010. Who Gets Blamed After a Collective Tragedy? The Role of Distress, Identification with Victims, and Time." *Journal of Loss & Trauma* 15(6):481–497.
Weakliem, David L., and Casey Borch. 2006. "Alienation in the United States: Uniform or Group-specific Change?" *Sociological Forum* 21(3):415–438.
Weaver, Scott R., and Hazel M. Prelow. 2005. "A Mediated-moderation Model of Maternal Parenting Style Association with Deviant Peers, and Problem Behaviors in Urban African American and European American Adolescents." *Journal of Child & Family Studies* 14(3):343–356.
Webb, James L. 2007. "Pragmatisms (Plural) Part I: Classical Pragmatism and Some Implications for Empirical Inquiry." *Journal of Economic Issues* 41(4):1063–1086.
Weber, Rene, Richard Huskey, and Britney Crayhead. 2017. "flow Experiences and Well-being: A Media Neuroscience Perspective." Pp. 183–196 in *The Routledge Handbook of Media Use and Well-being: International Perspectives on Theory and Research on Positive Media Effects*, edited by Leonard Reinecke and Mary Beth Oliver. New York, NY: Routledge.
Webster, Jeffrey Dean, Gerben J. Westerhof, and Ernst T. Bohlmeijer. 2014. "Wisdom and Mental Health across the Lifespan." *Journals of Gerontology Series B, Psychological Sciences & Social Sciences* 69(2):209–218.
Webster, Jeffrey Dean. 2010. "Wisdom and Positive Psychosocial Values in Young Adulthood." *Journal of Adult Development* 17:70–80.
Webster-Stratton, Carolyn, and Deborah Woolley Lindsay. 1999. "Social Competence and Conduct Problems in Young Children: Issues in Assessment." *Journal of Clinical Child Psychology* 28(1):25–43.
Wei, Hua and Meiting Liu. 2022. "Loving Your Parents and Treating Others Well: The Effect of Filial Piety on Cyberbullying Perpetration and Its Functional Mechanism among Chinese Graduate Students." *Journal of Interpersonal Violence* 37(11–12):NP8670–NP95.
Weiberg-Salzmann, Mirjam. 2014. "The Radicalisation of Buddhism in the Twentieth and Twenty-First Centuries: The Buddhist Sangha in Sri Lanka." *Politics, Religion & Ideology* 15(2):283–307.
Weimann, Gabriel, and Hans-Bernd Brosius. 1994. "Is There a Two-Step Flow of Agenda-Setting?" *International Journal of Public Opinion* 6(4):323–341.
Wein, Simon. 2007. "Is Courage the Counterpoint of Demoralization." *Journal of Palliative Care* 23(1):40–43.
Weinberg, Michael, Sharon Gil, Avi Besser, and Jasmin Bass. 2021. "Personality Traits and Trauma Exposure: The Relationship between Personality Traits, Ptsd Symptoms, Stress, and Negative Affect Following Exposure to Traumatic Cues." *Personality & Individual Differences* 177:110802.
Weine, Steven M., Elise Levin, Leonce Hakizimana, and Gonwo Dahnweih. 2012. "Has Prior Social Ecologies Shape Family Resilience amongst Refugees in U.S. Resettlement." Pp. 309–323 in *The Social Ecology of Resilience: Handbook of Theory and Practice*, edited by Michael Ungar. New York, NY: Springer.
Weiner, Bernard. 2012. "An Attribution Theory of Motivation." Pp. 135–155 in *Handbook of Theories of Social Psychology* (vol. 1), edited by Paul A.M. Van Lange, Arie W. Kruglanski and E. Tory Higgins. Los Angeles, CA: SAGE.
Weinstein, Netta, and Richard M. Ryan. 2010. "When Helping Helps: Autonomous Motivation for Prosocial Behavior and Its Influence on Well-being for the Helper and Recipient." *Journal of Personality & Social Psychology* 98(2):222–244.
Weinstein, Netta, Kirk W. Brown and Richard M. Ryan. 2009. "A Multi-Method Examination of the Effects of Mindfulness on Stress Attribution, Coping, and Emotional Well-Being." *Journal of Research in Personality* 43(3):374–85.
Weisberg, Herbert F. 2005. "The Structure and Effects of Moral Predispositions in Contemporary American Politics." *Journal of Politics* 67(3):646–668.

Welch, Michael R., David Sikkink, and Matthew T. Loveland. 2007. "The Radius of Trust: religion, Social Embeddedness and Trust in Strangers." *Social Forces* 86(1):23–46.
Welch, Michael, Charles Tittle, Jennifer Yonkoski, Nicole Meidinger, and Harold Grasmick. 2008. "Social Integration, Self-control, and Conformity." *Journal of Quantitative Criminology* 24(1):73–92.
Wells, Jennifer D., Steven E. Hobfoll, and Justin Lavin. 1999. "When It Rains, It Pours: The Greater Impact of Resource Loss Compared to Gain in Psychological Distress." *Personality & Social Psychology Bulletin* 9:1172–1182.
Welsch, Heinz. 2002. "Preferences over Prosperity and Pollution: Environmental Valuation Based on Happiness Surveys." *Kyklos* 55(4):473–494.
Welzel, Christian. 2013. *Freedom Rising: Human Empowerment and the Quest for Emancipation.* New York: Cambridge University Press.
Wen, Ming, Jessie Fan, Lei Jin, and Guixin Wang. 2010. "Neighborhood Effects on Health among Migrants and Natives in Shanghai, China." *Health & Place* 16(3):452–460.
Wen, Ming, Weidong Wang, Neng Wan, and Dejun Su. 2020. "Family Income and Student Educational and Cognitive Outcomes in China: Exploring the Material and Psychosocial Mechanisms." *Social Sciences* 9(12):225–23
Wen, Nainan, and Di Cui. 2014. "Effects of Celebrity Involvement on Young People's Political and Civic Engagement." *Chinese Journal of Communication.* 7(4):409–428.
Wen, Zhuoyi, Ka Ho Mok, and Padmore Adusi Amoah. 2022. "Productive Engagement and Ageing in Productivist Welfare Regimes: Questing for an Age-Friendly City in Hong Kong." *Ageing & Society* 42(11):2510–32 \102–304.
Wendt, Ronald F. 2001. The Paradox of Empowerment: Suspended Power and the Possibility of Resistance. Westport, CT: Praeger.
Wentzel, Kathryn R. 2003. "Sociometric Status and Adjustment in Middle School: A Longitudinal Study." *Journal of Early Adolescence* 23(1):5–28.
Wentzel, Kathryn, and Kathryn Caldwell. 1997. "Friendships, Peer Acceptance, and Group Membership: Relations to Academic Achievement in Middle School." *Child Development* 68(6):1198–1209.
Wenzel, Michael. 2000. "Justice and Identity: The Significance of Inclusion for Perceptions of Entitlement and the Justice Motive." *Personality & Social Psychology Bulletin* 26(2):157–176.
Werbner, Pnina. 1996. "The Enigma of Christmas: Symbolic Violence, Compliant Subjects and the Flow of English Kinship." Pp. 135–162 in *Consumption Matters: The Production and Experience of Consumption*, edited by Stephen Edgell, Kevin Hetherington, and Alan Warde. Oxford, UK: Blackwell.
Wessells, Michael G. 2018. "Supporting Resilience in War-Affected Children: How Differential Impact Theory Is Useful in Humanitarian Practice." *Child Abuse & Neglect* 78:13–18.
Western, Simon. 2017. "The Key Discourses of Coaching." Pp. 42–61 in *The SAGE Handbook of Coaching*, edited by Tatiana Bachkirova, Gordon Spence, and David Drake. London, UK: SAGE.
Westman, Mina, and Dalia Etzion. 1999. "The Crossover of Strain from School Principals to Teachers and vice versa." *Journal of Occupational Health Psychology* 4(3):269–278.
Wetterberg, Anna. 2007. "Crisis, Connection, and Class: How Social Ties Affect Household Welfare." *World Development* 35(4):585–606.
Whelan, Christopher T., and Bertrand Maitre. 2013. "Material Deprivation, Economic Stress, and Reference Groups in Europe: An Analysis of EU-SILC 2009." *European Sociological Review* 29(6):1162–1174.
Whelan, Christopher T., Richard Layte, and Bertrand Maitre. 2004. "Understanding the Mismatch between Income Poverty and Deprivation: A Dynamic Comparative Analysis." *European Sociological Review* 20(4):287–302.
Whigham, Stuart. 2019. "Nationalism, Party Political Discourse and Scottish Independence: Comparing Discursive Visions of Scotland's Constitutional Status." *Nations & Nationalism* 25(4):1212–37.

White, Ben. 2024. "A Structuralist Theory of Phenomenal Intentionality." *Inquiry*.

White, Brian, Simon Driver, and Ann-Marie Warren. 2008. "Considering Resilience in the Rehabilitation of People with Traumatic Disabilities." *Rehabilitation Psychology* 53(1):9–17.

White, Mathew A. 2014. "Positive Education at Geelong Grammar School." Pp. 657–668 in *the Oxford Handbook of Happiness*, edited by Susan A. David, Ilona Boniwell and Amanda Conley Ayers. Oxford, UK: Oxford University Press.

White, Melanie. 2006. "An Ambivalent Civility." *Canadian Journal of Sociology* 31(4):445–460.

White, Michael W., Nazia Khan, Jennifer S. Deren, Jessica J. Sim, and Elizabeth A. Majka. 2022. "Give a Dog a Bone: Spending Money on Pets Promotes Happiness." *Journal of Positive Psychology* 17(4):589–95.

White, Rachel E., Ethan Kross and Angela L. Duckworth. 2015. "Spontaneous Self-Distancing and Adaptive Self-Reflection across Adolescence." *Child Development* 86(4):1272–81.

Whitham, Monica M. 2012. "Community Connections: Social Capital and Community Success." *Sociological Forum* 27(2):441–457.

Whitton, Joy. 2018. Fostering Imagination in Higher Education: Disciplinary and Professional Practices. Abingdon, UK: Routledge.

Whynes, David K., and Tracey H. Sach. 2007. "WTP and WTA: Do People Think Differently?" *Social Science & Medicine* 65:947–957.

Whyte, Martin King, and Maocan Gao. 2009. "How Angry Are Chinese Citizens about Current Inequalities? Evidence from a National Survey." *Social Transformations in Chinese Societies* 5:17–54.

Wickham, Robert E. and C. Raymond Knee. 2012. "Interdependence Theory and the Actor–Partner Interdependence Model." *Personality & Social Psychology Review* 16(4):375–93.

Wickrama, Kas, Rand D. Conger, and Fredrick. O. Lorenz. 1995. "Work, Marriage, Lifestyle, and Changes in Men's Physical Health." *Journal of Behavioral Medicine* 18(2):97–112.

Widegren, Orjan. 1997. "Social Solidarity and Social Exchange." *Sociology* 31(4):755–771.

Widmer, Eric D. 2006. "Who Are My Family Members? Bridging and Binding Social Capital in Family Configurations." *Journal of Social & Personal Relationship* 26(3):979–998.

Wieloch, Neil. 2002. "Collective Mobilization and Identity Form the Underground: The Deployment of Oppositional Capital in the Harm Reduction Movement." *Sociological Quarterly* 43(1):43–72.

Wiest, Amber L., David L. Andrews, and Michael D. Giardina. 2015. "Training the Body for Healthism: Reifying Vitality in and through the Clinical Gaze of the Neoliberal Fitness Club." *Review of Education/Pedagogy/Cultural Studies* 37(1):21–40.

Wilcox, W. Bradford, and Jeffrey Dew. 2016. "The Social and Cultural Predictors of Generosity in Marriage: Gender Egalitarianism, Religiosity, and Familism." *Journal of Family Issues* 37(1):97–118.

Wilczenski, Felicia L., and Susan M. Coomey. 2007. A Practical Guide to Service Learning: Strategies for Positive Development in Schools. New York: Springer.

Wildemeersch, Danny. 2014. "Adult and Community Education in Complex Societies: Reconsidering Critical Perspectives." *International Journal of Lifelong Education* 33(6):821–31

Wilder, David H., Huhg F. McKeegan, and Robert M. Midkiffe, Jr. 2000. "A Factor-analytic Reinterpretation of the Clark-Trow Educational Philosophies." *Journal of College Student Development* 41(5):513–528.

Wiles, Janine L., Kirsty Wild, Ngaire Kerse, and Ruth E.S. Allen. 2012. "Resilience from the Point of View of Older People: There's Still Life Beyond a Funny Knee." *Social Science & Medicine* 74:416–424.

Wilhoit, Sarah A. and Jackson A. Goodnight. 2023. "Deviant Peer Affiliation Mediates the Prospective Association from Impulsivity to Alcohol Use in Late Adolescence." *Journal of Adolescence* 95(3):454–67.

Wilkinson, Derek. 2010. "Community Cohesion and Canadian Rural E-Mail Behavior." *American Behavioral Scientist* 53(9):1268–1282.

Wilks, Scott E., and Christina A. Spivey. 2010. "Resilience In Undergraduate Social Work Students: Social Support and Adjustment to Academic Stress." *Social Work Education* 29(3):276–288.
Williams, Bryan L., Sylvia Brown, and Michael Greenberg. 1999. "Determinants of Trust Perceptions among Residents Surrounding the Savannah River Nuclear Weapons Site." *Environment & Behavior* 31(3):354–371.
Williams, Christopher R. 2008. "Comparison, Suffering and the Self: A Moral Psychology of Social Justice." *Current Sociology* 56(1):5–24.
Williams, Colin C., and Jan Windebanh. 2000. "Beyond Social Inclusion through Employment: Harnessing Mutual Aid as a Complementary Social Inclusion Policy." *Policy & Politics* 29(1):15–28.
Williams, Emma, Michael Scott, and Colin Feltham. 2012. "Anger Management." Pp. 425–430 in The SAGE *Handbook of Counselling and Psychotherapy*, edited by Colin Feltham and Ian Horton. London: SAGE.
Williams, Helen, Stephen Palmer, and Nick Edgerton. 2018. "Cognitive Behavioural Coaching." Pp. 17–34 in *The Complete Handbook of Coaching*, edited by Elaine Cox, Tatiana Bachkirova, and David Clutterbuck. London, UK: SAGE.
Williams, Keith L., and Renee V. Galliher. 2006. "Predicting Depression and Self-esteem from Social Connectedness Support, and Competence." *Journal of Social & Clinical Psychology* 25(8):855–874.
Williams, Kevin J., John J. Donovan, and Tonya L. Dodge. 2000. "Self-Regulation of Performance: Goal Establishment and Goal Revision Processes in Athletes." *Human Performance* 13(2):159–80.
Williams, Lauren K., Jenny Veitch, and Kylie Ball. 2011. "What Helps Children Eat Well? A Qualitative Exploration of Resilience among Disadvantaged Families." *Health Education Research* 26(2):296–307.
Williams, Melissa J. and Jennifer L. Eberhardt. 2008. "Biological Conceptions of Race and the Motivation to Cross-Racial Boundaries." *Journal of Personality Social Psychology* 94(6):1033–47.
Williams, Philippa, and Barbara Pocock. 2010. "Building Community for Different Stage of Life: Physical and Social Infrastructure in Master Planned Communities." *Community, Work & Family* 13(1):71–87.
Williams, Terry, Eloise Dunlap, Bruce D. Johnson, and Ansley Hamid. 1992., "Personal Safety in Dangerous Places." *Journal of Contemporary Ethnography* 21(3):343–374.
Willis, Thomas A., Daryl B. O'Connor, and Lawrence Smith. 2008. "Investigating Effort-Reward Imbalance and Work-Family Conflict in Relation to Morningness-Eveningness and Shift Work." *Work & Stress* 22(2):125–137.
Willner, Tirza, Yuliya Lipshits-Braziler, and Itamar Gati. 2020. "Construction and Initial Validation of the Work Orientation Questionnaire." *Journal of Career Assessment* 28(1):109–27.
Wills, Thomas Ashby. 1997. "Modes and Families of Coping: An Analysis of Downward Comparison in the Structure of Other Cognitive and Behavioral Mechanisms." Pp. 167–193 in *Health, Coping, and Well-being: Perspectives from Social Comparison Theory*, edited by Bram P. Buunk and Frederick X. Gibbons. Mahwah, NJ: Lawrence Erlbaum.
Wilson, Franklin D., and Roger B. Hammer. 2001. "Ethnic Residential Segregation and Its Consequences." Pp. 272–303 in *Urban Inequality: Evidence from Four Cities*, edited by Alice O'Connor, Chris Tilly and Lawrence D. Bobo. New York: Russell Sage.
Wilson, George, and Berni Kelly. 2010. "Evaluating the Effectiveness of Said Work Education: Preparing Students for Practice Learning." *British Journal of Social Work* 40:2431–2459.
Wilson, John, and Marc Musick. 1997. "Who Cares? Toward an Integrated Theory of Volunteer Work." *American Sociological Review* 62:694–713.
Wilson, John. 2000. "Volunteering." *Annual Review of Sociology* 26:215–240.
Wilson, Sandra M., and Shann R. Ferch. 2005. "Enhancing Resilience in the Workplace through the Practice of Caring Relationships." *Organization Development Journal* 23(4):45–60.

Wilt, Joshua A., Joshua B. Grubbs, Kenneth I. Pargament, and Julie J. Exline. 2017. "Religious and Spiritual Struggles, Past and Present: Relations to the Big Five and Well-Being." *International Journal for the Psychology of Religion* 27(1):51–64.

Wiltermuth, Scott S., and Chip Heath. 2009. "Synchrony and Cooperation." *Psychological Science* 20(1):1–5.

Wiltgren, Layal Kasselias. 2014. "Youth Using National Symbols in Constructing Identities." *Journal of Youth Studies* 17(3):308–23.

Wiltshire, Jocelyn, Joshua S. Bourdage, and Kibeom Lee. 2014. "Honesty-Humility and Perceptions of Organizational Politics in Predicting Workplace Outcomes." *Journal of Business & Psychology* 29(2):235–51.

Windle, Michael, Carol Miller, Tutnauer, and Donna Domenico. 1992. "Alcohol Use, Suicidal Behavior, and Risky Activities among Adolescents." *Journal of Research on Adolescence* 2(4):317–330.

Wink, Paul, and Michele Dillon. 2003. "Religiousness, Spirituality and Psychological Functioning in Late Adulthood: Findings from a Longitudinal Study." *Psychology & Aging* 18(4):916–924.

Winkelmann, Rainer. 2009. "Unemployment, Social Capital, and Subjective Well-Being." *Journal of Happiness Studies* 10(4):421–430.

Winstock, Zeev, and Zvi Eisikovits. 2003. "Choice within Entrapment and Entrapment within Choice: The Challenge Facing Battered Women Who Stay." *Families in Society* 84(4):539–546.

Wintre, Maxine Gallander, and Mordechai Yaffe. 2000. "First-year Students" Adjustment to University Life as a Function of Relationships with Parents." *Journal of Adolescent Research* 15(1):9–37.

Wires, John W., Ralph Barocas, and Albert R. Hollenbeck. 1994. "Determinants of Adolescent Identity Development: A Cross-sequential Study of Boarding School Boys." *Adolescence* 29(114):361–378.

Wise, Jasmine and Robyn Driskell. 2017. "Tolerance within Community: Does Social Capital Affect Tolerance?" *Social Indicators Research* 134(2):607–29.

Wister, Andrew, and Zan Romeder. 2002. "The Chronic Illness Context and Change in Exercise Self-care among Older Adults: A Longitudinal Analysis." *Canadian Journal on Aging* 21(4):521–534.

Witkow, Melissa R. 2005. "Mutual Antipathies During Early Adolescence: More Than Just Rejection." *International Journal of Behavioral Development* 29(3):209–218.

Witt, Joshua, and William Revelle. 2009. "Extraversion." Pp. 27–45 in *Handbook of Individual Differences in Social Behavior*, Mark R. Leary and Rick H. Hoyle. New York, NY: Guilford.

Wojcieszak, Magdalena E., and Diana C. Mutz. 2009. "Online Groups and Political Discourse: Do Online Discussion Spaces Facilitate Exposure to Political Disagreement?" *Journal of Communication* 59:40–56.

Wojciszke, Bogdan, and Anna Struzynska-Kujolowicz. 2007. "Power Influences Self-esteem." *Social Cognition* 25(4):472–494.

Woldoff, Rachael A., and Seth Ovadia. 2009. "Not Getting Their Money's Worth: African-American Disadvantages in Converting Income, Wealth, and Education into Residential Quality." *Urban Affairs Review* 45(1):66–91.

Wolff, Jonathan. 2011. "Equality." Pp. 611–623 in *The Oxford Handbook of the History of Political Philosophy*, edited by George Klosko. Oxford, UK: Oxford University Press.

Wolff, Richard D. and Stephen A. Resnick. 2012. *Contending Economic Theories: Neoclassical, Keynesian, and Marxian.* Cambridge, MA: MIT.

Wollebaek, Dag, and Per Selle. 2002. "Does Participation in Voluntary Associations Contribute to Social Capital? The Impact of Intensity, Scope, and Type." *Nonprofit & Voluntary Sector Quarterly* 31(1):32–61.

Wollschleger, Jason. 2012. "Interaction Ritual Chains and Religious Participation." *Sociological Forum* 27(4):896–912.

Wong, Chack-kie, and Angela Wai-yan Shik. 2011. "Renewed Conception of Harmonious Society, Governance, and Citizenship: Evidence for the Study of Chinese Perceptions in Hong Kong." *Asian Social Work & Policy Review* 5:1–19.
Wong, Ipkin Anthony, and Iok Keng Veronica Lam. 2016. "A Multilevel Investigation of the Role of Retail Stores in Cross-Border Shopping." *Journal of Travel & Tourism Marketing* 33(6):837–853.
Wong, Jody Chin Sing, and Janet Zheng Yang. 2022. "Predicting the U.S. Public's Prosocial Responses during the COVID-19 Pandemic." *Journal of Health Communication* 26(9:597–607.
Wong, Kam C. 2007. "Studying Policing in China: Some Personal Reflections." *International Journal of the Sociology of Law* 35(3):111–126.
Wong, Kevin Tze-wai, Victor Zheng, and Po-san Wan. 2016. "The Impact of Cross-border Integration with Mainland China on Hong Kong's Local Politics: The Individual Visit Scheme as a Double-edged Sword for Political Trust in Hong Kong." *China Quarterly* 228:1081–1104.
Wong, Maria M. 2008. "Perceptions of Parental Involvement and Autonomy Support: Their Relations with Self-Regulation, Academic Performance, Substance Use and Resilience among Adolescents." *North American Journal of Psychology* 10(3):497–518.
Wong, Maria M., Leon I. Puttler, Joel T. Nigg, and Robert A. Zucker. 2018. "Sleep and Behavioral Control in Earlier Life Predicted Resilience in Young Adulthood: A Prospective Study of Children of Alcoholics and Controls." *Addictive Behaviors* 82:65–71.
Wong, Mathew Y. H. and Wing Hong Chui. 2017. "Economic Development and Subjective Well-Being: A Comparative Study of Adolescents in Hong Kong and Macau." *Child Indicators Research* 10(1):247–65.
Wong, Ngai-ying, and Sing Lau. 1993. "Effects of Self-Monitoring and Perceived Approval on Delinquent Behavior among Hong Kong Adolescents." *Journal of Youth and Adolescence* 22(2):191–200.
Wong, Peter Yih-Jiun. 2012. "The Music of Ritual Practice: An Interpretation." *Sophia* 51:243–255.
Wong, Rosa Sze Man, Frederick Ka Wing Ho, Wilfred Hing Sang Wong, Keith Tsz Suen Tung, Chun Bong Chow, Nirmala Rao, Ko Ling Chan, and Patrick Ip. 2018. "Parental Involvement in Primary School Education: Its Relationship with Children's Academic Performance and Psychosocial Competence through Engaging Children with School." *Journal of Child & Family Studies* 27(5):1544–1555.
Wong, Victor C.W., and Sammy W.S. Chiu. 1997. "Health-care Reforms in the People's Republic of China: Strategies and Social Implications." *International Journal of Public Sector Management* 10(1,2):76–92.
Wong, Yi-Lee. 2017. "Class Differentials in Getting Parental Assistance for Seeking a Second Chance of Getting into University: An Illustration of Community-College Students in Hong Kong." *Higher Education* 74(1):163–178.
Wong, Yin-Ling Irene, Jason Matejkowski, and Sungkyu Lee. 2011. "Social Integration of People with Serious Mental Illness: Network Transactions and Satisfaction." *Journal of Behavioral Health Services & Research* 38(1):51–67.
Wong, Yu Cheung, Chi Kwong Law, John Wat Chu. 2010. "Digital Divide and Social Inclusion: Policy Challenge for Social Development in Hong Kong and South Korea." *Journal of Asian Public Policy* 3(1):37–52.
Woo, Jean, Jason Leung, Samuel Wong, Timothy Kwok, Jenny Lee, and Henry Lynn. 2009. "Development of a Simple Scoring Tool in the Primary Care Setting for Prediction of Recurrent Falls in Men and Women Aged 60 Years and Over Living in the Community." *Journal of Clinical Nursing* 18:1038–1048.
Wood, Julia T. 2015. "Critical Feminist Theories: giving Voice and Visibility to Women's Experiences in Interpersonal Relations." Pp. 203–215 in *Engaging Theories in Interpersonal Communication: Multiple Perspectives*, edited by Dawn O. Braithwaite and Paul Schrodt. Thousand Oaks, CA: SAGE.
Wood, Lisa, Billie Giles-Corti, and Max Bulsara. 2005. "The Pet Connection: Pets as a Conduit For Social Capital?." *Social Science & Medicine* 61(6):1159–1173.

Wood, Lisa; Karen Martin, Hayley Christian, Andrea Nathan, Claire Lauritsen, Steve Houghton, Ichiro Kawachi, and McCune, Sandra. 2015. "The Pet Factor: Companion Animals as a Conduit for Getting to Know People, Friendship Formation and Social Support." *PLoS ONE* 10(4):1–17.

Woodard, Cooper R. 2010. "The Courage to Be Authentic: Empirical and Existential Perspectives." Pp. 109–123 in the *Psychology of Courage: Modern Research on an Ancient Virtue*, edited by Cynthia L.S. Pury and Bhane J. Lopez. Washington, DC: American Psychological Association.

Woodier, David. 2011. "Building Resilience in Looked after Young People: A Moral Values Approach." *British Journal of Guidance & Counselling* 39(3):259–282.

Woods, Kerri. 2014. *Human Rights*. Houndmills, UK: Palgrave.

Woods, Peter, Arthur Poropat, Michelle Barker, Ruth Hills, Ray Hibbins, and Sally Borbasi. 2013. "Building Friendship through a Cross-Cultural Mentoring Program." *International Journal of Intercultural Relations* 37(5):523–535.

Woodward, Lianne J., and David M. Fergusson. 1999. "Childhood Peer Relationship Problems and Psychosocial Adjustment in Late Adolescence." *Journal of Abnormal Child Psychology* 27(1):87–124.

Woolcock, Michael, and Deepa Narayan. 2000. "Social Capital: Implications for Development Theory, Research, and Policy." *World Bank Research Observer* 15(2):225–249.

Woolcock, Michael. 1998. "Social Capital and Economic Development: Toward a Theoretical Synthesis and Policy Framework." *Theory & Society* 27:151–208.

Woolcock, Michael. 2010. "The Rise and Routinization of Social Capital, 1988–2008." *Annual Review Political Science* 13:469–487.

Woollett, Nataly, Lucie Cluver, Abigail M. Hatcher, and Heena Brahmbhatt. 2016. ""To Be HIV Positive Is Not the End of the World": Resilience among Perinatally Infected HIV Positive Adolescents in Johannesburg." *Children & Youth Services Review* 70:269–75.

Worley, Timothy R. and Jennifer A. Samp. 2019. "Dyadic Power, Marital Status, Face Concerns, and Politeness in the Context of Relational Complaining." *Journal of Social & Personal Relationships* 36(4):1367–91.

Wright, Emily M., Gillian M. Pinchevsky, Michael L. Benson, Dana L. Radatz. 2015. "Intimate Partner Violence and Subsequent Depression: Examining the Roles of Neighborhood Supportive Mechanisms." *American Journal of Community Psychology* 56(3):342–356.

Wright, Erik Olin. 1997. *Class Counts: Comparative Studies in Class Analysis*. Cambridge, UK: Cambridge University Press.

Wright, Erik Olin. 2016. "How to Be an Anti-Capitalist for the 21st Century." *Journal of Australian Political Economy* 77:5–23.

Wright, John Pual and Matt DeLisi. 2016. *Conservative Criminology: A Call to Restore Balance to the Social Sciences*. New York, NY: Routledge.

Wright, Margaret O'Dougherty and Ann S. Masten. 2015. "Pathways to Resilience in Context." Pp. 3–22 in *Youth Resilience and Culture: Commonalities and Complexities*, edited by Linda C. Theron, Michael Ungar, and Liebenberg Linda. Dordrecht, Netherlands: Springer.

Wright, Robin, Lindsay John, Eric Duku, Giovani Burgos, Amanda, Krygsman, and Charlene Esposto. 2009. "After-school Programs as a Prosocial Setting for Bonding between Peers." *Child & Youth Services* 31:74–91.

Wright, Stephen C. 2001. "Restricted Intergroup Boundaries: Tokenism, Ambiguity, and the Tolerance of Injustice." Pp. 233–254 in *The Psychology of Legitimacy: Emerging Perspectives on Ideology, Justice, and Intergroup Relations*, edited by John T. Jost and Brenda Major. Cambridge, UK: Cambridge University Press.

Wrosch, Carsten, Isabelle Bauer, and Michael F. Scheier. 2005. "Regret and Quality of Life across the Adult Life Span: The Influence of Disengagement and Available Future Goals." *Psychology & Aging* 20(4):657–670.

Wrosch, Carsten, Jutta Heckhausen, Margie E. Lachman. 2000. "Primary and Secondary Control Strategies for Managing Health and Financial Stress across Adulthood." *Psychology & Aging* 15(3):387–399.

Wu, Homer C., Abby Liu, and Chih-Hung Wang. 2010. "Taiwanese University Students" Perceived Freedom and Participation in Leisure." *Annals of Leisure Research* 13(4):679–700.

Wu, Jinting, and Sou-Kuan Vong. 2017. "Macau Higher Education Expansion in Flux: A Critical Spatial Perspective." *Discourse: Studies in the Cultural Politics of Education* 38(6):937–954.

Wu, Joseph, and Dennis S.W. Wong. 2013. "Psychosocial Correlates of Friendship in School." Pp. 159–168 in *Friendships: Cultural Variations, Developmental Issues and Impact on Health*, edited by Sarah Kaufman and Viktor Meyer. New York: Nova.

Wu, Michael Shengtao, Xiaodan Yan, Chan Zhou, Yiwen Chen, Juan Li, Zhuohong Zhu, Xiangqin Shen, and Buxin Han. 2011. "General Belief in a Just World and Resilience: Evidence from a Collectivistic Culture." *European Journal of Personality* 25(6):431–442.

Wu, Qiaobing, Lawrence A. Palinkas, and Xuesong He. 2010. "An Ecological Examination of Social Capital Effects on Academic Achievement of Chinese Migrant Children." *British Journal of Social Work* 40(8):2575–2597.

Wu, Qinqin, Guangming Ran, and Qi Zhang. 2022. "Rejection Sensitivity and Trait Anxiety: The Indirect Effects of Regulatory Emotional Self-Efficacy and Shyness." *Current Psychology* 41(8):5481–90.

Wu, Zheng, and Lindy MacNeill. 2003. "Education, Work, and Childbearing after Age 30." *Journal of Comparative Family Studies* 191–212.

Wubbolding, Robert E., John Brickell, Lothar Imhof, Rose In-za Kim, Leon Lojk, and Basheer Al-Rashidi. 2004. "Reality Therapy: A Global Perspective." *International Journal for the Advancement of Counselling* 26(3):219–228.

Wulfhorst, J.D., and Richard S. Kranich. 1999. "Effects on Collective Morale from Technological Risk." *Society & Natural Resources* 12(1):1–18.

Wuthnow, Robert J. 2011. "Taking Talk Seriously: Religious Discourse as Social Practice." *Journal for the Scientific Study of Religion* 50(1):1–21.

Wuthnow, Robert. 2002. "Religious Involvement and Status-Bridging Social Capital." *Journal for the Scientific Study of Religion* 41(4):669–684.

Wuthnow, Robert. 2004. Saving America? Faith-based Services and the Future of Civil Society. Princeton, NJ: Princeton University Press.

Wyer, Robert S., Jr., and Dolores Abbarracin. 2014. "Belief Formation, Organization, and Change: Cognitive and Motivational Influences." Pp. 273–322 in *The Handbook of Attitudes*, edited by Albarracin Dolores, T. Johnson Blair and P. Zanna Mark. Mahwah, NJ: Psychology.

Wyman, Peter A. 2003. "Emerging Perspectives on Context Specificity of Children's Adaptation and Resilience: Evidence from a Decade of Research with Urban Children in Adversity." Pp. 293–317 in *Resilience and Vulnerability: Adaptation in the Context of Childhood Adversities*, edited by Saniya S. Luthar. Cambridge, UK: Cambridge University Press

Wypych, Murek et al. 2018. "Roles of Impulsivity, Motivation, and Emotion Regulation in Procrastination: Path Analysis and Comparison between Students and Non-students." *Frontiers in Psychology* 9:891.

Xi, Juan and Sean-Shong Hwang. 2011. "Relocation Stress, Coping, and Sense of Control among Resettlers Resulting from China's Three Gorges Dam Project." *Social Indicators Research* 104:507–522.

Xia, Zhichen and Fan Yang. 2020. "Ethical Leadership and Knowledge Sharing: The Impacts of Prosocial Motivation and Two Facets of Conscientiousness." *Frontiers in Psychology* 11:581236.

Xiang, Guangcan, Qingqing Li, Xiaoli Du, Xinyuan Liu, Mingyue Xiao, and Hong Chen. 2020. "Links between Family Cohesion and Subjective Well-Being in Adolescents and Early Adults: The Mediating Role of Self-concept Clarity and Hope." *Current Psychology* 41(1):76–85.

Xiao, Hong. 2000. "Structure of Child-rearing Values in Urban China." *Sociological Perspectives* 43(3):457–471.

Xiao, Jing Jian, Chunyi Tang, and Shim. 2009. "Action for Happiness: Financial Behavior and Life Satisfaction of College Students." *Social Indicators Research* 92:53–68.

Xie, Jia Lin. 1996. "Karasek's Model in the People's Republic of China: Effects of Job Demands, Control, and Individual Differences." *Academy of Management Journal* 39(6):1594–1618.

Xie, Qiuyuan and Daniel Fu Keung Wong. 2021. "Culturally Sensitive Conceptualization of Resilience: A Multidimensional Model of Chinese Resilience." *Transcultural Psychiatry* 58(3):323–34.

Xin, Ziqiang, Zhixu Yang, and Xihuan Ling. 2017. "Interdependent Self-Construal Matters in the Community Context: Relationships of Self-Construal with Community Identity and Participation." *Journal of Community Psychology* 45(8):1050–1064.

Xing, Linna, Sophia W. Deng, and Ghee W. Ho. 2024. "From Empathy to Resilience: The Mediating Role of Emotional Intelligence." *Psychological Reports.*

Xing, Xiaopei, Meifang Wang, Qing Zhang, Xiaorui He, and Wenzin Zhang. 2011. "Gender Differences in the Reciprocal Relationships between Parental Physical Aggression and Children's Externalizing Problem Behavior in China." *Journal of Family Psychology* 25(5):699–708.

Xu, Qian, Nan Yu and ,Yunya Song. 2018. "User Engagement in Public Discourse on Genetically Modified Organisms: The Role of Opinion Leaders on Social Media." *Science Communication* 40(6):691–717.

Xu, Wei, Marcus A. Rodriguez, Qian Zhang and Xinghua Liu. 2015. "The Mediating Effect of Self-Acceptance in the Relationship between Mindfulness and Peace of Mind." *Mindfulness* 6(4):797–802.

Xu, Yingjiao, Teresa A. Summers, and Bonnie D. Belleau. 2004. "Who Buys American Alligator? Predicting Purchase Intention of a Controversial Product." *Journal of Business Research* 57:1189–1198.

Xygalatas, Dimitris, Peter Maňo, and Gabriela Baranowski Pinto. 2021. "Ritualization Increases the Perceived Efficacy of Instrumental Actions." *Cognition* 215:104823.

Ya, Se. 2011. *Complete Works of the Classic of Changes.* Beijing, China: New World.

Yack, Bernard. 2012. *Nationalism and the Moral Psychology of Community.* Chicago, IL: University of University Press.

Yagci, Alper H. 2017. "The Great Recession, Inequality and Occupy Protests around the World." *Government & Opposition* 52(4):640–670.

Yahne, Carolina E., and William R. Miller. 1999. "Evoking Hope." Pp. 217–233 in *Integrating Spirituality into Treatment: Resources for Practitioners*, edited by William R. Miller. Washington, DC: American Psychological Association.

Yair, Gad. 2003. "Decisive Movements and Key Experiences: Expanding Paradigmatic Boundaries in the Study of School Effects." Pp. 124–142 in *The International Assessment of New Research and Theory*, edited by Carlos Alberto Torres and Ari Antikainen. Lanham, MD: Rowman.

Yakeley, Jessica. 2012. "Psychoanalytic Therapy." Pp. 268–272 in *The SAGE Handbook of Counselling and Psychotherapy*, edited by Colin Feltham and Ian Horton. London: SAGE.

Yamagishi, Toshio, Masako Kikuchi, and Motoko Kikuchi. 1999. "Trust, Gullibility, and Social Intelligence." *Asian Journal of Social Psychology* 2:145–167.

Yamagishi, Toshio, Yosake Makimura, Margaret Foddy, Masafumi Matsuda, Toko Kiysnari, and Michael J. Platow. 2005. "Comparisons of Australians and Japanese on Group-based Cooperation." *Asian Journal of Social Psychology* 8:173–190.

Yamaoka, Kazue. 2008. "Social Capital and Health and Well-being in East Asia: A Population-based Study." *Social Science & Medicine* 66:883–899.

Yang, Chao-Chin, Chin-Shen Wan, and Wen-Bin Chiou. 2010. "Dialectical Thinking and Creativity among Young Adults: A Postformal Operations Perspective." *Psychological Reports* 106(1):1–14.

Yang, Fan and Takashi Oka. 2022. "The Role of Mindfulness and Attachment Security in Facilitating Resilience." *BMC Psychology* 10(1).

Yang, Jie. 2017. "Virtuous Power: Ethics, Confucianism, and Psychological Self-Help in China." *Critique of Anthropology* 37(2):179–200.

Yang, Joyce P., Jane M. Simoni, Shannon Dorsey, Zhang Lin, Meiyan Sun, Meijuan Bao, and Hongzhou Lu. 2018. "Resilience Reducing Distress and Promoting Resilience: A Preliminary Trial of a Cbt Skills Intervention among Recently HIV-Diagnosed Msm in China." *AIDS Care* 30(SUP5):S39–S48.

Yang, Keming, 2019. *Loneliness: A Social Problem.* Abingdon, UK: Routledge.
Yang, Keming, and Christina R. Victor. 2008. "The Prevalence and Risk Factors for Loneliness among Older People in China." *Ageing & Society* 28:305–327.
Yang, Ming-Ching, Jen-Son Cheng, and Shu-Wen Yu. 2012. "Leisure Lifestyle and Health-Related Quality of Life of Taiwanese Adults." *Social Behavior & Personality* 40(2):301–317.
Yang, Shaohua, Salmi Mohd Isa, Hongyan Wu, Ramayah Thurasamy, Xi Fang, Yedan Fan, and Danping Liu. 2022. "Effects of Stores' Environmental Components on Chinese Consumers' Emotions and Intentions to Purchase Luxury Brands: Integrating Partial Least Squares-Structural Equation Modeling and Fuzzy-Set Qualitative Comparative Analysis Approaches." *Frontiers in Psychology* 13:840413.
Yang, Wen-Shan, and Pei-Chin Yen. 2012. "A Comparative Study of Marital Dissolution in East Asian Societies: Gender Attitudes and Social Expectations towards Marriage in Taiwan, Korea and Japan." *Asian Journal of Social Science* 39:751–755.
Yang, Xiaozhao Y. and Tingzhong Yang. 2020. "Pathways to Buying Sex among Migrant Labors: The Mediatory Role of Family Bonds and Peer Deviance on Social Network Homogeneity." *Sociological Quarterly* 61(4):768–86.
Yang, Xue. 2016. "Self-Compassion, Relationship Harmony, Versus Self-Enhancement: Different Ways of Relating to Well-Being in Hong Kong Chinese." *Personality & Individual Differences* 89:24–27.
Yang, Yuchen and Chunlei Wang. 2023. "Research on the Effects of Family Rituals on Subjective Well-Being of Chinese College Students." *Current Psychology* 42(32):28549–63.
Yao, Elvin, Yuhua Li, and Chunhui Wang. 2021. "The Fear of Being Associated with Sexual Minority Close Others: Socio-Cultural Predictors of Sexual Minority Affiliate Stigma." *Sexuality & Culture* 25(3):925–38.
Yao, Zhuojun, and Robert Enright. 2019. "Belief in Altruistic Human Nature and Prosocial Behavior: A Serial Mediation Analysis." *Ethics & Behavior* 30(2):97–111.
Yashima, Tomoko. 2010. "The Effects of International Volunteer Work Experiences on Intercultural Competence of Japanese Youth." *International Journal of Intercultural Relations* 34(3):268–282.
Yasuma, Naonori, Kazuhiro Watanabe, Mako Iida, Daisuke Nishi, and Norito Kawakami. 2019. "Personal Values in Adolescence and Psychological Distress in Adults: A Cross-Sectional Study Based on a Retrospective Recall." *PloS ONE* 14(11):e0225454.
Yates, Miranda, and James Youniss. 1996. "Community Service and Political-moral Identity in Adolescents." Journal of Research in Adolescence 6(3):271–284.
Ye, Feifei, and Tanner LeBaron Wallace. 2014. "Psychological Sense of School Membership Scale Method Effects Associated With Negatively Worded Items." *Journal of Psychoeducational Assessment* 32(3), pp. 202–215.
Ye, Wangqiong, Rolf Strietholt, and Sigrid Blömeke. 2021. "Academic Resilience: Underlying Norms and Validity of Definitions." *Educational Assessment, Evaluation & Accountability* 33(1):169–202.
Yeager, Leland B. 2001. Ethics as Social Science: The Moral Philosophy of Social Cooperation. Cheltenham, UK: Elgar.
Yeagley, Emily E., Linda M. Subich, and David M. Tokar. 2010. "Modeling College Women's Perceptions of Elite Leadership Positions with Social Cognitive Career Theory." *Journal of Vocational Behavior* 77:30–38. \
Yee, Der heuy, Kuo-shu Yang, and Barry K. Barnes. 1990. "An Inquiry into Confucian Socialization Related to the Development of Juvenile Delinquency." *Chinese Journal of Personality* 32:75–94.
Yee, Nick. 2006. "Motivations for Play in Online Games." *CyberPsychology & Behavior* 9(6):772–775.
Yeh, Kuang-Hui, Chin-Chun Yi, Wei-Chun Tsao, and Po-San Wan. 2013. "Filial Piety in Contemporary Chinese Societies: A Comparative Study of Taiwan, Hong Kong, and China." *International Sociology* 28(3):277–296.

Yetim, Nalan, and Ünsal Yetim. 2014. "Sense of Community and Individual Well-Being: A Research on Fulfillment of Needs and Social Capital in the Turkish Community." *Social Indicators Research* 115(1):93–115.

Yeung, W. Jean, Miriam R. Linver, and Jeanne Brooks-Gunn. 2002. "How Money Matters for Young Children's Development: Parental Investment and Family Processes." *Child Development* 73(6):1861–1879.

Yi, Chin-chun, and Ju-ping Lin. 2009. "Types of Relations between Adult Children and Elderly Parents in Taiwan: Mechanisms Accounting for Various Relational Types." *Journal of Comparative Family Studies* 40(2):305–324.

Yi, Chin-Chun, Chin-Fen Chang, and Ying-Hwa Chang. 2004. "The Intergenerational Transmission of Family Values: A Comparison between Teenagers and Parents in Taiwan." *Journal of Comparative Family Studies* 35(4):523–545.

Yienprugsawan, V., S. Seubsman, S. Kohamman, L.L.-Y. Lim, A.C. Sleigh, and the Thai Cohort Study Team. 2010. "Personal Wellbeing Index in a National Cohort of 87134 Thai Adults." *Social Indicators Research* 98:201–215.

Yin, Yizhen, Mengmeng Lyu, Yiping Chen, Jie Zhang, Hui Li, Huiyuan Li, Guili Xia, and Jingping Zhang. 2022. "Self-Efficacy and Positive Coping Mediate the Relationship between Social Support and Resilience in Patients Undergoing Lung Cancer Treatment: A Cross-Sectional Study." *Frontiers in Psychology* 13:953491.

Yip, Jeremy A., and Rod A. Martin. 2006. "Sense of Humor Emotional Intelligence and Social Competence." *Journal of Research in Personality* 40:1202–1208.

Yngfalk, Carl. 2016. "Bio-Politicizing Consumption: Neo-Liberal Consumerism and Disembodiment in the Food Marketplace." *Consumption, Markets & Culture* 19(3):275–95.

Yogeeswaran, Kumar, and Nilanjana Dasgupta. 2014. "Conceptions of National Identity In A Globalised World: Antecedents And Consequences." *European Review of Social Psychology* 25(1):189–227.

Yon, Kyu Jin, Ju-ri Joeng, and Michael Goh. 2012. "A Longitudinal Study of Career Maturity of Korean Adolescents: The Effects of Personal and Contextual Factors." *Asia Pacific Education Review* 13(4):727–739.

Yoon, Dalhee, Susan M. Snyder, and Susan Yoon. 2020. "Child Maltreatment Types and Adolescent Substance Use: The Role of Deviant Peer Affiliation." *Child & Family Social Work* 25(2):355–63.

Yoon, Jeongkoo, Shane R. Thye, and Edward J. Lawler. 2013. "Exchange and Cohesion in Dyads and Triads: A Test of Simmel's Hypothesis." *Social Science Research* 42(6):1457–1466.

Yoon, Jeongkoo. 2001. "The Role of Structure and Motivation for Workplace Empowerment: The Case of Korean Employees." *Social Psychology Quarterly* 64(2):195–206.

Yoos, George E. 2007. Reframing Rhetoric: A Liberal Politics without Dogma. New York: Palgrave.

Yorgason, Jeremy B., Fred P. Piercy, and Susan K. Piercy. 2007. "Acquired Learning Impairment in Older Couple Relationships: An Exploration of Couple Resilience Processes." *Journal of Aging Studies* 21:215–228.

Young, Anne F., Annette J. Dobson, and Julie E. Byles. 2001. "Determinants of General Practitioner Use among Women in Australia." *Social Science & Medicine* 53:1641–1651.

Young, Loretta, and Christopher Bagley. 1982. "Identity, Self-esteem and Evaluation of Colour and Ethnicity in Young Children in Jamaica and London." Pp. 191–211 in *Self-concept, Achievement and Multicultural Education*, edited by Gajendrak Verma and Christopher Bagley. London: Macmillan.

Young, Michael, and Peter Willmont. 1957. *Family and Kinship*. London: Routledge & Kegan Paul.

Youniss, James, and Miranda Yates. 1997. *Community Service and Social Responsibility in Youth*. Chicago, IL: University of Chicago Press.

Ysseldyk, Renate, S. Alexander Haslam, Kimberly Matheson, and Hymie Anisman. 2012. "Love Thine Enemy? Evidence That (Ir)Religious Identification Can Promote Outgroup Tolerance under Threat." *Group Processes & Intergroup Relations* 15(1):105–17.

Yu, Bin, Xinguang Chen, Amy L. Elliott, Yan Wang, Fang Li, and Jie Gong. 2019. "Social Capital, Migration Stress, Depression and Sexual Risk Behaviors among Rural-to-Urban Migrants in China: A Moderated Mediation Modeling Analysis." *Anxiety, Stress & Coping* 32(4):362–375.

Yu, Hong. 2020. "The Guangdong-Hong Kong-Macau Greater Bay Area in the Making: Development Plan and Challenges." *Cambridge Review of International Affairs* 34(3):481–509.

Yu, Lu, Mingyue Gu and Ko Ling Chan. 2023. "Hong Kong Adolescents" Participation in Political Activities: Correlates of Violent Political Participation." *Applied Research in Quality of Life* 18:1375–1405.

Yu, Meihua, Lingling Huang, Jiaqi Mao, Gese Dna, and Siyang Luo. 2022. "Childhood Maltreatment, Automatic Negative Thoughts, and Resilience: The Protective Roles of Culture and Genes." *Journal of Interpersonal Violence* 37(1–2):349–70.

Yu, Wei-hsin, and Chi-Tsun Chiu. 2016. "Growing Pains: Changes in Psychological Well-Being in Urban China." *Social Indicators Research* 129(3):1349–1382.

Yu, Xiaonan and Jianxin Zhang. 2007. "Factor Analysis and Psychometric Evaluation of the Connor-Davidson Resilience Scale (CD-RISC) with Chinese People." *Social Behavior & Personality* 35(1):19–30.

Yu, Xiaonan, Sunita M. Stewart, Iris K. F. Liu and Tai Hing Lam. 2014. "Resilience and Depressive Symptoms in Mainland Chinese Immigrants to Hong Kong." *Social Psychiatry & Psychiatric Epidemiology* 49(2):241–49.

Yu, Zhaoliang, Eddie M. W. Tong, Chi-Ching Leung, Elizabeth D. A. Chin, and Peiwei Lee. 2021. "Humility Predicts Resistance to Substance Use: A Self-Control Perspective." *Journal of Positive Psychology* 16(1):105–15.

Yuan, Hao. 2016. "Structural Social Capital, Household Income and Life Satisfaction: The Evidence from Beijing, Shanghai and Guangdong Province, China." *Journal of Happiness Studies* 17(2):569–586.

Yuan, Yue and Susan McNeeley. 2018. "Fear of Crime and Behavioral Adaptations: Testing the Effects of Fear of Violence on Unstructured Socializing with Peers." *Deviant Behavior* 39(12):1633–46.

Yucel, Deniz and Wen Fan. 2019. "Work–Family Conflict and Well-Being among German Couples: A Longitudinal and Dyadic Approach." *Journal of Health & Social Behavior* 60(3):377–95.

Yucel, Deniz. 2015. "What Predicts Egalitarian Attitudes Towards Marriage and Children: Evidence from the European Values Study." *Social Indicators Research* 120(1):213–28.

Yuchtman-Yaar, Ephraime. 2002. "Value Priorities in Israeli Society: An Examination of Inglehart's Theory of Modernization and Cultural Variation." *Comparative Sociology* 1(3-4):347–367.

Yue, Pengpeng, Aslihan Gizem Korkmaz, and Haigang Zhou. 2020. "Household Financial Decision Making Amidst the Covid-19 Pandemic." *Emerging Markets Finance & Trade* 56(10):2363–77.

Yuen, Gail. 2015. "Markets, Choice of Kindergarten, Mothers" Care Responsibilities, and the Voucher Scheme in Hong Kong." *Children & Youth Services Review* 48:167–176.

Yuji, Genda. 2007. "Jobless Youths and the NEET Problem in Japan." *Social Science Japan Journal* 10(1):23–40.

Zacher, Hannes, Antje Schmitt, Nerina L. Jimmieson. and Cort W. Rudolph. 2019. "Dynamic Effects of Personal Initiative on Engagement and Exhaustion: The Role of Mood, Autonomy, and Support. " *Journal of Organizational Behavior* 40(1):38–58.

Zalewski, Maureen, Stephanie F. Thompson, and Liliana J. Lengua. 2017. "Parenting as a Moderator of the Effects of Maternal Depressive Symptoms on Preadolescent Adjustment." *Journal of Clinical Child & Adolescent Psychology* 46(4):563–572.

Zamperini, Adriano, Marialuisa Menegatto, Miriam Mostacchi, Simone Barbagallo, and Ines Testoni. 2020. "Loss of Close Relationships and Loss of Religious Belonging as Cumulative Ostracism: From Social Death to Social Resurrection." *Behavioral Sciences* 10(6):99.

Zanin, Luca, Rosalba Radice, and Giampiero Marra. 2013. "Estimating the Effect of Perceived Risk of Crime on Social Trust in the Presence of Endogeneity Bias." *Social Indicators Research* 114(2):523–547.

Zanin, Luca. 2017. "Education and Life Satisfaction in Relation to the Probability of Social Trust: a Conceptual Framework and Empirical Analysis." *Social Indicators Research* 132(2):925–947.

Zanin, Luca. 2017. Education and Life Satisfaction in Relation to the Probability of Social Trust: A Conceptual Framework and Empirical Analysis." *Social Indicators Research* 132:925–47.

Zarean, Fahimeh and Zohreh Latifi. 2022. "The Effectiveness of Self-Healing (the Healing Codes) Training on Psychological Capital and Distress Tolerance in Women with Addicted Husbands." *Current Psychology* 41(6):3472–80.

Zarzeczna, Natalia, Bojana Većkalov, and Bastiaan T. Rutjens. 2023. "Spirituality and Intentions to Engage in Covid-19 Protective Behaviours." *Social & Personality Psychology Compass* 17(8):e12765.

Zautra, Alex J. 2014. "Resilience Is Social, After All." Pp. 185–196 in *The Resilience Handbook: Approaches to Stress and Trauman*, edited by Martha Kent, Mary C. Davis and John W. Reich. New York: NY: Routledge.

Zautra, Alex J., John Stuart Hall, and Kate E. Murray. 2010. "Resilience: A New Definition of Health for People and Communities." Pp. 3–29 in *Handbook of Adult Resilience*, edited by John W. Reich, Alex J. Zautra and John Stuart Hall. New York, NY: Guilford.

Zavala, Egbert, and Xavier Guadalupe-Diaz. 2019. "Testing Target Congruence Theory on Emotional Abuse Victimization Experienced by Heterosexual and LGBQ College Students." *Journal of Aggression, Maltreatment & Trauma* 28(9):1069–1090.

Zdrenka, Marco, Kumar Yogeeswaran, Samantha Stronge, and Chris G. Sibley. 2015. "Ethnic and National Attachment as Predictors of Wellbeing among New Zealand Europeans, Maori, Asians, And Pacific Nations Peoples." *International Journal of Intercultural Relations* 49:114–120.

Zee, Sze Yong. 2022. *What Will Be the Driving Force behind Humanity's Progress? The Chin Model and Chinese Power of Discourse vs The Western Model and Western Power of Discourse.* Hong Kong, China: Master Insight.

Zeidner, Moshe, and Gerald Matthews. 2011. *Anxiety 101.* New York: Springer.

Zeidner, Moshe, Gerald Matthews, and Richard D. Roberts. 2009. What We Know about Emotional Intelligence: How It Affects Learning, Work, Relationships, and Our Mental Health. Cambridge, MA: MIT.

Zeng, Guang, Hanchao Hou, and Kaiping Peng. 2016. "Effect of Growth Mindset on School Engagement and Psychological Well-Being of Chinese Primary and Middle School Students: The Mediating Role of Resilience." *Frontiers in Psychology* 7:1873.

Zeng, Hao, Lijing Zhao, and Shuai Ruan. 2020. "How Does Mentoring Affect Protégés" Adaptive Performance in the Workplace: Roles of Thriving at Work and Promotion Focus." *Frontiers in Psychology* 11:546152.

Zeon, David S. 1987. "The Relationship of Religious Involvement to a Variety of Indicators of Cognitive Ability and Achievement in College Students." *Adolescence* 88:883–895.

Zezelj, Iris and Ljiljana B. Lazarevic. 2019. "Irrational Beliefs." *Europe's Journal of Psychology* 15(1):1–7.

Zhan, Dongsheng, Mei-Po Kwan, Wenzhong Zhang, Li Chen, and Yunxiao Dang. 2022. "The Impact of Housing Pressure on Subjective Well-Being in Urban China." *Habitat International* 127:102639.

Zhan, Heying Jenny, Baozhen Luo, and Gehui Zhang. 2013. "Faith and Health: Meanings of Faith for Chinese Elders with Diverse Religious Backgrounds." *Ageing International* 38(4):343–63.

Zhang, Guoqing. 2006. In Search of Harmonious Society: From Politics to Political Sciences. Beijing, China: People.

Zhang, Jie, Sibo Zhao, David Lester, and Chengchao Zhou. 2014. "Life Satisfaction and Its Correlates among College Students in China: A Test of Social Reference Theory." *Asian Journal of Psychiatry* 10:17–20.

Zhang, Lening, and Steven F. Messner. 1994. "The Severity of Official Punishment for Delinquency and Change in Interpersonal Relations in Chinese Society." *Journal of Research in Crime and Delinquency* 31:416–433.

Zhang, Lening, William F. Wieczorek, John W. Welti, Craig Colder, and Thomas H. Nochajski. 2010. "Delinquency and Alcohol-impaired Driving among Young Males: A Longitudinal Study." *Journal of Criminal Justice* 38:439–445.

Zhang, Li-fang, and Robert J. Sternberg. 2012. "Cultured and Intellectual Styles." Pp. 131–152 in *Handbook of Intellectual Styles: Preferences in Cognition, Learning, and Thinking*. New York: Springer.

Zhang, Marina Yue with Bruce W. Stening. 2010. China 2.0: Transformation of an Emerging Superpower and the New Opportunities. Singapore: Wiley.

Zhang, Meng, and Susan E. Cross. 2011. "Emotions in Memories of Success and Failure: A Cultural Perspective." *Emotion* 11(4):866–880.

Zhang, Ning and Yun Kou. 2022. "Implicit Theories of Health, Consideration of Future Consequences, and Engagement in Health Protective Behaviors during the Covid-19 Pandemic in China." Journal of Health Psychology 27(6):1462–69.

Zhang, Shixin. 2003. Four Realms of Moral Education: Comparative Research on China's Ancient Moral Education. Hangzhou, China: Zhejiang Education.

Zhang, Shuwei, and Jie Zhou. 2018. "Social Justice and Public Cooperation Intention: Mediating Role of Political Trust and Moderating Effect of Outcome Dependence." *Frontiers in Psychology* 9:1381.

Zhang, Tony Huiquan. 2022. "Political Freedom, Education, and Value Liberalization and Deliberalization: A Cross-National Analysis of the World Values Survey, 1981–2014." *Social Science Journal* 59(3):357–74.

Zhang, Xia-jie, and Ai-ping Wang. 2011. "Development of a Psychosocial Adaptation Questionnaire for Chinese Patients with Visual Impairments." *Journal of Clinical Nursing* 20:2822–2829.

Zhang, Yi. 2005. *Legalist Great Wisdom*. Beijing, China: Overseas China.

Zhang, Yingqiang, and Tor Eriksson. 2010. "Inequality of Opportunity and Income Inequality in Nine Chinese Provinces, 1989–2006." *China Economic Review* 21(4):607–616.

Zhang, Yue, Muhammad Imran Rasheed, and Adeel Luqman. 2019. "Work-Family Conflict and Turnover Intentions among Chinese Nurses: The Combined Role of Job and Life Satisfaction and Perceived Supervisor Support." *Personnel Review* 49(5):1140–56.

Zhang, Zhaoduan. 2018. *The Knowledgeable Having No Doubt: Mohism, Guanzi, Legalism*, and Militarism. Beijing, China: Masses.

Zhang, Zhenmei, and Mark D. Hayward. 2001. "Childlessness and the Psychological Well-being of Older Persons." *Journal of Gerontology: Social Sciences* 56B(5):S311–S320.

Zhao, Kun, Eamonn Ferguson, and Luke D. Smillie. 2017. "Individual Differences in Good Manners Rather Than Compassion Predict Fair Allocations of Wealth in the Dictator Game." *Journal of Personality* 85(2):244–56.

Zhao, Meiju and Wangqian Fu. 2022. "The Resilience of Parents Who Have Children with Autism Spectrum Disorder in China: A Social Culture Perspective." *International Journal of Developmental Disabilities* 68(2):207–18.

Zhao, Ning. 2008. *Traditional Cultural Eloquence Intelligence*. Beijing, China: New World.

Zheng, Ping, Matt J. Gray, Wen-Jie Duan, Samuel M. Y. Ho, Mian Xia, and Joshua D. Clapp. 2020b. "Cultural Variations in Resilience Capacity and Posttraumatic Stress: A Tri-Cultural Comparison." *Cross Cultural Research* 54(2–3):273–95.

Zheng, Tiantian. 2008. "Commodifying Romance and Searching for Love Rural Migrant Bar Hostesses" Moral Vision in Post-Mao Dalian." *Modern China* 34(4):442–476.

Zheng, Xian, Zi-qing Yuan, and Xiaoling Zhang. 2020. "Does Happiness Dwell in an Owner-Occupied House? Homeownership and Subjective Well-Being in Urban China." *Cities* 96:102404.

Zheng, Yongnian, and Tok Sow Keat. 2007. "Beijing Responds to Hong Kong's Democratization Movement: From Bureaucratic Control to Political Leadership." *Asian Affairs* 33(2):235–255.

Zhong, Lena Y. 2009. Communities, Crime and Social Capital in Contemporary China. Cullompton, UK: Willan.

Zhong, Lena Y. 2010. "Bystander Intervention and Fear of Crime: Evidence from Two Chinese Communities." International Journal of Offender Therapy & Comparative *Criminology* 54(2):250–263.

Zhou, Bun. 2009. *Biblical Wisdom*. Huhehot, China: Distant Place.

Zhou, Shuangmei. 2008. Comparisons of Chinese and European American College Students on Individual Differences Variables Hypothesized to Predict Self-reported Interpersonal Competency. Doctoral Dissertation, University of Minnesota.

Zhou, Xiang. 2019. "Equalization or Selection? Reassessing the Meritocratic Power of a College Degree in Intergenerational Income Mobility." *American Sociological Review* 84(3):459–485.

Zhu, Yiting. 2003. *History of Chinese Traditional Ethical Thoughts*. Shanghai, China: Huadong Normal University.

Ziegler, John A. 1994. Experimentalism and Institutional Change: An Approach to the Study and Improvement of Institutions. Lanham, MD: University Press of America.

Ziemes, Johanna Fee, Hahn-Laudenberg Katrin, and J. Abs Hermann. 2019. "From Connectedness and Learning to European and National Identity." *Journal of Social Science Education* 18(3).1144.

Ziersch, Anna M., Fran E. Baum, Colin MacDougall, and Christine Putland. 2005. "Neighborhood Life and Social Capital: The Implications for Health." *Social Science & Medicine* 60:71–86.

Zietsma, Charlene, Madeline Toubiana, Maxim Voronov, and Anna Roberts. 2019. *Emotions in Organization Theory*. Cambridge, UK: Cambridge University Press.

Zimmer-Gembeck, Melanie J., and Ellen A. Skinner. 2015. "Adolescent Vulnerability and the Distress of Rejection: Associations of Adjustment Problems and Gender with Control, Emotions, and Coping." *Journal of Adolescence* 45:149–159.

Zimmerman, Jeffrey L., and Victoria C. Dickerson. 1996. *If Problems Talked: Narrative Therapy in Action*. New York: Guilford.

Zimmerman, Jennifer L., Christine Reyna. 2013. "The Meaning and Role of Ideology in System Justification and Resistance for High- and Low-Status People." *Journal of Personality & Social Psychology* 105(1):1–23.

Zimmerman, Marc A. 1995. "Psychological Empowerment: Issues and Illustrations." *American Journal of Community Psychology* 23(5):581

Zimmerman, Shirley L. 1992. Family Policies and Family Well-being: The Role of Political Culture. Newbury Park, CA: Sage.

Zimmermann, Marc A., and Jeffrey B. Bingenheimer. 2002. "Natural Mentors and Adolescent Resiliency: A Study with Urban Youth." *American Journal of Community Psychology* 30(2):221–243.

Zitek, Emily M. and Alexander H. Jordan. 2019. "Psychological Entitlement Predicts Failure to Follow Instructions." *Social Psychological & Personality Science* 10(2):172–80.

Ziv, Naomi. 2018. "Reactions to Patriotic and Protest Songs in Individuals Differing in Political Orientation." *Psychology of Music* 46(3):392–410.

Ziv, Naomi. 2019. "Pro-Peace or Anti-War: The Effect of Emotions Primed by Protest Songs on Emotions toward in-Group and out-Group in Conflict." *Journal of Applied Social Psychology* 49(12):778–95.

Zolkoski, Staci M., and Lyndal M. Bullock. 2012. "Resilience in Children and Youth: A Review." *Children & Youth Services Review* 34(12):2295–2303.

Zotti, Roberto, Nino Speziale, and Cristian Barra. 2016. "On the Causal Effect of Religiosity on Life Satisfaction Using a Propensity Score Matching Technique." *International Journal of Social Economics* 43(10):1031–1048.

Zsido, Andras N., Nikolett Arato, Andras Lang, Beatrix Labadi, Diana Stecina, and Szabolcs A. Bandi. 2021. "The Role of Maladaptive Cognitive Emotion Regulation Strategies and Social Anxiety in Problematic Smartphone and Social Media Use." *Personality & Individual Differences* 173:110647.

Zucker, Alyssa N. and Lina Y. Bay-Cheng. 2021. "Me First: The Relation between Neoliberal Beliefs and Sexual Attitude." *Sexuality Research & Social Policy* 18, 390–96.

Zukin, Sharon, and Jennifer Smith Maguire. 2004. "Consumers and Consumption." *Annual Review of Sociology* 30:173–197.

Zumbrunnen, John, and Amy Gangl. 2008. "Conflict, Fusion, or Coexistence? The Complexity of Contemporary American Conservatism." *Political Behavior* 30(2):199–221.

Zupancic, Maja, Luka Komidar, and Melita Puklek Levpuscek. 2014. "Individuation in Slovene Emerging Adults: Its Associations with Demographics, Transitional Markers, Achieved Criteria for Adulthood, and Life Satisfaction." *Journal of Adolescence* 37(8):1421–1433.

Zurbriggen, Eileen L. 2013. "Objectification, Self-Objectification, and Societal Change." *Journal of Social and Political Psychology* 1(1):188–215.

Zvi, Liza and Keren Cohen-Louck. 2023. "Exposure to Continuous Political Violence: Rational and Experiential Thinking Styles, Coping Styles and Post Traumatic Stress Symptoms." *Frontiers in Psychology* 14:1113608.

Zysberg, Leehu. 2012. "Loneliness and Emotional Intelligence." *Journal of Psychology* 146(1–2):37–46.

SPRINGER NATURE

# GPSR Compliance

*The European Union's (EU) General Product Safety Regulation (GPSR) is a set of rules that requires consumer products to be safe and our obligations to ensure this.*

*If you have any concerns about our products, you can contact us on ProductSafety@springernature.com*

In case Publisher is established outside the EU, the EU authorized representative is:

Springer Nature Customer Service Center GmbH
Europaplatz 3
69115 Heidelberg, Germany

The manufacturer's authorised representative in the EU is Springer Nature Customer Service Centre GmbH, Europaplatz 3, 69115 Heidelberg, Germany. If you have any concerns regarding our products, please contact ProductSafety@springernature.com

Printed and bound by CPI Group (UK) Ltd, Croydon, CR0 4YY
01/10/2026
02225909-0020